Mammographic Imaging:

A Practical Guide

Mammographic Imaging:

A Practical Guide

Fourth Edition

Shelly L. Lillé, BS, RT(R)(M)
Mammography Quality Management, LLC

Wendy J. Marshall, RT(R)(M)(QM)
Mammography Quality Management, LLC

. Wolters Kluwer

Philadelphia • Baltimore • New York • London
Buenos Aires • Hong Kong • Sydney • Tokyo

Senior Acquisitions Editor: Sharon Zinner
Senior Product Development Editor: Amy Millholen
Editorial Coordinator: Emily Buccieri
Marketing Manager: Leah Thompson
Production Project Manager: Marian Bellus
Design Coordinator: Holly McLaughlin
Compositor: SPi Global

9 8 7 6 5 4

Printed in the United States of America

Library of Congress Cataloging-in-Publication Data
Names: Lillé, Shelly, author. | Marshall, Wendy, 1956- author. | Preceded by (work): Andolina,
    Valerie. Mammographic imaging.
Title: Mammographic imaging : a practical guide / Shelly Lillé, Wendy Marshall.
Description: Fourth edition. | Philadelphia : Wolters Kluwer, [2019] | Preceded by
    Mammographic imaging / Valerie F. Andolina, Shelly Lillé. 3rd ed. c2011. | Includes
    bibliographical references and index.
Identifiers: LCCN 2018003393 | ISBN 9781496352026 (hardback)
Subjects: | MESH: Mammography—methods | Breast Diseases—diagnostic imaging |
    Radiography
Classification: LCC RG493.5.R33 | NLM WP 815 | DDC 618.1/907572—dc23 LC record
    available at https://lccn.loc.gov/2018003393

▌▌ DEDICATION

This book is dedicated with much love and gratitude to our mentors
Dr. Wende Logan-Young and Dr. Tamnit Ansusinha. By example,
you instilled in us a commitment to deliver the highest quality possible
for each examination and to treat each individual with dignity and respect.

We also dedicate this textbook to the technologists we have met along the way,
either as educators, students, or as coworkers. We have seen your dedication to this
profession. We are proud to be a part of this extraordinary group.

CONTRIBUTORS

Gerald R. Kolb, JD
President and Consultant
The Breast Group
Sunriver, Oregon

Avice M. O'Connell, MD, FACR, FSBI
Professor of Imaging Sciences
Chief, Breast Imaging
UR Medicine
Rochester, New York

Gale A. Sisney, MD, FACR
Executive Director
Global Radiology Outreach
Madison, Wisconsin

REVIEWERS

Crystal Bromeling, MBA, RT(R)(M) (ARRT)
Program Director
Radiologic Technology
Rasmussen College
Lake Elmo, Minnesota

Mary Carrillo, MBA/HCM, RT(R)(M)CDT
Program Director
Medical Radiography
GateWay Community College
Phoenix, Arizona

Mary F. Daniel, MAEd, RT-(R)(M)(BS)
Program Director Radiography/Breast Imaging
Pitt Community College
Winterville, North Carolina

Deborah Espen
Assistant Professor
University of Oklahoma Health Sciences Center
Oklahoma City, Oklahoma

Rebecca Farmer, RT(R)(M)(MSRS)
Associate Professor
Allied Health
Northwestern State University
Shreveport, Louisiana

Barbara Ferreira, BS, RT(R)(M)
Breast Imaging Clinical Instructor and Educator
Medical Imaging
Regis College
Weston, Massachusetts

Alicia Giaimo, MBA-HCM, MHS, RT(R)(M)(BD)(ARRT)
Clinical Associate Professor
Radiologic Sciences Diagnostic Imaging Department
Quinnipiac University
Hamden, Connecticut

Katie Gray, BS, RT(R)(M)(BD)
Mammography Education Coordinator/Mammography
Instructor
Department of Radiology
Saint Joseph Mercy Health System/Washtenaw Community
College
Ann Arbor, Michigan

Ann Hagenau, MS, RT(R)(M)
Associate Professor
Radiologic Technology and Medical Imaging
Clarkson College
Omaha, Nebraska

Julie Hall, MPH, RT(R)(CT)
Program Director
Radiologic Technology
Roane State Community College
Oak Ridge, Tennessee

Phyllis Hooi, MSRS, RT(R)(M)
Medical Radiography Professor
Medical Imaging Technology Program
San Jacinto College Central
Pasadena, Texas

Veronica Manning, EdS, RT(R)(M)
Assistant Professor/Clinical Coordinator
Department of Medical Imaging & Radiation Sciences
Arkansas State University
Jonesboro, Arizona

Debbie McCollam, RT(R)(M), MBA
Department Chair of Medical Imaging Technology
Professor in Radiologic Science
Oregon Tech
Klamath Falls, Oregon

Cynthia Meyers, BS
Professor, Radiologic Technology; Program Coordinator
Niagara County Community College
Sanborn, New York

Mary Potanovic, BS, RT(R)(M)
Assistant Professor
Medical Imaging
Hudson Valley Community College
Troy, New York

Mindy Smith-Amburgey, MA, BSRT(R)(M)RDMS, MBA
Department Chair, Medical Imaging
Program Director, Radiologic Science
University of Charleston
Charleston, West Virginia

Jennifer Wagner, MS, RT(R)(M)(QM), RDMS, RVT
Associate Professor
Allied Health
Fort Hays State University
Hays, Kansas

Richelle Weber, RT(M)(QM)
Adjunct Faculty
Department of Radiography
Cuyahoga Community College
Parma, Ohio

■ FOREWORD

It is a privilege for me to write the foreword to the fourth edition of *Mammographic Imaging: A Practical Guide,* by Shelly Lillé and Wendy Marshall. As a radiologist practicing in Madison, Wisconsin, I was instrumental in introducing the two authors in 1986. At the time, I could not have known that 21 years later, the three of us would reunite once again to provide mammography training to technologists on the other side of the world.

In 1986, our facility in Wisconsin was transitioning from xeromammography to screen/film imaging. The success of the pioneering Elizabeth Wende Logan-Young Breast Center in Rochester, New York, had been widely publicized, and I wanted the imaging techniques used by Logan-Young's technologists to be taught to our Madison technologists. Shelly, Dr. Logan-Young's chief technologist, agreed to come to Madison to work with our group. This would be the first meeting between Shelly and Wendy, one of the mammography technologists in our Madison group.

As a radiologist responsible for interpreting the mammographic study, I have always understood the importance of the technologist's role in executing this procedure. The detection of breast cancer requires excellence in imaging techniques, and for this reason, I have always advocated for the mammography technologist. Each patient encounter requires the technologist to expertly deliver the technical aspects of the examination while demonstrating genuine compassion to the patient. Dr. Logan-Young aptly described the essential attributes of the mammography technologist in the foreword of the second edition of this textbook:

> *"The role of the technologist remains as important and as difficult as ever...The technologist must win each woman's confidence, and treat her as if she is the most important person in the clinic. Once rapport is established, the patient and technologist can work together as a team to obtain the best possible mammogram...The radiologist knows more than anyone the importance of the technologist's role."*

While practicing in Madison, I continued to build upon my dream of returning to Thailand to set up a breast center.

In 1994, on a visit to Thailand, I was very fortunate to have a chance to present my idea to Somdech Phra Srinagarindra Boromarajajonani, known to the Thai people as Princess Mother, the mother of King Rama 9 of Thailand.

HRH Princess Mother advocated programs to improve the lives of Thai people and my presentation of the breast center fit well with her mission to help Thai women. She accepted my proposal to open a breast center, and in early 1995, I retired from Madison Radiologists SC to return to Bangkok and set up the first breast center in Thailand.

Later in 1995, Thanyarak Breast Center was opened at the Siriraj Hospital, Mahidol University in Bangkok, Thailand. My core belief in the importance of the technologist's role in this examination became a cornerstone of Thanyarak Breast Center, and to convey this value along with establishing the importance of the technologist's role within Thanyarak, I had Wendy travel to Thailand several times to mentor my technologists in all aspects of the mammography service.

It was from her initial experience training the technologists at Thanyarak that Wendy's career as a mammography instructor began. Upon her return to Madison, in addition to her lead mammography technologist role at the Dean Clinic (SSM Health), she provided training for new mammography technologists through mammography courses offered throughout the United States.

Soon after Shelly visited Madison to provide training to our technologists, she left her position at the Elizabeth Wende Logan-Young Breast Center to embark on a full-time career of providing mammography education to technologists. Since 1986, she has traveled extensively to share her mammography passion and expertise with hundreds of facilities and thousands of technologists, affectionately earning her the nickname, "Janey Appleseed."

The authors commitment to provide quality mammography education to technologists would eventually bring Wendy and Shelly together again in 2004, when they were asked to team teach an initial qualifications course in mammography throughout the United States. This partnership would bring the three of us together again after 21 years, when they traveled to the Thanyarak Breast Center in Bangkok to provide educational training to our technologists in 2007. Thanyarak has flourished since then, and our technologists are among the best in their profession.

Today, Thanyarak Breast Center is a state-of-the-art facility that currently provides mammography services to 65,000 women each year. Each day the Thanyarak staff perform 250 mammograms, 200 ultrasounds, and 10 biopsy procedures.

I have always had a very strong appreciation for Wendy and Shelly, both in the United States and in Thailand, and I am proud of them both for their efforts in the field and for updating this textbook. As in the mammography courses they have taught together over the last many years, the authors share their knowledge in all aspects of the mammography procedure and the patient experience inside the pages of this book.

It is invaluable how Wendy and Shelly share their expertise in the technical aspect of the examination, quality assurance and quality control, breast anatomy, and positioning and compression are just some of the subjects that satisfy the reader's desire to understand more about this challenging field. And because the authors have continued to practice mammography alongside their educational careers, they are able to bring practical solutions to the challenging techniques critical to image quality.

Thank you, Wendy and Shelly for continuing in your efforts to help provide the important foundations for practice to all current and future technologists.

To all the technologists who read this textbook, please know that I and every other radiologist are grateful to you for your role in providing each patient with quality imaging and for the compassionate care you impart to each individual. I applaud you all for your commitment to this significant medical imaging modality. It takes a special person to work in this discipline, someone who understands the meticulous requirements of creating the image, while also preserving the dignity of the patient.

My best wishes to you all throughout your career in this important field.

Tamnit Ansusinha, MD
Co-Founder, Madison Radiologists, Madison, Wisconsin
Secretary General, Thanyarak Foundation Under Patronage of Her Royal Highness Princess
Somdech Phra Srinagarindra
Chairman, Thanyarak Breast Center, Siriraj Hospital,
Mahidol University
Bangkok, Thailand

▍▍ PREFACE

The history of *Mammographic Imaging: A Practical Guide.*

1992, the first edition. Authors: Valerie Andolina, Shelly Lillé, Kathleen Willison. 300 pages.

2001, the second edition. Authors: Valerie Andolina, Shelly Lillé, Kathleen Willison. 500 pages.

2011, the third edition. Authors: Valerie Andolina and Shelly Lillé. 600 pages.

2019, the fourth edition. Authors: Shelly Lillé and Wendy Marshall. 608 pages.

Anyone who knows me knows my penchant for making analogies. While sitting at the kitchen table over my morning cup of coffee and contemplating what to write for the preface, I turned to my comfort zone—an analogy: writing a textbook is like buying a house. Growing up, one lives in a house—but this does not prepare you to purchase a house; similarly, one can read books, but this does not prepare you to write a book.

As young technologists, writing the first edition was like buying our first house. As a first-time home buyer, you must be educated in financial matters: that is, interest rates, closing costs; schooled in looking at home construction features: that is, cracked foundation walls, pitch of the roof; neighborhood scrutiny: that is, deed restrictions, school system; and learn to set and adhere to a budget before you actually start looking at houses. As authors, we had to learn about contracts and deadlines, artlogs, camera-ready art, galleys, references, permissions, and so much more. Then we had to decide which topics to consider, research these topics, and finally pick up a pen and actually start writing.

The second edition was so much easier to write because we were familiar with the entire process. The second edition was like remodeling our first house; we knew what we liked in our original house, and we knew what additions we wanted to make. In many respects, a new edition is like remodeling an old house; sometimes, it is painful to let things go that have sentimental value, but you do so because it is necessary to move on.

Edition 3 was nostalgic. Kathy Willison went to work in the commercial sector, so she opted out of involvement with this edition. It was like having one of the family members leave home to go off to college. The house got bigger for the two occupants left inside. We did some rearranging of the furniture and transformed the newly unused bedroom into a new living space.

With the fourth edition, I am moving into a brand new house. And I have a new co-owner of the house because Valerie Andolina retired from working… and from writing.

I am delighted to welcome Wendy Marshall. I have lectured with Wendy for more than 20 years. In our Initial Training course, she taught the art of positioning and unraveled the mysteries of QC, while I taught physics, anatomy, and pathology. Wendy has an innovative way of presenting positioning and compression. When she taught technologists just entering the field of mammography how to perform the CC and MLO projections, the students were well prepared when it came time for the hands-on positioning workshops. You will find the positioning chapters in this book to be user-friendly, and a helpful reference guide.

Wendy's true passion is QC. Analog QC was easier to teach than digital QC. In analog imaging, QC tests were standardized; whether you used Kodak film, or Agfa, or Fuji, all QC was the same. But with digital imaging, each manufacturer establishes their own QC requirements, plus the ACR offers an alternative version that attempts to standardize QC among all the manufacturers. I give much credit to Wendy for tackling this now convoluted topic.

A house can be built in 6 months; a textbook takes 2 years. With each of these textbook editions, it took a year and a half of researching and writing, followed by 6 months for the publisher to prepare the material for publication. We have already started our list of topics for the next edition to be published in 2029!

Wendy and I trust you will find this fourth edition to be a valuable resource.

Shelly Lillé

ACKNOWLEDGMENTS

With each edition of this textbook, the list of people I am indebted to grows longer. As I was making my list of acknowledgments for this fourth edition, I thought of the academy award shows on television, such as The Oscars, where the winning actors are on stage accepting their award...they take a piece of paper from their pocket and begin reading off a long list of names. The actors acknowledge the assistance of many others, without whose efforts there would be no award.

This textbook was not written by just Wendy and me, it is from all the interactions we've had with our mentors, teachers, medical physicists, service engineers, x-ray equipment company representatives, administrators, IT personnel, coworkers, patients, and our families. How do you thank all the people you have interacted with for decades? I have made my list and trust you all know how grateful I am for your willingness to explain concepts, for the time you expended on my behalf, and for your friendship.

Wende Westinghouse Logan-Young, MD. Even though you are now retired, you remain my mentor. Much gratitude to you for conducting mammography seminars beginning in the 1970s; this guided me to my career-long "Janey Appleseed" role.

Angie and (the late) Jack Cullinan. The impetus for writing the first edition. Without Angie's and Jack's encouragement, there never would have been a textbook.

The group from Wolters Kluwer:

   Jay Campbell—acquisitions editor
   Amy Millholen—product manager
   Emily Buccieri—editorial coordinator
   Bonnie Arbittier—photographer

I would be lost without the staff from WK to point the way. Jay: the extraordinary team leader. Amy: you did such fantastic work on third edition, thankfully we were reunited on the fourth edition. Thank you for all of your suggestions and solutions. Emily: you are fortunate to have Amy as a mentor; follow her lead and you'll be fantastic too. Bonnie: our nimble photographer who was able to contort herself in various positions in order to obtain photos from the correct perspective. And to our models for the positioning chapters, we are grateful to you for your patience in maintaining a pose until the photo was "just right."

Valerie Andolina and Kathy Willison. My original coworkers and coauthors. Thank you for establishing the foundation for this textbook. Wendy and I carry on your legacy.

The supportive team from Manatee Memorial Hospital in Bradenton, Florida:

   Amy Beaubien for discovering a method that saved me from months of searching for cases in PACS. Jason McLeod for reviewing and making suggestions for the MRI chapter. Mary Anne Edwards and Patricia Scruggs—it is impossible for me to put into words how much I value your support and needed your encouragement throughout this entire project. I managed to include you in photos in this book so that when I am old and gray and look at these pages, I will remember you both and all fun we had collecting cases.

   Marcy Adcox and Hologic, Inc. You have been a true friend and a valuable resource for almost every chapter in this book. How fortunate our paths crossed almost 40 years ago. Please "hang around" for the fifth edition, 10 years from now. Your e-mail in-box will again be flooded with requests for figures and information.

   Dr. Ed Barnes and Don Jacobson. Medical physicists. Thank you for expanding my knowledge base in mammography physics and for your willingness to share your information in my physics chapters. For 30 years, you have been my physics mentors.

My family. Joanne Lillé—artist. The creative one of the group. Thank you for the drawings; your art will live on through these textbooks. My sisters: Marlaya and Elizabeth. Your encouragement and taking over of daily chores freed up time to research, write, edit, rewrite, and edit some more.

Contributing author: Gerald Kolb, president of The Breast Group. Thank you for contributing the breast density section in Chapter 21. As always, your skill with a pen is logical, methodical, and factual.

Contributing author: Dr. Gale Sisney. Chapter 10 needed the perspective of a radiologist, so thanks to Wendy for volunteering you to write this chapter. Mark your calendar for 10 years from now for the three of us to undertake the fifth edition.

The Koning Corporation representatives: Roger Zhang and David Georges. Dave has had an impressive career in women's health care; he taught me about the business side. Contributing author: Dr. Avice O'Connell, University of Rochester Medical Center, for the section on Coned Beam Breast CT in Chapter 21. Thank you for your willingness to share your experience with this exciting technology.

My "bosom buddies": Rosalind Hall and Thelma. Ros, you have been a steadfast friend. Thank you for all the prayer chains. Thelma, I have told you more than a million times how thankful I am that we are life-long friends.

Ken Lillé. My rock. Steadfast, supportive, strong.

Shelly Lillé

Mammography has interested me since I was a student in radiology science. I was drawn to it because of its complex blend of science, art, and communication. It was my good fortune that an opportunity to work in this discipline arose early in my career, which has allowed me to spend almost 40 years continually learning about the breast imaging industry as it has evolved. Coauthoring this textbook has given me a unique opportunity to reflect on years of practice, objectives, and growth, and pull from them the knowledge and experiences that will provide the most value and meaning to those who wish to learn about this exciting and rewarding field. In doing so, I am reminded of the people and circumstances that have been so formative and influential throughout this journey. I have been fortunate to observe and learn from a number of professionals who have modeled the highest standards in quality and commitment to their craft. I am eternally grateful to those individuals who have "stood out" among the many; these are the colleagues and patients who have inspired my passion for this work, and whose valuable messages are imprinted in the pages of this book.

I am indebted to the many people who provided their expertise, advice, and assistance and to those who offered their steadfast support throughout this process. To all of these individuals, I would like to express my heartfelt appreciation.

To my husband Richard. Thank you for your never-ending patience, understanding, encouragement, and love. I am so lucky to share my life with you. To my three daughters, Lauren, Leah, and Lydia. The greatest privilege of my life has been being your mom. I have learned so much from you, thank you for teaching me.

To my mentor, Dr. Tamnit Ansusinha, whose example instilled in me the desire to learn and understand the science and art of mammography. He taught me that sharing knowledge is an obligation and an opportunity to empower others to improve patient care.

To the folks at Wolters Kluwer who entrusted the coauthorship of this textbook to me. My sincere thanks to Jay Campbell, Amy Millholen, and Emily Buccieri for their expertise and continual guidance throughout my foray into their world. Their advice will always be appreciated and their patience and professionalism always remembered. To Bonnie Arbittier, our unflappable photographer, we are grateful for your precision in capturing the artistic message in your photos.

To my friend and coauthor Shelly Lillé who so generously shared her knowledge and experience as an author with me throughout the entire process. I am so grateful for the privilege of working with Shelly. She is a wealth of knowledge and has a heart of gold. Many thanks to her husband Ken, who also lent his support in assisting me. They are friends for life.

To Kathy Willison and Valerie Andolina, the authors of the previous editions of this book. Although we have never met, I feel I know you. We share the same commitment to empowering the technologist. Thank you for framing the foundation of this book; your efforts provided a blueprint to build upon.

To SSM Health, Dean Medical Group, radiology administration. Thank you for cultivating an environment that encourages professional growth and fosters educational experiences. These endeavors promote the highest quality care for patients. Special thanks to Seth Teigen and Jolene Kent for their generous support during this process.

To Gale Sisney, MD, (Global Radiology Outreach) for her valuable contribution to the fourth edition. Her unique ability to educate technologists is shared in Chapter 15 through an exercise she designed to explain the medical audit. Chapter 10, Practical Applications in Problem Solving is described through the lens of Dr. Sisney's vast experience as a breast imaging specialist, providing the technologist a solid foundation for mammography imaging protocols. It has been my privilege to work with Dr. Sisney on many educational projects. She is a respected mentor to technologists, recognizing their valuable contribution to breast imaging, and committed to their success. Gale has been my teacher and my friend for many years, for which I am so grateful.

To Tom Aufdemberge, MS, DABR, (Medical Physics Consultants, Inc.), for helping me to understand the technical intricacies of achieving image quality in mammography. His willingness to provide answers to my endless questions and requests for explanations of mammography physics and equipment analysis over the past 16 years sparked in me a deep interest in quality improvement and mammography performance metrics that I would never have otherwise discovered. His advisement for Chapters 15 and 16 is greatly valued and appreciated. Thank you, Tom, for your generous gift of time and your incredible patience.

To my fellow technologists at SSM Health, Dean Medical Group, who supported me in so many ways throughout this process. They were always ready to lend me assistance whenever it was needed and for their kindness and support I will always be grateful. Special thanks go to Mary Klund, Chris Andrews, Cindy Pack, Ginger Anderson, Kathy Seltzner, Beth Mecum, Anne Koller, Dana Borgerding, Denise Konopacki, and Linda Smith for going above and beyond. You are the best!

Julie and Nicole Waner, Cindy Pack and Keith Schmudlach, and Linda Abel, my Waunakee friends, thank you for answering the call to contribute your time and efforts when they were needed. Your kindness will be remembered always.

The following individuals offered their assistance and advice in their area of expertise when it was needed:

Kari Sievert, Regional Coordinator, Wisconsin Well Woman Program (WWWP)
Leslie Christensen, SSM Health, Manager-Medical Library
Gregg Bogost, MD, Madison Radiologists, SC
Ronald Dolin, MD, Madison Radiologists, SC

Harold Bennett, MD, Madison Radiologists, SC

Thank you for your contribution to the fourth edition, your willingness to help made a difference and is greatly appreciated.

Wendy Marshall, RTR (M)(QM)

▌▌ USER'S GUIDE

This User's Guide introduces you to the helpful features of *Mammographic Imaging: A Practical Guide, Fourth Edition*, that enable you to quickly master new concepts and put your new skills into practice.

Creating the Digital Image

12

Objectives

Objectives help you focus on the most important information to glean from the chapter.

- List the key factors that made mammography the last x-ray procedure to convert to digital imaging.
- Explain the impact the ACRIN/DMIST study had on the acceptance of digital technology for mammography.
- Identify the components of a digital mammography system.
- Describe two methods of digital image production.
- Describe how a digital image is created and processed.
- Sequence the steps of image production and evaluation of the digital image.
- Explain the postprocessing features available to the radiologist at the reviewstation.
- **Define the terminology for digital image creation, storage, transmission, and retrieval.**

Key Terms

Key Terms for the most important concepts are listed at the beginning of the chapters, bolded at first mention in the chapter, and defined in the online Glossary.

- algorithms
- American College of Radiology Imaging Network/Digital Mammographic Imaging Screening Trial (ACRIN/DMIST)
- bit depth
- **detective quantum efficiency (DQE)**
- digital array
- Digital Imaging and Communications in Medicine (DICOM)
- direct conversion
- dynamic range
- **flat panel detector**
- hospital information system (HIS)
- indirect conversion

- Integrating the Healthcare Enterprise (IHE)
- matrix
- modality worklist (MWL)
- modulation transfer function (MTF)
- noise
- Picture Archival Communication System (PACS)
- pixel
- **postprocessing refinements**
- radiology information system (RIS)
- signal-to-noise ratio (SNR)
- window center
- window width

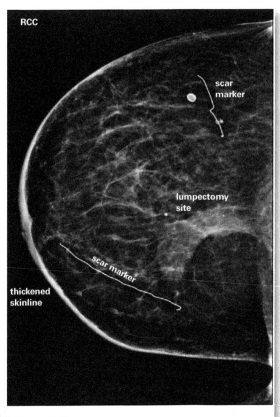

Figure 6-10
Skin thickening caused by lumpectomy with radiation treat-ment for breast cancer.

Helpful **Figures** and **Tables** throughout the text aid the visual learner.

Table 2-4 • Trends: Breast Cancer Death Rates for Females in the United States[a]

YEAR	RECORDED DEATHS
1989	43,391
1990	43,391
1991	43,583
1992	43,068
1993	43,555
1994	43,644
1995	43,844
1996	43,091
1997	41,943
1998	41,737
1999	41,144
2000	41,872
2001	41,394
2002	41,514
2003	41,620
2004	40,954
2005	41,116
2006	40,821
2007	40,460
2008	40,480
2009	40,170
2010	40,230
2011	39,970
2012	39,920
2013	40,030
2014	40,430
2015	40,730
2016	40,730

[a]Screening mammography begins in the United States in the mid 1980s. By the mid 1990s, we see the beginnings of a downward trend in mortality.
Source: U.S. Mortality Data, 1990–2016. National Center for Health Statistics, Center for Disease Control and Prevention; 2016.

Case Studies allow for practical application of chapter material.

Case Study **12-2**

Refer to Figure 12-19 and the text and respond to the following questions.

1. Which component contains the digital array?

2. Which component(s) does the technologist utilize?

3. Where is PACS physically located?

4. Why do all the components interact with "DICOM connectivity"?

Review Questions at the end of each chapter encourage critical thinking.

Review Questions

1. Why was mammography the last of the imaging modalities to go digital?

2. What conclusions came out of the ACRIN/DMIST study?

3. List the advantages of digital mammography.

4. The IHE Mammography Subcommittee is charged with improving connectivity issues between multiple vendor equipment. Why is this necessary?

5. What is the difference between the matrix, a pixel, and a TFT?

6. What function does flat-fielding provide?

7. Compare and contrast the indirect and direct-to-digital methods.

ADDITIONAL LEARNING RESOURCES

Valuable ancillary resources for both students and instructors are available on thePoint companion Website at http://thepoint.lww.com. See the inside front cover for details on how to access these resources.

Student Resources include a registry exam style question bank, glossary, PowerPoint slides, and case studies with situational judgment questions.

Instructor Resources include a test bank, PowerPoint slides, answers to chapter review questions and case studies, and answers to situational judgment questions.

CONTENTS

Mammography: Common Topic

History of Mammography

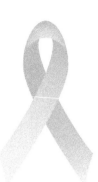

1

Those who cannot remember the past are condemned to repeat it.
—George Santayana

Objectives

- To relate the growth of mammography over its 95 years to 3 eras of development: a long and slow use of general x-ray units to serve only symptomatic patients (1925 to 1970), dedicated mammography units adopted with growing support for mammography specialization servicing asymptomatic women (1970 to 1990), and rapid professional and public support for screening mammography to connect with many imaging and treatment modalities (1990 through present)

- To identify early mammography practices that are no longer in use

- To gain an appreciation for the connection between scientific advances from technology and biology that made mammography what it is today

---

Key Terms

- analog mammography
- breast cancer
- dedicated mammography machine
- digital mammography
- screening mammography
- xeroradiography

INTRODUCTION

*"I remember the exact moment I found my breast cancer. Time stood still as my heart pounded. My brain tried to rationalize away this newfound lump in my breast," the woman sobbed. So many times, as the radiologic technologist performing a mammogram on such a woman, I've wanted to ask, "Why ... why did you **wait** to have a mammogram?"*

Breast cancer is emotional. Breast cancer is biologic. Mammography technologists must continue to search for a better understanding of both aspects of the disease to improve the technical skills necessary to detect disease and to strengthen interpersonal skills to help their patients.

This book addresses the biologic aspects of breast cancer from many viewpoints. These viewpoints include the etiology of breast disease and its appearance, the anatomy of the breast, how breast tissue affects and is affected by the design and performance of dedicated mammography machines, the appearance of breast tissue on a mammographic image, and positioning of the breast. Dealing with the emotional aspects of women who may/may not have breast cancer depends on your knowledge of the examination and your interpersonal skills. The radiologic technologist's focus is to help the patient progress through the mammogram. Firm breast compression and general anxiety worry most women. From the important initial meeting with the patient, through history taking and discussing breast health issues, the radiologic technologist allays the woman's fears. A patient's emotions can range from a mild case of embarrassment to hostile resistance. Mammographers have a responsibility to care about patients and to help them in a professional manner.

The history of mammography makes three points clear:

1. Breast cancer continues to be a major killer of women in the United States.
2. Early detection is necessary to improve the survival rate of women with breast cancer.
3. Knowledge of breast disease coupled with improved technical skills and a genuine concern for the health and well-being of your patients motivates the radiologic technologist to detect disease and to educate their patients about better breast care.

This book is written *by* radiologic technologists *for* radiologic technologists. The authors share their experiences, collect information about mammography, and present it from a practical viewpoint that is useful to the radiologic technologist.

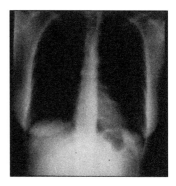

Figure 1-1
The outline of the breast is apparent on a chest x-ray. This realization triggered the first attempts to x-ray the breast for evidence of disease.

HISTORY

The Oldest Story in Mammography

Legend has it that the concept of mammography was first proposed in 1924 when a group of male radiologists in Rochester, NY, assembled around a viewbox "admiring" the chest x-ray of a buxom woman (Figure 1-1). After a brief discussion that included both playful and serious remarks, the radiologists' thoughts and discussions turned toward speculation about the ability to x-ray the breast to locate tumors. Stafford Warren, MD, published the first article on mammography in 1930.[1] Warren described the use of double-emulsion film and intensifying screens; a moving grid; a 60-kVp, 70-mA, 2.5-second exposure; and a 25-in. source-image detector distance. Articles detailing radiography of mastectomy specimens were published before 1930.

The Father of Mammography

It was not until the 1960s that the "father of mammography," Robert Egan, MD, then at M.D. Anderson Hospital in Houston, began teaching his mammographic technique. With his assistance, the American College of Radiology (ACR) established training centers for radiologists and technologists throughout the United States.

Not all in the medical community were as impressed with mammography and its potential as were those in the field of radiology. Many surgeons were concerned that a negative mammogram might delay or prevent an exploration suggested on clinical grounds. Experts ... protested that if a cancer was present, their fingers would find it, and that the "new-fangled" modality was not only unnecessary, but perhaps insidious. Many radiologists furtively attempting the new technique were effectively suppressed by blown x-ray tubes, less than 98% accu-

racy, and supercilious sneers of their surgical colleagues. However, a few radiologists persisted, excited by the potential of mammography. After all, there was a great need for improved diagnosis in breast disease, especially in that gray area of "fibrocystic disease." Also at times, cancer was detected when clinical findings were questionable and, even more remarkably, completely non-palpable cancers which turned out to have a high degree of no axillary nodal involvement were often discovered.[2]

We acknowledge and appreciate the efforts of the countless radiologists who valiantly maintained their belief in mammography. Any new procedure will be scrutinized and compared with current detection modalities. If the new procedure endures through initial doubts of its integrity, and the basic tenets upon which the examinations are proven to be sound, then those who helped evolve the examinations' principles deserve our gratitude.

The Vision: Early Detection

Early attempts in mammography were crude compared to the quality of images produced today. From mammography's advent in 1924 until the early 1980s, mammograms were done primarily on symptomatic patients who were referred to radiologists for the purpose of verifying breast disease before her appointment with a surgeon. The cancers were clinically obvious (Figure 1-2).

Few radiologists had any interest in mammography, yet all understood the futility of rendering a diagnosis for cancer in a later stage of development. The pioneers, men and women with a clear vision for change, developed screening mammography for asymptomatic women and pulled us into what wasn't possible in 1924 but was everywhere on earth before the end of the century.

Our resolute images today allow us to discover impalpable cancers; cancers so small that unless the interpreter remains ever vigilant, they easily can be overlooked. Radiologists need to maintain focused concentration while searching every image for these smaller indicators of disease and/or subtle changes in breast tissue when compared with prior images.

Earlier and Earlier

The ACR has always promoted efforts for change. Doctor Franklin Alcorn lauded their efforts in his 1971 paper, lamented that perhaps a physician assistant could help the radiologist, and called for his profession to do more to improve mammography.[3] During the 1970s, Doctor Lazlo Tabar and his colleagues in Sweden pioneered a three-county mammography screening trial of asymptomatic women as part of their country's national health program. In the United States, Doctors Philip Strax and Ferris Hall, forward-thinking clinicians, were moderators for a 1978 medical conference that featured papers and reports on early studies to detect breast disease in asymptomatic patients. Doctor Wende Logan-Young and others tested new special films for mammography and new dedicated mammography machines. Doctors Logan-Young and Edward Sickles pioneered magnification. In the 1980s, Doctors Lawrence Bassett and Stephen Feig worked on studies to improve the quality of mammograms. Doctors Young, Sickles, Tabar, Bassett, Feig, McLelland, Dowd, Alcorn, Strax, Hall, and countless other visionaries helped lay the groundwork with new techniques, positioning, and clinical practice to elevate mammography and women's health care to the levels we currently practice. Every visionary shared their passion for mammography and earlier breast cancer detection through innovations to their clinical practice, research, participation in professional and public efforts related to mammography, and in their publications. They shaped much of what is common today in mammography centers around the world. A closer look into one such medical practice provides us with an excellent example of this paradigm shift from imaging only symptomatic woman in the later stages of breast disease to screening asymptomatic women to detect breast disease earlier.

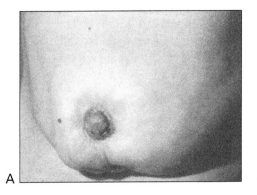 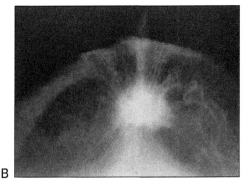

A   B

Figure 1-2
(A) Clinical signs of an advanced breast cancer. **(B)** With these clinically advanced cancers, the tumor is readily identified on the mammogram. Note the thickened, retracted skin line.

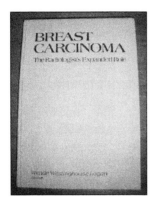

Figure 1-3
Breast Carcinoma: The Radiologist's Expanded Role, by Wende Westinghouse Logan. Published in 1977.

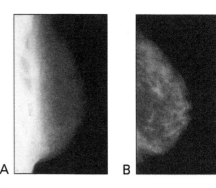

Figure 1-4
(A) Image taken with an all-purpose x-ray machine (circa 1960).
(B) The same breast imaged with a dedicated mammography machine (circa 1970).

Doctor Wende Westinghouse Logan-Young

In her 1977 book *Breast Carcinoma: The Radiologist's Expanded Role,* published 53 years after the start of mammography, Doctor Wende Westinghouse Logan-Young foretold the future: the creation of specialized breast care centers staffed by radiologists who actively participate in diagnostic mammography exams (Figure 1-3).

When Dr. Young opened her private practice breast center in Rochester, New York, in 1974, she participated in every patient's exam ranging from performing the clinical breast exam, ultrasound, cyst aspiration, ductogram, preoperative wire localization, and FNAC, and sometimes, she even positioned the woman for her mammogram! Before the woman left the center, Dr. Young always gave her the results of the mammogram.

Dr. Young realized imagers (radiologists) were in the best position to take charge of this image-directed diagnostic procedure. The radiologist is the diagnostician who is able to correlate the clinical breast exam with the findings on x-ray and ultrasound images, to focus on regions of interest during the diagnostic mammogram, and to perform a biopsy using ultrasound or x-ray guidance when required. Dr. Young's belief was that radiologists were in a unique position to become active participants in breast health care. Her philosophy had radiologists behaving as clinicians; up until this time, most were passive participants, isolated in the reading room. The reward for the breast imaging specialist is that they follow the patient from her screening mammogram to her final diagnosis. They are able to go full circle with patients and become more of a clinician.

Today, we find mammography centers throughout the world, staffed by radiologists who interact with their patients and who encourage their radiologic technologists to assist far beyond simply performing the mammogram. Radiologists have embraced their expanded role: once a screening exam becomes a diagnostic study, a radiologist actively participates in the exam.

I (SL') had the good fortune to work with and to learn from Dr. Logan-Young, to assist her in performing clinical breast exams, ultrasound, cyst aspiration, ductogram, preoperative wire localization, FNAC, mammograms, and other procedures. I came to share her passion for quality mammography and her focus on saving a woman's life. Her vision for the future was for radiologists to expand their role for better patient care; the authors' vision is for radiologic technologists to expand their role for earlier detection of breast disease and better patient care.

Improvements to mammography continue; it progresses while riding on the hopes of current visionaries. Compared with the 3D digital images we produce today, these initial attempts in mammography were of limited value and are considered archaic (Figure 1-4). But to put things in perspective, in the future when breast cancer is detected in its earliest, cellular stage, current mammography will be considered primitive.

In the Beginning

Doctor Warren produced his initial breast images in 1924 using the only x-ray machine in his facility (Figure 1-5). His all-purpose x-ray machine produced chest radiographs in the morning and mammograms in the afternoon. Tungsten target tubes with glass windows and aluminum filtration resulted in low-contrast mammographic images because of the high half-value layer (HVL) associated with this system. Initially double-emulsion film in conjunction with two intensifying screens captured the image. Due to poor contrast and resolution, this recording system yielded to the use of direct exposure single-emulsion medical or industrial film packaged inside a cardboard holder. Few physicians showed an interest in mammography over the next 35 years; it remained in the shadows of clinical medicine.

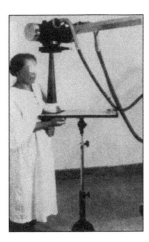

Figure 1-5
Initial attempts to image the breast (circa 1930). Photo courtesy of Pam Fulmer.

The Times They Were A-Changin': 1960s

The turbulent 1960s were a watershed for changes in society, feminist politics, and mammography. The clarion call sounded for mass screening and lower-dose mammography. Women saw the dramatic decrease in the number of deaths due to cervical cancer because the Pap smear was used in mass screening; they hoped **screening mammography** could replicate the success of the Pap smear and reduce the death rate from breast cancer.

During the early 1960s, the Haloid Corporation, with their principal investigator, John Wolfe, MD, began experimenting with a new recording system that eventually would become known as **xeroradiography** (Figure 1-6). X-ray facilities could continue to use their general all-purpose x-ray machine to produce breast images with xeroradiography by changing only the recording medium. The purchase of selenium plates to capture the latent image and the purchase of a processing and conditioning unit were required to produce these lower-dose, better

resolution images with its wonderful edge-enhancing capability. Xeroradiography became available commercially in 1971.

The Start of Modern Mammography

Meanwhile, on the other side of the Atlantic Ocean, Charles Gros, MD, and the CGR Company developed the first **dedicated mammography machine** in France in the mid-1960s. This was the first significant step in the development of mammography for mass screening.

The heart of the new unit, the molybdenum target tube, evolved from technology developed for quality control efforts in automobile and truck tire production. Tire manufacturing companies initially used the molybdenum target tube to produce high-contrast images of their tires to search for imperfections during final inspection. Until Gros adapted this invention, the ceiling-mounted, tungsten target diagnostic x-ray unit used for chest radiographs and other general radiologic studies was also used for mammography.

The new dedicated mammography unit, introduced commercially in the United States in 1969, incorporated a molybdenum target, utilized low kVp's, and had an integral device for compressing the breast (Figure 1-7). These three important contributions solved a major shortcoming of early mammography: low-contrast images. However, other problems persisted. Only direct exposure film (either medical or industrial) was available, and it required long x-ray exposure times and hand processing in the darkroom, both of which were time-consuming and cumbersome. Also, 8 to 12 R was a typical patient dose. Excessive radiation dose became an easy target for the early critics of mammography.

Meanwhile, xeroradiography flourished in the United States during the 1970s. By the mid-to-late 1980s, this method of imaging the breast was all but extinct. Frequent repairs to the conditioning and processing units along with a higher radiation dose contributed to the rapid demise of this modality. Screen–film (analog) imaging, introduced in

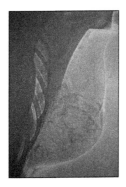

Figure 1-6
Xeromammography image displays as blue toner deposited on white paper. No viewbox required.

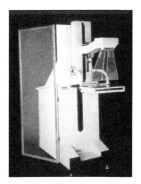

Figure 1-7
An early dedicated mammography machine (circa 1975).

1972, quickly surpassed xeroradiography as the preferred method of imaging.

Change, Change, and More Change

Xeroradiography, **analog mammography**, and **digital mammography** imaging systems have a common purpose: to x-ray the breast; but the similarities end there. The transition from xeroradiography to analog imaging was difficult for physicians and technologists because the two methods are dissimilar. Unfortunately, some misconceptions about mammography and some outmoded practices based on xeroradiographic principles still persist. It is important to recognize these outdated practices and to understand how they are often at odds with high-quality mammography of today.

The Major Differences

There are three major differences between xeroradiography and analog or digital imaging:

1. X-ray equipment and recording systems
2. Technical factors and radiographic physics
3. Patient positioning and radiographic landmarks

Various chapters in this book present information in each of these major categories as they apply to digital mammography. This section deals with the differences that confuse technologists even today (Table 1-1). The author assumes the reader is familiar with the principles of xeroradiography.

Case Study **1-1**

Refer to Table 1-1 and respond to the following questions:

1. Is positioning the breast the same in all three modalities?

2. Can the same mammography machine be used in all three modalities?

3. Is a distinctly separate processing unit used in all three modalities?

Nipple in Profile

"The nipple must always be imaged in profile" was a basic protocol and cardinal rule of xeroradiography. Toner robbing occurred on a xeromammogram when the nipple was projected into the breast (Figure 1-8). Analog and digital imaging do not have toner deposition problems.

The nipple is centrally located on the breast for most women; therefore, the nipple will be in profile or nearly in profile upon final compression. However, this is not the case for all women. Some women will be full either inferiorly (the bottom half of the breast), with little tissue in the superior aspect, or the opposite. When positioning these women for a xeromammogram, the technologist pulled posteroinferior or posterosuperior tissue, respectively, *off the image receptor* to image the nipple in profile.

Table 1-1 • Comparisons between Mammographic Systems

XERORADIOGRAPHY	ANALOG IMAGING	DIGITAL IMAGING
Major Differences		
Existing x-ray system (dedicated or overhead)	Dedicated mammography machine	Dedicated mammography machine
Tungsten target tube	Molybdenum/rhodium target tubes	Molybdenum/rhodium/tungsten target tubes
Selenium plate	Screen–film recording system	Digital detector
Specialized processing for selenium plates	Screen–film darkroom techniques	Electronic readout by computer
Blue and white images on paper	Black and white images on film	Black and white images on computer monitor
Curved compression device; kVp settings > 35	Straight-edge compression device; 25–32 kVp	Straight-edge compression device; 25–32 kVp
Minor Differences		
Nipple always in profile	Not required	Not required
Visualization of ribs	Not required	Not required
Laterally oriented CC projection	Medially oriented CC projection	Medially oriented CC projection
Lateral position	Oblique position	Oblique position
Visualization of the skin line	Not required, not visualized	Not required, but visualized
Use of sponges	Not required	Not required
No antiperspirant/powder	Not required	Not required
Breath holding	Not required	Not required

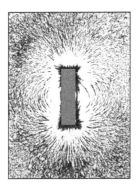

Figure 1-8
Xeromammography displays edge enhancement, a beneficial image-processing effect that highlights spiculation associated with architectural distortion, and also enhances the visualization of calcifications. The unwanted effect of edge enhancement: toner robbing. Toner robbing occurs when the nipple is not in profile (rather it is rolled into the breast), when skin folds are present, and when metallic particles associated with antiperspirant use are present in the high apex of the axilla. Toner robbing is a similar effect to iron filings attracted by a magnet; no filings are evident in the area surrounding the magnet. This same effect happens with blue toner deposited on the Xerox paper: there is no (*blue*) image surrounding the nipple, skin fold, or antiperspirant. (Image from Shutterstock, Inc.)

The nipple should, whenever possible, be projected tangentially. However, it is not always possible to observe this rule and at the same time include a maximal portion of the breast. In general, it is more important to visualize the posterior portion of the breast. It is usually not difficult to identify the nipple even if it is projected over breast tissue in one of the views.[4]

In mammography, there are three instances in which the nipple must be in profile:

1. Women who have spontaneous unilateral nipple discharge. Papillomas account for the vast majority of cases of nipple discharge and the vast majority of papillomas are within 1 cm of the nipple.
2. When performing a mammogram on a male. Males have rudimentary breast buds, as in an adolescent female. These tiny buds of tissue lie directly behind the nipple. The nipple must be in profile to visualize this small amount of tissue adequately. If this means removing some posterior "breast" tissue that you have captured on the image receptor, you are actually removing pectoral muscle because males have bigger, more developed muscles.
3. To determine the exact location of a region of interest (ROI) in order to perform triangulation for preoperative wire localization, fine-needle aspiration cytology (FNAC), or stereotactic core biopsy.

Mammography technologists work diligently to capture all the breast tissue on an image. Strict adherence to the outmoded xeroradiographic protocol of imaging the nipple in profile is counterproductive because it removes some tissue from the image.

Many think the nipple must be in profile to ascertain the location of a lesion. The nipple does not need to be perfectly in profile to do so. Craniocaudal (CC) views indicate whether the lesion lies in the medial half of the breast or in the lateral half. A nipple rolled into the breast tissue provides this same information. Lateral views (ML/LM) give superior or inferior location of a lesion relative to the nipple. Again a nipple rolled into the breast tissue provides this same information.

When the mammographer suspects a lump or lesion in the patient's nipple area, and the nipple does not fall in profile, she will take an additional image. Routine images should demonstrate as much breast tissue as possible; the extra image visualizes just the anterior portion of the breast with the nipple in profile. If possible, magnify the second image. The information obtained from magnifying the nipple and retroareolar region in profile will be far greater than that of the standard image.

Visualization of the Ribs

Technical differences between xeroradiography and analog mammography made it necessary to modify positioning and technique to meet the specific requirements of each modality. It was disconcerting to the technologist experienced in xeroradiography to exclude the ribs from the analog study. However, every position we subject the patient to will miss a portion of the breast, regardless of the imaging method—whether it is xeroradiography or analog or digital imaging and whether or not the ribs are included. The reason for this is that breasts attach to the rib cage, a curvilinear structure (Figure 1-9).

Xeroradiography demonstrated the retroglandular fat space and the ribs in the Lateral view. Early mammographers believed displaying these structures on a single image ensured all breast tissue was visualized. However, this belief created a false sense of security because the image visualized only the portion of the ribs and retroglandular fat space tangential to the x-ray beam. Posterolateral tissue that wraps around the curvature of the ribs was superimposed. Xeroradiography compensated for the nonvisualization of posterolateral breast tissue in the Lateral view by including this area on the laterally exaggerated CC view (Figure 1-10C).

Case Study **1-2**

Refer to Figure 1-10 and respond to the following questions:

1. A specific portion of the breast is missed in each position we do. What area does the CC view miss? The MLO view? The Lateral view?
2. Which view images the most breast tissue? What portion of the breast is not included in this view?

Xeroradiography

Screen/Film Imaging

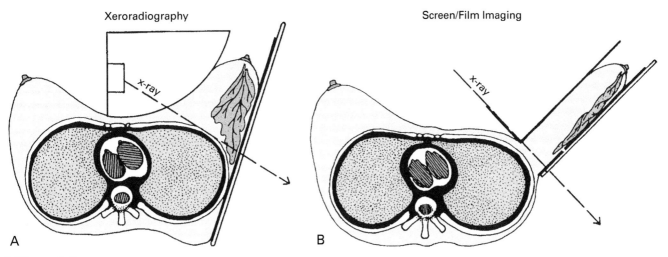

A

B

Figure 1-9
(A) In xeromammography, the central ray is directed tangentially across the rib cage. Because of the curve of the compression device and the need to visualize into the lung field, the breast cannot be pulled away and kept away from the ribs as compression is applied. Thus, posterolateral tissue is not visualized; however, the CC view will be laterally oriented to include this area. Medial tissue also is not included because of the divergence of the x-ray beam. **(B)** In analog and digital imaging, the chest wall edge of the image receptor is placed along the midaxillary line. The posterolateral portion of the breast is captured on the image because the IRSD "goes around the corner" of the rib cage. By going this far around the curve of the rib cage, medial tissue will be missed when applying compression. Thus, visualization of the medial portion of the breast is required on the CC projection. (Reprinted from Sinclair WK. *Mammography—A Users Guide*. NCRP Report No. 85. Bethesda, MD: National Council on Radiation Protection and Measurement; 1986, with permission.)

Analog and digital mammography have strengths and weaknesses as well. Visualization of one portion of the breast is "sacrificed" in each standard projection to completely capture other areas (Figure 1-10 A to C).

No single radiograph can ever display all the structures contained within a 3-dimensional object; nevertheless, it is the technologist's responsibility to visualize as much tissue as possible in every projection.

Lateral Versus Oblique Positioning

Before the design of the dedicated mammographic unit, mammographers used an x-ray table, a ceiling-mounted x-ray tube, and a suction cup compression device. Despite the constraints of this equipment, mammographers performed CC, Lateral, and axillary tail views. The 1965 development of the dedicated mammographic unit with an integrated compression device and C-arm design permitted versatility in positioning. Patients could stand or sit.

Xeroradiography receptors had the recording latitude to demonstrate the breast, from ribs to nipple, using a curved compression device. Analog recording systems do not offer this wide recording latitude and thus require an evenly compressed breast (Figure 1-11). Even compression of the breast means the ribs must be excluded. Exclusion of the ribs afforded analog and digital mammography the opportunity to position the breast in an oblique orientation, the direction in which the breast is attached to the body.

By the mid-1970s, Scandinavian mammographers reported advantages of a new position—the oblique view.[5] Breast compression applied in an oblique plane corresponds with the anatomical attachment of the breast to the body allowing more posterior tissue to be included on the oblique image than with a Lateral view (see Chapter 7).

When positioning for the Lateral view, the compression device "fights" against the muscular attachment of the breast to the body. Today, the Lateral position is a supplementary view relegated to the role of definitive lesion localization prior to preoperative wire localization or stereotactic core biopsy.

Visualization of the Skin Line

Another obsolete requirement from xeroradiography was to visualize the skin line. In high-contrast analog mammography, there is no need to show the skin line. Cancerous cells in the breast do not arise in the skin, and they do not arise from adipose tissue. "The primary focus of a breast cancer is rarely located in the subcutaneous fat zone. Thus, tumors with their epicenter in the subcutaneous tissue are, in all likelihood, benign and are usually inflammatory processes or hematomas. It should be noted that metastasis from cancers other than breast cancer may be located in the subcutaneous tissue."[4]

In high-contrast analog imaging, the skin line and the subcutaneous fat layer are considerably darker than

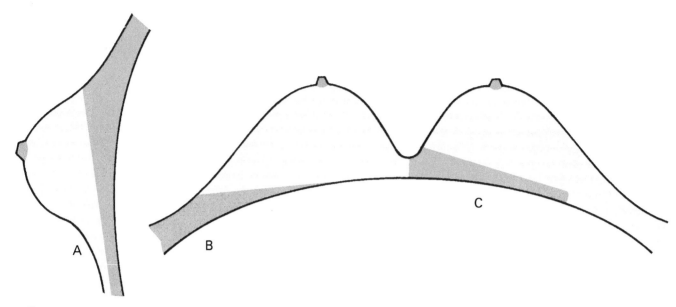

Figure 1-10
The "blind" areas of the standard mammography view. When the breast is compressed for the CC view, the superior–posterior portion of the breast is not imaged (*shaded area* in **A**). Furthermore, either a posteromedial or a posterolateral portion is not included, depending on how the patient is rotated (*shaded areas* in **B** and **C**). In the Lateral view, the posterolateral portion tends not to be imaged (**B**), whereas in the oblique view, the posteromedial portion of the breast tends not to be imaged (**C**). The CC projection can be either laterally or medially oriented. Usually, it is obtained so that the lateral posterior portion is included rather than the medial posterior portion. This is logical only if two views are used and the other view is the Lateral, which tends to omit the posterior lateral portion. If, on the other hand, the oblique view is used together with the CC view as a two-view standard, it might be wise to obtain the CC in a more medially oriented fashion. This is recommended since the oblique projection tends to miss the juxtathoracic medial portion of the breast. (Reprinted from Andersson, I. Mammography in clinical practice. *Med Radiogr Photogr.* 1986:62:2, with permission.)

the parenchyma of the breast in all cases except those of breasts that compress to approximately 2 cm or less and are composed primarily of adipose tissue. In direct opposition, xeroradiography used a low-contrast technique to allow for even densities on the resulting image from structures as radiolucent as the skin to structures as radiopaque as the ribs. It was this lack of contrast and density differentiation that trained xeroradiographers to look at the "halo" just outside the skin line to ascertain whether their radiographs were properly exposed. For xeroradiography, visualization of the skin line was

very important; for analog and digital mammography, it is not. It should be noted that only 2% of the skin line is visualized in tangent on a mammogram; thus, 98% remains hidden, superimposed on top or underneath the breast mound.

In the early days of film mammography, when the ability to find nonpalpable cancer was virtually nonexistent, the cancer that was confirmed by x-ray was already clinically evident; in fact, a prerequisite for having a mammogram in those days was a palpable mass. By the time the cancer had grown to an advanced stage and the person became symptomatic,

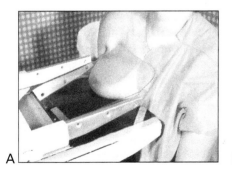
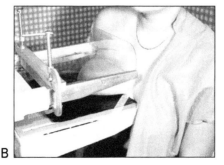
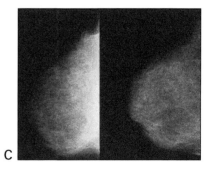

Figure 1-11
Compression devices. **(A)** A curved compression device allowed visualization of the ribs. **(B)** Straight chest wall edge compression device. **(C)** X-rays taken using the curved versus straight compression devices.

secondary signs such as skin thickening, skin dimpling, and nipple retraction were often present (Figure 1-2).

The mass ... has an irregular margin. In addition, there are spicules around its periphery, representing retraction of tissue strands toward the tumor. It is often referred to as scirrhous carcinoma. Microscopically, this type of cancer is characterized by retractive fibrosis. Thus, much of each tissue strand surrounding such a tumor represents thickened normal structures of the breast. The central lesion and the strands surrounding it undergo shortening (retraction), which is the basis for the skin dimpling and nipple retraction which is sometimes seen with these tumors. The skin is usually thickened in the area of retraction. This type of breast cancer usually feels larger than its radiographic size. (Leborgne Principle).[4]

Minimal breast cancers, which are unexpected clinically but have the best prognosis, will not exhibit the secondary signs of more advanced tumors. Diagnosis then relies primarily on evaluation of the mammogram. *"Retraction and thickening of the skin are secondary signs of cancer which may be helpful radiographically. Besides being non-specific, these signs are often not evident, or completely absent, with small tumors.* For the detection of small tumors, the demonstration of the mass and its primary characteristics on high-quality mammograms are crucial."[4]

With technical improvements in analog and digital mammography, cancerous tumors of minimal size (not clinically evident) are discovered. It is necessary to image the breast with high-contrast methods to detect these smaller lesions hiding within the glandular tissue. This means overexposing the skin line and subcutaneous fat with analog imaging. It is necessary in most cases to "bright light" the skin.

With the arrival of digital imaging in 2000, the dynamic range capability offered by the digital platform and computer monitor allows visualization of the skin, adipose tissue, and glandular tissue of the breast evenly. Digital systems can record and display approximately 16,000 shades of gray while analog systems capture about 100 shades. The extended dynamic range of digital imaging allows visualization of the breast and all of its internal structures evenly from the skin line to the base of the breast. Unlike xeroradiography, digital imaging does not need to sacrifice its contrast scale to do this. Using digital is like "having your cake and eating it too."

Use of Sponges

Mammographers used sponges as a positioning aid in xeroradiography to ensure the ribs were included on the image and to achieve the following:

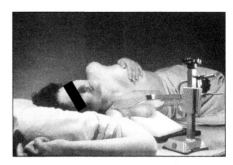

Figure 1-12
Sponges inserted between the breast and recording device.

1. Support the breast to match the thickness of the ribs so that the breast would not "disappear" around the curvature of the ribs as the woman lies on her side
2. Help form the breast into a relatively flat surface over which compression could be distributed evenly

Analog and digital mammograms do not visualize the ribs; therefore, the use of sponges is not necessary. By inserting a sponge between the breast and image receptor support device (IRSD), the imaged body part (the breast) moves away from the recording system (Figure 1-12). This results in geometric unsharpness.

Mammographers search for finite structures such as microcalcifications or the irregular borders of a mass, which require sharp images. The breast will always be in direct contact with the recording system in analog and digital imaging, which improves geometric resolution. Additionally, sponges may contain artifacts that imitate or obscure pathology.

Use of Antiperspirants and Powders

The use of antiperspirants and powders that contain aluminum, calcium, and zinc particles adversely affected a xeromammogram but should not interfere with the interpretation of an analog or a digital mammogram. Nevertheless, if a woman appearing for her exam has applied liberal amounts of powder or antiperspirant that has clumped in visible deposits along the moisture-prone inframammary fold (IMF) or in the axilla, ask her to clean that area before the mammogram is performed. Aluminum and zinc when clumped together can mimic microcalcifications. However, they will be found in the apex of the axilla where there are no ductal structures or glandular tissue, only lymph nodes (refer to Figure 1-13A).

Approximately 30% to 50% of primary breast cancers have mammographically detectable calcifications. These calcifications may be the only radiographic finding that suggests malignancy. When such neoplasms metastasize

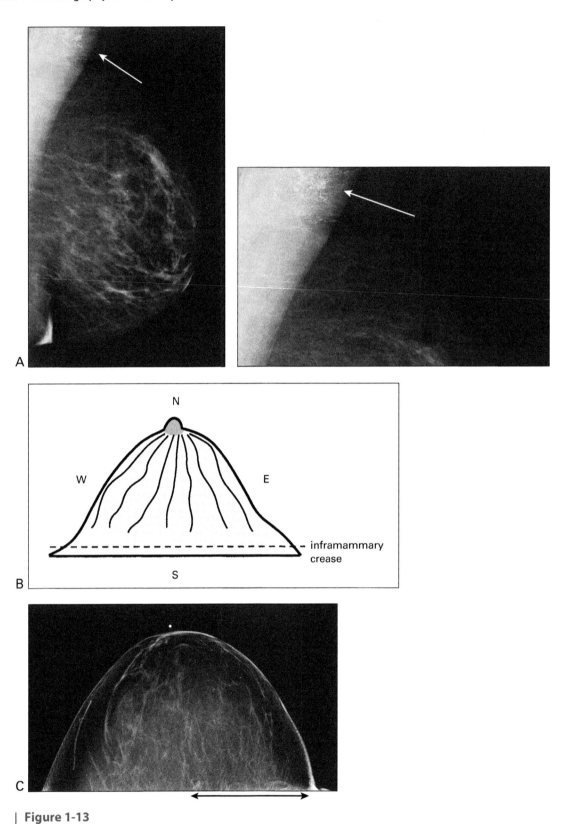

Figure 1-13
(A) Antiperspirant can be seen in the axilla. **(B)** Ductal structures align in a "north-to-south" direction; the IMF runs "east to west." **(C)** Powder in the IMF. An obvious artifact as it runs east to west in orientation, following the direction of the IMF.

to axillary lymph nodes, the nodes may appear dense but usually lack mammographically detectable calcifications or other abnormalities. Reports of calcified metastatic neoplasm in axillary nodes draining a primary breast cancer are rare.... Mammographically detectable calcifications in axillary lymph nodes usually are caused by previous inflammatory disease. Rarely they may be associated with metastatic breast carcinoma, especially in advanced cases. A recent report even suggests that punctate axillary nodal calcifications are more often indicative of intranodal gold deposits (in women treated for rheumatoid arthritis) than metastases.[6]

Talcum powder, which contains aluminum and calcium particles, is often applied over the entire surface of the breast but will tend to clump along the IMF, where the inferior half of the breast and the abdominal wall meet. This deposition of powder may be seen on the mammogram because efforts are made to include this area on the CC projection. Talcum powder can be distinguished from tumors when looking at the CC image because the IMF runs "east to west," whereas the ductal structures in which tumors would be found run "north to south" (Figure 1-13B and C).

Breath Holding

Because the ribs and lung field were included on a xeromammogram, which used considerably less compression than analog or digital imaging, respiration had to be suspended.

Because analog and digital imaging do not include the ribs or lungs, and because one of the objectives of compression is to immobilize the breast effectively, suspension of respiration is unnecessary except under the following circumstances:

1. The patient will not allow adequate compression of the breast.
2. The patient has implants and we perform the nondisplaced views.
3. The patient has emphysema or a similar respiratory problem.

Inadequate compression of the breast or excessive movement of the thorax invites motion; thus, some patients may need to suspend respiration.

Simply advise the patient to "stop breathing" rather than to hold her breath. A person tends to inhale a large volume of air to last for the duration of the x-ray exposure when advised to hold their breath. Inflating the lungs causes the rib cage to expand and the pectoral muscle to contract. Expansion of the ribs can cause the loss of posterior breast tissue on the mammogram because this bony structure

now offers serious opposition to the compression device. Contracting the pectoral muscle causes the breast to be held more tightly to the body; in turn, the compression will be more uncomfortable for the patient and the breast cannot easily be dislocated from the ribs.

TO SEE MORE CLEARLY: FIVE DECADES OF CHANGE AND STILL COUNTING

Significant changes in mammography occurred from 1965 to date. Innovators applied their research and advances from technology, medicine, electronics, and related fields to increase the effectiveness of the mammogram. Improvements came rapidly in equipment, accessories, compression devices, film, and techniques to better image glandular breasts and breast cancers.

1965

CGR developed the first dedicated mammography machine with a molybdenum target tube, use of low kVp, and an integral compression device and C-arm configuration.

1967

First commercial CGR Senographe unit was shown at RSNA.

1969

First CGR unit was sold in the United States.

1971

Although its use was reported in the literature as far back as 1960, xeroradiography was not introduced commercially until 1971. Many physicians preferred its lower x-ray dose (2 to 4 R) and its blue powder/white paper images to the available film systems. Xeroradiography also afforded the hospital the ability to use one of its existing diagnostic x-ray machines; thus, it was not necessary to purchase a special machine to perform mammography. However, specialized processing and conditioning units had to be acquired and maintained.

1972

R.E. Wayrynen, PhD, and the DuPont Company developed the LoDose I analog imaging system: a single calcium–tungstate–intensifying screen in conjunction with a single-emulsion film packaged in a polyethylene bag from which air was evacuated to achieve good screen–film contact. The radiation dose with this system was approximately 1 to 1.5 R, another improvement over existing systems. The development of this improved imaging system was needed to realize the potential benefits from dedicated mammography machines. Mass screening was considered by many to be on the horizon.

1973

Three manufacturers introduced new dedicated units: the Siemens' Mammomat, Philips' MammoDiagnost, and Picker's Mammorex.

1974

General Electric Healthcare (GE) introduced their dedicated MMX unit.

The 3M Company introduced the rare-earth phosphor generation of intensifying screens.

The variety of new dedicated mammography machines in the market and the availability of lower-dose analog imaging systems had a significant impact on mammography. Clinical practice began to change as xeroradiography and the new dedicated analog machines replaced the older equipment and methods for producing mammograms. The gap between mammographers who used dedicated machines versus those attempting mammography with standard x-ray equipment and industrial or medical film increased.

1976

Kodak introduced a low absorption cassette for use with a rare-earth screen and film combination—the Min-R system, with a dose measurement of approximately 0.08 R. At the same time, DuPont began to market their improved LoDose II system. Agfa-Gevaert also entered the film and cassette market during this period.

In response to concern about the x-ray dosage for mammography, those performing xeroradiography increased the filtration and recommended kVp settings to lower the dose to approximately 0.5 R.

1977

Techniques that allowed clearer, bigger, brighter, and better images were a major focus of equipment research and design at this time as clinicians and researchers sought to emulate successes in other types of imaging. In 1977, Xonics manufactured an x-ray machine that used electron

radiography. The Radiologic Science Inc. unit (later known as Pfizer and then as Elscint) introduced the microfocus tube (a 0.09-mm round focal spot) to allow for magnification. Systems that used the new electronics and computer-based technologies influenced the designs and directions taken by later generations of mammographic systems.

1978

Philips introduced a moving grid with special carbon fiber interspace material for low absorption of the soft x-ray beam necessary for analog mammography.

1984

Liebel-Flarsheim began marketing a fine-line stationary grid that was placed inside the cassette. This was an acceptable alternative for machines that could not be retrofitted with a moving grid.

LoRad Medical Systems introduced the high-frequency/constant-potential generation of dedicated mammography machines.

1986

Kodak introduced Min-R-T screens and film: two intensifying screens within a cassette combined with a double-emulsion film. This system increased speed and reduced dosage, but with slightly less resolution and contrast, for use with younger or infirm patients.

National Council on Radiation Protection and Measurement issued a mammography user's guide.

1991

ARRT offers advanced certification in mammography to technologists (M).

1992

Siemens developed the first multianode tube. The dual target is composed of molybdenum and tungsten. GE followed with another dual-target x-ray tube but incorporated molybdenum and rhodium (see Chapter 11).

Fischer and LoRad simultaneously introduced small-field digital mammography for use with stereotactic core biopsies (see Chapter 18).

DuPont (then Sterling, then Agfa) developed a new generation of film emulsion, a cubic grain film that provides another dimension to high-contrast images.

MQSA is signed into law: effective October 1, 1994.

1993

The FDA bans the use of silicone implants.

1995

LoRad marketed a new high-transmission cellular grid that improves contrast for thicker, glandular breasts (see Chapter 11).

1996

All manufacturers have added features to make mammography machines more "user-friendly." Technologists simply press the exposure button and the machine does the rest.

1998

The FDA approves CAD (computer-aided detection) equipment to be used only with analog mammography (see Chapter 11).

2000

GE receives FDA approval for full-field digital mammography (FFDM), although the images must still be printed on film.

2001

Fischer is the second company to gain FDA approval for their digital unit. Within 5 years, Fischer's slot scanning method of producing digital images will no longer exist; the company was purchased by a competitor and the slot technology phased out.

CAD is approved for use with digital mammography systems.

ACR begins the DMIST/ACRIN study to compare analog and digital imaging of women with glandular breasts.

2002

On October 28, the final MQSA equipment regulations take effect. The older noncompliant units are replaced primarily with analog units since the preliminary results from the DMIST/ACRIN study will not be published until 2005.

Hologic and Siemens Medical received FDA approval for their digital machines. The race for the digital market is on.

2005

Preliminary results from DMIST/ACRIN report that digital mammography is equivalent to analog imaging when dealing with an adipose breast; digital is superior when imaging the glandular breast.

U-Systems conducts studies using an automated breast ultrasound (ABUS) prototype.

2006

Fuji CR mammography was approved for use by FDA.

ACS no longer promotes BSE; CBE is still strongly recommended.

The FDA once again allows use of silicone implants.

2007

MRI of the breast is recommended as a screening test done in conjunction with mammography on women with a high risk for developing breast cancer.[6]

2008

The FDA approved tungsten target tubes for digital mammography.

Breast tomosynthesis enters the final phase of FDA acceptance.

2009

USPS Task Force issues controversial mammography guidelines. The ACS and almost all other medical organizations decry the task force recommendations.[7]

2011

Hologic receives FDA approval for digital breast tomosynthesis (DBT).

2014

GE receives FDA approval for digital breast tomosynthesis.

2015

Siemens receives FDA approval for digital breast tomosynthesis.

Koning Corp. receives FDA approval for coned beam breast CT, a diagnostic procedure.

ACS aligns with 2009 USPS Task Force guidelines. CBE is no longer promoted.[8]

Summary

The history of mammography began with good-natured discussion and scientific curiosity in 1924. From the start of modern mammography with Dr. Egan and his cohorts, the field progressed slowly during the 1950s and into the 1960s with help from the industrial sector. Mammography benefited greatly during the 30 years from 1970 through 2000 from rapid and remarkable technologic advances in electronics, computer sciences, plastics, and the emergence of other sophisticated medical imaging devices.

The interdependence between the recording system and x-ray system continues to be a major factor in producing the best image at the lowest dose. This relationship is central to the manufacturers' efforts to improve equipment, accessories, and image contrast and resolution as they strive to make the next breakthrough. Mammography capable of detecting breast cancers at an early stage could, with a regular screening program, reduce the mortality from breast cancer as dramatically as the Pap smear reduced the death rate from cervical cancer. The newer technologic advances in manufacturing, materials development and design, computer sciences (medical imaging without film), and biologic sciences (use of DNA technology) also have potential applications for the detection of breast cancer. Chapter 21 includes brief descriptions of alternative methods, some still in the research stage, that attempt to discover breast disease through cellular physiology.

One of the most powerful drives in humans is pleasure taken in their skills. They love to do what they do well, and having done well, work to do better. We see this process in every human endeavor. That bodes well for mammography too.

Review Questions

1. Name three differences in positioning and/or imaging between mammography done before and after dedicated machines were introduced.

2. List some advantages when using dedicated mammography machines rather than a general x-ray machine to produce an image.

3. How has the dose in mammography changed since it was first performed?

References

1. Warren SL. Roentgenologic study of the breast. *Am J Roentgenol.* 1930;24:113.
2. Strax P. Evolution in techniques in breast screening. In: Strax P, ed. *Control of Breast Cancer Through Mass Screening.* St Louis, MO: Mosby-Year book Inc; 1978:167.
3. Alcorn FS, O'Donnell EO, Ackerman LV. Training nonradiologists to scan mammograms. *Radiology.* 1971;99:523–529.
4. Andersson I. Mammography in clinical practice. *Med Radiogr Photogr.* 1986;62:2.
5. Lundgren B. The oblique view at mammography. *Br J Radiol.* 1977;50:626–628.
6. Helvie M, Rebner M, Sickles E, et al. Calcifications in metastatic breast cancer in axillary lymph nodes. *Am J Roentgenol.* 1988;151:921.
7. Barclay L. USPSTF issues new breast cancer screening guidelines. Medscape Medical News. November 16, 2009. Available at: Medscape.com
8. Simon S. American Cancer Society releases new breast cancer society guidelines. October 20, 2015. Available at: Cancer.org

Background: Need for Screening Mammography

2

▋▋ UPDATE

2011 Edition

Three changes during the 1990s demanded a complete revision of this chapter from our first edition (1992) to the second edition (2001). First was acceptance by health insurance companies and the medical community at large that screening mammography can visualize nonpalpable malignant breast tumors and effectively detect disease in its early stages. As the quality of mammograms improved, so did the ability to visualize small cancers. This was a significant paradigm shift regarding the efficacy of screening mammography. Second, the coupling of preventive medicine and consumer involvement in maintaining health became an accepted concept in the United States during this period. Finally, the statistics on breast cancer and medical treatment required an update.

With this, our third edition, we are pleased to report mammography remains an accepted screening procedure supported by the health care community, health insurance companies, and government programs. At imaging centers today, mammograms are as plentiful as chest x-rays. But most encouraging of all is that *screening* mammograms now account for approximately 80% of all mammograms done in the United States.

2019 Edition

The 2011 update mentions acceptance by health insurance companies and the medical community at large that screening mammography can visualize nonpalpable malignant breast tumors and effectively detect disease in its early stages, and that screening mammograms account for 80% of all mammograms that are done in the United States With this fourth edition, we find screening mammography has taken a step backward in time:

- In 2009, the U.S. Preventive Services Task Force (USP-STF) stunned the mammography community with reduced guidelines due to increased harms and reduced benefits associated with screening mammography
- In 2015, the American Cancer Society (ACS) changed its long-held guidelines concerning the age to begin screening mammography as well as changes in interval frequency
- We expect health insurance companies to align their policies with the new USPSTF/ACS guidelines.

For those in the mammography community who fought long and hard to gain acceptance for this screening exam, this change is a bitter pill to swallow.

▋▋ THE STARTING POINT FOR BREAST CANCER

The first written description of breast cancer was on ancient Egyptian papyrus.[1] The doctor described inflammatory breast cancer. He said treatment was futile and that the woman should be left alone. Ancient Greeks,[2] around 200 AD, thought an excess of black bile caused breast cancer. It was thought that the monthly menstrual flow naturally relieved women of this excess, which explained why breast cancer was more common after menopause.

Amazingly, this belief held until the early 1800s when Müller described the cellular nature of breast cancer; it consists of large, sticky cells. Today, research of the cause and behavior of various types of cancer has given us the knowledge that "Cancer results from a cascade of genetic changes in a single cell, all of which may be required for malignant conversion. Different changes, or combinations of changes, may result in different types of cancer ... Some cancers do, however, have a major genetic susceptibility component, making those strategies already developed for genetic testing in other diseases applicable to cancer."[3]

At Risk for Breast Cancer

In the year 2017, approximately 316,000 females and 2,500 males in the United States will develop breast cancer. According to these statistics, the most important risk factor is being a female. Next is having already been diagnosed and treated for breast cancer. A third risk factor is having a genetic predisposition to developing the disease based on a positive family history, such as a premenopausal mother, sister, or daughter. As always, bilateral cancer in such instances presents a higher risk than does unilateral cancer.

Unfortunately, according to Strax, a "statistical study by the ACS teaches us that less than 25% of cancers develop in women with any of these [risk] factors. The vast majority, up to 75% of breast cancer, occurs in women with none of the known risk factors. The sad truth is that we have to consider all women over the age of 30 at risk for this disease."[4] We must not wait until a woman meets certain risk profiles, nor should we wait until someone (the woman or her physician) feels something in the breast to justify having a mammogram. What are we *waiting* for?

Early Detection

Major considerations that support early detection include the following:

- The disease is important.
- It has a recognizable presymptomatic stage.

- Reliable tests exist that are acceptable in terms of risk, cost, and patient discomfort.
- Therapy in presymptomatic stages reduces morbidity and mortality more than does therapy initiated after the presence of symptoms.
- Screening programs should take precedence over other needs competing for the same resource money.
- Facilities are available for the diagnosis and treatment of patients with positive screening results.

Early detection of any type of cancer is critical to successful treatment and the quality of life. Screening mammograms of asymptomatic women are vital in the battle against breast cancer. However, before the discussion of *how* to obtain a good image begins, it must first be understood *why* technical expertise and interpretation are so vital in mammography.

White on White

Mammography images cancer in white—either as white microcalcifications or as a white mass that displays one of the following characteristics: (a) the borders of the mass are irregular, (b) the mass appears to be new when compared with previous mammograms, or (c) the mass has increased in size when compared with previous mammograms. The glandular tissue from which cancers arise also appears white on the mammogram. As women with varying parenchymal patterns age, all but one of these patterns experience a decrease in the amount of glandular tissue. Each pregnancy greatly displaces the amount of glandular tissue remaining, whereas each month during the menstrual cycle a much smaller scale of replacement occurs. The dark-appearing adipose tissue replaces the white-appearing glandular tissue. When looking for cancer in the typical young woman's more glandular breast, we are looking for a white dot on a white background. In the typical postmenopausal, adipose-replaced breast, we are looking for a white dot on a dark background. Use of hormone replacement therapy (HRT) throughout the postmenopausal years causes some of the glandular tissue to be retained.

Mammography is not appropriate for everyone. For women below the age of 40, routine mammography is not recommended for various reasons: first, younger women's breasts are more radiosensitive; second, the incidence is too low in this group to make screening cost-effective; finally, the white-on-white image in the younger woman's mostly glandular breast further compounds the inaccuracy rate. When a young woman is clinically symptomatic, she is better advised to see a surgeon before seeking a mammogram.

Detection of Breast Cancer

As women age, the likelihood of developing breast cancer increases. Table 2-1 illustrates the incidence rates of

Table 2-1 • 2016 Estimated Breast Cancer Incidence and Mortality, per Million Women per Year[a]

AGE	IN SITU	INVASIVE	TOTAL NO.	DEATHS
<40	1,610	11,160	12,770	990
40–49	12,440	36,920	49,360	3,480
50–59	17,680	58,620	76,300	7,590
60–69	17,550	68,070	85,620	9,420
70–79	10,370	47,860	58,230	8,220
80+	3,760	30,080	33,840	10,910
All ages	63,410	252,710	316,120	40,610

[a]Estimated breast cancer incidence and mortality segregated by:
- Age
- In situ
- Invasive
- Deaths

Source: National Center for Health Statistics. *Health, U.S. 2016 with Chartbook on Trends in the Health of Americans.* Hyattsville, MD: National Center for Health Statistics; 2017.

naturally occurring breast cancer cases per million women per year at various ages. Breast cancer is a disease directly related to age. Therefore, as women age, the need for mammography becomes more critical.

The data from Table 2-2, Breast Cancer Risk for U.S. Women, are correlated to the incidence data and U.S. Census population data for women aged 40 and over from 1950 through census projections for these age groups until 2030. The result is presented as a bar graph in Figure 2-1, which illustrates the dramatic increase in the incidence of breast cancer as we age. There are particularly sharp increases in the number of breast cancer cases occurring from the ages of 25 to 49. Indeed, 25% of all breast cancers occur in women below age 50. From age 50 on, the number of cases per 100,000 women continues to increase, but at a much slower rate.

Utilization

Mammography should be done on a screening basis, just as the Pap test is done, because the average time it takes for breast cancer to grow large enough to feel (approximately 1 cm) is 10 to 12 years.[4–7] If mammography is done well technically, with a qualified radiologist interpreting the

Table 2-2 • Breast Cancer Risk for U.S. Women[a]

AGE	RISK
20–29	1 in 1,674
30–39	1 in 225
40–49	1 in 69
50–59	1 in 44
60–69	1 in 29
70–79	1 in 26
Lifetime	1 in 8

[a]As women age, the likelihood of developing cancer increases.
Source: DevCan: Probability of Developing or Dying of Cancer Software, version 6.7.3. Statistical Research and Applications Branch, National Cancer Institute, 2015. Available at: www.srab.cancer.gov/decan.

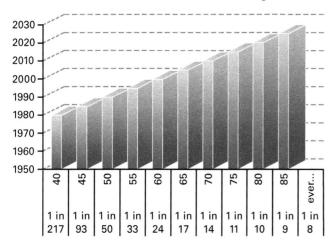

Risk for Breast Cancer Increases with Age

	40	45	50	55	60	65	70	75	80	85	ever...
	1 in 217	1 in 93	1 in 50	1 in 33	1 in 24	1 in 17	1 in 14	1 in 11	1 in 10	1 in 9	1 in 8

Figure 2-1

This is an example of how aging, increasing risk of breast cancer, and a life expectancy of age 85 would affect a woman. In our example, we track her entry into the screening mammography pool in 1986 and follow her increasing risk through the next 45 years to 2031, when she reaches age 85, the forecasted life expectancy for U.S. females. She enters the mammography suite at age 40 with a risk of 1 in 225 and ends at age 85 with a lifetime risk of 1 in 8.

images, the average malignancy should be detected 2 to 4 years before it becomes palpable.[8] Often, in this case, the cure rate approaches 95%.[9,10] A lead time of 1.7 years is reported in women aged 40 to 49 and between 2.6 and 3.8 years for women aged 50 to 74 years.[11]

People with health insurance are more likely to have screening examinations (Table 2-3). If there is no health insurance, then compliance rates decrease almost in half. When the woman has private health insurance, only 8% of breast cancer cases are later stages III or IV; 18% if uninsured; 19% if Medicaid provides health insurance coverage. The National Center for Health Statistics reports the utilization of preventive and screening services. In 2003, the rate for the Pap test for women aged 55 to 64 was 85.5%; in 2013, it was 75.9%. For mammography use in 2003, compliance was 76.9%, and in 2013, use was 71.3%.[12]

Reducing the mortality rate of breast cancer depends on early detection through mass screening, as proven in the use of the Pap test to reduce cervical cancer deaths. Cervical cancer mortality rates declined by 70% with the introduction of the Pap test in 1928. Between 1990 and 2010, breast cancer **mortality rates** fell from 33/100,000 per year to 21.3/100,000; a decline of 36%.[13]

Routine use of screening mammography begins in the United States in the mid 1980s, and within 10 years we see the beginnings of a reduction in mortality; breast cancer mortality rates have decreased approximately 2% each year beginning in the mid 1990s (Table 2-4). For women aged 50+ years, there is a 34% reduction in mortality; for 40- to 49-year-olds, there is a 51% reduction.[13]

Case Study 2-1

Refer to Table 2-4 and respond to the following questions:

1. When does the morality rate begin a downward trend?

2. In which year did the rules and regulations of MQSA take effect?

3. Could there be a cause-and-effect relationship between the signing of MQSA and the reduction in the number of deaths attributed to breast cancer?

This coincides with the increased use of screening mammography and the Federal government's enactment of the Mammography Quality Standards Act (MQSA) in October 1994.

It's a Plan

In Sweden, the United Kingdom, and other countries, where screening is a matter of official national policy in the context of a national health care delivery system, the support for breast and cervical cancer screening goes beyond recommendations for participation. This support

Table 2-3 • Use of Mammography among Women Aged 40 and Older, by Selected Characteristics, United States, Selected Years 1987 to 2015[a]

	1993	1994	2000	2003	2005	2008	2010	2013	2015
Age 40–64									
Uninsured	36.0	34.0	40.7	41.5	38.1	39.7	36.0	37.3	30.0
Insured	66.2	68.3	76.0	75.1	72.5	73.4	74.1	72.1	69.7
Private	67.1	69.4	77.1	76.3	74.5	74.2	75.6	73.4	72.2
Medicaid	51.9	54.5	61.7	63.5	55.6	64.2	64.4	63.5	57.7

[a]Women with health insurance are twice as likely to have a mammogram as women without health insurance.

Source: National Center for Health Statistics. *Health, U.S. 2016 with Chartbook on Trends in the Health of Americans.* Hyattsville, MD: National Center for Health Statistics; 2017.

Table 2-4 • Trends: Breast Cancer Death Rates for Females in the United States[a]

YEAR	RECORDED DEATHS
1989	43,391
1990	43,391
1991	43,583
1992	43,068
1993	43,555
1994	43,644
1995	43,844
1996	43,091
1997	41,943
1998	41,737
1999	41,144
2000	41,872
2001	41,394
2002	41,514
2003	41,620
2004	40,954
2005	41,116
2006	40,821
2007	40,460
2008	40,480
2009	40,170
2010	40,230
2011	39,970
2012	39,920
2013	40,030
2014	40,430
2015	40,730
2016	40,730

[a]Screening mammography begins in the United States in the mid 1980s. By the mid 1990s, we see the beginnings of a downward trend in mortality. Source: U.S. Mortality Data, 1990–2016. National Center for Health Statistics, Center for Disease Control and Prevention; 2016.

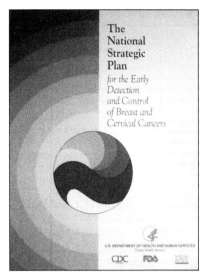

Figure 2-2
The National Strategic Plan. The U.S. initiative to provide the means to discover breast and cervical cancers early.

• Quality assurance: breast cancer screening
• Quality assurance: cervical cancer screening
• Surveillance and evaluation

Additional costs to the nation for breast and cervical cancer screening will be incurred with or without a Plan. The costs will be a shared responsibility of the public and private sectors and will increase gradually as more women take advantage of these lifesaving preventive services. However, these costs will be offset by treatment savings resulting from the detection of cancers of the breast and cervix at earlier stages of development.[14]

This Plan provided for screening examinations regardless of the woman's ability to pay. In 1991, $30 million was appropriated for this purpose; in 1992, $50 million; in 1993, $70 million; and in 2010, $100 million. Today, $169 million/year is allocated to this nationwide program. In 2016 the Plan:

• screened 290,095 women for breast cancer with mammography and diagnosed 2,639 invasive breast cancers and 829 premalignant lesions
• screened 140,073 women for cervical cancer with the Pap test and diagnosed 171 cervical cancers and 5,919 premalignant cervical lesions, of which 39% were high grade[15]

This Plan also provided support in several ways:

• It supported the ARRT's efforts to develop a competency examination in mammography for technologists.
• It encouraged continuing education in mammography for physicians and technologists.
• It provided money to standardize the training for medical physicists, radiologists, and radiologic technologists.
• It encouraged the manufacturing of high-quality mammography machines.

MQSA was an outgrowth of this plan.

includes resources for a system of elements necessary to both accomplish and realize the fullest benefits of early cancer detection. This system includes the following elements: promotion of screening, quality assurance, follow-up for women with abnormal findings, and routine monitoring of program effectiveness, costs, and benefits.[14]

In March of 1990, the U.S. government began development of the **National Strategic Plan for the Early Detection and Control of Breast and Cervical Cancers**. "Health services for breast and cervical cancers should be available to all women, regardless of age, geographic location, socioeconomic status, race, ethnicity, or cultural background ... the Plan is designed for use by public and private organizations at the national, state, and local levels in planning specific programmatic activities"[14] (Figure 2-2).

Six critical components formed the framework of this Plan:

• Integration and coordination
• Public education
• Professional education and practice

Table 2-5 • Cost of Medical Care[a]

	US GOV'T YLL (THOUSANDS)	MEDICARE SPENDS (MILLIONS)	NATIONAL SPENDING (BILLIONS)	LOST PRODUCTIVITY (BILLIONS)
Breast	761.3	1,375	13.886	10.879
Cervical	104.7	73	1.425	1.808
Prostate	267.4	2,294	9.862	3.538

[a]YLL = years of life lost. To calculate YLL, subtract age at death from life expectancy. YLL weighs severity of death by the age a person is killed.
Lost productivity is estimated from the present value of lifetime earnings of all people who die of this cancer this year.
Source: Carter A, Nguyen C, et al. A comparison of cancer burden and research spending reveals discrepancies in the distribution of research funding. *BMC Public Health*. 2012;12:526.

The Economics of Early Detection

The cost of medical care in America has become as important an issue as the need for care. Economic considerations fueled a renewed emphasis on disease prevention, patient participation in health decisions, and trade-offs in medical care. The true cost of treating a disease in its later stages is staggering. The economics of screening and early detection of cervical cancer through the Pap test are understood and accepted because these steps prevent future costs—in both lives and money. The cost of screening mammography is compared to other cancers (Table 2-5).

Managed care programs establish policies that encourage women to have mammograms. Outside of HMOs, women must be educated in the importance of screening mammograms. However, even insurance coverage does not automatically guarantee women will have this examination; approximately 64% of Medicare beneficiaries used this feature.

Barriers to having mammograms include the following[16–21]:

* No symptoms, therefore unnecessary
  Solution: medical organizations must educate the public on the need for mammograms
* Fear that cancer will be found
  Solution: reinforce that if cancer is found early, survival rates are higher and breast-conserving surgery may be possible
* Cost
  Solution: divide into less costly screening examinations versus more expensive diagnostic examinations; also encourage mandatory health insurance coverage

* Discomfort
  Solution: most women do not find the procedure uncomfortable
* Concern about overdiagnosis resulting in unnecessary biopsies
  Solution: radiologists must use problem-solving tree and audit results
* Time consuming and/or inconvenient
  Solution: mammograms are mostly an outpatient procedure with scheduled appointment times
* Radiation
  Solution: an earlier primary fear has been dispelled by public education about use of low-dose mammography systems

Women between the ages of 65 and 74 are most likely to comply. Almost half of the women who had not had a mammogram said their doctor never encouraged them to have it done.

Breast Cancer in America

Empirical data concerning breast cancer and mammography are both instructive and discomforting. The ACS estimates the risk of developing breast cancer for American women as 1 in 8, whereas the risk of dying from breast cancer is 1 in 37.[22] While the 1 in 8 statistic conveys the cumulative lifetime risk for women who live past the age of 85, perhaps more meaningful is stating the risk by decade. This risk never exceeds 1 in 26 in any single decade (Table 2-2). Age-adjusted **incidence rates** for breast cancer have been slowly rising over the past several decades[23] (Table 2-6). Incidence rates reflect the occurrence and frequency of breast cancer (Table 2-7).

Table 2-6 • Age-Adjusted Breast Cancer Incidence Rates in the United States by Cancer Site, 1990–2013 (Rates per 100,000)[a]

1990	1995	2000	2005	2009	2010	2011	2012	2013
129.4	130.9	134.2	124.3	127.4	122.9	126.2	126.3	126.2

[a]Experts believe the 10% decline in incidence rates that began in 2000 is due to the sudden decline in mammography compliance that began that year. With fewer women having screening mammograms, it is the delay in discovery that accounts for the apparent decline.
Source: National Center for Health Statistics. *Health, U.S. 2016 with Chartbook on Trends in the Health of Americans*. Hyattsville, MD: National Center for Health Statistics; 2017.

Table 2-7 • SEER 18 Incidence and Mortality of Breast Cancer, Age-Adjusted and Age-Specific Rates, by Race and Sex[a]

INCIDENCE	AGE	MORTALITY
27.0	30–34	2.7
60.4	35–39	6.5
122.2	40–44	13.1
189.2	45–49	20.3
224.9	50–54	30.4
263.4	55–59	40.4
339.7	60–64	52.7
424.2	65–69	65.9
447.0	70–74	78.7
451.3	75–79	96.5
418.4	80–84	122.4
350.1	85+	178.2

[a]Breast cancer is a disease of old age; as women age, the likelihood of developing this disease increases.
Rates are per 100,000 and are age-adjusted to the 2000 U.S. Standard Population.
Source: SEER Cancer Statistics Review 2009–2013.

1.5 million cases of breast cancer were projected worldwide in 2016. The year 2017 projections are 255,180 new cases of invasive breast cancer and 63,400 cases of ductal carcinoma in situ (DCIS) will occur in the United States, and an additional 40,610 people will die of this disease.[24] This means every 12 minutes, 6 American women will develop breast cancer and 1 will die (Figure 2-3). The median age at diagnosis is 62 years, while the median age at death is 68.

Case Study **2-2**

Refer to Figure 2-3 and respond to the following questions:

1. Women are most likely to develop which type of cancer?

2. How much more likely is a woman to develop breast cancer than the second most frequent cancer—lung cancer?

Between 1973 (with an incidence of 85 cases of breast cancer per 100,000 population) and 2000 (with 137 cases per 100,000 population), the incidence rose by 60%. Breast cancer incidence rates increased in Black women during the early 2000s; in 2012, the incidence rates for Caucasian and Black women converged.[25]

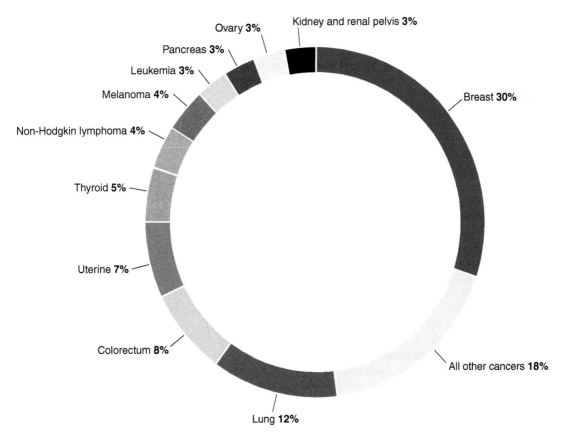

Figure 2-3
Breast cancer accounts for the highest proportion of cancer cases among women, more than double that of lung cancer. (Source: American Cancer Society. *Cancer Facts & Figures 2017*. ©2017 American Cancer Society, Inc.)

Table 2-8 • Breast Cancer Mortality Rates, USA: 1950–2015 (Age-Adjusted Death Rate per 100,000 Population)[a]

	1950	1960	1970	1980	1990	2000	2010	2012	2015
Rate	31.9	31.7	32.1	31.9	33.3	26.8	22.1	21.3	20.3

[a]The mortality rate from breast cancer steadily decreases from its peak in 1990.
Source: National Center for Health Statistics. *Health, U.S. 2016 with Chartbook on Trends in the Health of Americans.* Hyattsville, MD: National Center for Health Statistics; 2017.

The National Cancer Institute (NCI) announced breast cancer mortality rates decreased by an average of 37% between 1989 and 2012, from 32.9 cases per 100,000 women in 1984 to 20.7 cases in 2013.[13] Table 2-8 illustrates the long-term trend in mortality between 1950 and 2015. Screening for the detection of early breast cancer works.

Swedish Survival Statistics

Five mammography screening trials began in Sweden in the 1970s and ended in the 1980s. These were large, comprehensive, well-designed, and well-conducted studies.[26,27] After more than 30 years of follow-up, these screening trials show a 32% decrease in mortality.[28,29] While there are no comparable long-term screening trials in the United States, the results of the Swedish trials provide useful information about breast cancer and survival rates. A much smaller U.S. study, completed in 1989, found a 30% reduction in mortality.[30] The good news today is that 80% of women who develop this disease do not die of it.

From the Swedish studies, we see that tumors less than 15 mm received particular attention, while those less than 10 mm in size seem to be of a different breed altogether. Women with cancer detected at an early stage have excellent outcomes: survival rates of approximately 95% at 12 years.[29] The histologic grade of the tumor does not appear to matter when the cancer is tiny, nor does lymph node status or the woman's age, pre- or postmenopausal. Early detection at this stage means long-term survival.

Lesion Size and Survival Rates

By the time a nonpalpable 0.5 cm lesion increases in size to a palpable 1 cm, its mass has increased eight times (Figure 2-4). A 1-cm tumor contains from 100 million to 1 billion cells. By the time they reach 2 cm in size, these lesions often have metastasized. For patients with metastatic lesions, the median time of survival is 2 years. As the tumors increase in size, the cell types become more heterogeneous and respond less predictably to various drugs, radiation therapy, and biologic markers. In general, the duration of the patient's survival is inversely related to the size of the tumor; thus the larger the tumor, the lower the survival rate. This is why it is important to detect the smallest lesion possible.

An NCI medical audit stated that 73% of invasive cancers are invasive ductal carcinoma (IDC) and 9% are invasive lobular carcinoma (ILC), while 85% of in situ cancers are DCIS and 11.5% are lobular carcinoma in situ (LCIS).[31]

Survival rates of those women with lesions whose borders are smooth (such as mucinous carcinoma) are better than those whose lesions have irregular borders (such as the typical scirrhous carcinoma): 80% versus 38% at 10 years.

Case Study **2-3**

Refer to the text section "Swedish Survival Statistics" and respond to the following questions:

1. The histologic grade of a breast cancer has little effect on survival as long as the tumor is under _____ mm in size.

2. The Swedish screening trials show a long-term mortality reduction of _____ % after _____ years of follow-up.

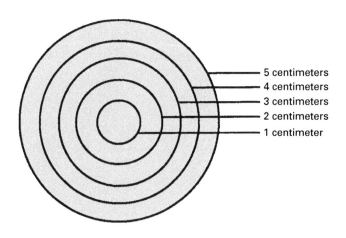

Figure 2-4
Size of breast lumps.

EVER-CHANGING GUIDELINES

During the authors' four decades of working in the field of mammography, they have seen mammography screening guidelines from national medical organizations change, always for the better ... until 2009 (Table 2-9).

In the 1970s, when the authors started working in this discipline, only diagnostic mammograms were performed; women with advanced clinical symptoms of advanced breast disease were imaged. Thanks to our European colleagues, particularly those from Sweden, our images improved in quality to a point that we began performing screening mammograms in the mid 1980s. In 1991, Medicare began coverage of annual mammograms for its beneficiaries. Once Medicare agrees to pay for a service, other insurance companies follow suit.

Once we begin performing routine screening exams, within a decade we see the beginnings of an ultimate 30% reduction in mortality due to earlier detection and improved treatments of those diagnosed with breast cancer. Since 1990, breast cancer mortality rates have decreased yearly by 2.3% overall and 3.3% for 40- to 49-year-old women.[32]

For the 50 years before screening exams were done in the United States, the mortality rate remained the same (Figure 2-5).

Old Guidelines

Old **guidelines** for mammography considered all women to be at equal risk for developing breast cancer; these old guidelines relied strictly on age. We now apply a different approach, one that considers age as well as the unique parenchymal pattern of each woman's breast tissue. Closer surveillance is recommended for women with more glandular breast tissue. Women whose tissue is adipose replaced may, if they so desire, extend this interval. Women at high risk are advised to have annual mammograms and an MRI.

Table 2-9 • USPSTF Guidelines and ACS Guidelines[a]

USPSTF GUIDELINES

• 1992–2002	• Baseline before age 50
	• Age 50–75 every 1–2 years
• 2002–2009	• Age 40+ every 1–2 years
• 2009 to present	• Age 50–74 every other year

ACS GUIDELINES

• 1976–1980	• Age 50+ annually
• 1980–1982	• Age 35–39 baseline
	• Age 40–49 talk with your doctor
	• Age 50+ annually
• 1983–1991	• Age 35–39 baseline
	• Age 40–49 every 1–2 years
	• Age 50+ annually
• 1992–1997	• Age 40–49 every 1–2 years
	• Age 50+ annually
• 1997–2003	• Age 40+ annually
• 2003–2015	• Age 40+ annually as long as in good health
• 2015 to present	• Age 40–44 talk with your doctor
	• Age 45–54 annually
	• Age 55+ every other year

[a]Ever-changing USPSTF and ACS mammography screening guidelines for the woman at average risk.

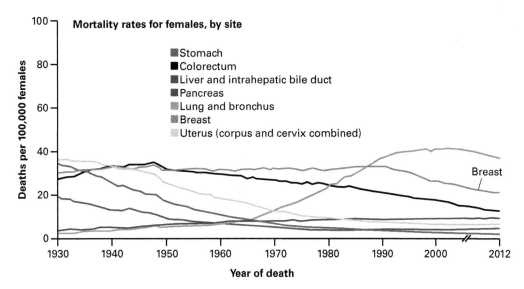

Figure 2-5
The first mammogram is performed in 1924. Screening mammography begins in the mid 1980s. Medicare begins annual coverage for this exam in 1991. Only after screening exams are widely utilized does the mortality rate decline. (Source: Siegel RL, Miller KD, Jemal A. Cancer statistics, 2016. *CA Cancer J Clin.* 2016;66(1):7–30; with permission of John Wiley and Sons.)

In the early 1980s the guidelines for screening mammography were altered to include younger women as our knowledge of the disease process became better defined. Cancer detected in women younger than 50 is usually more aggressive, with a faster growth rate.[8,33–35]

1980–1995 Guidelines

Mammography in its infancy (1924 to 1964) could find only clinically evident breast cancer. Indeed, the only women who had mammograms had lumps. In the late 1960s to early 1970s, use of general x-ray equipment and x-ray film gave way to dedicated mammography machines and specialized mammography recording systems. Gradually, as our positioning and radiographic physics techniques were refined, our ability to find smaller lesions (Table 2-10) resulted in the declaration from the ACS in 1976 to begin yearly screening mammograms on asymptomatic women aged 50 and older.[35] In 1980, a baseline exam, between ages 35 and 39, was added to provide

Table 2-10 • Cancer of the Female Breast, Incidence Rates, 1975–2013 by Age, In Situ versus Malignant All Races[a]

YEAR	IN SITU, AGES 20–49 RATE PER 100,000	MALIGNANT, AGES 20–49 RATE PER 100,000	IN SITU, AGES 50+ RATE PER 100,000	MALIGNANT, AGES 50+ RATE PER 100,000
1975	6.2629	67.2754	11.1923	273.8209
1976	4.4742	66.3327	12.0190	264.1082
1977	4.2363	64.7622	8.6756	262.4368
1978	3.9067	64.3321	9.7420	262.3760
1979	4.6579	62.9608	9.2101	269.9346
1980	4.9402	62.5704	9.6675	271.0606
1981	4.3403	64.9321	11.0521	282.1627
1982	4.5211	67.2004	12.0279	279.1434
1983	5.0223	66.6815	14.0912	296.7930
1984	7.9398	70.2240	18.6570	308.7479
1985	9.8047	73.4477	26.2363	333.4959
1986	11.2245	73.6946	31.5551	342.4351
1987	12.9614	75.4893	42.3906	367.4354
1988	13.5247	72.9163	42.2275	360.0659
1989	11.5867	71.8889	41.4865	346.7973
1990	13.8874	75.5561	47.3070	357.7299
1991	14.5519	78.2893	46.6169	360.6528
1992	14.9228	71.9636	53.9770	364.1563
1993	13.8442	71.0036	53.0393	355.3003
1994	14.4779	70.3187	57.8355	362.8670
1995	15.9547	71.5642	64.2399	367.0596
1996	16.2986	72.2378	66.0152	369.8252
1997	18.2610	72.0873	73.5655	385.4624
1998	19.8824	75.3364	87.1585	392.7757
1999	19.8515	72.5538	87.1354	397.2172
2000	19.5493	72.0511	87.9521	380.2615
2001	19.2019	72.8047	91.5652	387.1163
2002	19.7173	70.9739	92.0454	379.0462
2003	19.9360	71.8862	86.0912	346.1169
2004	21.1918	74.4162	86.6642	345.8531
2005	20.7326	73.0154	85.4709	342.7659
2006	22.9219	73.1502	84.1022	341.6874
2007	23.8289	74.9853	90.3565	345.3694
2008	23.3832	75.3520	96.3721	345.3946
2009	23.8649	75.2110	96.1673	354.3788
2010	21.7436	73.1880	88.2471	343.4571
2011	23.8821	75.1345	91.0761	351.9705
2012	22.6632	73.0695	85.3015	354.5614
2013	23.7936	75.0457	88.3743	353.1577

[a]There is a marked increase in in situ lesions in both the under- and over-age-50 groups. There is a slow but steady increase in malignant lesions in both the under- and over-age-50 groups.
Rates are age-adjusted to the 2000 U.S. Standard Population (19 age groups—Census P25-1103).
Source: SEER 9 areas.

images for future comparison. In 1983, the guidelines were changed to include screening every 1 to 2 years for women aged 40 to 49.

The battle in the 1990s was over what to do with women in their 40s. In 1993, the National Cancer Institute withdrew its support for screening mammograms for women younger than age 50. The NCI stated research had not shown a reduction in mortality rates for women who were screened in their 40s the way that it does for women older than 50 years of age.[36] Immediately after NCI's withdrawal of support for screening younger women, 18 other medical societies (ACS, ACR, AMA, ACOG, etc.) urged women to disregard this decision and to continue to follow the old guidelines of every 1 to 2 years for women in their 40s.[37,38]

To bolster support for screening women during the years 40 to 49, numerous articles appeared in print in the early 1990s. Statistics citing the benefits of screening came from the reevaluated Health Insurance Plan of New York (HIP) and Breast Cancer Detection Demonstration Project (BCDDP) studies in the United States, the Edinburgh Screening Trial, UCSF Service Screening Program, and Albuquerque Audit; the most important and impressive data came from the five Swedish screening trials regarding the efficacy of screening women in their 40s. Evidence quickly began to mount in favor of screening women annually beginning at age 40. By 1996, the battle between those for and those against screening mammograms of women aged 40 to 49 reached a climax.

1997 Guideline Controversy

At the urging of NCI Director Richard Klausner, MD, the National Institutes of Health (NIH) convened a conference to settle the issue of screening women in their 40s. For 3 days in January 1997, 32 speakers presented information to a panel of 13 (a major criterion for panel selection was an unbiased attitude concerning the screening issue as manifested by the absence of any articles or portions of articles addressing screening premenopausal women).[38] When the conference concluded, the panel issued a statement *against* recommending screening women younger than age 50. The panel suggested that women in their 40s should decide for themselves whether to be screened.

Immediately after the conference, media coverage of the panel's conclusions was unmerciful. A mockery was made of the panel's suggestion that women should decide for themselves (Figure 2-6). Public outcry against the decision was fueled by a hue and cry from many medical organizations. Even a Senate Appropriations Subcommittee hearing ensued. "NCI Director Richard Klausner, at whose

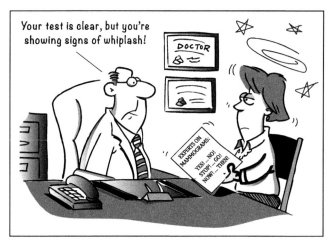

Figure 2-6
What's a woman to do? A mockery of guidelines. Drawing courtesy J. Lille[i]

urging the conference convened, publicly denounced the panel's findings, the first time in the history of the NCI that its Director has publicly disagreed with a consensus panel decision."[39]

Immediately after the panel's decision, the ACS and other medical groups announced their new guidelines: yearly mammograms for all women beginning at age 40.[40] Even Medicare announced annual coverage of mammograms beginning in 1998—not subject to satisfying the participant's yearly deductible. Shortly thereafter, the NCI/NIH altered their guidelines to recommend screening mammograms for women aged 40 to 49 be done every 1 to 2 years.

Use of mammography and clinical breast examination has increased significantly from the time of the first ACS recommendations in 1980. The number of women older than 40 years who have ever had a mammogram increased 200 percent during the 1980s ... Between 1985 and 1990, 44 states passed legislation requiring health insurance companies to cover the mammographic examination. In 1991, Medicare began reimbursement for screening mammograms every other year in women age 65 years and older.[35]

What a vindication for mammography.

2009 United States Preventive Services Task Force Recommendations

We were mystified when in 2009 the USPSTF issued their new recommendations for screening exams (Table 2-11). The USPSTF is an independent panel of primary care physicians funded and staffed by the Health and Human Services (HHS) Agency for Healthcare Research and Quality (AHRQ). Beginning in 2008, when determining what

Table 2-11 • USPSTF 2016 Final Recommendation Statement: Breast Cancer Screening[a]

Population Recommendation by Decade

Population	40–49	50–74	75+
Recommendation	Do not screen routinely; woman decides	Biennial	No recommendation
	Grade C	Grade B	Grade I (Insufficient)
Risk assessment	Average-risk woman	Average-risk woman	
Screening tests	Digital mammography	Digital mammography	
Timing		Evidence indicates biennial screening is optimal; preserves benefits of annual screening while reducing harms in half	
Benefits		Reduces mortality	
Harms	Moderate: psychological; false-positive results; additional medical visits; benign biopsies; overtreatment.	Moderate: psychological; false-positive results; additional medical visits; benign biopsies; overtreatment.	

Recommendations for All Women 40+

Population	40+	40+	40+	40+
Screening method	Digital mammography	With dense breasts, adjunctive modalities	CBE	BSE
Recommendation	Grade I	Grade I	Grade I	Grade D
Rational	Evidence lacking if DBT better than 2D FFDM	Evidence lacking if adjunctive modalities can substitute for 2D FFDM	Inadequate evidence of benefit	Does not reduce mortality

[a]False-positive findings are more common in the under-50 age group.
Number of biopsies performed is constant for all age groups.
False-negative findings are the same for all age groups.
Source: USPSTF Final Recommendation Statement: Breast Cancer Screening. Accessed January 30, 2018.

preventive services Medicare will cover, HHS is allowed to consider USPSTF recommendations; this is why the USPSTF recommendations are so vital: health insurance companies tend to follow Medicare's lead. Beginning in 2009, USPSTF evaluates the need for screening mammography using a new filter: harms versus benefits rather than the traditional filter: benefits. The USPSTF concludes mammography reduces breast cancer mortality in women aged 40 to 74 by 19%, with the greatest benefit for women aged 60 to 69, and the smallest benefit with women aged 40 to 49.[41]

USPSTF Recommendations

A "C" recommendation rating was issued for mammography use in women age 40 to 49. This C rating designates only a small benefit to screening women below the age of 50. It is *not* that mammograms are not recommended below age 50; rather the USPSTF states that women should weigh the harms versus the benefits and make a personal decision.

The "I" rating for women 75 years of age and above is a consequence of insufficient evidence from screening trial results whether or not there is a benefit in screening elderly women. Therefore, mammograms are not recommended for women above the age of 75.

The "B" rating for women aged 50 to 74 designates a benefit to screening for this age group; however, the USPSTF states that a large proportion of the benefits of screening mammography are maintained with biennial (every other year) screening. The USPSTF states that the harms of mammography screening are reduced by 50% by going to biennial rather than annual screening.

Clinical breast exam (CBE) is given a rating of "I," while breast self-exam (BSE) is rated "D." Digital mammography (2D FFDM), digital breast tomosynthesis (DBT), and breast MRI are given ratings of "I."

The USPSTF lists the harms of detection and early intervention to substantiate their B, C, D, and I ratings:

Psychological Harms

- Anxiety
- Unnecessary imaging tests: additional views, ultrasound, MRI
- Unnecessary biopsies in women without cancer
- Inconvenience of false-positive screening results (more common in women aged 40 to 49) (Table 2-12)
- Additional doctor appointments: family physician, surgeon, mammography facility

Table 2-12 • Harms of 1X Mammography Screening[a]

AGE	40–49	50–59	60–69	70–74
False positive	1,212	932	808	696
Biopsies	164	159	165	175
False negative	10	11	12	13

[a]False-positive findings are more common in the under-50 age group
Number of biopsies performed is constant for all age groups
False-negative findings are the same for all age groups
The following source must be cited when reproducing these data:
"Data collection and sharing was supported by the National Cancer Institute-funded Breast Cancer Surveillance Consortium (HHSN261201100031C). A list of the BCSC investigation and procedures for requesting BCSC data for research purposes are provided at: http://breastscreening.cancer.gov/."

Harms

- Treatment of noninvasive and invasive breast cancers that would not become clinically apparent during a women's lifetime (overdiagnosis; more common in older women)
- Unnecessary earlier treatment for breast cancer that would become clinically apparent but would not shorten a woman's life (overtreatment)
- False-negative (missed cancer) results provide false reassurance
- Effects of radiation exposure from a screening exam

The USPSTF recognizes that the benefit of screening mammography is equivalent for the age groups 40 to 49 and 50 to 59; however, the incidence of breast cancer and the consequences differ (Figure 2-7). More cancers are diagnosed in the 50 to 59 age group, so the harms are less, while fewer cancers are diagnosed in the 40 to 49 age group, so the harms are larger. The USPSTF states that the net benefit to the age 40 group is small; with the age 50 group, the benefit is moderate; for women in their 60s, the benefit is the greatest; women aged 70 to 74 have a moderate benefit; and for the woman aged 75+, there is insufficient data.

Response

More women in their 50s are diagnosed with breast cancer than those in their 40s, but younger women's cancers tend to be more aggressive.[42,43]

Twenty-five percent of women who die of breast cancer are diagnosed in their 40s.[44]

The 2010 Affordable Health Care Act did not support the 2009 USPSTF recommendations; "Obamacare" mandated that insurance companies cover screening mammography services beginning at age 40. This was reaffirmed by the Consolidated Appropriations Act, 2016 (H.R. 2029) in which Federal lawmakers extended that guarantee.

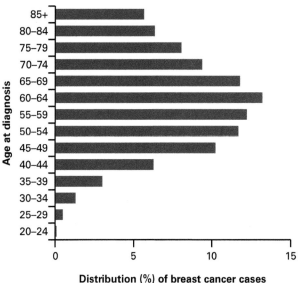

Figure 2-7
Breast cancer incidence by age. Advancing age places a woman at higher risk for developing this disease. (Source: National Center for Health Statistics. *Health, U.S. 2014 with Chartbook on Trends in the Health of Americans.* Hyattsville, MD: National Center for Health Statistics; 2015. National Cancer Institute Surveillance, Epidemiology, and End Results (SEER) 18 registries.)

2015 American Cancer Society Guidelines

October is breast cancer awareness month, the time each year that everyone gets "pink-ed"—from football players sporting pink sneakers and socks to pink lights on downtown landmark buildings. Everyone supports the pink cause: early detection.

It was a cruel turn of events for the ACS to announce their change in guidelines in October 2015, a policy shift that discounts the need for screening mammography. The new mammography screening guidelines were formulated after a committee was tasked with balancing the benefits versus the harms. The new 2015 ACS guidelines are not as extreme as those advocated by the USPSTF (Box 2-1).

According to the ACS, since the last guideline update in 2003, new studies have been published about the harms and drawbacks of screening mammography. Screening mammograms find something suspicious on the image: a BIRADS 0 classification; this requires further testing: additional views, ultrasound, or perhaps a biopsy, after which the suspicious area turns out to be (thankfully) benign. These additional tests carry risks: pain, anxiety, and other side effects. A recent screening trial conducted in the United Kingdom reported false-positive rates ranging from 0.9% to 6%, with higher rates for younger women and lower rates with older women.[45]

2015 American Cancer Society Recommendations for Early Breast Cancer Detection in Women without Breast Symptoms

- For women at average risk
- Women aged 40 to 44 should have the choice to start annual breast cancer screening with mammograms if they wish to do so.
- Women aged 45 to 54 should get mammograms every year.
- Women aged 55 and older should switch to mammograms every 2 years, or have the choice to continue yearly screening.
- Screening should continue as long as a woman is in good health and is expected to live 10 more years or longer.
- All women should be familiar with the known benefits, limitations, and potential harms associated with breast cancer screening. They should also be familiar with how their breasts normally look and feel and report any changes to their health care provider right away.

Source: https://www.cancer.org/content/cancer/en/healthy/find-cancer-early/cancer-screening-guidelines/american-cancer-society-guidelines-for-the-earlydetection-of-cancer.html. Reprinted by the permission of the American Cancer Society, Inc. www.cancer.org. All rights reserved.

In the United States, approximately 10% of screening mammograms are recalled for additional evaluation; this is the same recall rate as the Pap test. One to two percent are ultimately biopsied; 20% to 40% of biopsied lesions are cancer. The economic cost of recalls is estimated to be $1.6 billion.

The Mammography Community Responds To USPSTF Recommendations and ACS Guidelines

Mammography community leadership from the American College of Radiology (ACR) and the Society of Breast Imaging (SBI) formulated a response to this new risk-based assessment of the value of screening mammography used by the USPSTF and the ACS.[46]

The mammography community is "gravely concerned" about the new benefits versus harms assessment method that underestimates the benefits of screening mammography and overstates the harms associated with this exam. The ACR/SBI response addressed both written and insinuated points covered in the USPSTF guideline recommendations:

1. ***Task Force membership***
   No Task Force member is an expert in breast cancer diagnosis or care. In fact, a requirement for appointment to this Task Force was the total absence of any authoritative books, white papers, or articles on the topic of breast cancer.

Response
The ACR and SBI opinion is that formulation of guidelines with such important implications should be drafted by a multidisciplinary group representing all viewpoints of merit.

2. ***Statistical errors and assumptions***
   The Institute of Medicine (IOM), established in 1970, guides policy makers, health care professionals, the private sector, and the public in providing objective, evidence-based advice.

Response
The ACR/SBI stated that many of the types of significant statistical errors and inappropriate assumptions made by the USPSTF in formulating their recommendations were foreseen and could have been rectified by following the IOM document.[47]

3. ***Mortality reduction statistics***
   The USPSTF relied primarily on randomized clinical trial (RCT) data to compile statistics of a 19% mortality reduction (Table 2-13).

Response
RCT data results vary significantly between initiation-to-screen (invited versus not invited) versus exposure-to-screening (screened vs. nonscreened) trials. The former states a 25% reduction in mortality while the latter is 38%.[48]

The United States has limited current data with RCT studies. The United States performs opportunistic screening, while the European countries conduct screening programs. The majority of the RCT studies

Table 2-13 • Breast Cancer Deaths Avoided (95% CI) per 10,000 Women Screened by Repeat Screening Mammography over 10 Years: Data from Randomized, Controlled Trials[a,b] 2016 USPSTF Final Recommendation Statement

	AGES 40–49 Y	AGES 50–59 Y	AGES 60–69 Y	AGES 70–74 Y
Breast cancer deaths avoided	3 (0–9)	8 (2–17)	21 (11–32)	13 (0–32)

[a]All women did not have 100% adherence to all rounds of screening offered in the randomized, controlled trials.
[b]Over a 10-year period, screening 10,000 women aged 40–49 will result in 3 fewer breast cancer deaths; age 50–59 will result in 8 fewer; age 60–69 results in 21 fewer deaths.
Current as of: January 2018
Internet Citation: *Final Recommendation Statement: Breast Cancer: Screening.* U.S. Preventive Services Task Force. November 2016.
http://www.uspreventiveservicestaskforce.org/Page/Document/RecommendationStatementFinal/breast-cancer-screening

cited by the USPSTF were performed in the United States more than 40 years ago, using state-of-the art imaging techniques employed in those bygone eras; no current RCT studies employing modern imaging techniques are under way in the United States; therefore, we must look to our European colleagues for these statistics.

Results of opportunistic screening compare most closely to a more recent Euroscreen Working Group systematic review of 20 incidence-based trials, showing a 31% mortality reduction, plus 8 case-controlled studies with a 48% reduction.[48]

Opportunistic screening more closely aligns with exposure-to-screening (screened vs. nonscreened) programs. A Canadian study with 20 million person-years of follow-up shows a 40% mortality reduction with the screened versus nonscreened group.[49]

4. *Mortality reduction in women aged 40 to 49*

The data used by the USPSTF showed only a 12% reduction in mortality screening of women aged 40 to 49.

Response

The 2009 USPSTF failed to note a Swedish study of women aged 40 to 49 that showed a 26% mortality reduction for the screened versus nonscreened populations. An updated 2016 USPSTF paper mentions that the Task Force reviewed this study; their conclusion: more contemporary evidence using modern-day imaging is important to consider due to the age and obsolete technology used to gather the RCT data.

The Swedish study compared two matched groups of women in their 40s: those screened for breast disease and those not screened. Whether in the screened or the nonscreened group, all women diagnosed with breast cancer were given similar treatments. The screened group showed a 26% reduction in mortality versus the nonscreened group. This comparison showed there was no reduction in mortality for the nonscreened group who were diagnosed only when their cancer advanced

to a symptomatic stage; mortality reduction occurred only in the screened group.[50]

The Pan-Canadian Screening Study with 20 million person-years of follow-up showed the following mortality reduction based on exposure to screening (screened vs. nonscreened populations):

AGE	MORTALITY REDUCTION
40–49	44%
50–59	40%
60–69	42%
70–79	35%

The rate of mortality reduction is similar for each decade of life. Although the incidence of breast cancer increases with increasing age, early detection of disease benefits all age groups equally.[49]

A study conducted in England showed a mortality reduction of 48% in women aged 40 to 49, and 44% for the 40 to 69 age group.[51]

5. *"C" rating for women aged 40 to 49*

A "C" recommendation rating was designated by the USPSTF for screening mammograms of women between ages 40 and 49. Seventeen million women are in this age bracket in the United States. The Affordable Health Care Act of 2010 required that insurance companies include coverage for screening exams with a rating of "B" or above; the "C" rating given to mammography would exclude women from receiving the benefits of this exam. USPSTF advocates women in their 40s should decide for themselves whether or not to undergo screening mammograms by comparing the harms versus the benefits (Figure 2-6).

Response

Breast cancers in nonscreened women aged 40 to 49 still occur, only they will be advanced cancers with clinical signs and symptoms when discovered. A study by Webb et al. reported that most deaths from breast cancer occurred in nonscreened women (71%), and half of these deaths were in women younger than age 50.[52]

Table 2-14 • Cancer Rate (Per 1,000 Examinations) and Cancer Detection Rate (Per 1,000 Examinations) for 1,838,372 Screening Mammography Examinations from 2004 to 2008 by Age–based on BCSC Data through 2009

	NUMBER OF EXAMS	NUMBER OF CANCERS	CANCER RATE/1000 EXAMS	CANCER DETECTION RATE
18–39	44,339	136	3.07	2.35
40–44	222,292	590	2.65	1.95
45–49	271,698	988	3.64	3.00
50–54	294,922	1263	4.28	3.54
55–59	282,512	1319	4.67	4.00
60–64	220,259	1255	5.70	4.83
65–69	173,512	1062	6.12	5.28
70–74	136,528	923	6.76	5.84
75–79	105,115	744	7.08	6.26
80+	87,195	742	8.51	7.53

From Sinclair N, Littenberg B, Geller B, et al. Accuracy of screening mammography in older women. *AJR Am J Roentgenol*. 2011;197(5):1268–1273. Reprinted with permission from the American Journal of Roentgenology.

There are four major reasons to screen women aged 40 to 49: (a) it is effective; (b) cancer tends to have a rapid growth rate in women aged 40 to 49; (c) there is an increased incidence of developing cancer in women in their 40s; and (d) annual screening means a reduced mortality rate.

Screening of asymptomatic women in their 40s is effective in detecting small cancers.[27,28,30,35,53–62] Detecting cancer in its early stages offers a greater chance for recovery and more choices for intervention to stop the cancer from spreading beyond the breast tissue. Screening women annually beginning at age 40 will detect more cancers than by delaying annual screening to age 50. Newer techniques and equipment allow skilled technologists to image smaller malignant tumors and skilled physicians to perceive the subtle changes in these early growth stages.

Some malignant breast tumors progress faster from the early stages to their more advanced and deadly stages in women aged 40 to 49.[29,33,63,64] These aggressive tumors also take a significantly shorter time to develop in women of this age group, which strongly suggests the need for an annual mammogram. For now, the key to survival for women in their 40s is a quality mammogram every year, an accurate interpretation of their mammograms, and the detection of tumors under 10 mm in size.

In 2013, there were approximately 65,000 cases of breast cancer diagnosed in women younger than age 50.

6. *"I" rating for women age 75+*

An "I" recommendation rating was designated by the USPSTF for screening mammograms for women aged 75 and older. Not much data has been published on screening mammography outcomes for women in this age group. The "I" rating is due to insufficient data.

The USPSTF issued this policy to stop screening for all elderly women, regardless of their health status, due to their limited life expectancy and comorbidity likelihood.

Response

Ten million women in the United States are aged 75+. Actuarial tables provide life expectancy rates:

Women who live to age 75:

- 25% live another 17 years.
- 50% live another 12 years.
- 25% live another 7 years.

Data from a Breast Cancer Surveillance Consortium (BCSC) Screening Study, comprising over 4 million mammograms, done in the United States between 1996 and 2006 (Table 2-14) demonstrate a much higher cancer detection rate/1,000 women for the 70 to 80+ age groups than for the 60 to 69 age groups, which are the age groups the USPSTF states makes the most sense to screen.[65]

SEER data report that 30% of invasive breast cancer occurs in the 70+ age group. CISNET modeling data show that both age groups (70 to 74 and 75+) have similar incidence rates. The USPSTF gives a "B" rating for screening women age 70 to 74 and an "I" rating for age 75+.

Breast cancers in nonscreened women above age 74 still occur; only, they will be advanced cancers with clinical signs and symptoms when discovered.

7. *Annual versus biennial screening*

The USPSTF recommends biennial screening for women aged 50 to 74, a "B" recommendation rating (Table 2-15).

Response

Screening intervals are based on tumor sojourn time. Whether screening mammograms are done annually or biennially, the same ***total*** number of breast cancer cases are identified. The difference is in the size and stage of the tumor. A computer simulation method built

Table 2-15 • Lifetime Benefits and Harms of Annual versus Biennial Screening Mammography per 1,000 Women Screened: Model Results Compared with No Screening[a,b] 2016 USPSTF Final Recommendation Statement

VARIABLE	AGES 50–74 Y, ANNUAL SCREENING	AGES 50–74 Y, BIENNIAL SCREENING
Fewer breast cancer deaths, n	9 (5–10)	7 (4–9)
Life-years gained, n	145 (104–180)	122 (75–154)
False-positive tests, n	1798 (1706–2445)	953 (830–1325)
Unnecessary breast biopsies, n	228 (219–317)	146 (121–205)
Overdiagnosed breast tumors, n	25 (12–68)	19 (11–34)

[a]Values reported are medians (ranges).
[b]The rationale behind the new biennial versus annual guidelines. With biennial screening:
• There is a modest decrease in mortality
• There is a slight reduction in life-years gained
• False positives are reduced by half
• Biopsies are reduced almost by half
• There is a slight reduction in overdiagnosis
Current as of: January 2018
Internet Citation: *Final Recommendation Statement: Breast Cancer: Screening.* U.S. Preventive Services Task Force. November 2016. http://www.uspreventiveservicestaskforce.org/Page/Document/RecommendationStatementFinal/breast-cancer-screening

on breast cancer growth rates calculates that annual screening yields a 52% reduction in distant metastatic disease versus 27% with biennial screening.[66]

Annual screening finds cancers at a smaller size, more likely node-negative, at an earlier stage, with longer survival rates, with reduced treatment regimens, and with a reduction in mortality. The downside to annual screening is an increase in false-positive exams because it is more difficult to find early disease. Biennial screening has fewer false-positive findings because it is easier to identify more advanced cancers. The price to be paid for finding disease earlier is more frequent recalls of patients for additional views plus more biopsies.

CISNET modeling of annual screening of women aged 40 to 74 yields 46.5% more lives saved and 57% more life-years saved than when screening is delayed until age 50.

8. *Benefits of screening other than mortality reduction*
   • Screening detected (earlier stage disease) versus palpation detected (more advanced) breast cancer.
   • Earlier detection results in less surgery. Advanced cancers require extensive surgery: the Halsted radical mastectomy; screening detected cancers are smaller, resulting in less surgery: lumpectomy. Due to earlier detection of breast cancer, we rarely, if ever, perform Halsted radical mastectomies today. Modified radical mastectomies are performed today, but most screening detected cancers are treated with lumpectomy. Beginning in 1990, the NIH recommends breast conservation therapy (BCT) for early (stage I or II) breast cancer. Currently, approximately 65% of women choose lumpectomy.[67]
   • Chemotherapy: less frequent and less aggressive treatment regimes with fewer serious side effects

for screening detected cancer. Generally, if a tumor is under 1 cm in size, no chemotherapy is needed.
   • Increased anxiety for the 10% of incomplete exams (BIRADS 0); but 90% of women have decreased anxiety due to true negative results.
   • Decreased anxiety in women diagnosed with early-stage disease because they know early detection results in better survival rates with reduced therapies (surgery, radiation, chemotherapy). There is a certain peace of mind when cancer is found early.

OVERDETECTION, OVERDIAGNOSIS, OVERTREATMENT

Overdetection: Radiologist
Overdiagnosis: Pathologist
Overtreatment: Surgeon/Oncologist

The USPSTF refers to the harms of overdiagnosis of breast cancer; it is considered the most significant of all the harms associated with screening mammography. The USPSTF estimates overdiagnosis at 19%; in women below 50 years of age, the rate of overdiagnosis is between 20% and 40%.[68] The USPSTF estimates that 20 women/1,000 who undergo a lifetime of screening will be overdiagnosed; this is a 2% lifetime frequency.

Overdiagnosis of invasive carcinoma is virtually non-existent. Overdiagnosis generally deals with DCIS, especially low-grade tumors, which are 20% of DCIS cases. DCIS does not always progress to IDC; in fact, less than half of untreated DCIS advance to the invasive stage. Therefore, surgical removal with/without adjuvant therapy may represent overdiagnosis/overtreatment. The NCI recommends that DCIS should no longer be classified as breast cancer; instead, it should be considered as an indolent lesion.[69]

A study by Javitt reports that up to 30% of DCIS lesions treated only with local excision recur.[70]

In 1983, there were 4,900 cases of DCIS reported; in 2017, there are 63,400 cases projected.[71] DCIS has gone from 5% to 20% of findings on mammograms (Table 2-10). Forty percent of nonpalpable lesions detected at screening are DCIS. With appropriate treatment of DCIS, survival rates are 99.5%.[72]

Overdetection

Overdetection is a function of the radiologist; sensitivity and specificity rates are monitored by the annual medical outcomes audit. The sensitivity in mammography is between 77% and 95%, and specificity is 94% to 97%.[73,74]

Currently, it is impossible to determine if a screening detected cancer would have remained indolent, never causing a health care incident for which the woman is treated for cancer. This causes us to treat all screening detected cancers as malignant. Upon biopsy, we know if the DCIS tumor is low grade; it is this group of 20% that overdiagnosis impacts. But for 80% of cases that are the higher grade tumors, this is early detection. Early detection means less extensive treatment regimens.

Perhaps the best estimate of overdiagnosis is by Puliti et al., between 1% and 10%. The harm of overtreatment is removal of this lesion.[75]

Mitigate Overdetection

At this time, there do not appear to be any palatable methods to mitigate overdetection.

1. ***Raise the radiologist's threshold for considering findings sufficiently abnormal before recommending additional imaging as well as when to biopsy***
   This means waiting until a cancer advances in its growth until it clearly and unambiguously changes the architecture on an image. When the cancer advances and presents with classic radiographic characteristics of malignancy, there is no need for additional views, ultrasound, or any other ancillary procedures.

2. ***Delay the age for beginning screening mammography***
   In the 1980s, we performed a baseline mammogram between the ages of 35 and 39; this was abandoned. In 1992, the ACS guidelines changed to begin annual screening at age 40. In 2015, the ACS guidelines changed to begin at age 45; the USPSTF recommends beginning at age 50.

3. ***Lengthen the interval between screening exams***
   The USPSTF recommends biennial rather than annual exams for women aged 50 to 74.

4. ***Do not perform BSE/CBE***
   When we perform a physical examination of the breasts and feel "something," we take action to discover what it is: perform imaging (mammogram/ultrasound); interval follow-up in 6 months; refer the patient to a surgeon; and perhaps escalate to a biopsy. Most of the time the symptomatic area is not cancer. If we do not examine the breasts, then these "harms" would not happen.

5. ***Do not screen elderly women due to a comorbidity likelihood***

6. ***Do not treat screening-detected DCIS***
   Half or fewer of DCIS cases progress to invasive disease. Continue surveillance and treat only those cases that increase in size/symptoms.

There is not a single reported case of spontaneous disappearance of DCIS or invasive breast cancer happening without treatment. Conversely, there are thousands of examples of cancers visible in hindsight on previous exams, where the current exam shows the cancer has increased in size between the prior and current exams.

Nonscreened women still undergo false-positive tests due to clinical signs and symptoms. A study by Barton reported 16% of women (32% in their 40s) went to a physician for a breast "problem." Twenty-one percent had a biopsy, proving the symptomatic area was benign: in USPSTF terminology, an "unnecessary" biopsy.[76]

The USPSTF does not mention the harm of later detection of a breast cancer.

Since the advent of screening mammography in the United States in the mid 1980s, there are conflicting reports about the value of screening exams. This has led to confusion and mistrust on behalf of the public as well as those in the health care field who are asked by patients when is the correct age to begin screening, what age should this exam be discontinued, and what is the correct interval between exams.

What is the rationale behind this new policy? The ACS now aligns more closely with the findings of the 2009 USPSTF. The guidelines are beginning to align with those of our European colleagues. The baseline mammogram between ages 35 and 39 has long disappeared; annual exams no longer begin at age 40, and instead age 45 is the new recommendation; BSE has long been optional to perform; and now annual CBE is no longer recommended. No monthly BSE, no annual exam by your doctor, a delay until age 45 to begin mammography, and a reduction in the number of lifetime mammograms each woman undergoes—what impact will all these have on the strides we've made in early detection and a reduction in mortality rates? With the new guidelines just announced, we must wait years to learn the long-term effects.

Summary

The prevention, detection, and treatment of breast cancer continues to be a major goal in the health care of women. This disease strikes 1 in every 8 American women and is a major cause of death. We cannot prevent this disease at this time. We can, however, detect it at an earlier stage when the word "cure" can be more than something the woman hopes for. Mammography technologists promote breast health and inspire their patients to encourage their family members and friends to have mammograms. "You can survive breast cancer if it is detected early, and you can detect it early through monthly breast self-examination and periodic mammograms."[77]

Review Questions

1. Refer to Figure 2-2. What is the purpose of the National Strategic Plan for the Detection and Control of Breast and Cervical Cancers? When did this Plan begin? How much money is spent annually on this program?

2. Will the results of the Swedish screening trials apply to screening done in the United States?

3. Mammography guidelines are rewritten every few years. Why is this necessary?

4. Screening mammography has dramatically increased the detection of DCIS. What are the harms associated with detection of this stage of disease?

References

1. Breasted JH. *The Edwin Smith Papyrus*. Chicago, IL: University of Chicago Press; 1930:403–406.
2. Baum M. Breast cancer 2000 BC to 2000 AD—time for a paradigm shift? *Acta Oncol*. 1993;32(1):3–8.
3. Statement of the American Society of Human Genetics on genetic testing for breast and ovarian cancer predisposition. *Am J Hum Genet*. 1994;55:i–iv.
4. Strax P. Control of breast cancer. *Adm Radiol*. September 1989;30–36.
5. Dakins D. Diagnostic problem-solving takes a back seat in breast screening. *Diagn Imaging*. 1987;9(11):372.
6. Vinocur B. The breast cancer battle: screening with mammography. *Diagn Imaging*. 1986;8(7):84.
7. Self-exams, mammograms recommended. *USA Today*. October 19, 1987.
8. Gladwell M. How safe are your breasts? *New Republic*. October 24, 1994.
9. Subtle mammographic signs disclose presence of early breast cancer. *Radiol Today*. 1987;4(4):4.
10. Egan R. The new age of breast care. *Adm Radiol*. September 1989;9.
11. Tabar L, Vitak B, Chem JJ, et al. The Swedish 2 county trial 20 years later. *Radiol Clin North Am*. 2000;38:625–652.
12. National Center for Health Statistics. *Health, United States, 2014: With Special Feature on Adults Aged 55–64*. Hyattsville, MD: National Center for Health Statistics; 2015.
13. Narod SA, Javaid I, Miller AB. Why have mortality rates declined? *J Cancer Policy*. 2015;5:8–17.
14. CDC. The National Strategic Plan for the early detection and control of breast and cervical cancers. U.S. Department of Health and Human Services, Public Health Service, CDC, 1993.
15. National Breast and Cervical Cancer Early Detection Program. Centers for Disease Control and Prevention. Accessed October 18, 2017. Available at: https://www.cdc.gov/cancer/nbccedp/about.htm
16. Bassett LW. Screening strategies aim to increase compliance. *Diagn Imaging*. 1991;13:75–79.
17. Rebner M. Can government legislation improve screening mammography use? *Radiology*. 1996;198:636–637.
18. King A. Not everyone agrees with the new mammographic screening guidelines designed to end the confusion. *JAMA*. 1989;262(9):1154.
19. Rubin R. Study finds mammograms not as frequent as thought. *USA Today*. September 12, 2005:7D.
20. Song J. Women start mammography on time, but fail to followup. *Advance*. October 4, 2004:17.
21. Many women skipping breast exams. Available at: healthatoz.com. Downloaded November 1, 2007.
22. What are the key statistics for breast cancer? Available at: www.cancer.org. Accessed June 1, 2016.
23. National Center for Health Statistics. *Health, U.S. 2014 with Chartbook on Trends in the Health of Americans*. Hyattsville, MD: National Center for Health Statistics; 2015.
24. Siegel RL, Miller K, Jemal A. Cancer statistics, 2017. *CA Cancer J Clin*. 2017;67(1):7–30.
25. DeSantis CE, Fedewa SA, Sauer AG, et al. Breast cancer statistics, 2015: convergence of incidence rates between black and white women. *CA Cancer J Clin*. 2016;66(1):31–42.
26. Nystrom L, Rutqvist LE, Wall S, et al. Breast cancer screening with mammography: overview of Swedish randomized trials. *Lancet*. 1993;341:973–978.
27. Tabar L, Fagerberg G, Day NE, et al. Breast cancer treatment and natural history: new insights from results of screening. *Lancet*. 1992;339:412–414.
28. Tabar L, Dufy SW, Burhenne L. New Swedish breast cancer detection results for women aged 40–49. *Cancer*. 1993;72(4):1437–1448.
29. Tabar L, Vitak B, et al. Swedish two county trial: impact of mammographic screening on breast cancer mortality during 3 decades. *Radiology*. 2012;260(3):653–663.
30. Shapiro S. Determining the efficacy of breast cancer screening. *Cancer*. 1989;63:1873–1880.

31. Howlader N, Noone AM, Krapcho M, et al., eds. *SEER Cancer Statistics Review, 1975–2013*. Bethesda, MD: National Cancer Institute. Available at: http://seer.cancer.gov/csr/1975_2013/, based on November 2015 SEER data submission, posted to the SEER web site, April 2016.

32. Horner MJ, Reis LAG, Krapcho M, et al., eds. *SEER Cancer Statistics Review 1975–2006*. Bethesda, MD: National Cancer Institute; 2009.

33. Feig S. Determination of mammographic screening intervals with surrogate measures for women aged 40–49 years. *Radiology*. 1994;193:311–314.

34. Cancer Study Cites Rapid Growth. *Sarasota Herald Tribune*. July 3, 1996.

35. Mettein C, Smart C. Breast cancer detection guidelines for women aged 40–49 years: rationale for the American Cancer Society reaffirmation of recommendations. *CA Cancer J Clin*. 1994;44:248–255.

36. Cancer Agency Changes Mammogram Advice. *Sarasota Herald Tribune*. December 5, 1993.

37. Slantez P, Moore RH, Hulka CA, et al. Screening mammography: effect of national guidelines on current physician practice. *Radiology*. 1997;203:335–338.

38. D'Orsi C. NIH consensus development conference statement: breast cancer screening for women ages 40–49. *SBI News*. February 1997.

39. Linver M. *Summary: mammography outcomes in a practice setting by age: prognostic factors, sensitivity and positive biopsy rate. SBI News*. February 1997.

40. Leitch A. ACS guidelines for the early detection of breast cancer: update 1997. *CA Cancer J Clin*. 1997;47(3):150–153.

41. Siu AL; U.S. Preventive Services Task Force. Screening for breast cancer: US Preventive Services Task Force Recommendation Statement. *Ann Intern Med*. 2016;164(4):279–296.

42. Moskowitz M. Breast cancer: age-specific growth rates and screening strategies. *Radiology*. 1986;16(1):37–41.

43. Tabar L, Fagerberg G, Chen HH, et al. Efficacy of breast cancer screening by age. New results from the Swedish two county trial. *Cancer*. May 1995;75(10):2507–2517.

44. Buist DS, Porter PL, Lehman C, et al. Factors contributing to mammography failure in women aged 40–49 years. *J Natl Cancer Inst*. 2004;96(19):1432–1440.

45. Johns LE, Moss SM. False positive results in the randomized controlled trial of mammographic screening from age 40. *Cancer Epidermiol Biomarkers Prev*. 2010;19(11):2758–2764.

46. Monsees B, Monticciolo D, Murray R. *Electronic Response on Behalf of ACR and SBI to USPSTF Re: Draft USPSTF Recommendations on Breast Cancer Screening*.

47. Graham R, Mancher M, Miller Wolman D, et al., eds.; *Institute of Medicine of the National Academies. Clinical Practice Guidelines We Can Trust*. Washington, DC: National Academies Press; 2011.

48. Broeders M, Moss S, Nyström L, et al. The impact of mammographic screening on breast cancer mortality in Europe: a review of observational studies. *J Med Screen*. 2012;19(Suppl 1):14–25.

49. Coldman A, Phillips N, Wilson C, et al. Pan-Canadian study of mammography screening and mortality from breast cancer. *J Natl Cancer Inst*. 2014;106(11):261–263.

50. Hellquist BN, Duffy SW, Abdsaleh S, et al. Effectiveness of population-based service screening with mammography for women ages 40 to 49 years: evaluation of the Swedish

51. Wald NJ, Murphy P, Major P, et al. UKCCCR multicenter randomized controlled trial of one and two view mammography in breast cancer screening. *BMJ*. 1995;311:1189–1193.

52. Webb ML, Cady B, Michaelson JS, et al. A failure analysis of invasive breast cancer: most deaths from disease occur in women not regularly screened. *Cancer*. 2014;120(18):2839–2846.

53. American College of Radiology. News Releases. USPSTF Breast Cancer Screening Recommendations Could Endanger Women. News Release January 11, 2016. Available at: www.acr.org/Media Center. Accessed June 27, 2016.

54. Siedman H, Mushinski M. Breast cancer incidence, mortality, survival, prognosis. In: Feig S, McLelland R, eds. *Breast Carcinoma: Current Diagnosis and Treatment*. New York: Mason; 1983.

55. Benning T. Komen for the cure founder Nancy Brinker blasts proposed new mammography guidelines. *The Dallas Morning News*. November 23, 2009.

56. Ferrini R, Mannino E, Ramsdell E, et al. Screening mammography for breast cancer, American College of Preventive Medicine Practice Policy Statement. *Am J Prev Med*. 1996;12(5):340–341.

57. Mammography Screening Guidelines. American College of Obstetricians and Gynecologists. Available at: www.acog.org. Accessed April 21, 2010.

58. Newman J. Early detection techniques in breast cancer management. *Radiol Technol*. 1997;68(4):309–324.

59. Burkenne L, Burkenne H, Kan L. Quality oriented mass mammography screening. *Radiology*. 1995;194:185–188.

60. Baker L. BCDDP: 5 year summary report. *CA Cancer J Clin*. 1992;32:194–225.

61. Sickles E. Summary of presentation screening outcomes: clinical experience with service screening using modern mammography. *SBI News*. February 1997.

62. Sampson D; American Cancer Society. American Cancer Society report finds breast cancer death rate continues to drop. Breast Cancer Facts & Figures, September 25, 2007.

63. Pelikan S, Moskowitz M. Effects of lead-time, length bias, and false negative reassurance on screening for breast cancer. *Cancer* 1993;71:1998–2005.

64. Tabar L, Fagerberg G, Day NE, et al. What is the optimum interval between screening examination? An analysis based on the latest results of the Swedish two county breast cancer screening trial. *Br J Cancer*. 1987;55:47–51.

65. Sinclair N, Littenberg B, Geller B, et al. Accuracy of screening mammography in older women. *AJR Am J Roentgenol*. 2011;197(5):1268–1273.

66. Michaelson JS, Halpern E, Kopans DB. Breast cancer computer simulation method for estimation of optimal intervals for screening. *Radiology*. 1999;212:551–560.

67. Kummerow KL, Du L, Penson DF, et al. Nationwide trends in mastectomy for early stage breast cancer. *JAMA Surg*. 2015;150(1):9–16.

68. Allen JD, Blumethmann SM, Sheets M, et al. Women's responses to changes in US Preventive Services Task Force's mammography screening guidelines: results of focus groups with ethnically diverse women. *BMC Public Health*. 2013;13:1169.

Mammography Screening in Young Women (SCRY) cohort. *Cancer*. 2011;117(4):714–722.

69. Forbes LJ, Ramirez AJ. Expert group on information about breast screening. Offering informed choice about breast cancer screening. *J Med Screen.* 2014;21(4):194–200.

70. Javitt MC. Section editors notebook: breast cancer screening and over diagnosis unmasked. *AJR Am J Roentgenol.* 2014;202(2):259–261.

71. Nelson HD, Tyne K, Naika A, et al. *Screening for Breast Cancer: Systemic Evidence Review Updated for the U.S. Preventive Services Task Force.* Evidence synthesis No. 74. AHRQ Publication No. 10-05142-EF-1. Rockville, MD: Agency for Healthcare Research and Quality; 2009.

72. Feig SA. Screening mammography benefit controversies: sorting out the evidence. *Radiol Clin North Am.* 2014;52(3): 455–480.

73. Humphrey LL, Helfand M, Chan BK, et al. Breast cancer screening: a summary of the evidence for the U.S. Preventive Services Task Force. *Ann Intern Med.* 2002;137: 347–360.

74. Biesheuvel C, Barratt A, Howard K, et al. Effects of study methods and biases on estimates of invasive breast cancer overdetection with mammography screening: a systematic review. *Lancet Oncol.* 2007;(12):1129–1138.

75. Puliti D, Duffy SW, Miccinesi G, et al. Overdiagnosis in mammographic screening for breast cancer in Europe: a literature review. *J Med Screen.* 2012;19(Suppl 1): 42–56.

76. Barton MB, Elmore JG, Fletcher SW. Breast symptoms among women enrolled in a health maintenance organization: frequency, evaluation, and outcome. *Ann Intern Med.* 1999;130(8):651–657.

77. Silbner J. How to beat breast cancer. *US News & World Report.* July 1, 1988:52.

Patient Considerations

3

Objectives

- Understand the obligations of the health care system and individuals serving the patient to positively impact the patient experience
- To help the technologist better understand the patient's emotional needs and responses throughout the breast imaging process
- To empower the technologist through relevant information that provides emotional comfort, support, and relief to the patient
- Understand the importance of effective communication in reducing anxiety during the mammography patient experience
- Understand the patient preparation necessary for the mammography examination

Keywords

- decision aids
- Health Insurance Portability and Accountability Act (HIPAA)
- Hospital Consumer Assessment of Healthcare Providers and Systems Survey
- interpersonal skills
- patient-centered care
- patient experience
- shared decision-making

INTRODUCTION

Today's health care environment is immersed in strategies to ensure that the patient is satisfied over a wide range of services. These strategies are necessary due to the increasing requirements associated with health care reimbursement and the competitive health care market that exists today. There are several factors that contribute to assuring that excellence in health care is achieved across all service aspects. In 2006, the Centers for Medicare and Medicaid Services (CMS) implemented the **Hospital Consumer Assessment of Healthcare Providers and Systems Survey**, referred to as the Hospital CAHPS Survey (pronounced "H-caps"). The HCAHPS Survey is a standardized method developed by the CMS and the Agency for Healthcare Research and Quality to measure the patient's perspective of their hospital experience. Among other purposes, this survey is used to evaluate the perspective of the *inpatient* hospital experience allowing hospitals the opportunity to improve their quality of care.[1,2] The culture of measuring the quality of service in the health care industry has firmly taken root, with outpatient facilities also recognizing the need to ensure that exemplary care is delivered to their customers. The practice model of **patient-centered care**, health care that is organized around the patient, originally described the interaction and communication between the provider and the patient in an effort to satisfy the needs and the expectations of the patient.[3,4] Today, organizations recognize the need for patient-centered health care systems, where every employee of the organization has the responsibility to invest in the patient's quality of care.[5] These measures influence a change in the traditional medical imaging environment by calling for the radiologist to incorporate the patient-centered care model into the medical imaging practice and organizing radiology processes to address the needs and preferences of the patient.[3] This chapter discusses essential practices by the medical facility, medical imaging staff, radiologist, and technologist that serve to ensure a positive and safe **patient experience** throughout the mammography procedure.

COMPASSIONATE, COMFORTING CARE

Mammography is a sensitive and personal examination, generally causing some degree of discomfort to the patient.[6] This knowledge may commonly invoke feelings of nervousness, anxiety,[7] or, less common, frustration in the person reporting for the procedure. Each woman arriving for a mammogram carries within her different degrees of these feelings when she arrives for her appointment. According to many resources, the common fears and apprehensions that contribute to feelings of nervousness or anxiety associated with mammography include a combination of physical, emotional, and intellectual fears.[7–9]

Some fears associated with the mammography procedure:

- That breast cancer will be detected
- Pain or discomfort
- Embarrassment
- Modesty
- Body image
- Radiation
- Waiting for results
- Cost
- Competency/professionalism of the technologist
- That the procedure may cause cancer
- Previous unpleasant or bad experiences
- Frightening stories shared by friends or relatives
- Relatives or friends with a recent diagnosis of breast cancer
- First time mammography examination (baseline)

These are just *some* of the fears that may influence the emotional state of the patient arriving for a screening mammogram. Patients who have been called back for additional imaging generally report for their return mammography appointment with increased levels of anxiety. It should be noted that there are several preparatory provisions established to reduce patient anxiety in the screening and the diagnostic setting that are discussed later in this chapter. A perceptive mammography technologist understands the personal nature of the mammography examination and the potential for patients to harbor anxiety. There are significant reasons why the technologist should pay special attention to methods that help reduce patient anxiety during mammography. Technologists who understand the multipurpose necessity of ensuring patient relaxation and cooperation during the procedure allow the facility and the patient to benefit in these important aspects of the examination:

1. Demonstrating compassion and support to the anxious patient provides a positive patient experience in spite of their anxiety.
2. Patients perceive the quality of their experience with the facility through the professionalism and interpersonal skills of the staff. These experiences, whether positive or negative, are shared with others in the community.[10]
3. For the technologist, adequate capture of the posterior margin of the breast is the most challenging component of the mammography examination. In order to successfully *achieve capture and clarity* of tissue adjacent to the chest wall, the patient's chest wall muscles (thorax) must be completely relaxed.[9]

4. Generally, the posterior breast tissue adjacent to the chest wall can be captured *with reduced discomfort* to the patient when the muscles adjacent to the thorax are relaxed.

5. Research supports that the interaction between the technologist and the patient during the initial mammography procedure is an indicator of whether or not the patient will return for subsequent examinations.[8]

The fears associated with the mammography procedure are well documented, requiring the health care professional taking care of these patients to provide compassionate reassurance throughout the examination. Randi Gunther, PhD, in preparing for a presentation of "The Key Role of Mammogram Technologists in Mammogram Compliance," conducted in-depth interviews with radiologists, physicians, patients, and mammography technologists to better understand the role of the technologist in the breast imaging team. The results of her interviews demonstrated that mammography technologists share common personality characteristics with others working in a healing profession. According to Dr. Gunther, mammography technologists are more likely to be self-sacrificing individuals who have a greater interest in nurturing than in power, carry out their responsibility without complaint, are uncomfortable in confronting people in authority positions, and are interested in pleasing others.

The compassionate heart of a mammography technologist offers sincerity throughout the specific requirements of the patient experience. This essential element must be supported through additional efforts that are known to positively impact patient satisfaction and reduce anxiety. Mammography services that are knowledgeable about how patients perceive the care they have received are aware that the pain, discomfort, and distress associated with mammography negatively impacts patient satisfaction,[11] while in addition to these factors, satisfaction with the clinic service and health care provider are also important factors that influence the patient experience.[12] Researchers in Norway developed a questionnaire to measure patient satisfaction with mammography in an effort to better understand subsequent screening compliance. According to the researchers, assessment of the patient's mammography experience includes quality measures of four examination categories[11]:

• Structure: describes the convenience, accessibility, and physical environment of the patient experience during mammography
• Process: describes the information transferred between the patient and the mammography personnel, the interpersonal skills of personnel, and the perceived technical skills of personnel

• Discomfort: describes the physical and psychological discomfort experienced by the patient
• General satisfaction: describes elements that pertain to future mammography compliance

These important areas, examined to better understand patient adherence to breast screening, can also provide important feedback to the facility, medical imaging leadership, the mammography technologist team, and the individual mammography technologist who is interested in continuous quality improvement of the mammography service. An example of a patient satisfaction survey is illustrated in Figure 3-1. Each service category that influences the experience of the patient scheduled for a mammogram is discussed in this chapter.

FIRST IMPRESSIONS: PATIENT SCHEDULING AND REGISTRATION

In today's fast-paced society, scheduling medical appointments has become a sophisticated service demanding options for customers of varying age groups and varying abilities to access the Internet. Facilities need to project a convenient and positive "first impression" model of efficiency and friendliness whether the process is accomplished through face-to-face interaction, a phone call, or an automated process. During this interaction, sensitive information about the patient and her health history is collected. Whatever method is used to gather this information, the facility must abide by the regulations established by the **Health Insurance Portability and Accountability Act (HIPAA)** passed into law in 1996. This federal law establishes a set of national standards for the protection of certain health information through the Privacy Rule and establishes standards for the security of electronic protected health information (e-PHI) through the Security Rule.[13] Mammography personnel are expected to know and abide by these regulations.

Scheduling: Automated

The popularity of automated patient scheduling provides the 24-hour flexibility that an increasing number of customers prefer. The convenient access of automated information addresses a number of services surrounding the customer experience that include access to a secure Internet portal to schedule the examination, receive reminders of the appointment date and time, and access the examination results.[14] Like communication that addresses these services using a face-to-face or phone call method, the end

SUPERCARE MEDICAL GROUP
Harry B. Campbell, M.D.

Dear Patient: According to our records, you recently visited the **provider named above.** Please tell us your opinion about the service you received **from this provider.** Your responses will be kept strictly confidential. Thanks for your help.

PLEASE RATE THE FOLLOWING:

	Excellent	Very Good	Good	Fair	Poor	Does Not Apply
A. YOUR APPOINTMENT:						
1. Ease of making appointments by phone	5	4	3	2	1	N/A
2. Appointment available within a reasonable amount of time	5	4	3	2	1	N/A
3. Getting care for illness/injury as soon as you wanted it	5	4	3	2	1	N/A
4. Getting after-hours care when you needed it	5	4	3	2	1	N/A
5. The efficiency of the check-in process	5	4	3	2	1	N/A
6. Waiting time in the reception area	5	4	3	2	1	N/A
7. Waiting time in the exam room	5	4	3	2	1	N/A
8. Keeping you informed if your appointment time was delayed	5	4	3	2	1	N/A
9. Ease of getting a referral when you needed one	5	4	3	2	1	N/A
B. OUR STAFF:						
1. The courtesy of the person who took your call	5	4	3	2	1	N/A
2. The friendliness and courtesy of the receptionist	5	4	3	2	1	N/A
3. The caring concern of our nurses/medical assistants	5	4	3	2	1	N/A
4. The helpfulness of the people who assisted you with billing or insurance	5	4	3	2	1	N/A
5. The professionalism of our lab or x-ray staff	5	4	3	2	1	N/A
C. OUR COMMUNICATION WITH YOU:						
1. Your phone calls answered promptly	5	4	3	2	1	N/A
2. Getting advice or help when needed during office hours	5	4	3	2	1	N/A
3. Explanation of your procedure (if applicable)	5	4	3	2	1	N/A
4. Your test results reported in a reasonable amount of time	5	4	3	2	1	N/A
5. Effectiveness of our health information materials	5	4	3	2	1	N/A
6. Our ability to return your calls in a timely manner	5	4	3	2	1	N/A
7. Your ability to contact us after hours	5	4	3	2	1	N/A
8. Your ability to obtain prescription refills by phone	5	4	3	2	1	N/A

Client: 1234A   Provider: BQ   Site: AL   Specialty: S04

PLEASE COMPLETE THE OTHER SIDE ⟶

Figure 3-1

Example of a patient satisfaction survey. From MGMA AdminiServe Parner, Sullivan Luallin Healthcare Consulting. https://www.samhsa.gov/sites/default/files/programs_campaigns/samhsa_hrsa/patient-satisfaction-survey-sample.pdf

	Excellent	Very Good	Good	Fair	Poor	Does Not Apply
D. YOUR VISIT WITH THE PROVIDER: (Doctor, Physician Assistant, Nurse Practitioner)						
1. Willingness to listen carefully to you	5	4	3	2	1	N/A
2. Taking time to answer your questions	5	4	3	2	1	N/A
3. Amount of time spent with you	5	4	3	2	1	N/A
4. Explaining things in a way you could understand	5	4	3	2	1	N/A
5. Instructions regarding medication/follow-up care	5	4	3	2	1	N/A
6. The thoroughness of the examination	5	4	3	2	1	N/A
7. Advise given to you on ways to stay healthy	5	4	3	2	1	N/A
E. OUR FACILITY:						
1. Hours of operation convenient for you	5	4	3	2	1	N/A
2. Overall comfort	5	4	3	2	1	N/A
3. Adequate parking	5	4	3	2	1	N/A
4. Signage and directions easy to follow	5	4	3	2	1	N/A
F. YOUR OVERALL SATISFACTION WITH:						
1. Our practice	5	4	3	2	1	N/A
2. The quality of your medical care	5	4	3	2	1	N/A
3. Overall rating of care from your provider or nurse	5	4	3	2	1	N/A

WOULD YOUR RECOMMEND THE PROVIDER TO OTHERS?   Yes   1   No   2

IF NO, PLEASE TELL US WHY: _____

_____

IF THERE IS ANY OTHER WAY WE CAN IMPROVE OUR SERVICES TO YOU, PLEASE TELL US ABOUT IT: _____

_____

_____

SOME INFORMATION ABOUT YOU:

GENDER		**YOUR AGE**		**ARE YOU:**	
Male	1	Under 18	1	A new patient	1
Female	2	18-30	2	A returning patient	2
		31-40	3		
		41-50	4		
		51-60	5		
		Over 60	6		

Thanks very much for your help!

| **Figure 3-1** (*Continued*)

result must provide an organized solution that ensures the correct patient is scheduled for the correct exam at the correct time.[10,15] Technology used for the purpose of improving patient workflow must include the participation and input of the staff and physicians to ensure a successful outcome.[10]

Scheduling and Registration: Direct Patient Contact

The requirements of patient privacy due to the HIPAA regulations are common practices considered by facilities in today's health care environment. Direct patient contact either face-to-face or by a phone call is conducted through facility practices that limit the opportunity of other customers to overhear conversations intended to be private. Customers scheduling a mammography examination or checking in for a scheduled appointment expect privacy, professionalism, and efficiency when interacting with the health care staff in the reception area or on the phone.

Scheduling: Face-to-Face or Phone Call

Scheduling the mammography appointment requires the reception personnel to gather detailed information from the patient that ensures accuracy in selecting the correct patient for the correct mammography procedure. Friendly frontline staff who are aware of privacy concerns and considerate of the sensitive nature of the information being collected provide the patient with a positive experience. An example of the information necessary to schedule the mammography appointment includes:

- Name, address, and phone number
- Date of birth
- Name of the referring physician
- Previous breast health history (surgeries or diagnosis)
- Current breast health problems if applicable
- Whether or not the patient has breast implants
- Location of previous mammography studies (including ultrasound, MRI, other pertinent breast imaging studies if applicable)
- Date of her most recent mammography examination
- The patient's medical insurance information

Some of these questions may require the patient to divulge information to the receptionist that is uncomfortable or disconcerting to report. Additional information to discern whether the patient should be scheduled for a screening or a diagnostic examination may require the patient to answer questions that pertain to symptoms describing nipple discharge or the presence of breast lumps. Protocols developed by the facility to reduce patient discomfort, such as succinct written questionnaires capturing the patient's reasons for the appointment, do so limiting the need for a verbal answer for others to hear.

Determining the type of procedure the patient should be scheduled for is significant for two reasons:

- To ensure that the patient receives appropriate health care.
- Incorrectly scheduled procedures disrupt predicted scheduled workflows, affecting the service of other customers.

The symptomatic patient may conceal the fact that she has found a lump in her breast. She may think that if a lump exists, it will be revealed on the mammogram image. Because the overall sensitivity of mammography is approximately 84%, some breast cancers may not be detected by mammography; however, due to her symptoms, additional procedures such as ultrasound may be indicated. Any lump or other symptoms identified by the patient or her physician should be specifically addressed. Understanding the potential vulnerability of the patient, whether scheduling a mammography examination or arriving to have the procedure performed, requires the personnel assisting her to convey a courteous and patient demeanor.

Arrivals and Registration

The initial encounter between the patient and the health care staff throughout the check-in process is an important factor in the overall satisfaction of the patient experience. Patient satisfaction surveys for the mammography procedure include specific components of the registration process[3]:

- Efficiency and speed of the process
- Courtesy and helpfulness of the registration staff
- Cleanliness and comfort of waiting area
- Ease of facility navigation

The reception area represents the beginning of an experience in which the patient's feelings and privacy are respected, thereby contributing to her trust in the facility. To ensure that the patient experience begins with a good first impression, some health care organizations may provide a concierge service to greet the patient at the entrance of the facility and assist them through the check-in process. The concierge service offers many conveniences for customers who may need to have their car parked, require wheelchair transport, are unsure of how to find their provider's office, or simply just need to be greeted by a friendly smile.

THE EXAMINATION ENVIRONMENT

When a woman arrives for her first mammogram, she does not know what to expect. She may envision the mammography setting as similar to the traditional radiographic examinations that she has previously experienced: a cold, sterile room with a large intimidating machine, where she is left alone and exposed to radiation while the technologist retreats behind a lead wall. These thoughts alone may cause anxiety. Creating a comfortable and relaxed environment in both waiting and examination rooms can help to alleviate feelings of anxiety and embarrassment that are associated with mammography[10] (Figure 3-2). Room temperature, comfortable furniture, muted or soft colors, and soothing artwork all contribute to a more comforting, rather than clinical, setting. Soft lighting from table lamps, or recessed lighting, creates a more calming effect than harsh overhead fluorescent fixtures. Decaffeinated warm beverages and comfortable robes ward off chills and feelings of insecurity and immodesty and are extra personal touches that women appreciate. Modern breast imaging centers are designed with waiting areas resembling a cozier, home-like setting, while others create more of a spa-like atmosphere[9,16] complete with massage areas. Many have fresh flower arrangements, and some give patients a small memento to take home at the end of their appointment. These touches can make the environment feel more casual, soothing, and personable. Most women are more comfortable if they wait in an area separate from patients who are having other types of examinations; however, space constraints within a facility can make this expectation difficult to achieve. Patient-centered care encourages privacy throughout the examination process.[3] If patients wait in a general area after changing into their examination gowns, modesty is a concern. Thick gowns or capes in both small and large sizes that provide full coverage for all women are an important consideration.

The seating arrangement in the waiting room can also affect the comfort level and privacy consideration of the patient.[3,9] For this personal examination, many women feel more at ease if they have a sense of semi-seclusion, or "personal space." Style of the furniture, placement of leafy plants, and smaller seating groups within the room can help achieve this feeling. A fish tank can be soothing to patients and separates the room into smaller, more private seating arrangements. If a patient must breastfeed a child before her examination, a private, comfortable area should be available.

As important as these amenities are in ensuring that the patient is relaxed and comfortable throughout the mammography experience, there are other expectations that concern the patient when in a health care environment. Cleanliness was most often mentioned during focus groups conducted by the Picker Institute, with patients considering this aspect of health care to be a major failure if neglected.[3,17] Meeting patient expectations also may contribute to the satisfaction they feel about the physical environment of their health care facility. Patients expect the facility they select to use up-to-date equipment for mammography services capable of delivering the latest technology.[10,18] Patients also have expectations of the facility personnel that care for them throughout their mammography examination.

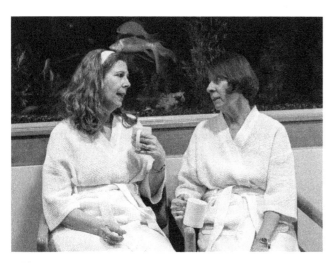

Figure 3-2
Creating a comfortable and relaxed environment in both waiting and examination rooms helps to alleviate feelings of anxiety and embarrassment associated with mammography.

INTERPERSONAL SKILLS: TECHNOLOGIST COMMUNICATION AND PATIENT INTERACTION

Although cleanliness and comfort are essential to the patient experience in a health care setting, other factors used to describe patient satisfaction include the overall quality of efficiency, punctuality, and flexibility experienced during the mammography visit.[10,18] The empathy, **interpersonal skills**, and professionalism of mammography personnel is factored into the perception of quality[10,18] the patient feels she has received during this highly personal and likely uncomfortable procedure. A formidable challenge for the mammography professional is balancing the restricted time that is allotted to deliver the mammography procedure with the requirements of high image quality standards.[19] These demands are discussed further in Chapter 15. Acknowledging this balance requires the mammography professional to strengthen communication and interpersonal skills that effectively convey understanding of the patient's emotional and physical needs. A study conducted at the University of Johannesburg, South Africa, observed personality traits of the mammography technologist and how these traits influence the perception of care the patient receives, providing insight into the significance of the patient–technologist interaction.[20] Based on this study, patients rated the approachable nature of the technologist, along with her honesty and gentleness, to be among the most important of personality traits. Table 3-1 describes the importance or unimportance of personality traits in mammography technologists that were rated by patients. These traits contribute to how the technologist is perceived by the patient in terms of[20]:

- Feeling safe
- Feeling trust
- Concern or interest (care) conveyed
- The communication skills of the technologist

Although the mammography appointment is complex in the variables that contribute to its success, a short amount of time may be allotted for its delivery. This requires that the technologist understand that the need for effective communication, both verbal and nonverbal, begins immediately upon greeting the patient. Assessment of the patient's physical and intellectual abilities is important as these qualities affect both the medical intake (history) component of the examination as well as the patient's ability to cooperate with the positioning/compression demands of the procedure. Facility workflow determines the amount of time the technologist spends with the patient prior to beginning the mammography procedure. Generally, the technologist greets and verifies the patient, communicating with her as they make their way to the changing area. This interval is an important factor in the examination process and should be used by the technologist to encourage feelings of trust and safety in the patient through a calm and reassuring demeanor. Within just a few minutes from this point, the examination will require the technologist to gather sensitive information from the patient while also ensuring that the patient is sufficiently relaxed for the purpose of obtaining superior quality images. During the imaging process, the technologist steps into the personal physical space of the patient; both verbal and nonverbal communication by the technologist is necessary to convey a sense of dignity and respect to the patient. A helpful tool developed by the Studer Group assists health care professionals in effective communication. The AIDET method provides the technologist with a communication strategy throughout the examination process, ensuring that essential communication skills are easily

Table 3-1 • Survey Results Indicating the Importance or Unimportance of Personality Traits of the Mammography Technologist

NUMBER	IMPORTANT TRAITS	%	UNIMPORTANT TRAITS	%
1	Approachable	97.5	Quiet	64.2
2	Honest	96.7	Inquisitive	56.5
3	Gentle	96.7	Talkative	47.3
4	Informative	96.6	Serious	39.1
5	Patient	96.6	Light-hearted	32.4
6	Friendly	95.5	—	—
7	Considerate	95.4	—	—
8	Dedicated	94.4	—	—
9	Attentive	93.9	—	—
10	Observant	93.5	—	—
11	Calm	93.1	—	—
12	Supportive	92.4	—	—
13	Positive (attitude)	92.3	—	—
14	Courteous	92.3	—	—
15	Reassuring	92.1	—	—
16	Sincere	90.9	—	—
17	Tolerant	90.2	—	—
18	Empathetic	88.7	—	—
19	Mature	80.2	—	—

Source: Louw, A., Lawrence, H. & Motto, J., 2014, 'Mammographer personality traits – elements of the optimal mammogram experience', Health SA Gesondheid 19(1), Art. #803, 7 pages. http://dx.doi.org/10.4102/hsag.v19i1.803

remembered. The acronym describes five foundations of effective communication[8,21]:

* Acknowledge
* Introduce
* Duration
* Explanation
* Thank you

Perhaps the most effective and immediate remedy for patient anxiety or apprehension is in the acknowledgment and introduction when greeting the patient. Feelings that result in shoulders tight with nervous tension and facial expressions of concern can be disarmed with reassuring actions by the technologist. Greeting the patient by name, introducing yourself, making eye contact and smiling are outward indications for the patient that you are approachable. Continued light conversation in a calm and unhurried manner provides added reassurance and distraction to the patient when in the vicinity of others, while ensuring the purpose of her visit to the facility remains protected until in a private setting.

Workflows differ from one facility to another. The designated room to acquire the patient's health history may not be the mammography procedure room. When the patient is settled and comfortable for the purpose of collecting the health history information (discussed in Chapter 4), provide her with an overview of the examination process and the estimated time it will take to complete her procedure. An explanation of the examination should take place in the mammography room so that the patient may view the equipment as the procedure is explained to her. Finally, inform the patient of the reporting process, ensuring that she understands how and when she will receive her examination result. Give her the opportunity to ask any questions she may have before sincerely thanking her for choosing your facility for her health care.

PATIENT PREPARATION FOR THE EXAMINATION

Patient-centered care provides a model of health care that considers and respects the values, needs, and preferences of the patient.[3,22] With this principle in mind, before the patient ever arrives for a mammography appointment, a discussion surrounding the benefits, harms, and risks of the examination has more than likely occurred between the patient and her health care provider. An important factor in patient-centered care is effective patient–provider communication and **shared decision-making**.[22] Shared decision-making involves communication between the patient and the provider that serves to inform the provider of the

patient's needs and preferences while informing the patient of the knowledge and experience of the provider in making medical decisions such as beginning medication, having a cancer screening examination, or elective surgery.[23] Additional educational tools used by providers to assist the patient in making medical decisions are called **decision aids**. Patients may be given booklets to read after visiting their health care provider's office or may be directed to their health care organization's Web site where they may find online resources explaining detailed information about the procedure or treatment being considered. Electronic information about tests or procedures may also be sent directly to the patient via their online chart portal from their provider. Sophisticated decision aids may be interactive, allowing the patient to have all of the pertinent information concerning a medical procedure at their fingertips. The Radiological Society of North America (RSNA) and the American College of Radiology (ACR) have developed an information Web site, RadiologyInfo (http://radiologyinfo.org), available to the public, radiology practices, and medical providers (Figure 3-3). The Web site may be viewed in both English and Spanish, offering explanations and photos of 200 radiologic procedures. The patient interested in learning more about having a mammogram is offered the following information when choosing to review this procedure:

* What is mammography?
* What are some common uses of the procedure?
* How should I prepare?
* What does the equipment look like?
* How does the procedure work?
* How is the procedure performed?
* What will I experience during and after the procedure?
* Who interprets the results and how do I get them?
* What are the benefits versus risks?
* What are the limitations of mammography?

Many of the questions included in educational material for the patient are discussed with their provider prior to making the procedure appointment. When the patient makes the decision to have the mammography procedure, health care facilities know that patients who are prepared for the examination and know what to expect experience less anxiety about the procedure.[24] A study published online in the Journal of the American College of Radiology, October 2015, describes the effects of providing a 1-hour educational session about the mammography examination by a specially trained radiologist to various community groups. Surveys were completed by the attendees prior to listening to the educational session and again after the session. Before listening to the presentation, complete with questions and

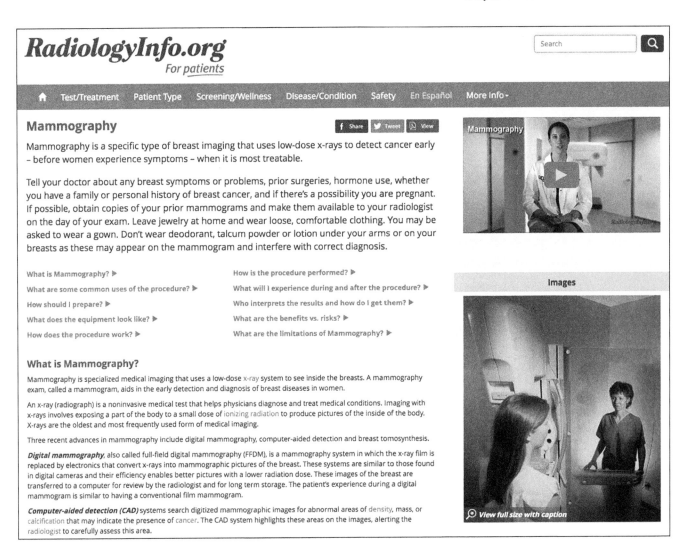

Figure 3-3
The introductory page of the Mammography Examination information developed by the American College of Radiology (ACR) and the Radiological Society of North America, Inc. (RSNA). Source: https://www.radiologyinfo.org/en/info.cfm?pg=mammo

answers, the attendees listed concerns that included the uncertainty about the procedure and whether or not it would be painful. After the informative session, the attendees were questioned about other factors, such as the need for breast cancer screening and anxiety. Researchers found that people who attended the presentation better understood why mammography was useful, suffered less anxiety concerning the procedure, and would more likely utilize mammography.[24] To ensure that patients are prepared for the examination, health care facilities at a minimum offer educational material on how to prepare for the mammography procedure (online and in paper form) and what to expect during their visit. This is reinforced by the mammography technologist or other health care staff throughout the patient experience. A variety of useful information is offered to patients depending on the facility they choose. Box 3-1A and B provides the

information included on the American Cancer Society Web site (cancer.org) under "How to prepare for your mammogram" and "Tips for getting a mammogram."[25]

A Word About Deodorants, Antiperspirants, Powders, Creams, and Lotions

Mammography technologists working in the field may notice that some facilities are more vigilant than others in ensuring the removal of deodorant or antiperspirant products. Figure 3-4A and B illustrates several varieties of deodorants and antiperspirants with a resulting digital radiographic image of the products. The image demonstrates that deodorants typically do not contain minerals that cause mammographic artifacts, while antiperspirants may or may not cause mammographic artifacts depending on the brand and how liberally it is applied. Antiperspirants and powders are usually seen on an image within skin folds or creases, where perspiration has caused them to become caked. These artifacts can usually be differentiated from calcifications that typify carcinoma. Caked talcum powder is usually seen as a line that runs in a lateral-to-medial direction, along the inframammary fold (Figure 3-5A, B) while cancer calcifications will orient in a linear ductal pattern toward the nipple. Caked antiperspirant will usually be found in the area of the axilla (Figure 3-5C, D). Occasionally, ointments or powders can also collect in the creases of a nevus or mole or in the nipple region. Unfortunately, the potential exists for any of these products to cause an artifact that may mimic microcalcifications or diminish tissue clarity, possibly resulting in a repeat exposure to the patient as well as adding time to the examination to ensure thorough cleansing of the axilla. Instructions addressing the preparation for mammography typically include the direction to abstain from using these types of products prior to the mammography procedure due to the potential of artifacts. It is common practice for mammography technologists to inquire about the patient's use of powders, deodorants, and lotions prior to the procedure. Single-use cleansing towelettes designed for the purpose of removing these types of products are made available in changing rooms when patients have not been informed or have forgotten this request. Providing amenities such as deodorant towelettes at the conclusion of their procedure is a courtesy gesture appreciated by the patient.

Case Study 3-1

1. Refer to Figure 3-4. Deodorant does not leave an artifact on the mammogram image; however, what other hygiene product may create an artifact? Depending on the formulation of this other product, an artifact may/may not be visible.

▌▌ PATIENT CONCERNS ABOUT DOSE

Some of the fears associated with the mammography procedure include (a) that cancer could be detected, (b) that the examination may be painful, and (c) that the exposure to radiation may cause cancer. The media hype of the 1970s that suggested mammography was dangerous remains a concern for some women in the general public, particularly older women. Fortunately, technological advances within the last few decades have shown that the benefits associated with mammography outweigh the potential harms. Today, patients are assured that

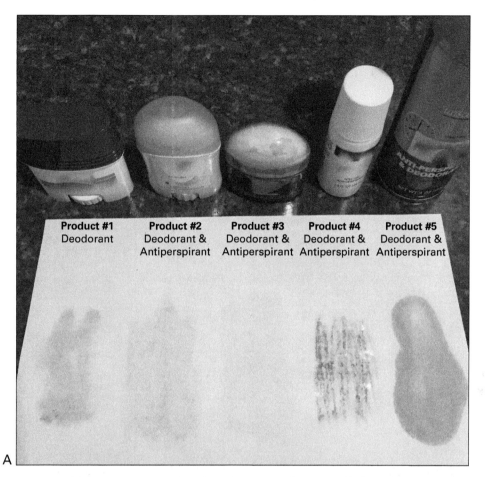

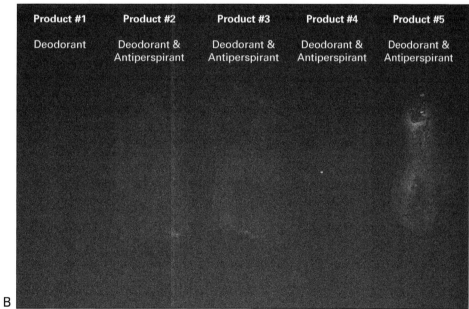

Figure 3-4
Several varieties of deodorants and antiperspirants **(A)**, illustrating resulting digital radiographic image of the products **(B)**.

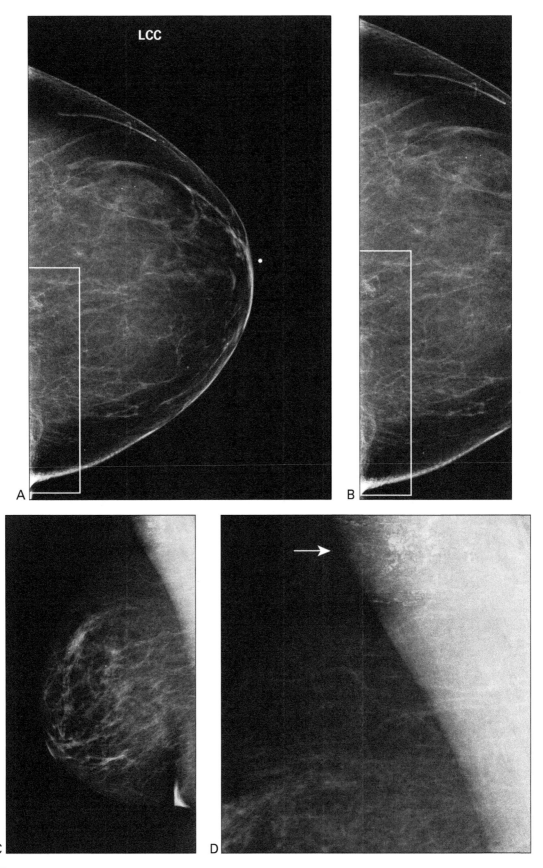

Figure 3-5
(**A** and **B**) Caked talcum powder is usually seen as a line that runs in a lateral-to-medial direction, along the inframammary fold (**A**), same radiograph enlarged to better appreciate the effect of talcum powder artifact (**B**). (**C** and **D**) Radiograph demonstrating caked antiperspirant usually found in the axillary area (**C**), same radiograph enlarged to appreciate antiperspirant artifact (**D**).

the amount of radiation involved in a mammography procedure is safe. According to the MQSA Final Rule, *"the average glandular dose delivered during a single craniocaudal view of an FDA-accepted phantom simulating a standard breast shall not exceed 3.0 milligray (mGy) (0.3 rad) per exposure. The dose shall be determined with technique factors and conditions used clinically for a standard breast."*[26]

Compared with the 8 to 12 rad measurement of exposure the patient received in the early 1970s, radiation dosage to the breast tissue has been reduced substantially throughout the decades.[27] The American Cancer Society reports that the average dose received for a mammography study that includes 2 views of each breast is approximately 0.4 mSv.[25] The International System of Units describes a Sv (Sievert) as a measurement of radiation, with the prefix "m" indicating "milli." Although these statistics are significant, to most patients, they would have little meaning. In order to put this dose into perspective for women who are concerned about radiation exposure, the exposure received from background radiation (radiation exposure to natural surroundings) to people in the United States each year is an average of approximately 3 mSv. This dose equals about the same dose that a person receives from her natural surroundings in a 7-week period.[25,28,29] As with any radiographic examination, unnecessary exposure to radiation should be avoided.

A Word about Thyroid Shielding

Until September, 2010, the subject of shielding a patient's thyroid during a mammography procedure would not have been included in a mammography textbook. Today, technologists should be aware of the ACR and Society of Breast Imaging (SBI) position regarding thyroid shielding for mammography: thyroid shielding is not necessary and its use is not recommended. The question of taking this precaution during mammography originated with a segment on a popular medical advice television show. During a segment discussing the possible reasons for an increase in thyroid cancer in women, the show's host discussed a study involving dental x-rays but further explained that the potential radiation exposure resulting from dental x-rays and mammography may have played a part in the increase. In speaking with the audience, the host expressed the wisdom in asking for a thyroid shield during the mammography procedure. This incident, assisted by social media, sparked an interest in patient's requesting thyroid shields for mammography across the nation.[30] In an effort to resolve this issue, the ACR and the SBI published a statement that addressed the safety of the mammography examination in regard to radiation exposure and to explain the potential that image quality could suffer needlessly through the practice of thyroid shielding. Mammography technologists should be aware of the recommendations made by the ACR and SBI in order to better serve the patient through education (Box 3-2). Technologists new to the field of mammography may wish to proactively discuss the subject of thyroid shielding requests and facility protocols that address this subject with mammography leadership.

BOX 3-2

The ACR and Society of Breast Imaging Statement on Radiation Received by the Thyroid from Mammography

Concern that the small amount of radiation a patient receives from a mammogram may significantly increase the likelihood of developing thyroid cancer simply is not supported in scientific literature.

The radiation dose to the thyroid from a mammogram is extremely low. The thyroid is not exposed to the direct x-ray beam used to image the breast and receives only a tiny amount of scattered x-rays (less than 0.005 mGy). This is equivalent to only 30 minutes of natural background radiation received by all Americans from natural sources.

For annual screening mammography from ages 40 to 80, the cancer risk from this tiny amount of radiation scattered to the thyroid is incredibly small (less than 1 in 17.1 million women screened). This minute risk should be balanced with the fact that thyroid shield usage could interfere with optimal positioning and could result in artifacts—shadows that might appear on the mammography image. Both of these factors could reduce the quality of the image and interfere with diagnosis.

Therefore, use of a thyroid shield during mammography is not recommended. Patients are urged not to put off or forego necessary breast imaging care.

For more information on this issue, please see Summary of Thyroid Cancer Risks Due to Mammography by R. Edward Hendrick, PhD, FACR.

For more information on why you should start annual mammograms at 40 years of age, please visit www. MammographySavesLives.org.

Source: Mammography Saves Lives: Home (http://www.mammography saveslives.org)

THE PREGNANT OR LACTATING PATIENT

Pregnant or lactating patients who present with a palpable mass are promptly evaluated using appropriate imaging modalities and necessary image-guided procedures supervised by a radiologist in an effort to provide a timely diagnosis. Depending on the individual needs of the pregnant patient, the radiologist may use ultrasound or ultrasound with mammography to provide a diagnosis. Depending on the individual needs of the lactating patient, the radiologist may use ultrasound, ultrasound with mammography, and possibly MRI to provide a diagnosis. When mammography is used to evaluate the lactating patient, the patient is asked to empty the breasts of any milk immediately before the procedure through nursing or pumping the breasts. Doing this helps to reduce the density associated with lactation as much as possible.[28] The care of a pregnant or lactating patient with a palpable mass commonly is initiated through provider to radiologist communication prior to the patient reporting to the mammography department.

MAMMOGRAPHY PATIENT ACCESS

In the late 1970s, the American Cancer Society (ACS) established the first breast cancer screening guidelines for the use of mammography.

Earlier research demonstrated that through adherence to regular screening mammography, the risk of dying from breast cancer was significantly reduced.[31] By 1983, ACS updated guidelines addressed using mammography to screen for breast cancer between the ages of 35-39 with a baseline mammogram; 40-49, every 1-2 years; and every year beginning at age 50. These guidelines would remain in effect for the next 14 years.[25] In spite of the published guidelines during these early years, data gathered in 1987 demonstrate that only about 25% of women age 50 and older received mammograms regularly, while poor and nonwhite women were less likely to be screened.[31,32] Efforts to initiate public education programs that partnered with communities for the purpose of increasing screening and awareness for women's health began. One such program was the Rhode Island Breast Cancer Project. The Rhode Island Department of Health partnered with communities to develop a program that successfully increased screening capacity and accessibility, educated the public concerning the need for screening, and reduced the false-positive/false-negative test results.[31] The Rhode Island project was successful in providing women with low-cost screening mammography. Other states implementing women's health initiatives included Colorado, Oklahoma, Maine, Washington, California, and the Navajo Nation. The states' women's health initiatives coincided with action from the Center for Disease Control and Prevention (CDC) in conducting research to understand the cause of various cancers. Several more projects would be funded by the CDC during the 1980s that served to provide the foundation for today's national cervical and breast cancer program. Successful progress made by the CDC-funded programs, along with support from state agencies and other influential organizations, paved the way for the Breast and Cervical Cancer Mortality Prevention Act that was signed into law on August 10, 1990.[31,33] The detail contained in this initiative that ensures underserved women receive appropriate health care services to detect breast and cervical cancer cannot be adequately explained in this chapter; however, a brief summary follows. The individuals, government offices, and organizations that shaped what is now the National Breast and Cervical Cancer Early Detection Program (NBCCEDP), funded by the CDC, sponsor programs in every state and territory in the United States, impacting thousands of lives. Although the CDC defines the eligibility and policies for the program, some flexibility is granted to each state. Federal guidelines direct services to uninsured or underinsured women at or below 250% of the federal poverty level. The services provided in each of the 50 states, the District of Columbia, 5 U.S. territories, and 11 American Indian/Alaska Native tribes or tribal organizations[34] funded by the NBCCEDP are allowed to determine the unique name of their program. The Wisconsin Well Woman Program portrays the intention of the NBCCEDP program funded by the CDC. Screening services are provided by a network of local hospitals and clinics. Covered screening services include a pelvic exam, Pap test, breast examination, and mammogram.[35] Diagnostic breast and cervical services may also be covered in some states.

This information is necessary knowledge for the technologist working in the field of breast imaging. Technologists may receive phone calls or inquiries from patients needing mammography services that they feel they cannot afford. Individual health care entities may also offer internal programs for patients that cannot afford to have a necessary medical procedure. Ensuring that frontline appointment and registration staff, along with all mammography personnel, are familiar with programs offering financial assistance to underserved patients is a responsibility that must be shared.

PATIENT COMMUNICATION BARRIERS

On any given day, mammography personnel care for patients arriving for the mammography examination with language barriers that may diminish their understanding and purpose of the procedure. Ensuring that "limited English proficiency" (LEP) patients are provided quality health care equal to that of English speaking patients is a serious obligation of the health care industry. This obligation requires that facilities comply with federal and individual state laws that ultimately protect its citizens from discriminatory practices. The authority of the 1964 Civil Rights Act provides the foundation in addressing language access to all patients receiving care. It is the responsibility of Health and Human Services (HHS) to ensure that federal dollars are not used to support discriminatory practices in health care settings through the oversight of the Office for Civil Rights. Health care facilities must also adhere to federal laws such as the Americans with Disabilities Act, and Health Insurance Portability and Accountability Act (HIPAA), as well as individual state laws when providing services for LEP patients.[36] Health care organizations have increasingly used language assistance services to address this obligation to LEP patients. Facilities may provide in-house medical language and medical sign language interpreters for patients to utilize during their health care appointments. When this solution is not practical, medical language interpreters are available by phone through companies specializing in this need. Recent technology available for patients who are deaf or hearing impaired is video remote interpreting (VRI). This technology uses video conferencing to provide a sign language interpreter to the patient and the technologist through the use of video conferencing equipment. Figure 3-6 shows that the sign language interpreter is connected remotely to the equipment in the mammography room and appears on a computer screen through webcam technology. The patient and the interpreter can communicate with each other using sign language as the interpreter relays the information to the technologist.

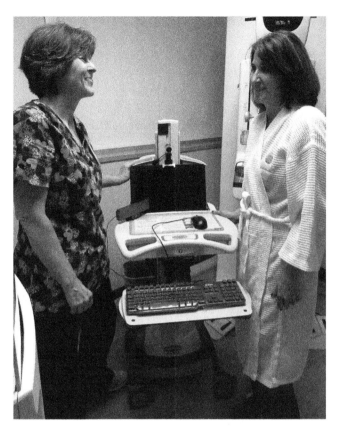

Figure 3-6
Video remote interpreting (VRI) technology available for patients who are deaf or hearing impaired. This technology uses video conferencing to provide a sign language interpreter to the patient and the technologist using video conferencing equipment.

PATIENT SUPPORT ORGANIZATIONS

Patients recently diagnosed with breast cancer or who have family members recently diagnosed are faced with an avalanche of emotions and unknowns. Fortunately, in many cases, health care facilities are prepared to help the patient as she navigates herself and her family through the maze of information she must familiarize herself with. Along with the services that the patient's health care system provides in answering questions the patient may have, support exists through a wide variety of services offered by many valuable organizations. Patients coping with breast cancer may need assistance to better understand the cancer diagnosis, various treatment options, sexuality, transportation for appointments, and financial concerns that impact their lives. Support blogs and legislative and public policy advocacy are also important components in offering support to patients diagnosed with breast cancer. The following organizations address these important aspects of patient support:

Case Study **3-2**

1. Refer to Figure 3-6. Discuss communication solutions for women who present with various disabilities, such as hearing or vision impairment and language barriers.

- American Cancer Society, www.cancer.org, 1(800) 227-2345
- Susan G. Komen, ww5.komen.org, 1-877, GO KOMEN 1(877) 465-6636
- National Cancer Institute, www.cancer.gov, 1(800) 4-CANCER
- Breastcancer.org, breastcancer.org, 120 East Lancaster Ave., Suite 201, Ardmore, PA
- National Breast Cancer Foundation, Inc., nationalbreast-cancer.org
- Look Good...Feel Better, lookgoodfeelbetter.org, 800-395-LOOK
- Mammography Saves Lives (Society of Breast Imaging), mammographysaveslives.org, 1(703)715-4390, e-mail: info@SBI.online.org
- National Breast Cancer Coalition (NBCC), breastcancerdeadline2020.org, info@breastcancerdeadline2020.org, 800-622-2838 or 202-296-7477
- National Alliance of Breast Cancer Organizations (NABCO), www.nabco.org, 888-80-NABCO, 212-719-0154
- Cancer Care, Inc., cancercare.org, 800-813-HOPE (4673)
- National Coalition of Cancer Survivorship (NCSS), www.canceradvocacy.org, (877) NCCS-YES, CancerbreastBreastcancer.org, 120 East Lancaster Avenue, Suite 201, Ardmore, PA 19003

▌ A WORD ABOUT THE MALE PATIENT

The American Cancer Society reports an estimate of 2,600 new cases of invasive breast cancer in men, with 440 male deaths from breast cancer in 2016. Other statistics relating to breast cancer in males include[25]:

- Breast cancer is about 100 times less common among men than among women
- A male's lifetime risk of developing breast cancer is about 1 in 1,000
- Breast cancer cases in men, relative to the ever-increasing population, have been fairly stable over the last 30 years.

Providing mammography services to males is not uncommon. Facilities and technologists should develop a workflow that considers the patient experience from the male's perspective when being cared for in an environment that usually accentuates female comfort. Many facilities are creative when addressing:

- Where the male patient may be comfortable waiting to have the examination
- Escorting the male patient back to an adjacent waiting area in close proximity to the mammography department

Male patients should be provided with the traditional professionalism the facility extends to any patient receiving mammography services. Due to the potential awkwardness or embarrassment the male patient may feel when requiring mammography, forethought of reducing these feeling should be considered by the facility.

▌ CHAPTER SUMMARY: A LETTER TO THE TECHNOLOGIST

Caring for the mammography patient in today's competitive health care setting requires the technologist to acquire strong interpersonal and communication skills (which includes the art of listening). Through verbal and body language expression to the patient, the technologist delivers care in a sensitive setting that is ultimately evaluated through the patient's perception. The satisfaction of the patient experience is impacted through two important factors: (a) facility practices and (b) the interaction of the patient and the technologist. A quality experience is more likely to be achieved when the technologist gives her full attention to the patient. Distraction is perceived by the patient when the technologist is multitasking while answering questions that the patient may have or when documenting patient health history. Time constraints imposed by the facility restricting adequate examination time impact not only the perception of the patient as being rushed through her appointment but also may impact resulting image quality. It is paramount in a successful mammography service to balance the intervals of the mammography schedule with the ability of the technologist to provide appropriate quality service to the patient. This subject is addressed further in Chapter 4. Chapter 3 focuses on the importance of the patient experience in today's health care market and factors that influence service delivery through the interpersonal skills of mammography personnel and the environmental setting of the facility. Although the measurement of this satisfaction is now a necessity in the health care service environment, consider this letter (modified only in the salutation and patient name) sent to a mammography facility in the 1980s describing the experience of the patient's mammography visit:

Dear Mammography Lead Technologist,

Yesterday, I had a baseline mammogram performed and I wanted to tell you that I was impressed with the technician. (She did introduce herself at the beginning of the appointment, but I am afraid I don't remember her name.)

I was nervous because I have heard a wide range of stories about the pain and discomfort other women have experienced. In fact, I had seriously considered canceling the appointment.

Some of the things that the technician did that impressed me were:

 1) She addressed me as Ms. Jones

 2) She thoroughly explained what was going to happen, when and why before beginning

 3) She talked to me throughout the entire procedure, not at me

 4) She stopped walking around the room and adjusting the machine, in the middle of the procedure, to look directly at me and answer a question

 5) She explained the follow-up, including her check for technical aspects, the radiologists actual review of the film, and that her department will notify me in about 2 weeks of the results (unless I hear from the physician)

 6) She discussed the possibility of being called back for a second or additional test, that I shouldn't assume something was wrong if I was called back and there would be an additional charge for a second test

The technician put me at ease with her high level of professionalism and competence. This is despite the fact that the appointment was at the end of the day and I wasn't shown to a changing room until 15-20 minutes after the scheduled appointment time. I believe the department was running late, but she didn't rush me and took the time to confirm that I understood what was happening. I left the clinic, later than I had anticipated, but glad that I had kept the appointment.

Please convey my appreciation for a job well done. Your mammography department should be proud of all employees who conduct themselves as she did.

The need to ensure basic human dignity does not change from decade to decade. Factors that influence patient experience expectations should be identified in each workflow unique to individual mammography services that include the balance of practical examination time intervals. Through this endeavor, authentic, genuine compassion, kindness, and skill expressed to every patient can be a realistic goal.

Review Questions

1. Patients may present for the mammography procedure nervous or anxious. What are some of the ways this is manifested in patients?

2. Explain the importance of the patient experience in health care and methods used to measure the process.

3. Explain what aspects of communication can be used to assist the patient in reducing the feeling of anxiety.

4. Discuss the technological advances in preparing the patient for the mammography examination, making appointments, and receiving reports.

5. What federal laws should be considered when caring for a patient with limited English proficiency?

References

1. HCAHPS Fact Sheet, June 2015. Baltimore, MD: Centers for Medicare and Medicaid Services (CMS). http://www.Hcahpsonline.org/Facts/aspx. Accessed January 18, 2017.
2. HCAHPS: patient's perspective of care survey. CMS.gov. Accessed January 18, 2017.
3. Itri JN. Patient-centered radiology. *Radiographics.* 2015; 35(6):1835–1846.
4. Beach MC, et al. The role and relationship of cultural competence and patient-centeredness in health care quality. The Commonwealth Fund; October 2006.
5. Gamble M. Developing a workforce strategy for patient-centered care: 6 key steps. *Beckers Hospital Review.* 2013. https://www.beckershospitalreview.com/hospital-management-administration/developing-a-workforce-strategy-for-patient-centered-care-6-key-steps.html. Accessed January 20, 2017.
6. *Minimizing Pain and Discomfort During Mammography (Dateline July 26, 2000).* Imaginis—The Women's Health and Wellness Resource Network; 2000. http://www.imaginis.com/breast-health-news/minimizing-pain-and-discomfort-during-mammography-dateline-july-26-2000. Accessed January, 2017.
7. Keller BR, Evans KD. Fighting anxiety in order to improve the quality of breast imaging for women. eRADIMAGING.com. Available at: https://eradimaging.com/site/article.cfm?ID=758#.WdvXA1tSzIU. Published December 15, 2010. Accessed January, 2017.
8. Arnold L. Patient care, communication, and safety in the mammography suite. *Radiol Technol.* 2016;88(1):33M–47M.
9. Randel S. Mammograms: reducing patient anxiety. *Radiol Technol.* 2016;87(6):707–709.
10. Johnson S, Johnson J. Managing a mammography center: a model to thrive. *Radiol Technol.* 2010;82(1):22–32.
11. Loeken K, et al. A new measure of patient satisfaction with mammography. Validation by factor analytic technique. *Fam Pract.* 1996;13:67–74.
12. Tang TS, et al. Women's mammography experience and its impact on screening adherence. *Psycho-Oncology.* 2009; 18(7):727–734.
13. United States Department of Health and Human Services (HHS.gov). Accessed January 18, 2017.
14. Manual vs. Automated Appointment Scheduling, Appointment-Plus, © Appointment-Plus, 2012.
15. Sharrock R. A well-appointed establishment. *Ind Eng.* 2007; 39(4):44–48.
16. Rimer BK, et al. Why women resist screening mammography: patient-related barriers. *Radiology.* 1989;172 (1):243–246.
17. Through the patient's eyes; understanding and promoting patient-centered care. In: Gerteis M, et al., eds. *Picker/Commonwealth Program for Patient-Centered Care.* San Francisco, CA: Jossey-Bass, 1993.
18. Hamilton EL, Barlow J. Women's views of a breast screening service. *Health Care Women Int.* 2003;24(1):40–48.
19. Morris N. When health means suffering: mammograms, pain and compassionate care. *Eur J Cancer Care.* 2015;24:483–492.
20. Louw A, et al. Mammographer personality traits—elements of the optimal mammogram experience, *Health SA Gesondheid.* 2014;19(1), Art. #803, 7 pages, http://dx.doi.org/10.4102/hsag.v19i1.803 © The Authors, 2014.
21. Rubin R. AIDET® in the Medical Practice: More Important than Ever. The Studer Group; 2014. A Huron Solution http://www.studergroup.com. Accessed January 18, 2017.
22. Institute of Medicine. Chapter 3. Patient-centered communication and shared decision making. In: *Delivering High-Quality Cancer Care: Charting a New Course for a System in Crisis.* Washington, DC: The National Academies Press; 2013. By the National Academy of Sciences. All rights reserved. For more information, see the Bookshelf Copyright Notice.
23. The Common Wealth Fund. Helping patients make better treatment choices with decision aids. *Quality Matters Archive*; 2012.
24. *Information Eases Anxiety About Screening Mammograms.* Breast Cancer.org. Published on November 16, 2015.
25. American Cancer Society Website/Cancer.org. Accessed January 17, 2017.
26. Fda.gov. Mammography Quality Standards Act/Guidance/Policy Guidance Help System (PGHS). Accessed January 18, 2017.
27. Andolina VF, Lille SL. *Mammographic Imaging: A Practical Guide.* 3rd ed. Philadelphia, PA: Wolters Kluwer/Lippincott Williams & Wilkins; 2011.
28. Vashi R. Breast imaging of the pregnant and lactating patient: imaging modalities and pregnancy-associated breast cancer. *AJR Am J Roentgenol.* 2013;200(2):321–328. Read more at http://www.ajronline.org/doi/full/10.2214/AJR.12.9814.
29. RadiologyInfo.org website. Patient safety: radiation exposure in X-ray and CT exams; 2012. Available at: www.radiologyinfo.org/en/safety/index.cfm?pg=sfty_xray. Accessed January 18, 2017.
30. Hardy K. Dr. Oz, Thyroid Shields & Mammography—the popular TV host sparks a debate with radiology. *Radiol Today.* 2011;12(6):18.
31. Lee NC, et al. Implementation of the National Breast and Cervical Cancer Early Detection Program: the beginning. *Cancer.* 2014;120(Suppl 16):2540–2548.
32. Centers for Disease Control and Prevention. *Health, United States, 2009: With Special Feature on Medical Technology.* Hyattsville, MD: Centers for Disease Control and Prevention, US Department of Health and Human Services; 2010.
33. Breast and Cervical Cancer Mortality Prevention Act of 1990. Pub L No. 301-354. [Accessed May 31, 2012]; Available at: http://www.cdc.gov/cancer/nbccedp/legislation/law.htm.
34. Centers for Disease Control and Prevention (CDC). Cancer screening—United States, 2010. *MMWR Morb Mortal Wkly Rep.* 2012;61(3):41–45.
35. Wisconsin Department of Health Services. Wisconsin Well Women's Program. dhs.wisconsin.gov. Accessed January 21, 2017.
36. Chen AH, et al. The legal framework for language access in healthcare settings: title VI and beyond. *J Gen Intern Med.* 2007;22(Suppl 2):362–367. Published online October 24, 2007. doi: 10.1007/s11606-007-0366-2.

The Role of the Technologist

4

Objectives

- To acknowledge the technologist's role in breast imaging
- To recognize the technologist's role in the health care team
- To understand the skills necessary to successfully perform the mammography procedure

---

Key Terms

- actual quality
- diagnostic mammogram
- exam management
- expected quality

- perceived quality
- risk factors
- screening mammogram
- soft skills

INTRODUCTION

Over the past several decades, the goal to detect breast cancer in its early stages has been assisted by the evolution of premium breast imaging options. For the majority of cases that require ancillary breast imaging modalities (discussed in Chapters 20 and 21), the process begins with the screening or diagnostic mammography examination. MQSA national statistics report 39,302,089 annual mammography procedures performed as of February 1, 2017 in the United States[1] (Table 4-1). Many of these mammography procedures were performed by the 49,426 ARRT-registered radiologic technologists who also acquired postprimary ARRT mammography certification[2] (Table 4-2).

In addition to these credentials, technologists performing mammography in the United States must adhere to strict Federal requirements of the MQSA, as well as State laws that govern the profession of radiologic technologists. Fulfilling these requirements prepares the technologist contemplating a future in breast imaging to understand the technical demands of mammography, as well as the emotional demands of serving a patient population often requiring expressions of genuine empathy and compassion. Needless to say, the challenge to accomplish the arduous task of preparing to join the mammography profession calls to those who do so because they are *motivated* to make a difference in the lives of the patient's who they serve.

The authors agree that the foundation of quality mammography rests on the technologist's ability to demonstrate empathy to the patient and to recognize the correlation of detecting early breast cancer through superior quality imaging. The mammography patient experience and image quality formula is seldom successful when a technologist is required to perform mammography when there is no interest in or desire to work in this discipline.

This chapter takes a closer look at the critical role of the mammography technologist in the breast health care service as she endeavors to meet professional expectations that include her responsibility to the patient and to other members of the patient's breast health care team.

THE TECHNOLOGIST ROLE IN THE BREAST HEALTH CARE TEAM

The mammography technologist is among the team of health care professionals who are responsible for providing breast health services to the patient. In many cases, outside

Table 4-1 • MQSA National Statistics

Certified facilities, as of October 1, 2016	8,741
Certification statistics, as of July 1, 2017	
Total certified facilities/total accredited units	8,730/17,656
Certified facilities with FFDM units/accredited FFDM units	8,605/12,739
Certified facilities with DBT[a] units/accredited DBT units	3,443/4,762
FY2017 inspection statistics, as of July 1, 2017	
Facilities inspected	5,925
Total units at inspected facilities	11,505
Percent of inspections where the highest noncompliance was a:	
Level 1 violation	0.8%
Level 2 violation[b]	10.7%
Certified facilities, as of October 1, 2016	8,741
Certification statistics, as of July 1, 2017	
Total certified facilities/total accredited units	8,730/17,656
Certified facilities with FFDM units/accredited FFDM units	8,605/12,739
Certified facilities with DBT[a] units/accredited DBT units	3,443 / 4,762
FY2017 inspection statistics, as of July 1, 2017	
Facilities inspected	5,925
Total units at inspected facilities	11,505
Percent of inspections where the highest noncompliance was a:	
Level 1 violation	0.8%
Level 2 violation[b]	10.7%
Level 3 violation	0.3%
Percent of inspections with no violation	88.3%
Total annual mammography procedures reported, as of July 1, 2017[c]	39,279,737

In this section of MQSA Insights, we present the most commonly requested national statistics regarding the MQSA program. These statistics are updated on the first of each month.

[a]Facilities with DBT also have FFDM, so the DBT facilities count is included within the FFDM facilities count.

[b]Based on an analysis of the violation rates for all MQSA citations, the FDA has decided to elevate the five remaining level 3 citations to level 2 citations. This change took effect on October 27, 2016. Since all level 3 citations, if repeated, could have been elevated to a level 2 with a requirement of a 30-day response to FDA, they should not be viewed as minor in nature, and they should be initially cited as a level 2. As a consequence, the level 3 violation rates will approach zero, and the level 2 violation rates may initially increase but should level off with time.

[c]This number is an aggregate of the total number of procedures performed annually as reported by facilities to their accreditation bodies at the time of their re-accreditation, which takes place once every 3 years. We have aggregated only the numbers reported by MQSA-certified, non-Veterans Hospital Administration facilities. The aggregate number may not reflect the current number of procedures performed at these facilities.

FFDM, full-field digital mammography unit; DBT, digital breast tomosynthesis.

Source: MQSA National Statistics published July 1, 2017. The FDA website, fda.gov, publishes this information on the first of every month. From: http://www.fda.gov

of the patient's primary provider, the technologist may be the first breast health care professional the patient comes in contact with. The expertise provided by the technologist not only is relied upon by the patient but also extends to other members of the patient's breast health care team.

Table 4-2 • Certificate Census by Location and Discipline

STATE/COUNTRY	RAD	NMT	THR	MRI	SON	MAM	CT	QM	BD	CI	VI	CV	VS	BS	RA	CERTs	TECHs
Alabama	5,314	76	297	514	34	673	972	17	34	21	15	55	6	13	1	8,042	5,480
Alaska	651	23	42	89	3	131	161	10	12	0	0	4	0	0	0	1,126	685
Arizona	5,944	215	394	637	14	888	1,264	23	104	38	79	78	0	33	5	9,716	6,233
Arkansas	3,642	140	203	249	3	476	585	13	15	16	33	69	3	15	14	5,476	3,801
California	21,575	1,013	1,620	2,306	29	3,380	5,110	59	99	62	244	209	6	76	18	35,806	23,248
Colorado	5,200	161	313	628	11	866	1,407	21	122	11	127	77	5	56	10	9,015	5,400
Connecticut	3,800	149	247	509	16	941	807	35	66	8	28	56	1	17	10	6,690	4,140
Delaware	1,030	48	56	158	1	174	234	6	5	0	11	10	0	9	0	1,742	1,098
District of Columbia	146	4	25	19	0	19	27	1	1	1	1	2	0	0	2	248	168
Florida	21,269	1,295	1,675	2,928	260	3,022	4,844	94	255	24	353	230	35	37	27	36,348	23,489
Georgia	9,896	343	724	977	28	1,375	1,874	45	60	14	97	96	5	32	13	15,579	10,411
Hawaii	1,006	41	73	120	2	207	218	1	7	13	25	20	0	4	0	1,737	1,048
Idaho	1,747	58	103	203	5	292	450	5	22	8	16	13	1	2	1	2,926	1,780
Illinois	13,411	464	941	1,513	14	2,080	2,426	35	104	37	83	93	2	53	5	21,261	14,127
Indiana	7,816	182	576	757	25	1,086	1,485	21	54	14	40	62	3	40	13	12,174	8,293
Iowa	3,859	135	192	340	4	811	789	17	52	16	36	54	3	6	2	6,316	3,951
Kansas	3,361	112	191	342	1	680	724	15	33	2	38	34	0	5	5	5,543	3,432
Kentucky	6,243	89	290	617	5	821	1,398	26	47	49	76	76	3	33	8	9,781	6,355
Louisiana	5,677	283	287	381	8	681	762	12	21	22	22	45	11	2	4	8,218	5,772
Maine	1,660	52	95	164	2	309	353	8	38	2	14	34	0	1	0	2,732	1,743
Maryland	5,590	228	401	778	10	1,045	1,155	35	50	17	52	127	3	7	5	9,503	6,111
Massachusetts	6,379	359	519	923	6	1,227	1,339	33	53	13	42	104	1	25	9	11,032	7,205
Michigan	9,769	426	827	1,140	22	1,729	1,976	27	121	16	114	100	17	44	6	16,334	10,863
Minnesota	5,755	75	421	675	5	1,182	1,207	32	131	15	60	59	2	25	2	9,646	5,974
Mississippi	3,958	177	201	234	4	418	527	6	16	4	38	40	7	5	8	5,643	4,010
Missouri	6,595	166	387	669	49	970	1,291	32	77	22	72	85	5	16	8	10,444	6,734
Montana	1,244	27	70	121	2	244	264	7	9	2	3	15	0	0	3	2,011	1,273
Nebraska	2,463	79	151	305	1	489	632	13	32	3	32	26	0	5	1	4,232	2,517
Nevada	2,101	131	165	258	4	318	457	11	10	6	45	19	1	0	2	3,528	2,279
New Hampshire	1,526	44	116	205	3	269	360	6	18	2	9	24	2	8	0	2,592	1,659
New Jersey	8,173	620	708	1,186	36	1,744	1,654	74	137	8	42	87	0	19	10	14,498	8,950
New Mexico	1,811	97	86	163	23	245	382	15	32	2	11	16	0	5	1	2,889	1,927
New York	14,934	862	1,249	1,919	8	2,991	3,387	73	204	26	91	99	5	30	22	25,900	16,882
North Carolina	10,986	432	751	1,296	49	1,682	2,432	68	152	48	135	183	12	33	23	18,282	11,565
North Dakota	997	7	59	79	1	186	168	10	8	5	14	16	0	0	3	1,553	1,006
Ohio	14,096	807	870	1,774	12	2,051	2,883	63	146	44	107	193	3	22	16	23,087	15,053
Oklahoma	3,886	138	309	330	5	535	819	14	16	15	17	46	1	18	10	6,159	4,177

(Continued)

Table 4-2 • Certificate Census by Location and Discipline (*Continued*)

STATE/COUNTRY	RAD	NMT	THR	MRI	SON	MAM	CT	QM	BD	CI	VI	CV	VS	BS	RA	CERTs	TECHs
Oregon	3,077	113	232	451	3	620	922	13	52	21	33	35	1	6	7	5,586	3,305
Pennsylvania	15,928	715	1,111	1,961	18	2,588	2,743	69	230	25	196	228	7	48	26	25,893	16,857
Rhode Island	1,214	56	59	203	3	287	249	6	7	0	10	13	0	0	3	2,110	1,276
South Carolina	5,328	234	291	545	21	787	1,096	15	34	5	42	65	11	24	5	8,503	5,608
South Dakota	1,166	26	83	79	3	245	261	6	17	0	10	18	0	5	0	1,919	1,196
Tennessee	8,009	269	490	729	13	1,011	1,528	16	93	11	67	78	2	33	12	12,361	8,237
Texas	22,795	885	1,425	2,465	199	3,048	5,491	99	152	43	156	185	32	80	18	37,073	24,381
Utah	2,616	127	174	341	0	329	533	3	14	4	33	10	0	4	4	4,192	2,691
Vermont	604	17	64	66	0	129	199	5	18	1	7	5	0	0	2	1,117	674
Virginia	8,023	219	578	768	53	1,251	1,462	40	92	16	130	129	3	39	13	12,816	8,436
Washington	5,747	126	491	723	8	1,010	1,513	17	56	15	73	85	0	12	12	9,888	6,161
West Virginia	2,761	93	127	227	4	375	381	14	19	13	24	36	0	7	3	4,084	2,803
Wisconsin	7,125	96	482	645	3	1,342	1,360	25	83	11	81	55	5	26	2	11,341	7,470
Wyoming	694	25	42	81	0	167	196	6	6	5	14	6	0	0	0	1,242	711
Subtotal	**308,597**	**12,559**	**21,283**	**34,790**	**1,033**	**49,426**	**64,757**	**1,317**	**3,236**	**776**	**3,098**	**3,504**	**204**	**980**	**374**	**505,934**	**328,645**
APO Miami	4	0	0	0	0	1	0	0	0	0	0	0	0	0	0	5	4
APO NY	158	4	6	12	1	18	30	0	1	0	0	0	0	0	0	230	167
APO Seattle/San Francisco	106	6	2	8	3	12	20	0	0	1	1	0	0	0	0	159	115
Subtotal	**268**	**10**	**8**	**20**	**4**	**31**	**50**	**0**	**1**	**1**	**1**	**0**	**0**	**0**	**0**	**394**	**286**
American Samoa	4	0	0	0	0	2	0	0	0	0	0	0	0	0	0	6	4
Canada	437	9	244	80	0	19	34	1	1	1	2	1	0	0	1	830	722
Guam	46	1	4	5	0	5	15	0	0	0	1	0	0	0	0	77	50
Other	273	19	37	46	0	37	53	1	1	2	0	0	0	1	0	470	327
Puerto Rico	181	6	7	25	0	10	40	0	2	0	0	1	0	0	1	273	191
Virgin Islands	34	1	6	6	0	4	9	0	0	0	0	2	0	0	0	62	38
Subtotal	**975**	**36**	**298**	**162**	**0**	**77**	**151**	**2**	**4**	**3**	**3**	**4**	**0**	**1**	**2**	**1,718**	**1,332**
Total	**309,840**	**12,605**	**21,589**	**34,972**	**1,037**	**49,534**	**64,958**	**1,319**	**3,241**	**780**	**3,102**	**3,508**	**204**	**981**	**376**	**508,046**	**330,263**

(Source: American Registry of Radiologic Technologists (ARRT) Census, last updated February 2017. Available at: http://www.arrt.org/about/census. Used with permission from The American Registry of Radiologic Technologists © 2018. The ARRT does not review, evaluate, or endorse publications or other educational materials. Permission to reproduce ARRT copyrighted materials should not be construed as an endorsement of the publication by the ARRT.)

The technologist may be asked to provide services in various situations with the patient as well as other medical professionals:

- The initial interview between the technologist and the patient documents important health information that is communicated to the radiologist; this information may help verify that appropriate mammography services are rendered to the patient.
- Providing the service of performing screening or diagnostic procedures requires the technologist to provide educational information about the examination and to answer questions patients may have about surveillance protocols or other breast imaging modalities.
- Contacting screening mammography patients to schedule additional imaging studies prompts compassionate and knowledgeable explanations by the technologist as she simultaneously searches for the next available appointment.
- Diagnostic studies may require the technologist to navigate the patient through ancillary breast imaging procedures such as ultrasound or MRI.
- A typical day for a mammography technologist may begin with performing quality control tests in the early morning before patients arrive, performing mammography throughout the rest of the morning, and providing core biopsy services in the afternoon.

All of these situations describe how the expertise of the technologist impacts the patient experience.

The technologist's performance also contributes to the patient's health care team in providing quality care to their in-common patient. Although the patient's interaction with the technologist during the mammography procedure lasts only a few minutes, the images produced during that short time frame are critical in determining what happens to the patient next. The quality images created by the technologist allow the radiologist, also a member of the patient's health care team, to determine whether the imaging information supports returning to screening mammography or if the imaging information indicates an abnormality.

If an abnormality is detected, the patient's health care team may expand to include the primary provider, an ultrasound technologist, an MRI technologist, the core biopsy team, a nurse navigator, a breast surgeon, a plastic surgeon, an oncologist, a radiation oncologist, and a counselor. Technologists working in association with hospital or outpatient services may also be called upon to assist members of the radiology and surgical team during the needle localization procedure prior to the patient's surgical biopsy.

Members of the patient's health care team may consult the mammography images acquired by the technologist as they determine appropriate treatment for the patient.

Each time the patient returns for future breast imaging follow-up services, the valuable archived images are reconstituted for comparison purposes during the radiologist's interpretation of the examination.

According to "Quality Management in the Imaging Sciences," the customer is defined as, "A person, department, or organization that needs or wants the desired outcome."[3] The technologist is a significant part of the health care team and is obligated to provide the best quality of care to the primary customer: the patient. It is also true that the breast health care team relies on the information created during the mammography procedure to make decisions on behalf of the patient. They too become the technologist's "customers," "wanting and needing a desired outcome" of accurate information and superior image quality.

Throughout the process of potential breast health care needs for the patient, the expertise of the technologist is depended upon. Although the patient is directly affected by the *quality of care* she receives from the technologist, other breast health care professionals rely on the *quality performance* of the technologist. The radiologic technologist who is called to be a mammography technologist thrives in a profession that requires strong communication, independent judgment, problem-solving capabilities, working as a team member, and the appreciation of a grateful patient.

DOCUMENTING PATIENT HEALTH INFORMATION

When a patient visits their health care provider in an outpatient setting, the patient is interviewed first by a nurse or medical assistant prior to the clinician meeting with the patient. The initial interview process provides the clinician with pertinent health information and the reason for the patient's visit. After reviewing the information gathered by the nurse or medical assistant, the clinician interacts with the patient to personally assess the patient and to provide care management.

In a medical imaging setting for screening or diagnostic mammography, it is the mammography technologist who gathers pertinent breast health information from the patient and documents the information in the patient's electronic chart.[4] Although practices vary throughout individual health care facilities, typically, screening mammography patients never come face to face with the radiologist who interprets their images. It *is* common practice for diagnostic mammography patients to have the opportunity to meet with the radiologist interpreting their breast imaging studies, but this event frequently occurs at the end of the examination when imaging has been finalized. It is therefore essential that the technologist interviewing the patient prior to performing the mammography procedure give her full attention to the task of gathering pertinent breast health information from the patient. This significant aspect of patient care is addressed by technologist professional organizations:

- American Society of Radiologic Technologists (ASRT), Mammography Practice Standards, "Mammography technologists are the primary liaison between patients, licensed independent practitioners, and other members of the support team. Mammography technologists must remain sensitive to the needs of the patient through good communication, patient assessment, patient monitoring and patient care skills."[4]
- American Registry of Radiologic Technologists (ARRT), Standard of Ethics document, Code of Ethics, #6, "The radiologic technologist acts as an agent through observation and communication to obtain pertinent information for the physician to aid in the diagnosis and treatment of the patient......."[5]

The importance of gathering accurate patient health information ensures that the patient receives the correct type of mammography procedure. Indications that determine a screening versus diagnostic mammogram are defined in the ACR Practice Parameter for the Performance of Screening and Diagnostic Mammography[6]:

- **Screening Mammogram:**
  - Examination performed annually for women age 40 and older who have an average risk of developing breast cancer
  - Examination performed on women younger than age 40 with various personal health history classifications that are associated with a higher than average risk of developing breast cancer
- **Diagnostic Mammogram:**
- Diagnostic mammography is performed when a problem has been identified by the patient, by her health care provider, or by screening mammography. A patient may present for a diagnostic mammogram when:
  - A clinical finding has been identified, such as a palpable lump, nipple discharge, persistent focal pain, or skin changes
  - Additional imaging is required when abnormal findings have been identified on a screening mammogram
  - A woman reporting for a screening mammogram indicates a breast symptom (requiring a conversion to a diagnostic mammogram following facility protocol)
  - Patients are recommended for short interval follow-ups based on previous imaging
  - Patients have a personal history of breast cancer (women with this history may opt to have screening mammography if offered by the facility)

Screening mammography appointments may be scheduled weeks in advance of the patient's arrival for their procedure. In the interim, breast symptoms may develop that the patient reports to the technologist during documentation of her breast health information. Incorrectly performing a screening mammogram on a patient requiring a diagnostic procedure could delay appropriate patient care or diagnosis. Clinical problems reported to the technologist during the heath information interview with the patient should be reported to the radiologist.[7,8] Corroboration of the patient's health information and the procedure order provided by the patient's health care provider should be verified by the technologist. Although this critical process is addressed through triage when the patient schedules her appointment with the facility, and again when the patient arrives at the facility to register for her services, it is the patient breast health interview conducted by the technologist that serves to confirm the type of mammography procedure the patient requires. In the event that a patient scheduled for a screening mammogram reports a symptom, the American College of Radiology (ACR) Practice Parameter For the Performance of Screening and Diagnostic Mammography states "The facility should have a process whereby screening mammography can be converted to diagnostic mammography."[6]

The patient health information interview begins with verification by the technologist that the correct patient is having the correct imaging procedure. The Joint Commission recommends that at least two patient identifiers be used for this purpose, such as the patient's name and birthdate.[9] The technologist should also verify with the patient that the correct electronic chart has been accessed prior to entering any health information. Establishing an atmosphere of calmness and reassurance helps the patient to focus on the process of answering the questions asked by the technologist and to offer information about breast symptoms that she may be fearful to disclose or embarrassed to discuss.

There are several verbal and nonverbal communication strategies used by the technologist to help enhance the interview process for the patient[10]:

- Address the patient by name throughout the interview process.
- Listen to the patient when she is speaking, without interrupting.
- Face the patient during the interview.
- Be aware of your voice tone, speed, and volume.
- Speak clearly.
- Be respectful.
- Accurately document information.

The health history obtained during the patient interview provides vital information to the interpreting radiologist as the patient's mammography images are evaluated.

The following information obtained from the patient must be available to the interpreting radiologist (Figure 4-1):

- Patient identification
- Exam identification

- Documentation of screening versus diagnostic examination
  - Baseline mammogram should be indicated.
- Information about previous studies
- Reason for the current examination

Additional View Exam Date _____
Technologist: _____

Date: _____

M.R. # _____

Technologist: _____   DOB: SX:
                            MRN:

Name: _____   Age: _____ B.D.: _____

M.D.: _____   Previous Mammogram: _____MMH
                                          Year: _____

Type of Study:

                                          Other: _____
Screen _____ Dx _____ F/U.: _____ R / L
     (check)   (circle)   _____

Reason for Exam: _____

_____

_____

# of pregnancies _____   age at 1st pregnancy: _____   age at 1st period: _____

Last Menstrual Period _____   Hormone Rx. _____

Family History of Breast Cancer: _____

I agree to contact my physician to obtain the mammogram results. I accept the responsibility for this "follow-up."

_____
Patient Signature   Date

To be filled out by the Technologist

Breast surface (moles, scars, etc:)

Nipples:
  Inverted? _____
  Discharge? _____
  How long? _____
Breast size discrepancy?
  Which: _____

Tech Comments: _____

_____

_____

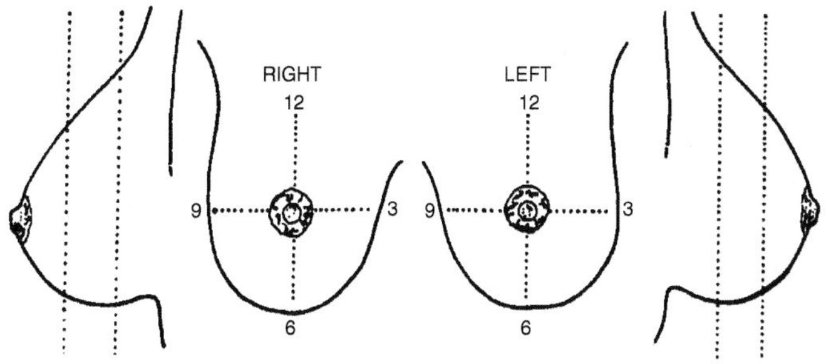

RIGHT   LEFT
12   12
9 ... 3 9 ... 3
6   6

Figure 4-1
The breast health history obtained during the patient interview provides vital information to the interpreting radiologist as she/he evaluates the patient's mammography images.

- Reported symptoms
- Risk factors
  - Personal
  - Family history
- Gynecological history
- Hormone history
- Breast surgical and treatment history
- Breast implant information

It is important that the technologist gathering information from the symptomatic diagnostic patient elicit specific descriptions about the complaints reported by the patient and to accurately document them for the interpreting radiologist. These descriptors assist the radiologist during their image evaluation and in the decision-making process of managing the patient's care. Information gathered by the technologist for the symptomatic patient should include seven descriptors[10,11]:

- Localization: define the location of the reported symptom
- Chronology: when symptoms began and how often they are noticed
- Quality: characteristic description of the symptom such as color of nipple discharge or size of breast lump
- Severity: intensity and extent of the symptom
- Onset: how the symptoms were made known to the patient
- Aggravating or alleviating factors: circumstances that modify or change the intensity of the symptom
- Associated manifestations: determining if other complaints the patient may report relate to the symptom

In mammography, an example of using this method to gather symptom specifics depends on the type of breast symptom being reported. For example, reporting breast pain as a symptom may require the technologist to inquire about the timing and frequency of the pain in relation to the menstrual cycle, if the patient is still menstruating, in addition to the more specific questions that describe the location, duration, and persistence of the pain.[7] The example of nipple discharge reported to the technologist also requires careful questioning of the patient to determine the amount, duration, color, and onset. Since there is greater significance to unilateral nipple discharge than bilateral, questions to the patient should include whether or not the discharge is observed in both breasts or is isolated to one breast.[7,12,13]

Physical Inspection

Prior to performing the mammography procedure, the technologist should inspect the skin for the presence of moles, scars, or other skin changes with a potential to be demonstrated on the mammographic image. The locations

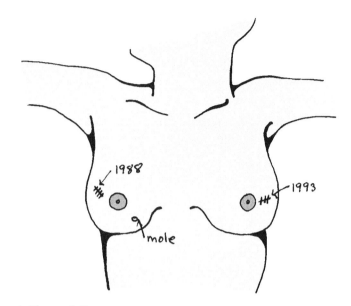

Figure 4-2
Documentation. Note skin changes (e.g., previous biopsies, moles, and scars) on a diagram to correlate with the mammogram.

of these skin conditions are transferred to a breast diagram that accompanies the health history information form Figure 4-2. Additionally, any clinical indications reported by the patient are documented on the breast diagram in the appropriate locations. The decision to use radiopaque breast markers on the skin to indicate moles, scars, or breast lumps is discussed in Chapter 7.

Risk Factors

The mammography breast health history form includes a section on breast cancer **risk factors** that provides the radiologist with pertinent information about the patient's breast cancer risk. This information is succinctly presented to the radiologist for immediate recognition of which risk factors apply to each patient (Figure 4-1).

A risk factor is anything associated with a greater likelihood of developing the disease. Several reliable resources such as the American Cancer Society, National Cancer Institute, and Susan G. Komen, among many others, provide comprehensive information about breast cancer including breast cancer risk factors. The Centers for Disease Control and Prevention Web site informs women that studies have demonstrated that the risk of developing breast cancer is due to a combination of factors. The CDC includes examples of breast cancer risk factors, shown in Box 4-1. Chapter 21, Breast Cancer Diagnostic Technologies: Today and Tomorrow, focuses on one specific breast cancer risk factor, which has gained increasing attention in the last few years: breast density.

BOX 4-1

What Are the Risk Factors for Breast Cancer?*

Studies have shown that your risk for breast cancer is due to a combination of factors. The main factors that influence your risk include being a woman and getting older. Most breast cancers are found in women who are 50 years old or older.

Some women will get breast cancer even without any other risk factors that they know of. Having a risk factor does not mean you will get the disease, and not all risk factors have the same effect. Most women have some risk factors, but most women do not get breast cancer. If you have breast cancer risk factors, talk with your doctor about ways you can *lower your risk* and about *screening* for breast cancer.

Risk factors include:

- **Getting older.** The risk for breast cancer increases with age; most breast cancers are diagnosed after age 50.
- **Genetic mutations.** Inherited changes (mutations) to certain genes, such as BRCA1 and BRCA2. Women who have inherited these *genetic changes* are at higher risk of breast and ovarian cancer.
- **Early menstrual period.** Women who start their periods before age 12 are exposed to hormones longer, raising the risk for breast cancer by a small amount.
- **Late or no pregnancy.** Having the first pregnancy after age 30 and never having a full-term pregnancy can raise breast cancer risk.
- **Starting menopause after age 55.** Like starting one's period early, being exposed to estrogen hormones for a longer time later in life also raises the risk of breast cancer.
- **Not being physically active.** Women who are not physically active have a higher risk of getting breast cancer.
- **Not being physically active.** Women who are not physically active have a higher risk of getting breast cancer.
- **Being overweight or obese after menopause**. Older women who are overweight or obese have a higher risk of getting breast cancer than those at a normal weight.
- **Having dense breasts**. Dense breasts have more connective tissue than fatty tissue, which can sometimes make it hard to see tumors on a mammogram. Women with dense breasts are more likely to get breast cancer.
- **Using combination hormone therapy**. Taking hormones to replace missing estrogen and progesterone in menopause for more than 5 years raises the risk for breast cancer. The hormones that have been shown to increase risk are *estrogen* and *progestin* when taken together.
- **Taking oral contraceptives (birth control pills).** Certain forms of oral contraceptive pills have been found to raise breast cancer risk.
- **Personal history of breast cancer**. Women who have had breast cancer are more likely to get breast cancer a second time.
- **Personal history of certain noncancerous breast diseases**. Some noncancerous breast diseases such as atypical hyperplasia or lobular carcinoma in situ are associated with a higher risk of getting breast cancer.
- **Family history of breast cancer**. A woman's risk for breast cancer is higher if she has a mother, sister, or daughter (first-degree relative) or multiple family members on either her mother's or father's side of the family who have had breast cancer. Having a first-degree male relative with breast cancer also raises a woman's risk.
- **Previous treatment using radiation therapy**. Women who had radiation therapy to the chest or breasts (like for treatment of Hodgkin's lymphoma) before age 30 have a higher risk of getting breast cancer later in life.
- **Women who took the drug diethylstilbestrol (DES)**, which was given to some pregnant women in the United States between 1940 and 1971 to prevent miscarriage, have a higher risk. Women whose mothers took DES while pregnant with them are also at risk.
- **Drinking alcohol**. Studies show that a woman's risk for breast cancer increases with the more alcohol she drinks.

Research suggests that other factors such as smoking, being exposed to chemicals that can cause cancer, and night shift working also may increase breast cancer risk.

From: Centers for Disease Control and Prevention (CDC). What are the risk factors for breast cancer? Available at: https://www.cdc.gov/cancer/breast/basic_info/risk_factors.htm.
*The Centers for Disease Control and Prevention (CDC) provides information on risk factors associated with the development of breast cancer.

Risk factors associated with developing breast cancer that are included on the mammography history form are generally known breast cancer risk factors recognized by researchers and medical professionals. The main risk factor for breast cancer is simply being a woman. Age is another important risk factor, as the likelihood of developing breast cancer increases as you get older.[14,15] Risk factors included on the mammography history form address the patient's personal health factors and family history that may increase her chances of developing breast cancer. Having a risk factor, or having several risk factors, does not guarantee that you will develop breast cancer. Some women who have several risk factors may never be diagnosed with breast cancer, while other women with no known major risk factors may develop the disease.[14,15]

Technologists working in the mammography discipline are continuously asked by their patients about risk factors associated with breast cancer and about mammography surveillance guidelines. It is essential that the technologist be familiar with the current breast cancer screening recommendations for women at average breast cancer risk and the recommendations for women at higher than average risk for developing breast cancer. Patients asking these questions should be directed to their health care provider to discuss what surveillance modalities and intervals are appropriate for them. Providing the patient inquiring about these important issues with information from reliable organizations allows them to be informed and prepared to ask knowledgeable questions prior to meeting with their physician for a better understanding of these subjects. The following organizations provide educational information about all aspects of breast cancer including explanations of breast cancer risk, risk assessment, and screening recommendations for mammography; this information is useful for the mammography technologist as well as her patient:

- American Cancer Society (ACS)
- Susan G. Komen
- MammographySavesLives.org
- National Cancer Institute
- Centers For Disease Control and Preventions (CDC)
- Breast Cancer.org

MASTERING THE BALANCING ACT: IMAGE QUALITY AND PATIENT SATISFACTION

It is well established that early detection of breast cancer affords the patient the greatest chance of successful treatment and long-term survival. Experts agree that breast cancer awareness and breast cancer screening, particularly utilizing mammography, have impacted the mortality rate associated with the disease. Statistics show a decline in deaths caused by breast cancer since 1989.[14] However, it is also recognized that mammography images are among the most difficult of radiographic images to interpret. Ensuring accuracy of the interpretation requires that the produced images be of high quality.

The consequences of poor image quality in mammography significantly impact the patient in ways that may affect their pocketbook, emotional health,[16] and their quality of life. Poor image quality may result in early indications of breast cancer that go undetected by the interpreting physician (IP). This type of report, called a "false negative," may delay important treatment of the disease, impact the patient's treatment options, or even contribute to a potential loss of life. Poor image quality in mammography may also result in the patient being asked to return for additional imaging when normal breast tissue is interpreted as an abnormality. This type of report, called a "false positive," may require the patient to undergo additional testing that causes increased anxiety, unnecessary discomfort, and additional cost.[17]

The significance of mammography image quality is addressed through the MQSA, which regulates mammography services in the United States. MQSA requirements ensure that equipment, personnel, and quality assurance meet established standards safeguarding the delivery of consistent, high-quality mammography to patients no matter where they may live.

There are two foundational components that produce or "create" the mammography image (discussed in detail in the following chapters of this book) that are distinguished in the MQSA standards. To ensure high-quality results for each acquired image, each of these components must perform at the level described by their MQSA standard. Figure 4-3 illustrates the two foundations that "create" the mammography image.

Both the equipment used for mammography imaging and the technologist creating the image must be "deemed" properly prepared to function in their ability to deliver high-quality service results. This responsibility does not pose an issue for the mammography equipment. Once the medical physicist approves the equipment for use, the technologist assumes operation for each individual exposure.

The technologist, however, is responsible for balancing two major components of the mammography examination:

- Producing a high-quality image
- Providing a positive patient experience

Balancing these two components introduces a conflict that she must learn to master for every patient interaction (Figure 4-4). This conflict may best be appreciated through the philosophy of Arthur C. Nielsen, who is recognized for developing methods to measure the audience of

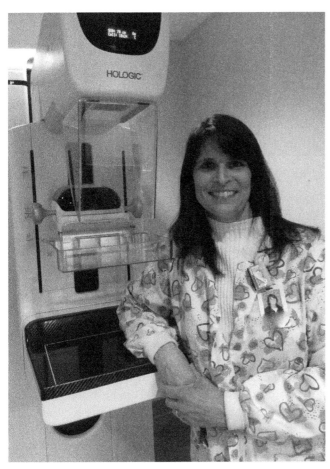

Figure 4-3
The two foundational components that "create" or produce the mammography image: the mammography equipment and the mammography technologist.

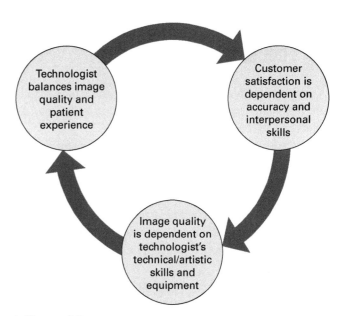

Figure 4-5
The quality of the mammography examination is dependent on the technologist's ability to continuously mingle technical skills and interpersonal skills.

between her knowledge and application of technical skills and her interpersonal interactions with the patient. The quality of the mammography examination is dependent on the continuous mingling of technical skills and interpersonal skills occurring simultaneously, not alternately, as illustrated in Figure 4-5.

Case Study **4-1**

1. Refer to Figure 4-4. Discuss workflow efficiencies and interpersonal skill development that a technologist should master in order to balance the image quality and the patient experience.

television programs, better known as the "Nielsen ratings." Mr. Nielsen stated simply, "Watch every detail that affects the accuracy of your work." A perceptive mammography technologist understands that the accuracy, or *precision* aspect of the work she creates, relies on the delicate balance

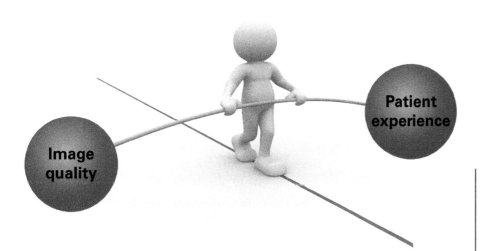

Figure 4-4
Every patient interaction requires the technologist to carefully balance the responsibilities of ensuring image quality and a positive patient experience. (Modified from Shutterstock, Inc.)

THE MAMMOGRAPHER'S DILEMMA

A factor that plays an important role in producing a quality image for the mammography examination is the "patient tolerance" of the procedure.

There is a wide variance of patient tolerance for the positioning maneuvers required to capture adequate breast tissue and for the application of compression required to obtain clarity in a quality image. The agility of the patient, along with their stamina for discomfort, must be considered and continuously monitored throughout the positioning and compression application process of the examination.

To understand the challenge of the technologist, Figure 4-6 illustrates the conflict inherent in the mammography examination. Quality/discomfort must be perfectly balanced with patient satisfaction, which is determined by patient tolerance. To successfully meet this expectation, the technologist must determine for each individual patient the precise point where both patient tolerance and image quality are achieved. The technologist's goal is a challenging one; she must repetitively produce quality mammographic images for a radiographic examination that inherently requires a degree of discomfort to the patient *while repetitively ensuring a positive patient experience.*

Unfortunately, and for various reasons (discussed later in this chapter), the equilibrium of quality/discomfort and patient satisfaction may not be achieved. Figure 4-7 illustrates the consequences of a disparity between quality/discomfort and patient satisfaction.

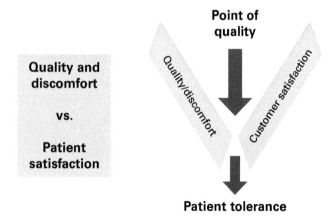

Figure 4-6
The technologist's commitment to quality presents a dilemma. The discomfort associated with high-quality mammography requires the technologist to accurately perceive patient tolerance in order to also achieve a satisfactory patient experience.

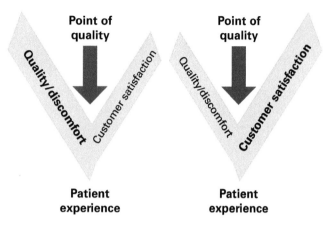

Figure 4-7
Circumstances associated with the examination may interfere with the technologist's ability to achieve equilibrium between quality/discomfort and patient satisfaction. When one factor dominates over the other, one goal of the examination is not met.

- In the first example, the quality/discomfort portion of the examination is exaggerated, while the patient satisfaction portion is minimized. This indicates that the patient's discomfort exceeded her point of tolerance. The illustration demonstrates that even if the accuracy goal of the examination was met, providing the patient with high-quality images, the patient's experience was less than satisfactory. This negative examination experience may influence the patient's future adherence to screening mammography and may cause the patient to discuss her negative experience with others in the community.

- In the second example, the patient satisfaction portion of the examination is exaggerated, while the quality/accuracy portion is minimized. Due to a variety of reasons, the examination may be subject to external circumstances that may compromise quality. Examples of this may include the following: the patient informed the technologist that she is unable to tolerate compression, or a patient has been added to the schedule affecting subsequent appointment time allotments. In these instances, consequences of unintentionally omitting breast tissue from the examination or inadequate compression of breast tissue may result due to attempts to appease the patient or remain on time. Although the patient experience may yield a very positive satisfaction result, the images produced during the examination may prohibit the detection of early indications of breast cancer.

These illustrations help reinforce the obligation of the technologist to also serve as an educator to the patient throughout the examination. When the patient is coached by the technologist as the positioning maneuvers are employed, explaining what is happening and why, the patient is invited into a "teamwork" process of reaching the procedure quality goals. The result of establishing a "teamwork" model through effective communication during the positioning/compression process serves to achieve the two goals required for the delivery of quality service:

1. Improving the image quality
2. Providing the patient with a satisfactory mammography experience

The technologist's contact with the mammography patient is approximately 10 to 20 minutes. In addition to serving as an educator to the patient, the technologist assumes the responsibility to simultaneously deliver the following requirements of the mammography procedure (Figure 4-8):

- Problem solve
- Adhere to facility policies
- Recall individual radiologist's expectations
- Ensure patient safety
- Compassionately meet the expectations of the patient

Fulfilling these responsibilities and also meeting expectations to produce superior image quality within the allowable time permitted may be challenging under some examination situations, requiring the technologist to suppress anxiety as she delivers quality patient care. This subject is addressed later in this chapter.

 # MEASURING QUALITY SERVICE

The technologist's ability to successfully balance the expectations of the patient experience and produce high image quality is one component of the mammography service. The mammography procedure serves to gather information providing an accurate representation of patient anatomy for skillful interpretation by the radiologist. The mammography service is completed when the IP provides an assessment to the patient and to the patient's referring health care provider. The entire process of the mammography service can be evaluated using three measurements of service quality (Figure 4-9):

1. **Perceived quality**

   Perceived quality is the impression the patient (customer) forms about the service they have received. Customer satisfaction is achieved when the patient feels that the actual quality received surpassed their expectation of quality.[18] Perceived quality is very subjective and is difficult to accurately calculate. Service factors such as the registration (check-in) process, how long they waited for the procedure, or their interpretation of how they were treated during the examination influence their perception of quality.[3] Perceived quality is a critical measurement of service quality as it represents customer satisfaction.[18] It is

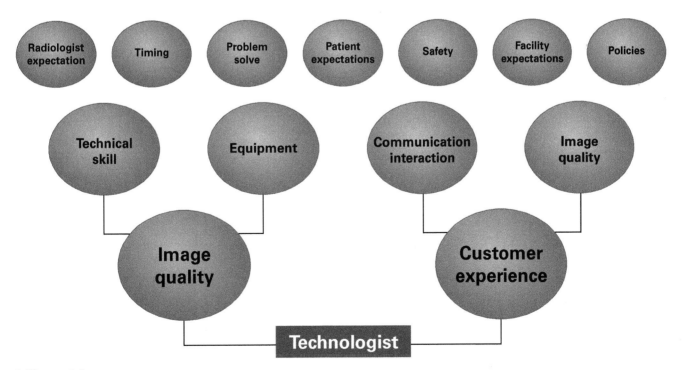

Figure 4-8
The technologist balances a variety of responsibilities during every mammography procedure she performs. The ability of the technologist to tailor the mammography examination to each individual patient and circumstance requires a perception of all factors that influence the procedure.

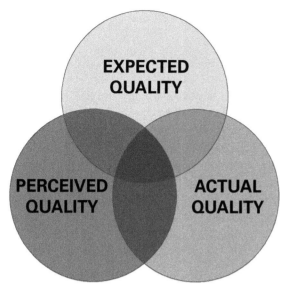

Figure 4-9
Service quality may be evaluated using three levels of measurement: perceived quality, expected quality, and actual quality.

important for the technologist to understand that their interaction with the patient has the greatest impact on perceived quality. This measure of quality may be more important that the actual quality, as it serves as the determining factor in whether or not customers return to the facility for future imaging services.[3]

2. **Expected quality**
Expected quality can be influenced by advertisements that the patient is exposed to, by word of mouth in the community, family member experiences, or other outside factors. When the customer has low expectations, they may go elsewhere for their services. In contrast, if the service expectations are too high, it may be difficult for the facility to meet them.[18] The customer's expectation of quality of service is formed prior to the service they receive, and therefore, the mammography technologist has minimal control over this measurement of quality.[3]

3. **Actual quality**
Actual quality is the true service that has been delivered to the customer and is demonstrated through statistical data.[18] Points of customer service, such as image quality, the accuracy of radiologist interpretation, and satisfaction of the referring health care provider, are measured through the use of survey results and computer collected data that provide the facility with factual outcomes of actual quality. This information is useful in comparing facility service outcomes to that of their competitors.[3]

Case Study **4-2**

1. Refer to Figure 4-9. Discuss the importance of service quality and the way service can be measured. Describe the significance of each measurement to the mammography facility.

QUALITY CHECKS AND BALANCES

Understanding the three measurements of service quality provides valuable information to the facility in establishing mechanisms that ensure service quality determinants are met. The facility, radiologist, senior technologist, and the technologist all play significant roles in ensuring the two critical elements of service: image quality and patient satisfaction are achieved. A closer look at each of these elements of the mammography examination and the specific factors that influence their quality are discussed further.

QUALITY FACTORS: ACHIEVING IMAGE QUALITY

Excluding equipment performance, there are two critical factors that ensure high-quality images are produced during the mammography procedure. The technologist acquiring images must be proficient in her ability to adequately capture breast tissue and to ensure visual clarity of the breast anatomy for accurate interpretation by the radiologist, *and* she must be provided adequate time to create quality images in a variety of patient situations.

Technologist Proficiency

Factors affecting technologist proficiency are influenced by:

- Technologist initial mammography education
- Radiologist's expectations, oversight, and guidance of image quality (includes ongoing feedback of technologist performance)
- Quality and length of time exposed to positioning/compression instruction (number of examinations supervised by qualified instructor)
- Imaging instruction and examination management guidance from senior mammography technologists
- Ensuring that periodic refresher positioning/compression techniques are included in continuing education

Image quality principles are developed by a fledgling technologist through expectations and guidance communicated to her by the interpreting radiologist and the senior technologists supervising her training. These expectations align with reduced radiation exposure in medical imaging initiatives introduced by the FDA and the ACR to ensure that appropriate image quality is achieved while observing a conscientious approach to patient dose.[6]

Passing the Baton

Mammography technologists who meet MQSA personnel requirements are considered "qualified instructors" by the FDA and are accountable for instructing novice technologists in the art and science of mammographic imaging. Currently, the ARRT reports 49,596 registered radiologic technologists with postprimary certification in mammography. Many of these technologists have been performing mammography since the 1970s and are considered a part of the "Baby Boomer" generation. According to research, Baby Boomers retire at a rate of 10,000 per day through at least 2030.[19] During the next decade, Baby Boomer technologists who were privileged to learn from and perform mammography under the guidance of physician, medical physicist, and technologist pioneers in mammography will pass the baton to the next generation (Figure 4-10). How best can these and other experienced technologists mentor a new generation of mammography technologists as they prepare to join the ranks of this unique profession?

Staging Instruction: An Important Prerequisite

Technologists preparing to legally perform mammography in the United States must fulfill personnel requirements established by MQSA. This requirement includes the performance of 25 mammography examinations performed under the direct supervision of a qualified instructor. The experienced technologist understands that this responsibility requires detailed positioning/compression instruction during an examination that may be considered "sensitive" by many patients. Perceptive technologists providing supervision for the examination recognize the importance of quality instruction to the novice while ensuring service satisfaction to the patient. This assurance begins with an explanation of the educational process to the patient and requesting her consent to allow the instruction to take place. Properly informing the patient of the technologist's professional credentials and the preparation requirements she has achieved allowing her to perform the procedure under supervision is critical to ensure that the patient experience and the instruction opportunity begin with respect.

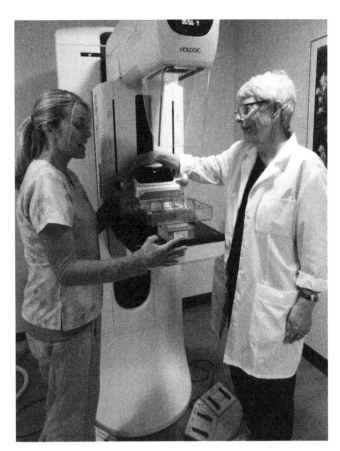

Figure 4-10
One of the most significant contributions to achieving image quality in the mammography service is the mentorship afforded to the fledgling technologist by the senior technologist and the interpreting radiologist.

The technologist providing mammography instruction must establish a professional environment for the educational experience, acknowledging its validity and inviting the patient into the process. Experienced technologists who mentor novice technologists utilizing training methods that demonstrate ideals and techniques to advance the goal of image quality are one of the most significant factors in perpetuating quality service in mammography.

Positioning/Compression Instruction

Supervising technologists providing positioning/compression instruction to beginning technologists should be familiar with and facilitate instruction using the Patient Positioning and Compression section of the ACR 1999 Quality Control Manual[20] and the concepts used to perform the standard and additional imaging projections, as well as appropriate compression application and evaluation. Additionally, supervising technologists should understand proper methods of instruction regarding spot compression, magnification, and implant imaging techniques as described in that same manual.[20]

Exam Management

For the majority of patients presenting for screening mammography, the examination is adequately managed utilizing the standard mammography projections, the craniocaudal and the mediolateral oblique, to complete the procedure. However, due to various limiting conditions, the patient's ability to cooperate with the positioning/compression maneuvers required for the standard projections may be compromised. Therefore, it is important for the novice technologist to be properly guided by a mentoring technologist in the art of exam management over a wide variety of situations. **Exam management** is the expertise of the technologist to recognize when the use of additional complementary or replacement views for the standard projections is necessary to adequately provide a quality examination (Figure 4-11). This ability is a

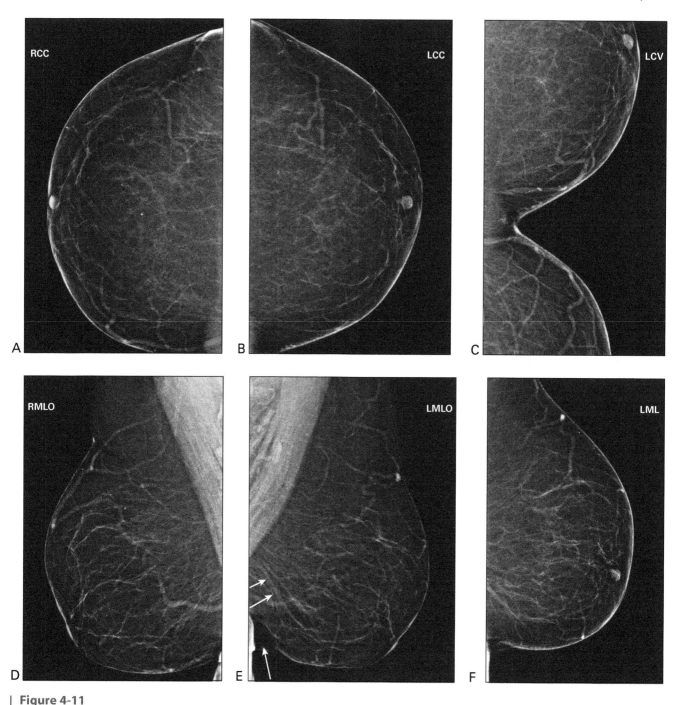

Figure 4-11

(A–F) An example of exam management by the technologist in determining which additional images elevate the image quality of the examination in a challenging circumstance: Figure 4-14 (**A** and **B**) demonstrates inadequate medial tissue capture on the RCC and LCC views due to the patient's breast size; this was improved by the additional CV projection (**C**). Part (**D**) demonstrates an adequate RMLO. Part (**E**) demonstrates inadequate support of posterior inferior tissue on the LMLO (*arrows*), with improvement noted on the additional LML acquired by the technologist (**F**).

quality determinant for the mammography examination and requires technologist competency in the following:

- Determining when to use problem-solving views
- Determining which views, or combination of views, provide a solution to achieving adequate breast tissue capture with clarity
- Consideration to conscientious radiation dose practices

The ACR Practice Parameter for the Performance of Screening and Diagnostic Mammography addresses the responsibility of all radiology professionals to ensure the radiation exposure to the staff and to the patient's they serve is "as low as reasonably achievable" (ALARA).[6] When faced with a challenging imaging situation, this goal is best achieved by using the movement of the mammography unit to benefit the patient's limitation. Technologists with this thoughtful insight are able to provide the patient with a positive experience and with a quality examination.

Chapters 7 and 8 describe various situations that may challenge achieving image quality when acquiring standard projections. A review of these chapters provides the technologist with examples of specific patient variables that impact image quality and specific problem-solving techniques used for improvement. It is important for the technologist to understand the broad application of image quality over a wide variation of patient cooperative abilities.

Adequate Examination Time

Producing a high-quality mammographic image is accomplished when the technologist is proficient in combining technical knowledge and artistic skills of precision. The images produced by the technologist are evaluated for quality by comparing specific features of the CC and the MLO projections to defined criteria established by accrediting bodies.

Published image criteria for the positioning/compression attributes, as described in the Clinical Image Quality section of the ACR 1999 Mammography Quality Control Manual, include the following[20]:

- Presence of pectoral muscle on the CC view
- Presentation of the pectoral muscle on the MLO projection (superior muscle width, muscle length, convexity of anterior border)
- Passing measurement of the posterior nipple line (PNL) rule
- Inclusion of inframammary fold (IMF) on the MLO view
- PNL direction on the CC projection
- Adequate support for breast structures in the MLO projection
- Adequate compression force

As with any skill, time and repetition are essential to acquire the proficiency necessary to ensure the presentation of these image quality features and to learn how to apply adequate compression force.

Digital imaging, compared to analog imaging, requires a shorter time to complete an exam. This time efficiency is due to the computer creating the digital image as opposed to waiting for a film taken into the darkroom to make its way through the film processor. However, whether creating an analog, digital, or DBT image, the time element to perform the artistic component of positioning the breast tissue and applying adequate compression force for each mammographic projection remains the same.

A study conducted at New York University in the early 2000s compared the time required to perform digital and analog screening examinations. A stopwatch was used to evaluate the time it took for the technologist to perform the examination, to interact with the patient, and to evaluate the images for each modality. Technologists performed 100 2-view/breast screening examinations using analog imaging and 100 2-view/breast screening examinations using digital imaging. The results confirmed that technologists needed 10 minutes and 29 seconds to perform and check the images of the analog examination compared to 6 minutes and 12 seconds for the digital examination.[21] The 4 minutes and 17 seconds decrease in time is indicative of the technological efficiencies of digital imaging over analog imaging. The length of time scheduled for the technologist to *create* the images is an extremely important factor that impacts image quality. Image quality is affected by two time conditions imposed on the technologist performing the examination:

- The time allowed by the facility to perform the screening mammography examination (example: examinations scheduled every 10, 20, or 30 minutes at the facility)
- Peer pressure: the nonverbalized "time" that technologists may impose on each other in the work environment (example: a technologist who performs mammography quickly expects other technologists to perform in like manner)

To accurately address time factors impacting image quality, it is necessary to know the average time it takes technologists to perform and check images that result in a *high-quality* screening examination at an individual facility and to know how long it takes to complete additional nonimaging workflow requirements of the examination. Digital mammography workflows are not standardized and are dependent on many information technology (IT) variables; these variables make it virtually impossible to compare one facility's workflow timing to another.

Knowing specific information about the technologist's performance quality and the facility's workflow requirements allows the facility to determine a realistic balance between quality and efficiency for patient scheduling. Additionally, this information provides the facility with opportunities to initiate continuous quality improvement (CQI) processes that identify methods to improve efficiency and staff performance.

Image Quality Checkpoints

Other factors that impact image quality can be collectively described as "viewbox quality checks." Image quality evaluation for analog mammography was consistently performed by technologists at the viewbox when the screening examination was completed. Image quality was evaluated by comparing available previous studies of the patient with the current study by placing them "back to back" on the viewbox. This method allowed the technologist to determine if the current study was equal or surpassed the quality of the previous study by evaluating and comparing the criteria for each standard projection. Additionally, the viewbox quality checks included the technologist's measurement of the PNL for the CC and for the MLO images to ensure that adequate posterior tissue had been captured.

If it was determined that image quality was substandard compared to the previous study, the technologist would repeat an image to improve the quality before allowing the patient to leave the department. These image evaluations were standardized for the analog examination and performed to ensure quality. In contrast, the digital workflow is not standardized. Today, these quality measures may be performed inside or outside of the digital mammography suite, using the acquisition monitor or a PACS monitor.

Although digital mammography equipment manufacturers have addressed image quality evaluation by providing electronic rulers to measure the PNL, and provide methods to compare current and previous patient studies, the authors have observed that the practice of performing these critical image quality measures by the technologist is not as consistently practiced in the digital environment. This may be a consequence of transitioning to digital mammography where:

- With a nonstandardized workflow, there is not a defined time or place when these quality measures should be done.
- The emphasis placed on efficiency in digital mammography.

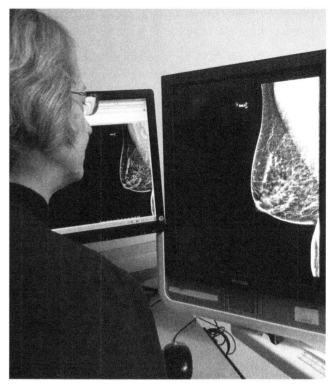

Figure 4-12
The current image (*right monitor*) is immediately compared to the previous image (*left monitor*) by the technologist to evaluate tissue capture and clarity. The current image should reflect equitable or superior image quality to the prior image unless limiting factors influence the procedure.

- There is lack of instruction for technologists regarding the use of electronic tools.

Performing "viewbox quality checks" is a factor that impacts image quality and should consistently be performed in the digital environment by the technologist. The value of comparing previous to current studies, and of measuring and comparing the standard projection PNLs (when applicable), is most effective in the digital workflow when:

- The previous patient study is available for review at the time of the current study acquisition (Figure 4-12). Example: The current RCC is immediately compared to the previous RCC to assess and compare positioning, compression, exposure, motion, and other imaging attributes. Note: current to previous comparison may be done after all standard projections have been completed as well.
- PNL rule should be applied to the current study (when applicable) while the patient is accessible to the technologist should repeat imaging be necessary (Figure 4-13).

According to the April 2016 MQSA Insight Article, "Poor Positioning Responsible for Most Clinical Deficiencies,

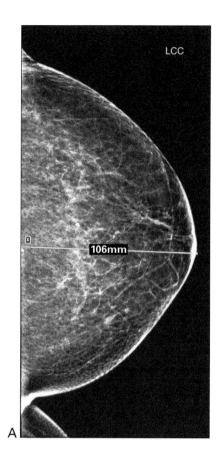
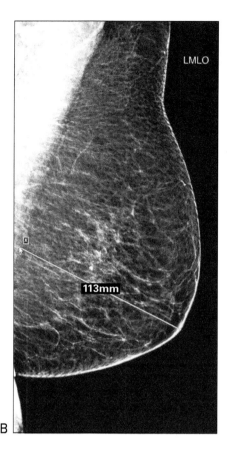

Figure 4-13
(A and B) A method commonly used by technologists to evaluate CC posterior tissue capture is the posterior nipple line rule. The standard projections are measured to determine the length of the PNL.

Failures," published on the FDA website, most clinical image deficiencies and most accreditation failures are due to poor positioning.[22] Establishing checkpoints to evaluate image quality for the mammography examination provides immediate performance feedback to the technologist that allows prompt corrective action for substandard quality while the patient is still in the department and accessible to the technologist.

Radiologist Supervision and Guidance

The role of the lead interpreting physician (LIP) and the role of the IP to safeguard image quality are strongly acknowledged by the MQSA and by the ACR. MQSA designates the LIP as the person responsible for the facility's mammography quality assurance program, the safeguard of image quality and safety for the patient[23]. The quality assurance program addresses every aspect of the mammography service including image quality[24]. MQSA also designates the IP's responsibility in safeguarding image quality[25] (Box 4-2).

Action taken by the FDA in September 2016 further establishes the emphasis on the interpreting radiologist to provide guidance to the mammography technologist when the radiologist is asked to interpret images of poor quality. The EQUIP initiative was announced in September 2016 and began in January 2017. EQUIP requires facilities establish mechanisms to review the image quality of each active radiologic technologist performing mammography and review the image quality accepted for interpretation of each active IP.[26] The ACR 2016 Digital Mammography Quality Control Manual provides an optional Radiologist Performance Feedback form for the purpose of notifying the technologist (a) when she has submitted images for interpretation that require quality improvement or (b) when the images are of exceptional quality[27] (Figure 4-14).

The role of the IP to establish image quality expectations in the mammography program is a key factor that affects significant aspects of the service. Consider the results cited by the FDA in the 2016 MQSA Insight article, "Poor Positioning Responsible For Most Clinical Image Deficiencies, Failures": in a 2002 study, the "sensitivity of mammography dropped from 84.4% among cases with passing positioning to 66.3% among cases with failed positioning."[28]

Radiologists and technologists who address image quality through respectful ongoing communication for the purpose of quality improvement participate in the most important professional obligation they share—to serve the mammography patient.

(A) Lead Interpreting Physician (Definition),* (B) Quality Assurance Program,† (C) Interpreting Physician Responsibilities‡ According to the MQSA

Lead Interpreting Physician (Definition)

Citation:

900.2(x) Lead interpreting physician means the interpreting physician assigned the general responsibility for ensuring that a facility's quality assurance program meets all of the requirements of section 900.12(d) through (f). The administrative title and other supervisory responsibilities of the individual, if any, are left to the discretion of the facility.

Quality Assurance Program

Citation:

900.12(d): Quality Assurance—general. Each facility shall establish and maintain a quality assurance program to ensure the safety, reliability, clarity, and accuracy of mammography services performed at the facility.

Interpreting Physician Responsibilities

Citation:

900.12(d)(1)(i),(ii)(A)(B): (1) Responsible individuals. Responsibility for the quality assurance program and for each of its elements shall be assigned to individuals who are qualified for their assignments and who shall be allowed adequate time to perform these duties.

(i) *Lead interpreting physician. The facility shall identify a lead interpreting physician who shall have the general responsibility of ensuring that the quality assurance program meets all requirements of paragraphs (d) through (f) of this section. No other individual shall be assigned or shall retain responsibility for quality assurance tasks unless the lead interpreting physician has determined that the individual's qualifications for, and performance of, the assignment are adequate.*

(ii) *Interpreting physicians. All interpreting physicians interpreting mammograms for the facility shall: (A) Follow the facility procedures for corrective action when the images they are asked to interpret are of poor quality, and (B) Participate in the facility's medical outcomes audit program.*

*MQSA designates the LIP as the person responsible for the facility's mammography quality assurance program, the safeguard of image quality and safety for the patient.
†The quality assurance program addresses every aspect of the mammography service, including image quality.
‡MQSA assigns responsibility to the IP to safeguard image quality by following the facility's corrective action protocol when asked to interpret images of poor quality. (Information for A–C taken from fda.gov website/Policy Guidance Help System (FDA).)

Image Quality: Continuous Quality Improvement

The Hawthorne effect traditionally has been used to describe the phenomenon that when an individual's performance is monitored, the result is a tendency of the individual to increase the quality of their performance.[29] Modern CQI methods demonstrate the importance of measuring performance periodically to establish processes that ensure the consistency of delivering a superior product. Since 1992, the MQSA has enforced strict standards for the equipment component of the image quality contribution in mammography, requiring acceptance quality control evaluation of the equipment by a qualified medical physicist as well as periodic quality control testing of the equipment by a qualified mammography technologist to comply with regulations designed to protect the patient. The technologist's proficiency in equipment operation and her artistic contribution to image quality is of equal importance and deserving of periodic performance review.

There are three areas of the technologist's performance that impact image quality. These areas consist of actions that take place:

- Preexposure: validation of correct patient, validation of correct procedure, and actions taken by the technologist to reduce patient anxiety in order to facilitate greater potential of posterior tissue capture

Optional - Radiologist Image Quality Feedback   *As Needed*

(For Quality Improvement)

Radiologist's Name _____

Date _____

Procedure	This report is to be completed by the Interpreting Radiologist when asked to interpret sub-optimal cases requiring the patient to be called back. The form may also be used to provide feedback on excellent quality. The radiologist should complete this form as needed for each case. A system should be in place for analyzing feedback and taking measures for improvement as necessary.

Objective   For the Radiologist to provide routine feedback to the technologists and manager on the quality of images.

Patient Identifier: _____
_____
Technologist's Name: _____
Date of Exam: _____

Overall Assessment

☐ Excellent   ☐ Good   ☐ Needs improvement, but do not repeat   ☐ Sub-Optimal, and should be repeated

Image Evaluation

	RCC	LCC	RMLO	LMLO	Other View	Other View
Positioning						
Missing tissue						
Laterally						
Posteriorly						
Medially						
Inferiorly						
Nipple not in profile						
Skin fold						
Pectoralis not down to PNL						
Tissue droopy (camel nose)						
Narrow/concave pectoralis						
Inframammary fold						
Not open						
Not shown						
Centering not correct						
Technical Issues						
Not enough compression						
Exposure Too Low (Excessive Noise)						
Exposure Too High (Image Saturation)						
Patient Motion						
Artifacts						
Incorrect Patient ID						
Other						

Additional Images Needed for Complete Breast Evaluation

Requested views   ☐ RCC   ☐ LCC   ☐ RMLO   ☐ LMLO   ☐ Other View _____

Action Limits	Recommended:	Patients should be called back for additional images if the quality is suboptimal according to the interpreting radiologist's request.
	Time frame:	Not applicable.

Figure 4-14
A method of preserving the standard of image quality in the mammography service includes continuous performance feedback to the technologist when submitted images are of exceptional quality or if improvement is warranted. (Source: Berns EA, Baker JA, Barke LD, et al. Digital Mammography Quality Control Manual. Reston, VA: American College of Radiology; 2016.)

- Acquisition of image: projections executed accurately, striving to meet ACR image quality objectives whenever possible, modifying the examination to best meet these objectives for patient conditions that may limit cooperative ability
- Postexposure: actions taken by technologist to immediately compare current projection image to previous study (same projection) to verify adequate or superior image quality has been achieved

The radiologist's medical audit, whether conducted individually or for the practice collectively, provides data about various accuracy aspects of the mammography service. This information can be compared among the group of IPs and to national benchmarks providing an opportunity for performance improvement if necessary. Similarly, effectively providing quality improvement opportunities to the technologist requires that information depicting performance patterns be collected and shared with her.

Factors that impact image quality that are specific to actions undertaken by the technologist include the following:

- Length of time taken to create the imaging requirements of the examination.
- Image execution accuracy (evaluating the mammography features of each projection to determine acceptance based on the patient's cooperative ability).
- Examination management (correct choice of projections included in the examination to adequately capture and accurately represent anatomy).
- Percentage of patients recalled for additional imaging.
- Percentage of technical recalls.
- Percentage of additional imaging performed to complete the screening examination.
- Overall compression accuracy (force/thickness used for examinations).
- Percentage of superior quality examinations produced by the technologist (screening examinations that could potentially be considered for accreditation purposes).
- Exposure accuracy (established manufacturer exposure factor parameters).
- Comparison to previous study quality, when available.
- The impact to image quality is dependent *on when and how, during the mammography workflow,* the current and prior images are compared. Preferably, this is performed, one image to one image, at the time of each acquisition (see Figure 4-12).

Collecting this information over time from many examination samples provides a pattern of the technologist's performance. Similar to the purpose of the radiologist's medical audit, providing the technologist with these aspects of her contribution to image quality and the effect her performance has on the mammography service as a whole is enlightening. The purpose of CQI is to evaluate processes and actions that negatively or positively impact cost, efficiency, quality, and accuracy of the mammography service. Meaningful CQI programs established to evaluate the balance of efficiency and quality fulfill the facility obligation to the patient and address the accountability of the technologist. Technologists who receive information providing specific patterns of performance and the ability to compare personal performance to that of her peers are afforded the greatest opportunity to make technical changes that benefit the care of future patients and to positively impact the mammography practice.

POSITIVE PATIENT EXPERIENCE: THE TECHNOLOGIST'S SPECIFIC ROLE

Several aspects of the technologist's role in ensuring a positive experience for the patient are discussed in Chapter 3. However, there are actions taken by the mammography technologist during her interaction with the patient that specifically affect image quality and that specifically serve to meet customer satisfaction. This chapter discusses three target areas of the mammography service that are affected by the technologist's interaction with the patient:

- **Image quality**—Prior to, as well as during, the procedure, the verbal and nonverbal communication between the technologist and the patient serves to effectively gain greater patient cooperation for mammography positioning/compression requirements. This communication results in higher image quality than when an examination is performed without using specific verbal or nonverbal prompts.
- **Patient examination experience**—How the patient perceives the care she receives from the technologist, from the time she is called from the waiting room until the end of the examination, is affected by behavior demonstrated by the technologist.
- **Patient satisfaction of future mammography service**—CQI involves more than just monitoring the quality of the image. CQI also includes an awareness of issues that contribute to customer *dissatisfaction* or that *cause anxiety* to the customer, issues that could be proactively managed through patient education.

TECHNOLOGIST'S SOFT SKILLS INFLUENCE ON IMAGE QUALITY

In Chapter 3, the patient experience discussion was focused on the ability of the facility and the mammography service to ensure that the patient felt satisfied with the care and treatment she received during her mammography visit. The importance of this discussion established that there is a necessary relationship between the patient and the facility:

- The facility must provide exceptional customer service to the patient.
- The patient needs to feel that exceptional customer service was provided by the facility.

There are a variety of skills that health care professionals deliver to the patient that impact the customer's perception of satisfaction. Hard skillsets have to do with technical knowledge and proficiency in performing the examination, while **"soft skills,"** otherwise known as "people skills," affect the emotional aspect of the examination.[30,31] Soft skills comprise an individual's ability to interact with others, work in a team environment, and communicate effectively. Successful mammography examinations require a strong blend of hard and soft skills to achieve quality and accuracy.[30]

Verbal and Nonverbal Communication

The simultaneous demands of positioning and compression require the patient to be an active participant and assist the technologist to capture and demonstrate the breast tissue with clarity.

For the mammography *procedure*, the technologist's ability to effectively communicate the requirements of positioning to the patient and to coach her through the discomfort that results from capturing tissue adjacent to the thorax and with sufficient compression *impacts the quality of the image*. Technologists have developed a scripted dialogue to inform the patient of each maneuver that is going to be performed and why, while using a slower, calming delivery gives the patient time to process what is being asked of them and to respond to the given direction. When what is being asked may cause discomfort, explaining why the maneuver is necessary helps them to understand that their participation contributes to a better image.

To provide an example of using effective communication, capturing the posterolateral tissue on the CC projection is discussed. The technologist needs to "wrap" her hand and fingers around the far lateral aspect of the patient's breast, lifting and shifting the posterolateral tissue forward onto the image receptor. For many women, this manipulation may cause discomfort, requiring the technologist performing the maneuver to properly prepare the patient prior to executing the maneuver. A simple explanation that includes both verbal and nonverbal instruction is suggested:

- Technologist: "The next step is to ensure that the outer breast is included on the image." (Spoken while the technologist wraps her hand around the tissue.)
- Technologist: While making eye contact with the patient, "This may be uncomfortable for you."
- Before performing the maneuver, allow the patient to respond either verbally by acknowledging she understood or nonverbally by a slight nod of her head or through eye contact.
- Performing the maneuver and noticing discomfort (usually through the facial expression of the patient), the technologist acknowledges the situation by responding in some form, "I know, I am so sorry, you are doing such a great job."

This communication takes just seconds, but accomplishes what is required by respectfully addressing human dignity in the goal to achieve image quality.

Another example of nonverbal communication that serves to ensure the patient feels secure is to execute maneuvers at a steady, calm pace. When it is necessary to reposition the patient's head, or to move her chin, techniques that are nonstartling help to maintain the patient's relaxation. Examples of nonstartling techniques to position the head include the following:

- Slowly move the back of the palm toward the patient's face.
- The technologist's hand travels upward toward the chin, close to the patient's body, out of her eyesight.

Chapter 7 thoroughly discusses the need for the patient to be relaxed throughout the mammography procedure to achieve the goals associated with adequate tissue capture and clarity. The verbal and nonverbal techniques developed by the technologist are important contributions in maintaining the established relaxation of the patient.

THE PATIENT NEEDS TO KNOW

Important aspects of the patient experience include imparting information regarding the mammography examination process that may be unfamiliar to the customer. Along with providing the service of executing the mammography procedure, it is the technologist's responsibility to prepare, educate, and inform the patient of processes that otherwise could cause anxiety. Many patients may have experienced the diagnosis of breast cancer in family members or friends. These experiences may contribute to a sense of anxiety that is possible to reduce when a courteous explanation of common mammography circumstances is proactively provided. Examples of common mammography circumstances that should be explained during the mammography visit include the following:

Baseline Examination

Patients who are scheduled for a baseline mammography examination do not know what to expect; before the examination begins, they should be informed how the examination is performed. Technologists who thoroughly explain the reasons for positioning maneuvers and the application of compression prepare the patient for the sensations they experience during the examination. Demonstrating how compression is applied and explaining how it is evaluated to ensure that adequate information is recorded on the image reduces the "fear of the unknown."

This communication invites the patient into a "teamwork" mindset that is necessary to produce high-quality mammography images and sets the stage for future mammography examinations the patient may have. After the first x-ray exposure is completed, the technologist should ask the patient how she tolerated the first image. Giving this time to provide feedback to the technologist further establishes the "teamwork" approach, especially noting any expressions of specific discomfort and providing an explanation of why this may have occurred. When the technologist understands the tolerance level of the patient, she may provide a solution to the problem if possible. An example of this may include: the patient that complains of her neck feeling "pulled" during the compression application of the CC projection. Having the patient provide this information after the first projection is completed allows the technologist to reexamine her performance of the maneuver to "reserve" tissue just superior to the clavicle prior to applying compression on the subsequent image in an effort to increase the comfort of the patient. Asking the patient how she tolerated the first image taken for the procedure and allowing feedback provides the technologist with valuable information in guiding the remainder of the examination. This communication technique benefits not only the baseline mammography patient, but is a courteous approach to all patients.

Explaining Additional Imaging

Being called back for additional imaging after a mammography procedure has been performed naturally elevates the anxiety level in almost all women.[16] The Breast Cancer Surveillance Consortium (BCSC) reports 10% of screening mammography patients are called back for additional imaging.[32] These statistics reflect the recall rate for women receiving 2D screening mammography (the rate is lower for 3D technology) and is higher than 10% for women receiving a baseline mammogram.[33]

Providing educational information to the patient about the need for additional imaging assists in reducing the anxiety in women who receive a positive mammogram result. A study showed that sending information about additional imaging along with the patient summary informing them of a positive mammography finding resulted in patients feeling more confident about their results than patients who did not receive the additional imaging information.[34]

At the conclusion of the mammography procedure, the patient should be informed about the additional imaging process and how that is managed at the facility where she has received her mammogram. Traditionally, this information is provided by the technologist at the conclusion of the mammography procedure, before the patient is informed of how and when she will receive the results of her mammogram. It is helpful to the patient to receive information that includes the National Cancer Institute BCSC recall rate, what type of imaging may be offered to her if she is called back for additional imaging, and how call back appointments are managed.

One additional note about additional imaging: A patient may undergo mammography for several years before ever being called back for additional imaging. Technologists commonly phone patients to schedule these additional imaging appointments. Occasionally the patient states, "I have been having mammograms for many years and this has never happened before. This year I had a different technologist perform my examination." It is possible to reduce the suspicion and anxiety associated with this positive mammography finding by thoroughly addressing additional imaging information to the baseline mammography patient at the time of her procedure. The baseline mammography patient provides a wonderful opportunity for the technologist to properly inform the patient about how the additional imaging process works, thus empowering the patient with knowledge.

Receiving Examination Results

According to MQSA, mammography patients must receive a written summary of their mammography procedure within 30 days of the examination date[35] (see Chapter 15 for further discussion). Facilities may fulfill this requirement through a variety of methods but must comply with the MQSA reporting standard. In today's environment of electronic information, patients have several options as to how they may receive their mammography result. Whether the patient receives their results by mail, through a facility online electronic chart service, or through their health care provider's office, informing them of all options and the timing of each option is an obligation of the mammography service.

Traditionally, the mammography examination is completed by the technologist providing this information to the patient. As an additional courtesy, the technologist may inquire whether the patient has any further questions regarding her procedure or the mammography process prior to her leaving the mammography suite. This last communication, accompanied by an expression of thanks for choosing this particular mammography facility, ensures that the patient feels that her service has ended on a satisfactory note.

Written Reinforcement

Verbal information communicated to the patient at the conclusion of the mammography examination regarding additional imaging and how results are received should be reinforced by providing this same information in a written summary to the patient before she leaves the mammography department.

RADIATION SAFETY

In April 2014, the American Association of Physicists in Medicine (AAPM) published a public position statement in response to media attention that discussed shielding during mammography. The positioning statement that addressed the general public did not recommend the use of thyroid shields, citing their potential interference with the mammography examination. The use of a lap apron for mammography is recommended if a woman is pregnant or thinks she may be pregnant.[36] Technologists performing mammography are obligated to know and to adhere to policies and procedures established by the facility where she works regarding the shielding of mammography patients and the established protocols for imaging a pregnant patient.

CREDENTIALS AND COMPLIANCE

It is the responsibility of the technologist to know and comply with all Federal and State requirements as well as professional registry (ARRT) requirements regarding the performance of mammography. Additionally, there may be individual facility requirements that are required for performing mammography.

MAMMOGRAPHY QUALITY CONTROL

It is the responsibility of the mammography technologist to understand her role in the quality control program established by the facility where she performs mammography.

Summary

The primary role of the mammography technologist is to produce radiographic images of the breast that are used to diagnose disease. Creating the mammographic image requires artistic precision and technical skill. Accomplishing this task can be challenging as the mammography procedure may generate feelings of anxiety in some women, requiring the caregiver to also impart genuine compassion as she carries out the technical examination requirements.

The mammography technologist is asked to perform a repetitive and tedious assignment in creating the mammography image, and each patient that she serves must be afforded the same focus and energy. Although this description may sound challenging, it draws to the profession committed individuals who are intrigued by the idea of making a positive difference among patients requiring breast health care.

The diversity of the breast care service offers the mammography technologist continuous personal and professional growth by being a part of a stimulating and challenging health care environment. The technologist's contribution to the breast care service is best captured by Randi Gunther, Ph.D., "The relationship between the patient and the [mammography] technologist in terms of quality communication, honest caring and confidence in technical expertise and knowledge provides the platform on which the positive [mammography] experience lies."

Review Questions

1. Explain the three levels of quality that are determined by the patient:

   Perceived quality

   Expected quality

   Actual quality

2. Explain the purpose of screening mammography and the purpose of diagnostic mammography.

3. Give specific examples of verbal and nonverbal communication that enhance the patient experience during the mammography examination.

References

1. FDA.gov/Mammography Quality Standards Act/MQSA Insights/MQSA National Statistics/. Accessed February 12, 2017.

2. American Registry of Radiologic Technologist/s/ARRT Website/consensus/. Accessed February 12, 2017.

3. Papp J. *Quality Management in the Imaging Sciences*. 4th ed. St. Louis, MO: Mosby Elsevier; 2010.

4. American Society of Radiologic Technologists/ASRT Website/. Accessed February 12, 2017.

5. American Registry of Radiologic Technologist's/ARRT Website/Code of Ethics/. Accessed February 12, 2017.

6. ACR Practice Parameter for the Performance of Screening and Diagnostic Mammography. Revised 2013 (Resolution 11)*.

7. Hendricks MM. Documentation for mammographers. *Radiol Technol.* 2007;78(5):396M–412M.

8. Homer JF, Berlin L. Malpractice issues in radiology: mammography and the patient information form. *AJR Am J Roentgenol.* 2002;178:307–310.

9. Joint Commission on Accreditation of Healthcare Organizations. *Hospital Accreditation Standards 2006*. Oakbrook Terrace, IL: Joint Commission Resources; 2006:113–123, 163–166, 338–344.

10. Arnold L. Patient care, communication, and safety in the mammography suite. *Radiol Technol.* 2016;88(1):33M–47M.

11. Adler A, Carlton R. Patient interactions. History taking. Safe patient movement and handling techniques. In: *Radiologic Imaging and Sciences and Patient Care*. 6th ed. St. Louis, MO: Elsevier; 2016:13–159.

12. Bland KI, Copeland EM. *The Breast: Comprehensive Management of Benign and Malignant Diseases*. 2nd ed. Philadelphia, PA: WB Saunders Co.; 1998:1–3, 370.

13. Saslow D, Hannan J, Ossuch J, et al. Clinical breast examination: practical recommendations for optimizing performance and reporting. *CA Cancer J Clin.* 2004;54:327–344.

14. Hartmann LC, Loprinzi CL. *Mayo Clinic Guide to Women's Cancers (Breast and Gynecologic Cancers Prevention, Treatment, Coping)*. Mayo Clinic Cancer Center; 2008.

15. American Cancer Society (ACS). Accessed February 12, 2017.

16. Keller BR, Evans KD. Fighting anxiety in order to improve the quality of breast imaging for women. Available at: http://eradimaging.com/site/printerfriendly.cfm?ID=758

17. Department of Health and Human Services/Food and Drug Administration/Code of Federal Register 21/Quality Mammography Standards; Final Rule.

18. Mears P, Voehl F. *The Executive Guide to Implementing Quality Systems*. 1st ed. CRC Press; 1995.

19. Insured Retirement Institute. Boomer expectations for retirement 2016. In: *Sixth Annual Update on the Retirement Preparedness of the Boomer Generation*. Washington, DC: IRI; 2016.

20. ACR Quality Control Manual. 1999.

21. Newstead GM. Digital mammography: cost and workflow issues. *Applied Radiology*, The Journal of Practical Imaging and Management FACR/Supplement to September 2006.

22. FDA/MQSA Insight Article/4-11-2016/. Poor Positioning Responsible For Most Clinical Image Deficiencies, Failures. Accessed February 12, 2017.

23. Fda.gov/MQSA/Guidance/Policy Guidance Help System/ Definitions/Lead Interpreting Physician/. Accessed February 12, 2017.

24. Fda.gov/MQSA/Guidance/Policy Guidance Help System/ General/Quality Assurance Program/. Accessed February 12, 2017.

25. Fda.gov/MQSA/Guidance/Policy Guidance Help System/ Policy Guidance Help System/General/Interpreting Physician Responsibilities/. Accessed February 12, 2017.

26. Fda.gov/MQSA/MQSA Insights Articles/EQUIP, Enhancing Quality Using the Inspection Program. Accessed October 21, 2016.

27. The ACR 2016 Digital Mammography Quality Control Manual.

28. Taplin SH, Rutter CM, Finder C, et al. Screening mammography: clinical image quality and the risk of interval breast cancer. *AJR Am J Roentgenol.* 2002;178:797–803.

29. The Economist. The Hawthorne effect. Nov. 2008/Online Extra/. Accessed February 12, 2017.

30. Balancing Hard and Soft Skills in Healthcare/HealthcareJobSite.com. Posted by Staff Editor, November 22, 2012.

31. Jacquelyn S. The 20 people skills you need to succeed at work. November 15, 2013. Accessed February 12, 2017.

32. Performance benchmarks for screening mammography. In: *Breast Cancer Surveillance Consortium (BCSC)*. National Cancer Institute.

33. Carroll D. *4 Reassuring Statistics About Abnormal Screening Mammograms*. Mammo Press; 2016. Accessed February 12, 2017.

34. Barton MB, Morley DS, Morre S, et al. Decreasing women's anxieties after abnormal mammograms: a controlled study. *J Natl Cancer Inst.* 2004;96:529–538.

35. Fda.gov/MQSA/Guidance/Policy Guidance Help System/ Medical Records and Reports/Communication of Results to Patients.

36. American Association of Physicists in Medicine. Public and Media/Public Position Statements/AAPM Response to Use of Lead Aprons in Mammography/April 14, 2011.

Breast Anatomy and Physiology

5

Objectives

- Link the external landmarks of the breast with the internal structures
- Delineate the internal composition of the breast and match tissue types to their radiographic appearance
- Recognize the internal and external changes to the breast as women age

---

Key Terms

- apex
- base
- breast
- Cooper ligaments
- estrogen
- inframammary fold

- parenchyma
- progesterone
- retroglandular fat space
- retromammary fat space
- terminal duct lobular unit

ANATOMY OF THE BREAST

The **breast** is a well-differentiated apocrine sweat gland of the same type found in the axilla and elsewhere in the body. These glands have evolved into an organ that produces and secretes milk during lactation.

External Appearance

External Landmarks

Breast size and shape vary individually. The external landmarks of the breast include the nipple, **inframammary fold**, and axilla (Figure 5-1). The **base** of the breast is the portion adjacent to the chest wall; the **apex** is the nipple (Figure 5-2). Four named quadrants describe location in the breast:

- Upper outer quadrant
- Upper inner quadrant
- Lower inner quadrant
- Lower outer quadrant

Clock time further refines location (Figure 5-3). (See Chapter 9 for further discussion.)

Skin

The skin covering the breast is thickest at the base of the breast (about 2 mm thick)[1,2] and becomes thinner as it approaches the nipple (0.5 mm). The skin of the nipple–areola complex measures 4 to 5 mm (Figure 5-4). Sweat glands, sebaceous (oil) glands, and hair follicles that open

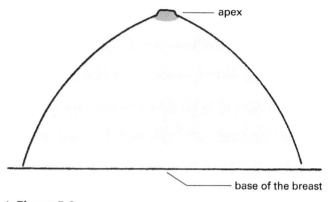

Figure 5-2
Base and apex of breast. The base of the breast is adjacent to the chest wall and the apex is the nipple.

to form skin pores occupy the skin of the body and the breast.[1] The skin pores are sometimes evident mammographically as tiny multiple lucencies across the mammogram (Figure 5-5). The sebaceous glands are prone to infection and may imitate carcinoma radiographically.

Nipple and Areola

At the breast's most distal point (the apex) are the areola and nipple (Figure 5-4). The placement of the areola and nipple again varies individually, but the nipple is the center point and provides a reference to describe location of normal anatomy and pathology. The areola is a smooth, circular darkening surrounding the nipple. Occasionally, small protrusions on the surface of the areola are visible, especially during pregnancy and lactation. The protrusions are

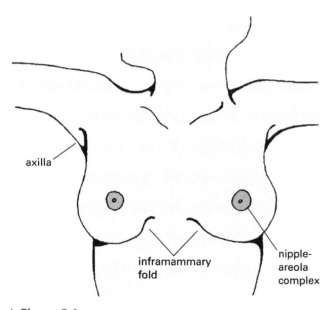

Figure 5-1
External appearance and landmarks. Breast size and shape vary individually. External landmarks include the nipple, axilla, and inframammary fold.

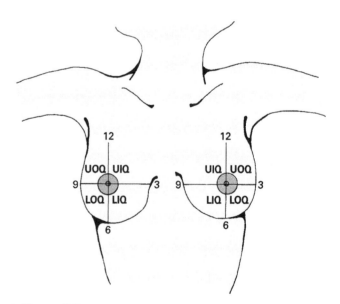

Figure 5-3
Clock time and quadrants. Four named quadrants and clock time describe location in the breast.

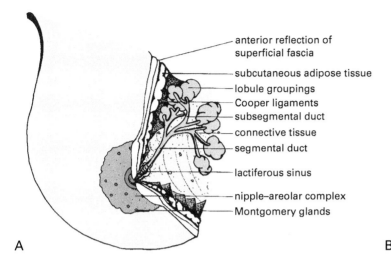

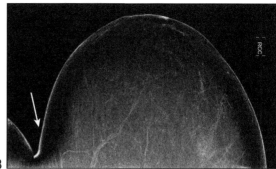

A

B

Figure 5-4
(A) The skin. The cutaway exhibits the thinning of the skin as it approaches the nipple, the thicker areolar complex, and internal breast structures. **(B)** The mammogram shows the thicker skin reflection *(arrow)* where the breast attaches to the sternum. This is a radiographic landmark when positioning for the CC view.

called Montgomery glands (named for the doctor who first described them). These glands are a specialized sebaceous type providing lubrication during lactation. The nipple is a raised, darkened, circular extension with multiple crevices. Within these crevices are five to seven orifices (collecting ducts)[3] that transfer milk from the lactiferous ducts.[4] Most often, the nipple protrudes from the breast. Unilateral or bilateral inverted nipple(s) occur occasionally. However, sudden inversion or flattening of the nipple can indicate underlying malignancy.

Each breast usually exhibits one nipple, but one or more accessory nipples can occur anywhere along the mammary ridge, which is present during our embryonic development. A common location for accessory nipples is the 6:00 o'clock position near or below the inframammary fold. Accessory nipples may have attached glandular structures and therefore are susceptible to developing cancer. For this reason, it is important to inspect for and screen accessory nipples during mammography.

Internal Anatomy

The breast lies anteriorly to the pectoralis major muscle, which runs in an oblique line from the humerus to midsternum (Figure 5-6). A layer of adipose tissue and connective fascia (not distinguishable from other breast structures on the mammogram) separate the breast from the pectoral muscle, forming the **retromammary fat space**. (Do not confuse this structure with the mammographic landmark, the **retroglandular fat space**, discussed later in this chapter.) The posterior fascia and the anterior superficial fascia of the skin completely envelope the breast (Figure 5-7).

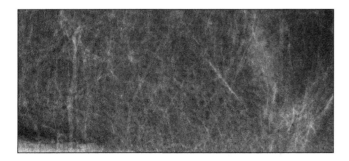

Figure 5-5
Skin pores dilate and trap air, evident as multiple lucencies across the mammogram. They appear like leopard spots on the mammogram.

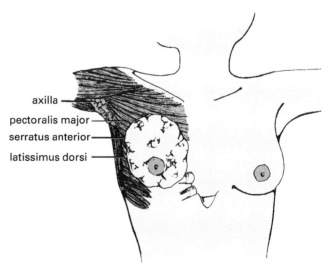

Figure 5-6
The margins of the breast. The breast lies anterior to and courses along the pectoral muscle. Its margins can reach the clavicle superiorly, the latissimus dorsi muscle laterally, and the sternum medially; it extends into the axilla.

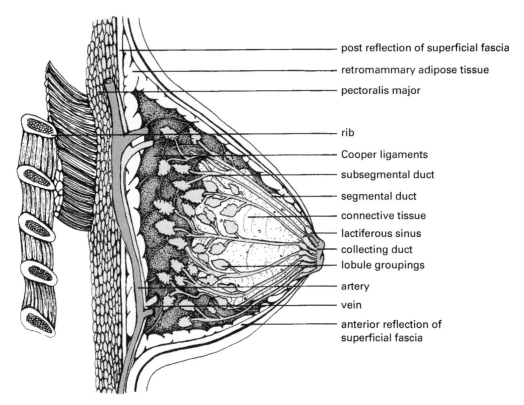

post reflection of superficial fascia

retromammary adipose tissue

pectoralis major

rib

Cooper ligaments

subsegmental duct

segmental duct

connective tissue

lactiferous sinus

collecting duct

lobule groupings

artery

vein

anterior reflection of superficial fascia

Figure 5-7
Normal anatomy of the breast.

Breast tissue covers a wider area than its outward appearance. The organ can reach as far superiorly as the clavicle (level of the second or third rib) and inferiorly to meet the abdominal wall at the level of the sixth or seventh rib (called the inframammary fold or crease). The breast tissue may also extend laterally to the edge of the latissimus dorsi muscle and medially to midsternum (Figure 5-6).[5] The organ reaches into the axilla (the Tail, axillary tail, or the Tail of Spence).[6,7] The anatomic extent of the breast tissue is critical knowledge for efficient mammographic positioning.

Internally, the breast includes a varying mixture of fatty tissue and the **parenchyma**. The parenchyma consists of the following:

- Glandular components
- Lymphatic network
- Blood vessels
- Connective and supportive stroma (Figure 5-7)

Connective and Supportive Stroma

The supportive structures of the breast are **Cooper ligaments**.[1] They are fibrous membranes that incompletely sheathe but support the lobes of the breast. The ligaments attach at the base of the breast and extend outward, attaching to the anterior superficial fascia of the skin. Figure 5-8 illustrates these structures and their distribution. Cooper

ligaments are not individually appreciated on the mammogram but are of particular significance because of their notable effect on the glandular tissue. Cooper ligaments are not elastic, like breast tissue.[8] Once stretched, for example, when the breast increases in size during pregnancy or by weight gain followed by a loss of weight, the pendulous presentation is referred to as "Cooper droop."

Other tissues that give the breast structures support consist of the extralobular and intralobular stroma. The extralobular stroma holds the larger ductal structures. The intralobular stroma is specialized tissue that gives the

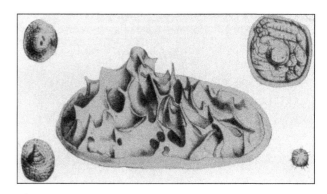

Figure 5-8
Cooper ligaments. Notice the outward projection from the base of the breast. (Drawing from Cooper SA. *Anatomy and Diseases of the Breast*. Philadelphia, PA: Lea & Blanchard; 1845.)

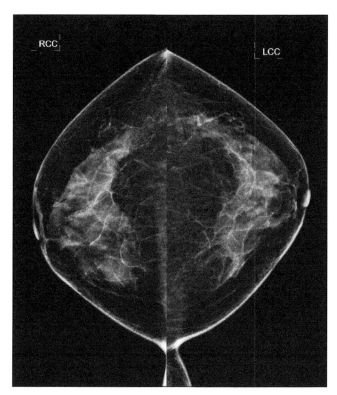

Figure 5-9
Pattern distribution. Bilateral CC mammograms demonstrating the pattern of centrally and laterally dispersed glandular tissue. Notice the symmetry of breast tissue distribution between breasts.

The Glandular Parenchyma

Distribution of Glandular Tissue

The pattern and distribution of the glandular tissue is essentially the same bilaterally. The tissue from one breast will "mirror" the opposite breast with minor variations. The majority of this tissue lies centrally and laterally within the breast. This distribution is recognizable mammographically (Figure 5-9). The total amount of glandular tissue increases and decreases with hormonal fluctuation, administration of synthetic hormones (Figure 5-10), pregnancy (Figure 5-11), lactation, menopause, and subsequently atrophies with age (Figure 5-12). Weight gain or loss also affects the radiographic appearance (Figure 5-13).

Atrophy of glandular tissue begins medially and posteriorly, working its way to the nipple. This is an important point when interpreting the mammogram, because "new" tissue or growth of tissue in these areas in an aging woman may signal the presence of malignancy.

Breast Architecture

The glandular tissue or "parenchyma" consists of 15 to 20 lobes that extend from the nipple in a radial pattern. Consequently, the ductal flow will follow this radial pattern forming the *normal architecture* of the breast (Figure 5-14). Changes in this radial pattern or architecture can indicate pathology. However, blood vessels that meander through the lobes in no apparent pattern, and Cooper ligaments, which attach to the anterior fascia, often oppose this normal ductal flow and may mammographically imitate pathologic processes.

lobule its shape and definition.[9] An extensive capillary network allows the exchange of hormones into and secretions out of the lobule and is in close contact with the lymphatic system. This intimate contact also provides for transmission of cancer cells to the lymphatic network and blood stream.

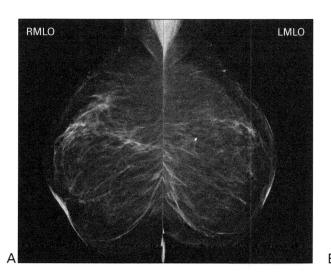

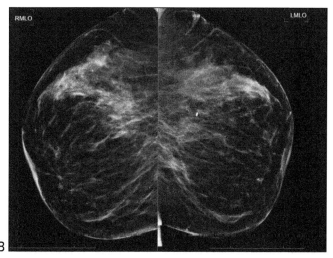

Figure 5-10
Effect of synthetic hormones. **(A)** MLO images of a patient prior to use of synthetic hormones. **(B)** Same patient after starting hormone replacement therapy. (Images courtesy Avice O'Connell, M.D., University of Rochester Medical Center. Rochester, NY.)

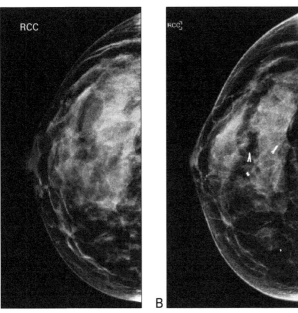

Figure 5-11
Visual effect of pregnancy. **(A)** Patient is pregnant. Presents with a 1.5-cm palpable lump at 7:00. **(B)** Patient is no longer pregnant. Had a lumpectomy due to cancer. (Images courtesy Avice O'Connell, M.D., University of Rochester Medical Center. Rochester, NY.)

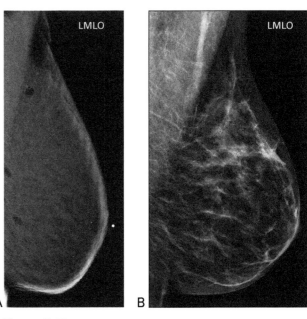

Figure 5-13
Weight change. A dramatic example of how weight gain or loss affects the proportion of glandular to fatty tissue in the breast. **(A)** MLO mammogram of a woman with anorexia nervosa. **(B)** MLO mammogram of same woman after weight gain and recovery.

The Lobes and Ductal Structures

Each of the 15 to 20 lobes contains a tree-like pattern of ductal structures (Figure 5-15). Two layers of epithelial cells of many differing types line the lumen of the ducts and smaller ductal structures.[9] Beneath the epithelial layer is a layer of

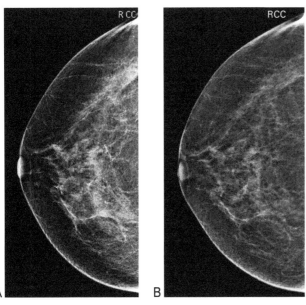

Figure 5-12
Menopause atrophy. **(A)** A more prominent glandular tissue pattern; heterogeneously dense (BIRADS B). **(B)** Four years later, after entering menopause, the glandular tissue islands are sparse; scattered fibroglandular (BIRADS C).

myoepithelium. This myoepithelium is a type of smooth muscle that contracts the acini and ducts to empty these structures of milk produced during lactation. The outer layer is the basement membrane (Figure 5-16). The changes that take place in the breast mostly occur at the level of the epithelial cell; however, the myoepithelium and the basal membrane respond to hormonal changes. These changes occur in the expected normal physiologic conditions as well as in pathologic situations.

Extending from the nipple orifice, the duct starts as a collecting duct that immediately widens into the lactiferous sinus (ampulla), a pouch-like structure that again narrows

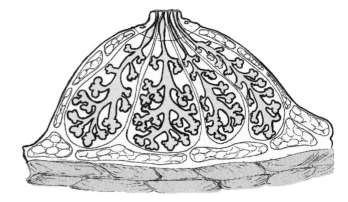

Figure 5-14
Normal architecture. The lobes extend from the nipple in a radial pattern. The ductal structures follow this flow, forming the normal architecture of the breast.

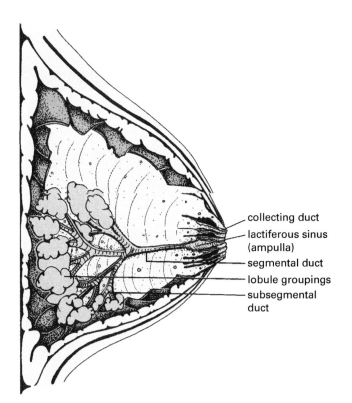

Figure 5-15
The lobe. The anatomic structures of a single lobe.

as it joins one or more segmental ducts.[3] The larger, main segmental duct branches into many medium-sized subsegmental ducts. These further branch and divide, until coming to the lobule. The lobule is the minute (1 to 2 mm) portion of the duct that holds the milk-producing elements of the breast. A single lobe contains many lobule groupings.

The small duct just outside and leading to the lobule is the extralobular terminal duct. Once inside the lobule, this duct divides into the intralobular terminal ducts. The intralobular terminal ducts end at the terminal ductules, numbering

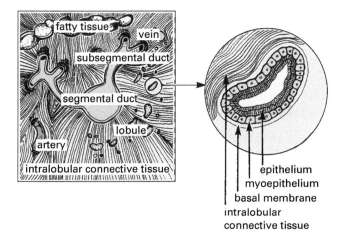

Figure 5-16
The duct. Cross-section of the breast with an enlargement to show cellular makeup of ductal walls.

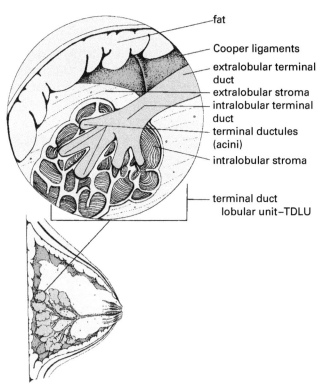

Figure 5-17
The lobule and TDLU. Enlargement of a single lobule exhibiting the intralobular stroma (a highly specialized tissue) and other structures. The terminal duct lobular unit (TDLU) begins at the extralobular terminal duct and ends at the terminal ductules.

anywhere from 10 to 100 in any lobule. The terminal ductule is a blind ending to the ductal pattern corresponding to the acinus (plural—acini), the sac-like, functional, milk-producing unit of the breast. Most authorities believe that acini form only during pregnancy, reach full maturity during lactation, and disappear at its completion.

The portion of the ductal structure starting at the extralobular terminal duct and ending at the terminal ductules is the **terminal duct lobular unit** (TDLU) (Figure 5-17). The TDLU is the critical hub of the functioning breast and is responsible for milk production and hormonal and nutritional exchange. The TDLU increases and decreases in *number* and *size* depending on life cycle changes, menstrual cycle, and hormone fluctuation. Most pathology, including most types of cancer, arises from the TDLU.

▮▮ PHYSIOLOGY OF THE BREAST

To discuss physiology of the breast, it is first necessary to define the "resting breast." In this case, "resting" means that there is no pregnancy or lactation. However, the breast is never truly resting. A constant state of change exists due to menstrual cycle superimposed over life cycle changes. These changes range from proliferation of cells or ductal structures to involution, regression, and atrophy of these same structures. In addition, many of these structures fail to completely regress or involute, or there can be early atrophy. This variation in duct appearance causes difficulty for pathologists attempting to define "normal" breast anatomy.

Hormonal Influences during the Life Cycle

At about the age of 17 years, and in response to earlier hormonal stimuli, the formation of the ductal structures, including the lobule, is complete.

Influencing the normal physiologic changes of the breast are many hormones. The two most prominent hormones active in breast physiology are **estrogen** (responsible for ductal proliferation) and **progesterone** (responsible for lobular proliferation and growth). Prolactin is another significant hormone but is present only during initial breast growth, pregnancy, and lactation. Abnormal growth and change in the breast are partially due to the over- or underproduction of hormones. Inconsistencies in hormone levels from one menstrual cycle to another can also produce aberrant changes.

Menstrual Cycle Changes

The following changes occur during the menstrual cycle:

1. During the first phase of the menstrual cycle, estrogen stimulates epithelial proliferation and enlargement within the larger ductal structures.
2. During ovulation, epithelial cells proliferate in the lobule in response to progesterone,[1] forming new TDLUs. The lobules enlarge and the terminal ductules are more apparent. An increase in blood flow and interstitial fluid retention leads to premenstrual lumpiness and tenderness.
3. At the onset of menstruation, estrogenic influences cause involution and regression of the terminal ductal lobular unit and the lobules.[9] This regression can take several weeks.[10] Not all the lobules regress or involute, leaving some fully formed lobules behind.

Pregnancy and Lactation

Changes within the breast are evident within several weeks of conception. These changes are secondary to the increase in estrogen, progesterone, and prolactin production.[5] At this time, the epithelial cells again proliferate, increasing the size and number of TDLUs (Figure 5-18). The lobules enlarge and the acini fully form for the production of milk. After birth, the epithelial cells of the acini undergo secretory changes as a result of the hormonal influence of prolactin, allowing for the production and secretion of milk. Milk production causes ductal dilation.

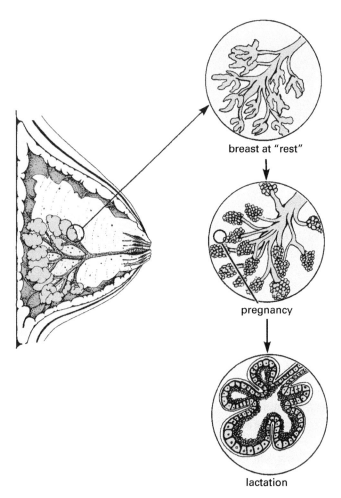

Figure 5-18
Development of the TDLU. The development of the TDLUs from a "resting" state to pregnancy and lactation.

When lactation ends, the structures begin to involute and regress. Hoeffken and Lanyi[1] stated, "The degree of involution following lactation is variable. It can be quite extensive with almost total replacement of stromal and parenchymal tissue by fat with only fibrous septa, ducts, and vessels remaining. In spite of this, however, the breast retains its ability to redevelop parenchyma and secrete milk during any subsequent pregnancy."

Menopause Atrophy

Menopause atrophy of mammary tissue commences at menopause and ceases 3 to 5 years later. Atrophy begins medially and posteriorly, then laterally, working its way to the nipple. In addition, atrophy can be spotty within one breast—one lobule may disappear, while an adjacent one does not. Menopausal atrophy may also be asymmetric from one breast to the other. The breast will lose its supportive tissue to fat, producing a smaller breast or a larger, more pendulous breast. This replacement by fat can occasionally give rise to a lump, physically imitating carcinoma; mammography is useful in these cases. The epithelial cells of the lobules will flatten and the basement membrane will become indistinguishable from the atrophied specialized connective tissue. Once this occurs, the lobule loses its definition and eventually disappears completely. The smaller ducts involute; however, the larger ducts may remain (Figure 5-12).

Postmenopausal Hormone Replacement Therapy

Some post- and/or perimenopausal women elect to receive hormone replacement therapy (HRT). The benefits of HRT include alleviation of post- and perimenopausal symptoms and a decrease in risk or improvement of osteoporosis.[11]

Contraindications for HRT are family or personal history of breast cancer, particularly if immunoassays of the original tumor were estrogen receptor positive. Studies on HRT suggest an increase in risk for breast cancer with long-term use.[12] Additionally, HRT can influence the growth of an existing tumor.[13] Still, the benefits of HRT in most cases outweigh the potential risk, as long as women follow the recommended regimen of yearly mammograms, routine physical examinations, and breast self-examinations.

If the woman has had a hysterectomy, HRT may only include estrogen. If she still has her uterus, then her doctor will prescribe a combination of estrogen and progesterone. The addition of progesterone prohibits the proliferation of the uterine lining, reducing the risk of associated endometrial cancer.

Hormones come in many pill forms, a skin patch, or a vaginal cream. Dosages vary depending on the presence or severity of postmenopausal symptoms and the severity of side effects of HRT. Side effects influencing the breast may include breast enlargement, pain and lumpiness, and fibrocystic changes, including cysts. Adjustment of the dosage depends on the required benefits versus the tolerated side effects.

A change is immediately noticeable in the breast at the inception of HRT, especially in those women completely through menopause. The breast tissue reblossoms, in its entirety, from larger ducts to the smaller ductal structures, causing an overall increase in glandular tissue. Additionally, interstitial fluids may increase.

▌▌ MAMMOGRAPHIC ANATOMY

Symmetry and Distribution

The American College of Radiology[14] details descriptive terminology for the ratio of fatty to glandular tissue in the breast. Figure 5-19 describes these terms, which replace the descriptive Wolfe classifications (N, P1, P2, DYS). Viewing

Tissue Composition   Terminology

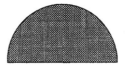
fatty—predominately fatty composition

fibro-fatty—more fat than glandular tissue

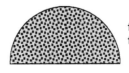
fibro-glandular—more glandular than fatty tissue

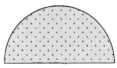
glandular—predominately glandular composition

Figure 5-19
American College of Radiology—Descriptive Terminology. This figure details the terminology from the American College of Radiology to describe the ratio of glandular to fatty tissue in the breast.

the four-view mammogram back to back (Figure 5-20), there is an apparent symmetry with minor variation in the distribution of the glandular tissue from right to left. If one breast is larger than the other, even slightly, then the parenchyma will present a greater volume in that breast. This is normal variation. Asymmetric breast tissue is not uncommon and may be a normal variant. However, asymmetric tissue, especially when it is a new finding as opposed to a stable appearance confirmed by a previous study, may indicate the presence of carcinoma.

Case Study **5-1**

Refer to Figure 5-19 and the text and respond to the following questions:

1. Most women who have mammograms have which type of breast tissue composition?

2. Why does the composition of breast tissue change during our different decades of life?

3. Which type of tissue composition allows us to detect breast cancer easily?

4. What is the function of glandular tissue?

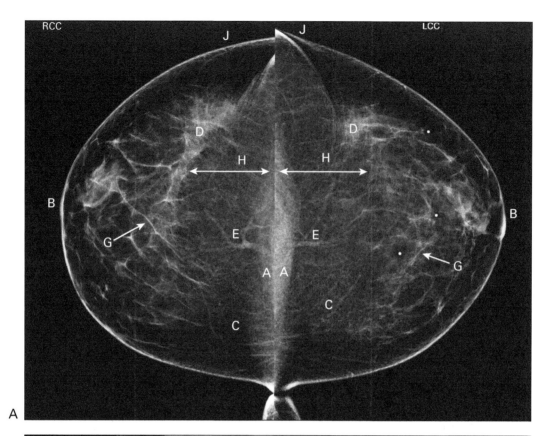

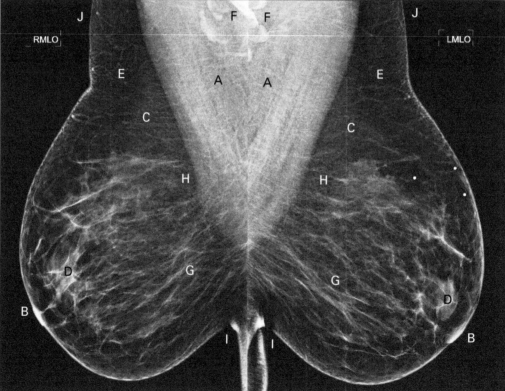

Figure 5-20

Mammographic anatomy landmarks and symmetry. Back-to-back **(A)** CC and **(B)** MLO projections demonstrating both anatomical structures and mammographic landmarks useful for positioning purposes and as descriptive aids. (*A*) Pectoral muscle. (*B*) Nipple. (*C*) Adipose tissue. (*D*) Glandular tissue. (*E*) Blood vessel. (*F*) Lymph node. (*G*) Cooper ligaments. (*H*) Retroglandular fat space. (*I*) Inframammary fold. (*J*) Axilla. Note that the distribution of breast tissue, with minor variation, is symmetrical from right to left.

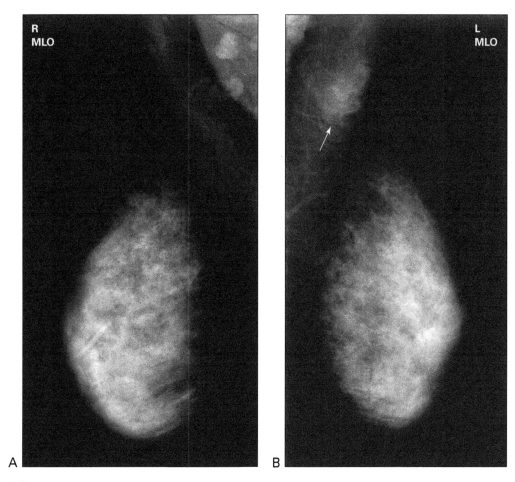

Figure 5-21
Ectopic tissue. Ectopic tissue occurs most often in the low axillary region. It may be **(A)** symmetric in its distribution or **(B)** asymmetric in occurrence and distribution (*arrow*) from one breast to the other.

Case Study 5-2

Using Figure 5-20, and without reading the figure legend, list as many radiographic landmarks (labeled A–J) as you can.

Occasional ectopic tissue appears bilaterally, high in the upper outer quadrants of the breast and in the low axillary area[3] and is quite normal. The appearance is usually symmetric but in some cases may be of greater volume in one breast or may appear in one breast only (Figure 5-21). The technologist must include this low axillary region during positioning of the oblique view, as cancer does occur in this ectopic tissue, although it is rare.

Normal Anatomy

Many individual anatomic breast structures are evident on the mammogram, while others are only recognizable by the effect or pattern they form. Additionally, named mammographic landmarks are useful descriptive aids for discussing location within, and positioning of, the breast (Figure 5-20).

The nipple, when in profile, and its surrounding areola produce an increased radiographic density along the skin line due to the thickness of the areolar complex (Figure 5-22A). If the nipple is not in profile, the mammogram often shows the nipple as a well-circumscribed radiopaque density (Figure 5-22B) that may imitate a mass. Extending posteriorly from the nipple is the glandular tissue, which appears as a radiopaque "sheet" (the white or "denser" areas).[15] Adipose tissue (fat) appears as radiolucent areas (black, grayer, less dense areas) on the mammogram. Fatty tissue surrounds and is dispersed among the glandular structures. The retroglandular fat space (Figure 5-20) is a landmark useful for positioning purposes and indicates the band of fatty tissue lying posteriorly to the glandular sheet (this should not be confused with the retromammary fat space, an anatomic structure not evident on the mammogram).

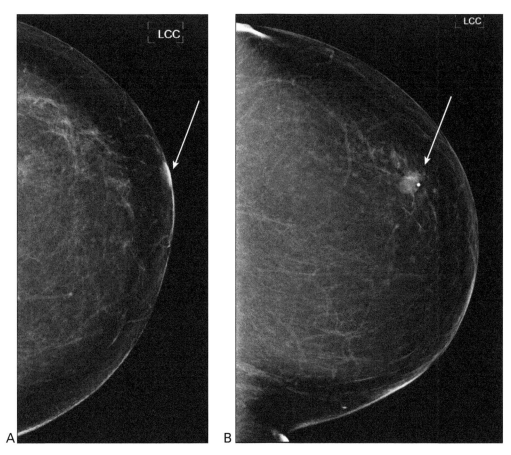

Figure 5-22
The nipple (*arrows*) **(A)** shown in profile as an increase in density along the skin line and **(B)** demonstrating a well-circumscribed density when not in profile; marked with a metallic BB.

This glandular "sheet" consists of blood vessels, the lymphatic network, supportive and connective tissue (stroma), and the various ductal structures. The ductal structures are not individually evident, but form a pattern of radial lines extending from the nipple. This ductal pattern is recognizable with ductography (Figure 5-23). Blood vessels are apparent as separate structures, especially when arteries characteristically calcify (Figure 5-24). During ductography, a filled lymphatic network may be evident, but usually the lymphatic

channels are indistinguishable on the plain mammogram. In contrast, lymph nodes of varying number are apparent both in the axilla and often within the breast (intramammary lymph nodes) (Figure 5-25). They appear as smoothly outlined isodense masses, usually with telltale lucency within the borders.[3] The only portions of the connective stroma discernible mammographically are Cooper ligaments. They present as thin curved convex lines leading to the subcutaneous adipose tissue (Figure 5-20). These structures can imitate architectural distortion, a distinctive sign of carcinoma.

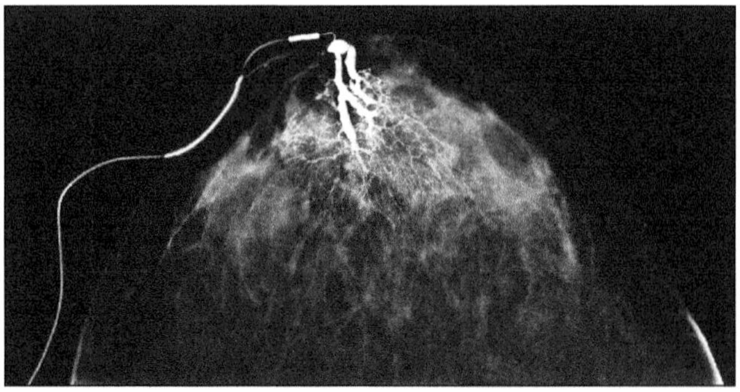

Mammographic Changes due to Life Cycle and Hormonal Influences

Pregnancy and Lactation

The mammographic appearance of the breast during pregnancy (Figure 5-11) and lactation (Figure 5-26) shows increased density due to physiologic changes, milk production, and increased blood supply. The increased density can reduce the accuracy of mammography. Mammography may be useful for the symptomatic pregnant or lactating woman, but screening is usually reserved until lactation ends. An

Figure 5-23
Ductal pattern. CC projection ductogram showing the radial pattern of the ductal structures.

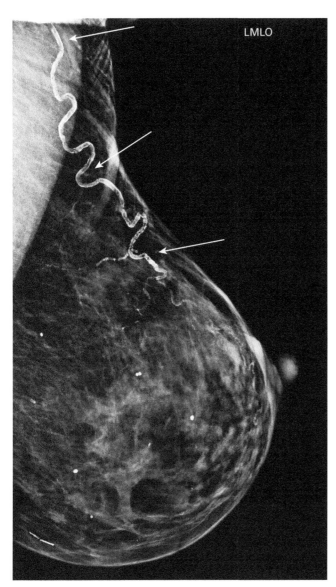

Figure 5-24
Arterial calcifications. MLO projection demonstrating characteristic calcification of an artery (*arrows*).

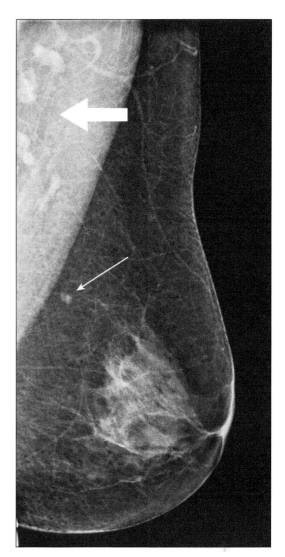

Figure 5-25
Lymph nodes. MLO mammogram showing lymph nodes in the axilla (*large arrow*) and an intramammary lymph node (*small arrow*) trailing into the breast.

exception is if the woman is at high risk for breast cancer (history of personal breast cancer, family history of mother or sister with premenopausal breast cancer). The total length of pregnancy and lactation, in these cases, may exceed recommended screening intervals for high-risk women. This woman should schedule her screening mammogram sometime after the birth of her child. Any lactating woman should nurse just before the mammogram. The removal of the super imposed milk improves visualization of the breast tissue.

Menstruation

An increase in overall density of the breast tissue during menstruation is usually not evident on a mammogram (however, Haagensen describes difficulty and discrepancies in physical examination during the premenstrual phase).[5] During

the premenstrual period tolerating the vigorous compression necessary for mammography may be more difficult for some women. Extreme tenderness may limit compression. The best time to perform mammography is during the week after the menses. In large-scale screening programs, this type of scheduling is extremely difficult; however, the patient can make an informed decision about scheduling if she has a regular menstrual cycle. Advising women to decrease caffeine 2 weeks before the mammogram (caffeine adds to the hormone effect) may help prevent extreme discomfort during the compression stage of mammography.

Menopausal Changes

The menopausal breast will often be of greater fatty content on the mammogram (Figure 5-12). Asymmetric tissue may be due to uneven atrophy.

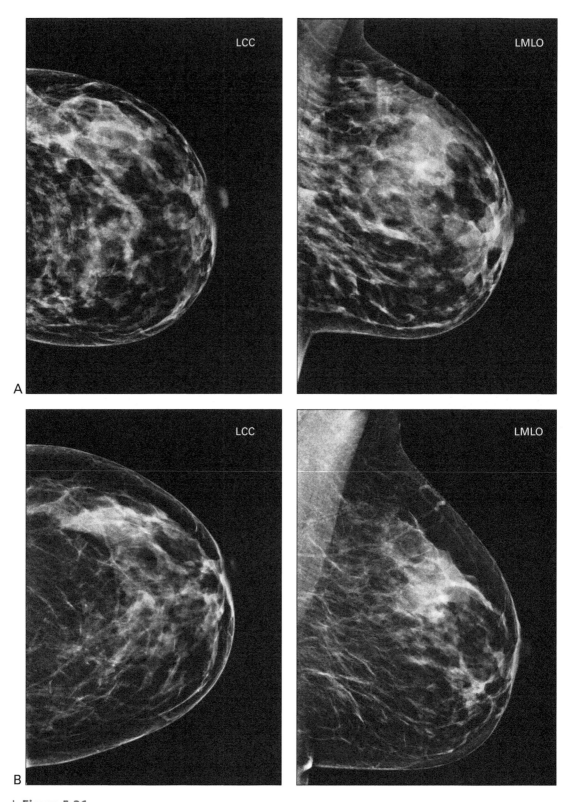

Figure 5-26
Visual effect of milk production. **(A)** The lactating breast; increased tissue density due to fluid production. **(B)** The normal breast. (Images courtesy Avice O'Connell, M.D., University of Rochester Medical Center Rochester, NY.)

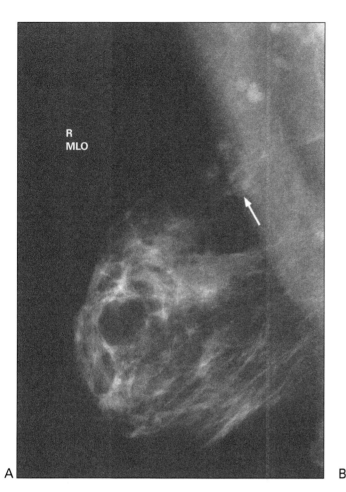 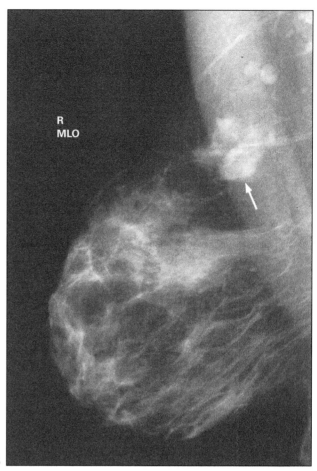

Figure 5-27
HRT. Mammographic changes due to HRT can be uneven from one breast to the other, often requiring special views and workup to prove hormone effect. This ectopic glandular tissue **(A)** (*arrow*) has increased in size and density **(B)** (*arrow*) due to HRT.

Postmenopausal Hormone Replacement Therapy

The effects of HRT are apparent mammographically, especially in those women who were completely through menopause before implementing an HRT program (Figure 5-10). In comparison to previous mammographic studies, the mammogram will show an increase in density of the parenchyma, requiring greater technique. The breast may show fibrocystic changes. Additionally, glandular structures may cover a wider area requiring the technologist to pay special attention to positioning. The patient's breast may increase in size secondary to side effects of HRT and/or weight gain. She may not compress as easily and may not tolerate vigorous compression due to increased discomfort.

Studies demonstrate that HRT probably does not affect the sensitivity of the mammogram but may reduce the specificity.[6,16] The rejuvenation of the glandular structures can be spotty and uneven, adding to the difficult chore of interpretation (Figure 5-27). The initial mammogram after starting HRT is the most critical and may require supplementary views and a workup to prove hormonal effect. However, it is not unusual to see continuing mammographic changes in subsequent years of therapy.

Review Questions

1. How do we describe the location of a region of interest: In general? Specifically?

2. Identify the superior, inferior, medial, and lateral borders of the breast. Which are mobile margins and which are fixed?

3. Describe the location of a terminal duct lobular unit. What is the significance of this structure?

References

1. Hoeffken W, Lanyi M. *Mammography*. Philadelphia, PA: WB Saunders Company; 1977.
2. Shaw-de Parades E. *Atlas of Film-Screen Mammography*. Baltimore, MD: Urban & Schwarzenberg; 1989.
3. Logan-Young W, Hoffman NY. *Breast Cancer: A Practical Guide to Diagnosis*. Vol. I. Rochester, NY: Mt. Hope Publishing Company; 1996.
4. Azzopardi JG. *Problems in Breast Pathology*. London, UK: WB Saunders; 1979.
5. Haagensen CC. *Disease of the Breast*. Philadelphia, PA: WB Saunders Company; 1986.
6. Laya MB, et al. Effect of postmenopausal hormonal replacement therapy on mammographic density and parenchymal pattern. *Radiology*. 1995;196:433–437.
7. Egan RL, McSweeney MB. The normal breast. In: Harper P, ed. *Ultrasound, Mammography*. Baltimore, MD: University Park Press; 1985.
8. Cooper SA. *Anatomy and Diseases of the Breast*. Philadelphia, PA: Lea & Blanchard; 1845.
9. Page DL, Anderson TJ. *Diagnostic Histopathology of the Breast*. Edinburgh: Churchill Livingstone; 1987.
10. Gallager HS. Pathology of benign breast disease. In: Harper P, ed. *Ultrasound, Mammography*. Baltimore, MD: University Park Press; 1985.
11. Kopans DB. *Breast Imaging*. 2nd ed. Philadelphia, PA: Lippincott–Raven; 1998.
12. Colditz GA, et al. The use of estrogens and progestins and the risk of breast cancer in postmenopausal women. *N Engl J Med*. 1995;332:1589–1593.
13. Harvey SC, et al. Marked regression of nonpalpable breast cancer after cessation of hormone replacement therapy. *Am J Roentgenol*. 1996;167:394–395.
14. D'Orsi C, et al. *ACR Breast Imaging Reporting & Data System*. 4th ed. Reston, VA: American College of Radiology; 2003.
15. National Council on Radiation Protection and Measurements. Mammography—A Users Guide. NCRP report No. 85. Bethesda, MD: National Council on Radiation Protection and Measurements; 1986.
16. Thurfjell EL, et al. Screening mammography: sensitivity and specificity in relation to hormone replacement therapy. *Radiology*. 1997;203:339–341.

Bibliography

Egan RL. *Breast Imaging Diagnosis and Morphology of Breast Diseases*. Philadelphia, PA: WB Saunders Company; 1988.

Logan-Young WW, Hanes-Hoffman NY. *Breast Cancer: A Practical Guide to Diagnosis*. Vol. I. Rochester, NY: Mt. Hope Publishing Company; 1996.

Stomper PC, et al. Mammographic changes associated with postmenopausal hormone replacement therapy: a longitudinal study. *Radiology*. 1990;174:487–490.

Tabar L, Dean PB. *Teaching Atlas of Mammography*. 2nd ed. New York: Thieme Inc.; 1985.

Wolfe JN. *Xeroradiography of the Breast*. Springfield, IL: Charles C. Thomas; 1972.

Mammographic Pathology

6

Objectives

- Describe the pathologist's contributions to a diagnosis when a biopsy is requested
- Recognize the radiographic appearance of:
  - Benign breast disease
  - Malignant disease
- Report the external condition of the breast to the radiologist

Key Terms

- carcinoma in situ
- epithelial hyperplasia
- genes
- initiation
- invasive carcinoma
- progression
- promotion
- staging

MAMMOGRAPHY AND BREAST DISEASE DIAGNOSIS

For most patients, the radiologist makes a diagnosis at the time of her visit: "I'll see you next year for your annual screening mammogram," or "I want you to come back in 6 months," or "We need to schedule a biopsy." This diagnosis is based on information and experience in the detection of breast disease. The information comes from imaging studies performed by the technologist and may include a mammogram, an ultrasound examination, MRI, nuclear medicine study, patient breast history form, information from a technologist who observed the patient during the exam, and from the physician's clinical breast examination (CBE).

Detection and diagnosis, the twin pillars of a medical investigation, are improved with specialized knowledge, diligence, and clinical experience. Yet for all our tests and observations, there are some indeterminate cases where the radiologist recommends a biopsy in order to provide a definitive diagnosis. For these cases, we must investigate what is happening *inside* the breast, at the cellular level, to verify observations made during interpretation of the images in order to understand the condition of the tissue. When the radiologist recommends a biopsy, it is the pathologist who makes the ultimate diagnosis.

This chapter focuses on three areas of interest to a radiologic technologist:

1. A brief explanation of breast disease development, its etiology (progression from healthy tissue to nonfunctional tissue with uncontrolled growth), and how the pathologist contributes to the process
2. Aspects of the detection process by the radiologist and the radiologic technologist prior to a diagnosis
3. A suggested approach the radiologic technologist can use during the detection of breast disease.

For the technologist, improved knowledge of breast disease and experience in observing the physical indications for these conditions leads to better quality mammograms and earlier disease detection. This chapter summarizes the diagnostic implications of various physical and visual presentations.

THE ROLE OF THE PATHOLOGIST

How Does the Pathologist Contribute to the Diagnostic Process?

The pathologist is the person who makes the diagnosis when the radiologist recommends a biopsy. The evidence from a microscopic examination of the tissue at the cellular

Table 6-1 • Cancer Types in Ductal and Lobular Carcinoma

DUCTAL	LOBULAR
Intraductal	In situ
Invasive	Invasive
Comedo	
Inflammatory	
Medullary	
Mucinous	
Papillary	
Scirrhous	
Tubular	

level reveals information not available to the radiologist from the radiographic study. Let's take a brief look at what the pathologist does.

A brief generic job description includes the following:

Professional Education
- Completed advanced study of human tissues
- Demonstrated ability to identify and study function, morphology, and pathology of difficult-to-identify cells, fibrous, and connective tissues
- Trained in diagnosis of lesions
- Trained in cyto (nuclear studies) analysis of human tissues
- Trained in identifying types of cancers, progression, variations, and related causes (Table 6-1)
- Trained in radiographic studies

Professional Experience
- Performs microscopic examination to detect changes in cell structures indicative of disease
- Prepares or supervises preparation of biopsied tissue for microscopic study
- Devises or directs use of special stains for isolating, identifying, and studying pathology
- Makes comparisons with controls and standard references
- Makes notations of the prevalence of lesions through studies and autopsy specimens
- Looks for features (size, border, calcifications, distance between features, etc.) that may predict recurrence, relative risk, and as the basis for recommendations for additional therapy or surgery
- Follows specified pathways for a suspected disease

Diagnostic Reporting
- Provides data to delineate the cause and progress of disease that impairs bodily functions
- Indicates evidence of staging, using evidence from examined slides (Table 6-2)

Table 6-2 • Staging: General Categories and Characteristics of Breast Cancer

STAGE	TUMOR SIZE	AXILLARY METASTASES	DISTANT METASTASES	CONDITION OF METASTATIC NODES/OTHER CHARACTERISTICS
Stage 0	Carcinoma in situ	No	No	Not applicable
Stage I	≤2 cm	No	No	Not applicable
Stage II	>2 cm but <5 cm	Yes	No	Microscopic involvement of lymph nodes
Stage III	Any size	Yes	No	Lymph nodes are fixed together in a matted axillary mass; invasion of chest wall; skin involvement
Stage IV	Any size	Yes	Yes	Any condition

- Makes a diagnosis in accordance with criteria that is both quantitative and qualitative
- Makes recommendations for additional therapy or surgery
- Rates suspected tissue as benign or equivocal, suspicious or malignant

Pathology Report

A pathologist's report presents a picture from the inside to better serve the case.[1]

- **Specimen:** Tissue samples taken from the breast, lymph nodes, or both.
- **Clinical history:** A short description of the patient and how the breast abnormality was found. It also describes the kind of surgery (if any) that was done.
- **Clinical diagnosis:** This is the preliminary diagnosis physicians (referring physician, radiologist, oncologist) were expecting before the breast tissue sample was tested.
- **Gross description:** A description of the tissue sample(s). It includes physical features as size, weight, texture, and color for each sample.
- **Microscopic description:** A description of how cancer cells look under the microscope. This is where the pathologist's specialized knowledge and skills (recognizing disease types and abnormalities in the cell, the use of stains to better visualize abnormalities, and use of standards and references for cancer's appearance) pay big dividends in shaping the report recommendations.
- **Special tests or markers:** This section of the report describes the results of tests for proteins, **genes**, and how fast the cells are growing.
- **Summary or final diagnosis:** This is a short description of all the important findings for each tissue sample.

Biopsied tissue (Figure 6-1) is prepared and studied by a pathologist who is familiar with breast cancer and skilled at recognizing changes in cell structure at various stages of breast disease.

The cytopathologist/histopathologist identifies the type of disease in the examined cells and the condition or function of its cells along the same continuum from healthy to dying. This analysis appears in the diagnosis for the examined cells.

ETIOLOGY OF BREAST CANCER

Breast cancers are masters of disguise, ever changing, taking on various forms, yet always relentless in leading healthy breast tissue toward the death of its host.

Breast tissue evolves as a result of monthly and life cycle changes (Figure 6-2). The ever-changing radiographic appearance of breast tissue presents a challenge to the radiologist trying to detect disease. Radiologists must recognize not only normal involutional patterns as the woman ages but also radiographic patterns of malignancy.

Distinguishing progressive changes in cells from normal to benign, through premalignant stages, and finally into malignant conditions is the essence of ongoing imaging and diagnostic development. The ability to observe, measure, and record subtle changes in the breast during

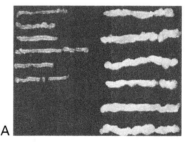

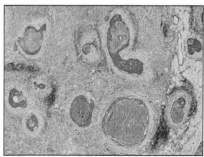

Figure 6-1
(A) Biopsied breast tissue. **(B)** Stained slide, as viewed through the pathologist's microscope.

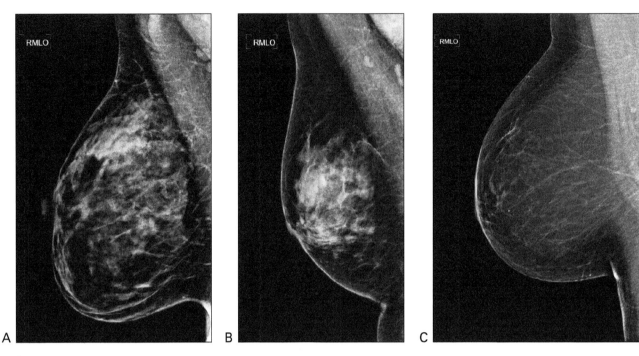

Figure 6-2
The composition of breast tissue changes as we age, have children, and go through menopause. **(A)** The younger woman's more glandular breast is firm and "perky." **(B)** A middle-aged woman's breast. She is approximately equal in glandular to adipose tissue ratio. The breast feels softer and has lost some of its perkiness. **(C)** The typical postmenopausal breast; soft and droopy.

the progression of a disease is not only useful for diagnosis, it also results in a more definitive study that is important for patient prognosis and treatment.[2]

A series of defects occur in a cell before it becomes cancer. There are three phases for the development of breast cancer[3–5]:

1. **Initiation**: A mutation occurs. A carcinogenic agent triggers the beginning by damaging and changing DNA in a cell. Genes 17 (BrCA1), 13 (BrCA2), and 22 (CHEK2) are among the better-known locations in breast cells where cancer originates.[6] These genes, programmed to repair defective cellular damage, become modified and are unable to produce the required proteins and enzymes to continue normal cell functions. Proteins and enzymes are the necessary chemical switches that turn a gene on or off, allowing it to perform its designated job.

2. **Promotion**: A process where mutant-damaged cells can be further weakened by any number of agents such as cigarettes, some household chemicals, injury, or exposure to carcinogenic agents. These agents by themselves may not be enough to initiate a cancer, but over time, they promote the uncontrolled growth and proliferation of mutated cells.

3. **Progression**: In this third phase, cells lose all normal functions except the ability to grow more abnormal cells—they metastasize; they break through outer walls of the duct or lobule and spread the out-of-control,

fast-growing cancerous cells without their functioning DNA to nearby tissue or organs. In breast disease, the favored carriers of metastatic cancer cells are the lymphatic system and blood circulatory system.

Breast Cancer (BrCA): It's in the Genes

Breast cancer is a multifactorial disease, meaning a variety of factors contribute to the biological processes involved in carcinogenesis. Some of these factors are genetic changes in oncogenes and in tumor suppressor genes, growth factor imbalances, enzyme production, and telomerase activity. Once initiation begins, neoplastic changes evolve in a single cell line resulting in a progressively dysplastic cellular appearance, deregulated cell growth, and ultimately a cancer.

Genes carry the DNA code to produce the necessary proteins and enzymes that guide the cell to function as a normal/healthy cell. Genes signal the cell to turn on or off at appropriate times according to their unique code, to transfer and exchange necessary chemicals within the cell's cytoplasm, to differentiate cell/tissue types (as skin, blood, bone, nerve, breast, etc.), control growth, and repair and replace functioning specialized breast cells. Damage to genes results in mutations; mutations change the cells they control. Cancers are the result of uncontrolled growth of cells that have lost their ability to function as normal cells; no longer can they reproduce themselves with an exact copy of their normal predecessors (transcription or translation of DNA), nor can they carry on their specialized activities.

Tumor suppressor genes (BrCA1, BrCA2, CHEK2) control growth factor imbalances and produce specialized proteins and telomerase, a key enzyme. When the tumor suppressor gene is not activated because telomerase is not available, life as we know it has changed for that cell.

Oncogenes (genes with mutations known to initiate cancer) are responsible for hereditary breast cancers BrCA1 and BrCA2, accounting for 5% to 10% of all breast cancers.[7] For the other 90% to 95% of breast cancers, the cause is a mutation to genes in healthy breast cells. These changes are generated by a myriad of possible factors such as lifestyle, occupation, injury, aging, and a host of other "life's little insults."

Most breast cancers originate in the epithelial cells that line the ducts and the lobules. Epithelial carcinogenesis is a multistage process that may take a decade or longer before clinical signs are evident.

Diseases of the Breast

The majority of benign and malignant breast disease occurs in the terminal duct lobular unit (TDLU). They arise predominantly from the epithelial cell layer; however, the fibrous or connective tissue also plays a role. Pathologic changes also can occur in the larger ducts. Rarely, breast disease involves the skin or the nipple. Figure 6-3 illustrates various types of breast disease and their common site of origin.

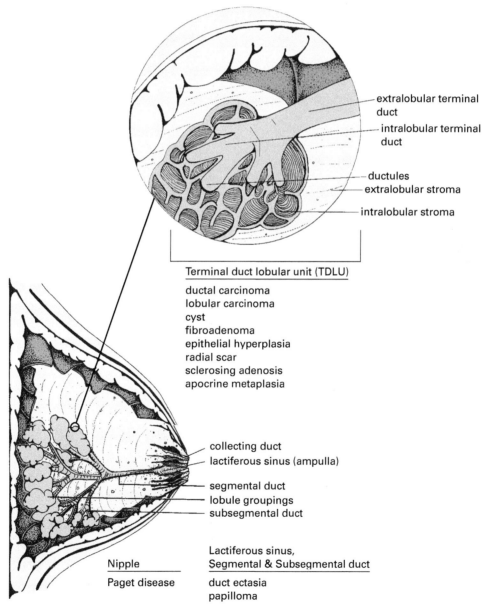

extralobular terminal duct

intralobular terminal duct

ductules
extralobular stroma

intralobular stroma

Terminal duct lobular unit (TDLU)

ductal carcinoma
lobular carcinoma
cyst
fibroadenoma
epithelial hyperplasia
radial scar
sclerosing adenosis
apocrine metaplasia

collecting duct
lactiferous sinus (ampulla)

segmental duct
lobule groupings
subsegmental duct

Nipple	Lactiferous sinus, Segmental & Subsegmental duct
Paget disease	duct ectasia papilloma

Figure 6-3
Various breast diseases and their most common site of origin.

The majority of breast cancers, approximately 95%, arise in the TDLU. The extralobular terminal duct is the site of *ductal carcinoma* and the intralobular terminal duct the site of *lobular carcinoma*. However, the terms "ductal" and "lobular" also describe a cell type rather than a site of origin. In addition, other types of cancer, although small in number, arise from the stromal tissue and at the site of the nipple, as in the case of Paget disease. Inflammatory carcinoma, another type of breast cancer, involves invasion of the skin lymphatics evident by skin erythema and edema. Some breast cancers do not fit any category or cell type; these are *carcinoma NOS* (not otherwise specified).[8]

Ductal and lobular carcinomas are classified into specific types of cancer depending on the changes that occur in the epithelial cells, as well as other characteristics (Table 6-1). The most common form of breast cancer is *invasive (infiltrating) ductal carcinoma NOS*. Approximately 65% of breast cancers are invasive ductal carcinomas, 20% are ductal carcinoma in situ (DCIS), and 10% to 13% are lobular.[9,10]

There are 21 distinct histological subtypes of breast cancer, and four different molecular subtypes. The molecular subtypes are:

1. Luminal A (HR+/HER2−): The slow-growing, less aggressive types of breast cancer. These cancers respond favorably to hormone therapy.
2. Luminal B (HR+/HER2+): Characterized by actively dividing cells. These cancers are higher grade and more aggressive than the luminal A types.
3. Triple negative (HR−/HER2−): More common in African American women, in premenopausal women, and in women with the BrCA1 gene mutation. There are no targeted therapies for these tumors.
4. HER2 enriched (HR-/HER2+): There are no hormone receptors on the surface of the breast cancer cell; instead, there are many HER2 receptors; the cancer cells produce an excess of the HER2 protein. The HER2 proteins control growth and replication of the cell; with an overabundance of HER2 receptors, these cells rapidly reproduce themselves in an uncontrollable fashion. These cancers are very aggressive, with an increased rate of recurrence. Long-term prognosis is poor.

Epithelial Hyperplasia

Most experts believe that malignant disease develops through a process that starts with **epithelial hyperplasia**, sometimes referred to as epitheliosis or papillomatosis. Epithelial hyperplasia is the increase in number, over the normal amount, of epithelial cells lining the duct. Certain degrees of epithelial hyperplasia may be premalignant.

Benign breast conditions are categorized into three groups, depending on whether they are an increased risk for later development of breast cancer.

1. Nonproliferative lesions: These do not affect breast cancer risk. Examples are fibrocystic changes, mild hyperplasia, adenosis of the nonsclerosing variety, a single papilloma, fat necrosis, duct ectasia, periductal fibrosis, squamous and apocrine metaplasia, epithelial-related calcifications, lipoma, and hamartoma.
2. Proliferative lesions without atypia: Associated with an excessive growth of the epithelial cells that line the ducts and lobules, this has a 1.5X-2X increase in later development of breast cancer. Some examples of this condition are ductal hyperplasia without atypia, fibroadenoma, sclerosing adenosis, papillomatosis, and radial scar.
3. Proliferative lesions with atypia: An excessive growth of epithelial cells that line the ducts and lobules, with some abnormal cells present. Associated with a 4X-5X increased risk for later development of breast cancer. Examples include atypical ductal hyperplasia and atypical lobular hyperplasia.

The three grades of epithelial hyperplasia are mild, moderate, and florid. Epithelial hyperplasia can progress to atypical hyperplasia in which the epithelial cells increase and change in a way that is abnormal for these cells. At this stage, the process may be reversible. The next step is **carcinoma in situ**, where there is no invasion of the abnormal cells outside the lobule or the duct (LCIS, DCIS). At this stage, the process is irreversible, and at some time, the condition will progress. The next stage is infiltrating or **invasive carcinoma**, where the cancer cells break out of the lobule or duct walls, invade stromal tissue, and have access to the lymph channels and blood vessels.[3–5]

As cells devolve, they lose their healthy functioning structure. Figure 6-4 illustrates this loss.

Malignant Disease

Breast cancer arises from the glandular tissue, the majority of which lies centrally and laterally in the breast. This accounts for the uneven occurrence of carcinoma by quadrants (Figure 6-5). Carcinoma of the breast predominantly occurs in women, but a small percentage of males will develop breast malignancies. Gender does not affect the development of the disease. However, males tend to have a poor prognosis due to delayed discovery and attention.[9,11] Males develop ductal cancers; they rarely develop lobular.

Gynecomastia

Gynecomastia is a benign proliferation of tissue in the male breast (Figure 6-6). Gynecomastia does not increase the

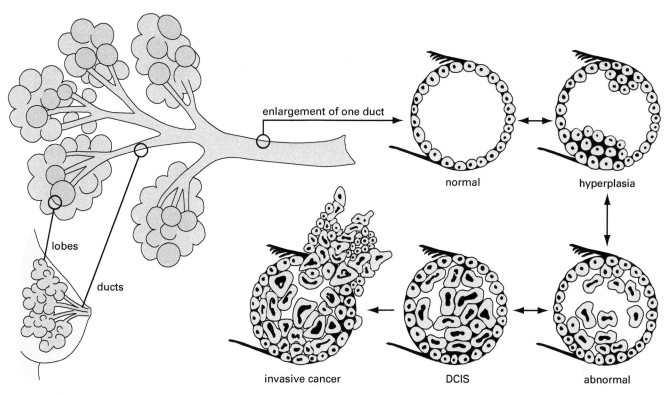

Figure 6-4
Notice the loss of structure as a cell devolves until only uncontrolled growth/proliferation of cells without function invades nearby tissue.

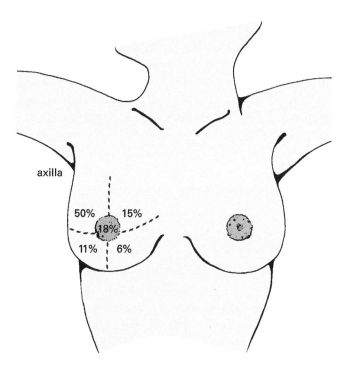

Figure 6-5
Breast cancer occurrence by quadrant.

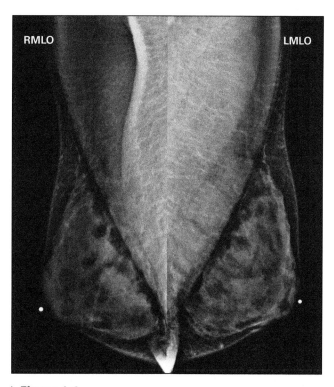

Figure 6-6
Gynecomastia. Male patient presented with bilateral breast enlargement and sensitivity. A side effect of medication he was taking. Gynecomastia can appear as a mass or a prominence of the ductal pattern, can be bilateral or unilateral.

risk of breast carcinoma for the male patient. It presents clinically as a palpable mass, an area of pinpoint tenderness, or there can be nipple discharge. Gynecomastia usually occurs bilaterally but is often more pronounced in one breast. The etiology of gynecomastia can be due to many conditions:

- Medication
- Habitual marijuana use
- Aging
- Obesity
- Liver disease
- Hyperthyroidism
- Androgen deficiency states (age, chronic renal failure)

Breast Cancer Staging

Staging is based on the size of the tumor, whether lymph nodes are involved, and whether the cancer has spread beyond the breast.[12]

Staging of breast cancer is useful to the clinician to identify the appropriate treatment for a patient. Table 6-2 illustrates the staging of breast cancer. In general, the higher the stage, the poorer the prognosis. However, today, more women are surviving breast cancer at all stages due to improved treatment regimes.

The degree of aggression of the tumor, affecting treatment and prognosis, is rated by histopathologic and nuclear grade. The pathologist rates the tumor by histopathologic grade: well differentiated, moderately differentiated, poorly differentiated, and finally undifferentiated. Tumors that are well differentiated offer a better prognosis. Additionally, the pathologist determines the tumor's nuclear grade as I, II, or III; grade III is the most aggressive tumor. It is possible to have DCIS, a small tumor that does not invade the duct walls, with a high nuclear grade.

Pathologists consider all this and a lot more when preparing a report and rendering a diagnosis. A pathologist's report contributes in part to the diagnosis as well as a breast cancer treatment plan. Notice that a report includes both qualitative and quantitative information.

▮▮ RADIOLOGIST DETECTION PROCESS

Radiologists interpret mammograms, comparing current and prior exams in conjunction with ancillary imaging studies. They relate this information to the CBE, patient history form, and observations from technologists and referring physicians. Physical inspection can often indicate both benign and malignant processes. Radiologists depend partly on the clinical and physical presentation to make a diagnosis (and/or recommendation for biopsy).

Radiologists look for mass lesions, calcifications, and other changes such as architectural distortion and asymmetry. Shape, density, size, location in the breast, and distribution of anomalies are always considered and can influence a diagnosis. The radiologist, as clinician, takes charge coordinating patient care by using all of the tools available for improved detection, diagnosis, and, when required, interventional procedures and a treatment plan.

Recognizing subtle changes to breast tissue on a mammogram requires great skill. Experienced mammographers find 24% more cancers on diagnostic mammograms than general radiologists.[13] Sorting out a judgment between benign conditions and possible malignant conditions further tests the knowledge and skills of a mammographer. According to the PIAA, the insurance industry association representing domestic and international medical professional liability insurance companies, breast cancer claims are the costliest of all cancer claims: recent payments exceed $296 million. With radiologists as the top physician specialty named in lawsuits, diagnostic errors (delay in diagnosis, failure to diagnose, and misdiagnosis) result in payment 44% of the time. "Having a high-quality systematic process for the performance and interpretation of all breast imaging examinations is essential to minimizing avoidable error."[14]

Improved knowledge of breast disease and experience in observing the physical indications for these conditions can lead to better quality mammograms and earlier detection. While this detection process urges technologists to understand the distinctions between conditions that are benign, or benign with a potential for further progression toward malignancy, and/or malignant, it is not an invitation to diagnose a mammogram. Only the radiologist can interpret a mammogram and other imaging exams to make the diagnosis.

Skin Problems

External visual clues are an easy and important starting place for breast disease detection. These visual observations noted by the technologist should be included on the history form that accompanies the images.

Skin Changes Appearing as Mass Densities

Abnormalities of the skin can appear mammographically as mass densities. They may even calcify. Applied ointments may imitate calcifications.

Skin Mole (Nevus)

Some skin moles are dense enough to attenuate x-ray photons and present mammographically with a density similar to that of surrounding glandular tissue; occasionally, they can appear more dense. Often, there is a lucency that surrounds these raised moles as a result of air being trapped between the image receptor and the skin or compression device and the skin. Labeling of skin moles on a diagram that accompanies the completed mammogram helps avoid confusion for the radiologist (Figure 6-7).

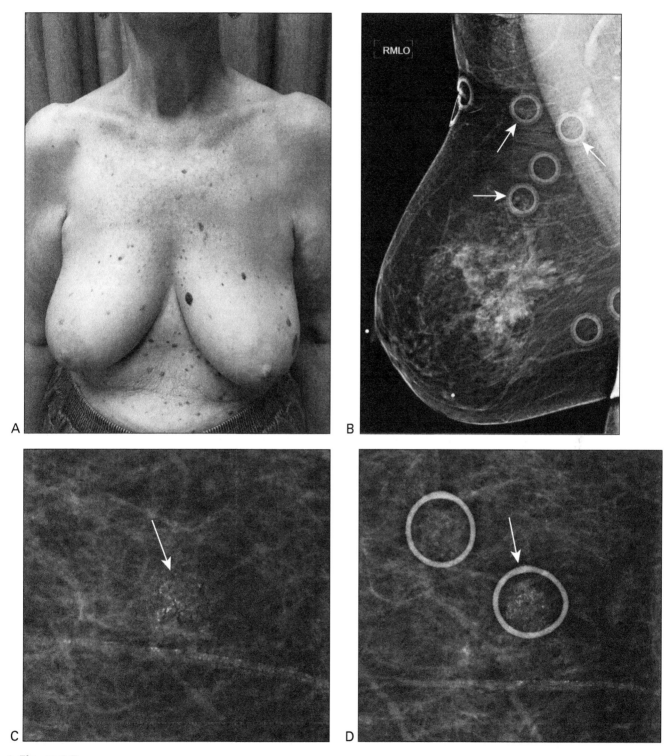

Figure 6-7
Skin moles. **(A)** Some moles are dense enough that they need to be marked for the radiologist. **(B)** Of all the moles marked, only three (*arrows*) are seen on the mammogram. **(C)** Radiologist detects suspicious calcifications (*arrow*) and has patient brought back for a diagnostic workup. **(D)** Fortunately, this turned out to be a mole with powder trapped in the crevices.

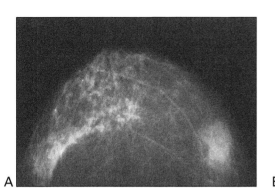 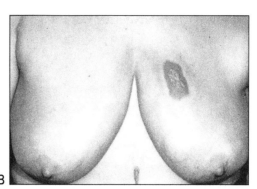 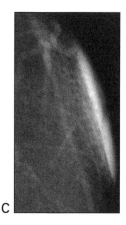

Figure 6-8
Keloid scar. **(A)** Keloid is visible in the medial aspect on this left CC view. **(B)** Keloid scar secondary to Mediport implantation. **(C)** Tangential view.

Keloid Scar

Keloid scars may form on the surface of the skin after surgical biopsy. They are evident on the skin as a thick, darker pigmented irregular area (Figure 6-8). Mammographically, the keloid scar may appear as an irregular mass of varying density, sometimes above the skin surface (Figure 6-8C). Correlation between physical appearance and the mammogram is necessary to rule out breast disease.

Sebaceous Cyst

Sebaceous cysts occur in the oil glands of the skin. They may be radio*lucent* and well circumscribed with a smooth border, which may characteristically calcify (Figure 6-9). When infected, the sebaceous cyst may imitate carcinoma mammographically. Infected sebaceous cysts appear smooth in outline and more dense than glandular tissue. In some cases, with "bright lighting" the mammogram, a sinus to the skin is evident. Physical inspection almost always reveals a "pimple-like" raised area on the skin corresponding to the mammographic density.

Edema (Skin Thickening)

Edema is the retention of fluid within the skin and interstitial spaces, causing skin thickening (Figure 6-10). Occasionally, the skin takes on the appearance of an orange peel (peau d'orange). This peau d'orange presentation most often indicates either an infection (mastitis) or carcinoma; however, edema may occur with systemic diseases that manifest with fluid retention in the breast. Inflammatory carcinoma is one type of breast cancer that presents with edema. Edema may also be present following radiation treatments for cancer of the breast.

Redness (Erythema)

Erythema of the skin may be local or extensive, including just a segment of the breast or the entire breast. Infection, abscess, and inflammatory carcinoma may present with redness of the skin. However, redness is possible with other types of carcinoma and with benign processes such as a large tension cyst. Erythema may also be present after radiation treatments for breast cancer (Figure 6-11).

Nipple Changes

The nipple is an important radiographic landmark. Radiologists use it as a reference point to identify the location of an ROI. Disease processes can involve the nipple and areolar complex.

Nipple Inversion

An inverted nipple(s) can be developmental; however, sudden inversion can indicate the presence of a tumor. Many decades ago, when cancers were detected only because they were clinically evident, nipples were often retracted as a consequence of the advanced disease state. Today, however, we predominately perform screening exams; thus, no clinical symptoms are present. The occult tumors found today will not involve the nipple as advanced cancers from the past did (Figure 6-12).

Paget Disease

Pay particular attention to the woman who comes to the mammography room and has some of the following symptoms: red nipple (looks like a skin infection), scaling/flaking of the skin of the nipple (looks like eczema), itching/tingling/burning sensations in the subareolar complex, and nipple discharge. This woman may have Paget disease (Figure 6-13).

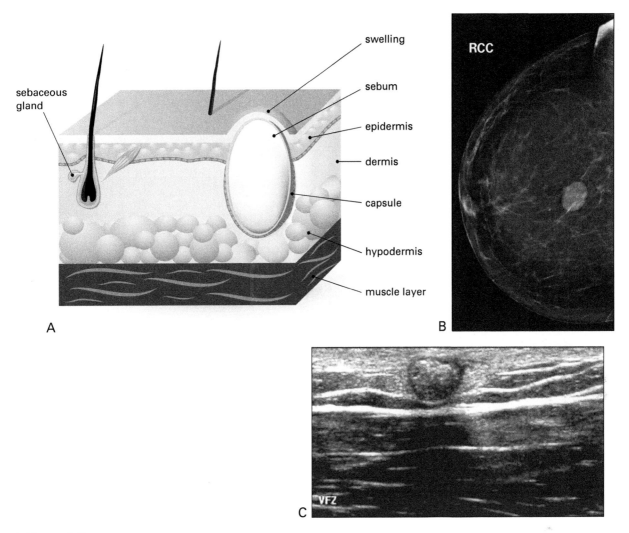

Figure 6-9
Sebaceous cyst. **(A)** Sebaceous cyst. (Image from Shutterstock, Inc.) **(B)** Correlates to the mass on the CC projection.
(C) Ultrasound demonstrates this mass is located at the skin level.

Five percent of the women with Paget disease have only Paget disease while 95% have Paget with an underlying intraductal breast cancer. It is thought this disease starts in the ductal system and spreads out to the nipple, but this does not account for the 5% who have Paget of the nipple only.

Because the symptoms are innocuous and on the surface of the skin of the nipple, most women experience a delay of 6 to 8 months before a diagnosis is made. The average age for developing this type of cancer is 57. This type of carcinoma constitutes just 2% to 4% of all breast carcinomas.

Eczematous Changes

Eczematous changes are most often due to benign conditions such as allergy. However, reddening, flaking, and crusting of the nipple can also be symptoms of Paget disease of the nipple, a carcinoma that may accompany an underlying intraductal carcinoma of the breast.

Nipple Discharge

Most nipple discharge is benign. The color of the discharge is *less* important than its occurrence in one or both breasts and whether the discharge occurs spontaneously or is expressed. A unilateral spontaneous discharge always requires further study. An expressed or bilateral discharge is most often the result of hormonal imbalances or benign conditions such as duct ectasia or other fibrocystic condition. Discharge can vary in color. Yellow, white, green, and brownish discharges are usually an indication of fibrocystic changes or hormonal fluctuations. Bloody or clear watery discharge is most indicative of papilloma (benign tumor of epithelial cells) or carcinoma; *clear watery discharge is more an indication of carcinoma than any other color*[15] (Figure 6-14).

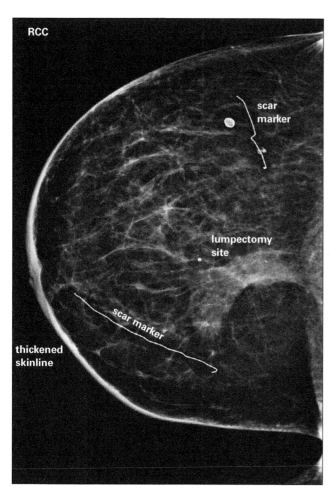

Figure 6-10
Skin thickening caused by lumpectomy with radiation treatment for breast cancer.

Papilloma Papillomas occur in the breast in one of two ways (Figure 6-15). One type occurs in the larger ducts near the nipple, producing a unilateral spontaneous discharge. These are only evident with ductography. Removal is necessary to end the discharge.

A papilloma may also occur deep in the breast, appearing mammographically as a mass. Both are benign epithelial growths with or without a connective tissue

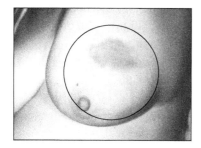

Figure 6-11
Inflammation in the breast (mastitis) causes erythema on the skin.

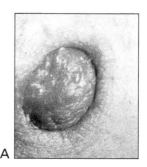

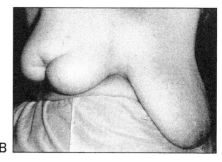

Figure 6-12
(A) Inverted nipple due to benign etiology. **(B)** Autoamputation from an advanced cancer.

Figure 6-13
Paget disease of the nipple can mimic a skin infection.

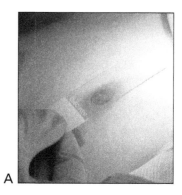

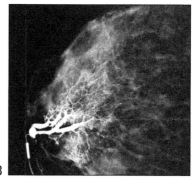

Figure 6-14
(A) Nipple with discharge. **(B)** Ductogram helps identify the source of the discharge.

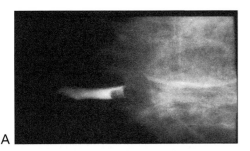

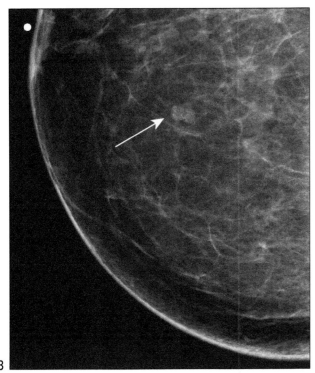

B

Figure 6-15
(A) Ductography reveals a papilloma in close proximity to the nipple. **(B)** A papilloma that has grown large enough to be visible with mammography, exhibiting a typical "raspberry"-like configuration (*arrow*).

stalk emerging from the wall of larger ducts. Papillomas that grow large enough to be mammographically visible appear as smoothly outlined, lobulated masses of approximately the same density as surrounding glandular tissue. They sometimes have a "raspberry"-like configuration[11] and, because of the lobulation, may exhibit small fatty lucencies.

Shape, Size, and Motion

Look for symmetry of the breasts; they should be mirror images. The contour of the breasts should be smooth and flow naturally and easily with movement. Size should not differ much, although there are natural size differences. During pregnancy, there can be significant size differences.

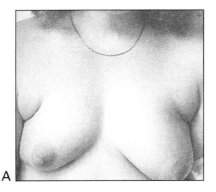

A

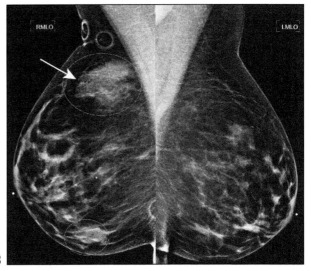

B

Figure 6-16
Asymmetry. **(A)** External. Asymmetric size of breasts. This is a normal variant of development. **(B)** Internal. This asymmetric area (*arrow*) is a normal variant of development.

Asymmetry: External and Internal

Minor differences in size between the left and right are normal, with most left breasts slightly larger than the right. Gross differences may be developmental; however, a shrinking or enlarging breast, unilaterally, can indicate underlying carcinoma. Just as outwardly the breasts are mirror images, the same premise holds true for the "inward" appearance of the breasts (Figure 6-16).

Asymmetry is the radiologist's greatest aid in determining abnormalities, both benign and malignant. The breasts are mirror images; mammographically, the distribution of the glandular tissue should appear the same, with minor variation from one breast to the other. If one breast is physically larger than the other, then mammographically, the glandular composition will be greater. Often, asymmetry is a result of anatomic variations due to uneven development or prior surgery. However, a disproportionate amount of tissue in one area of one breast needs further evaluation.

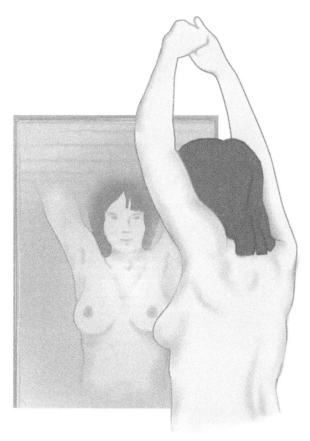

Figure 6-17
Our breasts are mirror images of one another. Whichever way one moves, the other should replicate that movement.

Difference in Movement

The breasts should move symmetrically when slowly raising the arms. Differences can indicate underlying pathologic processes, including carcinoma. When performing breast self-examination, women look for differences in behavior from one breast to the other: when raising arms up, when bending forward from the waist, and when flexing the pectoral muscle (Figure 6-17).

Lump

An asymmetric palpable lump can present with carcinoma or benign processes. Carcinoma in its early stages may exhibit benign characteristics. It can feel smooth and soft and can move freely (mobile) rather than fixed to the skin or underlying tissue. In addition, some benign lesions can feel much like an advanced carcinoma—hard, irregular in outline, and fixed to the skin. Any new lump requires investigation.

Nodularity

Nodularity, lumpiness occurring bilaterally, is a normal presentation for the breast but may also present with

malignant conditions. Women should be familiar with the natural "lumpiness" of their own breast tissue so that if a new nodule is detected, they can bring this change to the attention of their physician.

Pain

When a woman indicates she experiences intermittent pain bilaterally, it is usually due to hormonal fluctuations or other systemic functions. Pain or other sensation, however, is common,[1] even with early carcinoma, and should not be dismissed. Pinpoint tenderness is more disconcerting than overall breast pain (Figure 6-18).

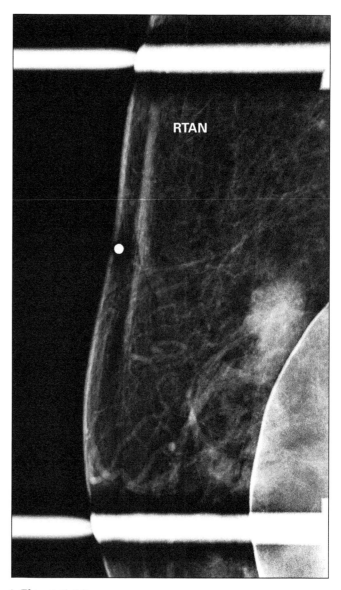

Figure 6-18
Patient complained of pinpoint pain. A metallic BB was placed on the skin to draw the radiologist's attention to the specific area of pain.

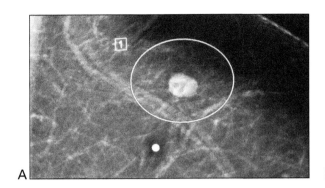

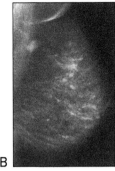

Figure 6-19
Lymph nodes. **(A)** Close-up of a lymph node: oval, fatty hilum, close to blood vessel. **(B)** Lymph nodes in the Tail of Spence.

Lymph Nodes

Lymph nodes in the axilla as well as intramammary lymph nodes are common (Figure 6-19). They are smoothly outlined, sometimes lobulated, with a zone of lucency corresponding to the hilus. Their density is usually that of surrounding glandular tissue. However, lymph nodes can appear more dense, especially when superimposed over the pectoral muscle. Axillary lymph nodes are usually larger in size (in fact, they might be as large as 2 in.) but of the same composition of intramammary lymph nodes, with greater fatty replacement. *Reactive* (i.e., nodes reacting to systemic disease such as rheumatoid arthritis, infection, leukemia, lymphoma, or acquired immune deficiency disease) or *metastatic* lymph nodes (from breast or other cancer) will remain smooth in outline but increase in size and density, usually losing the fatty component. Metastatic nodes (from breast cancer) occur unilaterally on the affected side. Occasionally, metastatic nodes will be the only indication of an occult carcinoma within the breast. Reactive lymph nodes usually occur bilaterally; however, unilateral occurrence is possible secondary to infection on the ipsilateral side.

▌ MAMMOGRAPHIC PRESENTATION OF PATHOLOGY

Pathology displays mammographically as (a) calcification, (b) mass, and (c) diffuse accentuation of the glandular tissue. These manifestations may only be apparent by the following indicators: *asymmetry, architectural distortion,* and/or *changes in contour* of the parenchyma. Other mammographic signs of disease, although secondary, are dilated ducts, dilated veins, and skin thickening. The presence of these indicators or secondary characteristics serves as a "flag" to be attentive to this area for further study rather than an absolute assurance of underlying disease.

As a practical matter, few mammograms, about 4 to 5 out of every 1,000 screening mammograms, have a finding of cancer. These odds make it all the more important for you, the technologist, to create a quality mammogram to visualize the disease for the radiologist.

Calcifications

Calcifications in the breast can occur with both benign and malignant processes. About 40% to 50% of calcifications represent malignant disease; the rest are a result of inspissated secretions (i.e., secretions within the ductal structures that have become thickened and dried) or as a result of necrotic processes (Figure 6-20).

Case Study 6-1

Refer to Figure 6-20 and the text and respond to the following questions.

1. Is Figure 6-20A benign or malignant calcification? Is Figure 6-20B benign or malignant?

2. Describe several visual characteristics of benign calcifications.

3. Describe several visual characteristics of malignant calcifications.

4. If the calcifications are not clearly benign or malignant, how do you classify them?

5. What procedures are utilized when dealing with calcifications from question #4 to ultimately determine benign versus malignant?

Radiologists consider certain mammographic characteristics of the calcifications *with* clinical and historical information to determine the necessity for biopsy. The radiologist classifies calcifications as benign, malignant, or indeterminate. Table 6-3 summarizes the characteristics of obviously benign and malignant calcium. Indeterminate calcifications exhibit properties of both. Needle core biopsy, open biopsy, or surveillance mammography is useful for indeterminate calcium.

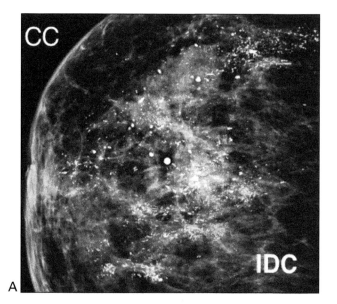

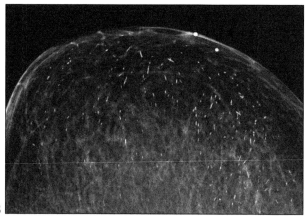

Figure 6-20
Calcifications. **(A)** Malignant calcifications; invasive ductal carcinoma. (Reprinted with permission from Georgian-Smith D, Lawton T. *Breast Imaging and Pathologic Correlations: A Pattern-Based Approach.* 1st ed. Wolters Kluwer; 2014.) **(B)** Benign calcifications; plasma cell mastitis.

Skin Calcifications

Characteristically, skin calcifications are smooth in outline with radiolucent centers, usually scattered throughout the medial half of the breast (Figure 6-21). However, they may be fully radiopaque and present as a tight cluster, unilaterally. In this instance, workup is necessary to insure that the cluster is not a more worrisome process.

Arterial Calcifications

Arterial calcifications result from arterial atherosclerosis. They may be easily identifiable within the blood vessel, especially when well developed (Figure 6-22). However, in the early stages or if the vessel is not easily identifiable, arterial calcifications may imitate carcinoma.

Milk of Calcium

Milk of calcium occurs in microcysts when the cyst contains radiopaque particles mixed with the fluid. On the CC projection, they appear faint, ill-defined, and smudgy (Figure 6-23A). A Lateral projection (and sometimes the mediolateral oblique [MLO] projection) reveals the true characteristics of milk of calcium (Figure 6-23B). As the particles settle to the dependent portion of the microcyst, the crescent shape milk of calcium is evident. These calcifications are clustered or scattered, may be multifocal, and may occur bilaterally.

Popcorn-Type Calcifications

Large, thick, dense, popcorn-shaped calcifications are a result of involuting fibroadenomas and occasionally other benign processes (Figure 6-24).

Fibroadenoma

A fibroadenoma can present as lobulated and may exhibit a halo sign because it displaces surrounding structures.

Table 6-3 • Mammographic Characteristics of Calcifications

	BENIGN	MALIGNANT
Shape	Round, ring-like	Varying shapes
Density	Same density	Varying densities
Distribution	Scattered. Benign Ca⁺⁺ can also be clustered.	Clustered
Definition	Well-defined borders	Poorly defined borders
Unilateral or bilateral	If the same type of calcifications occur in both breasts, they are more likely benign.	Unilateral
Surrounding tissue	If the calcium is seen within a benign-appearing mass or if the tissue surrounding the calcium appears normal, this is a benign indicator.	If there is architectural or parenchymal distortion associated with calcium, malignancy must be considered.
Increasing in number from prior mammogram	Can be benign	Not an indicator alone but, when considered with other characteristics, can indicate malignancy
Size	Can be large or small	Most often small

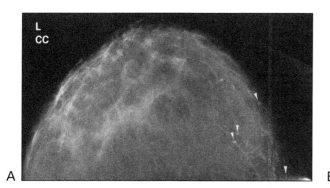

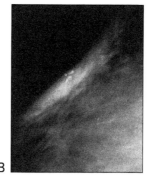

Figure 6-21
Skin calcifications. **(A)** Skin calcifications (*arrowheads*), often appearing medially, are typically ring-like with radiolucent centers. **(B)** Tangential view of skin calcium.

A fibroadenoma also may present as a mammographically benign-appearing, oval, well-circumscribed mass (Figure 6-25). Its density is normally that of surrounding glandular tissue. Fibroadenomas may respond to cyclical hormonal changes, growing and regressing in size, and can characteristically calcify. It may be palpable if large enough. This abnormality is a benign overgrowth of the fibrous tissue of the lobule. Because it contains epithelial tissue, the fibroadenoma can respond to cyclical hormonal changes. Calcifications may develop. After menopause, the

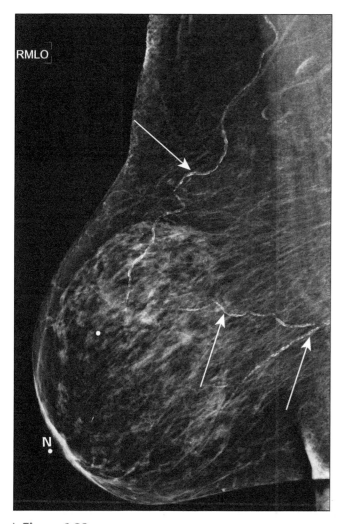

Figure 6-22
Arterial calcification (*arrows*) evident within blood vessels. If these calcifications were ductal, they would be heading toward the nipple (*N*).

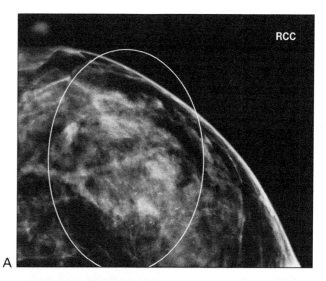

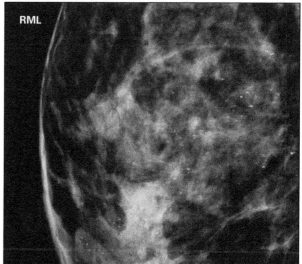

Figure 6-23
Milk of calcium. **(A)** Smudgy-appearing calcifications on the CC projection that **(B)** exhibit layering on the Lateral projection.

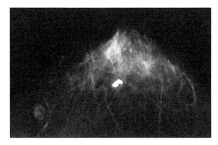

Figure 6-24
Typical popcorn calcification found in a degenerating fibroadenoma.

fibroadenoma will atrophy along with the rest of the breast tissue, leaving the calcifications behind. A fibroadenoma will rarely develop a tumor—it does contain epithelial components; however, it is not premalignant, nor does its occurrence increase the risk for breast cancer.

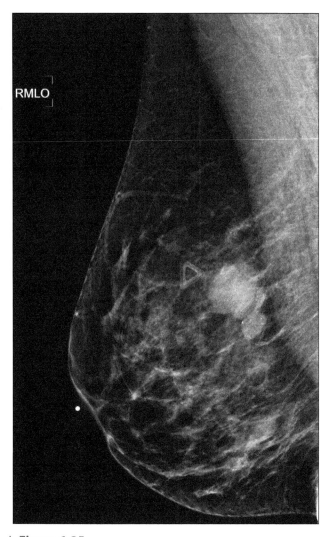

Figure 6-25
Triangular shape skin marker indicates to radiologist the patient has a palpable lump. Upon diagnostic workup, this proved to be a fibroadenoma.

Rim Calcifications

Rim calcifications occur along the border of a benign mass. Cysts, oil cysts, and sebaceous cysts may all calcify like this. Difficulty arises in the early formation of rim calcium, which can appear as unilateral, fine, irregularly shaped calcifications imitating carcinoma.

Fat Necrosis/Oil Cyst

Oil cysts form as a result of fat necrosis. Fat necrosis is death of fatty tissue. Most often, fat necrosis occurs after biopsy or injury, when blood supply to that portion of the breast is disrupted. However, spontaneous fat necrosis may occur for unknown reasons. When fatty tissue dies, it changes to oil. The body, protecting itself, collects and organizes the oil and builds a capsule around it creating an oil cyst. An oil cyst is a smoothly outlined, well-encapsulated radiolucent mass. An oil cyst may only be evident after it characteristically calcifies. An oil cyst may be palpable and can feel hard, especially as it calcifies. Fat necrosis and oil cysts are benign (Figure 6-26).

Masses

Mass densities that visualize on the mammogram can be either benign or malignant. The radiologist considers certain mammographic characteristics of a mass in conjunction

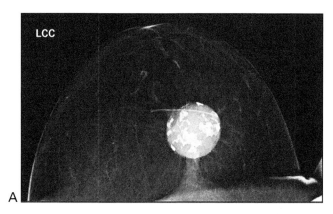

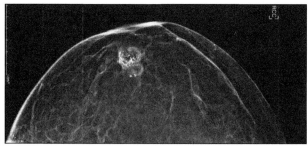

Figure 6-26
(A) An oil cyst forms as a result of fat necrosis. May be palpable, especially as it calcifies. **(B)** Fat necrosis. Not all fat necrosis results in formation of an oil cyst; oftentimes, it remains as fat necrosis.

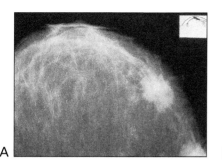 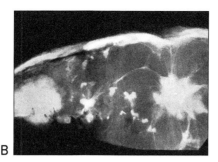 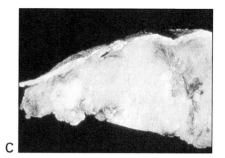

Figure 6-27
(A) A malignant mass is usually denser than surrounding glandular tissue and has spiculated borders. **(B)** X-ray of a specimen. **(C)** Photo of the specimen.

with the clinical and breast history information, as well as breast ultrasound, to determine a recommendation for biopsy. These characteristics include the border, density, and tissue makeup of the mass and the presence or absence of a capsule, halo, or silhouette sign. Again, the presence or absence of any one of these indicators does not necessarily determine the likelihood of disease but rather serves as a "flag" to pay attention to this area.

Malignant Masses

The typical malignant mass is spiculated and usually of greater density than surrounding glandular tissue. However, a malignant mass may also be smooth in outline,

isodense, or of lesser density than surrounding structures (Figure 6-27).

Architectural Distortion

The ductal structures, while not individually evident mammographically, present a pattern of radial lines that converge at the nipple. This is the normal architecture of the breast. *Architectural distortion* is the interruption of this pattern, lines that *oppose* this natural flow of ducts to the nipple. Although architectural distortion is a strong indicator of malignancy (Figure 6-28), other breast structures can imitate architectural distortion. Blood vessels and Cooper ligaments often run askew of the ductal architecture. These

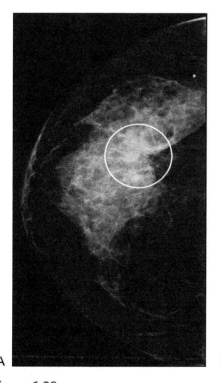 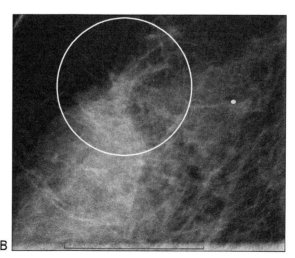 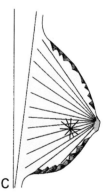

Figure 6-28
Architectural distortion. **(A)** Architectural distortion, interruption of the normal flow of ductal structures to the nipple, is difficult to see on this CC image. **(B)** With a special view, the architectural distortion is more apparent. **(C)** The ductal structures of the breast are seen as a pattern of radial lines that converge at the nipple. This is understood as the normal architecture. When *lines* appear that oppose this natural flow, it is termed "architectural distortion."

contribute to a "pseudo (false) carcinoma effect," as can overlapped ductal structures. Architectural distortion may be present with both benign and malignant disease processes, occurring with both mass and calcifying lesions. Serving as a flag for the mammographer to pay attention to the area, architectural distortion may be the only indication that an otherwise obscured mass is present. Surgical intervention, resolving hematoma, injury, and radial scar can also be evident as architectural distortion.

Probably Benign Masses

Many benign masses occur in the breast. All masses present in various ways with different characteristics. Radiologists use visual clues to sort out the benign/malignant classification.

Clues for Detection

Experienced investigators have identified specific conditions, patterns, locations, and mammographic clues that may aid in the detection process.

Composition

The tissue composition of a mass can indicate whether it is benign or malignant:

Fatty—always benign
Fatty and glandular mix—usually benign
Glandular or fibrous—benign or malignant

Contour Change

Externally, the shape of both breasts should be symmetrical, with minor variations. Bulging, dimpling, or retraction of the skin can indicate an underlying process, either benign or malignant (Figure 6-29A).

Internally, the radiologist looks at the contour of the glandular tissue on the mammogram. Smooth borders and rounded contours are preferred shapes; conversely irregular borders and sharply angled contours are more worrisome and warrant a closer examination (Figure 6-29B).

Density

This particular attribute is becoming less dependable as the technical attributes of mammography improve allowing visualization of carcinomas earlier in the disease process. In most cases, a carcinoma will be of greater density or the same density as the surrounding glandular tissue; however, low-density carcinomas do occur.

Capsule

A capsule appears mammographically as a thin radiopaque line surrounding a mass.[11] An encapsulated mass is most often benign; rarely, this can occur with malignancy.

Halo

A halo appears as a thin, radiolucent curved line on the mammogram that represents the edge of a mass compressing the

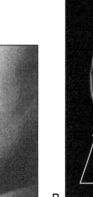

A

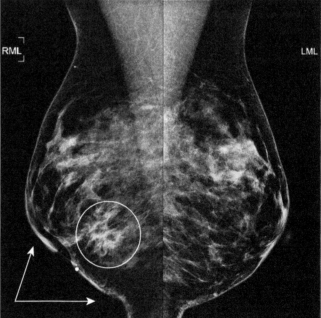

B

Figure 6-29
Contour change. A change in the outline of the inside/outside of the breast. **(A)** External. The contour of the breast is no longer smooth and round. This is due to an advanced breast cancer. **(B)** Internal. A *circle* is drawn around a large cancer. The contour of the left breast is smooth while that of the right breast (between the *arrows*) is flattened and retracted.

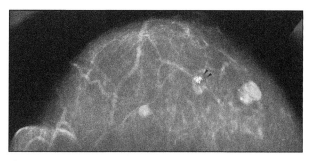

Figure 6-30
A thin radiolucent line, or "halo sign" (*arrowheads*), surrounds this fibroadenoma. Note also the silhouette sign (lines appearing to extend from the borders of these three masses can actually be followed into and out of the abnormalities). Both the halo and the silhouette signs are indicators of benign disease. Benign masses are usually smooth in outline and are likely to be oval or lobulated in shape.

surrounding fatty tissue[8,11] (Figure 6-30). A halo sign usually occurs with benign abnormalities but can occur rarely with a malignant mass.

Silhouette Sign

The silhouette sign can help the mammographer discern whether an abnormality has a spiculated border. If a mass is truly spiculated, the lines radiating from it will disappear in the middle of the abnormality; this is a strong indicator of malignancy. If the reader can follow each line into, through, and out of the mass, then these lines represent silhouetted structures in front of or behind the mass (Figure 6-31).

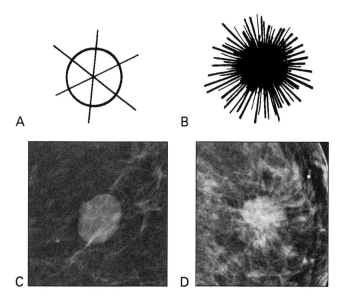

Figure 6-31
A "silhouette sign" **(A)** occurs when a low-density mass superimposes other breast structures. Lines can be followed into and out of the mass. A true spiculated mass **(B)** will have lines that disappear into the center of the abnormality. **(C)** X-ray of a benign mass. **(D)** X-ray of a cancer.

Case Study 6-2

Refer to Figure 6-31 and the text and respond to the following questions.

1. Which figures are indicative of benign masses?

2. Which figures are indicative of malignant masses?

3. Describe several visual characteristics of benign masses.

4. Describe several visual characteristics of malignant masses.

Border and Shape

The border of a mass may be spiculated or smooth; its shape is round, oval, or lobulated. A spiculated border is a strong indicator of carcinoma but can also occur with benign conditions such as hematoma and tension cyst. A smooth (or well-circumscribed) border, especially when the mass is oval or lobulated, is a strong indicator of a benign abnormality. However, a malignant mass may present with a smooth border as well; 5% of breast cancers have smoothly marginated borders.

Benign Breast Masses

The following lesions can be identified on a mammogram but are benign in nature.

Lipoma

A lipoma presents mammographically as a benign-appearing, radiolucent, well-circumscribed, encapsulated abnormality (Figure 6-32). A lipoma can feel soft and easily movable but occasionally can have the physical attributes of an advanced carcinoma (hard and fixed). A lipoma is a fatty tumor with no epithelial component. It is benign and has no potential for malignancy, and its occurrence does not increase the risk for breast cancer.

Hamartoma

A hamartoma is an island of glandular tissue separated from the normal ductal structures. Some experts believe that this is a variant of development, a vestigial breast (as a developing embryo, we have 16 "breasts") that does not disappear when it should. The two types of hamartoma are fibroadenolipoma and fibrous hamartoma (Figure 6-33). Fibroadenolipomas consist of a mixture of glandular, fibrous, and fatty tissue; the fibrous hamartoma is

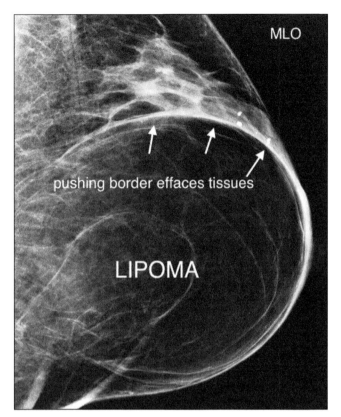

Figure 6-32
Example of a well-encapsulated fatty tumor known as a lipoma (*arrows*). (Reprinted with permission from Georgian-Smith D, Lawton T. *Breast Imaging and Pathologic Correlations: A Pattern-Based Approach*. 1st ed. Wolters Kluwer; 2014.)

predominantly glandular and fibrous in composition. The risk of developing carcinoma in a hamartoma is the same as for other glandular components. Hamartoma is not a premalignant condition.

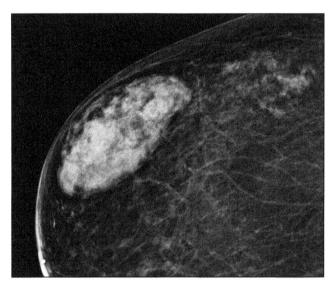

Figure 6-33
Hamartoma: fibroadenolipoma—smoothly outlined, well-encapsulated mixture of fatty and glandular components. The fatty component can increase and decrease with weight fluctuations.

A hamartoma presents mammographically as a benign-appearing, well-encapsulated, smoothly outlined mass. Hamartomas are soft upon palpation and may be indistinguishable from the surrounding breast tissue. They can be quite large and usually respond to hormonal changes in the body. The radiologist may mistake a hamartoma for a new mass as technical improvements of the mammogram make them more distinct in comparison to the surrounding parenchyma.

Fibrocystic Changes

Various breast changes that fall under the term "fibrocystic disease" are currently defined more specifically. Histologically, the phrase "fibrocystic disease" is falling by the wayside. Histopathologists are trying to be more specific in their description of benign processes, determining their likelihood to become cancerous, and the degree to which their presence indicates increased risk. Some of these processes are adenosis, sclerosing adenosis, fibrosis, cysts, apocrine metaplasia, radial scar, epithelial hyperplasia, and duct ectasia.[8,11,16–18]

Fibrocystic changes can cause physical pain, a lump, and/or discharge. Mammographically, they may appear as mass, calcification, and prominent ductal patterns. Occasionally, the pathology demonstrates an abnormality in isolation, but more often, they present together.[8]

Adenosis Adenosis is the enlargement and/or proliferation of new lobular units. It may be a "normal" change, as with the "adenosis of pregnancy" (Figure 6-34), or pathologic when involved with other processes. Adenosis is not premalignant.

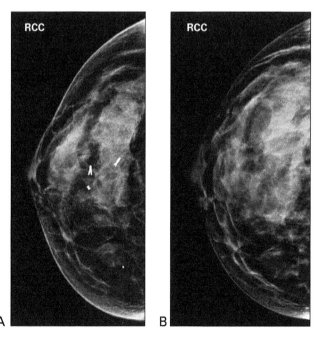

A   B

Figure 6-34
Adenosis of pregnancy. **(A)** The normal state. **(B)** Pregnant state.

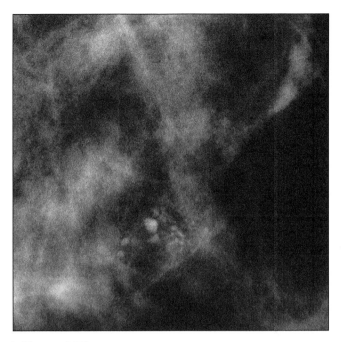

Figure 6-35
Sclerosing adenosis typically presents with fine calcifications, sometimes associated with a mass but oftentimes not.

Sclerosing Adenosis Sclerosing adenosis is adenosis with sclerosing (hardening) of the intralobular stroma. This condition may present as a calcification or a mass, is benign, and is not a premalignant condition (Figure 6-35).

Fibrosis Fibrosis is the formation of fibrous tissue stemming from the connective and supportive stroma. It is a benign condition.

Cyst A cyst occurs in the TDLU when the extralobular terminal duct becomes blocked. Accumulation of fluid occurs when the resorption rate of the normal ductal secretions is less than the production rate. The fluid accumulates in the TDLU, increasing the pressure. This causes the TDLU to lose its shape, forming a cyst. Cysts vary in size and respond to hormonal fluctuation. According to Wellings et al.,[19] there are three types of cysts. The cell type found in the lining of the cyst defines its type. An epithelial cyst is lined by epithelial cells; a stromal cyst is an epithelial cyst that has lost its epithelial component; and finally, the apocrine cyst is a cyst where the epithelial cells display apocrine metaplasia. Rarely, an intracystic carcinoma or papilloma can arise from the epithelium of the wall of a cyst. However, the presence of cysts alone does not increase the risk of subsequent carcinoma, unless there is significant family history. The combination of cysts and family history slightly increases the risk for breast cancer.

A cyst presents mammographically as a well-circumscribed mass (Figure 6-36). Its density is usually that of surrounding glandular tissue; however, it can also be of greater density. When a cyst is under great pressure

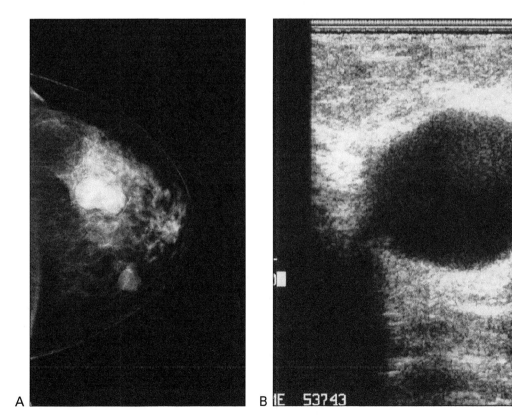

Figure 6-36
(A) Large, smoothly outlined masses that were proven to be fluid-filled cysts with ultrasonography. **(B)** Ultrasound of a cyst.

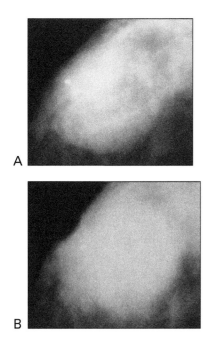

A

B

Figure 6-37
(A) Large smoothly outlined cyst, proven with ultrasound.
(B) The same cyst 1 year later, under tension, exhibiting ragged borders.

(termed a "tension cyst"), its borders can look ragged, similar to a carcinoma (Figure 6-37). A cyst can also demonstrate a halo sign because it compresses structures around it. While mammography can be suggestive of a cyst, only ultrasonography, needle aspiration, or biopsy can diagnose it. Cysts vary in size and physical attributes. They may be quite large and still not be palpable if not under pressure. Conversely, a cyst can be small in size and present as a hard lump upon physical examination.

Apocrine Metaplasia (Apocrine Change)

Apocrine metaplasia is a change occurring in the epithelial cells where they exhibit characteristics of apocrine sweat glands. By itself, apocrine metaplasia does not increase the risk of breast cancer; however, it may occur with other more worrisome processes.

Radial Scar

The radial scar (also known as infiltrating epitheliosis, black hole, etc.) has a "central fibrous core"[5] with radiating arms made up of benign epithelial growth and sclerosis. It can mimic cancer both mammographically and histologically. It is unclear whether a radial scar signals premalignancy or the likelihood of the breast tissue to develop carcinoma subsequently.

Radial scars are unrelated to surgical scars. They present as a wide area of architectural distortion, mimicking

carcinoma. Radial scars are sometimes distinguishable from malignancy by their small multiple radiolucencies at the center (Figure 6-38). Additionally, radial scars often appear on one mammographic view and seem to disappear on the opposing projection. Despite their usual large size, they are rarely palpable. The radiologist will almost always recommend biopsy for a radial scar because of its mammographic similarities to carcinoma.

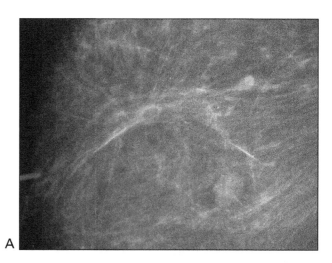

A

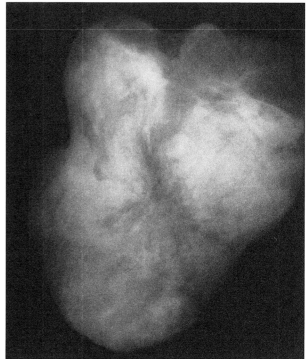

B

Figure 6-38
(A) Radiating lines extending from a zone of radiolucency are typical of a radial scar. **(B)** Radiograph of a surgical specimen of a radial scar exhibiting radiating lines from a radiolucent center.

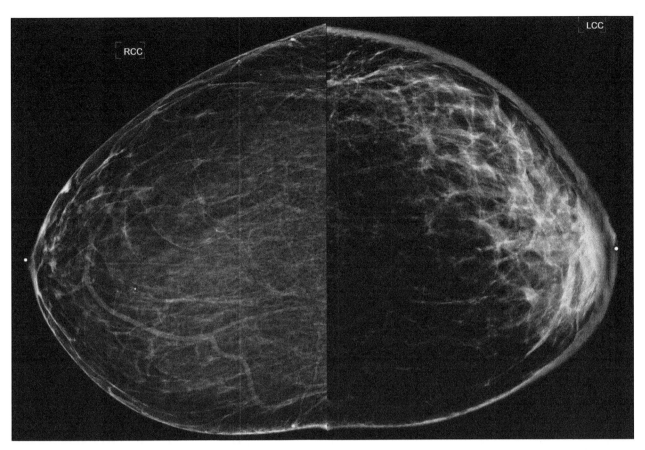

Figure 6-39
Bilateral CC projections. Diffuse accentuation of the glandular tissue of the right breast is due to infection. The breast tissue returns to normal after treatment with antibiotics.

Diffuse Accentuation of Glandular Tissue

Prominent Ductal Pattern Breast disease is complex; it is often the result of the little battles we endure as we age. These effects either cause or promote changes to the glandular tissue, and these changes may present as an overall prominence of the ductal pattern (Figure 6-39). In some processes, both benign and malignant, the breast may appear red, edematous, and with skin thickening.[8,16,17] The following causes can result in diffuse accentuation mammographically:

- Infection
- Trauma (contusion)
- Effects of medications
- Effects of caffeine
- Systemic disease
- Carcinoma
- Inflammatory carcinoma
- Radiation therapy

Duct Ectasia Occurring in the larger ducts, ectasia is a benign process consisting of widened ducts containing thickened material. Inflammation surrounds the ducts. Its cause is unknown. However, its presence does not increase risk for breast cancer (Figure 6-40).

Abscess An abscess is a localized infection. An abscess presents mammographically as a well-circumscribed mass with a density greater than surrounding glandular structures. It is usually palpable and may have associated skin erythema and tenderness.

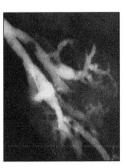

Figure 6-40
Ductogram depicts the dilated ducts in the subareolar complex.

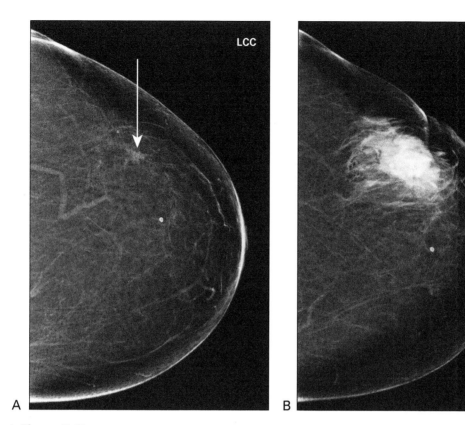

Figure 6-41
Hematoma. **(A)** *Arrow* points to a suspicious mass that was biopsied. Pathology results were benign.
(B) Post biopsy, the patient developed a hematoma.

Hematoma (Contusion) A hematoma can occur following injury or surgery when there is bleeding within the breast (Figure 6-41). The body is excellent at protecting itself; it organizes, collects, and encapsulates the blood, forming a walled mass. A *new* hematoma is rounded, well circumscribed, and denser than surrounding glandular structures. A resolving hematoma can appear dense and spiculated and may calcify over time, imitating carcinoma. Hematomas may fully resolve or remain stable for many years.

Summary

The description of mammographic pathology in this chapter is by no means all-encompassing; rather, it is an introduction to pathologic patterns. Tabar and Dean,[11] Shaw-de Parades,[18] Kopans,[16] Salkowski,[17] and Logan-Young and Hoffman[8] give excellent descriptions in their atlases concerning mammographic findings. Page and Anderson,[2] Azzopardi,[3] Wellings et al.,[19] Haagensen,[4] and Lanyi[20] are good sources of information concerning etiology, development, and histology of breast disease.

To become more adept at perceiving contrary mammographic patterns, investigate the normal patterns of breast tissue (see Chapters 5 and 7). In addition to the available outstanding texts and atlases (see references), the technologist can learn normal mammographic patterns and patterns of pathology in several ways:

1. Work side by side with the radiologist during patient workup. In this way, the technologist will also become aware of what the radiologist recognizes as suspicious and in need of further study.
2. In many clinics, the radiologist includes the technologist during the reading of the mammogram, indicating not only pathology but also findings that would indicate an extra view. At many of these clinics, the radiologist depends on the technologist for correlative physical findings and patient information.
3. In-service programs and inclusion of the technologist in tumor board meetings.

Review Questions

1. How does the diagnosis by a radiologist differ from that of a pathologist?

2. What is the progression of a cell from normal/healthy into a cancer? Is the cell progression the same or different for ductal and lobular carcinomas?

3. What is symmetry/asymmetry of a breast?

References

1. Your Pathology Reports. Ardmore, PA: Breastcancer.org. Accessed June 26, 2008.
2. Page DL, Anderson TJ. *Diagnostic Histopathology of the Breast.* Edinburgh: Churchill Livingstone; 1987.
3. Azzopardi JG. *Problems in Breast Pathology.* London, UK: WB Saunders; 1979.
4. Haagensen CC. *Diseases of the Breast.* Philadelphia, PA: WB Saunders Company; 1986.
5. Hoeffken W, Lanyi M. *Mammography.* Philadelphia, PA: WB Saunders Company; 1977.
6. Cavelli LR, et al. Loss of heterozygosity in normal breast epithelial tissue and benign lesions in BRCA1/2 carriers with breast cancer. *Cancer Genet Cytogenet.* 2004;149(1):38–43.
7. Kamm B. The genetics of sporadic and inherited breast cancer. *Radiol Technol.* 1998;69(4):299–311.
8. Logan-Young W, Hoffman N. *Breast Cancer: A Practical Guide to Diagnosis.* Rochester, NY: Hope Publishing Company, Inc.; 1994.
9. Kopans DB. *Breast Imaging.* 2nd ed. Philadelphia, PA: Lippincott–Raven; 1998.
10. http://www.cancer.org/cancer/breastcancer/typesofbreastcancer. Accessed August 6, 2016.
11. Tabar L, Dean PB. *Teaching Atlas of Mammography.* 2nd ed. New York, NY: Thieme Inc.; 1985.
12. Fleming ID, et al. *Manual for Staging of Cancer: American Joint Committee on Cancer.* Philadelphia, PA: Lippincott–Raven; 1997:171–180.
13. Sickles EA, et al. Performance benchmarks for diagnostic mammography. *Radiology.* 2005;235:775–790.
14. News release from PIAA Nov 22, 2013. *New PIAA Study Analyzes Diagnosis and Treatment of Breast Cancer.* https://piaa.us
15. *Sartorious*
16. Kopans DB. *Breast Imaging.* Philadelphia, PA: JB Lippincott Co.; 1989.
17. Salkowski L. *Rad cases: Breast Imaging.* New York, NY: Thieme; 2014.
18. Shaw-de Parades E. *Atlas of Film-Screen Mammography.* Baltimore, MD: Urban & Schwarzenberg; 1989.
19. Wellings SR, et al. An atlas of subgross pathology of the human breast with special reference to possible precancerous lesions. *J Natl Cancer Inst* 1975;55:231.
20. Lanyi M. *Breast Calcifications.* New York, NY: Springer-Verlag; 1986.

Mammography
Examination

Mastering the Mammography Examination

▌▌▌ PART 1
MASTERING THE STANDARD PROJECTIONS

Objectives

- Understand the appropriate use of the mammography equipment for the examination and the equipment operator's influence to affect image quality.

- Understand the artistic and technical skills required for critical positioning and compression techniques used in the routine mammography examination and how they are accomplished.

- Understand the interdependency of positioning and compression and its effect on image quality.

- Understand established image criteria for the standard mammographic projections: craniocaudal and the mediolateral oblique.

- Understand the image assessment process for the standard mammographic projections: craniocaudal and mediolateral oblique.

- Understand the positioning and compression strategies that correlate to established standard imaging criteria.

Key Terms

- compression
- exam management
- glandular distribution
- image quality
- ipsilateral

- mobile borders
- mosaic
- motion
- respiration
- standard projections

INTRODUCTION

Producing a quality mammographic image while providing a positive patient experience is a complicated process requiring a blend of performance reliability between two basic components: equipment and technologist. The technologist is expected to master equipment operation and projection execution under challenging circumstances for the screening and diagnostic setting. The projections used in the mammography service are divided into two groups. The **standard projections**, the craniocaudal (CC) and the mediolateral oblique (MLO), are the backbone of the mammography examination. They are the primary projections used in the screening setting and require the technologist to meet image quality criteria established by the facility's accrediting body. The second group, problem-solving views, consists of various projections and techniques that are used to improve the visualization of breast tissue. Problem-solving projections may be used to complete the screening examination, to provide further information for the diagnostic examination, or to complement or replace the standard projections for the nonconforming patient. The technologist's skill in the use of all mammography projections, combined with the essential knowledge of basic mammography principles, contributes to the service as a whole and therefore cannot be isolated from the other. This requires that a substantial amount of information surrounding the preparation of the technologist to perform mammography be provided in one chapter, an ambitious undertaking for the reader. To solve this problem, this chapter is divided into two smaller subchapters, Part 1 and Part 2. Part 1 highlights the standard projections and the quality measures used to ensure superior imaging, while Part 2 highlights the problem-solving projections and their purpose. Each part includes basic mammography principles and helpful suggestions that apply to all circumstances in which image quality and patient satisfaction are influenced. It is the hope that although the information is supplied to the reader in parts, the message is clear that through the intermingling of their value, the goal to detect early indications of breast cancer is accomplished.

A CHALLENGING MISSION

Assuming equipment performance has been verified, technologists in the field of medical imaging agree that the major factors affecting image quality are determined by technologist performance and the compliance capability of the patient. Each of these important distinctions plays a significant role in the outcome of the study. Successful **image quality** outcomes initiated by the technologist

relate to the combined knowledge and expertise in technical proficiency (equipment/computer operation), breast anatomy, and positioning/compression techniques. The patient qualities impacting successful image quality outcomes are related to body habitus, glandular tissue distribution, breast pliability, and the physical, cognitive, and emotional conditions for exam compliance. Due to a wide range of subject variability, achieving superior image quality for all patients can be challenging and sometimes unobtainable for the technologist.

From its inception, countless authorities acknowledge the challenges associated with mammography and the critical contribution of the technologist. This belief was substantiated by the adoption of rules and regulations to perform mammography as established by the Mammography Quality Standards Act (MQSA) in 1992. Mammograms were recognized among the radiographs most difficult to interpret, acknowledging the need for superior image quality to ensure interpretation (*assessment*) accuracy.[1] Technologists performing mammography would now be required to obtain specialized training prior to producing mammography images, the only imaging modality requiring this regulation under federal law. Summarizing the difficulty of the technologist's responsibilities, Ward Parsons, MD, wrote, "Mammography technologists are crucial to the production of useful x-ray images of the human breast; their tasks are far from simple."[2] All medical imaging procedures require advanced technical skills and knowledge to produce images critical to the diagnosis of disease and appropriate treatment. Technologists who do not specialize in mammography may wonder why additional certification is required by the FDA prior to performing this study. What makes mammography different? Early pioneers described mammography as being a blend of science and art. Technologists performing mammography must have a comprehensive understanding of the interdependency of positioning, compression, and exposure technique. Positioning the breast is an artistic skill that requires the technologist to customize learned maneuvers for each individual patient. Adequate compression is dependent on the combination of positioning techniques and breast pliability, while resulting exposure techniques are dependent on both positioning and compression.

Defining the Challenge

Typically, in medical imaging procedures, the technologist directs and assists the patient with placing the appropriate anatomy within the x-ray exposure field. Patient response to direction indicates the degree to which the technologist needs to provide assistance to achieve the desired goal. For example, the technologist directs a patient lying supine on the table to roll onto their side in order to prepare the patient for a lateral lumbar spine exposure. The technologist may or may not have to assist the patient in performing this task. Depending on subject ability, the technologist may utilize imaging tools such as sandbags, foam support, etc. to ensure compliance. In contrast to the lumbar spine example, the breast is a skin appendage incapable of following instructions; instead, we rely on instructions that result in the body being synchronized to breast anatomy for effective capture with clarity by the technologist. In addition, the use of compression to immobilize and ensure thickness uniformity is an application that is interdependent with intricate manipulations of the breast. Although positioning/compression techniques are repetitive in mammography, no body, breast, or patient ability is identical, requiring each study to be customized to the individual patient. All of these described attributes are most successfully achieved when the patient's upper body is relaxed, in spite of the fact that most patients present for the exam with some degree of anxiety and are unable to relax on demand. Compassion and effective communication skills are necessary attributes in mammography technologists due to the sensitivity of the examination. Ask any technologist practicing this complex modality today, and she will agree that the artistic and scientific components of mammography cannot be separated.

The Artistic Component

Mammography is a labor-intensive art requiring precision and fine motor skills. It can be compared to artistry that requires years to master depending on the investment the artist makes to the craft. Jewelry making, cake decorating, and quilting are just a few examples of art requiring precision and fine motor skills. Beginning quilters first sign up for an introductory course to become familiar with what they need in order to complete a quilt. Equipment and materials are purchased, allowing the process of learning to begin. Techniques, color arrangement, and patterns are introduced to the novice, and slowly, the student grasps understanding, putting what has been learned into practice. Becoming proficient in the different aspects of quilting can take years as each new pattern provides experience in mastering new skills that eventually build on each other. Mammography's skills are mastered in much the same way. Technologists take courses to familiarize and prepare themselves for the process of learning how to perform mammography. Additional supervised hands-on training introduces them to the basics of breast capture, compression, and clarity. Each unique individual and unique circumstance

provides experience for the technologist to progress in mastering the intricate art of positioning/compression, image quality, and communication. The process of mastering mammography comes with continued education, guidance, experience, and investment of the artist. Be patient with the process.

THE SCIENTIFIC COMPONENT

Tools of the Trade

Image Receptor

Under MQSA, two different sized image receptor support devices (IRSDs) were required for analog mammography.[1] The different sized Buckies were designed to benefit positioning/compression techniques for smaller or larger breasts. These standardized IRSDs were designed to accommodate the 18 × 24-cm cassette for smaller breasts and the larger 24 × 30-cm cassette for larger breasts. Compression devices matching the measurements of each IRSD were used for the examination. This important feature in mammography equipment design benefited image quality by managing breast tissue capture, adequate breast compression, patient dose, and enhanced patient comfort. Computed radiography (CR) full-field digital mammography (FFDM) is the only digital technology that uses the same size IRSD as analog imaging. Early direct ray (DR) FFDM design accommodated only the smaller breast size, as the initial IRSD measured 19 × 23 cm. Larger breast sizes required additional overlapping images to visualize all of the tissue. Today, mammography machine manufacturers offer one large DR FFDM IRSD to accommodate both small and large breast sizes and include two standard size compression devices. The DR FFDM design for the larger breast size is manufacturer specific (close to 24 × 30 cm), and the smaller size remains 18 × 24 cm. When operating DR FFDM units, the radiation field and light field correspond to the compression device size that is selected. Some DR FFDM manufacturers include a shifting compression device design for the 18 × 24 cm size paddle (Figure 7-1). This feature allows flexibility in positioning the smaller breast primarily for the MLO projection, reducing the need to elevate the arm above the shoulder, which negatively effects image quality. The flexibility of the 18 × 24 cm size shifting compression device design is also beneficial in providing versatility when performing the CC or exaggerated craniocaudal lateral (XCCL) projections being done for a wheelchair patient or when positioning a very small breast. The importance of selecting the correct compression device size for the exam will be discussed later in this chapter.

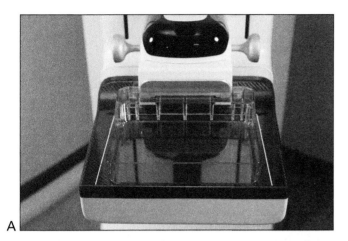

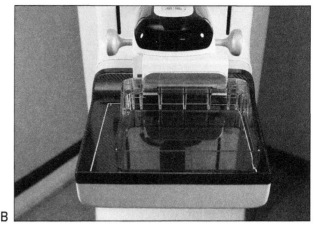

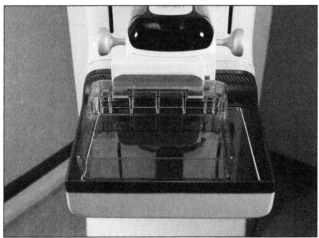

Figure 7-1
A 18 × 24-cm-size shifting compression device. **(A)** Center position used for CC projection. **(B)** Shifted to the right for RMLO, right Lateral projections. **(C)** Shifted to the left for LMLO, left Lateral projections.

Magnification Mammography

Magnification is an invaluable technique used to increase the resolution of breast tissue. Its purpose is to provide further definition of features indicating possible breast cancer detected on standard images, confirming suspicious areas requiring biopsy, and to determine the extent of disease. Any mammographic view can be performed using magnification, but the amount of tissue that can be imaged is confined to a much smaller area. Generally, the entire breast cannot be imaged in one view with this method due to limitations in the image receptor size. In addition, specialized compression devices are also used with magnification. These include quadrant and spot compression sizes, which allow better compression of a smaller area of tissue, increasing resolution by reducing scatter through decreased breast thickness, and improved penetration of denser tissue. Magnification technique is commonly used for the following indications:

- To better delineate the borders of a mass
- To characterize or search for calcifications (Figure 7-2)
- For proving similar calcifications in the contralateral breast

- Specimen radiography
- Imaging of lumpectomy surgical sites

Magnification is achieved by modifying the image receptor with a specially designed platform (the "magnification stand" or "mag stand") (Figure 7-3). Magnification eliminates the need for a grid due to an airgap. Placing the mag stand on the image receptor introduces an airgap (distance) between the breast and the recording system. The small focal spot must be employed because the breast is no longer in contact with the IRSD. Additional information on magnification techniques can be found in Chapter 11.

Compression Device

Standard compression devices are designed for large area contact projections and promote uniform compression of the breast. In addition to the 18 × 24-cm and (approximate) 24 × 30-cm compression devices, additional specialty compression devices of varying sizes and shapes are included with each mammography unit. Although the majority of compression devices on the market have been designed for a specific purpose, technologists should be creative when confronted with technically challenging situations. Problem-solving

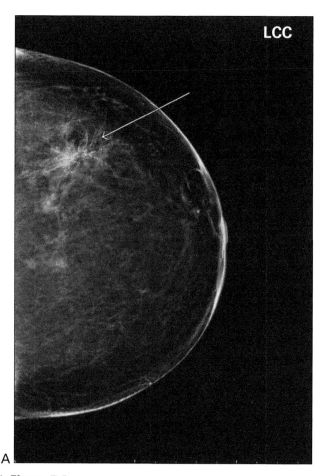

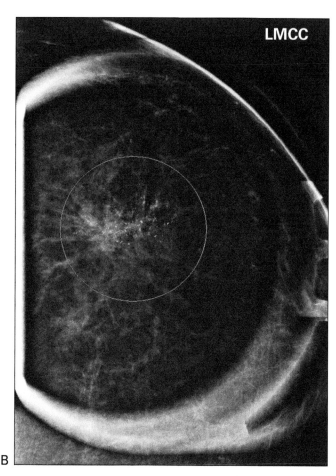

Figure 7-2
Magnification mammography for a calcifying lesion. **(A)** Contact CC projection; *arrow* points at a ROI. **(B)** Magnified spot compression image demonstrates enhanced lesion characteristics.

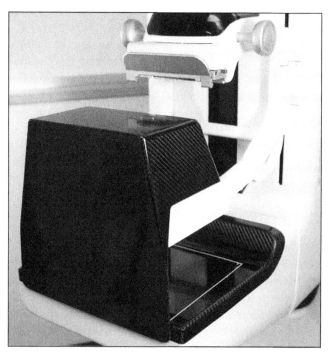

Figure 7-3
Magnification platform installed on the mammography machine.

techniques using some of the specialty compression devices that allow adequate capture of desired breast anatomy to benefit the patient are included in this chapter.

Contact Compression Devices

18 × 24-cm Standard Compression Device Standard contact compression device is used for imaging smaller breast sizes. This compression device is smaller than the surface of the IRSD; therefore, most FFDM manufacturers who utilize one large IRSD for all breast sizes allow this compression device to shift from center to the right and from center to the left primarily for positioning the MLO projections (Figure 7-1).

24 × 30-cm Standard Compression Device Standard contact compression device is used for imaging larger breast sizes. This compression device is the same size as the active area of the IRSD, so no shifting to the right or left is necessary when performing the MLO projections. It is acknowledged that the large standard contact compression device differs slightly among manufacturers measuring approximately 24 × 30 cm. For simplicity, the standard

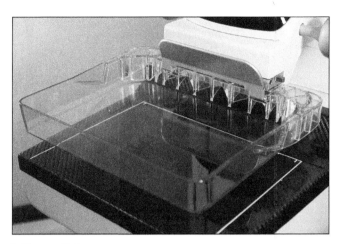

Figure 7-4
A 24 × 30-cm contact compression device, used for imaging larger breast sizes.

large compression device is referred to as the "24 × 30 cm" size in this book (Figure 7-4).

Standard Compression Device, Tilt Paddle Design (available in both 18 × 24 cm and 24 × 30 cm sizes): Used for contact imaging, this unique compression device design provides a more uniform compression result from the thicker base of the breast to the thinner apex, especially when applying compression to a breast that is minimally compressible. The compression device conforms to the varying breast thickness as compression is applied, tilting toward the thinner anterior breast when posterior compression has been achieved. The compression device design benefits uniformity, increased sharpness, patient comfort, as well as reducing the need for additional anterior compression (AC) in the standard projection views to complete the exam (Figure 7-5).

Small Breast Compression Device Sometimes referred to as the half paddle, this contact compression device is a modification of the standard 18 × 24-cm device, with the compression surface measuring only 9 cm from the

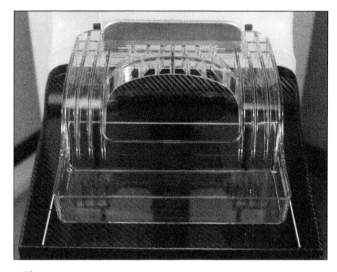

Figure 7-6
Small-breast compression device, sometimes referred to as the half paddle.

chestwall edge. Advantageous when positioning small breasts, extremely thin breasts, males, and patients with implants, this compression device allows more control with almost 9 cm of compression surface area removed for positioning access (Figure 7-6).

Contact Compression Device (15 cm) This contact compression device is slightly smaller than the 18 × 24 cm size, very close to being square in shape (15 × 18 cm). It is not commonly used but provides another choice of contact compression devices and is available from manufacturers if desired.

Contact Compression Device (10 cm) Sometimes referred to as a "quad" paddle, this is an in-between compression device size: smaller than the standard 18 × 24-cm compression device but larger than the 7.5-cm spot compression device. This smaller contact paddle can be used creatively when the use of the full compression

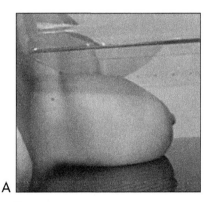

A

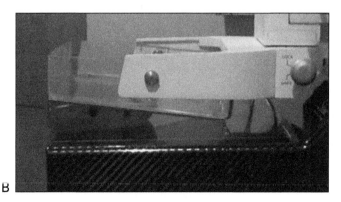

B

Figure 7-5
"Tilt" compression device. **(A)** A noncompressible breast; there is no compression to the front half of the breast.
(B) The "tilt" design allows anterior compression to a breast with nonuniform thickness. Note the red line indicating the compression tapering from the breast base to the apex.

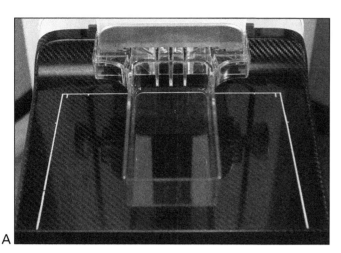
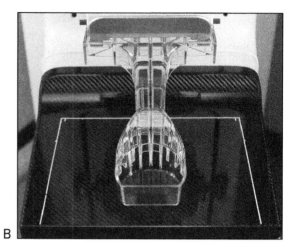

Figure 7-7
Reduced FOV contact compression devices. **(A)** A 10-cm contact compression device, sometimes referred to as a "quad" paddle. **(B)** A 7.5-cm true spot contact compression device.

device size is prohibitive to capture the desired anatomy. Although this smaller contact paddle is used over a smaller volume of tissue, thus increasing compression and reducing breast thickness, it may not provide the same focal compression value as the true spot (7.5 cm) size for feature definition. Radiologists may have a preference regarding the use of the 10-cm contact compression device (Figure 7-7A) or the 7.5-cm spot contact compression device for lesion definition.[3]

Spot Contact Compression Device (7.5 cm) True spot compression device (Figure 7-7B) is used for further lesion definition. This technique is invaluable in determining lesion characteristics by spreading out overlapping tissue (superimposition) and bringing the ROI (region of interest) closer to the image receptor resulting in increased sharpness. See Spot Compression Technique.

Magnification Compression Devices

Spot Magnification Device (7.5 cm) True spot magnification device is used to evaluate the presence of microcalcifications and/or other ROIs identified on the original screening examination. It is the most commonly used of the magnification compression devices (Figure 7-8A).

Magnification Compression Device (10 cm) This magnification device has multiple uses: specimen radiography, occasionally for ductography,[2] further defining calcifications and mass lesions, and some instances when imaging

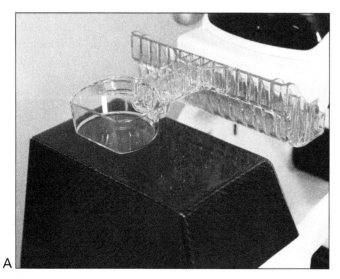
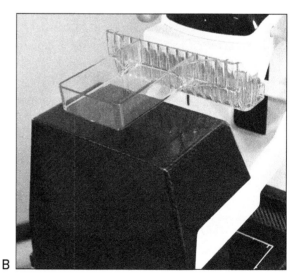

Figure 7-8
Magnification compression devices. **(A)** A 7.5-cm true spot magnification compression device. **(B)** A 10-cm magnification compression device, sometimes referred to as a "quad" paddle.

postsurgical patients. Radiologists may have a preference regarding the use of the 10-cm magnification compression device (Figure 7-8B) or the 7.5-cm spot magnification compression device for lesion definition.

Localization Paddles
Perforated or Open Localization Compression Device
The localization compression device design (perforated or open) is used for examinations where breast access is necessary, such as needle localization, core biopsy, FNAC, and evaluation of skin calcifications. These specially designed compression devices (Figure 7-9) display alphanumeric coordinates for exact location of a ROI. See Tangential view for verifying skin calcifications.

Collimation

Unlike general x-ray, which collimates the x-ray exposure field to within an inch of the body part, close collimation to the breast is not allowed in mammography.[1] Exposing the entire image receptor provides for black opacity surrounding the breast and prevents ambient light from the computer monitor from degrading image contrast during interpretation. Additionally, the use of antiscatter grids and digital technology provides the image contrast necessary for interpreting conditions. Collimation regulations are addressed by the medical physicist in the Mammography Equipment Evaluation required by the FDA.[4]

Automatic Exposure Control

Digital detector design permits the automatic exposure control (AEC) to determine tissue composition based on a sample preexposure in order to select an appropriate target/filter combination, as well as kVp and mAs. The smart AEC is programmed to determine the appropriate dose necessary to ensure a strong signal with minimal noise to the final image. Each manufacturer describes the use of the AEC function as it relates to their particular design. Generally, AECs operate by the information they receive as photons pass through the tissue and reach the AEC electronics. For projections where there may be insufficient tissue covering the AEC, a manual technique must be used. Implant-displaced views and a cleavage view are examples when a manual technique may be required. It is the responsibility of the equipment operator to understand the intricacies of how the manufacturer intends the AEC to function.

Adequate Exposure Assessment

Technologists should familiarize themselves with the mammography equipment they use to produce an image. Manufacturers have specific operational methods that are unique to their equipment, including target/filter combinations, kVp range, compression device advantages, compression force display, and image acceptance dose thresholds. Each manufacturer defines its own dose acceptance threshold in their own unique language: EI number, DEI number, REX number, or S number. For more information on this subject, see Chapter 11. Much like driving a car, the delivery process of the mammography examination is affected by the familiarity and smoothness of the operator.

Compression

Compression is essential to the quality outcome of the mammography image. Gradually applied, vigorous compression allows for dose and scatter reduction, decreased

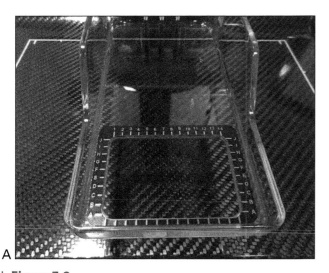
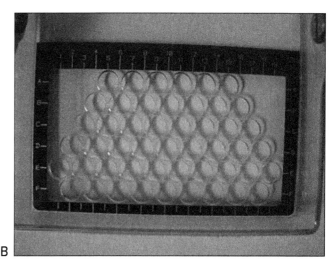

Figure 7-9
Localization compression devices. **(A)** A 10-cm rectangular opening localization device. **(B)** A 10-cm concentric circle localization device.

motion and geometric unsharpness, increased contrast, and the separation of breast structures.[5] Additionally, adequate compression allows a homogeneous thickness from the nipple to the chestwall, preventing under- or overexposure of breast tissue. Ensuring breast tissue uniformity allows for better assessment of mass lesions as the radiologist uses relative density to perceive potential abnormal tissue that may only be apparent as subtle density differences amidst normal glandular structures.[6] For best technical results, the compression device *should* remain parallel to the image receptor unless otherwise specified by the manufacturer's design[1] (Figure 7-10). Standard compression devices with tilt design are described earlier in this section. **Compression** is influenced by the knowledge, application, and judgment of the technologist in each unique mammography examination. Achieving adequate breast compression is accomplished through a blend of each technologist's communication and technical skills impacting both image quality and the patient experience. The importance of the technologist's role cannot be overstated in the delivery of this crucial task. Inadequate compression results in poor image quality as well as introduces the potential to exclude anatomy due to the breast not being secured properly.

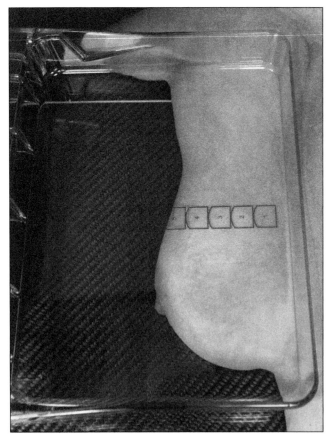

Figure 7-10
Nontilt compression device. When the breast compresses evenly from the apex to the base, the use of a tilting compression device is not necessary.

Overzealous compression does not improve image quality and if too uncomfortable may deter patient compliance with future mammography examinations. Compression device design and performance requirements addressed by MQSA are discussed further in Chapter 11.

Adequate Compression

Adequate compression is described as the breast feeling "taut" to the touch. This tautness is dependent on the composition of the breast and the elasticity of the skin surrounding the breast. As compression is applied, the breast tissue spreads outward as its thickness is reduced.[7] Technologists should monitor the breast as compression is applied, tapping the skin to determine when tautness has been achieved[8] (Figure 7-11). This is evaluated on the medial and lateral aspects of the breast for the CC projection and superior and inferior aspects for the MLO and Lateral projections. For most patients, compressing the breast until taut seems to correlate with the amount of compression they can actually tolerate. In the event that adequate compression was not used for the exam, an accurate description of the reasons why adequate compression was not tolerated should be documented on the patient history form.

Application of Compression

Most patients present for the mammography examination with some degree of apprehension and anxiety. Mammography is an examination that benefits from patients who are relaxed and cooperative as more tissue can be captured with adequate compression applied. Technologists with strong communication and interpersonal skills who prepare the patient for the exam, including the role of compression, will benefit with superior quality results. For patients who present for their first mammography examination (BASELINE), a thorough explanation should be given prior to the exam, complete with a demonstration of how the compression device works and what it sounds like. Letting the patient know approximately how long they remain in compression and that the compression device automatically releases when the exposure is complete provides them with knowledge that helps reduce anxiety. Compression is applied after the breast has been positioned satisfactorily on the image receptor. The technologist activates the automatic compression mode using a foot pedal (Figure 7-12A) for continuous compression until breast tissue is reached. Continuous compression should stop and be replaced with intermittent compression as the technologist slides her hand away from the chestwall toward the nipple and the compression device replaces her anchoring hand. When the breast is secured, with the patient unable to pull out of compression, the technologist checks for positioning accuracy, for skinfolds, and for artifacts in the field of view. *Final compression is*

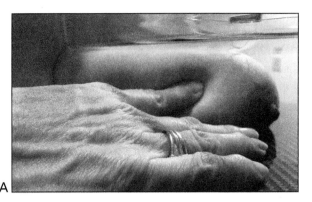
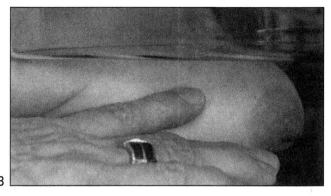

Figure 7-11
Technologist evaluation of compression force. **(A)** Indentation of the skin demonstrates undercompression. **(B)** Tapping the skin while compression is applied assists the technologist to determine appropriate tautness.

accomplished using the manual compression mode (Figure 7-12B) *while communicating with the patient and tapping of the skin for tautness evaluation.* During a routine examination, the equipment automatically releases compression when the exposure is completed. It should be noted that the compression device can be set for manual release for procedures such as needle localization, imaging patients unsteady on their feet, ruling out dermal calcifications, etc. Compression is generally not painful during mammography, and although not a comfortable procedure, it should be tolerable for most patients. If a patient complains of pain during the procedure, ensure that the compression device or image receptor is not pressuring bony structures of the thorax or that skin is not being unduly stressed or pinched. Further discussion involving anxiety and pain during mammography is included in Chapter 3.

Additional Tips for Compression Application

After the first exposure is completed, ask the patient how she "tolerated" the first image. This gives the patient an opportunity to let the technologist know if specific positioning/compression components exceeded the patient's expectations of tolerance for the first projection. Having this information gives the technologist an opportunity to determine if the patient requires further education to continue achieving adequate compression throughout the remainder of the exam or the need to adjust the force delivery due to patient intolerance.

Respiration

There are differing opinions as to whether the patient should be instructed to stop breathing during mammography. Many technologists believe that adequate compression and instructing the patient to "remain still" reduce the occurrence of motion, obviating the need for patients to hold their breath. Others believe that having the patient suspend breathing minimizes the likelihood of motion. Mammography equipment AEC determines dose and exposure time. Exposures exceeding 2 seconds in length are not as common today, reducing the probability of motion occurrence. Given the fact that motion observed on any area in the mammography image significantly degrades the

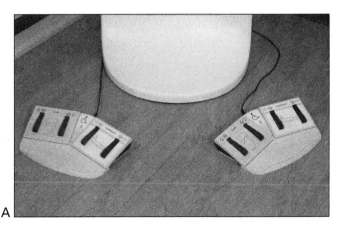
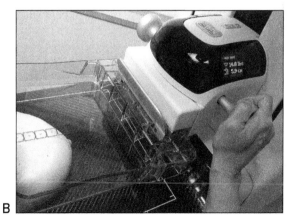

Figure 7-12
Two modes of compression application. **(A)** The automatic mode is operated by foot control pedals. **(B)** A knob located near the compression device allows the technologist to control the application of compression in the manual mode.

quality and the potential ability to detect early indications of breast cancer, consider the following when making the decision to have the patient hold their breath during the exposure:

- There is a low probability of motion when the patient suspends breathing during the procedure.
- Technologists evaluate postexposure images on acquisition workstation monitors; these monitors may not have the technical capability to detect subtle motion due to reduced resolution (megapixel design).
- If motion is detected on an image, it is necessary to repeat the exposure, increasing the dose to the patient.
- Asking the patient to suspend breathing during the exposure is generally accomplished with little effort.

If the technologist elects to have the patient suspend breathing, it is best to instruct the patient to "stop breathing," rather than "hold your breath." When instructing a patient to "hold your breath," many women may take in a deep breath, expanding the thorax as they do so. This may cause the patient to move slightly from the position she has just painstakingly been secured in, potentially excluding tissue at the chestwall.[9]

Skin Assessment: Mammography Examination Skin Markers

Prior to performing the mammogram, the technologist communicates with the patient, thoroughly documenting any medical history relating to the patient's breast health. A discussion of documenting patient history for the mammography examination is found in Chapter 4. Following the process of documenting the patient's history, the technologist turns her attention to the surface of the breast. The technologist inspects the skin covering the breast for:

1. The presence of raised moles, sebaceous cysts, or surgical scars that may be visible on the mammogram.
2. The nipple is an important feature visualized on the mammogram. To denote the location of the nipple for the purpose of localization measurements and to distinguish the nipple from glandular tissue, should it be presented out of profile, radiologists commonly require the nipple location be identified during imaging.

Radiologist protocols may require the technologist to use radiopaque skin markers noting the locations of moles, scars, and the nipple location (Figure 7-13A,B). In

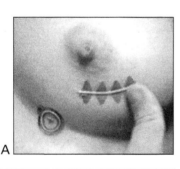

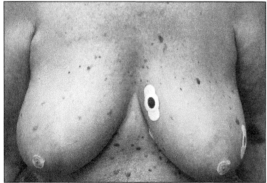

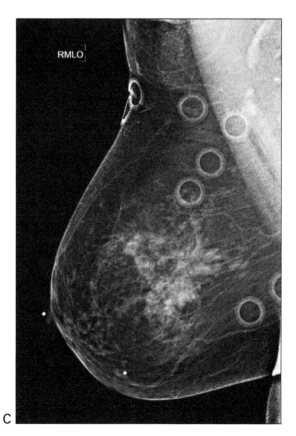

Figure 7-13
Specialized skin marking system for mammography. **(A)** A scar marker (*line*) and mole marker (*circle*). **(B)** Mole markers and nipple location markers. **(C)** These translucent markers are shown on the mammogram but do not obscure pathology within the tissue.

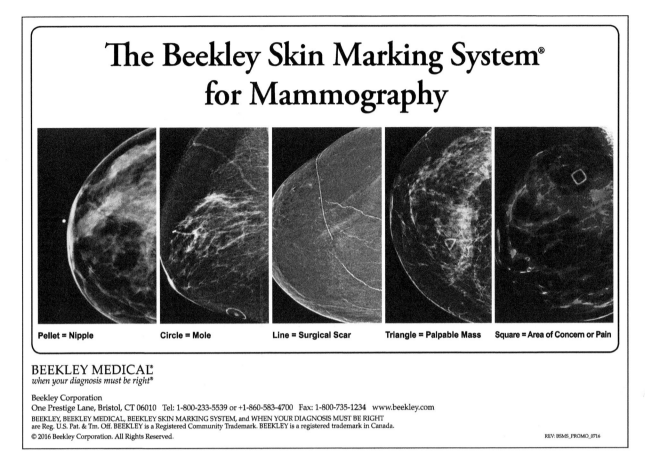

The Beekley Skin Marking System®
for Mammography

| Pellet = Nipple | Circle = Mole | Line = Surgical Scar | Triangle = Palpable Mass | Square = Area of Concern or Pain |

Figure 7-14
The Beekley Skin Marking System standardizes the shapes used to mark the breast: the BB/pellet marks the nipple, the *circle* is used to advise the radiologist of a skin mole (nevus), *lines* are used to indicate surgical scars, the *triangle* is used to mark palpable masses, and the *square* denotes an area of concern or point of pain. (Images courtesy Beekley Corp., Bristol, CT.)

addition to the radiopaque markers, technologists transfer the location of any skin conditions to the diagram on the history form used by the facility. However, the use of radiopaque markers can be distracting on the image (Figure 7-13C); therefore, some radiologists prefer the location of skin conditions to be documented only on the history form diagram. Patients presenting for mammography with breast symptoms, such as a palpable lump or pinpoint tenderness, require the use of a radiopaque marker to identify the exact location in the breast. There are several companies that supply skin markers for mammography. One company has devised a complete system of lower-density markers designed specifically for 2D FFDM and DBT mammography. Beekley Medical (Bristol, CT) offers a skin marking system consisting of five types of markers: the N-SPOT for marking the nipple; the O-Spot for marking moles; the S-Spot, which is actually a bendable wire, for marking surgical scars; the A-Spot, a triangle, for marking palpable masses; and a square-shaped marker used to indicate nonpalpable areas of concern such as

pain (Figure 7-14A–E). The lower density of these markers designed for digital and tomosynthesis applications prevents areas beneath the marker from being obscured, is less distractive to the reader, and reduces the potential of marker artifacts.

▌▌ EXAMINATION PROJECTION PRINCIPLES

Standard Projections: Craniocaudal and Mediolateral Oblique

Two mammography projections, the CC and the MLO, make up the routine mammographic study[10] (Figure 7-15A,B). When properly performed, these standard projections provide complementary images resulting in adequate capture and representation of as much breast tissue as possible for most patients. The MLO projection is considered the primary view in screening mammography because when

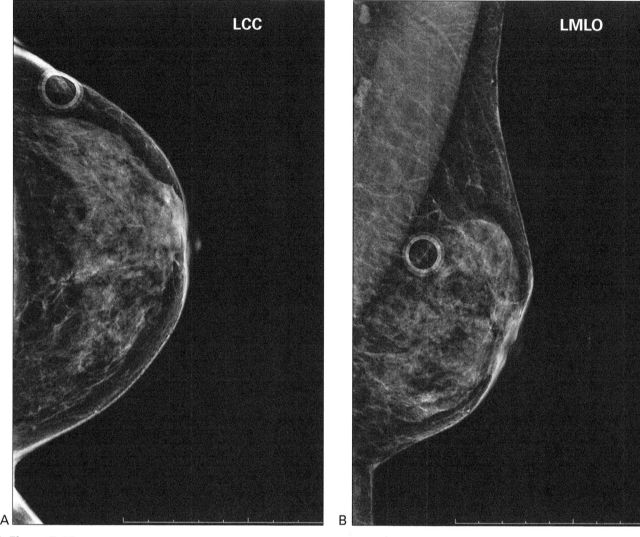

Figure 7-15
Two mammography projections make up the routine mammographic study. **(A)** The craniocaudal (CC) projection. **(B)** The mediolateral oblique (MLO) projection.

properly positioned, it demonstrates the greatest amount of breast tissue in a single view[11–13] and demonstrates a higher number of breast cancers, thereby designating it as the most useful of the two standard projections.[13] Although the MLO view includes the greatest amount of breast tissue, and is the only projection to completely capture the axillary tail, the MLO may not image the far medial breast tissue satisfactorily[13] for two reasons. Even when properly performed using the principle of breast mobility, the MLO (a) has the potential to exclude medial breast tissue because the compression device moves beyond the medial margin in order to reach adequate compression[7]; or (b) if included in the image, medial breast tissue may suffer from geometric unsharpness due to its distance from the IRSD[6] (Figure 7-16). The CC projection complements the

MLO view in its ability to visualize the far medial aspect of the breast, but it is unreliable in capturing the superior tissue and excludes the far lateral tissue from the image[12] (Figure 1-8). Although the use of additional images to complete a screening mammogram is not routine, not every breast is adequately captured with clarity using only the CC and MLO projections. Approximately 15% of patients (about 3 of 20) require an additional view to image tissue that was missed on the two-view mammogram.[14]

Exam Management and Image Execution

The goal of routine mammographic imaging is to portray an accurate representation of breast tissue (anatomy) through adequate capture with clarity (on the image).

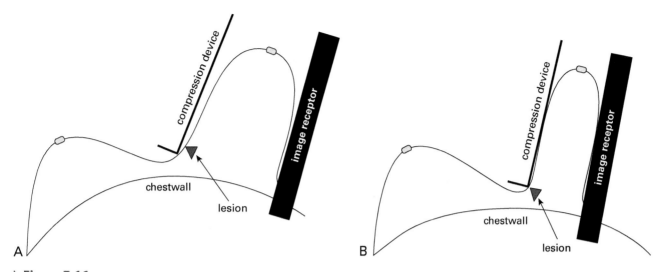

Figure 7-16
The MLO projection may exclude tissue adjacent to the sternum even when the mobile lateral margin of the breast was sufficiently moved toward the fixed medial margin by the technologist. **(A)** Note the location of the posteromedial lesion (*triangle*) *before* compression is applied. **(B)** Movement of the compression device laterally across the thorax may exclude far medial tissue once adequate compression is achieved. (Modified from Eklund GW, Cardenosa G. The art of mammographic imaging. *Radiol Clin North Am.* 1992;30(1).)

This goal is achieved through **exam management**: *the technologist's ability to evaluate imaging compliance during the performance of the standard projections, whether the use of replacement or complementary projections will assist in achieving this goal, and the selection of specific projection(s) to accomplish the objective of adequate capture with clarity resulting in the least amount of dose to the patient* (Figure 7-17). Throughout the process of positioning and caring for the patient, the technologist performing the procedure makes exam management decisions as the exam proceeds. Only she is able to evaluate adequate visualization and clarity of the combined final images to determine whether the exam is complete. Extensive knowledge in breast anatomy, mammographic projections, and technical problem-solving skills are necessary to navigate through each procedure (Figure 7-18). Assessment of the final images in the examination demonstrates the technologist's understanding of *image execution: knowledge of each projection, its intended purpose, inclusion of expected anatomy, and positioning techniques for each specific projection* (Figure 7-19). Technologists knowledgeable in breast anatomy and competent in their technical skills are confident in making the decisions required for satisfactory tissue capture, adequate compression, and adequate exposure of final images using minimal dose. Understanding the location of breast margins, glandular tissue distribution, and breast mobility is essential for determining exam management and image execution. As mentioned earlier, approximately 15% of patients require additional imaging to complete the screening examination. For these patients, it is the technologist's responsibility to customize the examination for each patient, intricately balancing subject cooperative ability with the obligation of capture with clarity of breast tissue. This approach offers the best opportunity to visualize as much breast tissue as possible, producing an accurate representation of the breast from the mammographic perspective.

Adequate Capture

Breast Margins, Glandular Distribution, and External Positioning Landmarks

The technologist must have comprehensive knowledge and understanding of the location and extent of the external margins of breast anatomy in order to satisfy adequate capture for each patient. The margins of the breast extend:

1. Superiorly to the clavicle (level of the second or third rib) and inferiorly to the sixth or seventh rib.
2. Laterally, the breast margin extends to the edge of the latissimus dorsi muscle. This significant landmark for positioning the lateral breast margin is referred to as the midaxillary line and is described by imagining a line drawn from the hollow (or center) of the axilla, straight downward.
3. The medial margin of the breast extends to the sternum.

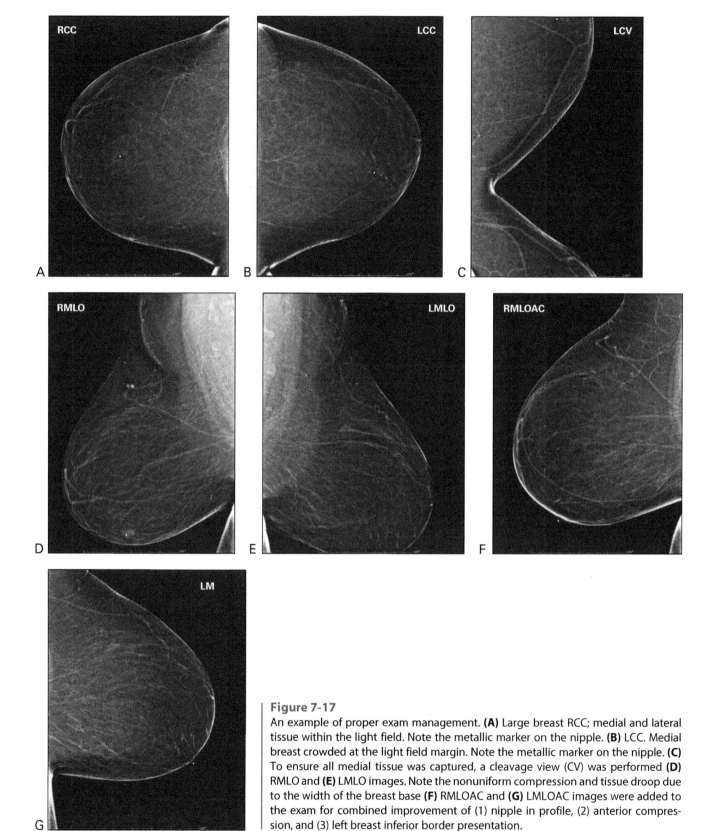

Figure 7-17

An example of proper exam management. **(A)** Large breast RCC; medial and lateral tissue within the light field. Note the metallic marker on the nipple. **(B)** LCC. Medial breast crowded at the light field margin. Note the metallic marker on the nipple. **(C)** To ensure all medial tissue was captured, a cleavage view (CV) was performed **(D)** RMLO and **(E)** LMLO images. Note the nonuniform compression and tissue droop due to the width of the breast base **(F)** RMLOAC and **(G)** LMLOAC images were added to the exam for combined improvement of (1) nipple in profile, (2) anterior compression, and (3) left breast inferior border presentation.

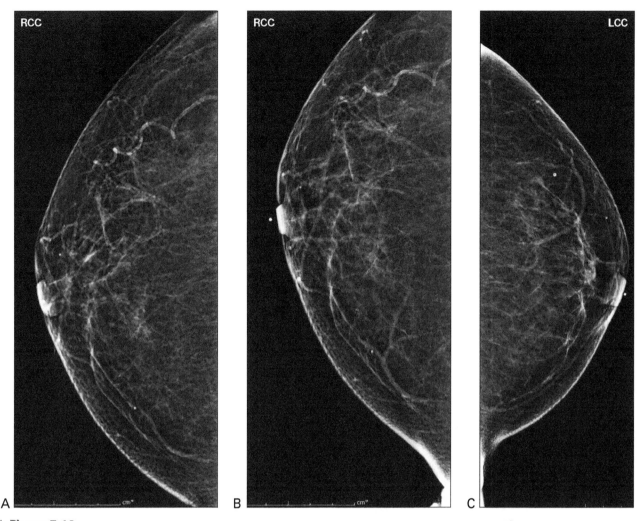

Figure 7-18
An example of poor exam management. **(A)** Incorrect compression device size selection; a wide breast is positioned in the center of an 18 × 24-cm compression device. Both medial and lateral tissues are excluded. **(B)** Repeat RCC, again using 18 × 24-cm compression device, again excludes lateral tissue; the medial tissue margin is crowded at the light field. **(C)** A 24 × 30-cm-size compression device is selected for the LCC and includes both lateral and medial breast margins.

4. The inferior border of the breast, marked by the junction of the inferior breast and superior abdominal wall, is known as the inframammary fold (IMF), a landmark used extensively in positioning.

5. The breast lies anterior to the pectoralis major muscle with glandular tissue distribution commonly located centrally and laterally, with the tail of the breast extending into the axilla.

6. The axilla includes three significant external landmarks used in positioning:
   - Pectoral muscle
   - Midaxilla
   - Latissimus dorsi muscle

Understanding these physical boundaries of the breast significantly contributes to the success of adequate capture when combined with the knowledge of breast mobility described in the next section. For extensive coverage of this topic, refer to Chapter 5, Breast Anatomy. A review of breast margins, **glandular distribution**, and external positioning landmarks is included in Figure 7-20.

Breast Composition

The American College of Radiology BIRADS Atlas Fifth Edition describes four categories of breast tissue composition[15]: (a) almost entirely fatty, (b) scattered areas of fibroglandular density, (c) heterogeneously dense, and (d) extremely dense (Figure 7-21). In addition to the external landmarks that determine breast tissue capture, technologists should also be familiar with the four different types of defined tissue compositions. The four tissue compositions may affect the pliability of the breast as well as its compressibility. Experience is the best teacher for identifying how each tissue composition category, combined with various skin envelope elasticities, responds to positioning techniques.

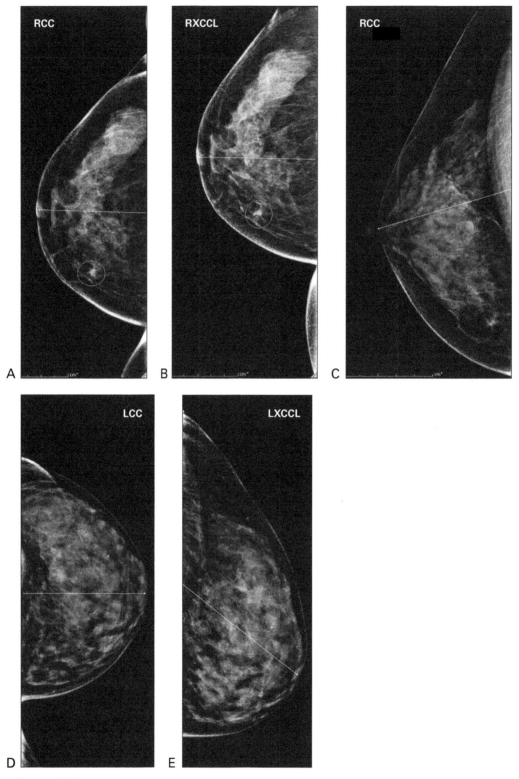

Figure 7-19
Image execution. **(A)** RCC; note PNL direction. **(B)** Same patient as in **(A)**. The image is labeled RXCCL and mimics positioning of the RCC due to insufficient lateral rotation of the patient for the XCCL image. **(C)** Image is labeled RCC; however, it mimics a RXCCL. The patient is reclined laterally toward the image receptor resulting in exaggerated capture of lateral tissue; note the pectoral muscle laterally positioned on the image and the direction of the PNL. **(D)** Correct positioning for the image labeled LCC; note the PNL direction. **(E)** Same patient; correct positioning for the image labeled LXCCL. Note the PNL direction.

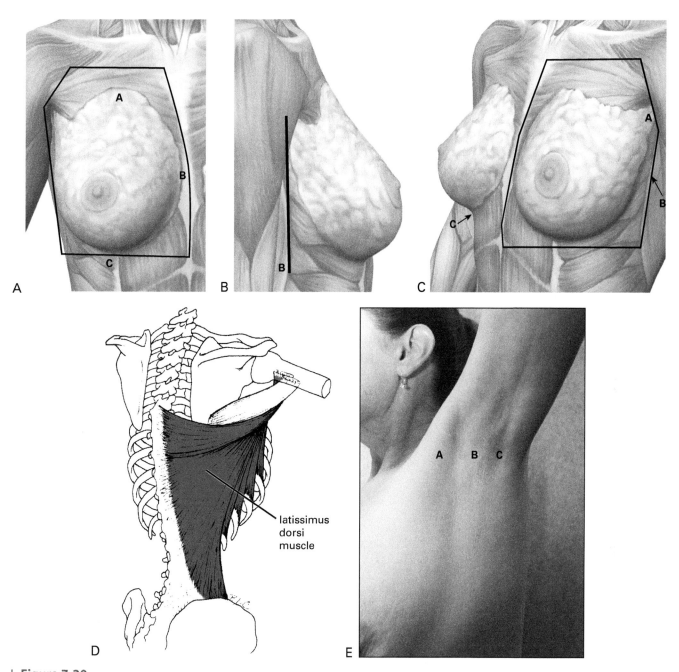

Figure 7-20

Breast margins and glandular tissue distribution. **(A)** Breast tissue extends: superiorly to the clavicle (level of the second or third rib) (labeled *A*), medially to the midsternum (labeled *B*), inferiorly to the sixth or seventh rib (labeled *C*), and **(B)** laterally to the midaxillary line (labeled *B*). **(C)** Mammographic positioning landmarks: tail of Spence (labeled *A*), latissimus dorsi muscle margin (labeled *B*), and inframammary fold (IMF) (labeled *C*). **(D)** Latissimus dorsi muscle. **(E)** Axillary positioning landmarks: pectoral muscle (labeled *A*); midaxilla (labeled *B*); label *C* indicates the location of the anterior latissimus dorsi muscle, which is positioned on the superior corner of the IRSD for the MLO projection. (D, Adapted from Simons DG, et al. *Travell & Simons' Myofascial Pain and Dysfunction: The Trigger Point Manual*. Vol. 1. 2nd ed. Philadelphia, PA: Lippincott Williams & Wilkins; 1998.)

Breast Mobility

A fundamental principle of breast positioning is understanding the advantages afforded by the natural mobility of the breast in capturing and compressing tissue. The **mobile borders** of the breast are lateral and inferior, while the fixed borders are superior and medial[8,16] (Figure 7-22). Moving the mobile borders toward the fixed borders at the beginning of the positioning process allows for maximum inclusion of the fixed breast tissue adjacent to the chestwall. In addition to this advantage, moving the mobile borders toward the fixed borders minimizes the distance

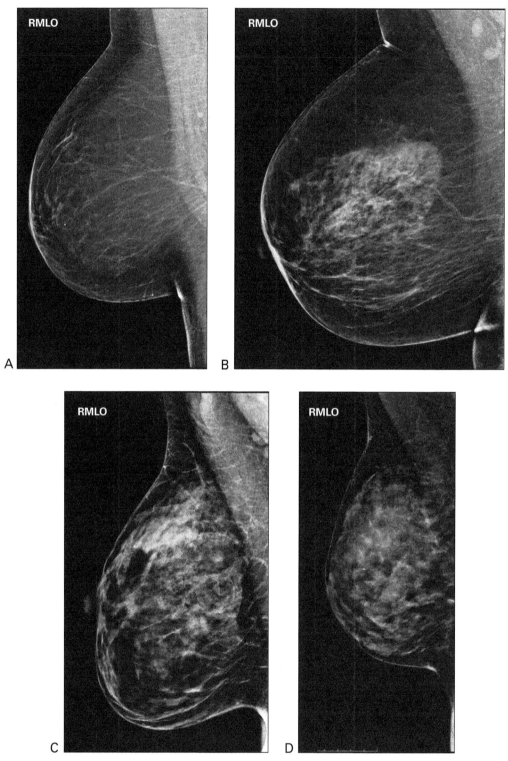

Figure 7-21
Breast tissue composition categories. **(A)** Almost entirely fatty. **(B)** Scattered areas of fibroglandular density. **(C)** Heterogeneously dense. **(D)** Extremely dense.

the compression device travels across the chestwall before reaching adequate compression, allowing for greater patient comfort during the procedure.[8,16] The advantage of using breast mobility when positioning will be further described in each projection.

Developing Your Technique

Mastering positioning/compression techniques for mammography begins by understanding the concept of capture with clarity. Basic rules apply for the process of tissue

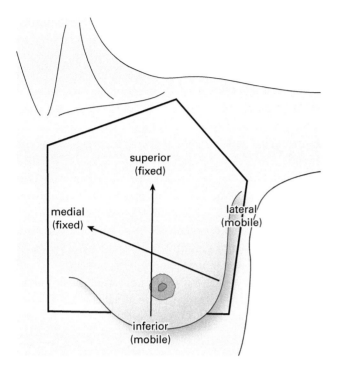

Figure 7-22
Breast mobility describes: lateral and inferior tissue as mobile borders; superior and medial tissue as fixed borders.

capture that involves learned positioning maneuvers and compression techniques. Each learned maneuver results in capturing specific features of the breast on the image. These features must then be adequately compressed, ensuring detail through appropriate exposure techniques affecting image sharpness, contrast, and patient dose. Additionally, the technologist is instructed in the art of minimizing skin-folds and eliminating artifacts on the final image. This basic instruction for positioning/compression is understood and practiced collectively by all mammography technologists. Beyond that foundational knowledge, positioning/compression is an art that each technologist uniquely develops as her own. Influences that determine the technologist's technical style depend upon her physical strengths and weaknesses, height, agility, mentoring (supervising technologist's knowledge), length of hands-on training time, further educational opportunities, and mammography experience. Each opportunity she has to glean insight from radiologists, other technologists, or educational forums provides a platform to assimilate new techniques into strategies that work with her personal strengths and eliminate those that do not. It has been said many times by novice technologists learning from experienced mentors, "She makes that look so easy!" In reality, the experienced technologist has repeated the maneuvers necessary to create a superior image so many times that there is no longer any break in her positioning maneuvers, an illusion formed from dedicated practice.

Establish Patient Partnership

Much has been written about the need to establish rapport with the patient during the mammography procedure. For the purposes of obtaining the projections, it is helpful to again note that successful imaging of the breast is increased when the patient is relaxed, specifically the upper body, shoulders, and thorax. Positioning techniques, compression, patient tolerance, and final image outcome are all affected by the ability of the patient to relax for the procedure. Mammography is a collaborative effort between the technologist and the patient. Using a team approach, enlist the patient as a partner in the positioning/compression techniques required to benefit her imaging.

- *Give the patient control*
  Mammography is a "contact sport" that requires the technologist to invade the personal space of her patient. In addition, the procedure may also cause discomfort to the patient. These exam characteristics describe a sensitive procedure that may potentially be problematic for the patient who perceives she has not been properly informed about the procedure or who feels she is not in control. Simply letting the patient know prior to positioning the first image that she may stop the exam at any time or for any reason creates an equitable atmosphere for her and promotes a teamwork approach.
- *Provide exam purpose and clear instructions*
  Superior quality breast imaging requires capturing the challenging posterior tissue adjacent to the chestwall. Ensuring that the patient has been properly informed about what will take place during the mammography procedure is essential before beginning the exam. Positioning techniques always require relaxation of the patient's thorax and, sometimes, require an awkward body stance or a difficult to maintain head, neck, hip, and knee position. It is absolutely necessary for the technologist to provide clear and concise instructions to the patient and to ensure that what is being requested is physically possible for the patient to do *before they are directed or physically guided to do so.*
- *Listen to the patient*
  Listening to the patient begins immediately after calling her name in the waiting area. Body language as she walks toward you may be an indicator of her present emotional state. Any number of possibilities may contribute to observed anxiety, providing the opportunity for you to connect with her as you walk her to the next destination. Continue to listen and observe her body language throughout the procedure providing factual information combined with compassionate care as needed in each unique encounter. This purposeful practice may sometimes reveal clues that lead to the detection of cancer that may not otherwise have been found.

Selecting the Compression Device Size

DR FFDM mammography machine manufacturers offer one large IRSD to accommodate both small and large breast sizes and include two standard size compression devices. The size of the compression device corresponds to the size of the light field and resulting radiation exposure to the image receptor. This is the first important decision the technologist makes affecting image quality and exam management during the procedure. In the majority of cases, the choice of one compression device size is sufficient for both standard projections: the CC and the MLO. However, the primary factor in choosing the size of the compression device (the radiation field) is determined by ensuring all margins of the breast are included in the field of view (Figure 7-23). This is evaluated by the width of the base of the breast for the CC projection, the length of the base of the breast for the MLO projection, and the distance from the base of the breast to the apex.

Selecting the larger compression device when imaging a smaller breast can negatively affect positioning and adequate compression and is also detrimental to the digital detector as this causes saturation of the pixels not covered by breast tissue (Figure 7-24). For example, positioning the MLO using the larger compression device size for a smaller breast excessively raises the patient's arm beyond the recommended shoulder level and forces the thorax away from the image receptor, resulting in tissue exclusion. Additionally, an excessive amount of shoulder and upper axilla under the compression device prohibits adequate compression of the breast. Most, but not all, DR units allow shifting of the 18 × 24-cm compression device toward the axilla when positioning the patient for the MLO and Lateral views. This equipment design feature allows the technologist to position the breast so that the arm is not raised above shoulder level, ensuring the pectoral muscle remains relaxed.

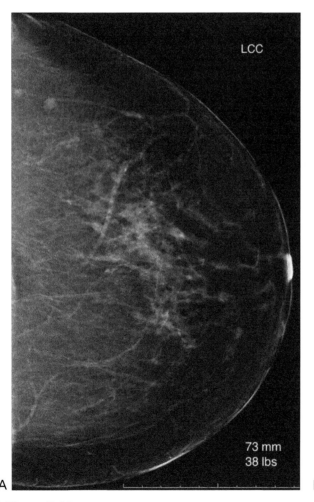
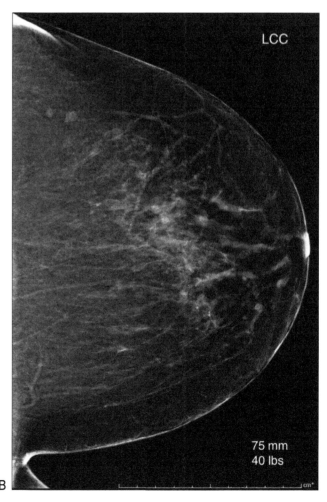

Figure 7-23
Selection of compression device size; same patient in **(A)** and **(B)** images. **(A)** Incorrect selection: using 18 × 24-cm compression device size for a larger breast: note exclusion of posterior, medial, and lateral margins. **(B)** Improved image quality. The use of the 24 × 30-cm-size compression device includes posterior and medial margins sufficiently, while the lateral margin extends to the edge of the light field.

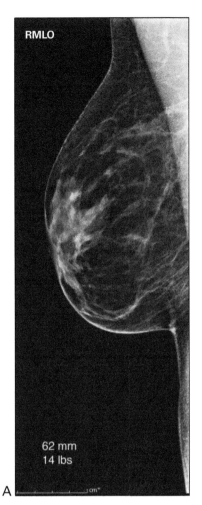
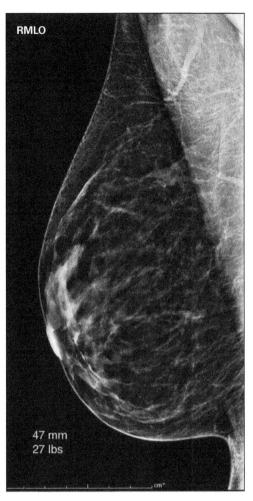

Figure 7-24
Selection of compression device size; same patient in **(A)** and **(B)** images. **(A)** Incorrect selection; using 24 × 30-cm-size compression device for a smaller breast: note abdomen length included on image. Compressed thickness: 62 mm, compression force: 14 lb. **(B)** Improved image quality using the 18 × 24-cm-size compression device; note compression thickness: 47-mm compression force: 27 lb.

Mosaic or Tiling Breast Imaging

Occasionally, patients present for mammography requiring overlapping images of the same projection to visualize all of the tissue due to breast size; the breast is larger than the active area of the digital detector. This is referred to as "**mosaic**" or "tiling" imaging, as the tiles are fitted together to form a complete picture (Figure 7-25).

▊ MAMMOGRAPHIC PROJECTIONS

A standardized labeling system developed by the ACR is used to describe individual mammography projections and their abbreviations.[8] By defining these standards for identification, the ACR intended to reduce confusion for patient care across all facilities. Labeling of laterality, projections, and techniques follows a specified order. Laterality,

always listed first, describes either the right or the left breast, followed by the projection. In most cases, the projection is described by the direction of the x-ray beam. Additional modifiers describe an imaging technique such as magnification or implant displacement. Some modifiers are listed prior to the projection, and others are listed following the projection. Table 7-1 lists the ACR standardized terminology and abbreviations for mammography projections. In addition to the list of ACR standardized projections, this chapter includes a description of historical projections developed by pioneers in mammography whose creativity solved positioning challenges still experienced today. These problem-solving projections are addressed later in this chapter.

The order of maneuvers and positioning directives included in this chapter for each projection are given as examples for technologists ensuring that breast anatomy and breast margins are included with clarity on the image. It is acknowledged that each technologist should develop

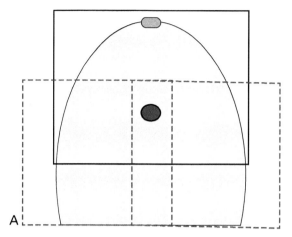

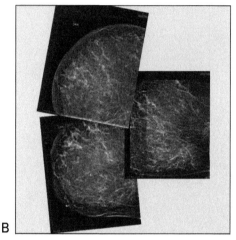

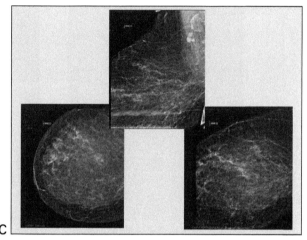

Figure 7-25
When the breast tissue is larger than the image receptor, multiple exposures of the same projection ("mosaic imaging") are required to visualize all the tissue. **(A)** Schematic of three mosaic images in the CC projection, using a metallic marker placed at breast center for image orientation. **(B)** Demonstrates three mosaic images of the CC projection to visualize anteromedial, anterolateral, and posterior tissue. **(C)** Demonstrates mosaic images of the MLO projection to visualize inferoposterior, anterior, and posteroaxillary tissue.

positioning strategies using the inherent strengths of her physical abilities. Each radiographic image for the CC, MLO, and several problem-solving projections is evaluated using established industry criteria. Technologists should develop their own order and style of positioning techniques to meet those defined image quality standards.

The Mediolateral Oblique Projection

Application

A properly positioned MLO projection demonstrates specific pectoral muscle features and the inclusion of the six regions of the breast (Figure 7-26):

1. **Pectoral muscle**[8]
   - Wide superior pectoral muscle width.
   - Gradual narrowing of the pectoral muscle from superior to inferior border.
   - Anterior pectoral muscle border convex in appearance.
   - Length of the pectoral muscle reaches to the posterior nipple line (PNL) or below (ACR states approximately 80% of the time).

2. **Breast regions**
   - **Superiorly**: from the high apex of the axilla, including the tail of Spence.
   - **Centrally**: the mound of the breast, nipple presentation.
   - **Inferiorly**: to the sixth or seventh rib, which includes the external landmark of the IMF.
   - **Laterally**: to the midaxillary line, demonstrated by a line drawn from the center of the axilla down to just below the IMF.
   - **Medially**: to the sternum. This area is included on the MLO by ensuring the mobile lateral portion of the breast is adequately moved toward the fixed medial portion and that the patient's hips and pelvis

Table 7-1 • This Table Provides a Quick Reference for Each of the ACR Standardized Projections Used in Mammography, Detailing Indications for Their Use and Tissue Best Visualized by Each View

PROJECTION	ACR ID	C-ARM ANGLE	IMAGE RECEPTOR PLACEMENT	TISSUE BEST VISUALIZED	APPLICATIONS
Mediolateral Oblique	MLO	30°–60°		Posterior, upper outer quadrant, axillary tail, lower inner quadrant	Routine
Craniocaudal	CC	0°		Subareolar, central, medial, and posteromedial tissue	Routine
Mediolateral	ML	90°		Lateral, central, superior, and inferior	True orthogonal to CC for lesion localization, opens tissue for structural overlap
Lateromedial	LM	90°		Medial, central, superior, and inferior	True orthogonal to CC for lesion localization, opens tissue for structural overlap
Exaggerated Craniocaudal Lateral	XCCL	0°–5°		Posterolateral	Posterolateral tissue adjacent to the thorax
Cleavage	CV	0°		Posteromedial	Extreme medial tissue, slippery medial lesions
Axillary Tail	AT	60°–80°		Posterolateral, axillary tail	Localizing abnormality

(Continued)

Table 7-1 • This Table Provides a Quick Reference for Each of the ACR Standardized Projections Used in Mammography, Detailing Indications for Their Use and Tissue Best Visualized by Each View (*Continued*)

PROJECTION	ACR ID	C-ARM ANGLE	IMAGE RECEPTOR PLACEMENT	TISSUE BEST VISUALIZED	APPLICATIONS
Tangential	TAN	0°–90°	Example illustrates TAN for lesion in UOQ or LIQ.	All	Palpable abnormality, to visualize borders with better detail; often used in conjunction with magnification
Rolled Medial	RM	0°		Subareolar, central, medial, and posteromedial tissue	Separation of superimposed glandular tissue
Rolled Lateral	RL	0°		Subareolar, central, medial, and posteromedial tissue	Separation of superimposed glandular tissue
Rolled Inferior	RI	90°		Lateral, central, superior, and inferior	Separation of superimposed glandular tissue
Rolled Superior	RS	90°		Lateral, central, superior, and inferior	Separation of superimposed glandular tissue
Caudocranial	FB	180°		Central and medial, high on the chestwall	Nonconforming pt., superior lesion not seen on CC
Lateromedial Oblique	LMO	90°–180°		Posterior, medial, upper outer quadrant, lower inner quadrant	Can replace MLO in pts with pacemakers, open heart surgical scars
Superolateral to Inferomedial Oblique	SIO	1°–90°		Posterior, medial, upper inner quadrant, lower outer quadrant	Additional view for encapsulated implants, nonconforming pt., orthogonal to MLO for localization

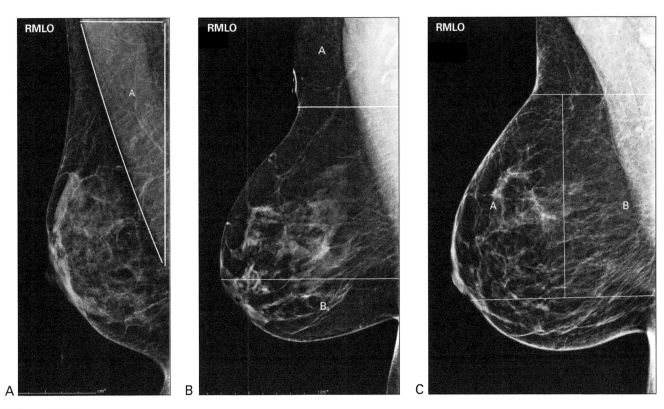

Figure 7-26
A properly positioned MLO projection demonstrates: **(A)** pectoral muscle (labeled *A*); wide superior muscle width; gradual narrowing of the muscle from the superior to inferior border; anterior pectoral muscle border convex in appearance; length of the muscle reaches to the PNL or below (ACR states approximately 80% of the time) **(B)** superiorly (labeled *A*): from the high apex of the axilla, including the tail of Spence; inferiorly (labeled *B*): to the sixth or seventh rib, which includes the external landmark of the IMF **(C)** anterocentral (labeled *A*): the mound of the breast including the subareola and nipple features; posterocentral (labeled *B*): including the chestwall margin, the pectoral muscle mid to inferior insertion, and the retroglandular fat space.

are rotated squarely to face the unit. Even with the best positioning skills, far medial anatomy has the potential to be excluded on the MLO due to the fixed tissue at the sternum and as the compression device moves laterally across the thorax to achieve adequate compression.

- **Posteriorly**: to the chestwall margin, including the pectoral muscle, retroglandular fat space and IMF.

Of the two projections used for routine mammography, the MLO projection (Figure 7-27) best visualizes the extreme posterior and upper outer quadrants of the breast. This is intrinsic to the anatomy of the breast, which lies anterior to and follows the line of the obliquely coursing pectoral muscle. By positioning the breast parallel to this oblique line, which follows the breast's natural course of tissue, it is possible to demonstrate most of the glandular tissue. The MLO is referred to as the primary view because between the two standard projections (CC and MLO), it includes the greatest amount of tissue. However, even

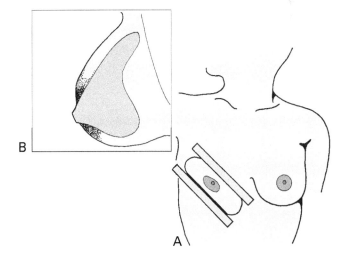

Figure 7-27
MLO projection. **(A)** Schematic of the orientation of the breast to the image receptor for the MLO projection. **(B)** Schematic demonstrating the "glandular island" usually evident with this projection.

though the MLO images the breast in its entirety, it does so with much structure overlap of anterior structures.[6]

Performing the Mediolateral Oblique Projection

The C-arm is rotated for a superomedio–inferolateral beam direction. The appropriate degree of obliquity is based on the natural angle of the pectoral muscle for each individual.[8] The degree of the angle averages approximately 45°, but varies from 30° to 60° depending on the patient's body habitus. Patients who are longer and thinner from shoulder to waist have pectoral muscles with a steeper angle requiring a steeper IRSD angle. Patients with a shorter, stockier build have a more horizontal presentation of the pectoral muscle, requiring a shallower IRSD angle. Patients of average shoulder to waist length measurement require the IRSD angle at approximately 45° (Figure 7-28). These established ACR guidelines assist in determining which angle works best for specific body types, but the technologist should be flexible, using the equipment design to benefit the patient. By customizing the angle of the IRSD to the patient, the pectoral muscle is more relaxed, suspending tissue forward naturally, demonstrating breast tissue as far posteriorly as possible, with increased comfort during compression.

Customizing the IRSD Angle

The angle can be identified by having the patient move their elbow slightly away from the body, hand resting on the upper thigh, and pectoral muscle relaxed. Keeping the arm at the side of the patient to customize the angle retains the muscle in a relaxed position. Using this technique to find the natural angle of the muscle ensures the breast suspends forward onto the image receptor with the least resistance allowing the capture of maximum posterior tissue. The technologist places her flat hand against the portion of the pectoral muscle that extends from the thorax to the axilla. With fingers gently inserted into the axilla, flat hand supporting the pectoral muscle, the technologist lifts and moves the muscle anteriorly and medially defining its specific angle. Using the

customized angle of the patient's pectoral muscle, rotate the IRSD parallel to this angle (Figure 7-29). Although this method is described in the ACR manual to locate the natural angle of the pectoral muscle,[8] another guideline commonly used is to draw an imaginary line from the patient's shoulder to midsternum, rotating the C-arm parallel to this angle.[6]

> Determine the C-arm Angle
> Short torso measurement, stockier build = 30° to 40° angle
> Average patient height and torso length = 40° to 50° angle
> Tall patient, longer torso measurement = 50° to 60° angle

IRSD Height

When the C-arm angle has been determined, the patient's arm should be returned to its natural position. With the patient standing in close proximity to the image receptor, the appropriate height of the IRSD can be easily adjusted by the technologist.

Determining the correct height of the image receptor for the MLO projection is critical for inclusion of the high apex of the axilla. With the correct image receptor height:

- Most of the tail of Spence is visible with good presentation, and uniform compression of the tail and the breast mound is possible.
- With the image receptor height properly positioned, the superior chestwall corner of the compression device should rest in the natural depression that forms where the clavicle and the humeral head intersect.

Initially position the height of the IRSD at the relaxed level of the axilla; this needs to be further adjusted for each patient during axillary placement maneuvers (Figure 7-30A). Placement too low excludes superior tissue in the axillary tail (Figure 7-30B). Raising the IRSD too high excessively elevates the arm and stretches the pectoral muscle, causing difficulty in pulling the breast into view, excluding posterior tissue (Figure 7-30C). The arm position for the MLO affects the ability of the pectoral muscle to relax. Raising the arm above the shoulder forces the pectoral muscle to tense, inhibiting the desired effect that

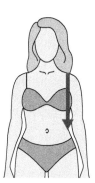 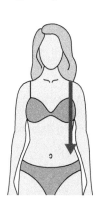 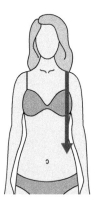

Figure 7-28
Schematic of body habitus examples depicting established guidance for MLO projection C-arm angle. **(A)** Shorter shoulder to waist measurement; shallower angle, 30° to 40°. **(B)** Average shoulder to waist measurement; average angle, 40° to 50°. **(C)** Longer shoulder to waist measurement; steeper angle 50° to 60°. (Adapted from Shutterstock.)

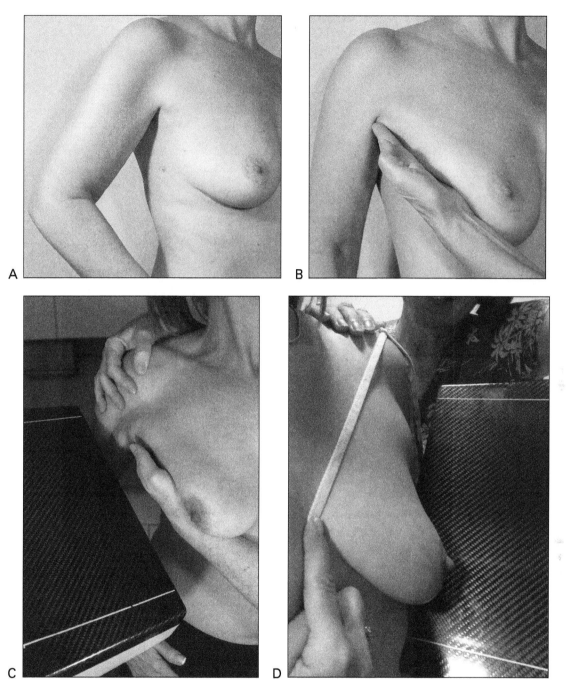

Figure 7-29
Customizing the IRSD angle. **(A)** Position the patient's elbow slightly away from her body, with hand resting on the upper thigh and pectoral muscle relaxed. Keeping the arm at the side of the patient to customize the angle retains the muscle in a relaxed position. **(B)** To identify the angle, the technologist places her flat hand against the portion of the pectoral muscle that extends from the thorax to the axilla. **(C)** With fingers inserted into the axilla, flat hand supporting the pectoral muscle, the technologist lifts and moves the pectoral muscle anteriorly and medially to define its specific angle, rotating the image receptor parallel to this angle. **(D)** Another commonly used method for defining the pectoral muscle angle is to imagine a line drawn from the patient's shoulder to midsternum, rotating the C-arm parallel to this angle.

relaxation provides during positioning. Ensuring the arm is not elevated above the shoulder allows for increased posterior capture as the breast naturally falls forward onto the image receptor. Additionally, too much upper axilla captured under the compression device prohibits adequate compression on the lower portion of the breast. Excessive superior placement of the breast may also cause exclusion of the inferior breast tissue and IMF. Appropriate

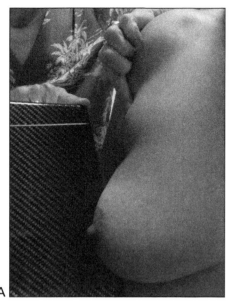
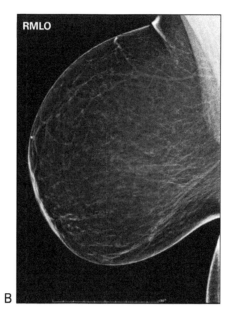
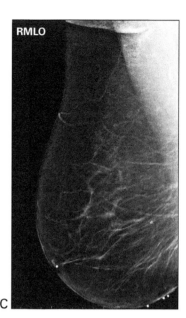

Figure 7-30
(A) To determine the height of the IRSD for the MLO projection, initially position the IRSD at the relaxed level of the axilla; this needs to be further adjusted for each patient during axillary placement maneuvers. **(B)** The IRSD positioned too low excludes superior tissue, excluding the most superior portion of the axillary tail. **(C)** The IRSD positioned too high excessively elevates the arm, stretching the pectoral muscle, impeding the capture of posterior tissue. The IRSD positioned too high additionally may exclude the IMF region and affect adequate compression.

positioning of the MLO includes tissue from high in the axilla to below the IMF, taking up most of the "real estate" of the field of view. Developing a positioning method that includes desired superior breast anatomy, while not excessively elevating the arm for the MLO view, requires artistic expertise by the technologist.

Patient Stance

Where the patient stands for the remainder of the MLO maneuvers is extremely important as the position of her feet and pelvis placed in relation to the IRSD determines the capture of the superior, inferior, and posterior breast margins. In order to ensure these margins are satisfactorily included on the MLO projection, the patient should stand:

1. With her feet and pelvis facing the unit.
2. With the pelvis offset to the inferior edge of the image receptor. This position places the IMF region (junction of the inferior breast and superior abdomen) in front of the IRSD (Figure 7-31A) as the patient leans laterally onto the image receptor for the MLO projection.
3. The patient's abdomen must be in contact with the chestwall edge of the image receptor at a level comfortably below the IMF region. For the MLO projection, there should not be a space between the image receptor and the patient (Figure 7-31B).

Axillary Placement

Proper placement of the axilla on the IRSD determines the width of the pectoral muscle superiorly on the image and posterior tissue inclusion. The axilla contains three significant landmarks used to position the MLO projection (Figure 7-20C).

1. The pectoral muscle is included in the image and lies anterior to the hollow of the midaxilla.
2. The midaxilla (hollow) and the line drawn inferior to the midaxilla identify the lateral edge of the breast tissue.
3. The latissimus dorsi muscle is located posterior to the midaxilla.

Ensuring the lateral margin of breast anatomy is demonstrated on the image requires placement of the IRSD beyond the midaxillary line to the landmark just anterior to the latissimus dorsi muscle.[8] Additionally, the width of the superior pectoral muscle is determined by proper placement of the axilla and follow-through of patient rotation toward the image receptor medially. When axillary placement maneuvers are successfully completed, with adequate rotation of the patient until her sternum touches the compression device, the landmark of the anterior axillary skinline projects toward the approximate center of the light field on the image receptor (Figure 7-32).

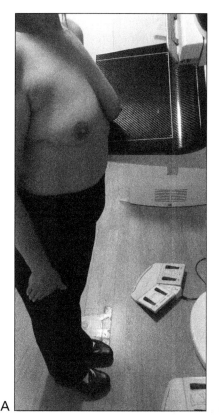 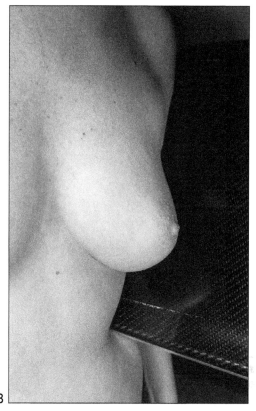

A   B

Figure 7-31
Where the patient stands in relation to the IRSD for the MLO projection determines sufficient capture of the superior, inferior, and posterior breast margins. **(A)** The patient should stand with her feet and pelvis facing the unit and offset to the inferior edge of the image receptor, engaging the IMF region in front of the IRSD. **(B)** The patient's abdomen must be in contact with the chestwall edge of the image receptor and extend comfortably below the IMF region.

This is an indication of satisfactory superomedial tissue inclusion and is demonstrated by a wide superior pectoral muscle on the radiographic image.

Superior Breast Maneuvers

Standing at the superior aspect of the IRSD, the technologist faces the patient and elevates the patient's **ipsilateral** arm so that the axilla is in view. Determine the landmark posterior to the midaxillary line, just anterior to the latissimus dorsi muscle in the axilla (Figure 7-33A). Using one hand to support the patient's arm and the other to ensure that the entire length of the breast is captured in front of the IRSD, guide the patient to place or "plant" the posterior axillary landmark at the corner of the IRSD (Figure 7-33B). Ensure that the patient allows her axilla to sink into the IRSD corner capturing the anatomy deep into the axilla. As the posterior axilla makes contact with the IRSD, guide the patient's arm, gently stretching and draping the shoulder and arm *in a forward direction* over the superior edge of the IRSD, simultaneously rotating the triceps muscle

posteriorly and superiorly to position any excess arm tissue behind the IRSD. This maneuver minimizes the thickness of the upper breast and axilla under compression and also eliminates skinfolds and arm artifacts in the superior aspect of the MLO image. The ipsilateral arm continues its forward motion to rest along the side of the C-arm, elbow flexed, extremity completely relaxed, and hand resting on the unit throughout the remainder of the positioning maneuvers (Figure 7-33C).

Standing at the superior aspect of the IRSD provides the technologist with an advantageous angle to preview three building blocks of the MLO projection: the angle, the height, and the placement of the IRSD. From this vantage point, evaluation of an axillary airgap, potential skinfolds, and posterior breast inclusion are more readily identified in order to make minor adjustments to the IRSD (Figure 7-33D). This location also affords the ability for eye contact with the patient, connecting with her if the arm and shoulder are tense, requiring further IRSD height adjustment or additional coaching for relaxation if needed. Explaining the necessity for a relaxed shoulder

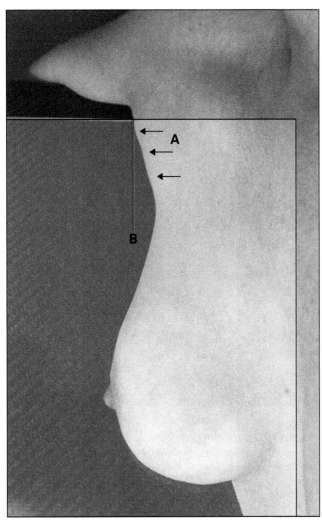

Figure 7-32
Inclusion of posteromedial breast margins requires adequate patient rotation toward the image receptor. This maneuver will direct the skinline of the tail of Spence (labeled A) toward the center of the image receptor/light field (labeled B).

and thorax is of utmost importance as this controls the relaxation of the pectoral muscle, which influences its presentation on the image and impacts the comfort of the exam. The final maneuvers for capture of the superior breast tissue are to ensure that both the patient's pelvis and feet rotate until they face the unit. This final maneuver ensures the medial aspect of the breast is included on the image. Lean the patient's thorax and head laterally toward the IRSD while reminding her to relax and slouch her body. This maneuver brings the sternum parallel to the IRSD, while bringing her head closer to her shoulder collapses the fanned pectoral muscle, making it pliable to allow for uniform compression and increased comfort (Figure 7-34). When the patient rotates her feet to face the unit, and she completely relaxes her hand, arm, shoulder, and pectoral muscle, a "slope" or "dip" can be identified

anterior to the sternum and inferior to the clavicle and humeral head junction. This feature indicates the patient is relaxed and ready for the next positioning maneuvers.

Relaxation of the Pectoral Muscle

Relaxation of the pectoral muscle impacts several aspects affecting image quality on the MLO projection; therefore, before the technologist turns her attention to the posterolateral positioning maneuvers, it is critical she take the time necessary to ensure the patient's shoulder and thorax are as relaxed as possible. The relaxation of the pectoral muscle is controlled by the relaxation of the patient's shoulder, the arm, and the thorax. Image quality factors (Figure 7-26) negatively affected by a tense pectoral muscle include:

1. Convex anterior pectoral muscle presentation
2. Maximum posterior tissue inclusion
3. Adequate compression

Posterolateral Maneuvers

During the following posterolateral maneuvers, the use of good communication while intermittently inspecting the axilla and shoulder placement ensures that the patient does not move the superior aspect of her breast away from the IRSD. The technologist moves to the opposite side of the patient, positioning herself in close proximity to both the surface of the image receptor and the contralateral side of the patient (Figure 7-35). In this location, the technologist can easily view the medial aspect of the breast on the image receptor. *When performing a RMLO* view, the technologist positions her *left flat hand* between the lateral breast and the IRSD, placing the fifth finger in contact with the posterolateral breast at approximately the landmark of the midaxillary line. Using the *right hand*, the technologist places the flat palm in contact with the chestwall edge of the IRSD. The technologist's arms encircle the patient's thorax for maximum control over posterolateral capture. Gently lift the patient's thorax slightly away from the image receptor capturing and guiding the posterolateral aspect of the breast forward (slightly medial and anterior) (Figure 7-36A,B). The technologist's left hand controls capture of the lateral margin of breast tissue, while the right hand manages several other important positioning details. The technologist's right hand makes contact with the posterolateral margin of the breast, easing tissue securely downward, ensuring that from the axilla to the IMF, skinfolds are smoothed away and breast tissue is not excluded. Additionally, the fingers verify correct lateral capture, ensuring posterolateral tissue inclusion, while also ensuring no "extra" back tissue extending beyond the

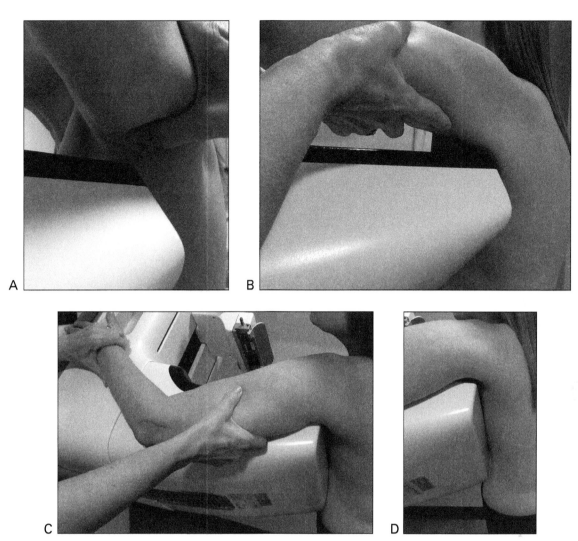

Figure 7-33
Axillary placement determines the superior width of the pectoral muscle and posterior tissue inclusion. **(A)** The patient's ipsilateral arm is elevated to view the axillary landmarks. **(B)** Guide the patient onto the image receptor and place or "plant" the landmark just anterior to the latissimus dorsi muscle over the corner of the IRSD. **(C)** Continue to guide the patient's arm, draping the shoulder and arm *in a forward direction* over the top of the IRSD, simultaneously rotating the triceps muscle posteriorly and superiorly to position excess upper arm tissue behind the IRSD. **(D)** Standing near the superior aspect of the breast allows the technologist a thorough evaluation of the completed axillary placement maneuvers: verifies posterior breast inclusion without axillary airgap or potential skinfolds.

latissimus dorsi line is captured on the image (Figure 7-37). Both hands work simultaneously at their positioning tasks, sometimes meeting and working together. When the lateral posterior tissue has been properly captured and smoothed, it is anchored to the image receptor at the anterior latissimus dorsi line to complete the maneuver (Figure 7-38). With the lateral posterior breast secured against the image receptor, the hands now sandwich the breast and pull the breast straight out and away from the chestwall (Figure 7-39). In the sandwich scenario, the left hand is in contact with the lateral half of the breast, while the right hand is in contact with the medial half of the breast.

The scenario in this section described the hand positions used for the *right* MLO projection. *When positioning the left breast, the hand positions should be reversed.*

Inferior Maneuvers

Ensure that the patient's pelvis, hips, and feet are facing the unit, with the tissue supported approximately 90° from the chestwall. When the inferior breast and superior abdomen (IMF) are properly positioned in front of the IRSD, the supported breast demonstrates an open IMF (Figure 7-40). Slide the hand in contact with the lateral breast out, supporting the medial tissue straight out from the chestwall, preventing

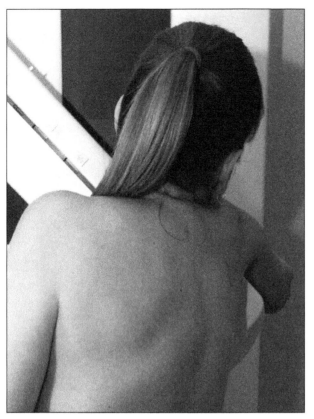

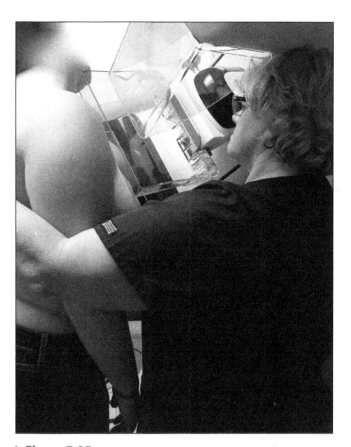

Figure 7-34
Leaning the patient's thorax and head laterally toward the IRSD brings the sternum parallel to the image receptor, collapsing the fanned pectoral muscle, making it pliable for uniform compression, and increasing comfort to the patient.

Figure 7-35
The technologist moves to position herself on the medial side of the breast in order to address posterolateral, inferior, and the out-and-up positioning maneuvers.

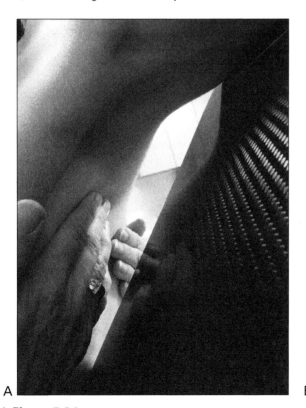

A

B

Figure 7-36
(A) The technologist uses two hands to address posterolateral tissue capture: lifting the patient's thorax slightly away from the image receptor, the technologist uses one hand to capture and guide posterolateral tissue forward and the other to smooth tissue in a downward direction, eliminating skinfolds. **(B)** The mobile posterolateral tissue is moved medially and anteriorly toward the fixed medial tissue, and once moved, the posterior breast margin is anchored against the chestwall edge of the IRSD.

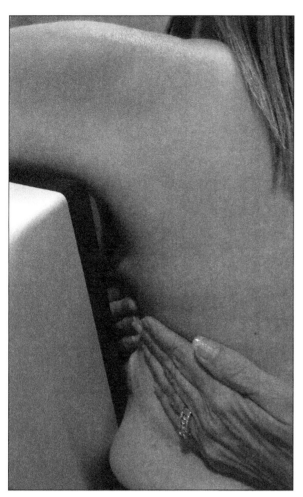

Figure 7-37
The technologist verifies correct posterolateral capture, ensuring "extra" back tissue extending beyond the latissimus dorsi line is not included.

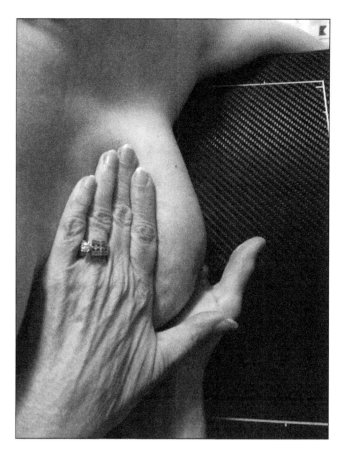

Figure 7-39
When the breast has been secured against the image receptor, the technologist sandwiches the breast between her hands and pulls the tissue away from the chestwall, ensuring the posterior structures are positioned approximately 90° from the thorax.

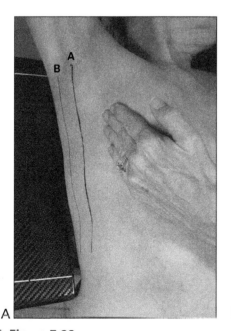

A

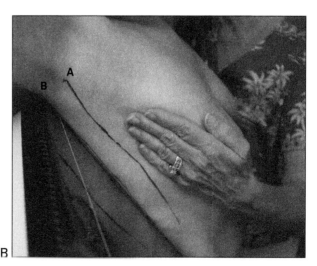

B

Figure 7-38
The technologist should be familiar with two positioning landmarks and why they are important to posterolateral tissue capture. **(A)** The midaxillary line (labeled *A*) is drawn downward from the midaxilla, indicating the lateral border of the breast. The latissimus dorsi line (labeled *B*) is drawn downward from the axillary point just anterior to the latissimus dorsi muscle. **(B)** Posterolateral tissue is anchored to the image receptor beyond the lateral breast margin at the latissimus dorsi line (labeled *B*) ensuring all posterolateral tissue is included on the image.

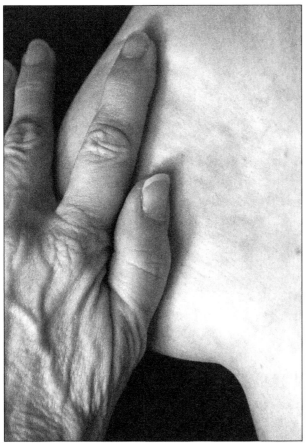

Figure 7-40
When the breast and superior abdomen (IMF) are properly positioned anterior to the IRSD, with the patient's pelvis, hips, and feet facing the unit, the sandwiched tissue supported approximately 90° from the thorax demonstrates an open IMF.

the tissue from drooping (Figure 7-41A,B). Prior to activating compression, verify that the lateral posterior tissue is secured on the image receptor and the patient's sternum, pelvis, hips, and feet are rotated toward the image receptor to include the inferior breast and IMF. Excluding the IMF prevents posterior breast tissue from being visualized. The IMF should be in an "open" position on the image, without evidence of creasing. Supporting the medial breast tissue outward and upward away from the chestwall at approximately 90° accomplishes this open IMF appearance. With your fingers, smooth out the medial and lateral tissue of the IMF to eliminate skinfolds, and ensure tissue contact with the image receptor and compression device, eliminating airgaps (Figure 7-41C).

Compression Application

Rotate the patient toward the unit to prepare her for compression; this action brings medial breast tissue onto the image receptor. The chestwall edge of the compression device first comes into contact with the sternum as it skims across the thorax. Continue to support the breast at all times, outward and away from the thorax at approximately 90° from the chestwall. Do not allow the medial tissue to droop while applying compression to ensure visualization of posterior tissue and the IMF. Lower the compression device just enough to hold the posterior portion of the breast in place, sliding the supporting hand anteriorly toward the nipple as the compression device takes over holding the breast in place. This prevents the breast from drooping and anchors posterior tissue more securely. Maintain support of the breast until the compression device replaces the

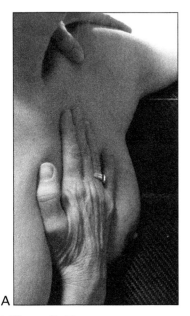

A

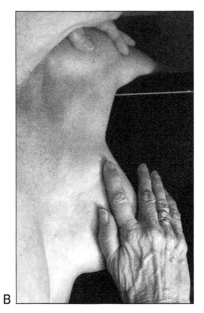

B

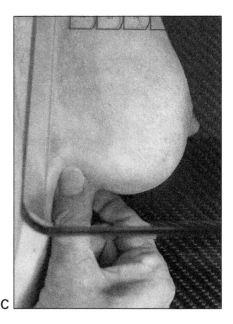

C

Figure 7-41
The breast is anchored to the image receptor using specific positioning maneuvers during compression application: slide the hand in contact with the lateral breast straight out from the chestwall. **(A)** Anchor the breast using one hand near the sternum. **(B)** Continue to move the anchoring hand straight out away from the chestwall as compression is applied, supporting the breast straight out from the chestwall, not allowing medial tissue to droop. **(C)** The technologist uses her fingers to smooth out medial and lateral tissue at the IMF eliminating skinfolds and to ensure tissue contact with the image receptor and compression device eliminating airgaps.

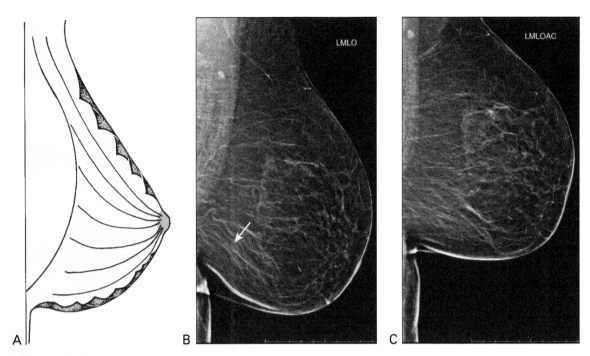

Figure 7-42
Breast architecture. **(A)** Ductal structures that are allowed to droop will overlap making detection of architectural distortion more difficult if not impossible. **(B)** When drooping occurs (*arrow*), the silhouette of the breast appears as a camel's face, earning it the nickname of "camel's nose." **(C)** The breast should be supported at approximately 90° from the thorax with adequate compression to properly demonstrate ductal structures and alleviate tissue overlap. If this cannot be accomplished on the standard MLO projection, the MLOAC projection is necessary.

anchoring hand to ensure proper presentation of ductal structures. Ductal structures run in straight lines toward the nipple; if the breast is allowed to droop, the detection of architectural distortion, a common sign of cancer, is more difficult, if not impossible to discern[6] (Figure 7-42). The superior chestwall corner of the compression device rests in the hollow between the humeral head and the clavicle as compression is applied (Figure 7-43). The patient may have to gently hold the contralateral breast out of the way (without pulling the medial ipsilateral breast from view) to avoid superimposition (Figure 7-44).

Summary of MLO Positioning

The step-by-step processes of patient positioning for the MLO projection are listed here.

Beginning: Preparation
Addressing IRSD Angle, IRSD Height, and Proper Feet Placement
1. Choose the appropriate size compression device.
2. Customize the angle of the C-arm to the patient. The patient stands with the lateral aspect of her breast near the IRSD and arms relaxed at her side.

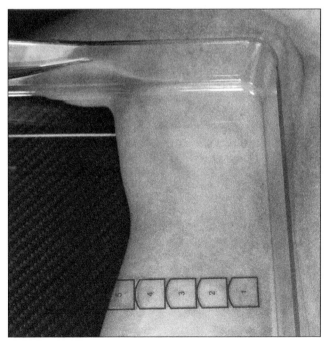

Figure 7-43
Proper positioning of the MLO to include posteromedial breast tissue places the superior chestwall corner of the compression device in the hollow between the humeral head and the clavicle as compression is applied.

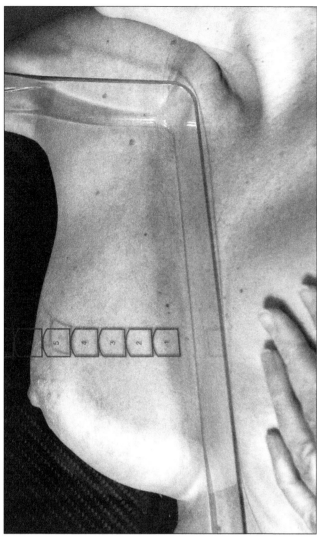

Figure 7-44
When compression is completed, the patient holds the contralateral breast out of the way (without pulling the medial ipsilateral breast from view) to avoid superimposition. Instructing the patient to elevate the contralateral breast as it is secured from the FOV directs the posteromedial tissue upward reducing the introduction of skinfolds in the IMF region.

3. Instruct the patient to slightly bend her elbow away from her body.
4. The technologist places her flat hand against the portion of the pectoral muscle extending from the axilla.
5. With the technologist's fingers into the patient's axilla, and with her hand supporting the pectoral muscle, lift the pectoral muscle medially, defining its specific angle.
6. Adjust the angle of the image receptor parallel to the pectoral muscle angle.
7. The height of the IRSD is approximately at the level of the relaxed axilla.
8. *Turn the patient, with her feet and pelvis directly facing the mammography machine.*

9. Sidestep the patient away from the IRSD until her ASIS is aligned with the inferior corner of the IRSD. This action places the IMF region (inferior breast and superior abdomen junction) in front of the IRSD. *Ensuring IMF inclusion on the image places the abdomen in contact with the chestwall edge of the image receptor at a level comfortably below the junction of the IMF region.*

Superior Breast Maneuvers

10. Elevate the patient's arm, placing the corner of the IRSD posterior to the midaxilla hollow, just anterior to the latissimus dorsi.
11. Continue to guide the arm in a forward direction, draping the shoulder and axilla over the top of the IRSD. The patient's arm and hand, with elbow flexed, are relaxed and resting on the C-arm.
12. Ensure the triceps muscle is rotated posterior and superior, eliminating folds and arm artifact.
13. Rotate the patient medially toward the image receptor, projecting the anterior axillary skinline toward the approximate center of the light field on the image receptor.
14. Ensure that the patient's thorax, shoulder, and pectoral muscle are relaxed.

Anterior to Posterior Maneuvers

15. Ensure the patient does not move the superior aspect of her breast away from the image receptor during the following maneuvers.
16. With a flat and open hand, capture the lateral breast using the midaxillary line as a landmark guide.
17. Lift the breast away from the IRSD while moving the far lateral tissue anteriorly and medially to capture lateral tissue to the latissimus dorsi line.
18. Using both hands, sandwich the breast, firmly grasping and pulling the breast out and away from the chestwall at an approximate 90° angle.
19. Slide the hand in contact with the lateral aspect of the breast out.
20. Using one hand, anchor the breast out and away from the chestwall at an approximate 90° angle.

Inferior Breast Maneuvers

21. The feet and pelvis should be directly facing the unit.
22. The IMF region is engaged in front of the image receptor.
23. Continue to pull the breast out and away from the chestwall at an approximate 90° angle while simultaneously supporting the medial tissue upward.

Compression Maneuvers

24. Begin compression: slowly lower the compression device, skimming the chestwall surface; gradually remove the supporting hand as the compression takes over holding the breast in position.
25. Monitor compression contact with the bony structures of the thorax, including the clavicle, sternum, and

ribs. Patient relaxation and good communication are essential for patient comfort.

26. Complete compression until device adequately supports and compresses breast from the chestwall to the nipple.

27. Ensure IMF is open and free of skinfolds and airgaps by using fingers to sweep medial and lateral breast tissue downward.

The Craniocaudal Projection

Application

The craniocaudal (CC) projection best visualizes all medial (with emphasis on the posteromedial), posterior, anterior, central, and as much lateral breast tissue as possible (Figure 7-45). The nipple placement on the image is also an important indicator of adequate tissue capture and should follow a perpendicular path from the chestwall with minimal exaggeration either laterally or medially[8] (Figure 7-46). The CC image of the breast is one of the two complementary projections that make up the routine mammographic study.[10] Because the posteromedial region of the breast has the potential to be excluded on the MLO projection, its inclusion on the CC projection is critical (Figure 7-47). For this reason, the technologist stands on the medial side of the breast during positioning for the CC projection,[8] giving her a greater advantage of ensuring appropriate attention to this region. Additionally, the patient's face is turned in the direction of the medial breast, allowing the technologist to have eye contact with her during much of the procedure.

Performing the Craniocaudal Projection

Position the C-arm at 0°: the image receptor is parallel to the floor. The x-ray beam is directed superiorly to inferiorly through the breast. Create a comfortable stance for the patient, making sure she is stable. The patient's body faces the unit, the pelvis is squared to the image receptor, and arms are at her side. The thorax, including arms and shoulders, is as relaxed as possible. The patient steps back slightly away from the unit and bends forward at the waist just enough to allow the breast to naturally fall forward[6,7] (Figure 7-48). Allow about a hands width between the image receptor and the patient's abdomen; however, the degree to which the patient bends forward and the distance between the patient's abdomen and the image receptor will require further adjustment for each patient. Positioning the anterior border of the patient's thorax in a vertical position is advantageous for superior and posterior tissue

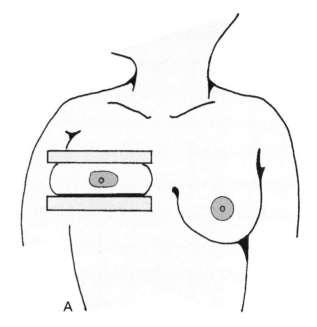

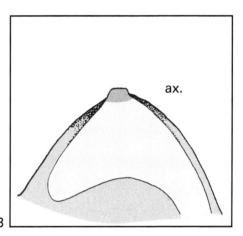

Figure 7-45
Craniocaudal projection. **(A)** The orientation of the breast to the C-arm for the craniocaudal projection. **(B)** Schematic demonstrating the amount of the "glandular island" imaged with the CC projection.

capture on the image (Figure 7-49A,B). Standing at the side of the patient allows the technologist to view the anterior ribs in a vertical straight line as the patient bends forward (Figure 7-49C). Envisioning her skeletal structure from this vantage point allows the technologist to:

• Determine the degree each patient must bend forward for her thorax to reach a vertical position.

• Determine the patient's feet placement for appropriate distance between her abdomen and the chestwall edge of the image receptor.

As she leans forward, instruct the patient to relax or to droop her shoulders.

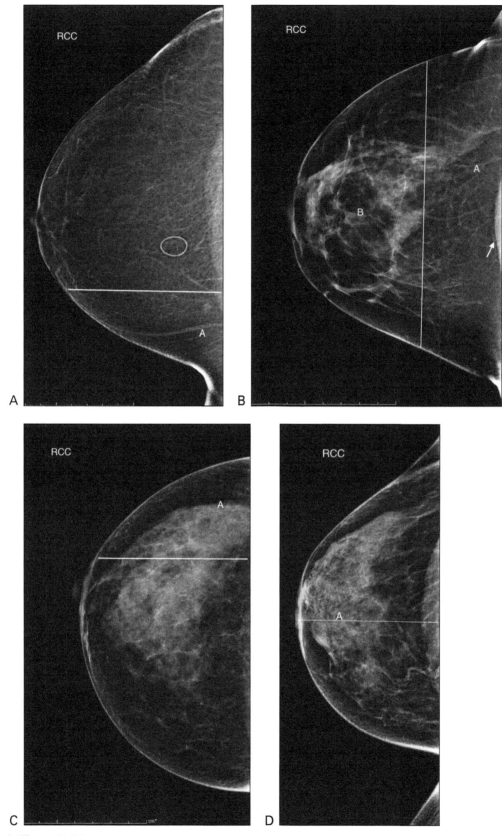

Figure 7-46
The properly positioned CC projection demonstrates: **(A)** all medial tissue (labeled *A*) with emphasis on posteromedial; **(B)** posterior (labeled *A*), *arrow* indicating pectoral muscle; anterior (labeled *B*), including the subareolar features and nipple; **(C)** as much posterolateral tissue (labeled *A*) as possible; and **(D)** the PNL (labeled *A*) indicates that the nipple direction follows a perpendicular path from the chestwall with minimal exaggeration laterally or medially.

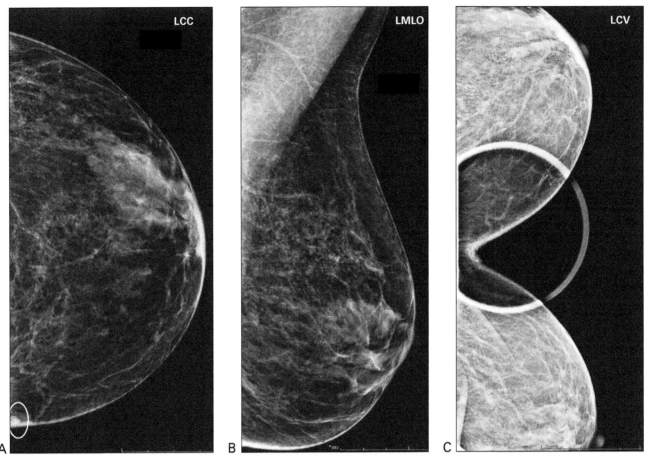

Figure 7-47
The posteromedial region of the breast has the potential to be excluded on the MLO projection; its inclusion on the CC projection is critical. **(A)** Posteromedial lesion captured on the CC projection (*circle*). **(B)** Far posteromedial breast tissue not visualized on the MLO projection. **(C)** Additional CV spot compression projection reveals normal glandular tissue.

Height of the Image Receptor

Select the appropriate height of the receptor:

- The technologist places her flat hand, palm up on the undersurface of the breast at the junction of the inferoposterior breast and the superior abdominal wall (IMF).
- With a flat hand against the patient's thorax, the technologist firmly skims the anterior ribcage in an upward direction elevating the IMF until there is natural resistance.
- Adjust the C-arm height, bringing the image receptor to the level of the elevated IMF (Figure 7-50).

Eklund[9,16] describes this maneuver as taking advantage of the more mobile inferior aspect of the breast. By moving the mobile inferior breast toward the fixed superior tissue, greater capture of the superior and posterior breast tissue is achieved, resulting in more tissue visualized (Figure 7-22). The appropriate height of the image receptor is indicated by the resistance the technologist senses as she elevates the breast. Be attentive to this technical detail. Raising the image receptor too high prohibits the patient from leaning forward and relaxing into position and eliminates posterior and inferior breast tissue (lower outer and lower inner quadrant) from view. In contrast, when the image receptor is positioned too low, the breast tissue droops, which excludes superior and posterior tissue as compression is applied[6] (Figure 7-51).

Posterior and Central Breast Maneuvers

When the height of the image receptor has been adjusted to match the elevated breast, the technologist should sandwich the breast firmly between both hands, with the flat portion of her hands as far posterior on the chestwall as possible in order to control the posterior margin of the breast. Gently "dislocate" the pectoral muscle away from the thorax. Using both hands, guide the breast onto the image receptor as the patient's upper abdomen comes in contact with the chestwall edge of the image receptor

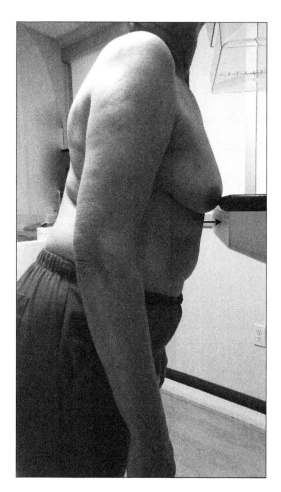

Figure 7-48
The patient's head is turned toward her contralateral breast with her body facing the unit pelvis squared to the image receptor, arms at her side, as relaxed as possible. Allow an approximate hands-width distance from the abdomen to image receptor (*arrow*) as the patient bends slightly forward at the waist ensuring posterosuperior tissue capture.

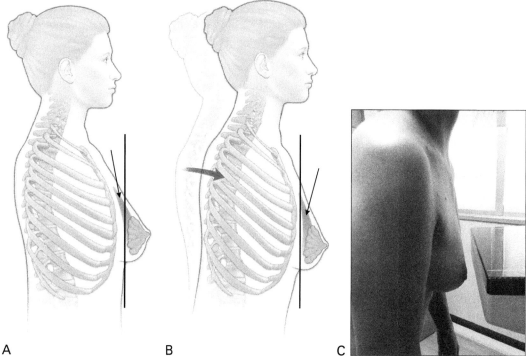

A   B   C

Figure 7-49
CC projection: patient stance. **(A)** Schematic of erect patient stance demonstrates posterosuperior breast tissue (*arrow*) excluded from radiation field (*black vertical line* to the nipple). **(B)** Schematic of patient stance leaning forward placing the anterior chestwall in a vertical position allowing capture of posterosuperior tissue (*arrow*) within radiation field (*black vertical line* to the nipple). **(C)** Standing on the medial side of the breast being positioned allows the technologist to view the anterior ribs in a vertical straight line as the patient bends forward to determine appropriate thorax angle and feet placement.

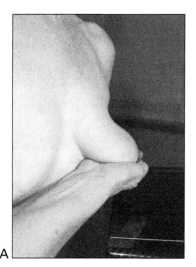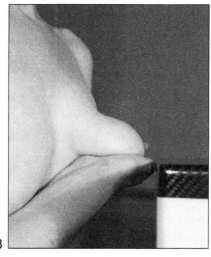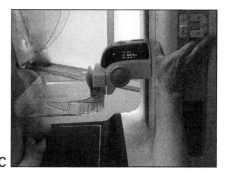

Figure 7-50
Determining image receptor height. **(A)** The technologist places her flat hand, palm up on the undersurface of the breast at the IMF. **(B)** With a flat hand against the patient's thorax, elevate the IMF until natural resistance is sensed. **(C)** Adjust the C-arm height, bringing the image receptor height to the level of the elevated IMF.

(Figure 7-52). Continue to encourage relaxation, as elevated shoulders apply tension to the pectoral muscle, which in turn results in a loss of breast tissue, and a pectoral muscle under tension prohibits adequate compression.

When the patient's inferior breast is secured on the image receptor, the technologist slides the hand positioned inferiorly on the breast out, following the straight pathway of the nipple from the chestwall to anterior breast (Figure 7-53). Sliding the hand out medially rather than straight out from the nipple causes torqueing of the parenchymal structures. The visual effect of torqueing resembles a spider web spun

on top of the image and, depending on the severity, may interfere with visualization of finite structures, especially architectural distortion (Figure 7-54). From this point in the examination until the compression device assumes this responsibility, superior breast tissue is secured to the image receptor by the technologist's "anchor hand" (Figure 7-55). Each technologist decides for herself which is the anchor hand that secures the breast during the following maneuvers. The hand on the superior breast is continually working to dislocate the pectoral muscle away from the chestwall and to secure posterior tissue onto the image receptor. If the

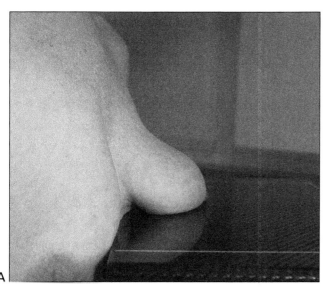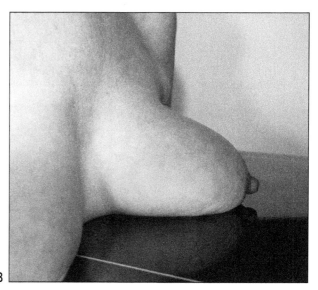

Figure 7-51
Appropriate image receptor height is critical for the CC projection. **(A)** Positioning the image receptor too low allows the breast to droop, resulting in posterosuperior tissue exclusion while introducing posteroinferior skinfolds. **(B)** Appropriate receptor height places the inferior aspect of the breast in intimate contact with the image receptor, resulting in maximum posterior tissue capture, while reducing the introduction of posteroinferior skinfolds.

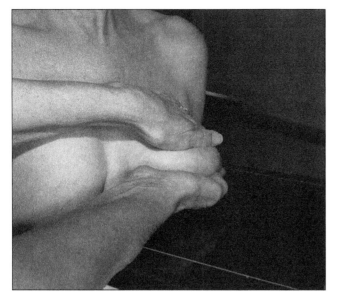

Figure 7-52
The technologist captures the breast firmly between both hands at the chestwall, controlling the posterior breast margin as the pectoral muscle is gently "dislocated" from the thorax.

anchor hand releases its grip before the compression device takes control of the breast, the pectoral muscle escapes out of the field of view, risking posterior tissue exclusion. An analogy is that dislocating the breast away from the ribs is like stretching a rubber band. Once the rubber band is stretched, if the anchor hand relaxes its grip, the rubber band returns to its natural flaccid state.

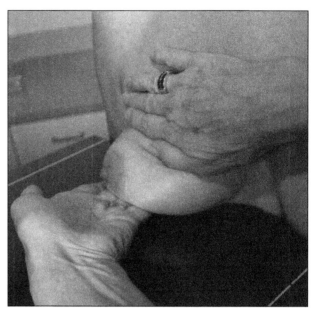

Figure 7-53
With the breast securely anchored to the image receptor, the technologist slides the hand positioned inferiorly on the breast outward, following a perpendicular path from the chestwall to the nipple.

Medial Breast Maneuvers

Twenty-three percent of breast cancers arise in the medial half of the breast. During MLO positioning, even when the technologist makes every effort to include medial tissue, there is potential for far medial breast anatomy to be

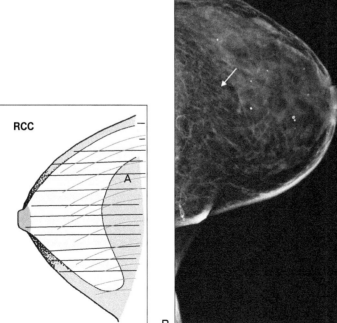

Figure 7-54
(A) Sliding the hand in contact with the inferior breast out medially rather than straight out from the nipple causes torqueing (labeled *A*) of the parenchymal structures. The lines representing torqueing are curvilinear in appearance. **(B)** The visual effect of torqueing resembles a spider web spun on top of the image (*arrow*) and, depending on the severity, may interfere with visualization of finite structures, especially architectural distortion.

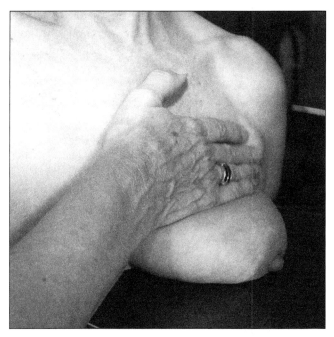

Figure 7-55
Controlling the posterior breast margin during positioning of the CC projection requires an "anchor hand" to continually secure the superior tissue, posterior tissue, and pectoral muscle on the image receptor until the compression device assumes this responsibility.

sacrificed due to the application of compression. In order to reach adequate compression for support of breast structures on the MLO projection, the compression device often skims laterally beyond the midsternum, thus eliminating visualization of this far medial tissue[7] (Figure 7-16). If posteromedial tissue is not visualized on the MLO view and the technologist fails to capture this tissue on the CC projection, medial tissue is excluded from both projections. Therefore, the emphasis of the CC projection is placed on the medial aspect of the breast, ensuring the inclusion of posteromedial features.[8,17] With the focus of the CC projection on the medial aspect, it is suggested the technologist stand on the medial side of the breast being positioned. The technologist uses two hands to bring the breast onto the image receptor, emphasizing capture of medial and posterior tissue. Due to the technologist standing on the medial side of the breast being positioned, and due to using both hands to dislocate the breast and place it on the image receptor, the technologist's own forearm may impede the medial portion of the breast from coming in contact with the edge of the receptor (Figure 7-52). To adequately bring the medial tissue of the breast onto the image receptor, it is necessary to rotate the patient's thorax medially toward the image receptor until the sternum is flush against the image receptor and comes into contact with the chestwall rise of the compression device (Figure 7-56).

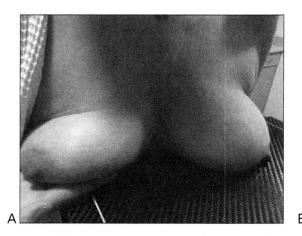

A

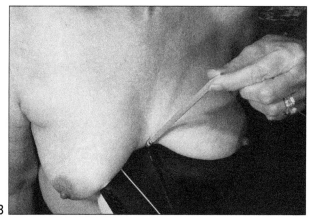

B

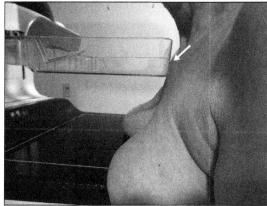

C

Figure 7-56
To adequately bring medial breast tissue onto the image receptor for the CC projection. **(A)** Elevate the contralateral breast while rotating the patient's thorax medially toward the image receptor. **(B)** Position the sternum and thorax flush against the image receptor draping the contralateral breast across the IRSD chestwall corner. **(C)** The thorax and sternum are in contact with the chestwall rise of the compression device as compression is applied.

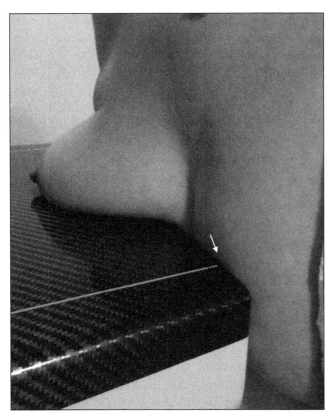

Figure 7-57
Allowing the contralateral breast to remain in its natural position between the image receptor and the patient's thorax causes discomfort during the procedure and additionally acts as a "spacer" (*arrow*) preventing the inclusion of posteromedial tissue.

These maneuvers provide the best visualization of the medial and posterior tissue and are accomplished simultaneously as the contralateral breast is elevated and draped over the medial corner of the IRSD. It is important that the contralateral breast is not allowed to remain in its natural position (between the image receptor and the patient's thorax) as the IRSD corner causes increased discomfort to the patient. Additionally, the contralateral breast resting on the chestwall acts as a "spacer" prohibiting inclusion of posteromedial tissue on the breast being imaged (Figure 7-57). Rotating the patient's body medially may mean the loss of some far lateral tissue, which is best imaged with the MLO view.

It is important to address the patient's head and neck posture to ensure patient comfort and to ensure she does not pull tissue away from the image receptor. By bringing the patient's head and neck slightly around the face shield, toward the unit, medial breast tissue is further secured in place and discomfort of the neck position is decreased (Figure 7-58). The patient's chin is positioned at a natural level, not looking excessively down or up, as these positions draw the chestwall away from the image receptor. The final medial maneuver is to secure the tissue by having the patient rest her contralateral hand on a handle or on the side of the unit, ensuring medial tissue remains in place while the technologist addresses the lateral aspect of the breast (Figure 7-59). Bringing the contralateral hand forward to secure medial tissue placement should not force

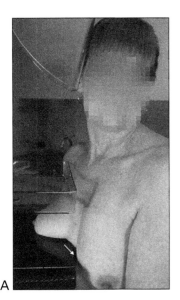
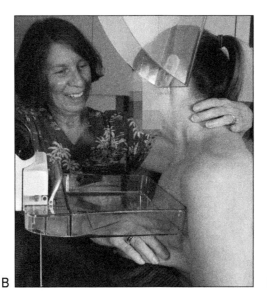
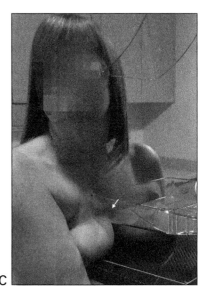

A   B   C

Figure 7-58
Head and neck posture. **(A)** Placing the head and neck upright behind the face shield prevents medial breast tissue inclusion on the image receptor (*arrow*). **(B)** Positioning the head and neck toward the medial edge of the face shield allows thorax rotation, which places the posteromedial tissue in contact with the image receptor while also relieving discomfort to the neck. **(C)** Position the patient's chin at a natural level, not looking excessively down or up, as these positions draw the chestwall away from the image receptor; note the inclusion of the medial and contralateral breast tissue (*arrow*) under the compression device.

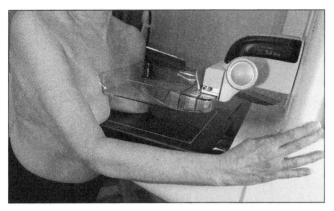

Figure 7-59
With medial positioning maneuvers completed, place the patient's contralateral hand on the side of the unit or the handle to secure medial tissue in place (*arrow*) during subsequent lateral positioning maneuvers.

the contralateral breast to come in contact with the breast being imaged at the cleavage. If possible, try to maintain separation of the breast tissue at the cleavage (Figure 7-60). All medial breast maneuvers are accomplished with the anchor hand remaining on the breast, securing the posterior tissues and nipple direction in place. Performing the

medial maneuvers properly provides the reflection of the cleavage and a small amount of the contralateral breast in the field of view (Figure 7-61). This expectation is not achieved for all patients due to the variations of the sternum, rib skeletal structures, and breast size. Due to the improvement in positioning of the posteromedial breast region, occasionally, the sternalis muscle may be present on the CC image[18] (Figure 7-62). Located at the sternal edge, its appearance as a rounded density is familiar to radiologists and most often can be differentiated between an abnormality and a normal variance of anatomy.

Lateral Breast Maneuvers

Including as much lateral breast tissue as possible on the CC projection requires specifically addressing the lateral tissue prior to compression. The anchor hand keeps the medial, anterior, central, superior, and posterior tissues and nipple direction secure, while the fingers of the opposite hand move beyond the edge of the image receptor to capture far lateral tissue. Place the fingers beneath the lateral posterior breast, grasping the lateral breast margin, slightly lifting and freeing it from the image receptor. Bring the lateral tissue forward in a straight path

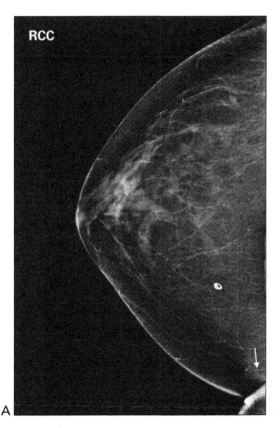

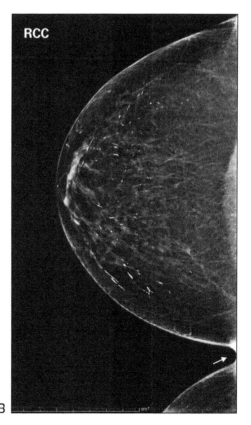

Figure 7-60
(A) The contralateral hand placement on the unit handle or the side of the detector should not force superimposition of the contralateral breast at the cleavage (*arrow*). **(B)** If possible, try to maintain separation of the breast tissue at the cleavage (*arrow*).

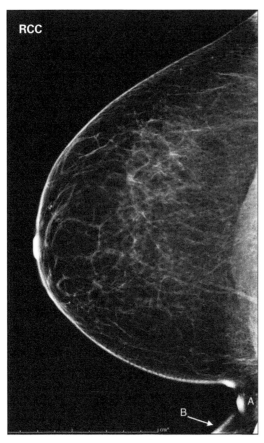

Figure 7-61
Proper positioning of medial breast tissue visualizes the (A) reflection of the cleavage and (B) a small amount of the contralateral breast in the field of view. This expectation is not achieved for all patients due to the variations of the sternum, rib skeletal structures, and breast size.

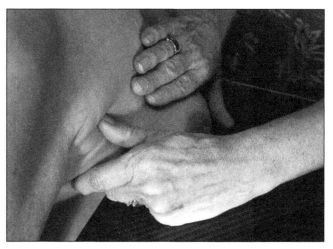

Figure 7-63
Lateral breast capture, CC projection: the anchor hand keeps the medial, anterior, central, superior, and posterior tissues and nipple direction secure, while the fingers of the opposite hand move beyond the edge of the image receptor to capture far lateral tissue.

ensuring no torqueing occurs as this additional tissue is brought into the field of view (Figure 7-63). This lateral tissue maneuver compensates for any tissue lost during performance of the medial capture maneuvers and is commonly referred to as the "lateral pull" (Figure 7-64). A very small skin crease in the far posterolateral aspect of the breast may be evident on the CC image indicating the "lateral pull" was included in the positioning maneuvers[3] (Figure 7-65).

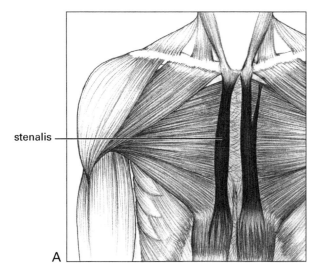

stenalis

A

Figure 7-62
(A) Improved positioning of the posteromedial breast region occasionally includes visualization of the sternalis muscle on the CC image. **(B)** Located at the sternal edge, its appearance as a rounded density (*arrow*) is familiar to radiologists and can be differentiated between an abnormality and a normal variance of anatomy. (**A**, Adapted from Simons DG, et al. *Travell & Simons' Myofascial Pain and Dysfunction: The Trigger Point Manual.* Vol. 1. 2nd ed. Philadelphia, PA: Lippincott Williams & Wilkins; 1998.)

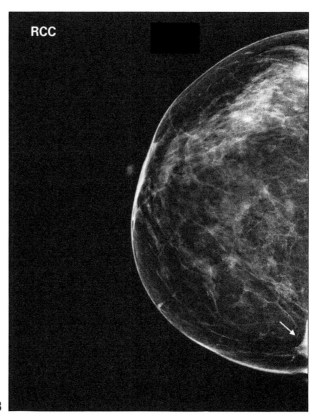

B

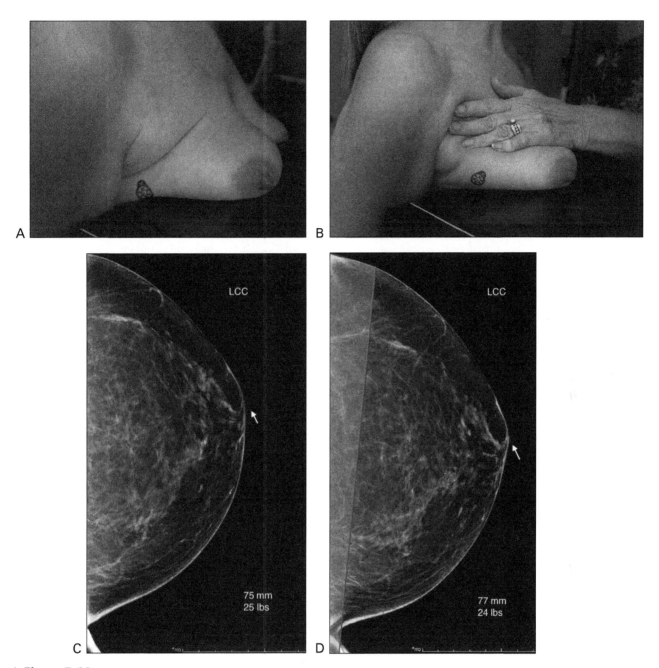

Figure 7-64
The maneuver used to visualize as much lateral tissue as possible on the CC projection is commonly referred to as the "lateral pull." **(A)** Note the metallic marker location at the lateral breast prior to performing the lateral pull maneuver. **(B)** Note the metallic marker location and increased inclusion of posterolateral tissue after performing the lateral pull maneuver. **(C)** LCC image without benefit of lateral pull maneuver; note lateral nipple exaggeration (*arrow*) and exclusion of posterolateral tissue. **(D)** LCC of same patient demonstrating greater posterolateral tissue capture and correction of the PNL direction (*arrow*) using the "lateral pull" technique.

Compression Maneuvers

Prior to beginning compression, the technologist places her arm around the patient, resting her hand on the patient's shoulder while reminding her once again to relax. Frequently, the patient slowly and involuntarily raises her shoulders during the positioning maneuvers; reminding the patient once again to relax usually results in a noticeable slump of the entire thorax. Using the fingers of your hand resting on her shoulder, slide a small amount of skin up and over the clavicle to reduce the "pulling" sensation in the patient's neck as compression is applied (Figure 7-66). This tissue is released during the initial compression phase.

The compression device contact point begins just below the clavicle. As the compression device skims down the superior ribcage, pressure is placed on the patient's chest

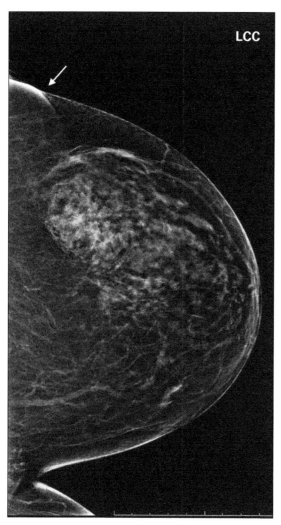

Figure 7-65
A very small skin crease in the far posterolateral aspect of the breast (*arrow*) may be evidence that the "lateral pull" was included in the positioning maneuvers on the CC image.

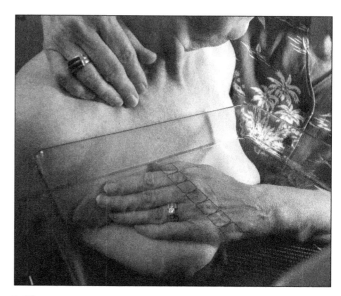

Figure 7-66
Compression preparation. The technologist uses the fingers of her hand resting on the patient's shoulder to slide a small amount of skin up and over the clavicle to reduce the "pulling" sensation in the patient's neck as compression is applied.

wall, potentially pushing the posterior breast from the field of view. To counteract the pressure placed against the patient's chestwall, and to prevent natural movement away from the compression device, the technologist uses the elbow of the hand and arm resting on the patient's shoulder to gently apply pressure to the patient's back, encouraging her to remain close to the unit.

As compression is applied, position the palm of the anchor hand on the center of the breast mound. This placement leaves the fingers free to fan out lateral skinfolds as the compression device meets the breast tissue (Figure 7-67A). Taller technologists additionally benefit by using the

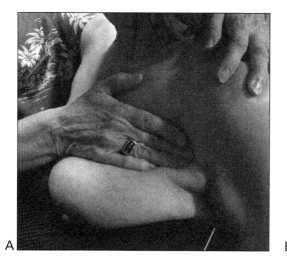

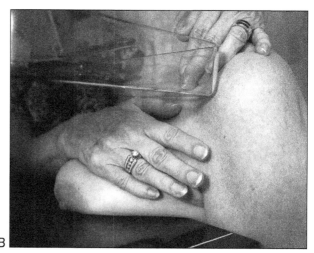

A   B

Figure 7-67
(A) Positioning the palm of the anchor hand on the center of the breast mound leaves the fingers free to fan out lateral skinfolds as compression is applied. **(B)** Taller technologists benefit by using the opposite hand positioned at the patient's shoulder to meet the fingers of the anchor hand at the junction of the lateral breast, axilla, and compression device to control posterolateral tissue and skinfolds during compression.

opposite hand currently positioned at the patient's shoulder to meet the fingers of the anchor hand at the junction of the lateral breast, axilla, and compression device, allowing control over final breast adjustments for tissue inclusion and skinfold elimination (Figure 7-67B). As compression is applied, hold the breast in place, smoothing skinfolds out toward the nipple. As compression gradually stabilizes the breast in place, slide the anchor hand out toward the nipple.

Apply firm compression, evaluating the medial and lateral breast for tautness. In some women, an axillary fat pad may overlap the lateral tissue as compression is applied. To counteract this large skinfold, finalize the CC positioning maneuvers by externally rotating (supinating) the ipsilateral hand; this may reduce the amount of the skinfolds, and this maneuver also flattens the anterior axilla area, moving the rounded portion of the humeral head out of the field of view (Figure 7-68). A properly positioned CC projection visualizes tissue extending from the medial margin, where the chestwall edge of the compression device comes in contact with the patient's medial chestwall (sternum), to the lateral margin where the chestwall edge of the compression device comes in contact with the junction of the lateral breast/axilla (Figure 7-69).

Craniocaudal Projection Summary

The step-by-step processes of patient positioning for the CC projection are listed here.

Beginning: Preparation
1. Select the appropriate size compression device.
2. *The technologist stands on the medial side of the breast being imaged.*
3. The patient stands facing the IRSD:
   * Feet facing forward.
   * Ribcage approximately a hands width away from IRSD.
   * Patient relaxed, arms at sides, and shoulders slouched.
   * Patient's head turned toward the technologist.
   * Instruct the patient to lean the upper body slightly forward; pelvis remains back.

Addressing the IMF
4. Technologist's flat hand is placed on the inferior tissue of the breast, making firm contact with the ribcage.
5. With a flat hand, palm up, firmly pressed against the patient's thorax, the technologist skims the ribcage as she elevates the IMF upward until natural resistance is felt.
6. IRSD height is adjusted to the level of the elevated IMF.

Addressing the Posterior Tissue
7. The technologist places her opposite hand in firm contact with the chestwall and the superior tissue of the breast.

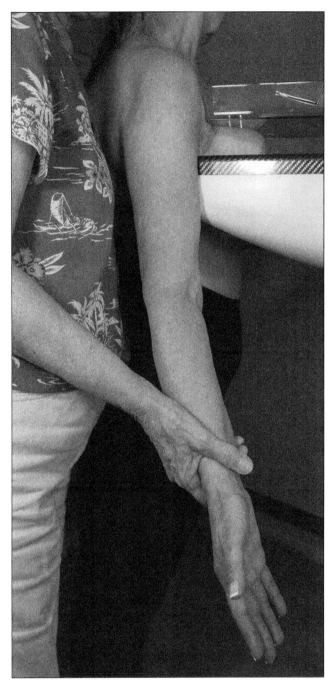

Figure 7-68
The ipsilateral hand of the patient is rotated externally to remove the rounded portion of the humeral head from the FOV and to reduce skinfolds in the posterolateral tissue.

8. Using two hands, simultaneously lift the breast forward onto the image receptor as the patient leans forward and her ribs come in contact with the IRSD.
9. The technologist slides the hand in contact with the inferior breast tissue out from underneath the breast following the path of the nipple.
10. The technologist's hand located superiorly on the breast continues to anchor the tissue and secure the pectoral muscle onto the image receptor.

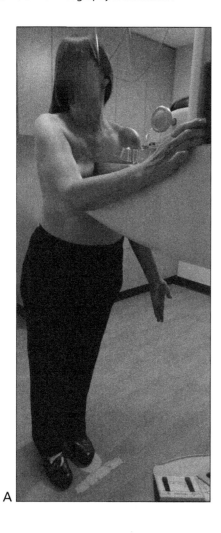

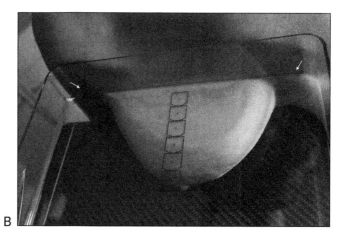

Figure 7-69
Completion of the CC projection. **(A)** Patient stance after completion of all CC positioning/compression maneuvers. **(B)** A properly positioned and compressed CC projection places the chestwall edge of the compression device in contact with the patient's medial chestwall (sternum) and in contact with the junction of the posterolateral breast/axilla (*arrows*).

11. The breast is continuously anchored to the image receptor during the remaining CC positioning maneuvers in order to ensure posterior tissue remains in the field of view. Technologists may choose to switch anchor hands, alternating between the right and the left hands.

Addressing Medial Breast
12. Bring the patient's head and neck around the face shield, slightly rotating the sternum medially toward the IRSD.
13. Elevate the contralateral breast.
14. Complete rotation of the patient's body medially until the thorax and sternum are flush against image receptor.
15. Drape the contralateral breast over the corner of the IRSD.

Addressing Lateral Breast: Lateral "Pull"
16. The technologist positions her hand on the lateral margin of the breast, wrapping her fingers around the lateral tissue. Lift the breast slightly, pulling the posterolateral tissue in a forward direction for inclusion of as much lateral tissue as possible on the image receptor.

Compression
17. The technologist places her arm around the patient, resting her hand on the shoulder of the breast being imaged, reminding the patient to relax her shoulders.
18. Place the fingers of the hand resting on the patient's shoulder along the clavicle. Gently slide the tissue upward toward the neck, reserving a small amount of skin above the clavicle. This reduces the pulling sensation in the neck as compression is applied.
19. Begin compression, gradually letting go of the reserved skin at the clavicle as compression is applied.
20. The compression device skims the superior chestwall as compression is applied. The compression device ultimately replaces the anchor hand and holds the breast in place.

Completion of the CC Projection
21. Place the patient's hand, opposite of the breast being imaged, onto the handle or side of the unit to secure medial tissue on the image receptor (tip: perform this maneuver prior to leaving the medial location of the patient, ensuring the cleavage presentation remains in an open position).

22. Moving to the lateral side of the patient, relax the patient's ipsilateral arm by her side, externally rotating her hand, ensuring the humeral head is removed from the field of view.

23. Complete compression using the manual mode, evaluating breast tissue for tautness by tapping a finger on the lateral breast.

24. Gently smooth skinfolds without sacrificing breast tissue.

▐▐ COMMON IMAGING PROBLEMS

The Use of Modifiers

Nipple in Profile Modifier

Unlike diagnostic imaging of the breast, technologists performing screening mammography do not have an indication of which patient, which breast, or what location within a breast may have a detectable sign of cancer. For these reasons, it is important that the primary objective for the CC and MLO projections is to include as much breast tissue as possible from the chestwall to the nipple. Projecting the nipple in profile (NP) is desirable whenever possible, but only if this can be accomplished without sacrificing breast tissue. For most women, the nipple is centrally located on the breast and will naturally fall into profile in at least one view. Repositioning the breast to bring the nipple into profile generally results in posterior tissue being excluded[8,16] either superiorly or inferiorly and medially or laterally depending on the projection and location of the nipple on the breast. Tissue excluded to place a NP may not be captured on the standard complementary view, contributing to undetected cancer.[7] For these reasons, it is more important to include as much breast tissue as possible rather than to image the NP. The ACR reports the nipple should be in profile in at least one standard view.[8] If this is not possible, an additional view of the anterior breast with the NP can be performed (modifier label: NP) (Figure 7-70). For additional value, using the spot compression device over the retroareolar region is also acceptable. Individual radiologists determine this specific protocol. Since the modified images for positioning the NP

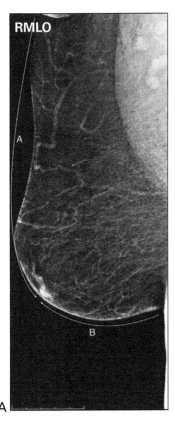
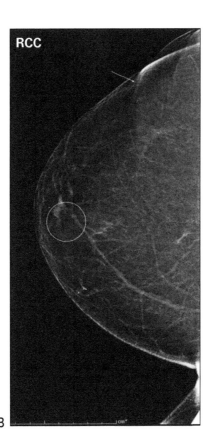
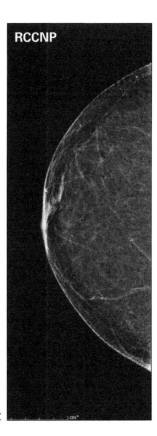

Figure 7-70
Nipple in profile (NP) modifier: tissue sacrificed to present the NP may contribute to undetected breast cancer. **(A)** RMLO of patient demonstrates longer measurement from the clavicle to nipple (labeled *A*); shorter measurement from the nipple to IMF (labeled *B*). **(B)** RCC same patient: adequate posterior tissue inclusion results in nipple rolled inferiorly on the image (*circle* identifies nipple location); note nonuniform compression due to thick breast base (*arrow*). **(C)** An additional RCCNP presents the NP with adequate compression of the anterior breast.

are a repeat of a standard image, the label options include RCCNP, LCCNP, RMLONP, and LMLONP. Indications for taking an additional view with the NP should be considered: when the nipple is indistinguishable from a mass (for further discussion, see Chapter 8), for triangulation purposes, when imaging a male patient, or for a suspected subareolar abnormality including patients presenting with nipple discharge.

Anterior Compression Modifier

For patients who present with a base of the breast circumference that is thicker, tapering to an apex of the breast that is much thinner, uniform compression from the chestwall to the nipple region may not be possible with standard compression techniques. Nonuniform compression degrades image quality through inadequate separation of glandular structures, increasing dose and scatter radiation, decreasing sharpness and contrast, the inability to control motion, and over- or underexposure. This discrepancy in thickness from base to nipple can also result from pectoral muscle prominence in the patient, producing the same problem of nonuniform compression. The technologist must problem solve to achieve both adequate capture of the posterior breast margin and to deliver adequate compression that ensures appropriate exposure and sharpness. When using a standard compression device (without "tilt" option), first, image the entire breast to capture all margins, including posterior tissue to the chestwall. If satisfactory compression is not achieved, an additional view of the anterior portion of the breast should be included (Figure 7-71). This modification of the standard projection provides compression to the anterior portion of the breast to ensure

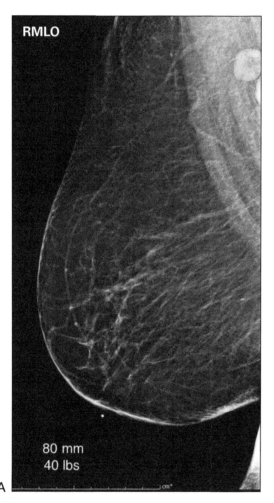
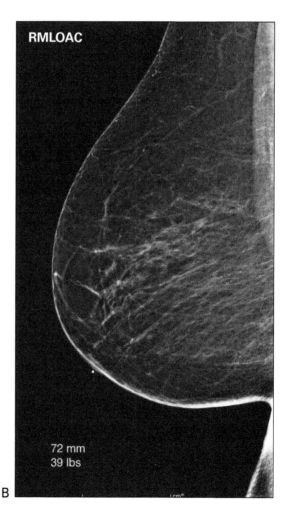

Figure 7-71

Technologists must problem solve to achieve both adequate capture of the posterior breast margin and to deliver adequate compression for the patient with a breast base circumference that is thicker, tapering to a much thinner apex. Uniform compression from the chestwall to the nipple region may not be possible with standard compression techniques, requiring two images to satisfy image quality. **(A)** RMLO demonstrating adequate pectoral muscle presentation, nonuniform compression, inadequate breast tissue support, and inferoposterior tissue exclusion. **(B)** Same patient, additional RMLOAC demonstrating inferoposterior tissue inclusion, posterior–anterior breast structures adequately supported and compressed, improving separation of breast tissue.

image quality when the two projections are combined. The image taken to improve compression to the anterior breast uses the modifier AC in conjunction with the standard projection taken: RCCAC, LCCAC, RMLOAC, LMLOAC, RMLAC, LMLAC, RLMAC, and LLMAC. The option to use the tilt compression device designed for standard imaging reduces, but does not completely eliminate, the need for additional AC views.

Compromised Inferior (IMF) Breast Tissue

Including posterior breast tissue on the CC projection requires a series of positioning maneuvers that stress the skin at the junction of the inferior breast and superior abdomen (IMF region). For patients with healthy skin in the IMF region, these maneuvers are tolerated without incident to the inferior tissue. Patients with delicate skin conditions in the IMF region may experience a "tearing" or "separation" of the skin when compression is applied. This compromised tissue is occasionally observed in patients with pendulous breasts that promote moisture accumulation in the IMF region further complicated by irritation such as skin infection. When breast elevation is combined with pulling the breast tissue forward onto the image receptor, this delicate tissue is susceptible to injury. Although no guarantees can be offered, additional cautionary positioning methods used by the technologist during the CC projection can help minimize if not eliminate the problem of injury to the IMF region for these patients.

- Inspect the breast tissue prior to the examination for signs of irritation in the IMF.
- Allow communication time for the patient. Patients with prior experience of skin tears in the IMF region usually are forthcoming with this information to the technologist.
- If possible, use a procedural aid such as the MammoPad or the Bella Blanket.
- As the breast is pulled forward onto the image receptor, use the fifth finger positioned against the inferior breast to hold and reserve tissue toward the chestwall as the breast makes contact with the IRSD.
- When compression is applied, instruct the patient to slightly bend her knees (slowly and gently, only by millimeters).

Skinfolds

Skinfolds may interfere with accurate tissue representation; thus, an effort is made to reduce or minimize their appearance. Skinfolds can present as:

1. Expected small posterolateral folds, indicating the lateral tissue has been addressed and pulled onto the field of view (CC projection).

2. Torqueing of breast tissue, demonstrating parenchymal striations interrupting natural tissue patterns. This positioning artifact occasionally appears posteriorly on the CC projection as a result of the technologist (a) using both hands to bring the breast forward onto the image receptor sliding the hand in contact with the inferior breast out in the medial direction rather than following the path straight out toward the nipple or (b) torqueing may appear when the technologist performs the lateral pull maneuver and allows the lateral tissue to be rotated medially rather than directed straight forward.

3. Large skinfolds interfering with adequate compression and visualization. It is impossible to eliminate all skinfolds for all patients during routine imaging in mammography. For the vast majority of patients, the technologist uses methods to minimize and eliminate skinfolds by smoothing the skin of the breast forward, gently working the tissue toward the nipple, *not by pulling the tissue out posteriorly, removing it from the field of view.* Removing breast tissue captured under the compression device to solve skinfold problems should be avoided as this eliminated tissue may also be omitted on the complementary projection. Skinfolds can occur as a result of the image receptor being positioned too low for the CC projection or by the use of an incorrect angle for the MLO projection. In the case of the CC projection, when the patient presents with excessive superolateral tissue compromising image quality due to a large axillary skinfold, the tissue may have to be excluded in order to capture the breast with adequate compression and clarity (Figure 7-72).

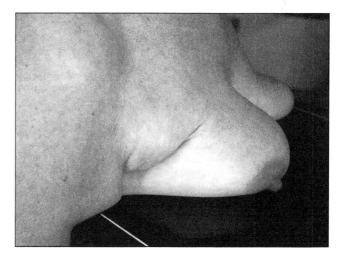

Figure 7-72
Large axillary skinfolds may compromise image quality in the CC projection requiring the technologist to exclude lateral tissue from the original image to improve compression and clarity. This excluded tissue can be visualized by adding the XCCL projection to the exam, reducing the skinfold effect on the image and providing adequate compression to the tissue.

In this situation, the technologist should add an additional projection, such as an XCCL, to capture the lateral tissue excluded from the original image and to smooth out skinfolds with adequate compression. (See Problem-Solving Projections.) Images with skinfolds should be evaluated by the technologist to determine if tissue representation has been compromised. Repeated images should be reserved for skinfolds that truly interfere with interpretation. The decision to repeat an image due to a skinfold artifact is directed by radiologist protocol and can be evaluated by determining if breast structures can be visualized into, through, and out of the skinfold.

Airgap

Like skinfolds, airgaps on a mammogram range in severity of image degradation. Airgaps are caused when skin does not come in smooth contact or is not flush against either the image receptor surface or the compression device surface. Airgaps most often appear on the medial aspect of the breast on the CC projection due to the curved shape of the medial breast meeting the flat surface of the image receptor (Figure 7-73). On the MLO projection, airgaps are commonly seen in the IMF region due to trapped air sandwiched on the undersurface of the breast between the image receptor and skin; MLO airgaps also occur in the axillary tail area in patients whose axillary tissue does not adequately fill the superior lateral region—the breast mound is thicker than the tail of Spence. Additionally, airgaps are often present adjacent to skinfolds; as the skinfold increases in severity, so does the airgap, making it more prominent on the image. Like skinfold artifacts, airgaps are impossible to completely eliminate; however, their effects can be minimized on most images. The decision to repeat an image due to airgap artifact is directed by radiologist protocol and can be evaluated by determining if breast structures can be visualized into, through, and out of the airgap.

Motion

Motion, blurring that results from patient movement during the x-ray exposure, degrades image quality for interpretation. Motion may exist across the entire image, or in just one area. It may be readily apparent, but more often it is subtle, perceived when compared with another mammogram (Figure 7-74). Patient movement during the exposure can be controlled by the technologist through procedural behaviors that help to prevent motion occurrence and increase image quality.

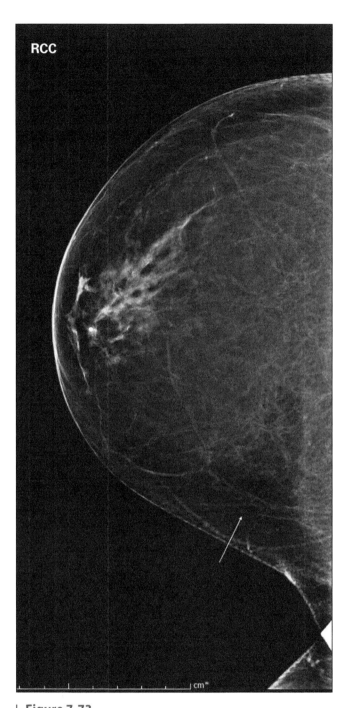

Figure 7-73
Airgaps are caused when skin does not come in intimate contact or is not flush against either the image receptor surface or the compression device surface. On the CC projection, airgaps most often appear on the inferomedial aspect of the breast (*arrow*) due to the curved shape of the medial breast meeting the flat surface of the image receptor.

Compression

The use of vigorous compression is essential for immobilizing the breast during the x-ray exposure and preventing patient movement. In addition to stabilizing

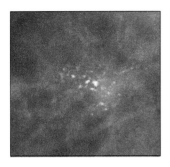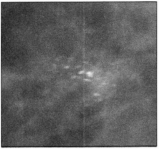

Figure 7-74
Motion, blurring that results from patient movement during the x-ray exposure, degrades image quality for interpretation. Motion may exist across the entire image or in just one area. It may be readily apparent, but more often it is subtle, perceived when compared with another mammogram. (Images courtesy of Hologic, Inc. and affiliates.)

the breast, compression uniformly decreases the thickness of the tissue, reducing the time of the exposure, which also reduces the potential for motion on the image. Technologist's attention to the use of adequate compression force is critical and can be evaluated by reviewing the compression factors between the same projections of the right and the left breasts on the image. Inconsistencies noted between centimeter thickness and compression force for the same projections in an exam may indicate the technologist is not properly evaluating breast tissue tautness routinely for every projection.

Patient Stability

In order to adequately capture the posterior aspect of the breast for mammography, patients are sometimes positioned in awkward stances that can be difficult for them to maintain stability. The technologist can control this problem by ensuring the patient is properly aligned with the image receptor for the projection, her body is supported through even weight distribution, and she is adequately stabilized using the equipment hand placements prior to exposure. Effective communication with the patient informs the technologist of physical limitations the patient may have such as joint replacements, back problems, or other medical conditions affecting balance. Asking the patient if she feels stable prior to leaving her to take the exposure not only prevents the potential for motion but also assures her safety during the procedure as well. Patients who indicate that balance may be problematic during the mammography procedure may be seated for the examination.

Respiration during the Exposure

Instructing the patient to stop breathing during the exposure may reduce the incidence of motion on the image. Further discussion about **respiration** is included earlier in this chapter.

Technologist Assessment of the Image for Motion

When inspecting the mammogram for motion, look for feature sharpness across the image including linear structures, calcifications, blood vessels, and Cooper ligaments. Sharpness of features in one area of the image compared with a slight blur of features in another is an indication of motion. Motion blur is more often detected on the MLO projection due to inadequate compression than on the CC projection.[8] The regions of the breast most vulnerable to motion on the MLO projection are the posterior/inferior and the anterior/central aspect. Feature sharpness of the subareolar tissue, anterior border of the pectoral muscle, and linear structures in these susceptible areas should be included in the technologist's inspection for motion. Subtle areas of motion may be difficult for the technologist to detect due to the reduced resolution of the acquisition monitor she uses compared to the 5-mp monitor used by the radiologist for interpretation. Using the zoom feature on the acquisition workstation can help the technologist better perceive motion if it is suspected.

Exposure Factors

Digital detector design permits the AEC to determine tissue composition based on a sample pre-exposure in order to select an appropriate target/filter combination, as well as kVp and mAs selection. This equipment capability delivers an exposure to the breast using exposure factors that address tissue composition, contrast, patient dose, and length of exposure time. Exposure times lasting longer than 2 seconds are no longer a common problem in mammography, reducing the potential of motion due to length of exposure time. When phototiming a patient with a labored breathing condition (i.e., emphysema, COPD), select an AEC mode that allows the kVp to be increased so the resulting exposure time is shortened. This results in a trade-off of contrast versus motion, but with window/leveling, the contrast index can be retrieved. When the technologist is required to use manual techniques for mammography, length of the exposure time should be considered in choosing the exposure factors.

QUALITY ASSESSMENT FOR POSITIONING AND COMPRESSION OF THE ROUTINE OR STANDARD PROJECTIONS

▮▮ MEDIOLATERAL OBLIQUE AND CRANIOCAUDAL PROJECTIONS

Introduction

The technologist should understand that superior image quality in mammography is critical and that her performance in obtaining the images for the exam impacts both interpretation accuracy and appropriate health care decisions for the patient. Image quality in mammography affects sensitivity (how often are abnormalities detected) and specificity (once detected, how often is the diagnosis correct/incorrect) of the exam. As recent as April 2016, the FDA Web site posted an MQSA Insight document reminding facilities of the importance of superior image quality citing a 2002 study, which demonstrated an 84% sensitivity for images that passed positioning criteria compared to a 66% sensitivity with exams that failed positioning.[19] Poor positioning has been identified as the leading problem associated with accreditation deficiencies and with not passing the clinical image evaluation process.[20] Substandard positioning/compression practices result in an inaccurate representation of breast tissue on the image, which may require the patient to return for additional imaging. Being recalled for additional imaging due to inferior image quality causes anxiety to the patient,[21] is an interruption to the patient's schedule that should not have happened, and is a non–revenue-producing appointment slot for the facility. The most serious consequence of inferior quality imaging can be the delay in the detection of disease,[1] which in turn affects timeliness of treatment and treatment options for the patient as well as potential life lost. Therefore, positioning and compression assessment of image quality, defined by two factors, capture and clarity, is an essential skill in mammography. This section describes appropriate mammography image assessment using established criteria for positioning and compression for the standard projections, as well as additional helpful tips that assist in the process of obtaining superior quality images for common challenging conditions.

Posterior Nipple Line Measurements

PNL measurements are used to determine posterior tissue inclusion, the most challenging tissue to capture and adequately visualize on the CC or MLO image. PNL measurements involve the MLO and the CC projections. The defined measurements for each projection are provided initially in this section, as they may be referenced in this, as well as subsequent chapters in describing superior quality achievement in specific imaging categories.

Mediolateral Oblique Projection PNL Measurement

The PNL on the MLO projection is drawn from the skinline at the nipple to the pectoral muscle or the edge of the image, whichever is reached first when making the measurement. The line is drawn at an approximate perpendicular angle to the pectoral muscle[8] (Figure 7-75).

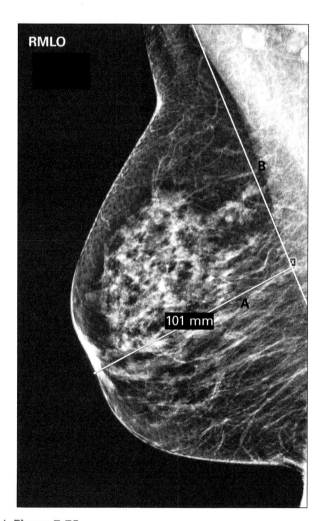

Figure 7-75

The posterior nipple line (PNL) (labeled *A*) on the MLO projection is drawn from the skinline at the nipple to the pectoral muscle or the edge of the image, whichever is reached first when making the measurement. The PNL is drawn at an approximate perpendicular angle to the pectoral muscle (labeled *B*).

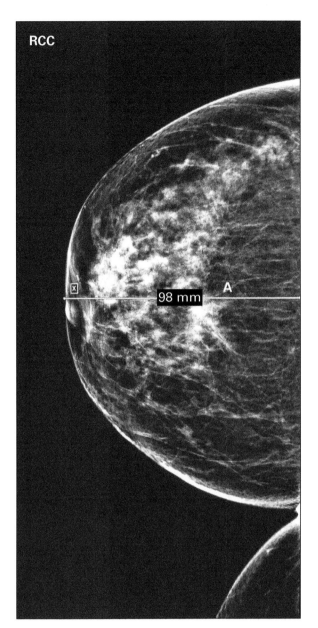

Figure 7-76
The posterior nipple line (PNL) (labeled *A*) on the CC projection is drawn from the skinline at the nipple to the posterior edge of the image.

Craniocaudal Projection PNL Measurement

The PNL on the CC projection is drawn from the skinline at the nipple to the posterior edge of the image. Whether the pectoral muscle is visible or not, the measurement is made from the nipple to the chestwall edge of the image[8] (Figure 7-76).

MEDIOLATERAL OBLIQUE PROJECTION ASSESSMENT

The MLO projection is assessed by dividing the MLO projection into six regions of evaluation. The regions include the superior and inferior breast margins, the anterior and posterior breast margins, the pectoral muscle presentation, and compression.[22] Each region is discussed for the MLO projection. The technologist should understand what features of the breast are demonstrated in each region and what positioning maneuvers are used to ensure the features are visible on the image.

MLO Projection Image Quality Criteria

The following bullet points describe the MLO image quality criteria included in Figure 7-77:

* The breast is imaged from high in the axilla at the superior margin to the inferior margin at the sixth or seventh rib to include the IMF.
* Wide superior pectoral muscle width.
* Gradual narrowing of the pectoral muscle from superior to inferior border.
* Length of pectoral muscle reaches to the PNL or below (ACR criteria suggest approximately 80% of the time).[8]
* Anterior pectoral muscle border convex in appearance.
* Open IMF is present on the image.
* Posterior tissue demonstrates visible retroglandular fat space (the retroglandular fat space may not be visible in patients with tissue composition of entirely adipose tissue or of extremely dense glandular tissue).
* Posterior structures directed at an approximate 90° angle from the chestwall.
* Anterior breast supported out from the chestwall, ensuring medial tissue is supported.
* Compression demonstrates sharpness of structures, with compression force and centimeter thickness proportional to the MLO of the contralateral breast compression factor results.

Four Building Blocks

C-arm angle
Receptor height
Axillary placement
IMF placement

The four building blocks of the MLO projection are related to the angle of the C-arm, height of the image receptor, placement of the axilla on the image receptor, and placement of the IMF region anterior to the image receptor. Additional positioning/compression maneuvers contribute to image quality on the final image. If any of these building blocks or positioning maneuvers are neglected, there will be a negative effect on image quality. The MLO Fix-It Table, Table 7-2, lists appropriate positioning maneuvers used to correct common problems associated with image quality when performing the MLO projection.

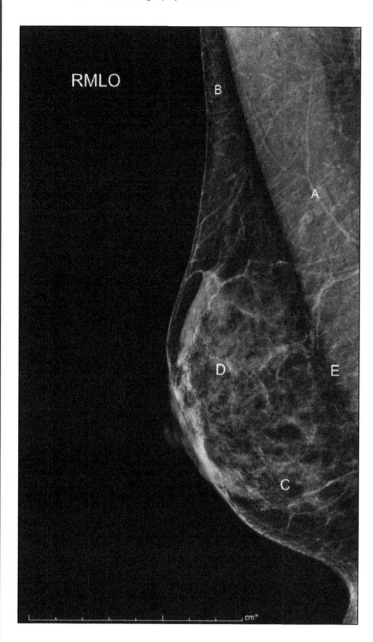

Figure 7-77
The MLO projection is assessed by dividing the breast into regions: presentation of the pectoral muscle (labeled *A*); the superior region (labeled *B*); the inferior region (labeled *C*); the anterior region (labeled *D*); and the posterior region (labeled *E*). Also included in the assessment for the MLO projection is compression evaluation.

Table 7-2 • MLO Fix-It Table: Positioning/Compression Maneuvers Used for the MLO Projection

FIX-IT NUMBER	FIX-IT MANEUVER
1	Compression device size is congruent to the light field and radiation field size and should include all breast margins
2	Customize angle of the image receptor to the natural angle of the pectoral muscle
3	Initially adjust the height of the image receptor to the level of the relaxed axilla to ensure capture of superior tissue; additional adjustment may be necessary for each patient as the arm is guided up and over the IRSD, and specific axillary placement is identified
4	Feet and pelvis must be positioned facing the unit, off set to the chestwall edge of the image receptor. This position places the IMF region (junction of the inferior breast and superior abdomen) in front of the IRSD as the patient leans laterally onto the image receptor for the MLO projection.
5	The patient's abdomen must be in contact with the chestwall edge of the image receptor at a level comfortably below the IMF region for the MLO projection. There should not be a space between the image receptor and the patient.
6	To include deep superoposterior tissue, axillary placement requires the superior chestwall edge corner of the IRSD to come in contact with the anatomical landmark just anterior to the Latissimus Dorsi muscle.

Table 7-2 • MLO Fix-It Table: Positioning/Compression Maneuvers Used for the MLO Projection (*Continued*)

FIX-IT NUMBER	FIX-IT MANEUVER
7	Rotate the patient toward the x-ray unit to capture the posteromedial aspect of the breast on the image. This is observed by the medial breast and sternum coming in contact with the chestwall rise edge of the compression device. The patient's feet point toward the unit.
8	Completed rotation of the patient to include medial tissue places the landmark of the anterior axillary skinline toward the approximate center of the light field superiorly, and the landmark of the IMF on the image receptor inferiorly.
9	Adequate capture of the posterolateral breast margin necessitates moving the mobile lateral aspect of the breast towards the fixed medial aspect. Capturing and anchoring the breast to the image receptor beyond the lateral mid-axillary margin to the line descending from the point just anterior to the Latissimus Dorsi muscle, posterior to the mid-axilla, ensures adequate posterolateral tissue inclusion on the image
10	With a flat hand in contact with the lateral aspect of the breast, position the fifth finger on the mid-axillary line, and move the breast anteriorly and medially toward the fixed medial border.
11	With a flat hand placed at the lateral margin, fifth finger at the mid-axillary line, starting superiorly at the axilla and moving inferiorly to the level of the IMF, ease lateral tissue downward smoothing out the skin. Skin that is "caught" superiorly is adjusted to its natural position as lateral tissue is eased downward.
12	Anchor the lateral breast to the image receptor at the line descending from the axillary landmark of the point just anterior to the Latissimus Dorsi muscle.
13	Relaxation of the pectoral muscle (controlled by relaxation of the shoulder and extremity)
14	Relaxation of the thorax
15	An open IMF is dependent on the position of the feet and pelvis of the patient squarely facing the unit, without rotation of the thorax
16	Sandwich the breast firmly, pulling tissue away from chestwall. Secure the lateral breast against the image receptor, sliding the hand supporting the lateral breast straight out following the path of the nipple. Simultaneously anchor the breast against the image receptor while supporting the medial tissue upwards, not allowing it to droop.
17	Directing the posterior tissue outward at an approximate 90° angle from the chestwall while supporting the medial tissue upward ensures the IMF remains open until compression replaces the supporting hand
18	After compression is completed, open the IMF by sweeping your fingers in a downward direction between the medial tissue and the compression device and between the lateral tissue and the image receptor to eliminate skinfolds and airgaps
19	Use a "tilt" compression device if available. If anterior tissue is not supported out and away from the chestwall, take an additional view of the anterior breast to achieve adequate compression: anterior compression (AC) view
20	Visual verification of inclusion of the superior breast margin that includes the Tail of Spence anatomy is to view the contact point of the compression device with the patient's chestwall. The superior chestwall edge corner of the compression device should rest in the natural depression that forms where the clavicle and the humeral head intersect.
21	Compression skims medially to laterally across the chestwall until the breast offers active resistance and tapping the skin indicates it is taut
22	When performing the superior tissue and axillary placement maneuvers, rotate the triceps muscle and excess arm skin posteriorly, positioning it behind the IRSD to remove arm artifact from the image.
23	When positioning a patient with a protruding abdomen at the IMF, tip the ASIS of the ipsilateral breast downward. This action orients the superior abdomen in a downward direction, placing its anterior border parallel with the image receptor edge. Removing abdominal tissue by tipping the pelvis downward opens the IMF without excluding inferior posterior tissue and achieving adequate compression
24	Using fingers inserted beneath the apex of the axilla, wrap the hand around the pectoral muscle pulling and smoothing both lateral and medial skinfolds forward in an effort to minimize their appearance on the image
25	As final compression is applied, the technologist taps the skin of the breast to gauge tautness superiorly or inferiorly, and communicates with the patient regarding compression tolerance. For the MLO view, adequate compression anchors the breast at an approximate 90° direction away from the chestwall.

Source: Mammography Quality Management (MQM, LLC), Waunakee, WI, W. J. Marshall, S. L. Lille.

Match the "Fix-It Number" that describes the "Fix-It Maneuver" corrections with the number listed under each problem in the MLO Projection Assessment section to improve image quality for that specific mammographic feature.

Pectoral Muscle Presentation on the MLO Projection

The presentation of the pectoral muscle on the MLO projection is considered a critical criterion due to the anatomy that is visualized through the muscle: far lateral, superior, medial, and the axillary tail. When the angle of the image receptor is customized to the patient's pectoral muscle angle, and the muscle has been coached to relaxation, it is possible to capture the maximum amount of breast tissue on the image. Additional positioning maneuvers are required to visualize pectoral muscle features that affect breast tissue visualization. Several problems associated with adequate presentation of the pectoral muscle on the

MLO projection are discussed in this section. Image quality suffers when these maneuvers are not executed properly or are omitted by the technologist.

Features Visualized

- Wide superior pectoral muscle width.
- Gradual narrowing of the pectoral muscle from superior to inferior border.
- Length of pectoral muscle reaches to the PNL or below.
- Anterior pectoral muscle border convex in appearance.

Pectoral Muscle Presentation Problem #1: Superior Pectoral Muscle Not Sufficiently Wide

Figures 7-78 and 7-79 illustrate insufficient image quality for superior pectoral muscle width and overall muscle presentation along with images demonstrating improved image quality for this feature. Capture of the posterior tissue high into the apex of the axilla ensures visibility of

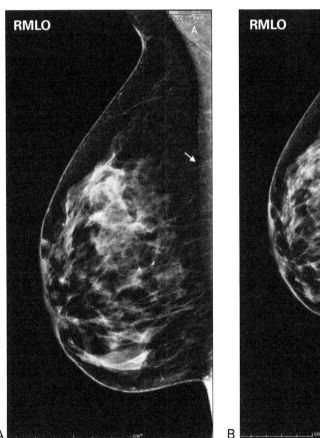
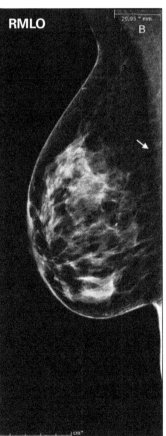
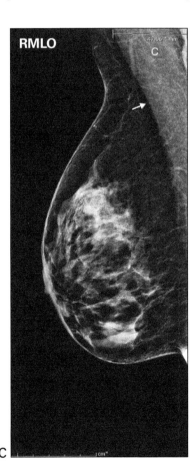

Figure 7-78
Axillary placement on the image receptor affects the superior width of the pectoral muscle presentation, an indication of adequate superior–posterior tissue capture. Three RMLO projections of the same patient demonstrating three different measurements of superior muscle width: **(A)** superior muscle width of 22.6 mm (labeled *A*); insufficient pectoral muscle presentation, vertical appearance (*arrow*); **(B)** superior muscle width of 29.9 mm (labeled *B*); (improved superior measurement, insufficient pectoral muscle presentation, vertical appearance (*arrow*); **(C)** improved superior measurement of 47.0 mm (labeled *C*); slightly concave pectoral muscle presentation (*arrow*), improved superior–posterior tissue capture.

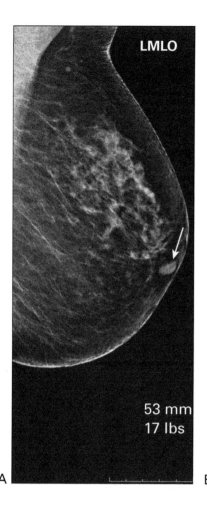

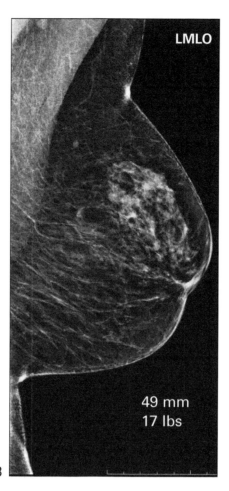

Figure 7-79
Axillary placement on the image receptor combined with rotation of the patient medially toward the image receptor affects capture of superior, posterior, and medial breast tissue. Two LMLO projections of the same patient; **(A)** demonstrating insufficient superior, posterior, and medial visualization; note nipple out of profile (*arrow*) and **(B)** improved positioning techniques for axillary placement combined with sufficient medial patient rotation captures superior, posterior, and medial breast tissue; note nipple presentation.

the tail of Spence and axillary lymph nodes. Two factors affecting the success of superior tissue visibility are the height of the image receptor and the axillary placement of the patient on the IRSD ensuring posterolateral tissue capture. Additionally, rotating the patient toward the image receptor to include medial tissue ensures a wide superior muscle presentation on the image.

Fix-It Problem #1: Superior Pectoral Muscle Not Sufficiently Wide

Refer to Table 7-2: 2, 3, **6**, 7, **8**, 12, 20, 22
(Bold numbers have the greatest impact on this positioning feature.)

Additional Tips for Axillary Placement on the Image Receptor

1. To find the landmark just anterior to the latissimus dorsi for axillary placement on the image receptor, reach across your own thorax into the axilla using "pinching" fingers. With your fingers, pinch the thick latissimus dorsi muscle in the posterior margin of the axilla. The thumb location is resting just anterior to the latissimus dorsi muscle, the placement for the image

receptor corner when positioning the superior tissue for the MLO projection (Figure 7-80).

2. FFMD detectors accommodating both large and small breast sizes may have white lines indicating the light field margins at the side edges of the detectors. These image receptor light field indicators are useful for assessing the appropriate height of the image receptor to the anatomical landmark of the external axilla, ensuring adequate superior capture (Figure 7-81).

Pectoral Muscle Presentation Problem #2: Inadequate Pectoral Muscle Length Presentation

When the MLO projection has been properly performed, the length of the pectoral muscle indicates the inclusion of posterior tissue (Figure 7-82). Keeping the pectoral muscle relaxed for this projection is of primary importance, as a tense muscle works against the goal of capturing deep tissue at the chestwall. When the image receptor is angled parallel with the patient's natural pectoral muscle angle, the breast easily dislocates onto the receptor, capturing posterosuperior tissue from the axilla to the inferior IMF. Successful positioning of this region is influenced by the angle selected for the C-arm and is assessed by the length of the pectoral muscle on

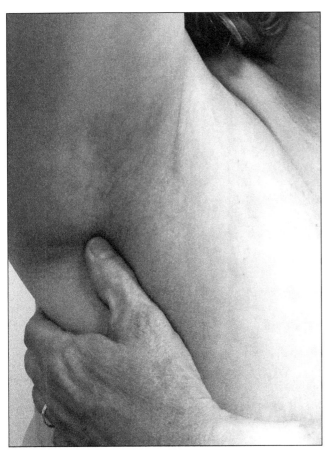

Figure 7-80
Sufficient superior–posterior tissue is included on the MLO projection by placing the axilla on the image receptor corner just anterior to the latissimus dorsi muscle. To find this landmark, reach across your own thorax into the axilla using "pinching" fingers. Pinch the thick latissimus dorsi muscle in the posterior margin of the axilla. The thumb location rests just anterior to the latissimus dorsi muscle, posterior to the midaxilla.

the image. Identify the PNL on the MLO projection. Determine if the PNL reaches to or below the pectoral muscle to assess posterior tissue inclusion (Figure 7-83). This assessment strategy is accurate only if the muscle presentation is sufficiently wide superiorly and gradually narrows to the inferior border. *Established criteria by the ACR report the pectoral muscle should extend to or below the PNL in approximately 80% of patients.* The ability to visualize the pectoral muscle to the level of the PNL or below is not possible with all patients, particularly patients with a history of breast reduction and patients with a shorter, stockier body habitus.

Fix-It Problem #2: Inadequate Pectoral Muscle Length Presentation

2, 3, 4, 5, **6, 7,** 8, 9, 10, 12, 14, 20, 21
(Bold numbers have the greatest impact on this positioning
    feature.)

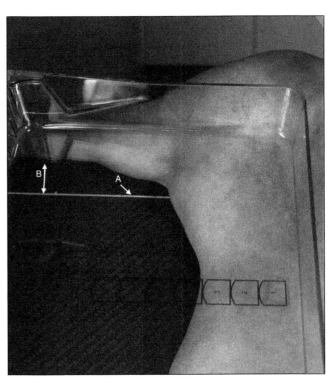

Figure 7-81
A FFDM detector may have *white lines* indicating the light field margin (labeled *A*) at the side edge of the detector for assessing the appropriate receptor height to the anatomical landmark of the external axilla. Technologists should be aware of the electronic dead space (*vertical arrow* labeled *B*) at the side edge of the detector when positioning the superior breast for the MLO projection.

Pectoral Muscle Presentation Problem #3: Narrow/Vertical Pectoral Muscle Presentation

Figure 7-84 illustrates insufficient pectoral muscle presentation influenced by incorrect placement of the axilla on the IRSD.

    Adequate capture of breast tissue is indicated by the shape of the pectoral muscle on the image. The muscle should demonstrate a generous width superiorly, gradually narrowing as it descends to the inferior border (see Figure 7-26A). This shape describes adequate visualization of the superior, anterior, and posterior breast margins and is influenced by axillary placement on the IRSD, sufficient posterior tissue capture, and patient rotation toward the image receptor.

Fix-It Problem #3: Narrow/Vertical Pectoral Muscle Presentation

Figure 7-85 illustrates image quality improvement for pectoral muscle presentation when the following positioning/compression maneuvers are employed from Table 7-2.

2, 3, 4, 5, **6**, **7**, 8, **9**, 10, 12, 13, 14, 20, 21
(Bold numbers have the greatest impact on this positioning
    feature.)

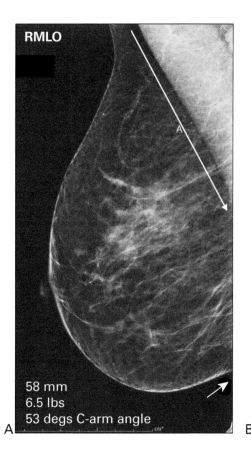

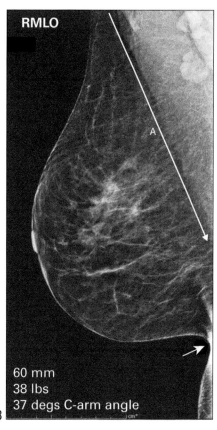

Figure 7-82
Adequate visualization of pectoral muscle length and its impact on posterior tissue capture and visualization is affected by the C-arm angle. Two RMLO images of the same patient comparing C-arm angle and resultant posterior tissue visualization. **(A)** Shorter pectoral muscle length (labeled *A*) corresponds to 53° C-arm angle; note compression force of 6.5 lb, and IMF exclusion (*arrow*). **(B)** Longer pectoral muscle length (labeled *A*) corresponds to a 37° C-arm angle; note compression force of 38 lb and IMF inclusion (*arrow*).

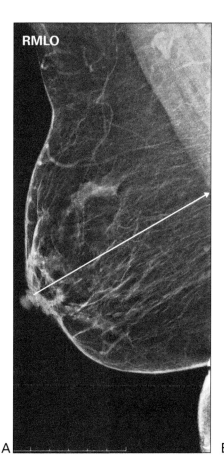

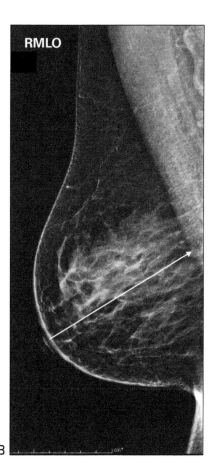

Figure 7-83
According to established criteria, the pectoral muscle should extend to or below the PNL in approximately 80% of patients. Determine if the PNL extends *to* the pectoral muscle **(A)** or *below* the pectoral muscle **(B)** to assess posterior tissue inclusion.

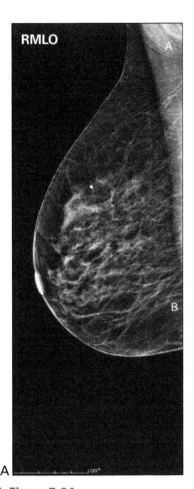

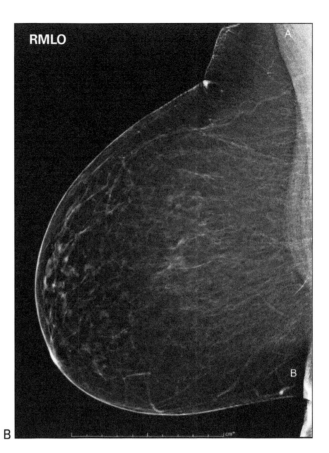

Figure 7-84

The pectoral muscle shape is affected by adequate capture of breast tissue and relaxation. The muscle should demonstrate a generous width superiorly, gradually narrowing as it descends to the inferior border. Both RMLO projections demonstrate a vertical pectoral muscle presentation. **(A)** Demonstrates the axilla placed too anteriorly on the image receptor (labeled *A*), which affects posterior capture, preventing adequate superior pectoral muscle width and inferior tissue inclusion (labeled *B*). **(B)** Demonstrates the axilla placed too anteriorly on the image receptor (labeled *A*) and insufficient capture of posterior tissue, which affects pectoral muscle anterior border presentation and introduces airgaps (labeled *B*).

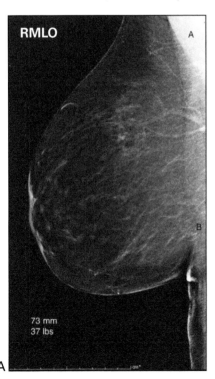

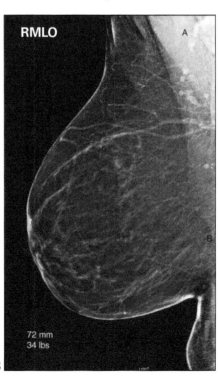

Figure 7-85

RMLO images of the same patient demonstrating pectoral muscle presentation. **(A)** Demonstrates exclusion of superoposterior tissue (labeled *A*) due to axillary placement and insufficient capture of posterior tissue, which also affects inferior region capture (labeled *B*). **(B)** Accurate placement of the axilla on the image receptor combined with medial rotation of the patient toward the image receptor demonstrates a generous amount of superior pectoral muscle (labeled *A*) gradually narrowing to the inferior border (labeled *B*) affecting visualization of superoposterior, posterior, and inferior tissue; note also the improved breast support in **(B)**.

Pectoral Muscle Presentation Problem #4: Anterior Pectoral Muscle Border Not Convex

Figure 7-86 illustrates a concave anterior border of the pectoral muscle influenced by several factors including the patient's ability to relax and the height of the IRSD.

It is desirable for the anterior border of the pectoral muscle to appear convex as it is an indication that the muscle is relaxed, thereby affording the ability to capture deep posterior tissue, and to enhance comfort as compression is applied. It is not possible to visualize a convex anterior border of the pectoral muscle in all patients, even when the muscle and thorax have been coached to relaxation. With some patients, the anterior border of the pectoral muscle presents as a straight line, while others may have a very slight concave appearance. Visualizing a convex-to-straight line appearance of the anterior border of the pectoral muscle on the MLO projection is possible in the majority of patients (Figure 7-77).

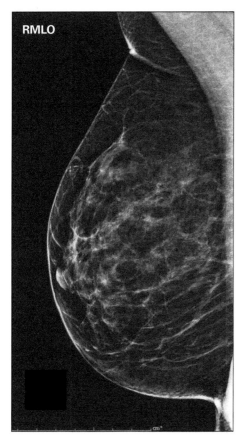

Figure 7-86
When the patient's shoulder, arm, and thorax have not been coached to appropriate relaxation, the pectoral muscle will appear concave rather than convex. A convex presentation is desired as this affords the ability to capture deep posterior tissue and to enhance comfort as compression is applied.

Fix-It Problem #4: Anterior Pectoral Muscle Border Not Convex

Figure 7-87 illustrates image quality improvement for anterior border pectoral muscle presentation when the following positioning/compression maneuvers are employed from Table 7-2.

2, **3**, 4, 6, 7, 8, 9, **13, 14**, 20
(Bold numbers have the greatest impact on this positioning feature.)

MLO Pectoral Muscle Presentation is Affected By:

- Customize angle of the image receptor to the natural angle of the pectoral muscle
- Height of the image receptor
- Axillary placement on the image receptor
- Adequate posterolateral capture
- Adequate medial rotation of the patient toward the image receptor
- Relaxation of the pectoral muscle and thorax

Superior Tissue

Features Visualized

- Apex of the axilla
- Tail of Spence

Superior Tissue Presentation: Breast Placement on the Image Receptor

The MLO projection uses the entire "real estate" of the image receptor to include the length of the breast from high in the axilla to the inferior border at the sixth or seventh rib, including the IMF region. These external landmarks describe inclusion of breast tissue superiorly to inferiorly when visualized on the MLO projection (Figure 7-88).

Superior Tissue Presentation Problem #1: Breast Placed Too Low on the Image Receptor

Figure 7-89 illustrates insufficient image quality when the superior to inferior breast borders have been incorrectly positioned on the IRSD. When the breast is positioned too low on the image receptor, the following features may be observed on the MLO image:

1. Pectoral muscle is stressed by raising the arm higher than the shoulder, moving the patient away from the image receptor, excluding posterior tissue.
2. Vertical pectoral muscle presentation.

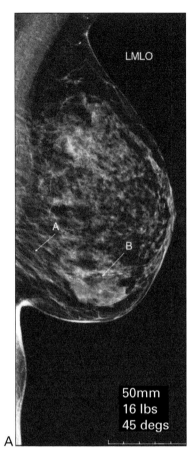

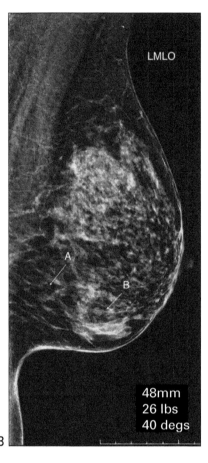

Figure 7-87
The anterior border of the pectoral muscle is affected by adequate capture of the posterior tissue and relaxation of the patient. **(A)** Demonstrates an unrelaxed pectoral muscle and insufficient posterior tissue capture; note tissue droop (*arrow A*) and inadequate glandular separation (*arrow B*), compression thickness, compression force, and C-arm angle. **(B)** demonstrates a relaxed pectoral muscle with adequate posterior capture; note improved tissue support (*arrow A*), and glandular separation (*arrow B*), compression thickness, compression force, and C-arm angle.

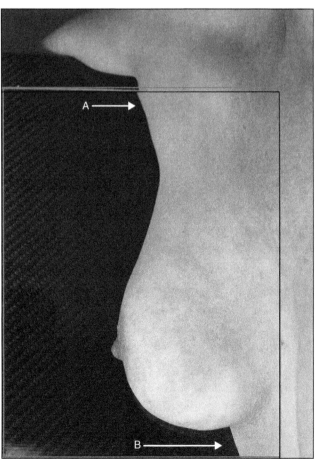

Figure 7-88
The MLO projection uses the entire "real estate" of the image receptor to include the length of the breast from high in the axilla (*arrow A*) to the inferior border at the sixth or seventh rib (*arrow B*), including the IMF region.

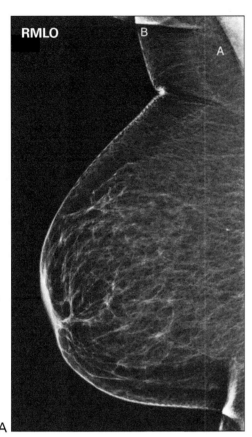

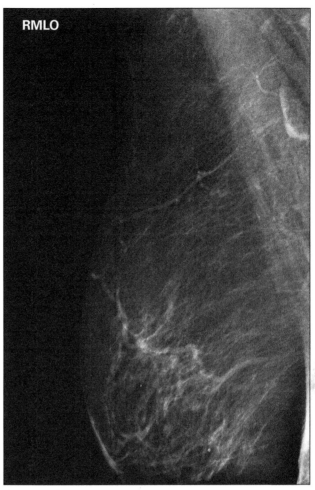

Figure 7-89
Both RMLO projections demonstrating breast placed too low on the image receptor. **(A)** Stresses the pectoral muscle (labeled *A*) by raising the arm higher than the shoulder, excluding posterior tissue. Additionally, including arm artifact (labeled *B*) affects the delivery of adequate compression. **(B)** Positioning the breast too low on the image receptor may exclude inferior breast tissue.

3. Includes arm artifact and introduces skinfolds.
4. Results in inadequate compression of the mound of the breast.
5. May exclude IMF from image.

Superior Tissue Problem #2: Breast Placed Too High on the Image Receptor

Figure 7-90 illustrates insufficient image quality when the superior to inferior breast borders have been incorrectly positioned too high on the IRSD. This positioning error includes the following observations for the MLO projection:

1. A common problem associated with digital imaging due to detector electronic dead space at each side edge of the IRSD affecting superior tissue inclusion on MLO projection
2. Excludes superior tissue from the image, including the tail of Spence
3. Excessive abdomen included on the image

Fix-It Problems #1 and #2: Proper Breast Placement on the Image Receptor

Figure 7-91 illustrates image quality improvement for adequate demonstration of the superior and inferior breast borders. Correct breast placement on the image receptor is achieved when the following positioning/compression maneuvers are employed from Table 7-2.

1, 2, **3, 6,** 7, 8, 12, **20**
(Bold numbers have the greatest impact on this positioning feature.)

Superior Tissue Presentation is Affected By:

• Selection of the compression device size
• Breast placement on the image receptor
• Receptor height

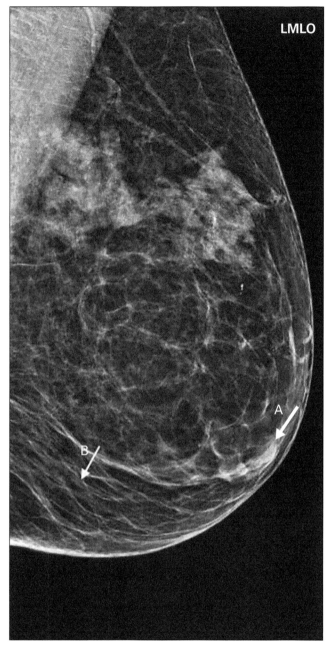

Figure 7-90
RMLO projection demonstrating breast placed too high on the image receptor resulting in superior tissue exclusion; note nipple out of profile due to patient rotated away from the image receptor (*arrow A*), tissue droop (*arrow B*), and exclusion of IMF region.

- Axillary placement of the corner of the image receptor
- Compression device placement at the superior–posterior breast margins

Additional Tips for MLO Breast Placement

1. To find the landmark just anterior to the latissimus dorsi for axillary placement on the image receptor, reach across your own thorax into the axilla using "pinching" fingers. With your fingers, pinch the thick latissimus dorsi muscle in the posterior margin of the axilla. The thumb location is resting just anterior to the latissimus dorsi muscle, the placement for the receptor corner when positioning the superior tissue for the MLO projection (Figure 7-80).

2. FFMD detectors accommodating both large and small breast sizes may have white lines indicating the light field margins at the side edges of the detectors. These image receptor light field indicators are useful for assessing the appropriate height of the image receptor to the anatomical landmark of the external axilla, ensuring adequate superior capture (Figure 7-81).

3. The entire "real estate" of the light field should be used for the MLO projection: the superior capture is observed by the placement of the chestwall corner of the compression device at the clavicle and humeral head junction; the inferior breast margin is located a few centimeters from the image receptor lower edge (Figure 7-88).

Inferior Tissue

Features Visualized

- Inferior breast
- Inframammary fold

Inferior Tissue Presentation Problem #1: IMF Excluded from Image

The inferior border of the breast, including the IMF, is challenging to capture on the MLO projection. Very thin patients present a particular challenge in including the IMF on the image due to the 4- to 7-mm electronic dead space at the chestwall edge of the digital detector (Figure 7-92); however, there are many examples of an open IMF included on MLO projections of thin males. Adequate rotation of the patient's thorax toward the image receptor resolves this particular issue for the majority of thin patients. Patients with a protruding abdomen present the opposite challenge in capturing the IMF on the image as the inferior breast/superior abdomen junction (IMF) is difficult to separate and compress adequately. For the vast majority of patients, incorrect feet placement in relation to the image receptor, rotation of the patient's thorax away from the image receptor, proximity of the patient's abdomen to the image receptor (comfortably below the IMF), and incorrect C-arm angle are the primary reasons why the IMF is excluded from the image. When the IMF is excluded from the image, the posteroinferior tissue is also

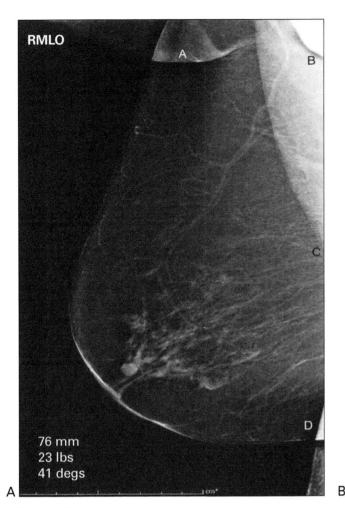

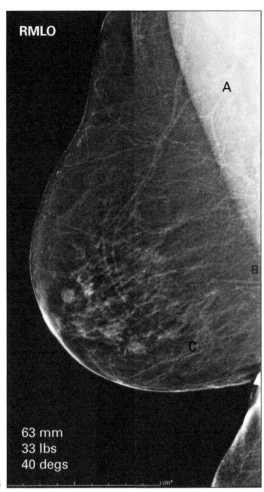

Figure 7-91
RMLO projections of the same patient resulting in image quality differences due to breast placement on the image receptor. **(A)** Breast positioned too low results in inclusion of arm artifact (labeled *A*) affecting adequate compression thickness and force: 76 mm, 23 lb; axilla artifact affects breast thickness (labeled *B*); also note insufficient posterior tissue capture resulting in shorter muscle length (labeled *C*) and insufficient support of posterior structures resulting in IMF skinfold (labeled *D*). **(B)** Improved axillary breast placement combined with medial rotation of the thorax toward the image receptor results in adequate pectoral muscle presentation (labeled *A*), improved posterior capture and muscle length (labeled *B*), and improved support of breast structures (labeled *C*) affecting compression thickness and force: 63 mm, 33 lb.

excluded. There are several positioning maneuvers that affect visualization of the IMF on the image. The following problems describing IMF exclusion assume the height of the image receptor and the placement of the breast on the receptor have been addressed.

Inferior Tissue Presentation Problem #2: Patient Stands with Her Feet and Pelvis Directly in Front of or Slightly Toward the Underside of the Image Receptor

Positioning the patient facing the unit with the image receptor centered to the patient's pelvis or positioning the pelvis slightly to the underside of the image receptor does not allow the IMF region of the abdomen to be included on the final image. The IMF region is not engaged in front of the image receptor, and inferior breast tissue is excluded from the image (Figure 7-93).

Inferior Tissue Presentation Problem #3: Patient's Thorax From the Superior to Inferior Chestwall Margin Is Not in Contact with Image Receptor

The patient is positioned standing slightly back from the image receptor and leans forward, resulting in adequate to excessive capture of superior tissue, with the breast directed downward, excluding posteroinferior breast tissue and the IMF region from the image (Figure 7-94).

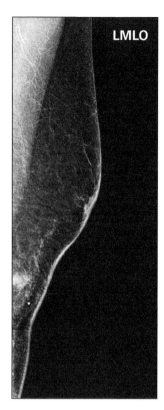

Figure 7-92
LMLO projection demonstrates IMF visualization of a male being evaluated for a breast lump (indicated by metallic marker). The 4- to 7-mm electronic dead space at the chestwall edge of the digital detector presents a particular challenge when imaging very thin female patients and males. Positioning techniques that include placing the abdomen in front of the image receptor combined with sufficient medial rotation of the thorax toward the image receptor allows visualization of the IMF in these patients.

Inferior Tissue Presentation Problem #4: Inadequate Posterolateral Capture

Visualization of the IMF requires adequate capture and control of the posterolateral tissue bringing the IMF onto the image receptor. Technologists must incorporate maneuvers designed specifically for adequate posterior tissue capture of the posterolateral breast into their positioning techniques for the MLO projection (Figure 7-95).

Fix-It Problems 1, 2, 3, and 4: Inferior Tissue and IMF Presentation

Figures 7-96 and 7-97 illustrate image quality improvement for IMF presentation when the following positioning/compression maneuvers are employed from Table 7-2.

1, 2, **4**, **5**, 7, 8, **9**, 10, 12, 20
(Bold numbers have the greatest impact on this positioning feature.)

Capture of IMF onto the Image Receptor Is Affected By:

- Selection of correct size compression device
- Patient's feet and pelvis facing the unit, IMF engaged anterior to the IRSD
- Abdomen in contact with the image receptor comfortably below the IMF region: no distance between the patient and the equipment
- Posterolateral tissue capture of the breast and IMF region

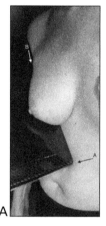
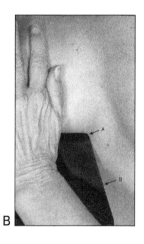
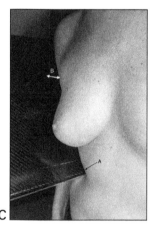
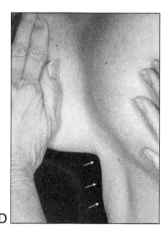

A   B   C   D

Figure 7-93
Capturing adequate inferior breast tissue that includes the IMF on the MLO projection is dependent on the feet and pelvis placement in relation to the image receptor. **(A)** Incorrect feet and pelvis placement resulting in the lower IRSD corner (labeled A) positioned at the center of the patient's abdomen just above the umbilicus; note the close contact of the lateral breast to the image receptor (labeled B). **(B)** Incorrect feet and pelvis placement demonstrated in **(A)** does not allow capture of the IMF region (labeled A); note the abdomen positioned behind the IRSD chestwall edge preventing superior abdominal tissue capture (labeled B). **(C)** Correct feet and pelvis placement resulting in the IMF region engaged to the front of the IRSD; note the position of the lower IRSD corner (labeled A) is now directly above the ASIS; note the space present between the lateral breast and the image receptor (labeled B). **(D)** Correct feet and pelvis placement positions the IMF region (*arrows*) in front of the image receptor.

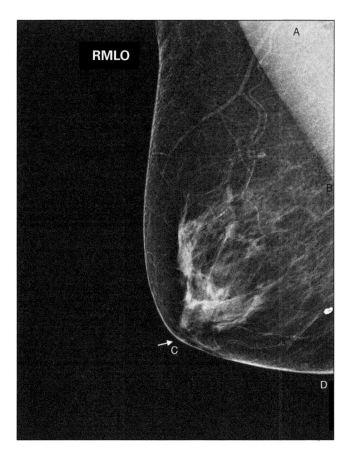

Figure 7-94
Capturing adequate posterior–inferior tissue on the MLO projection requires the abdomen to be in contact with the image receptor throughout the positioning maneuvers. RMLO demonstrating a wide superior pectoral muscle (labeled A) with inadequate muscle length (labeled B); the nipple pointing excessively downward (labeled C) excluding inferoposterior tissue and the IMF region (labeled D); these feature presentations indicate space between the chestwall edge of the image receptor and the patient's superior abdomen, requiring her to lean her upper body forward directing the breast in a downward direction.

Inferior Tissue Presentation Problem #5: IMF Is Present but Not Open

For some women, the pliability of the inferior breast attachment does not allow the breast to be pulled away from the chestwall to open the IMF (Figure 7-98). For these patients, the IMF region can be captured on the image, but the IMF will not be completely open. For the majority of women, there are several positioning maneuvers that affect the visualization of the open IMF on the image.

Inferior Tissue Presentation Problem #6: Patient's Feet and Pelvis Are Not Facing the Unit

Rotation of the patient's thorax away from the unit, even slightly, introduces creases or skinfolds in the

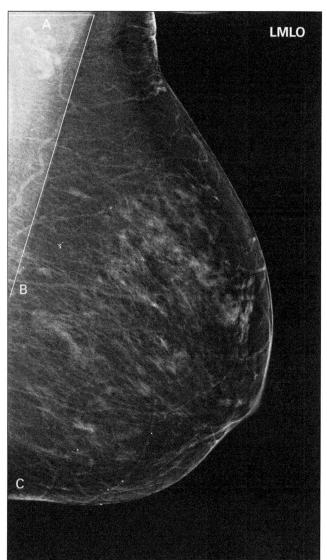

Figure 7-95
Inferior tissue visualization requires adequate capture and control over the inferoposterior breast to bring the IMF into the FOV. LMLO demonstrates superior breast features adequately included on the image: muscle width (labeled A) and muscle length (labeled B), with sufficient rotation of the patient toward the image receptor. Only the inferior breast was not captured on the image, excluding inferoposterior tissue and the IMF (labeled C).

posteroinferior region that obscure the visualization of the IMF (Figure 7-99).

Inferior Tissue Presentation Problem #7: Medial Tissue Allowed to Droop

As positioning maneuvers are completed for the MLO projection, the technologist's hand anchors the breast straight out from the chestwall. Allowing the medial tissue to droop places a crease in the IMF (Figure 7-100).

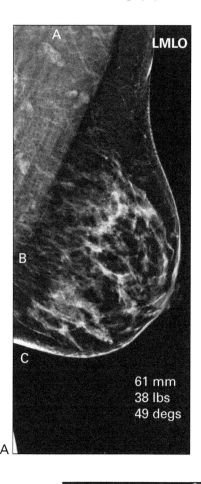

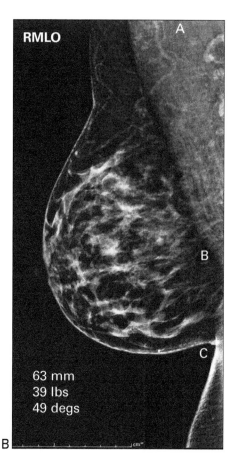

Figure 7-96
MLO images of the same patient. **(A)** LMLO demonstrates adequate muscle width (labeled *A*) and muscle length (labeled *B*) but exclusion of inferior breast tissue and the IMF region (labeled *C*) due to insufficient inferoposterior breast capture. **(B)** RMLO breast adequately positioned on the image receptor visualizing inferoposterior tissue and the IMF region (labeled *C*); note adequate muscle width (labeled *A*) and muscle length (labeled *B*).

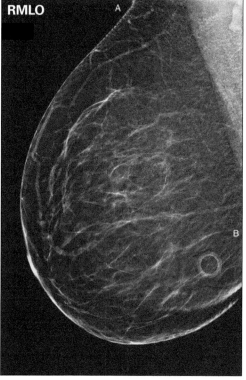

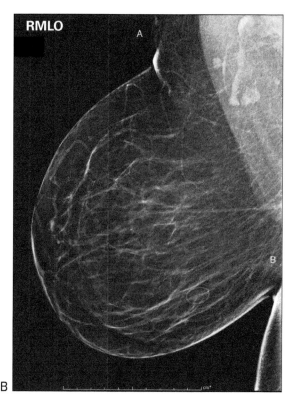

Figure 7-97
Visualization of inferoposterior tissue on the MLO requires attention to feet and pelvis placement, abdomen in contact with the IRSD, and adequate inferior tissue capture. RMLO images of the same patient. **(A)** Demonstrates insufficient capture of the inferoposterior region (labeled *B*); note insufficient inclusion of superior tissue above the breast mound (labeled *A*). **(B)** Demonstrates adequate capture of inferoposterior region and IMF (labeled *B*); note improved superior inclusion above the breast mound (labeled *A*).

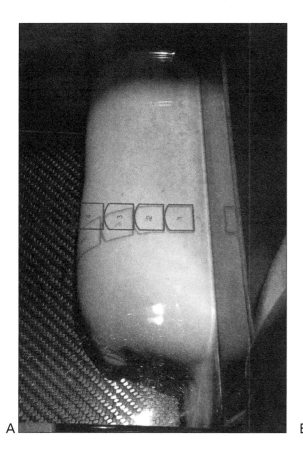

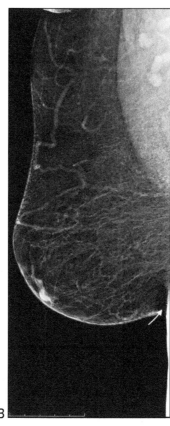

Figure 7-98
For some women, the pliability of the inferior breast attachment does not allow the breast to be pulled away from the chestwall to open the IMF region. For these patients, the IMF region can be captured on the image, but the IMF will not be completely open. **(A)** Patient with IMF tissue attachment that does not allow sufficient open IMF presentation. **(B)** Image of the same patient with tissue attachment preventing an open IMF presentation (*arrow*).

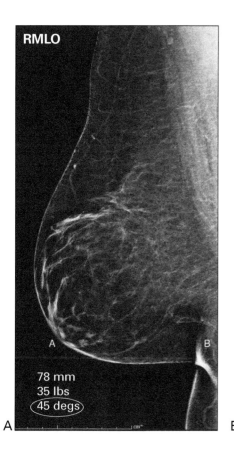

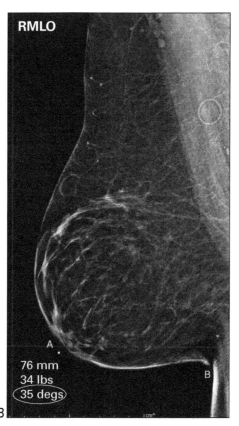

Figure 7-99
Open IMF: even slight rotation of the patient's thorax away from the unit introduces creases or folds at the IMF region that obscure visualization of the IMF. **(A)** RMLO with very slight rotation away from the image receptor indicated by nipple slightly out of profile (labeled *A*) resulting in skinfolds at IMF region (labeled *B*); note 45° C-arm angle. **(B)** RMLO of same patient without rotation of the thorax indicated by nipple presented in profile (labeled *A*) resulting in an open IMF region (labeled *B*); note 35° C-arm angle.

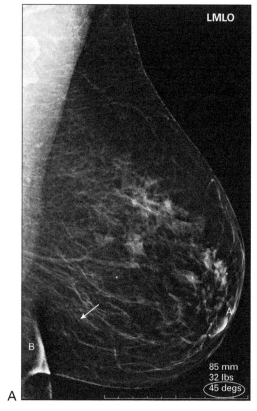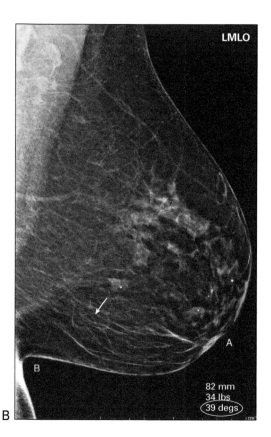

Figure 7-100
The technologist's hand anchors and supports the breast tissue approximately 90° away from the thorax in preparation for compression. LMLO projections of the same patient. **(A)** Patient rotated away from the image receptor indicated by nipple out of profile (labeled *A*); inadequate support of the breast allowing medial tissue droop (*arrow*), nonsupport of posterior breast structures introduces IMF fold (labeled *B*). **(B)** LMLO demonstrates improved breast support indicated by outward direction of posterior linear structures (*arrow*), no rotation of the thorax indicated by nipple presented in profile (labeled *A*) and open IMF region (labeled *B*).

Inferior Tissue Presentation Problem #8: Skinfolds

Positioning the MLO can naturally create skinfolds medially and laterally in the IMF. The lateral skinfolds are often undetected by the technologist because they occur on the undersurface of the breast between the skin and image receptor.

Fix-It Problems 5, 6, 7, and 8: IMF Presentation

15, 16, **17**, **18**, 21, **25**
(Bold numbers have the greatest impact on this positioning feature.)

Inferior Tissue Presentation Problem #9: Protruding Abdomen in IMF Region

For patients presenting with a larger, protruding abdomen, positioning of the IMF region with an open presentation is challenging. Successful opening of the IMF region is dependent on the degree of softness of the abdomen. For patients with a softer abdomen, adjustments in the positioning of the pelvis and excess abdomen or an additional SIO projection may suffice to correct the problem. For patients presenting with a very firm abdomen, oftentimes as a consequence of a medical condition causing an accumulation of fluid in the abdomen, an additional Lateral projection may assist in visualizing the inferoposterior breast tissue.

Fix-It Problem #9: Open IMF Presentation for Patients with Protruding Abdomen

Figure 7-101 illustrates image quality improvement for patients with a protruding abdomen in the IMF region when the following positioning/compression maneuvers are employed from Table 7-2.

19, 23
(Bold numbers have the greatest impact on this positioning feature.)

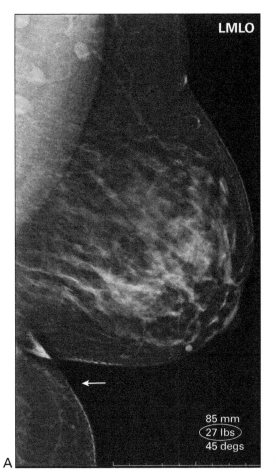
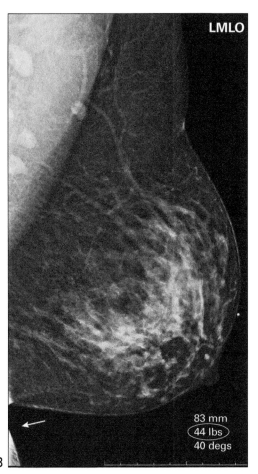

Figure 7-101
(A) For patients presenting with a larger, protruding abdomen, positioning of the IMF region with an open presentation is challenging (*arrow*) and may result in inadequate compression (27 lb). **(B)** Removing protruding abdominal tissue by tipping the patient's pelvis downward opens the IMF region (*arrow*) and allows for adequate compression application (44 lb).

Inferior Tissue and Open IMF Are Affected By:

- Pelvis and feet placement squarely facing the unit
- Anchoring the breast securely to the image receptor, preventing medial tissue from drooping
- Removing medial and lateral skinfolds using a downward finger sweep
- Adequate compression
- Protruding abdomen

Additional Tips for Inferior Tissue and Open IMF Presentation

- When the patient leans her upper torso laterally toward the image receptor for the MLO projection, the IMF region "buckles," placing skinfolds at the junction of the superior abdomen and the inferior breast tissue. Due to the length of the digital detector, elongating the thorax to more efficiently match the image receptor length encourages the IMF region to open. This is done by bending the ipsilateral knee of the patient and telling her to "slouch" while adjusting the angle of her thorax to match the angle of the image receptor. Combining this tip with Fix-it #11 adjusts the lateral tissue downward to assist in opening the IMF region (Figure 7-102).
- Prior to making the exposure for the MLO projection, the final positioning maneuver is to have the patient hold her contralateral breast out of the field of view. For patients with small to average size breasts, this has no effect on the presentation of the open IMF. For patients with larger, pendulous breasts, the posteromedial tissue can be directed downward by the weight of the contralateral breast, introducing a fold at the IMF. For these patients, elevate the contralateral breast prior to having the patient hold it from the field of view. This maneuver lifts and opens the posteromedial tissue in the IMF region.
- When additional imaging is necessary for further definition in the IMF region, an SIO projection may be beneficial for patients with softer, pliable abdomens.

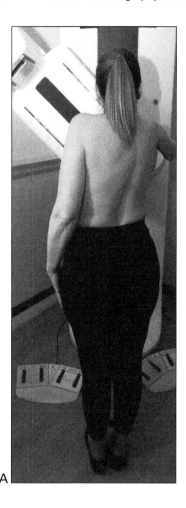

A

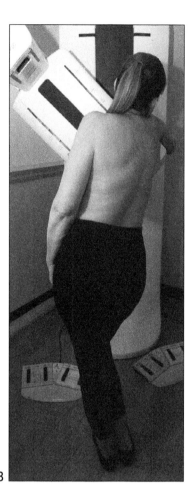

B

Figure 7-102
(A) Keeping the hips and pelvis in a vertical position for the MLO causes the IMF region to "buckle" as the thorax meets the image receptor. **(B)** Elongating the thorax to match the image receptor length encourages the IMF region to open. This is accomplished by bending the ipsilateral knee of the patient and telling her to "slouch" while adjusting the length of her thorax to match the length of the image receptor.

• Adjusting the C-arm to a shallower angle for the MLO projection distributes the weight of the breast more evenly across the image receptor.

Anterior Tissue

Features Visualized

• Nipple presentation
• Anterior and central breast
• Subareolar region

Anterior Tissue Presentation Problem #1: Anterior Tissue Sagging, Demonstrating Tissue Droop

Anterior Tissue Presentation Problem #1A: Patient Presents with Thick Base of the Breast, Tapering to a Thinner Apex

Anterior tissue on the MLO projection demonstrates structures directed at an approximate 90° angle from the chestwall. Uniform compression for all patients is not possible due to varying thicknesses from the base of the breast to the nipple. For patients who present with thickness variation from the chestwall to the nipple, where uniform compression cannot be achieved on the MLO projection, imaging strategies using the "tilt" compression device design are beneficial. When the anterior tissue is not supported and compressed and adequately on the MLO projection, an additional MLOAC projection is warranted.

Fix-It Problem #1A: Patient Presents with Thick Base of the Breast, Tapering to a Thinner Apex Figure 7-103 illustrates image quality improvement for tissue demonstration through adequate capture and breast compression when the following positioning/compression maneuvers are employed from Table 7-2.

1, 2, 11, 16, **17**, 18, **19**, 22, 23, 25
(Bold numbers have the greatest impact on this positioning feature.)

Anterior Tissue Presentation Problem #1B: Technologist Does Not Effectively Support Breast Outward and Upward

Positioning/compression maneuvers used to support and secure the anterior structures out and away from the chestwall additionally assist in ensuring the IMF is open.

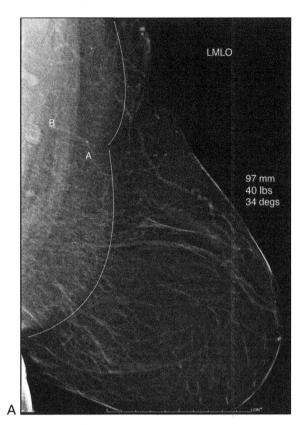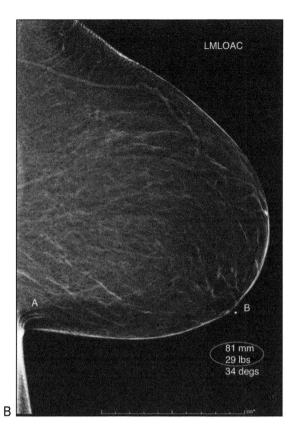

Figure 7-103
When uniform compression cannot be achieved on the MLO projection due to thickness variation from chestwall to nipple, the anterior tissue structures are not accurately represented on the image. **(A)** LMLO projection of patient with thick breast base tapering to thinner apex. Compressed base of the breast (indicated behind white lines labeled *A*) includes pectoral muscle (labeled *B*). Anterior tissue in front of white lines inadequately compressed as indicated by tissue droop; note compression thickness of 97 mm and compression force of 40 lb. **(B)** LMLOAC projection of the same breast optimizing anterior breast tissue including nipple (labeled *B*) and IMF region (labeled *A*); note compression thickness of 81 mm and compression force of 29 lb.

Fix-It Problem #1B: Technologist Does Not Effectively Support Breast Outward and Upward Figure 7-104 demonstrates effective breast support and compression for a patient with a large breast when the following positioning/compression maneuvers are employed from Table 7-2.

16, **17**, **19**, 21, **25**
(Bold numbers have the greatest impact on this positioning feature.)

Anterior Tissue Sagging Is Affected By:

1. Larger, pendulous breasts, with a thicker base and thinner apex
2. Anterior breast adequately supported outward from the chestwall; medial tissue adequately supported, not allowing droop (technologist technique)
3. Availability of "tilt" compression device design

Additional Tip for MLO Anterior Presentation and Breast Support

"*Support the medial breast in an approximate 90° direction, outward and upward from the chestwall.*"[8] This critical maneuver for accurate breast positioning and compression describing the "out and up" maneuver warrants further explanation. Technologists can infer this to mean the entire breast mound must be directed "up" toward the superior distal corner of the image receptor. Doing this exacerbates skinfolds in the superior aspect of the breast mound/inferior tail of Spence junction and introduces skinfolds. Supporting all breast tissue, both laterally and medially, projecting from the chestwall at an approximate 90° angle, demonstrates the tissue as it naturally travels in the posterior to anterior direction. Excessive force, directing the medial breast upward in an unnatural projection from the chestwall, may alter the natural tissue pattern extending from the thorax to the nipple (Figure 7-105).

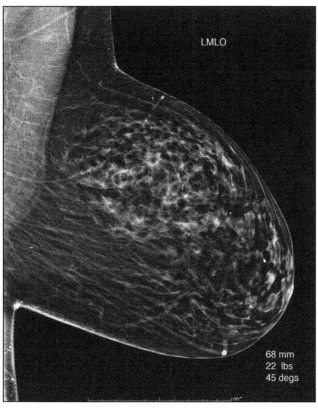

Figure 7-104
LMLO projection of larger breast demonstrating technologist's use of good positioning techniques to position and adequately compress breast tissue approximately 90° from the thorax, additionally assisting in visualizing an open IMF.

Posterior Tissue

Features Visualized

- Retroglandular fat space
- Pectoral muscle extending to or below the PNL
- IMF
- Posterior tissue adjacent to the thorax directed approximately 90° from the chestwall

Posterior Tissue Presentation Problem #1: Posterior Breast Excluded from Image

Even when sufficient positioning has been achieved to include the posterior breast margin, the retroglandular fat space may not always be visualized. This is true for patients with extremely dense glandular tissue extending to the posterior margin of the chestwall and for patients with entirely adipose breast tissue (Figure 7-106). For these patients, indicators of posterior tissue capture are adequate length of pectoral muscle (when superior muscle width is sufficiently wide, with gradual narrowing to the inferior border), visibility of the IMF, and measurement of the PNL. There are several positioning maneuvers that ensure the capture and visibility of the posterior breast margin, all of which are interdependent on each other for superior image quality.

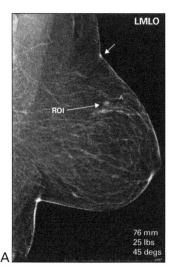
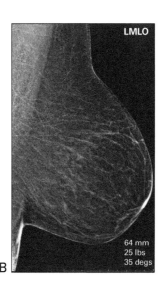
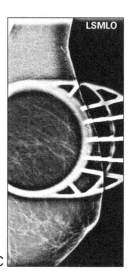
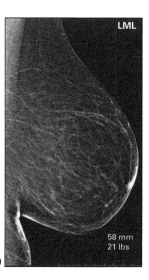

Figure 7-105
Supporting the tissue approximately 90° from the thorax demonstrates the tissue as it naturally travels in the posterior and anterior direction. Excessive upward direction and support of *only the medial* breast may inaccurately represent tissue on the image. **(A)** LMLO projection indicates stressed tissue at breast mound/inferior tail of Spence junction (*arrow*), rotated tissue (labeled *A*), ROI indicated by radiologist (*ROI arrow*); note 76-mm compression thickness, 45° C-arm angle. **(B)** Repeat of LMLO demonstrates breast structures directed posterior to anterior revealing normal glandular tissue at ROI; note 64-mm compression thickness, 35° C-arm angle. **(C)** LSMLO reveals normal glandular tissue. **(D)** LML reveals normal glandular tissue.

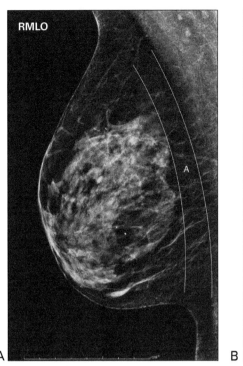
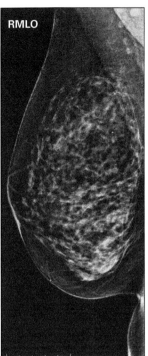
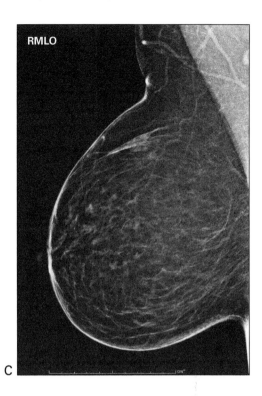

Figure 7-106
(A) The retroglandular fat space is visualized on the MLO projection in the posterior region of the breast (labeled *A*). The retroglandular fat space may not always be visualized. **(B)** This is true for patients with extremely dense glandular tissue extending to the posterior margin of the chestwall and **(C)** for patients with entirely adipose breast tissue.

Fix-It Problem #1: Posterior Breast Excluded from Image

Figure 7-107 illustrates image quality improvement for capture of posterior breast margin when the following positioning/compression maneuvers are employed from Table 7-2.

2, 3, **4**, 5, **6**, 7, 8, **9, 10, 12**, 13, **20**
(Bold numbers have the greatest impact on this positioning feature.)

Posterior Tissue Presentation Problem #2: Patient Is Rotated Away from the Image Receptor

Assuming posterolateral capture is accomplished, two factors affect the visibility of the retroglandular fat space. The patient must directly face the unit, and the x-ray beam must be directed perpendicular to the retroglandular fat space. If one of these conditions is not met, the retroglandular fat space is unable to be observed on the MLO image. Indications that the patient is rotated away from the image receptor on the MLO projection include: inferoposterior

tissue excluded from the image, inferoposterior tissue is superimposed over the retroglandular fat space, exclusion of IMF, or the nipple presenting out of profile.

Fix-It Problem #2: Patient Is Rotated Away from the Image Receptor

Figure 7-108 illustrates the resulting image when the patient that is rotated away from the image receptor along with the resulting image demonstrating improved posterior tissue presentation when the following positioning/compression maneuvers are employed from Table 7-2.

4, 5, **7**, 8, **20**, 21
(Bold numbers have the greatest impact on this positioning feature.)

Posterior Tissue Visualization Is Affected By:

1. Ensuring IMF is engaged in front of the image receptor.
2. Capturing posterolateral breast beyond the margin of the midaxilla.
3. Rotating the patient toward the x-ray unit, capturing medial tissue in the field of view.
4. Feet and pelvis directly facing the mammography unit.

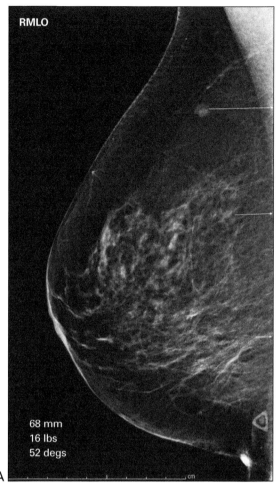

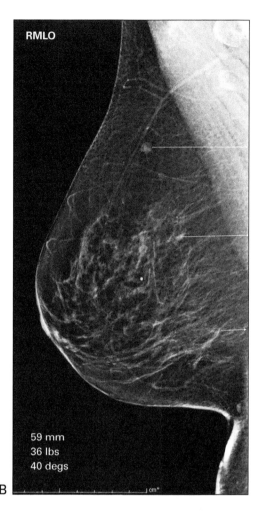

Figure 7-107
Positioning maneuvers used to capture posterior tissue are interdependent: feet and pelvis placement, axillary placement, lateral capture to the latissimus dorsi line, and adequate medial rotation of the thorax to the image receptor all are required for adequate posterior tissue visualization. **(A)** RMLO projection excludes posterior tissue from the superior to the inferior breast margins; note breast structures indicated by *arrows* and their distance from the posterior margin of the image. **(B)** RMLO of the same patient using positioning techniques described in the MLO Fix-It Table to maximize posterior tissue capture and visualization; note same breast structures indicated by *arrows* and their distance from the posterior margin of the image.

Compression

Compression is critical to the mammography image, ensuring separation of breast structures for better visualization, increasing sharpness, and reducing the dose to the patient. Evaluation of technical factors such as centimeter thickness of the compressed breast and compression force utilized should be reviewed by the technologist. Ensuring these factors are similar between the right and left breast projections is an indication that attention was given to techniques used for adequate compression application. Patients presenting with size differences between the right and the left breast require documentation on the history form for the interpreting physician.

Features Visualized

1. Blood vessels, microcalcifications, anterior border of pectoral muscle, and Cooper ligaments
2. Adequate separation of tissues
3. Fibrous structures directed approximately 90° from the chestwall

Compression Problem #1: Undercompression, Possible Motion, and Compression Inconsistencies

Adequate compression results in separating islands of glandular tissue and increasing sharpness of detail, two critical

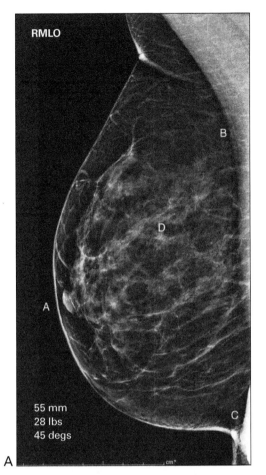
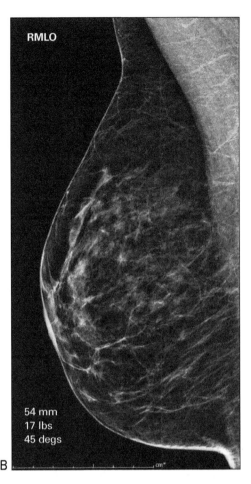

Figure 7-108
Patient rotation affects the visibility of the retroglandular fat space. The patient must directly face the unit ensuring no rotation of the breast structures from the chestwall to the nipple, and the x-ray beam must be directed perpendicular to the retroglandular fat space. **(A)** RMLO projection demonstrating patient rotated away from image receptor indicated by nipple out of profile (labeled *A*), insufficient pectoral muscle presentation (labeled *B*), IMF skinfold (labeled *C*), and glandular tissue rotated into the retroglandular fat space (labeled *D*). **(B)** RMLO of same patient directly facing the unit improving presentation of nipple, pectoral muscle, IMF, and retroglandular tissue.

elements for detecting the earliest indications of breast cancer. Of the two projections, it is more likely that inadequate compression is observed on the MLO view, the most common reason being the technologist's use of inadequate compression force. Adequate compression on the image is observed by separation of tissues, sharpness of linear structures, blood vessels, and microcalcifications. The subareolar tissue, the IMF region, and the anterior border of the pectoral muscle are all primary areas for evaluation of sharpness. Looking closely at the entire image, with these areas in particular, to evaluate sharpness may reveal motion on the image.

Compression Problem #1A: Undercompression and Use of Inadequate Force

Adequate compression can be influenced by the correct selection of the compression device size. Adequate compression is evaluated by the tautness of the skin enveloping the breast. This evaluation can only be done by the technologist performing the exam. The final maneuver to complete compression requires the use of manual compression that is completely under the control of the technologist.

Fix-It Problem #1A: Undercompression and Use of Inadequate Force Figure 7-109 illustrates image quality improvement for adequate compression of breast tissue when the appropriate size compression device has been selected and when the following positioning/compression maneuvers are employed from Table 7-2.

1, 19, 21, **25**
(Bold numbers have the greatest impact on this positioning feature.)

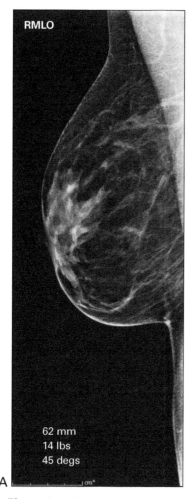
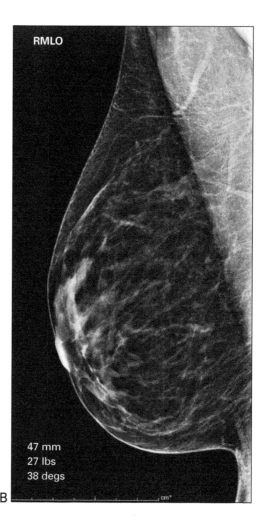

Figure 7-109
Adequate compression is influenced by the selection of the compression device size and the technologist's evaluation of the skin's tautness by tapping the breast as compression is completed using the manual mode of operation. **(A)** RMLO projection using 24 × 30-cm-size compression device for a small breast; 62-mm compression thickness, 14 lb compression force. **(B)** Same patient using 18 × 24-cm-size compression device; 47-mm compression force, 27 lb compression force.

Compression Problem #1B: Undercompression, Additional Body Parts Included on Image

Figure 7-110 illustrates insufficient compression influenced by body parts other than breast tissue included in the field of view. To obtain adequate compression of the breast, only the breast margins should be included in the field of view. Visible arm artifact and abdominal artifact included on the image are usually accompanied by large skinfolds and airgaps indicating compromised compression force.

Fix-It Problem #1B: Undercompression, Additional Body Parts Included on Image   Figure 7-91 illustrates image quality improvement through adequate compression application. This quality can be achieved by ensuring only the breast tissue is included under the field of view

while incorporating the following positioning/compression maneuvers from Table 7-2.

1, **22, 23**, 25
(Bold numbers have the greatest impact on this positioning feature.)

Compression Is Affected By:

- Selection of the correct size compression device for the patient.
- Including only the breast and pectoral muscle under the compression device.
- Relaxation of the patient.
- Patient tolerance.
- Use of the "tilt" compression device when available.
- When the "tilt" compression device is not available, add an AC view, which captures only the anterior portion of

facilitates uniform compression to the breast. Lean the patient's head near her shoulder to ensure the collapse of the pectoral muscle. Slightly elevate her chin to avoid contact with the compression device as it is lowered as well as when it is automatically released upon completion of the exposure.

- Bend the ipsilateral knee; this action results in the patient slouching onto the image receptor, further relaxing the breast tissue adjacent to the thorax and slightly increasing the movement of the posterolateral breast margin toward the fixed medial margin.

- When applying compression for the MLO projection, the use of breathing techniques can be beneficial as their affect further reduces the tension of the pectoral muscle and the relaxation of adjacent tissues of the thorax. With a firm grasp securing the breast to the image receptor, use the automatic compression mode to lower the compression device until it rests just above the sternum. Ask the patient to take in a breath. Simultaneously tell the patient to exhale her breath while continuing compression. Because the patient relaxes the tissue adjacent to the thorax when she exhales, the technologist can easily manipulate the compression device past sternum and clavicle, without scraping the compression device against the bony structures of the sternum and ribs while capturing deep posterior tissue. Final compression is applied using the manual compression mode, resulting in satisfactory compression and increased comfort to the patient (Figure 7-111).

Skinfolds

Skinfolds on the MLO projection are introduced by adjacent tissues not adequately smoothed away from each other, resulting in compression of overlapping skin. Eliminating all skinfolds from every MLO image is simply not possible. Skinfolds commonly found on the MLO image appear in the IMF region, in the axillary region, and in the junction of the superior breast mound and the lower axilla. The technologist evaluates each image to determine the degree of degradation to image quality due to skinfolds. Skinfolds are generally acceptable if breast tissue can be visualized into, through, and out of the fold and compression is not compromised. Maneuvers that minimize and control skinfolds help to provide an accurate representation of breast tissue on the final image. Careful consideration should be given to exam management when problem solving for skinfolds. Radiologists may have repeat protocols regarding the threshold of acceptability in their practice for the presence of skinfolds on the image.

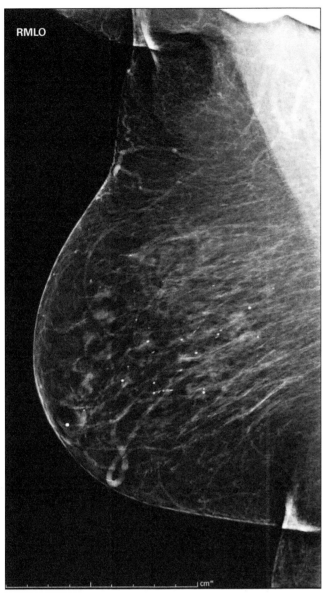

Figure 7-110
To achieve adequate compression, only breast tissue should be included in the field of view. Visible arm artifact and abdominal artifact included on the image are usually accompanied by large skinfolds and airgaps indicating compression has been compromised.

the breast, excluding the pectoral muscle and the thick base of the breast.
- Compression application evaluation by the technologist ("tautness" check).

Additional Tips for Adequate Compression

- Lean the patient's upper thorax toward the image receptor to ensure the sternum is parallel to the receptor edge; this reduces the thickness of the pectoral muscle and

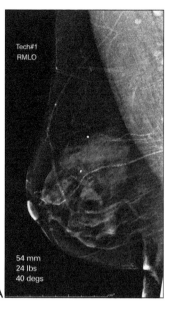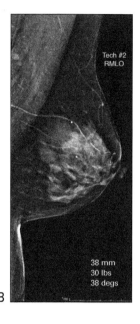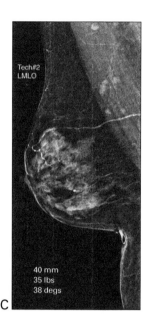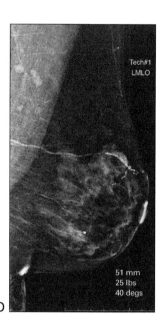

Figure 7-111

When applying compression for the MLO projection, the use of breathing techniques can be beneficial. These techniques help to further reduce the tension of the pectoral muscle and assist in relaxation of adjacent tissues of the thorax. **(A)** RMLO demonstrates 54-mm compression thickness and 24 lb compression force using traditional compression technique for Technologist #1. **(B)** Same patient RMLO demonstrates 38-mm compression thickness and 30 lb compression force when Technologist #2 employs MLO breathing technique during compression application. **(C)** LMLO demonstrates 40-mm compression thickness and 35 lb when Technologist #2 employs MLO breathing technique during compression application. **(D)** Same patient LMLO demonstrates 51-mm compression thickness and 25 lb compression force using traditional compression technique for Technologist #1.

Skinfold Problem #1: Axillary Skinfolds

Axillary skinfolds are commonly visualized on the MLO image in patients of all body types, requiring specific positioning strategies to minimize and hopefully eliminate them. For the very thin patient, skinfolds are particularly challenging in the axillary region as there is minimal tissue present to fill the area, introducing folds that are difficult to reach and to eliminate. For very thin patients to satisfactorily image the axillary area, two images may be required. Managing skinfolds in the axilla is possible through positioning strategies designed to minimize and control them.

Fix-It Problem #1: Axillary Skinfolds

Figure 7-112 illustrates quality improvement of the axillary skinfolds when incorporating positioning/compression maneuvers from Table 7-2.

3, 4, **6**, 7, **8**, 11, 12, 13, 14, 20, 22, **24**
(Bold numbers have the greatest impact on this positioning feature.)

Skinfold Problem #2: Superior Breast Skinfolds, "Smile Crease"

Skinfolds are commonly visualized on the MLO image of larger pendulous breasts where the anterior/superior breast mound intersects with the lower axilla. Sometimes referred to as "smile" creases or folds, these skinfolds are naturally introduced by patient body habitus on the image. Technologist's positioning techniques should include properly addressing the lateral aspect of the breast to reduce the effect of this type of skinfold and to ensure the breast mound is not excessively directed upward prior to compression.

Fix-It Problem #2: Superior Breast Skinfolds, "Smile Crease"

Figure 7-113 illustrates image quality improvement for superior breast skinfolds when the following positioning/compression maneuvers are employed from Table 7-2.

2, 4, 6, **7**, 8, 9, 10, **11**, 12, 13, 14, 16, 17, 19, 20, 25
(Bold numbers have the greatest impact on this positioning feature.)

Skinfold Problem #3: Inferior Breast Skinfolds (IMF)

Skinfolds in the IMF region are commonly seen on the MLO image. Introduced by rotation of the patient's thorax, or by insufficient support of the breast outward and upward by the technologist, or by a combination of the two, these skinfolds are easily corrected by positioning

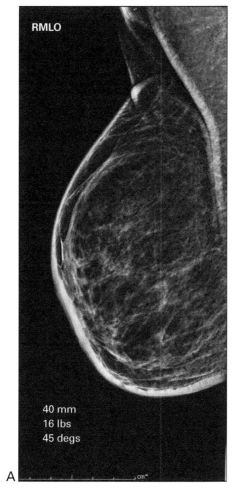

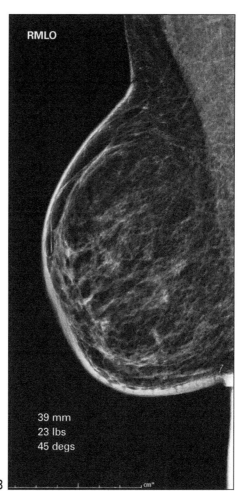

Figure 7-112
For the very thin patient, axillary skinfolds are particularly challenging as there is minimal upper outer tissue fullness present to fill the area, introducing skinfolds that are difficult to reach and to eliminate. **(A)** RMLO demonstrating large axillary skinfold. **(B)** RMLO of the same patient with skinfolds eliminated when combining positioning maneuvers #6, #8, and #24 from the MLO Fix-It Table.

strategies specifically designed to open the IMF (Figures 7-99 through 7-101).

Fix-It Problem #3: Inferior Breast Skinfolds (IMF)

2, 4, 5, 7, 11, **15**, 16, **17**, **18**, 25
(Bold numbers have the greatest impact on this positioning feature.)

Additional Tips for IMF Skinfold Elimination

1. When the patient leans her upper torso laterally toward the image receptor for the MLO projection, the IMF region "buckles," placing skinfolds at the junction of the superior abdomen and the inferior breast tissue. Due to the length of the digital detector, elongating the thorax to more efficiently match the image receptor length encourages the IMF region to open. This is done by bending the ipsilateral knee of the patient and telling

her to "slouch" while adjusting the angle of her thorax to match the angle of the image receptor. Combining this tip with Fix-it #11 adjusts the lateral tissue downward to assist in opening the IMF region.

2. For patients with "heavy" pendulous breast tissue, consider a shallower C-arm angle, allowing the image receptor to assist with breast support.

Airgap

Airgaps in the MLO projection result from lateral tissue not resting flush against the image receptor or medial tissue not resting flush against the compression device. They are commonly introduced as a consequence of skinfolds and range in degrees from minimal airgaps that do not compromise image quality to a noticeably uneven distribution of plus and minus densities degrading the appearance of the image. The technologist evaluates each image to determine the degree

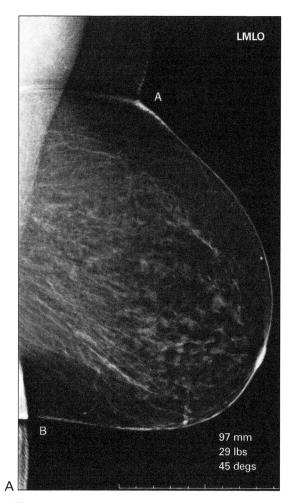

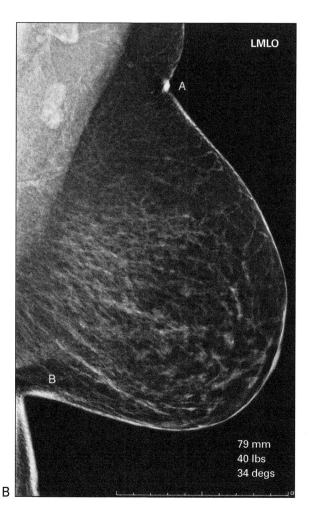

Figure 7-113

Skinfolds are commonly visualized on the MLO image of large pendulous breasts where the lower axilla intersects with the anterior/superior breast mound. These skinfolds are reduced or eliminated by using #11 on the MLO Fix-It Table, which suggests easing lateral tissue in a downward direction from the axilla to the IMF. **(A)** LMLO demonstrating "smile" crease (labeled *A*) and IMF skinfold and airgap (labeled *B*); note 97-mm compression thickness 29 lb compression force. **(B)** LMLO same patient demonstrating improved image quality when lateral tissue has been readjusted to its natural position on the thorax; elimination of superior skinfold (labeled *A*), and improved visualization of IMF region (labeled *B*); note 79-mm compression thickness, 48 lb compression force.

of degradation to image quality due to airgaps. Airgaps are generally acceptable for image quality if breast tissue can be visualized into, through, and out of the airgap and compression is not compromised. Positioning maneuvers can be incorporated to minimize and control airgaps on the image. Careful consideration should be given to exam management when problem solving for airgaps. Radiologists may have repeat protocols regarding the threshold of acceptability in their practice for the presence of airgaps on the image.

Airgap Problem #1: Axillary Airgap, Very Thin Patient, and Small Breast

Superior airgaps can be introduced from insufficient tissue filling the axillary space in very thin patients with a smaller breast size (Figure 7-114). At the opposite end of the spectrum, in patients with excessive upper outer quadrant breast tissue, large skinfolds can easily be introduced resulting in adjacent airgaps.

Fix-It Problem #1: Axillary Airgap, Thin Patient, Small Breast

Figure 7-115 illustrates image quality improvement for axillary airgaps when the following positioning/compression maneuvers are employed from Table 7-2.

1, 2, 3, 6, 7, 8, 11, 12, 13, 14, 20, 22, **24**
(Bold numbers have the greatest impact on this positioning feature.)

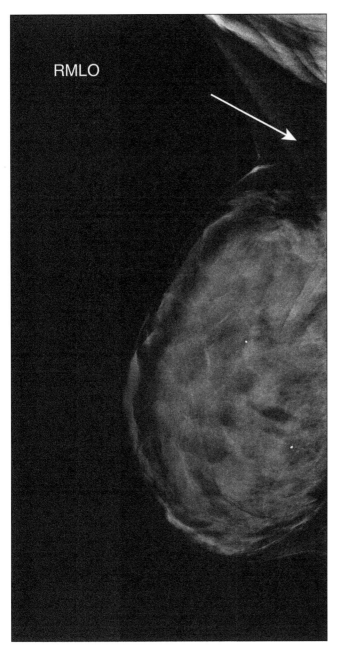

Figure 7-114
Airgaps located superiorly (*arrow*) can be caused by insufficient tissue filling of the axillary space in very thin patients with a smaller breast size.

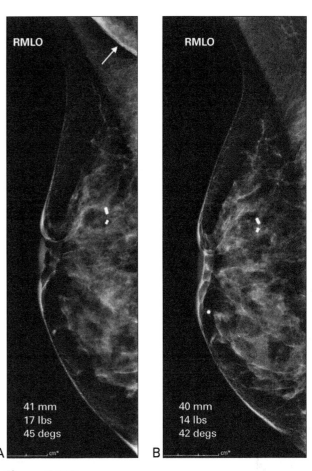

Figure 7-115
(A) Airgaps introduced by skinfolds in the axilla (*arrow*) can be controlled by using the "half paddle" designed specifically for the small breast and by ensuring the point of contact when positioning the axilla is placed just anterior to the latissimus dorsi muscle. **(B)** RMLO of the same patient using suggested techniques for the smaller breast.

Additional Tips for Managing Airgaps in the Axillary Region

1. Use the half contact paddle specifically designed for imaging the smaller breast whenever possible (Figure 7-6).
2. When positioning the axilla on the image receptor corner for the axillary placement maneuver, ensure the point of contact is anterior to the latissimus dorsi muscle.

Airgap Problem #2: Superior Breast Airgap

Airgap Problem #2A: Superior Breast Airgap, Addressing Lateral Tissue

Airgaps are commonly introduced on the MLO image between the skin of the lateral breast and the image receptor in the superior lateral region. The technologist should apply techniques that reduce or eliminate them. When the patient's thorax is brought into position to meet the image receptor with a lateral leaning movement as the axilla is placed in position on the image receptor corner, the lateral breast skin does not automatically come into contact with the image receptor from superior tissue to inferior tissue. During this action, the lateral skin may "catch" upward on the image receptor as contact is made forming airgaps (Figure 7-116). The technologist is unable to see this problem and must

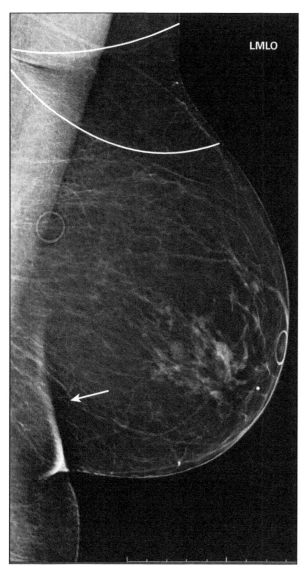

LMLO

Figure 7-116
Airgaps between the skin of the lateral breast and the image receptor may be naturally introduced on the MLO image when the patient's thorax leans laterally onto the image receptor. The superolateral skin may "catch" on the image receptor as contact is made forming airgaps. This airgap is demonstrated within the white lines and is caused by the superior skinfold located at the chestwall edge; note additional airgap at IMF (*arrow*).

verify that the lateral skin is in contact with the image receptor using her fingers to reposition the lateral breast tissue in a downward direction.

Fix-It Problem 2A: Superior Breast Airgap, Addressing Lateral Tissue Figure 7-117 illustrates image quality improvement for superior breast airgaps when the following positioning/compression maneuvers are employed from Table 7-2.

2, 3, 4, 7, 9, **11**
(Bold numbers have the greatest impact on this positioning feature.)

Airgap Problem #2B: Superior Breast Airgap, Excessive Upper Outer Quadrant Tissue

Figure 7-118 illustrates airgap problems associated with skinfolds on patients with excessive breast tissue in the upper outer quadrant. Patients who present for mammography with this particular issue may require two images to satisfy image quality for the axillary region. The first image satisfies the requirement of capturing all superoposterior tissue, while the second image smooths out the skinfold and airgap to satisfy adequate visibility and compression.

Fix-It Problem #2B: Superior Breast Airgap, Excessive Upper Outer Quadrant Tissue Figure 7-119 illustrates image quality improvement for superior airgaps for patients with excessive upper outer quadrant tissue when the following positioning/compression maneuvers are employed from Table 7-2.

1, 2, 3, 6, 7, 8, **11**, 12, 13, 14, **19**, 20, 22, 24
(Bold numbers have the greatest impact on this positioning feature.)

Airgap Problem #3: Inferior Breast (IMF) Airgap

Figure 7-120 illustrates airgap problems associated with skinfolds in the IMF region.

Airgaps in the IMF region on the MLO projection are introduced when lateral tissue is not flush against the image receptor or medial tissue is not flush against the compression device. This can occur when the thorax is rotated from the image receptor, when the breast tissue is not properly supported outward from the chestwall, when skinfolds have not been appropriately addressed by the technologist, or when the patient is extremely thin.

Fix-It Problem #3: Inferior Breast (IMF) Airgap

Figure 7-99 through Figure 7-101 illustrate image quality improvement for airgaps in the IMF region when the following positioning/compression maneuvers are employed from Table 7-2.

2, 4, 7, 8, 11, **15**, 16, 17, **18**, 20, 23, 25
(Bold numbers have the greatest impact on this positioning feature.)

Additional Tip for IMF Airgap Elimination

1. When the patient leans her upper torso laterally toward the image receptor for the MLO projection, the IMF region "buckles," placing skinfolds at the junction of the superior abdomen and the inferior breast tissue. Due to the length of the digital detector, elongating the thorax

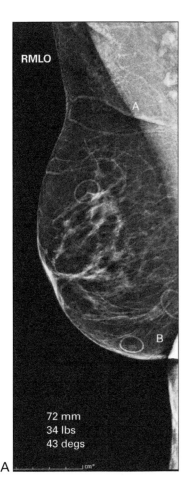

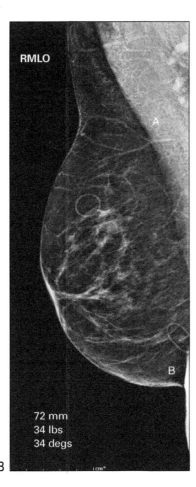

Figure 7-117
(A) Common skinfold with airgap in the superior aspect (labeled *A*); note IMF skinfold with airgap (labeled *B*). The same maneuvers used to eliminate superiorly located skinfolds resulting in airgaps also may reduce or eliminate skinfolds and airgaps in the IMF region. **(B)** Same patient demonstrating improved image quality when #11 on the MLO Fix-It Table is employed.

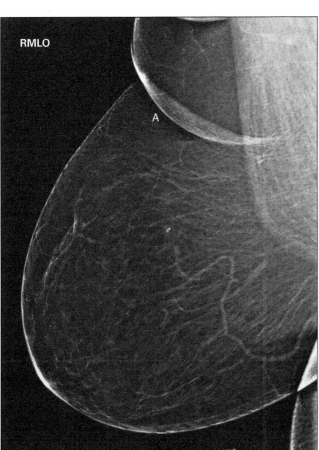

Figure 7-118
Patients with excessive breast tissue in the upper outer quadrant introduce a skinfold with airgap resulting from compression to the extra "fat pad" in the superior region of the breast on the MLO projection (labeled *A*).

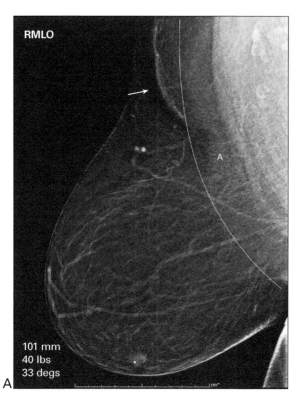

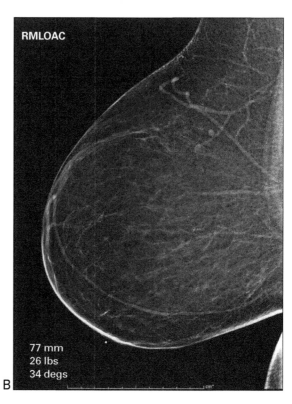

Figure 7-119

Excessive breast tissue in the upper outer quadrant may require two images to satisfy image quality for the MLO projection. **(A)** The first image satisfies the capture of superoposterior tissue; tissue posterior to the white line (labeled *A*) is adequately compressed; *arrow* indicates airgap. **(B)** The second image smooths out the skinfold and airgap to satisfy adequate visibility and compression of the breast mound and anterior tissue. Note compression thickness and compression force differences between RMLO **(A)**, 101 mm, 40 lb, and RMLOAC **(B)**, 77 mm, 26 lb.

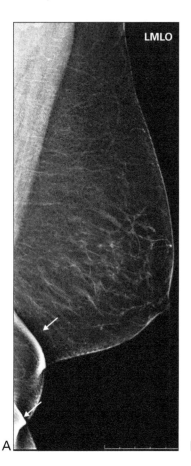

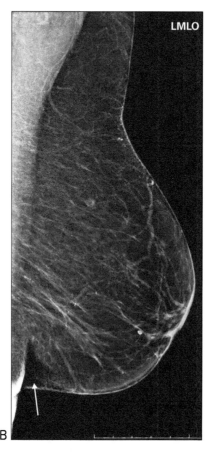

Figure 7-120

Airgaps in the IMF region on the MLO projection are introduced when lateral tissue is not flush against the image receptor or medial tissue is not flush against the compression device. Common examples of airgaps resulting from skinfolds in the IMF region include **(A)** skinfolds and airgaps (*arrows*) introduced by rotation of the thorax or **(B)** skinfolds and airgaps (*arrow*) introduced when posterior breast structures are not adequately supported and when posteromedial or posterolateral tissue at the IMF is not in intimate contact with the image receptor or compression device when compression is completed.

to more efficiently match the image receptor length encourages the IMF region to open. This is done by bending the ipsilateral knee of the patient and telling her to "slouch" while adjusting the angle of her thorax to match the angle of the image receptor. Combining this tip with Fix-it #11 adjusts the lateral tissue downward to assist in opening the IMF region.

CRANIOCAUDAL PROJECTION ASSESSMENT

The CC projection is assessed by dividing the CC image into five regions of evaluation. They include the posterior and anterior breast margins, the medial and lateral breast margins, and compression.[22] Each region is discussed for the CC projection. The technologist should understand what features of the breast are demonstrated in each region and what positioning maneuvers are used to ensure the features are visible on the image.

Craniocaudal Projection Image Quality Criteria

The following bullet points describe the CC image quality criteria included in Figure 7-121:

1. Pectoral muscle visible (established ACR criteria = 30% to 40% of the time).
2. Retroglandular fat space visible.
3. All medial breast tissue included:
   - Desirable feature: reflection of the cleavage.
   - Desirable feature: small amount of contralateral breast at medial corner.
   - Desirable feature: skin thickening toward the cleavage of the breast. The skin at the base of the breast is thick and tapers as it approaches the nipple–areola complex.
4. Lateral breast includes visible retroglandular fat if applicable (evidence of lateral pull).
5. Anterior breast demonstrates nipple centered on the image: direction follows a PNL path as close as possible to perpendicular with the chestwall.
6. Compression demonstrates sharpness of structures with force and centimeter thickness proportional to the CC of the contralateral breast compression factor results.

Six Building Blocks

- Elevation of IMF
- Image receptor height
- Patient stance: leaning the upper body forward
- Two hands to control the breast
- Rotating the sternum to the image receptor
- Lateral pull for posterolateral tissue inclusion

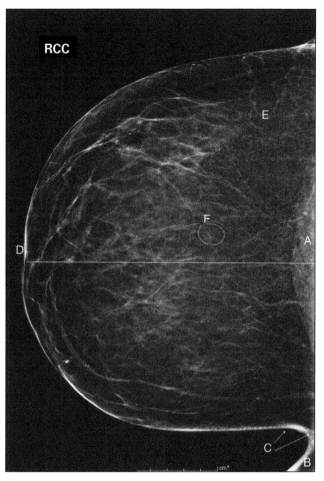

Figure 7-121
CC projection with mole marker (labeled *F*) demonstrating mammographic features that describe image quality: pectoral muscle presentation (labeled *A*), small amount of contralateral breast (labeled *B*), posteromedial skin thickening and reflection of cleavage (labeled *C*) PNL perpendicular to the chestwall (labeled *D*), and posterolateral retroglandular fat presence (labeled *E*), if applicable.

The six building blocks of the CC projection emphasize the capture of posterior tissue, which is the most challenging breast tissue to visualize on a mammogram. The six building blocks include elevation of the IMF, alignment of the height of the image receptor to the elevated IMF, the forward leaning stance of the patient, use of two hands to "dislocate" the pectoral muscle, addressing the posteromedial breast, and with final attention given to posterolateral breast tissue inclusion. Additional positioning/compression maneuvers contribute to image quality on the final image. If any of these building blocks or positioning maneuvers are neglected, a negative effect on image quality will be observed. The CC Fix-It Table, Table 7-3, lists appropriate positioning maneuvers used to correct common problems associated with image quality when performing the CC projection. Match the "Fix-It Number" that describes the "Fix-It Maneuver" corrections to the number listed under each problem in the CC Projection Assessment section to improve image quality for that specific mammographic feature.

Table 7-3 • CC Fix-It Table: Positioning/Compression Maneuvers Used for the CC Projection

FIX-IT NUMBER	FIX-IT MANEUVER
1	Compression device size is congruent to the light field and radiation field size and should include all breast margins
2	Patient distance from the image receptor: approximately a hands width away from the unit, but customize for each patient.
3	Patient stance: relaxed; slightly leaning forward from the waist, just enough for the technologist to envision the chestwall edge of the thorax in a vertical position. The amount the patient leans forward is specific to each patient and is determined by the envisioned vertical edge of the chestwall.
4	Elevate the IMF until natural resistance is felt
5	Adjust the image receptor to match the height of the elevated IMF
6	With two flat hands, firmly sandwich the breast at the chestwall margin
7	Pull, or "dislocate," the pectoral muscle from the chestwall
8	Using two flat hands pull the breast tissue onto the image receptor until the thorax comes in contact with the chestwall edge of the image receptor. Only the patient's upper body should move forward
9	The hand in contact with the inferior breast slides out following the PNL path perpendicular to the chestwall edge of the image receptor
10	Do not remove the hand anchoring superior breast tissue throughout the remaining CC positioning maneuvers
11	Rotate the patient medially toward the image receptor while elevating the contralateral breast
12	Ensure the sternum and thorax make contact with the image receptor, draping the elevated contralateral breast over the medial corner
13	Medial light field includes the cleavage reflection and small amount of contralateral breast (when possible)
14	The nipple path (PNL) is perpendicular to the chestwall edge of the image receptor
15	The anchor hand secures the medial and central tissue to the image receptor while maintaining the dislocated pectoral muscle away from the thorax, while also maintaining the nipple direction
16	After completing the medial breast tissue maneuvers, inspect the inferior tissue ensuring contact with the image receptor: no airgap should be visible; medial tissue should be in intimate contact with the image receptor
17	If inferomedial tissue is not flush against the image receptor, insert the index finger between the image receptor edge and posteromedial breast tissue. Gently ease the tissue posteriorly and inferiorly by pressing your index finger against the thorax to bring the inferior breast into intimate contact with the image receptor. Pressing against the thorax as this maneuver is accomplished is beneficial. Communicate clearly with the patient when performing this maneuver as this area is sensitive to discomfort. Ease, rather than pull on this tissue, due to the delicate composition of the skin. The skin at the junction of the inferomedial breast and the sternum can easily separate when stressed.
18	The technologist uses her free hand to wrap the fingers around the lateral aspect of the breast extending beyond the chestwall edge of the image receptor
19	Gently lift the lateral breast slightly off the image receptor, pulling the lateral tissue onto the receptor. When performing this maneuver, direct both superior and inferior lateral tissue straight forward onto the image receptor. This maneuver requires precision; if not properly positioned, it is easy to torque the posterior tissue medially. When the lateral pull is performed, a small posterolateral skinfold is commonly visualized on the image.
20	With the breast secured on the image receptor, the technologist places her arm around the patient, resting her hand on the patient's shoulder, and reminds the patient once again to relax her shoulder and thorax
21	The technologist places her fingers against, or just above, the clavicle, gently lifting the skin covering the clavicle superiorly, reserving additional tissue in the neck region, countering resistance the patient may feel during the application of compression
22	As compression is applied to the breast, slowly release the tissue reserved at the clavicle
23	The technologist initially applies compression using the automatic mode (controlled with the foot pedal), stopping when the compression device comes in contact with the breast
24	Place the palm of the hand, rather than the fingers, on the breast mound during positioning maneuvers for the CC projection; this leaves the fingers free to control the lateral tissue

Table 7-3 • CC Fix-It Table: Positioning/Compression Maneuvers Used for the CC Projection (*Continued*)

FIX-IT NUMBER	FIX-IT MANEUVER
25	Control lateral breast tissue inclusion and minimize posterolateral skinfolds by fanning the fingers as compression is applied
26	Use the fingers resting on the patient's shoulder to reach the lateral breast for additional control of lateral tissue as compression is applied
27	Intermittent compression, controlled by tapping the foot pedal, allows the technologist to slowly apply additional compression while ensuring only breast tissue is included under the compression device
28	Place the patient's contralateral hand onto the handle or side of the unit to secure medial tissue on the image (tip: ensure the cleavage presentation remains in an open position)
29	Relax the patient's ipsilateral arm by her side, externally rotating her hand, ensuring the humeral head is removed from the field of view
30	Slight bending of the patient's knees contributes to equal compression of superior and inferior tissue and posterior tissue inclusion (this is an optional technique)
31	Initial compression is accomplished with the automatic mode, however final compression should be done using the manual mode as it affords the technologist the incremental precision necessary to gauge adequate compression
32	The junction of the humerus and axilla should be in contact with the chestwall rise of the compression device
33	Compression force is evaluated by tapping the skin of the medial or lateral aspect of the breast for tautness (note: the lateral breast has a greater volume of tissue)
34	Compare current centimeter thickness and compression force results to prior exam information. This information helps the technologist to determine her performance patterns.
35	Compare current centimeter thickness and compression force results to each other as exposures are taken. This information helps the technologist to determine her performance patterns.
36	Assuming the right and the left breast are similar in size, the centimeter thickness and the compression force results for the CC projections should be similar, centimeter thickness and compression force results for the MLO projections should be similar

Source: Mammography Quality Management (MQM, LLC), Waunakee, WI, W. J. Marshall, S. L. Lille.

Posterior Tissue

The pectoral muscle should be present on the CC image between 30% and 40% of the time. This structure is a radiopaque density of varying size and often mirrors itself when apparent bilaterally. With emphasis on medial tissue inclusion, the sternalis muscle may be visualized on the CC projection. The sternalis muscle can imitate a medial breast lesion and is occasionally displayed (Figure 7-122). A superolateral to inferomedial oblique (SIO) of 5° to 20° may better demonstrate this density to rule out cancer.

Features Visualized

- Pectoral muscle
- Retroglandular fat space

Posterior Tissue Presentation Problem #1: Pectoral Muscle Not Visualized

The pectoral muscle is visualized on the CC projection 30% to 40% of the time according to criteria established by the ACR.

Posterior Nipple Line (PNL) Rule[8]:

When the pectoral muscle is not present on the CC image, the comparison between the CC PNL measurement and the MLO PNL measurement assists to determine if adequate posterior tissue has been visualized on the CC projection. For an acceptable assessment of posterior tissue visualized on the CC projection, the CC PNL measurement must be within 1 cm of the MLO PNL measurement. One important caveat to this rule requires the MLO image used for measurement must reflect proper positioning/compression established criteria (Figure 7-123).

Mediolateral Oblique Projection PNL Measurement

The PNL on the MLO projection is drawn from the skinline at the nipple to the pectoral muscle or the edge of the image, whichever is reached first when making the measurement. The line is drawn at an approximate perpendicular angle to the pectoral muscle.

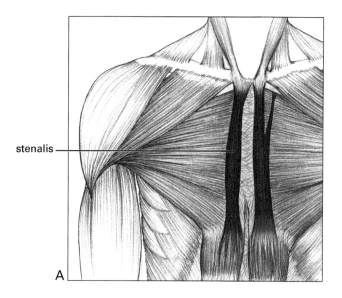

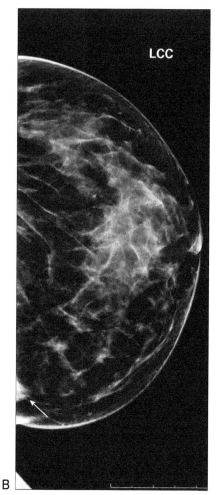

Figure 7-122
(A) With emphasis on medial tissue inclusion, the sternalis muscle may be visualized on the CC projection. **(B)** The sternalis muscle can imitate a medial breast lesion and is only occasionally displayed (*arrow*). (**A**, Adapted from Simons DG, et al. *Travell & Simons' Myofascial Pain and Dysfunction: The Trigger Point Manual.* Vol. 1. 2nd ed. Philadelphia, PA: Lippincott Williams & Wilkins; 1998.)

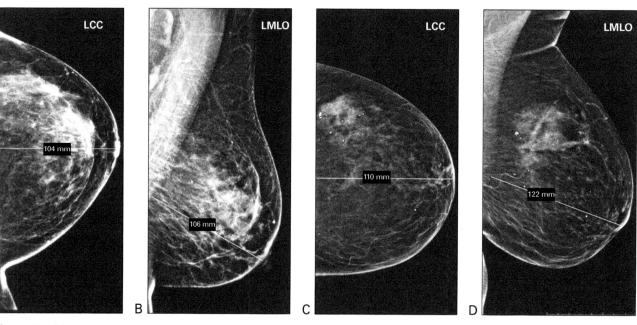

Figure 7-123
Two mammography examinations demonstrate the PNL rule and its use to determine if adequate posterior tissue has been included on the CC projection when the pectoral muscle is not present. Examination one: **(A)** LCC projection, PNL measures 10.4 cm. **(B)** LMLO projection, PNL measures 10.6 cm. The CC PNL measurement is within 1 cm of the MLO PNL measurement indicating sufficient posterior tissue has been included on the CC image. Examination two: **(C)** LCC projection, PNL measures 11.0 cm. **(D)** LMLO projection, PNL measures 12.4 cm. The CC PNL measurement does not fall within 1 cm of the MLO PNL measurement indicating that insufficient posterior tissue has been included on the CC image.

Craniocaudal Projection PNL Measurement

The PNL on the CC projection is drawn from the skinline at the nipple to the posterior edge of the image. Whether the pectoral muscle is visible or not, the measurement is made from the nipple to chestwall edge of the image.

Fix-It Problem #1: Pectoral Muscle Not Visualized

Several positioning maneuvers ensure visualization of the pectoral muscle on the CC image. Figure 7-124 illustrates image quality improvement for presentation of the pectoral muscle when the following positioning/compression maneuvers are employed from Table 7-3.

1, **2, 3, 4, 5, 6, 7, 8,** 9, **10,** 15, 16, 30, 32
(Bold numbers have the greatest impact on this positioning feature.)

Posterior Tissue Presentation Problem #2: Retroglandular Fat Space Not Visualized, Patient Stance

The retroglandular fat space is visualized in the posterior aspect of the breast on the CC image; this space is located posterior to the glandular tissue and anterior to the pectoral muscle (Figure 7-125A). For patients with entirely adipose replaced breast tissue or those with extremely dense glandular tissue extending to the chestwall, the retroglandular fat space is not able to be identified (Figure 7-125B,C). The primary factors affecting the visualization of the retroglandular fat space on the CC projection are the upper body stance of the patient and adequate posterior tissue capture. Leaning the upper body (above the waist) forward until the anterior border of the thorax is in a vertical position places the retroglandular fat space perpendicular to the x-ray

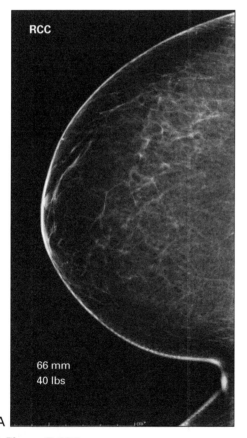
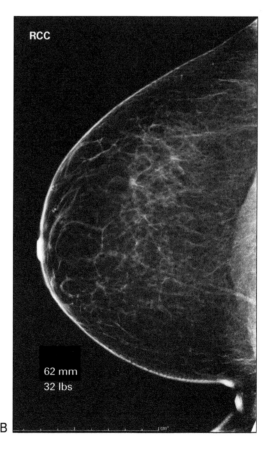

Figure 7-124
To increase posterior and superior tissue visualization, incline the thorax slightly forward to position the anterior chestwall in a vertical position. **(A)** LCC projection with the patient standing too erect, indicated by the nipple presentation and posterior tissue exclusion. **(B)** Same patient, with the thorax brought into a vertical position. Note the improved posterosuperior tissue visualization as indicated by the nipple presentation and the presence of the pectoral muscle.

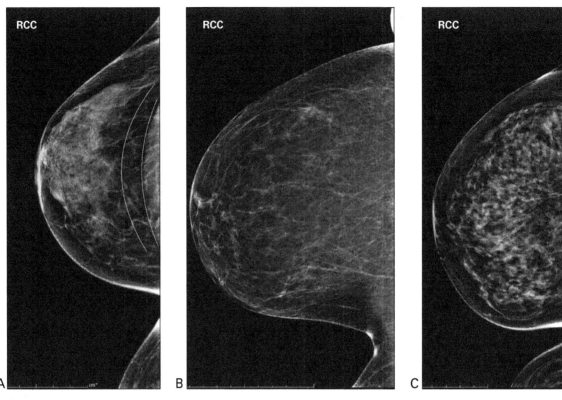

Figure 7-125
(A) The retroglandular fat space is located posterior to the glandular tissue and anterior to the pectoral muscle on the CC image (between *white lines*). **(B)** For patients with entirely adipose replaced breast tissue or with **(C)** extremely dense glandular tissue extending to the chestwall, the retroglandular fat space is not able to be identified.

beam (Figure 7-126). When the upper body is erect during positioning of the CC projection, superior–posterior tissue is excluded from the image, or it is superimposed over the retroglandular fat space (Figure 7-127A).

Fix-It Problem #2: Retroglandular Fat Space Not Visualized, Patient Stance

Figure 7-127B illustrates image quality improvement for presentation of the retroglandular fat space when the following positioning/compression maneuvers are employed from Table 7-3.

1, **2, 3, 4, 5, 6, 7, 8**, 9, **10**, 15, 16, 30, 32
(Bold numbers have the greatest impact on this positioning feature.)

Visualization of Posterior Tissue Is Affected By:

1. Patient stance: relaxed and a forward angle of the upper body placing the anterior chestwall in an approximate vertical position.
2. Patient distance from the image receptor.
3. Elevation of the IMF.
4. Image receptor height.

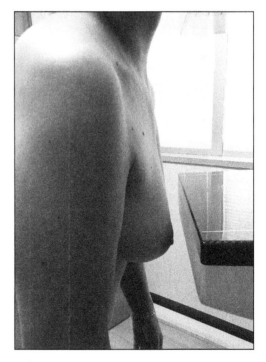

Figure 7-126
CC projection: having the patient lean forward places the anterior chestwall in a vertical position, which allows capture of posterosuperior breast tissue.

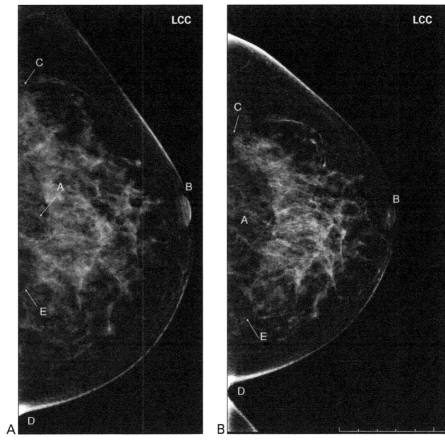

Figure 7-127
Accurate representation of the retroglandular fat space, located posteriorly on the CC projection, requires the patient to bend forward slightly at the waist as the breast is brought onto the image receptor. **(A)** LCC erect patient stance indicated by superimposed glandular tissue onto the retroglandular fat space (labeled *A*) and nipple presentation (labeled *B*). Note exclusion of posterolateral (labeled *C*) and posteromedial glandular tissue (labeled *E*) and exclusion of cleavage and contralateral breast (labeled *D*). **(B)** LCC same patient, forward stance indicated by visualization of retroglandular fat space (labeled *A*), nipple presentation (labeled *B*). Note capture of posterolateral (labeled *C*) and posteromedial glandular tissue (labeled *E*) and visualization of cleavage reflection and contralateral breast (labeled *D*).

5. Two hands control the posterior breast margin.
6. Address posteromedial and posterolateral tissue.

Additional Tip to Visualize the Pectoral Muscle and the Retroglandular Fat Space

1. After the IMF comes into contact with the image receptor, use the ipsilateral ASIS to tip the pelvis in a slightly forward direction; do not allow the patient to step backward when performing this maneuver. This action slightly rolls the ribs in contact with the image receptor downward (in millimeters) allowing greater posterior tissue inclusion and enhanced comfort for the patient.
2. See CC projection compression tips in this section, bending the patient's knees.

Medial Tissue

Features Visualized

- All medial tissue
- Reflection of the cleavage
- Contralateral breast
- Posteromedial skin thickening

Medial Tissue Presentation Problem #1: Posteromedial Tissue Excluded from the Image

Due to the potential exclusion of posteromedial breast tissue from the MLO projection, it is essential that all tissue in this region be included on the CC projection. For patients who present with chestwall anomalies, it is challenging to include this region on the CC projection. For these examinations, it may be necessary to use complementary projections such as the exaggerated craniocaudal medial (XCCM) or the cleavage (CV) projection. For the majority of patients, several common positioning maneuvers ensure capture of the posteromedial aspect of the breast. Radiographic landmarks that verify maximum medial tissue inclusion on the CC projection are posteromedial skin thickening, cleavage reflection, and a small amount of contralateral breast tissue (Figure 7-128).

Fix-It Problem #1: Posteromedial Tissue Excluded from the Image

Figure 7-129 illustrates image quality improvement for posteromedial tissue presentation when the following positioning/compression maneuvers are employed from Table 7-3.

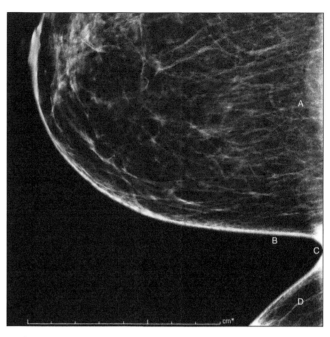

Figure 7-128
Radiographic landmarks that verify maximum medial tissue inclusion on the CC projection are posteromedial skin thickening (labeled *B*), cleavage reflection (labeled *C*), and a small amount of contralateral breast tissue (labeled *D*); note pectoral muscle presentation (labeled *A*).

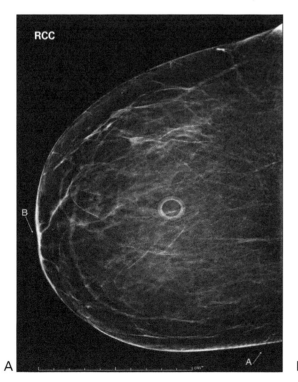

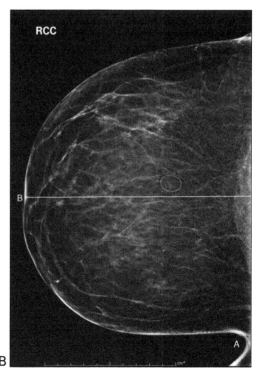

Figure 7-129
Positioning maneuvers that include rotating the patient medially to place the sternum and thorax in contact with the chestwall edge of the image receptor assist in capturing all medial tissue. **(A)** RCC demonstrating slight medial exaggeration of nipple (labeled *B*) resulting in no evidence of posteromedial skin thickening and posteromedial tissue exclusion (labeled *A*). **(B)** RCC same patient demonstrating PNL perpendicular to the chestwall (labeled *B*) with visualization of cleavage reflection, posteromedial skin thickening, and contralateral breast (labeled *A*).

1, 3, 4, 5, 6, **11, 12, 13,** 14, 15, 28
(Bold numbers have the greatest impact on this positioning
feature.)

Medial Tissue Visualization Is Affected By:

- Selection of the correct compression device size
- Chestwall presentation of the patient
- Chestwall anomalies
- Elevated contralateral breast, rotation of the thorax medially toward the image receptor (Figure 7-130)
- The thorax positioned flush against the image receptor
- The contralateral breast draped across medial chestwall edge of the image receptor if applicable

Additional Positioning Tip to Visualize the Posteromedial Breast Tissue

Use the contralateral scapula as a steering wheel to finalize the patient rotation toward the unit.

Lateral Tissue

Features Visualized

- Posterolateral tissue
- Retroglandular fat visualized posterior to posterolateral glandular tissue (Figure 7-131)
- Evidence of lateral tissue pull

Lateral Tissue Presentation Problem #1: Posterolateral Tissue Not Visualized on Image

When positioning to visualize the medial and posterior central aspects of the breast is completed, attention is

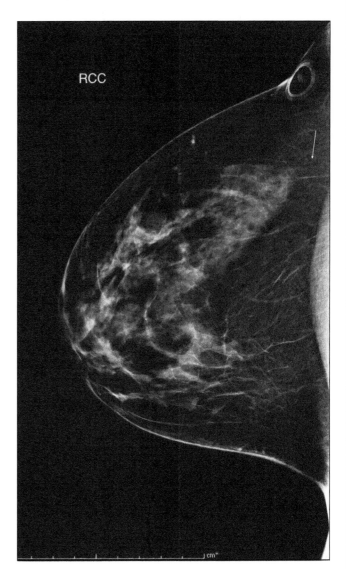

Figure 7-131
The CC projection emphasizes inclusion of all medial tissue, but does not neglect lateral tissue, including as much as possible. Using techniques such as the "lateral pull" maneuver assists in visualizing retroglandular fat posterior to the posterolateral glandular tissue (*arrow*). Note mole marker (*circle*).

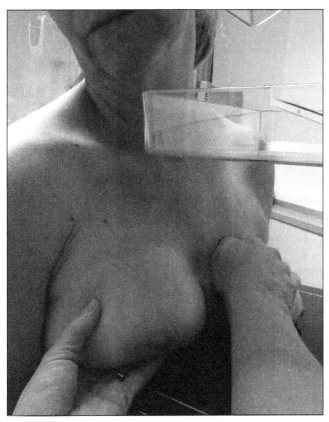

Figure 7-130
Sufficient elevation of the contralateral breast and medial rotation of the patient toward the IRSD places the thorax in contact with the chestwall edge of the image receptor, draping the contralateral breast across the medial corner.

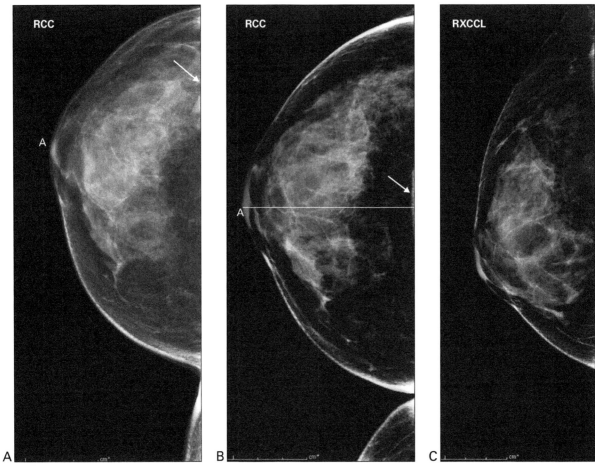

Figure 7-132
Posterolateral tissue capture on the CC projection; same patient. **(A)** Prior RCC demonstrates nipple exaggeration later-ally (labeled *A*) resulting in posterolateral tissue exclusion (*arrow*). **(B)** Subsequent RCC demonstrates PNL perpendicular to chestwall (labeled *A*), again demonstrating incomplete capture of posterolateral tissue; note small amount of pectoral muscle on image (*arrow*). **(C)** RXCCL added to the examination to visualize far posterolateral tissue.

directed toward including as much lateral tissue as pos-sible prior to engaging compression. Even when the best positioning efforts have been applied, all of the posterolat-eral tissue may not be captured and visualized on the image (Figure 7-132). The need for additional imaging due to pos-terolateral tissue exclusion is determined by:

1. Inspecting the nipple direction on the CC projection, ensuring the PNL is perpendicular to the chestwall edge of the image receptor
2. Inspecting the CC projection for evidence of the "lateral pull"
3. Inspecting the MLO image, ensuring visualization of the retroglandular fat space if applicable

Fix-It Problem #1: Posterolateral Tissue Not Visualized on Image (Using the Lateral Pull Maneuver)

Figure 7-133 illustrates image quality improvement for posterolateral tissue presentation when the following positioning/compression maneuvers are employed from Table 7-3.

1, 4, 5, 8, 18, **19**, **24**, 25, 26, 29, 32
(Bold numbers have the greatest impact on this positioning feature.)

Additional Tip for Visualizing Posterolateral Tissue

Some women, even after the "lateral pull" maneuver has been employed, have glandular tissue that extends postero-laterally beyond the IRSD. Approximately 10% of patients have extremely dense breast tissue extending to the chest-wall, wrapping laterally around the thorax. Even with the best positioning capabilities, the tissue is excluded from the CC projection because the tissue location is beyond the capture of the lateral chestwall edge of the image recep-tor. For these patients, it is appropriate to add an additional XCCL projection to complete the examination ensuring visualization of the far lateral tissue.

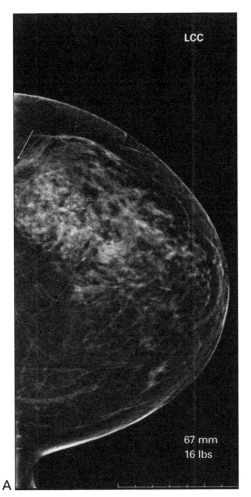 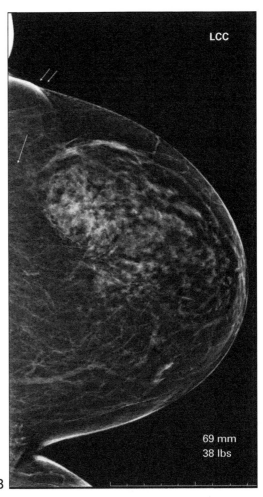

Figure 7-133
Posterolateral tissue capture on the CC projection using the lateral pull maneuver is demonstrated. **(A)** LCC projection with adequate visualization of all medial tissue, but excludes posterolateral tissue (*arrow*). **(B)** same patient demonstrates adequate medial tissue; inclusion of the lateral pull technique by the technologist captures posterolateral tissue, visualizing retroglandular fat (*arrow*); note evidence of lateral pull maneuver (*double arrows*).

Lateral Tissue Visualization Is Affected By:

- Selection of the correct compression device size
- Use of the "lateral pull" maneuver
- Distribution of glandular tissue in the posterolateral region
- Patient body habitus

Anterior Tissue

Features Visualized

Nipple profile
Nipple direction
Central breast tissue
Subareolar tissue

Anterior Tissue Presentation Problem #1A: Nipple Presentation, Not in Profile

Capturing all posterior breast tissue on the CC image may result in the nipple presenting out of profile. Generally, this is the case in patients with a longer measurement from the clavicle to the nipple and a shorter measurement from the nipple to the IMF (Figure 7-134). Conversely, patients who present with a history of breast reduction generally have superior breast tissue measuring a shorter distance from the clavicle to nipple and a longer measurement from the nipple to the IMF (Figure 7-135). Addressing appropriate exam management to visualize the NP without sacrificing posterior breast tissue is explained using the NP-modified views (Figure 7-70).

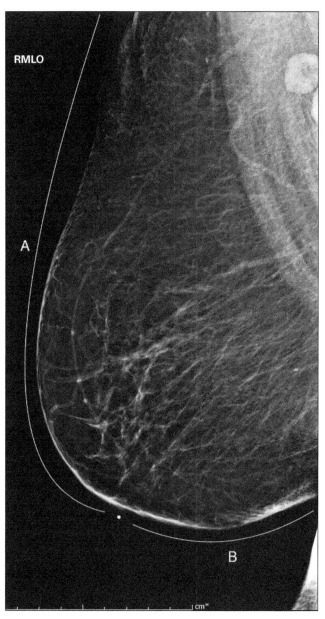

Figure 7-134
For patients who present with a longer measurement from the clavicle to the nipple (labeled *A*), and a shorter measurement from the nipple to the IMF (labeled *B*), the nipple may not be presented in profile on the CC projection when all superior and inferior tissue to the chestwall has been included.

Anterior Tissue Presentation Problem #1B: Nipple Direction from the Chestwall Is Exaggerated Medially

There are several positioning behaviors that may contribute to the nipple being exaggerated medially on the CC image (Figure 7-136).

1. The breast is brought onto the image receptor with a slight medial nipple exaggeration due to:

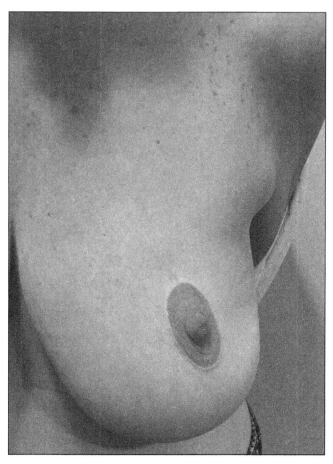

Figure 7-135
Patients who present with a history of breast reduction generally have superior breast tissue measuring a shorter distance from the clavicle to nipple, and a longer measurement from the nipple to the IMF, which may prevent nipple presentation in profile on the CC projection.

  a. The technologist standing at the medial aspect of the breast for positioning the CC projection and

  b. When using two hands to guide the breast onto the image receptor, the technologist's forearm angle prohibits the breast from approaching the image receptor with the PNL perpendicular to the chestwall edge of the image receptor.

  c. Positioning corrections are necessary to counteract actions a and b; rotate the thorax medially to come in contact with the image receptor while ensuring the contralateral breast is elevated and draped over the medial corner of the image receptor.

2. When performing the lateral pull maneuver to include as much lateral breast tissue as possible on the image, the technologist does not properly anchor the medial and central breast to the image receptor, allowing the thorax to rotate medially (Figure 7-63).

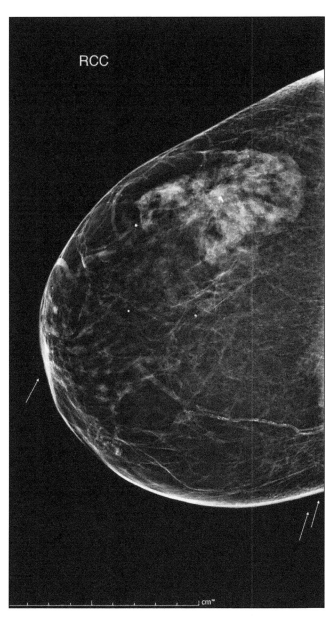

Figure 7-136
A general rule when the nipple is exaggerated on the CC projection: a nipple exaggerated medially indicates the exclusion of medial tissue; a nipple exaggerated laterally indicates the exclusion of lateral tissue. This RCC image demonstrates medial nipple exaggeration (*arrow*), with medial tissue excluded from the image (*double arrows*).

3. The technologist allows the patient to recline laterally toward the image receptor in an attempt to capture all lateral glandular tissue for the CC projection (Figure 7-137).
4. Appropriate knowledge and understanding of the focus for the CC projection:
   • Medial tissue may be excluded on the MLO image, making it a priority for visualization on the CC projection.
   • It may not be possible to include all lateral glandular tissue on the CC projection; reclining the patient

laterally to include this tissue and rotating the thorax laterally to capture lateral tissue are incorrect positioning maneuvers for the CC projection.
5. The technologist controls the patient's upper body direction as the breast is guided forward onto the image receptor. The goal is to bring the breast onto the image receptor with the PNL directed perpendicular to the chestwall edge of the image receptor (Figure 7-121). There are several positioning maneuvers to ensure the nipple is centered on the image receptor.

Fix-It Problem #1B: Nipple Exaggeration Medially

5, 8, 9, 10, **11, 12, 13, 14, 15,** 28
(Bold numbers have the greatest impact on this positioning feature.)

Anterior Tissue Presentation Problem #1C: Nipple Direction from the Chestwall Is Exaggerated Laterally

Lateral nipple exaggeration (Figure 7-138) is a common problem affecting image quality in the routine mammogram. This can occur for two reasons:

1. The CC projection emphasizes the capture of the medial tissue. When positioning maneuvers are employed to ensure medial tissue visualization, such as rotating the patient's thorax medially until the sternum is in contact with the chestwall edge of the image receptor, lateral nipple exaggeration can occur as the result.
2. Positioning strategies for the CC projection that do not include the "lateral pull" maneuver do not appropriately address nipple direction, resulting in a lateral exaggeration on the image.

For the majority of patients who present for routine mammography, specific positioning strategies for the CC projection that address both medial and lateral breast tissue capture also incorporate securing nipple direction, which results in the PNL presenting perpendicular to the chestwall edge of the image receptor (Figure 7-121).

Fix-It Problem #1C: Nipple Exaggeration Laterally

Figure 7-139 illustrates image quality improvement for posterolateral tissue presentation when the following positioning/compression maneuvers are employed from Table 7-3.

15, 18, 19, 24, 26, 32
(Bold numbers have the greatest impact on this positioning feature.)

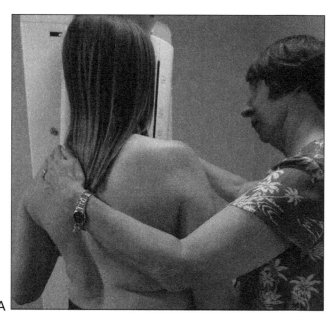
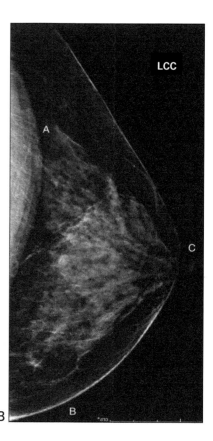

Figure 7-137
(A) Slight medial exaggeration of the nipple can occur when CC positioning techniques allow the patient's thorax to lean laterally toward the image receptor to ensure visualization of all lateral glandular tissue. **(B)** Incorrect positioning of the LCC projection allowing the patient to lean laterally toward the image receptor indicated by pectoral muscle presentation demonstrated laterally on the image (labeled *A*), exclusion of medial breast tissue (labeled *B*), and medial nipple exaggeration (labeled *C*).

Additional Tips for Nipple Exaggeration

Nipple exaggeration in either the lateral or medial direction is an indication that tissue is excluded on the image. CC images with the nipple exaggerated medially indicate medial tissue is excluded. When the nipple is exaggerated laterally on the image, some lateral tissue is excluded from the image. Occasionally, patients may present with slightly lateral or slightly medial placement of the areola on the breast. Documenting this information on the history form along with any additional images included to complete the exam is helpful to the radiologist.

Nipple Exaggeration on the Image Is Affected By:

- Chestwall anomalies such as pectus excavatum or pectus carinatum
- The use of specific positioning maneuvers to ensure the PNL is perpendicular to the chestwall edge of the image receptor

  ○ Rotation of the patient medially toward the image receptor until the sternum is flush against the chestwall edge of the image receptor
  ○ Addressing the lateral breast tissue ensuring the PNL is perpendicular to the chestwall edge of the image receptor using the "lateral pull" maneuver

Compression

Compression is essential to the quality of the mammography image, ensuring separation of breast structures, increasing sharpness, and reducing dose to the patient. Separating overlapping structures and increasing sharpness are critical elements for detecting the earliest indications of breast cancer on the mammography image. The application of compression is controlled by the technologist and is dependent on the tolerance level of the patient. Adequate compression applied to the breast is evaluated by the sharpness of linear structures, blood vessels, and microcalcifications; look closely at posterior, anterior,

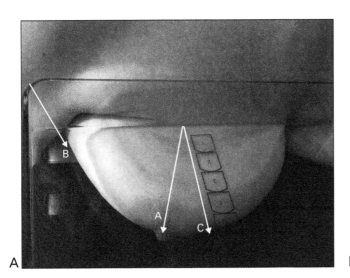
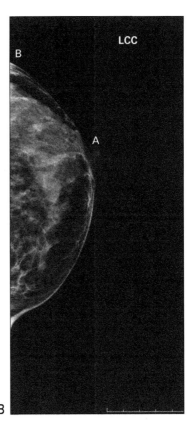

Figure 7-138

Nipple exaggeration indicates posteromedial or posterolateral tissue excluded from the CC image. CC positioning techniques that secure nipple direction perpendicular to the chestwall while capturing lateral and medial tissue onto the image receptor prevent nipple exaggeration. **(A)** Illustrates incorrect positioning of the CC projection: note lateral nipple exaggeration indicated by PNL (labeled *A*), gap between the lateral chestwall edge of the image receptor and the junction of the lateral breast/axilla (labeled *B*). Label C indicates correct PNL perpendicular to the chestwall. **(B)** LCC projection illustrating incorrect positioning indicated by lateral nipple exaggeration (labeled *A*) and posterolateral tissue exclusion (labeled *B*).

lateral, and medial regions with particular attention to the subareolar section. Signs of decreased sharpness in any of these regions may indicate that inadequate compression was used and additionally may reveal motion on the image.

Features Visualized

- Sharpness of structures
- Blood vessels, microcalcifications, anterior border of pectoral muscle, and Cooper's ligaments
- Adequate separation of tissues
- Subareolar region

Compression Problem #1A: Undercompression and Compression Inconsistencies

The use of inadequate compression or inconsistent compression by the technologist reduces the opportunity to detect fine detail on the image. Consistent, adequate

compression should be assured for every projection, correlated to the degree of tolerance for each patient. Several behaviors throughout the examination process ensure consistent use of compression by the technologist.

Fix-It Problem #1A: Undercompression and Compression Inconsistencies

Figure 7-140 illustrates image quality improvement for breast tissue presentation in the CC projection due to adequate and uniform compression application. This image improvement along with observed increased posterior breast tissue capture is demonstrated in Figure 7-140B when the following positioning/compression maneuvers are employed from Table 7-3.

1, 20, **23, 27**, 30, **31, 33, 34, 35, 36**
(Bold numbers have the greatest impact on this positioning feature.)

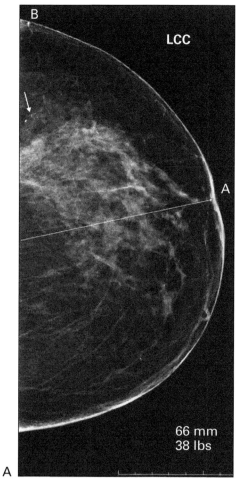

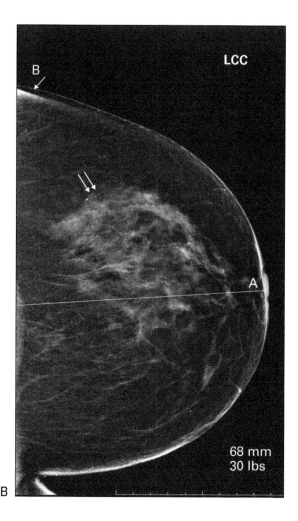

Figure 7-139
(A) LCC projection demonstrating lateral nipple exaggeration (labeled *A*), with posterolateral tissue excluded from the image (labeled *B*); note location of calcifications (*arrow*). **(B)** Specific positioning strategies for the CC projection that address both medial and lateral breast tissue captures also incorporate securing nipple direction. LCC same patient demonstrating improved nipple direction (labeled *A*) and inclusion of posterolateral tissue (labeled *B*) when incorporating the lateral pull technique; note the location of calcifications (*double arrows*).

Compression Problem #1B: Undercompression, Neck Tissue Has Reached Maximum Resistance

Compression for the CC projection is initiated at the level of the second or third rib, located just inferior to the clavicle. Capturing the breast tissue at this location introduces resistance when the tissue from the neck has reached its capacity to stretch, impeding the completion of compression. CC positioning maneuvers used to address the neck tissue assist in avoiding this problem altogether.

Fix-It Problem #1B: Undercompression, Neck Tissue Has Reached Maximum Resistance

Prior to beginning compression:
20, 21, 22

Compression Is Affected By:

- Including only the breast under the compression device.
- Relaxation of the patient.
- Patient tolerance.
- Use of the "tilt" compression device.
- When the "tilt" compression device is not available, add an AC view, which captures only the anterior portion of the breast, excluding the pectoral muscle and the thick base of the breast.
- Resistance of neck tissue.
- Equal application to the superior and inferior breast.
- Compression evaluation by the technologist.

Additional Tips for Adequate Compression

- Patients presenting with size differences between the right and the left breast result in discrepancies for

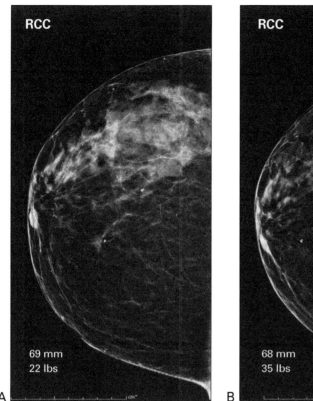
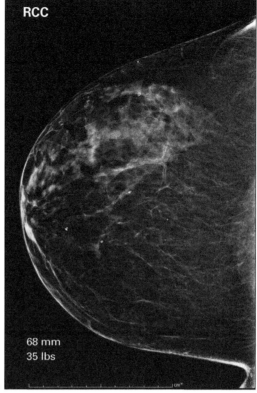

Figure 7-140
RCC projections of the same patient demonstrate the importance of adequate compression to image quality; inspect each image for separation of lateral glandular tissue. **(A)** RCC compression thickness, 68 mm, and compression force, 22 lb. **(B)** RCC compression thickness, 68 mm, and compression force, 35 lb.

centimeter thickness and compression force used for each breast. Appropriate documentation should be included on the history form for the interpreting physician regarding these differences.

- Achieving uniform compression on patients with a large discrepancy between the thickness at the base of the breast and the thinness of the apex is challenging. When available, use of the "tilt" compression device provides a solution to this common problem in mammography. When a "tilt" compression device is not available, an additional AC view of the breast, including only the breast anterior to the pectoral muscle, is required to achieve adequate compression (Figure 7-141).

- A design feature on older mammography equipment assisted in the application of compression. This older equipment compressed the breast the same way we do today, with one modification. After compressing the breast in the usual manner, the technologist could then use a foot pedal device to activate the Bucky to move the inferior breast in an upward motion. This action created slack to the superior breast allowing additional compression

using the compression device. When resistance was again detected, the process could be repeated. This method moved the breast in millimeters as it was compressed, eventually locating a neutral position on the chestwall where the superior and inferior breast tissues were compressed equally; using the maximum degree of compression while providing the greatest comfort to the patient (Figure 7-142). These maneuvers increase the ability to capture and visualize posterior tissue, including the pectoral muscle and the retroglandular fat space. The natural anatomy of the posterior chestwall adapts beautifully to this concept; the retromammary fascia located at the posterior margin of the breast meets the prepectoral fascia of the thorax, allowing movement between the two (Figure 7-143). The older concept of moving the Bucky toward the fixed superior tissue can still be accomplished when using equipment without this function by having the patient slightly bend her knees; this provides slack to the superior breast. This action must be done with precision as the patient may move her upper body backward when bending her knees. Keep an arm around

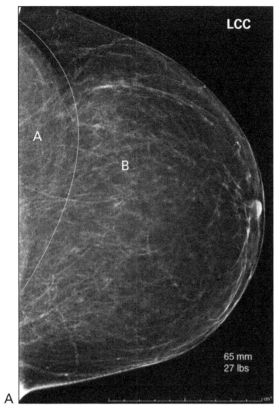

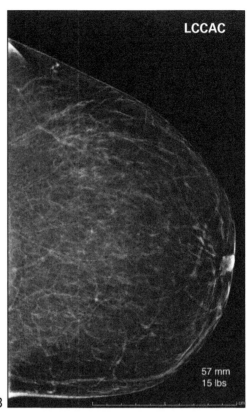

Figure 7-141
Achieving uniform compression on patients with a large difference between the thickness at the base of the breast and the thinness of the apex is challenging. **(A)** LCC projection of a patient with a thick breast base; tissue posterior to line (labeled *A*) is compressed while tissue anterior to line (labeled *B*) is not adequately compressed. **(B)** When a "tilt" compression device is not available, an additional anterior compression (AC) view achieves adequate compression to the anterior portion of the breast. (Note compression thickness and force on each image.)

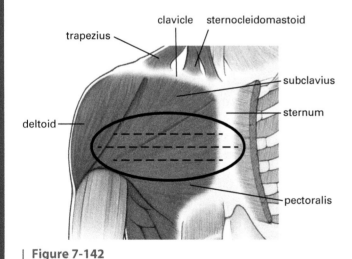

Figure 7-142
Compression methods that assist in locating the neutral position of the breast on the chestwall ensure that the superior and inferior breast tissues are equally compressed for the CC projection, allowing the maximum degree of compression with the greatest comfort to the patient. Location of the neutral breast position for each individual varies and will fall within the area of the *dotted lines* when compression is completed. (Adapted from Detton AJ. *Grant's Dissector*, 16th ed. Philadelphia, PA: Wolters Kluwer, 2017.)

the patient, securing her against the image receptor while watching the posterior margin of the field light to ensure the posterior tissue remains in the field of view. As in any radiology procedure, ensure the patient can safely tolerate this maneuver prior to adding it to the exam. Give instructions choosing words that describe a slow movement from the patient such as "slowly bend your knees a little bit." This ensures a response the technologist can monitor, keeping the movement of the patient to a minimum.

Skinfolds

Skinfolds on the CC projection are introduced by adjacent tissues not adequately smoothed away from each other, resulting in compression of overlapping skin. Eliminating all skinfolds from mammography imaging is simply not possible. Maneuvers that minimize and control skinfolds provide an accurate representation of breast tissue on the image. Careful consideration should be given to exam management when problem solving for skinfolds. Radiologists

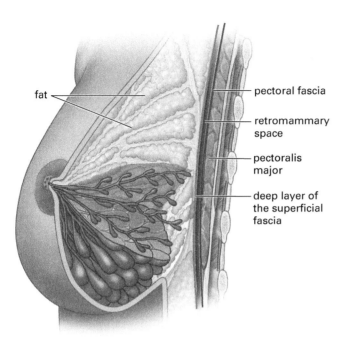

fat

pectoral fascia

retromammary space

pectoralis major

deep layer of the superficial fascia

Figure 7-143
The anatomy of the posterior chestwall conforms to the concept of the patient bending her knees very slightly as compression is applied; the retromammary fascia located at the posterior margin of the breast meets the prepectoral fascia of the thorax, allowing movement between the two. This CC positioning technique can increase posterior tissue capture while providing more comfort to the patient. (Illustration adapted with permission from Moore KL, Dalley AF, Agur AM. *Clinically Oriented Anatomy*. 8th ed. Philadelphia, PA: Wolters Kluwer; 2017.)

may have repeat protocols regarding the threshold of acceptability in their practice for the presence of skinfolds on the image.

Medial Breast Skinfolds

Medial skinfolds on the CC image range from small superior tethering type folds that do not compromise image quality to large hidden skinfolds on the undersurface of the breast unaddressed by the technologist. Larger skinfolds are usually accompanied by adjacent airgaps that further degrade the image. There are several positioning behaviors that ensure medial skinfolds are minimized on the final image.

Skinfold Problem #1A: Tethering Medial Skinfolds

Small medial skinfolds (Figure 7-144) can be a result of tissue tethered from the sternum to the medial breast. These skinfolds are usually minor and difficult to eliminate. They do not result in compromising airgaps further degrading the image and generally do not require an image to be repeated.

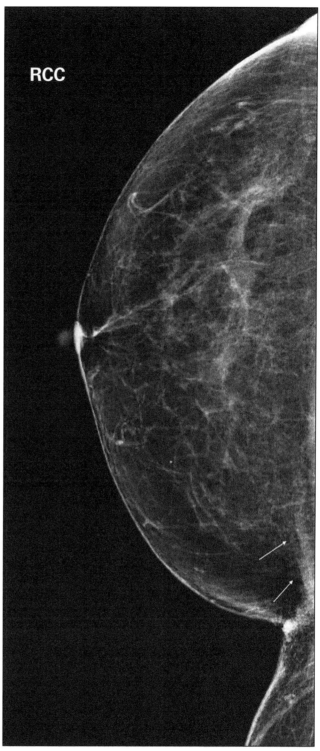

RCC

Figure 7-144
Small medial skinfolds can be a result of tissue tethered from the sternum to the medial breast (*arrows*). These skinfolds are usually minor and difficult to eliminate. They generally do not require an image to be repeated.

Skinfold Problem #1B: Medial Skinfolds

Skinfolds in the medial aspect of the breast can be naturally introduced on the image from positioning maneuvers that elevate the IMF and bring the breast tissue onto the image receptor. Appropriately inspecting the inferomedial tissue to ensure it is in intimate contact with the image receptor from chestwall to nipple can eliminate skinfolds in this region.

Fix-It Problem #1B: Medial Skinfolds Figure 7-145 illustrates image quality improvement for posteromedial tissue presentation when the following positioning/compression maneuvers are employed from Table 7-3.

3, **4, 5**, 6, 8, 9, 11, 12, 13, 15
(Bold numbers have the greatest impact on this positioning feature.)

Medial Skinfolds Are Affected By:

- Elevation of the IMF
- Height of the receptor
- Stance of the patient
- Control of the inferomedial tissue by the technologist
- Inspection of the inferomedial tissue for intimate contact to the image receptor

Additional Tips for Medial Breast Skinfolds

- Stance of the patient: the thorax must approach the image receptor with as little rotation as possible and with only the upper body being brought forward onto the image receptor. The pelvis and feet remain at a slight distance from the chestwall edge of the image receptor.

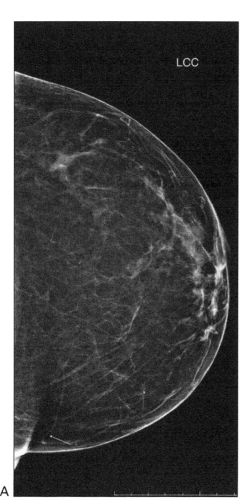
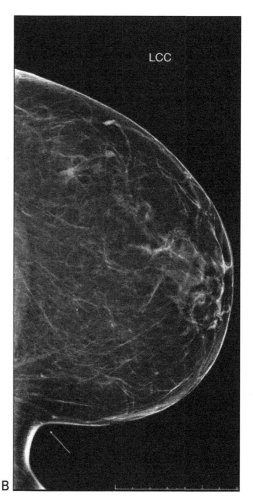

Figure 7-145
Left CC projections, same patient. **(A)** Skinfolds in the medial aspect of the breast (*arrow*) can be naturally introduced on the image from positioning maneuvers that elevate the IMF and bring the breast tissue onto the image receptor. **(B)** Inspection of the inferomedial tissue to ensure it is in intimate contact with the image receptor from the chestwall to the nipple can eliminate skinfolds in this region (*arrow*).

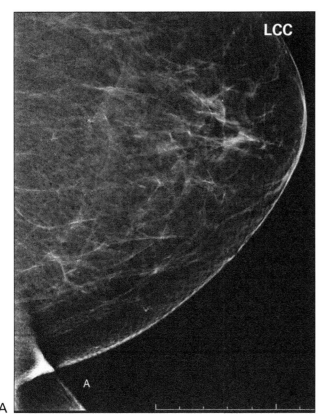

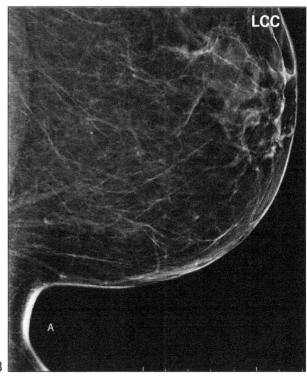

Figure 7-146
(A) When draping the contralateral breast over the medial corner of the image receptor, ensure separation of the tissue (labeled *A*) at the cleavage. **(B)** When possible, look for a "u"-shaped space (labeled *A*) between the right and the left breasts, without overlap of tissue from one breast to the other.

- Control the tissue as it is placed on the image receptor. Allowing the breast to be placed on the receptor, rolled either laterally or medially, introduces skinfolds.
- When draping the contralateral breast over the medial corner of the image receptor, ensure separation of the tissue at the cleavage. When possible, look for a "u"-shaped space between the right and the left breasts, without overlap of tissue from one breast to the other (Figure 7-146).

Posterior Skinfolds

Inferoposterior skinfolds are common in mammography and are the result of the inferior tissue not resting flush against the image receptor. This occurs when:

- The patient is allowed to stand in too vertical of a position and in too close proximity to the image receptor at the beginning of the exam.
- Excessive elevation of the IMF region results in a small amount of superior abdomen included in the image. When the breast is compressed, this overlap of breast

and abdominal tissue is usually accompanied by an adjacent airgap.
- Exacerbation of posterior skinfold problems occurs when the image receptor is positioned too low for the exam.

Skinfold Problem #1A: Inferoposterior Skinfolds

Figure 7-147 illustrates how skinfolds are introduced in the posterior breast tissue if the IRSD is positioned too low and is not accurately adjusted to match the elevated IMF for the CC projection. This lack of precision results in the creation of inferoposterior skinfolds as a result of abdominal tissue being included in the image as the IMF is elevated and brought forward onto the image receptor. These skinfolds can imitate the presence of the pectoral muscle (Figure 7-148). Although it is sometimes difficult to differentiate between the pectoral muscle and this type of skinfold on the radiograph, the skinfold is usually accompanied by an adjacent airgap and does not "blend" into the breast as the pectoral muscle does.

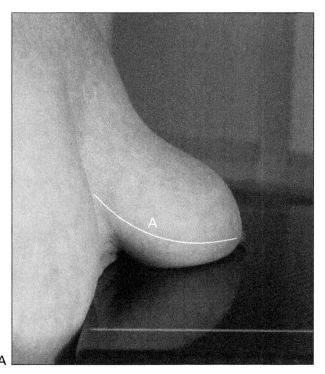

A

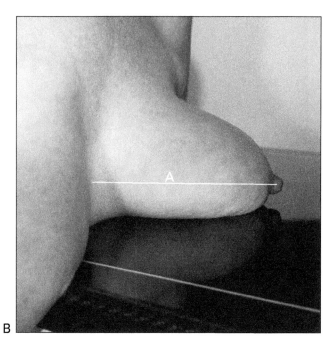

B

Figure 7-147
Inferoposterior skinfolds are common in mammography and are most often the result of the inferior tissue not resting flush against the image receptor. **(A)** Exacerbation of posterior skinfold problems occurs when the image receptor is positioned too low for the exam; note the drooping PNL (labeled *A*) not parallel to the image receptor. **(B)** Intimate contact between the inferior breast tissue and the image receptor is possible with careful attention to elevation of the IMF, image receptor height, and control over posterior tissue capture; note the line (labeled *A*) is now parallel to the image receptor.

Fix-It Problem #1A: *Inferoposterior Skinfolds*
2, **3, 4, 5,** 6, 7, 8, 9, 10, 16, 17, 30
(Bold numbers have the greatest impact on this positioning feature.)

Skinfold Problem #1B: Torqueing Skinfolds

Torqueing of the breast is most commonly detected in the posterior aspect, but it may also be detected centrally on the breast mound. To understand how torqueing affects image quality, first it is necessary to understand how breast structures are portrayed on the CC projection. When positioning the CC projection, the technologist pulls the superior and inferior breast tissue from the chestwall of the thorax onto the image receptor in a straight forward direction to accurately demonstrate their linear pattern. This pattern can be interrupted when the technologist allows "shifting" (torqueing) to occur either on the inferior or superior aspect of the breast during positioning (Figure 7-149). There are two opportunities for torqueing to occur when positioning for the CC projection:

- To ensure a linear demonstration of breast structures, the technologist uses two flat hands to capture the breast at the chestwall and bring it straight forward onto the image receptor. The hand in contact with the inferior aspect of the breast must be removed in a straight forward direction from the underside of the breast. If the technologist removes the hand positioning the inferior breast toward herself (medially), rather than in a straight forward direction, a "shifting" of only the inferior aspect of the breast occurs interrupting the linear pattern. This interruption introduces "torqueing," a slight roll of only one portion of the breast.
- Torqueing can be introduced on the CC projection during the lateral pull by bringing the posterolateral tissue onto the image receptor and unintentionally rolling the superior tissue medially as the breast is secured onto the image receptor.

Fix-It: Problem #1B: Torqueing Skinfolds
6, 8, 9, 10, 18, 19
(Bold numbers have the greatest impact on this positioning feature.)

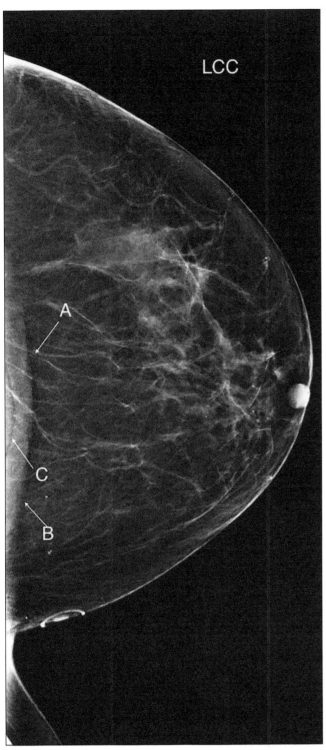

Figure 7-148
Inferoposterior skinfolds on the CC projection are the result of abdominal tissue being included as the IMF is elevated and brought forward onto the image receptor. These skinfolds can imitate the presence of the pectoral muscle. LCC image with abdomen skinfold extending from posterior–central tissue (labeled A) to posterior–medial tissue (labeled B). Pectoral muscle presentation (labeled C).

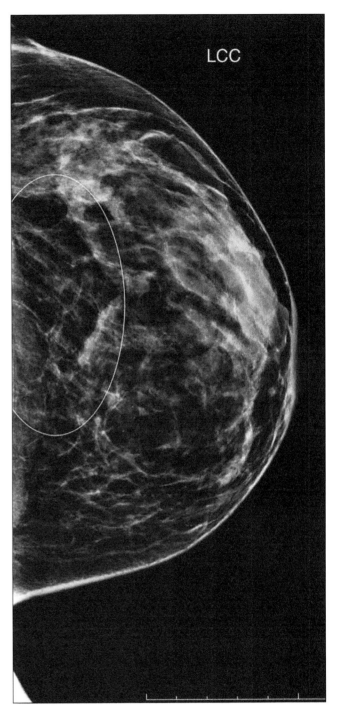

Figure 7-149
Torqueing of the breast is most commonly detected in the posterior region of the CC projection (circle). It can result when the technologist allows "rotation" to occur in either the superior or inferior tissue as she brings the breast onto the image receptor, interrupting the orientation of the linear pattern that extends from the chestwall to the nipple.

Posterior Skinfolds Are Affected By:

- Elevation of the IMF.
- Height of the image receptor.
- Patient stance.
- Control of the posterior breast structures while directing the breast forward onto the image receptor.
- The hand positioning the underside of the breast is removed following a perpendicular path from the chestwall edge of the image receptor.
- Inspection of the inferior aspect of the breast for intimate contact to the image receptor.
- Ensuring the "lateral pull" maneuver is executed with a straight forward motion.
- Ensuring the abdomen is not included posteriorly on the image.

Lateral Breast Skinfolds

Skinfold Problem #1A: Lateral Skinfolds

Lateral skinfolds on the CC image (Figure 7-150) are naturally introduced as the upper outer quadrant of the breast contains more tissue when compared to the medial aspect plus the compression device is applied *not with but rather against* the pectoral muscle fiber direction. Final positioning maneuvers used for the CC image involve techniques to remove the humeral head from the field of view; this action also aids with removal of the natural lateral skinfolds. Final positioning maneuvers for the CC projection include:

1. The patient's arm is at her side and shoulder relaxed prior to compression.
2. Compression is applied.
3. Ask the patient to externally rotate her hand.

For skinfolds that remain after these final positioning maneuvers, strategies exist to control and minimize them.

Fix-It Problem #1A: Lateral Skinfold, Finger Roll Strategy Figure 7-151 illustrates the finger roll strategy used to reduce or eliminate posterolateral skinfolds on the CC projection. After initial compression is applied to immobilize the breast, but final compression is not yet completed[8]:

1. Place the index finger on the skinfold.
2. Press down on the skinfold.
3. Roll the finger out laterally as manual compression is applied.

Fix-It Problem #1A: Lateral Skinfold, Palm Placement Strategy (Author's Choice) Figure 7-152 illustrates the palm placement strategy used to reduce or eliminate posterolateral skinfolds on the CC projection. After all medial and lateral positioning maneuvers have been

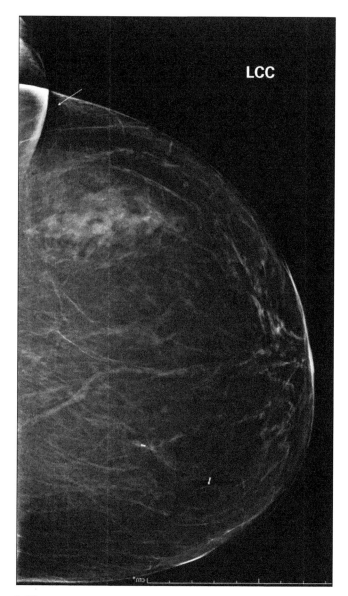

Figure 7-150
Lateral skinfolds on the CC image are naturally introduced as the upper outer quadrant of the breast contains more tissue when compared to the medial aspect; additionally, the compression device is applied *not with* but rather *against* the direction of the pectoral muscle bundle fibers.

completed, address lateral skinfolds prior to compression. Placing the palm of the hand, rather than the fingers, on the breast mound during positioning maneuvers for the CC projection allows continual control of the lateral tissue as compression is applied. This position assists in eliminating skinfolds by fanning the fingers to spread and minimize the folds while monitoring lateral tissue inclusion.

20, 21, **24, 25, 26,** 27
(Bold numbers have the greatest impact on this positioning feature.)

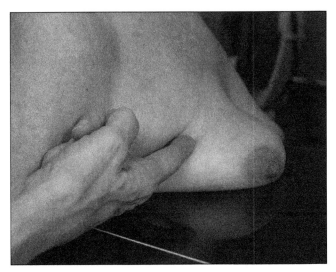

Figure 7-151
After initial compression to immobilize the breast is applied, but final compression is not yet completed: (a) place the index finger on the skinfold; (b) press down on the skinfold; and (c) roll the finger out laterally as manual compression is applied.

Skinfold Problem #1B: Excessive Thickness Upper Outer Quadrant, Lateral Breast

For patients who present with excessive breast tissue in the upper outer quadrant, adequate positioning and compression can be challenging due to (a) large and

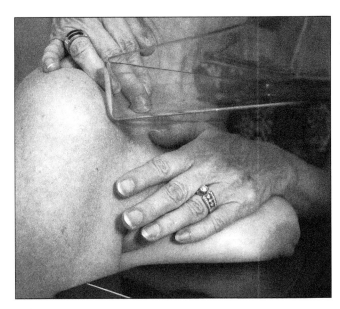

Figure 7-152
Placing the palm of the hand, rather than the fingers, on the breast mound during positioning maneuvers for the CC projection allows continuous control of the posterolateral tissue as compression is applied. This position assists in lateral tissue inclusion while simultaneously controlling skinfolds by fanning the fingers to spread and minimize or eliminate the folds.

unmanageable skinfolds in the lateral aspect of the CC projection and (b) difficulty in the delivery of uniform compression. This excessive tissue is the result of patient body habitus. Purposely excluding breast tissue to eliminate skinfolds is not recommended as there are several positioning behaviors to improve the problem without sacrificing tissue. However, when recommended skinfold removal strategies are not effective and compression is compromised due to excessive upper outer quadrant fullness, measures should be taken to ensure that adequate capture with clarity of the posterolateral tissue is achieved.

Fix-It Problem #1B: Excessive Thickness Upper Outer Quadrant, Lateral Breast Figure 7-153 illustrates improved image quality for lateral tissue presentation attributed to the following exam management solution for the patient with excessive thickness in the upper outer quadrant:

- Two images are taken. The first CC image includes all medial tissue and as much lateral tissue as possible, ensuring adequate compression and visualization of breast tissue by reducing the visual effects of the superolateral skinfold as much as possible.
- Additionally, an XCCL projection is included to capture superolateral tissue that was excluded from the original CC projection.

Lateral Skinfolds Are Affected By:

- Natural amount of breast tissue in the upper outer quadrant
- Control of the posterior breast tissue by the technologist
- Strategies used to control the posterolateral breast tissue as compression is applied
- Patient body habitus

Medial Airgap

Airgaps on the CC projection commonly result from inferior tissue not resting flush against the image receptor. Occasionally, an airgap can be introduced superiorly when the breast does not rest flush against the compression device; this should be addressed by the technologist during positioning. When minor airgaps are introduced on the image from either one of these two reasons, acceptable image quality may still be achieved. Airgaps are generally acceptable for image quality if breast structures can be visualized into, through, and out of the airgap. Airgaps range from minimal airgaps that do not

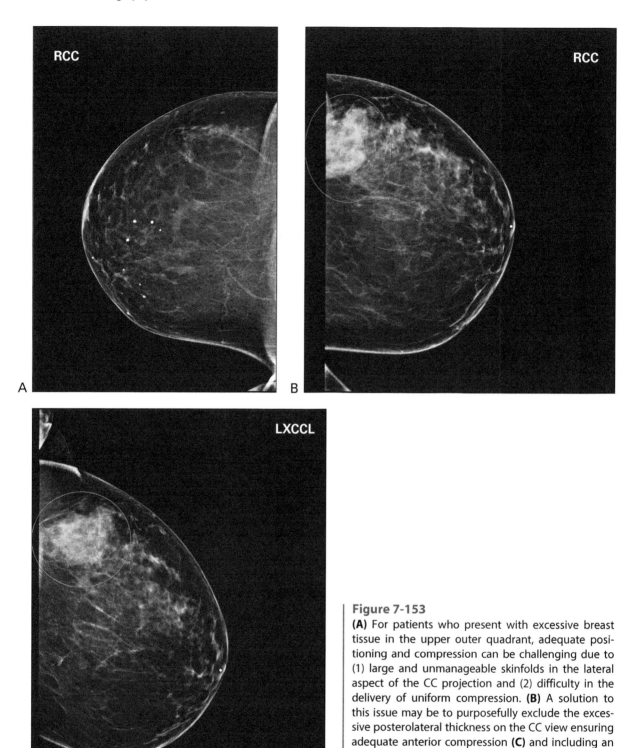

Figure 7-153

(A) For patients who present with excessive breast tissue in the upper outer quadrant, adequate positioning and compression can be challenging due to (1) large and unmanageable skinfolds in the lateral aspect of the CC projection and (2) difficulty in the delivery of uniform compression. **(B)** A solution to this issue may be to purposefully exclude the excessive posterolateral thickness on the CC view ensuring adequate anterior compression **(C)** and including an additional XCCL projection to capture the excluded posterolateral tissue.

compromise image quality to a noticeably uneven distribution of plus and minus densities degrading the appearance of the image. The technologist evaluates each image to determine the degree of degradation to image quality due to airgaps. Positioning maneuvers can be done to minimize and control airgaps on the image. Careful consideration should be given to exam management when problem solving for airgaps. Radiologists may have repeat protocols regarding the threshold of acceptability in their practice.

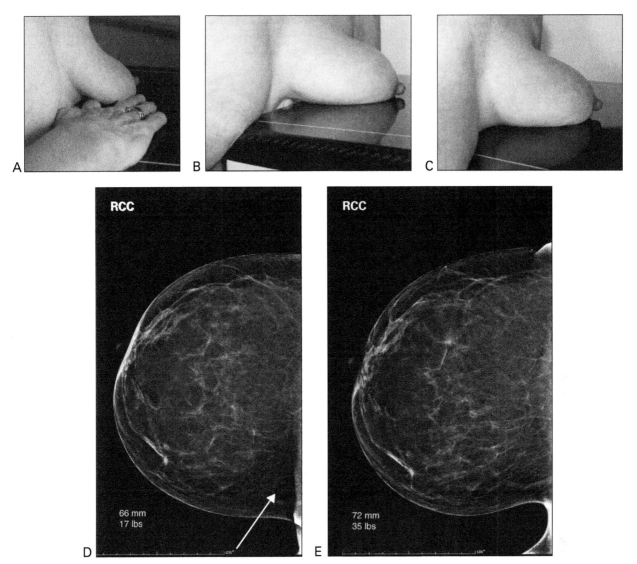

Figure 7-154
Airgaps in the CC projection are naturally introduced in the inferomedial region as the breast is elevated to capture superior and posterior tissue. **(A)** For the majority of patients, positioning behaviors must be incorporated to address airgaps in the inferomedial region of the breast on the CC projection. **(B)** The technologist uses her index finger placed between the image receptor and the thorax to gently eliminate the airgap. **(C)** Elimination of posteromedial airgap indicated by intimate contact of the skin to the image receptor. **(D)** RCC projection demonstrating large posteromedial airgap (*arrow*). **(E)** RCC same patient after positioning techniques were applied to eliminate posteromedial airgap.

Medial Airgap Problem #1: Inferomedial Airgap

Airgaps in the CC projection are naturally introduced in the inferomedial region as the breast is elevated to capture superior and posterior tissue. The inferomedial breast contour is rounded, while the surface of the image receptor is flat. When the elevated breast is brought forward to rest on the image receptor, an airgap is introduced at this rounded contour because the inferior breast tissue is not in contact with the image receptor. Consequently, for the majority of patients, positioning behaviors must be incorporated to address airgaps in the inferomedial

region of the breast on the CC projection. Airgaps in the inferomedial breast can be exacerbated by excessive IMF elevation.

Fix-It Problem #1: Inferomedial Airgap

Figure 7-154 illustrates image quality improvement strategies for inferomedial airgaps when the following positioning/compression maneuvers are employed from Table 7-3.

2, **3, 4, 5, 6, 8**, 9, 11, 12, 13, 15, 16, 17
(Bold numbers have the greatest impact on this positioning feature.)

Additional Tip for Eliminating Inferomedial Skinfolds and Airgaps

- Throughout the positioning process of the CC projection, the patient unconsciously allows her pelvis to migrate forward, coming in contact with the image receptor. This action brings her upper body erect, introducing an airgap and possible posterior skinfolds to the inferomedial aspect of the breast. When an airgap is noticed in this region, first check the position of the pelvis, directing it backward at the ASIS if it has migrated forward.

Inferomedial Airgap Is Affected By:

- Elevation of the IMF
- Height of the image receptor
- Patient stance
- Control of the posterior breast by the technologist
- Inspection of inferomedial tissue ensuring intimate contact to the image receptor
- Inspection for skinfolds that may introduce an adjacent airgap

Summarizing Image Quality in Routine Mammography

Under a variety of imaging circumstances, the technologist strives to meet established quality standards ensuring as much breast tissue as possible is captured with as much detail as possible on the image for every patient. Technologists who have a comprehensive understanding of image quality assessment customize this approach to the many anatomical differences from one patient to another and even from one breast to another on the same patient. However, even with the best positioning and compression efforts made by the technologist, one or all of these quality positioning indicators may be absent on images in an examination. Understanding the concepts of breast margins, mobility, and landmarks assists the technologist in problem solving when these quality standards cannot be met. The technologist should use discretion in adding subsequent images to the exam, determining their necessity by evaluation of the patient's ability to comply with adequate capture with clarity of breast tissue. Quality indicators can be used to measure the technologist's positioning/compression performance. When images demonstrate repetitive problems in meeting established criteria for image quality, the technologist should consider refining the techniques she uses to increase her abilities in meeting those standards.

Review Questions, Chapter 7, Part 1

1. Describe the complementary relationship between the craniocaudal and mediolateral oblique projections in their ability to capture as much breast tissue as possible for the routine mammography examination.

2. Describe positioning of the craniocaudal view. What subtle nuances are performed within the positioning to maximize the amount of glandular tissue seen?

3. Describe positioning of the mediolateral oblique view. What subtle nuances are performed within the positioning to maximize the amount of glandular tissue seen?

4. Image receptor height is critical when positioning the breast. Describe how the image is affected when the image receptor is placed too high for the CC projection. Describe how the image is affected when the image receptor is placed too low for the CC projection.

5. Image receptor height is critical when positioning the breast. Describe how the image is affected when the image receptor is placed too high for the MLO projection. Describe how the image is affected when the image receptor is placed too low for the MLO projection.

6. Describe the established image criteria for the craniocaudal projection that indicates the patient has been properly positioned and compressed.

7. Describe the established image criteria for the mediolateral oblique projection that indicates the patient has been properly positioned and compressed.

8. Explain the posterior nipple line (PNL) rule used for the routine or standard projections and what specific feature it evaluates.

PART 2
MASTERING PROBLEM-SOLVING PROJECTIONS

Objectives

- Understand the purpose for using complementary or replacement imaging for the mammography examination and the value they contribute to the interpreting physician.

- Understand the versatility of the mammography equipment to accomplish challenging imaging techniques while ensuring patient tolerance.

- Understand the execution of additional projections used to further define or complete the routine projections.

- Understand the mammographic requirements and techniques used for imaging patients with breast implants.

- Understand the MQSA requirements for mammography image identification.

Key Terms

- axillary tail
- encapsulated
- implant displaced
- magnification
- milk of calcium

- orthogonal
- spot compression
- superimposition
- tangential
- triangulation

ADDITIONAL MAMMOGRAPHIC PROJECTIONS (PROBLEM SOLVING)

The routine screening mammogram consists of two standard projections, the MLO and the CC. When properly performed, they complement one another in terms of their ability to accurately represent the breast in its entirety.[10] There are circumstances when two projections do not completely capture breast tissue with sufficient information for the interpreting physician to make a final diagnosis. Further information can be obtained to define, localize, and adequately capture breast tissue for patients with special examination considerations using a variety of problem-solving projections designed for these purposes. These projections, sometimes called supplemental, diagnostic, special, and additional views, all share a common purpose in that they provide further information to assist the radiologist in determining a final assessment for the patient and to define appropriate patient care. Table 7-1 describes additional projections used for problem solving in breast imaging.[8] The technologist who possesses a strong understanding of the projections used for additional imaging and their purpose also possesses the ability to manage the mammography examination with confidence. This level of understanding requires technical skills associated with equipment operation as well as problem-solving skills correlating to breast anatomy. Possession of these skills is critical for additional imaging purposes as some projections and situations may produce discomfort to the patient. The technologist who is familiar with equipment operation and problem-solving projections manages the requirements of tissue capture with clarity while minimizing patient discomfort:

1. For patients with limited physical ability, chestwall anomalies, or implanted medical devices within the breast margins, problem-solving projections can be used to modify the examination by replacing standard projections or providing complementary projections to complete the exam.
2. For screening examinations that do not sufficiently demonstrate breast tissue for final interpretation, patients are recalled for further projections that better define and localize the area of concern. When using 2D FFDM technology, approximately 10% of patients are called back for further imaging.[23] When employing digital breast tomosynthesis (DBT), studies show that the rate for patients needing further imaging is reduced by approximately 40%.[24–27]
3. Symptomatic patients presenting for diagnostic mammography may require additional views tailored to their specific area of concern.

Lateral Projections: Mediolateral (ML) and Lateromedial (LM)

Applications of the Lateral Projections

The Lateral projection is the most commonly used additional view for problem solving in mammography, with the x-ray beam entering either the medial or lateral side of the breast. The name of each projection (ML or LM) indicates the direction of the entrance and exit of the x-ray beam. The Lateral projection is performed when the radiologist believes he/she is dealing with:

1. Milk of calcium: Calcifications detected on the standard views that have a smudge-like appearance and are thought to be benign **milk of calcium** are further defined on the Lateral projection, which is often combined with a magnification spot compression technique (Figure 7-155). These tiny deposits found within microcysts in the breast are calcifications that eventually layer out on the bottom of the cyst wall, reflecting its curved form, sometimes called "tea cupping."
2. Real versus superimposition: Another common use for the Lateral projection is to determine if a lesion seen on only one standard projection is "real." When the Lateral projection confirms the presence of an abnormality that has also been identified on one of the original standard images (CC/MLO), this confirms the ROI is not due to superimposition of breast structures (Figure 7-156). When the Lateral projection demonstrates normal breast tissue, this indicates an overlapping of breast tissue on the original standard image (CC/MLO), which is commonly referred to as "superimposition of normal tissue" (Figure 7-157).
3. **Triangulation**: Because the Lateral projection is an **orthogonal** projection to the CC view, it is used to triangulate the exact location of a lesion for preoperative needle localizations and for determining the approach for core biopsy. For accurate measurements when using the Lateral for localization purposes, the nipple should be projected in profile.

Case Study 7 Part **2-1**

1. Refer to Figures 7-155 through 7-158. The Lateral projection serves many purposes. Describe the various reasons why a Lateral projection would be added to a patient examination. In addition, why would an ML projection be selected versus an LM—and vice versa.

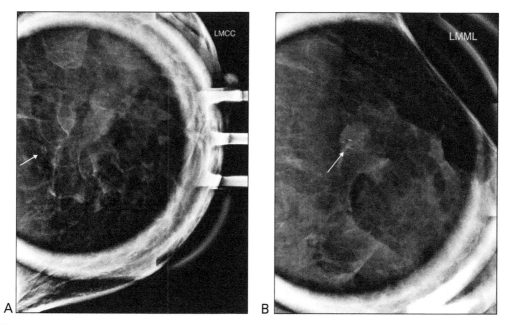

Figure 7-155
Milk of calcium **(A)** LMCC projection demonstrating calcifications with a smudge-like appearance; detected on the standard CC view and thought to be benign milk of calcium **(B)** calcifications are further defined on the Lateral projection combined with magnification spot compression technique confirming milk of calcium.

When a lesion is seen on only the MLO standard projection and is not seen on the CC projection, the Lateral projection helps locate the lesion by following the movement of the lesion from the MLO projection to the Lateral projection.

- Lesions that move upward on the Lateral from the MLO projection are located in the medial aspect of the breast. Technologists remember this general rule by remembering "the sun rises in the morning," referring to the upward movement and the medial location (the word "morning" begins with an "M") (Figure 7-158).

- Lesions that move downward on the Lateral from the MLO projection are located in the lateral aspect of the breast. Technologists remember this general rule by noting the common phrase "down and out," referring to the downward movement and the lateral location (Figure 7-159).

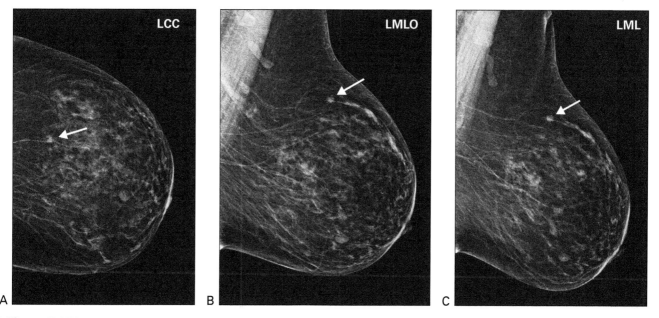

Figure 7-156
Screening examination reveals a ROI detected on the **(A)** LCC and the **(B)** LMLO. The ROI is still visible on the **(C)** LML projection, confirming the presence of a "real" lesion; this is known as focal asymmetry.

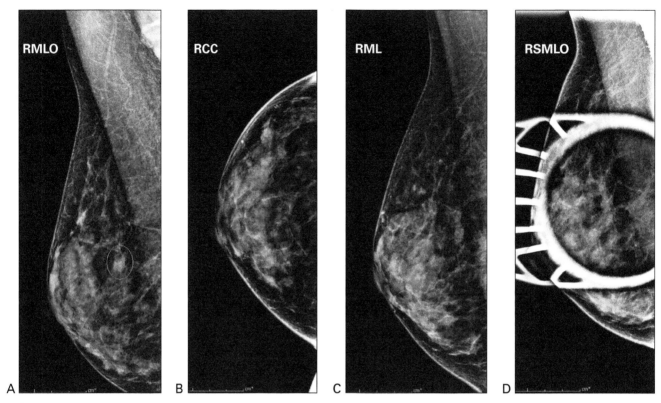

Figure 7-157
Screening examination, **(A)** RMLO and **(B)** RCC projections, reveals a ROI detected on the RMLO (*circle*). **(C)** The Lateral projection is used to determine if a lesion seen on only one standard projection is "real." When normal breast tissue is demonstrated on the Lateral projection, this confirms superimposition (tissue overlap) on the original image; this is known as asymmetry. **(D)** A RSMLO was included in the additional imaging examination further revealing normal glandular tissue. This exam was assessed BIRADS 2.

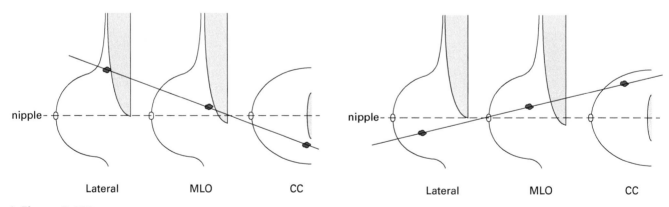

Figure 7-158
The Lateral projection is the orthogonal projection to the CC view; it is used to triangulate the exact location of a lesion for preoperative needle localizations and the approach for core biopsy. Lesions that move upward on the Lateral from the MLO projection are located in the medial aspect of the breast. (Modified from Cardinosa G. *Breast Imaging Companion*. 3rd ed. Wolters Kluwer/Lippincott Williams & Wilkins, 2001.)

Figure 7-159
The Lateral projection is the orthogonal projection to the CC view; it is used to triangulate the exact location of a lesion for preoperative needle localizations and the approach for core biopsy. Lesions that move downward on the Lateral from the MLO projection are located in the lateral aspect of the breast. (Modified from Cardinosa G. *Breast Imaging Companion*. 3rd ed. Wolters Kluwer/Lippincott Williams & Wilkins, 2001.)

- Lesions that are centrally located in the breast have minimal movement from the MLO projection to the Lateral.

Mediolateral (ML) Projection

Applications Specific to the Mediolateral Projection

For the mediolateral (ML) projection, the x-ray beam enters the medial aspect of the breast at 90°. The lateral breast is in contact with the image receptor, providing the best resolution for lesions located in the lateral breast due to reduced object-to-image receptor distance (Figure 7-160).

Mediolateral Projection Summary

1. The C-arm is rotated 90° placing the lateral aspect of the breast in contact with the image receptor.
2. The patient stands facing the unit.
3. The patient's arm is raised to a level slightly above the shoulder for the technologist to identify the midaxillary landmark.
4. The patient steps forward, posterolateral breast in contact with the chestwall edge of the image receptor, as the arm is guided forward placing the midaxilla in contact with the superior corner of the image receptor (for deep posterior lesions, place the corner of the image receptor posterior to the midaxilla) (Figure 7-161).
5. Gently stretch and rest the patient's arm across the top edge of the image receptor, elbow bent, hand resting on the C-arm. The chestwall edge of the image receptor rests against the lateral edge of the breast, and the thorax is relaxed.

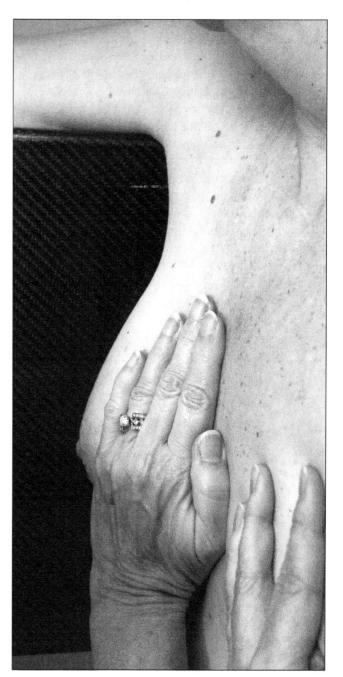

Figure 7-161
The ML projection positions the posterolateral breast in contact with the chestwall edge of the image receptor and places the midaxilla in contact with the superior corner of the image receptor.

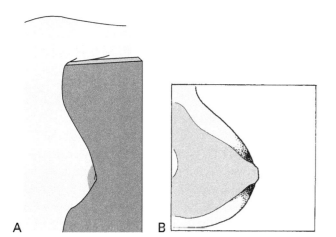

A   B

Figure 7-160
The ML projection. **(A)** 90° orientation of the C-arm to the breast. **(B)** Schematic of the amount of the "glandular island" usually included with this projection.

6. Adjust the patient's thorax position, ensuring the bony structures are excluded from compression by placing a hand on the ipsilateral ASIS of the patient and gently tilting the pelvis forward/downward to control rib placement against the image receptor. This action removes the prominent ribs of the thorax from compression without excluding inferolateral tissue from the image.

7. Capture the lateral edge of the breast by using a flat hand and placing the fifth finger against the lateral breast margin at the midaxillary line. Move the lateral breast anteriorly and medially (Figure 7-162).

8. Using two hands, sandwich the lateral and medial breast tissue, pulling the breast straight out away from the chestwall (Figure 7-163).

9. Slide the hand in contact with the lateral breast out; use the opposite hand to anchor the breast tissue securely against the image receptor, out and away from the chestwall at approximately 90°, while supporting the medial breast tissue upward.

10. Using the ipsilateral scapula as a "steering wheel," rotate the patient toward the unit, ensuring the pelvis and feet are facing forward, capturing medial tissue to the sternum (Figure 7-164). This action presents the nipple in profile and places the pectoral muscle on the image,

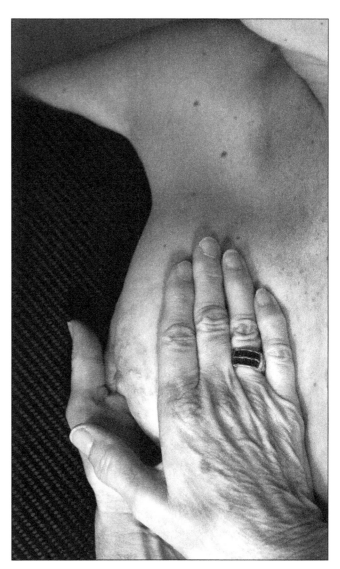

Figure 7-163
The breast tissue is directed 90° from the thorax for the ML projection. Using two hands, firmly sandwich and control the lateral and medial tissue at the posterior breast margin as it is pulled forward.

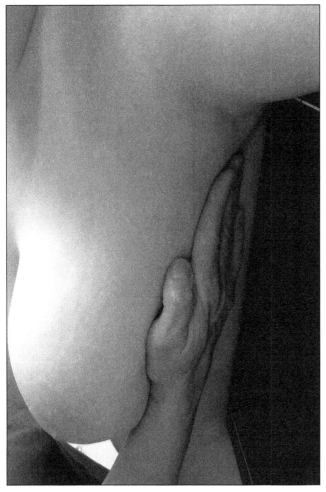

Figure 7-162
Ensuring visualization of the posterolateral tissue on the ML projection requires the technologist to position her flat hand at the posterolateral breast margin as she captures and moves the breast anteriorly and medially prior to securing the tissue against the image receptor.

although the appearance is narrow and vertical when compared to the MLO pectoral muscle presentation.

11. Final positioning maneuvers place the superior light field margin at the level of the axilla.

12. Pull the breast tissue outward and anchor the tissue approximately 90° from the chestwall, ensuring the medial tissue is supported upward until adequate compression is reached.

13. As compression is applied, the patient's thorax remains relaxed, allowing the technologist to skim the compression device across the thorax in the medial to lateral direction. This must be done while monitoring the posterior margin of the thorax, ensuring only the soft tissue of the breast, not the skeletal component of the medial or lateral

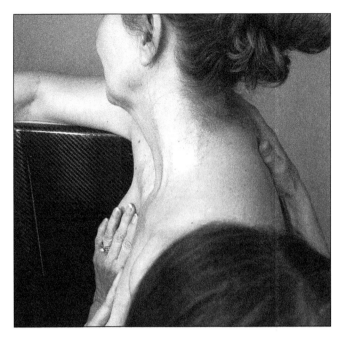

Figure 7-164
Capturing adequate medial tissue on the ML projection relies on the maneuvers used to sufficiently rotate the thorax toward the image receptor. The ipsilateral scapula provides a steering wheel that gives the technologist control over the patient's upper body as it is directed toward the image receptor. With adequate rotation of the patient's thorax medially, the pectoral muscle will be present on the ML projection.

ribcage, is included under compression. Monitoring compression ensures increased comfort to the patient, providing adequate compression to the posterior margin of the breast. The compression device gradually replaces the hand anchoring the medial breast until adequate compression is reached (Figure 7-165).

14. For lesion location purposes, ensure the nipple is in profile.

Lateromedial (LM) Projection

Applications Specific to the Lateromedial Projection

For the lateromedial (LM) view, the x-ray beam enters the lateral aspect of the breast at 90°. The medial breast is in contact with the image receptor, providing the best resolution for lesions located in the medial breast due to reduced object-to-image receptor distance (Figure 7-166).

The LM projection can be used as a replacement or complementary view to complete the examination when the MLO projection cannot be performed or is inadequate for capture with clarity due to patient physical limitations, chestwall anomalies, or implanted medical devices. Although some posterior tissue is sacrificed due to the use of the 90° angle instead of the customized pectoral muscle angle, the LM choice benefits the limited study

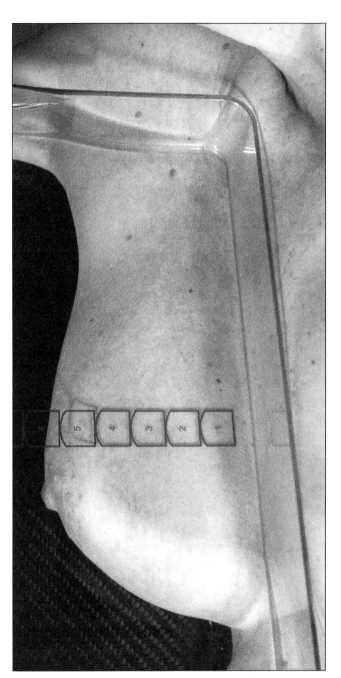

Figure 7-165
As compression is applied, monitor the posterior margin of the thorax, ensuring only the soft tissue of the breast, not the skeletal component of the medial or lateral ribcage, is included under compression. Monitoring compression ensures increased comfort to the patient while providing adequate compression to the posterior margin of the breast.

due to its flexibility. The face shield of the mammography unit can be removed when performing lateral to medial projections as there are no extraneous body parts in the field of view resulting in artifact on the image. Removal of the face shield facilitates technologist positioning due to an increase in the workspace. The LM projection is advantageous when performing mammography on patients in

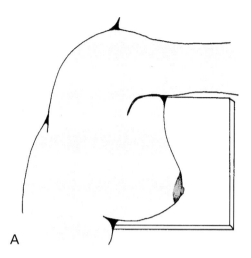

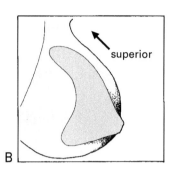

Figure 7-166
The LM projection. **(A)** Schematic of the 90° orientation of the C-arm to the breast. **(B)** Schematic of the amount of the "glandular island" usually included with this projection.

a wheelchair, as this position allows for a less restrictive workspace for the technologist. For patients with limited mobility, the LM projection allows for slight medial rotation toward the image receptor as compression is applied, capturing additional lateral tissue on the final image.

Additionally, the LM projection is useful to image suspected abnormalities located medially, high on the chestwall, or those that are extremely posterior in the inferior half of the breast.

Lateromedial Projection Summary

1. The C-arm is rotated 90°, placing the medial aspect of the breast in contact with the image receptor.
2. The height of the image receptor places the superior light field at the approximate level of the suprasternal notch.
3. The patient stands facing the unit, feet forward, with the chestwall edge of the image receptor very slightly off center to the midsternum, toward the contralateral breast. Slightly off centering the patient to the image receptor ensures that the medial breast tissue in closest proximity to the sternum will more likely be included on the image.
4. Raise the ipsilateral arm; guide it up and over the image receptor toward the contralateral shoulder until the arm rests on the superior aspect of the image receptor; elbow bent as the hand rests on the contralateral shoulder.
5. Place the patient's contralateral hand on the top edge of the image receptor. Lean the patient forward, bringing the superior sternum in contact with the image receptor. The patient's head is brought forward, chin resting on the contralateral hand for additional comfort, securing posterior/superior tissue onto the image receptor (Figure 7-167A).
6. Using a flat hand to capture the medial breast, place the fifth finger against the image receptor chestwall

edge, gently pulling and freeing any medial tissue caught under or behind the image receptor.
7. *The flat hand, used to capture the medial tissue, now rotates its position, coming in contact with the lateral breast, in order to capture and pull the lateral tissue outward, approximately 90° from the chestwall.*
8. With a flat hand, anchor the breast against the image receptor, supporting the tissue in the outward and upward position to open the IMF as compression is applied; the patient's feet and pelvis should be facing the unit (Figure 7-167B).
9. Use fingers to sweep the medial and lateral IMF region downward, eliminating skinfolds and airgaps.
10. Upon completion of positioning maneuvers and compression, the superior margin of the compression device is positioned just anterior to the latissimus dorsi muscle (Figure 7-167C).
11. Lateral to medial projections allow additional rotation of the patient's thorax toward the image receptor as compression is applied for maximum capture of posterolateral tissue.

Laterally Exaggerated Craniocaudal (XCCL) Projection

Applications

The laterally exaggerated XCCL projection is used to image the outer aspect of the breast for better visualization of deep posterolateral tissue (Figure 7-168).

Some women have glandular tissue that extends laterally beyond the capture of the CC projection, even though the "lateral pull" maneuver was performed. Adding the XCCL to the screening examination allows for complete evaluation of this far lateral extension of glandular tissue, including as much of the **axillary tail** as possible (Figure 7-169). For diagnostic purposes, the XCCL projection is useful to

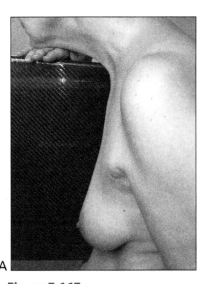
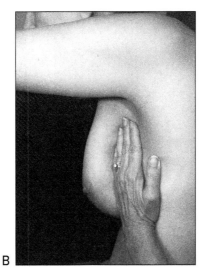
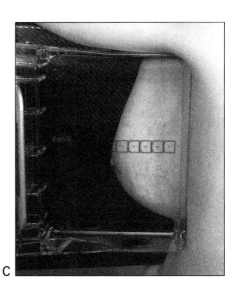

A　　　　　　　　B　　　　　　　　C

Figure 7-167
The LM projection relies on specific positioning maneuvers to adequately visualize breast tissue: **(A)** superoposterior tissue is visualized by bringing the upper thorax in contact with the image receptor; **(B)** after securing capture of posteromedial tissue, posterolateral tissue is brought forward at approximately 90° from the thorax as the breast is anchored to the image receptor; **(C)** upon completion of positioning maneuvers and compression, the superior corner of the compression device is positioned just anterior to the latissimus dorsi muscle.

capture deep lateral lesions near the chestwall and can be combined with spot compression (Figure 7-170).

Laterally Exaggerated Craniocaudal Projection Summary

1. The C-arm can be angled 0° to 5° for the XCCL projection.
2. The x-ray beam is directed superiorly to inferiorly, as with the CC projection.

3. Initially the patient stands facing the unit.
4. Elevate the IMF using a flat hand, palm up, placed firmly against the patient's ribcage—ensuring the capture of the outer breast margin.
5. Adjust the image receptor height to the level of the elevated outer breast.
6. Rotate the patient's body and feet approximately 45° from the image receptor, placing the posterolateral (outer) breast in contact with the image receptor

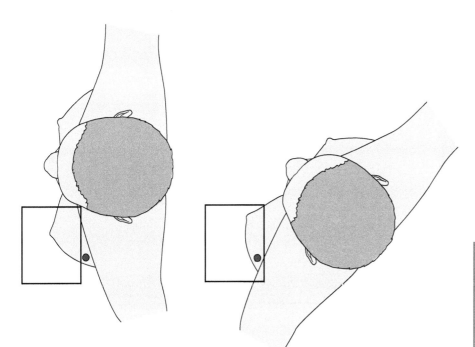

Figure 7-168
The XCCL is used to image the outer breast for better visualization of posterolateral tissue. Schematic illustrating the value of the XCCL projection to visualize posterolateral breast tissue not able to be included on the CC projection.

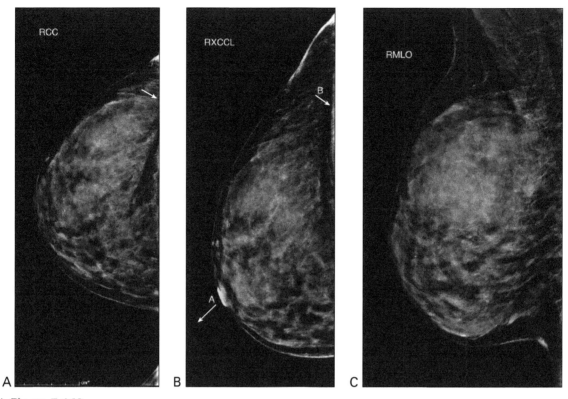

Figure 7-169
(A) Approximately 10% of women have glandular tissue that extends laterally beyond the capture of the CC projection (*arrow*). **(B)** Adding an XCCL to the screening examination includes as much lateral and axillary tail tissue as possible; note the diagonal direction of the nipple (labeled *A*) and pectoral muscle (labeled *B*) parallel to the image receptor. **(C)** RMLO projection included to demonstrate dense breast tissue extending to the chestwall.

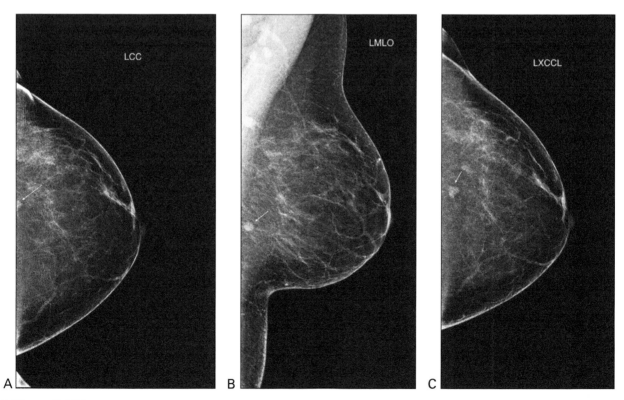

Figure 7-170
For diagnostic purposes, the XCCL projection is useful to capture deep lateral lesions near the chestwall. **(A)** LCC projection demonstrates slightly lateral posterior lesion, margins not completely visualized (*arrow*). **(B)** RMLO projection with *arrow* indicating posterior lesion. **(C)** RXCCL projection with posterior lesion margins adequately visualized (*arrow*).

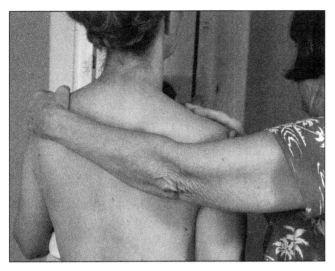

Figure 7-171
The patient's ipsilateral shoulder should not lean toward the image receptor, but remains equal to the height of the contralateral shoulder throughout positioning maneuvers for the XCCL.

chestwall edge. In this orientation, when the breast is brought onto the image receptor, the nipple is directed to the far medial corner.

7. The patient's ipsilateral shoulder should not recline toward the image receptor, but remains equal to the height of the contralateral shoulder throughout positioning maneuvers for the XCCL (Figure 7-171).

8. With the breast elevated, bring the posterolateral breast tissue onto the image receptor until the thorax meets the chestwall edge of the receptor. Anchor the tissue onto the image receptor, ensuring deep posterolateral tissue is positioned in the field of view.

9. Apply compression ensuring that the compression device avoids coming into contact with the humeral head.

10. Hold the breast in place, continuing to anchor the posterior breast tissue onto the image receptor until the compression device replaces the anchoring hand.

Additional Tips for the XCCL Projection

- If the compression device is obstructed by the shoulder, the C-arm may be rotated up to 5° in the same orientation as the MLO projection. When properly positioned, minimal pectoral muscle is visualized at the margin of the image.[28]
- In order to maximize the contact of the compression device against the chestwall for deep capture of tissue adjacent to the thorax, position the lateral chestwall compression device rise just to the inside of the humeral head.
- For patients with physical limitations such as a frozen shoulder or who are kyphotic, it may be necessary to angle the C-arm more than 5°. The C-arm angulation used is indicated on the image as the radiologist may use

this view to localize an abnormality. A generous convex pectoral muscle presentation indicates that the patient is reclined laterally toward the image receptor or that an excessive angle has been placed on the C-arm or a combination of these actions.

- To visualize deep posterolateral tissue when using the 18 × 24-cm compression device to perform the XCCL projection, one of the two methods could be employed:
  1. Shift the compression device to the right position on the image receptor when performing a RXCCL and to the left position when performing a LXCCL. Position the lateral chestwall compression device rise just to the inside of the humeral head (Figure 7-172).
  2. Place the compression device in the center of the IRSD. Position the patient off-center to the IRSD. Positioning the patient in this way allows the lateral chestwall compression device rise to be placed just inside of the humeral head.

Cleavage (CV) Projection

Application

The cleavage projection is used to demonstrate deep posteromedial breast tissue and is performed by placing both breasts on the image receptor (Figure 7-173). Imaging this area of the breast securely is difficult due to the inability to freely move the fixed superior and medial borders. For patients with large breasts requiring tiling or mosaic imaging to complete the exam, the cleavage view may be useful for exam management in capturing both the right and the left medial breast margins on one image (Figure 7-174). When attempting to capture a lesion deep in the posteromedial breast, using the 10-cm contact compression device may aid in this process (Figure 7-175). The cleavage view may also be used as a complementary projection for patients with chestwall anomalies.

Exposure Preparation

Slightly offsetting the affected breast from the center of the image receptor allows the use of phototiming. Manual technique should be used if offsetting the breast tissue from center is not done or if there is insufficient tissue to cover the AEC detector.

Cleavage Projection Summary

1. Position the C-arm at 0° for the cleavage projection.
2. The patient stands facing the image receptor, approximately a hands-width distance from the receptor. Positioning the area of interest slightly off center on the image receptor enables the use of the AEC.

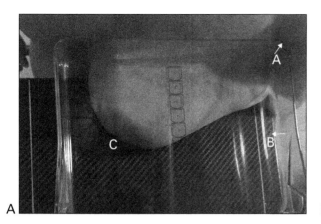

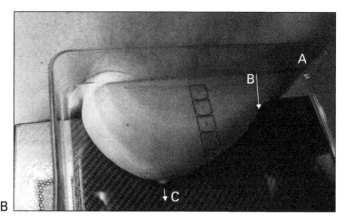

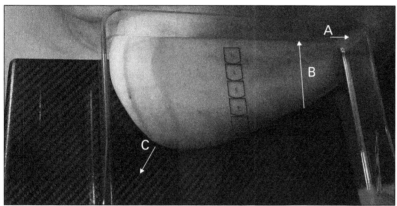

Figure 7-172

Three examples of positioning the LXCCL projection. The technologist must be mindful of the electronic dead space located at the side edges of the IRSD and potential tissue that may be excluded. **(A)** Larger breast positioned using the 24 cm × 30-cm-size compression device; note the placement of the lateral chestwall corner of the compression device positioned just inside the humeral head (labeled A), the electronic dead space at the image receptor side edge (labeled B), and the diagonal nipple direction (labeled C). **(B)** Smaller breast using the 18 × 24-cm-size compression device positioned in the center of the IRSD; note the placement of the lateral chestwall corner of the compression device positioned on the outside of the humeral head (labeled A) preventing deep capture to the thorax depth of posterolateral tissue captured (labeled B) and the nipple direction perpendicular to the chestwall (labeled C). **(C)** Smaller breast with the 18 × 24-cm compression device shifted to the left position on the image receptor; note the placement of the lateral chestwall corner of the compression device positioned just inside the humeral head (labeled A), depth of posterolateral tissue capture (labeled B), and diagonal nipple direction (labeled C).

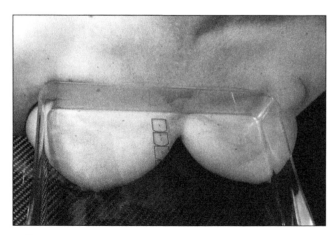

Figure 7-173

The CV projection is used to demonstrate deep posteromedial breast tissue and is performed by placing both breasts on the image receptor.

3. Turn the patient's head away from the affected breast. The technologist may stand either behind or in front of the patient.

4. Elevate both breasts, leaning the patient's upper body forward. Initially, adjust the height of the image receptor to meet the level of the cleavage, although refinement of the image receptor height is necessary for each patient. The height of the image receptor is critical in capturing cleavage anatomy and should be carefully adjusted during positioning. An image receptor positioned too low excludes superomedial tissue, while positioned too high excludes inferomedial tissue. For a lesion already identified in the cleavage area from a screening exam, the height of the image receptor is determined by its location.

5. Guide both breasts onto the image receptor until the thorax meets the receptor, head positioned around the

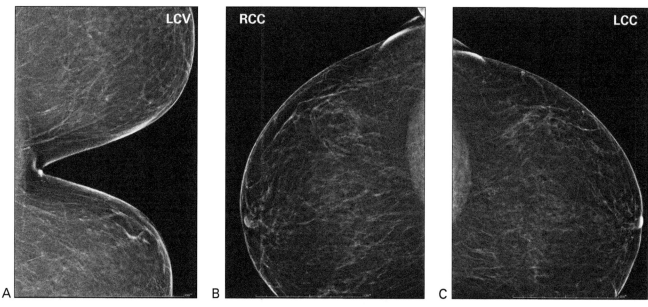

Figure 7-174
For patients with large breasts requiring tiling or mosaic imaging to complete the exam, **(A)** the CV may be useful for exam management in capturing both the right and the left medial breast margins on one image. **(B)** RCC and **(C)** LCC projections include the lateral breast margins.

face shield. If possible, demonstrate the cleavage in an open position, separating the breasts to prevent tissue overlap.

Axillary Tail (AT) Projection

Application

The AT projection is performed to demonstrate the entire AT and includes most of the superolateral aspect of the breast. It is used primarily for visualization of glandular breast tissue very high in the axilla that is inadequately

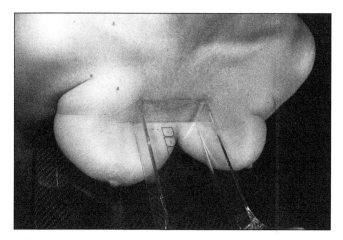

Figure 7-175
The 10-cm contact compression device may be useful for difficult-to-capture lesions located in the posteromedial aspect of the breast.

imaged on the MLO. The AT projection uses a C-arm angle that is customized to parallel the angle of the patient's AT angle. This angle is determined for each patient by imagining an oblique line drawn from the nipple to the axilla.

Axillary Tail Projection Summary

1. The C-arm angle is customized for each patient. To find the angle, imagine an oblique line from the nipple to the axilla. Using two hands to sandwich the breast along this imaginary line assists in defining each patient's obliquity and to envision the angle the image receptor should be rotated parallel to.

2. Rotate the C-arm parallel to the natural angle defined by the "line" sandwiched between the technologist's two hands (Figure 7-176). The degree varies from one patient to another, but will generally be angled between 60° and 80°.

3. The image receptor is placed just below shoulder level, with the patient's body slightly rotated away from the unit. The AT projection does not replicate the MLO projection and requires the patient's body be placed in more of an anterior to posterior position on the image receptor rather than the patient's feet and pelvis directly facing the unit as required by the MLO projection.

4. Drape the patient's ipsilateral arm over and behind the image receptor, with elbow flexed and the hand resting on the C-arm.

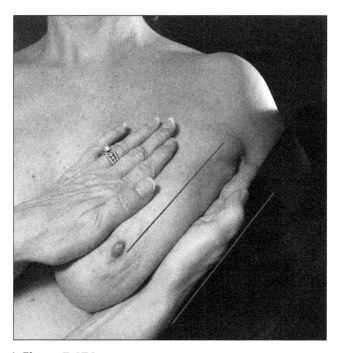

Figure 7-176
For the AT projection, the C-arm is rotated parallel to an angle determined from the nipple to the axilla for each individual patient. This "angle" can be found by sandwiching these two points between the technologist's hands and imagining a straight line connecting the nipple and the axilla.

5. Gently pull the AT of the breast out and away from the chestwall, anchoring the lateral aspect of the breast against the image receptor.
6. Secure the AT in place until the compression device replaces the flat hand (Figure 7-177).
7. The AT projection includes anatomy high into the axilla. When positioning the AT projection, be attentive to the tissue visualized within the light field and mindful of the electronic dead space located superiorly on the DR FFDM detector.

Tangential (TAN) Projection

Application

The tangential (TAN) projection, first described by Logan Young,[10] directs the x-ray beam **tangential** to the area of interest (Figure 7-178). This view is primarily used to evaluate palpable abnormalities surrounded by dense glandular tissue or to determine if calcifications detected on the mammography image are located within the skin.

Palpable Abnormalities

A metallic BB is placed on the skin in the location of the palpable abnormality. The tangential view skims the metallic marker, projecting the area of interest within the subcutaneous fatty layer of tissue, differentiating this tissue from that of the surrounding tissue. The tangential view affords

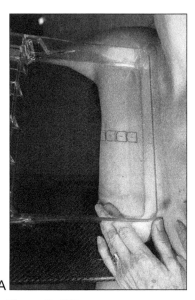
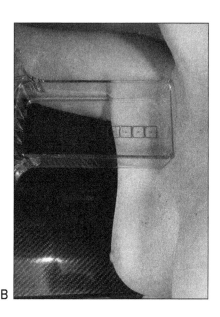
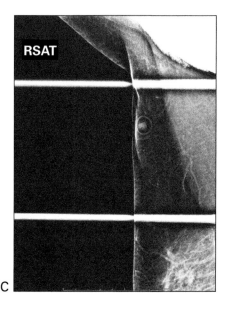

A   B   C

Figure 7-177
The AT projection does not replicate the MLO projection and **(A)** requires the patient's body be placed in more of an anterior to posterior position on the image receptor rather than the patient's feet and pelvis directly facing the unit as required by the MLO projection. The image receptor is placed just below shoulder level, with the patient's body rotated away from the unit. **(B)** The 10-cm contact compression device may be useful for difficult-to-capture lesions located in the axillary tail region. **(C)** Using the 10-cm contact compression device, the AT projection verifies the presence of a mole in the axilla.

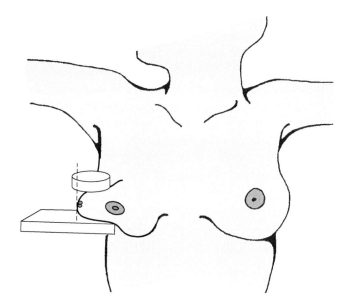

Figure 7-178
The TAN projection directs the x-ray beam tangential to the area of interest. This view is primarily used to evaluate palpable abnormalities surrounded by dense glandular tissue or to determine if calcifications detected on the mammographic image are located within the skin.

the best image of a suspected abnormality, projecting it free of **superimposition** and often bringing it closer to the image receptor for optimum detail.

This view is especially useful for visualizing palpable abnormalities that remain occult on the two-view mammogram and for demonstrating areas of interest in a dense breast. Projecting the abnormality adjacent to subcutaneous adipose tissue results in an increase in subject contrast to enhance radiographic characteristics. The 7.5-cm compression device is commonly used for the tangential view, providing additional benefit for evaluation.

Tangential Projection Summary

Palpable Abnormality

- The angle of obliquity is dependent on the location of the palpable abnormality in the breast. To determine the angle of obliquity, imagine a line drawn from the nipple to the palpable abnormality. Using two hands to sandwich the breast from the nipple to the palpable abnormality assists in defining the obliquity and to envision the angle the image receptor should be rotated parallel to. Rotate the C-arm so that the image receptor parallels the imagined line. Rules of thumb for determining the rotation of the C-arm are:
  - Abnormalities in the upper inner or lower outer quadrant require an SIO of some degree, depending on the location of the abnormality (Figure 7-179A).

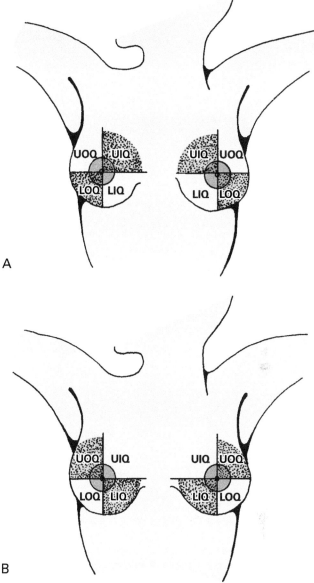

A

B

Figure 7-179
Appropriate projections for tangential view. **(A)** ROI in the upper inner quadrant (UIQ) or lower outer quadrant (LOQ) requires a SIO of some degree when performing the TAN projection. **(B)** Areas in the upper outer quadrant (UOQ) or lower inner quadrant (LIQ) require an MLO of some degree when performing the TAN projection.

  - Abnormalities in the upper outer or lower inner quadrant require a MLO of some degree, depending on the location of the abnormality (Figure 7-179B).
  - A Lateral projection best visualizes abnormalities that approximate 12:00 or 6:00.
  - A CC projection or (variation of the CC) best visualizes abnormalities that approximate 3:00 or 9:00.

Figure 7-180 illustrates correlation of the location of the abnormality with the appropriate angle of the C-arm,

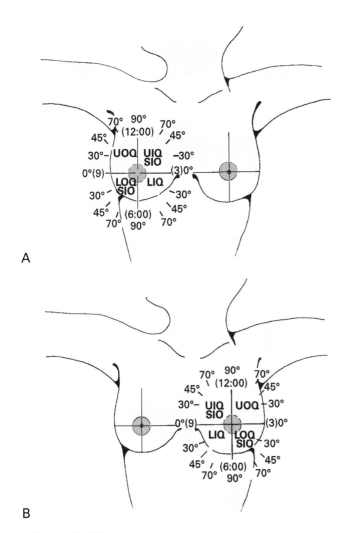

A

B

Figure 7-180
Degree of angle for the TAN projection. Correlate the location of the abnormality with the degree of rotation of the C-arm; note that an angle of the C-arm will demonstrate both an upper quadrant and a lower quadrant abnormality tangentially. Note the right breast (**A**) and the left breast (**B**) schematics for the TAN projections.

and Figures 7-181 through 7-185 illustrate the application of tangential positioning. The projection and angle of the C-arm should always be marked on the TAN image to document the location of the lesion being imaged.

Skin Calcifications

Calcifications detected on screening mammography may have characteristics suggesting they are benign dermal calcifications located within the skin. Place a metallic BB on the suspected skin calcifications. Use the appropriate tangential projection to image the metallic marker to verify whether or not the calcifications are in the skin, saving the patient from the anxiety and stress of a biopsy.

1. Proving skin calcifications on the image requires the use of a localization compression device.
2. Evaluate the screening mammogram projections (CC and MLO) identifying the calcifications on each projection. Based on the location of the calcifications on the breast surface (superior, inferior, medial, or lateral), determine which approach provides the easiest access to the calcifications.
3. Using the localization compression device, choose the projection that allows accessibility to the surface of the breast containing the calcifications: CC, FB*, ML, and LM.
4. It is helpful to have the patient seated for the initial exposure, ensuring her safety should a vasovagal reaction occur.
5. Compress the breast placing the localization compression device against the surface of the breast containing the calcifications.
6. With the compression automatic release function disabled, make an exposure.
7. Evaluate the alphanumeric coordinating points to locate the calcifications on the breast, marking first with a skin marker and then applying the metallic BB over the marked skin (this ensures the location of the calcifications should the metallic BB accidentally be removed during the following positioning maneuvers) (Figure 7-186).
8. Release compression after calcifications have been marked with the metallic BB.
9. Imagine a line drawn from the nipple to the metallic BB, rotating the C-arm parallel to the imagined line. Using two hands to sandwich the breast from the nipple to the metallic BB assists in defining the obliquity and to envision the angle the image receptor should be rotated parallel to.
10. Using magnification, position the BB in profile on the magnification stand. Ensuring the calcifications are projected in profile can be done with the assistance of a white sheet of paper to optimize visualization of the metallic BB. Tuck the paper just under the edge of the breast, casting the shadow of the metallic BB onto the paper. When the metallic BB is projected in profile, compress the breast using the 7.5-cm magnification compression device. Remove the paper prior to exposure (Figure 7-187).
11. With the BB imaged in profile using the tangential projection, the location of the calcifications is verified (Figure 7-188).
12. For access to skin calcifications located inferiorly on the breast, lay the patient on her side on a cart, rotating the C-arm to the FB (from below) approach. This FB approach places the superior breast in contact with the image receptor and the localization device in contact with the inferior breast. Resume following steps 9 to 11. *Additional information on the FB projection is explained later in this chapter.

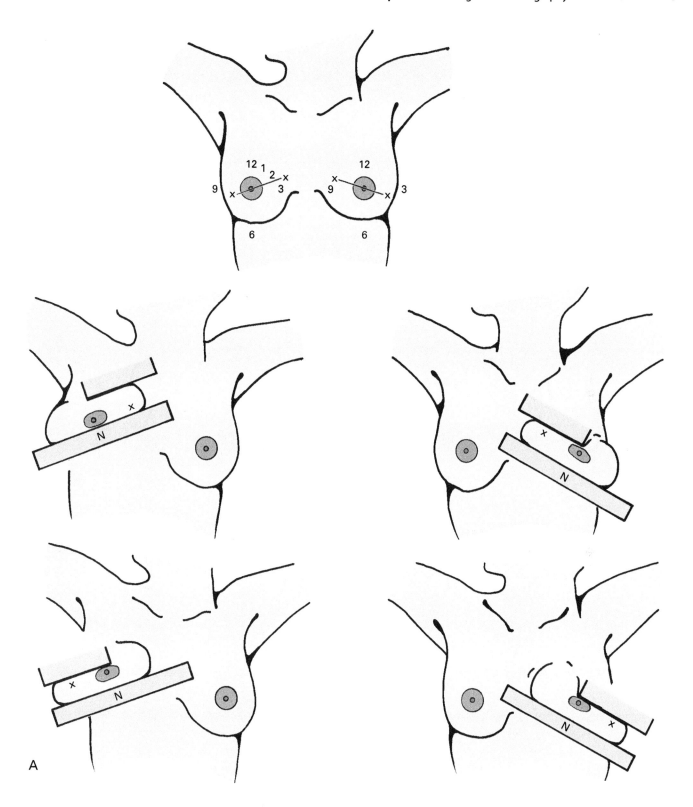

A

Figure 7-181
TAN projection. **(A)** If the lesion lies at 2:30 or 8:30 in the right breast or 9:30 or 3:30 in the left breast, then a SIO projection of about 15° will demonstrate these areas tangentially. Again, note that a certain C-arm angle illustrates both an upper quadrant and lower quadrant abnormality tangentially.

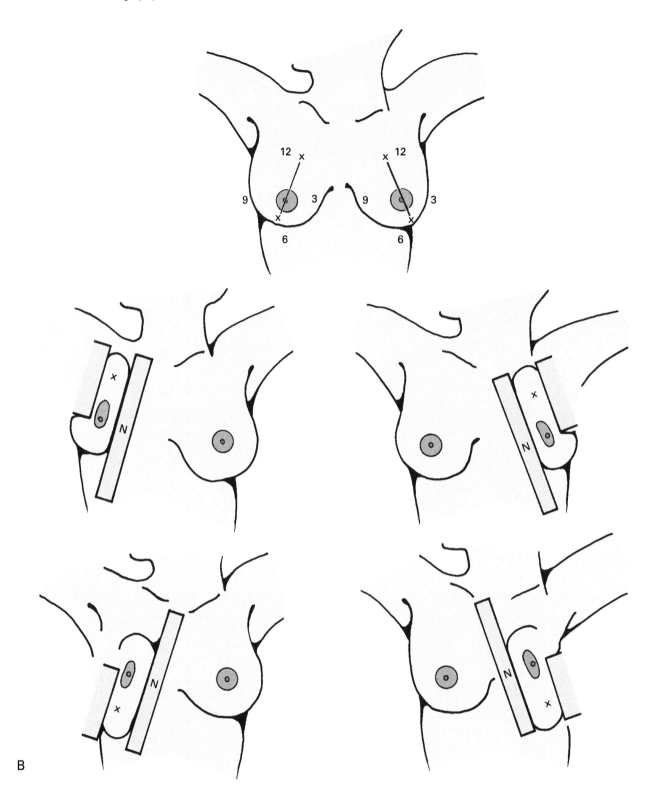

B

Figure 7-181 (*Continued*)
(B) If the lesion lies at 1:00 or 7:00 in the right breast or 11:00 or 5:00 in the left breast, then a SIO projection of about 70° will demonstrate these areas tangentially.

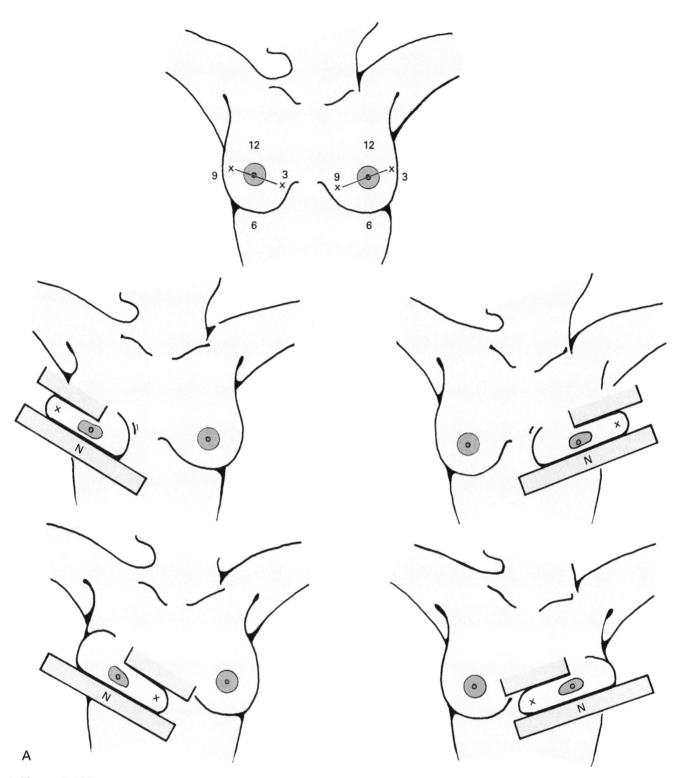

A

Figure 7-182
TAN projection. **(A)** If the lesion lies at 9:30 or 3:30 in the right breast or 8:30 or 2:30 in the left breast, then an MLO projection of about 15° will demonstrate these areas tangentially. Again, note that a certain C-arm angle illustrates both an upper quadrant and a lower quadrant abnormality tangentially.

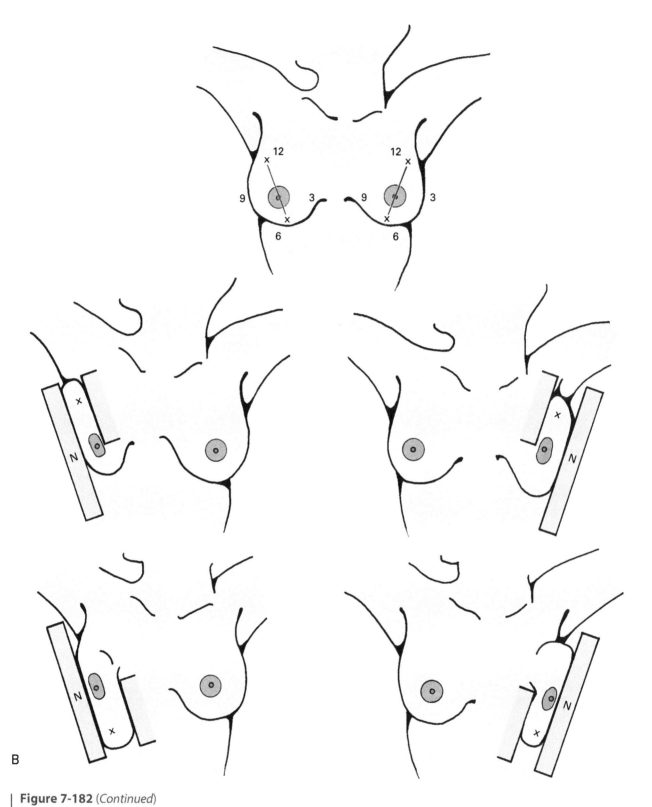

B

Figure 7-182 (*Continued*)
(B) If the lesion lies at 11:00 or 5:00 in the right breast or 1:00 or 7:00 in the left breast, then an MLO projection of about 70° will demonstrate these areas tangentially.

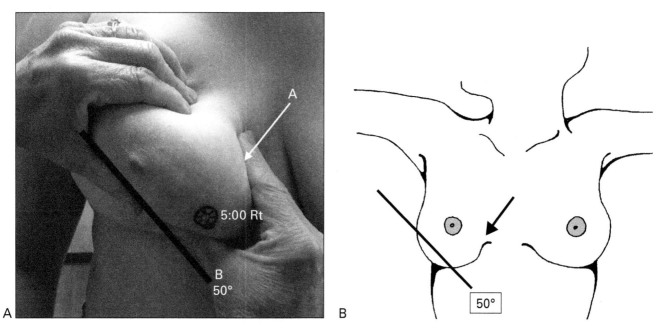

Figure 7-183
TAN projection. **(A)** Finding the angle for the TAN projection when the abnormality lies at 5:00 in the right breast: x-ray beam (labeled *A*) is perpendicular to the image receptor (labeled *B*); image receptor positioned parallel to an imaginary line drawn from the nipple to the metallic marker. **(B)** Schematic illustrating that a 50° MLO angle demonstrates the 5:00 area of the right breast in tangent.

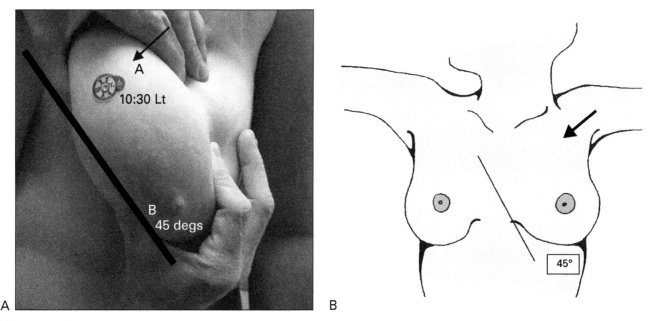

Figure 7-184
TAN projection. **(A)** Finding the angle for the TAN projection when the abnormality lies at 10:30 in the left breast: x-ray beam (labeled *A*) is perpendicular to the image receptor (labeled *B*). Image receptor is positioned parallel to an imaginary line drawn from the nipple to the metallic marker. **(B)** Schematic illustrating that a 45° SIO angle demonstrates the 10:30 area of the left breast in tangent.

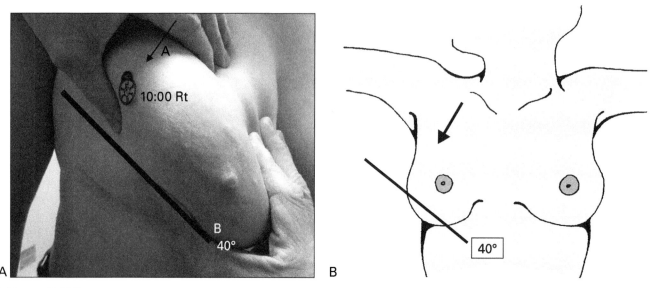

Figure 7-185
TAN projection. **(A)** Finding the angle for the TAN projection when the abnormality lies at 10:00 in the right breast: x-ray beam (labeled *A*) is perpendicular to the image receptor (labeled *B*). Image receptor positioned parallel to an imaginary line drawn from the nipple to the metallic marker. **(B)** Schematic illustrating that a 40° MLO angle demonstrates the 10:00 area of the right breast in tangent.

Rolled Projection (RM, RL, RI, RS)

Application

The rolled projection is performed to evaluate areas of breast tissue that give the impression of a suspected abnormality (asymmetry), but may simply be the result of superimposed tissue. Confirming the presence of a true lesion is done by rolling the breast in opposite directions. When the breast tissue presentation is altered from the original image using the rolled technique, superimposed (overlapping) breast structures separate, no longer demonstrating the suspected abnormality (Figure 7-189). Lesions that persist after the rolled views are performed continue to be investigated using various projections and techniques such as triangulation, discussed earlier in this chapter, to specifically locate the area of concern in the breast. It is possible to broadly determine

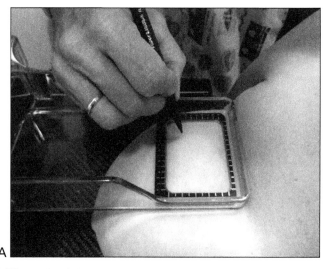

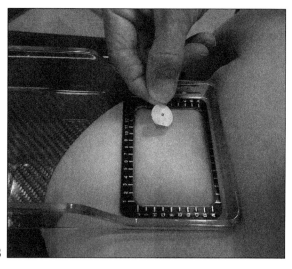

Figure 7-186
Using the TAN projection and the localization compression device to prove skin calcifications. **(A)** Assess the alphanumeric coordinate points on the mammogram image to locate the calcifications on the breast, marking first with a skin marker. **(B)** Apply the metallic BB over the marked skin. This sequence ensures the location of the calcifications should the metallic BB accidentally be removed during the remaining positioning maneuvers.

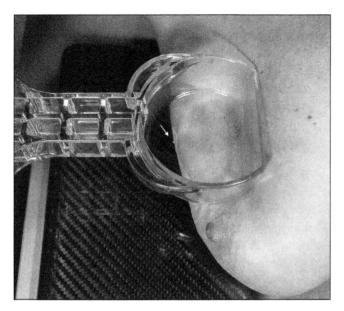

Figure 7-187
Using the TAN projection combined with spot magnification technique to prove skin calcifications: after determining the correct angle for the C-arm to place the abnormality in tangent, the metallic BB is positioned in profile on the magnification stand. Using the 7.5 spot compression device, compress the breast tissue ensuring the shadow of the metallic BB is projected onto image receptor.

lesion location within the breast using the rolled projections depending on the ratio of fatty versus dense glandular tissue and the tissue distribution. If it is possible to observe the suspected lesion when rolled into the fatty area of the breast,

the location may be indicated by the direction of the rolled tissue. The rolled projection can be done using the CC, MLO, or Lateral projections. The use of rolled projections to define, confirm, or locate an abnormality is determined by radiologist guidance and/or protocol and may include the projection performed in both directions or a singular direction (Figure 7-190). The projection summary example used in this section describes the use of the rolled views in the CC position.

Rolled Medial Projection Summary

1. The C-arm is positioned at 0° for the RM (rolled medial) projection.
2. The patient stands facing the unit as for the CC projection.
3. The thorax is positioned approximately a hands width from the image receptor.
4. Standing on the medial side of the patient, elevate the IMF using a flat hand in firm contact with the chestwall. Adjust the image receptor height to the elevated IMF. Place the opposite hand on the superior breast in firm contact with the chestwall.
5. The patient leans her upper body forward, relaxing the shoulders and thorax.
6. Using both hands, firmly grasp the breast, simultaneously rolling the superior breast medially and the inferior breast laterally. Hold the breast securely in the rolled position while bringing the thorax in contact with the image receptor, guiding the breast onto the receptor. The hand in contact with the inferior breast tissue follows the path

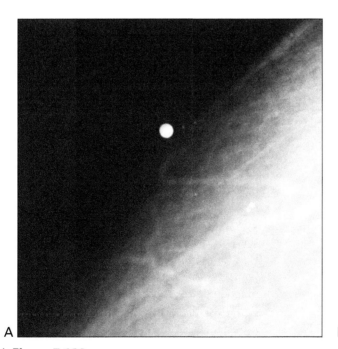
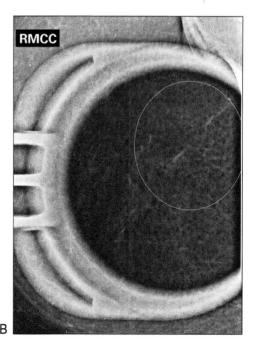

A   B

Figure 7-188
(A) With the metallic BB imaged in profile using the tangential projection, the location of the calcifications is verified.
(B) LMCC projection demonstrating calcifications originally detected on the screening examination.

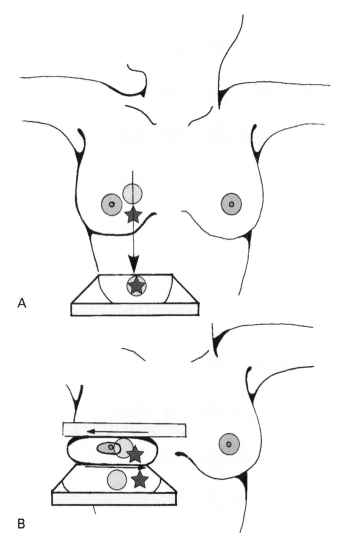

A

B

Figure 7-189
Rolled projection concept. **(A)** "Rolled" projections can solve the dilemma of overlapping structures or superimposed breast tissue. **(B)** Rolling the top half of the breast in one direction and the bottom half in the opposite direction separates superimposed tissue by projecting them away from each other.

of the lateral direction as it relinquishes contact with the breast, leaving the hand securing the superior tissue to anchor the breast in the medially rolled position.

7. Apply compression as the anchoring hand securing the superior breast slides out in a medial direction, continuing to ensure the superior breast is rolled medially until the compression device replaces the anchor hand. The projection is labeled RCCRM or LCCRM (right craniocaudal rolled medial or left craniocaudal rolled medial).

Rolled Lateral Projection Summary

1. The C-arm is positioned at 0° for the RL (rolled lateral) projection.

2. The patient stands facing the unit as for the CC projection.

3. The thorax is positioned approximately a hands width from the receptor.

4. Standing on the lateral side of the patient, elevate the IMF using a flat hand in firm contact with the chestwall. Adjust the image receptor height to the elevated IMF. Place the opposite hand on the superior breast in firm contact with the chestwall.

5. The patient leans her upper body forward, relaxing the shoulders and thorax.

6. Using both hands, firmly grasp the breast, simultaneously rolling the superior breast laterally and the inferior breast medially. Hold the breast securely in the rolled position while bringing the thorax in contact with the image receptor, guiding the breast onto the receptor. The hand in contact with the inferior breast tissue follows the path of a medial direction as it relinquishes contact with the breast, leaving the hand securing the superior tissue to anchor the breast in the laterally rolled position (Figure 7-191).

7. Apply compression as the anchoring hand securing the superior breast slides out in a lateral direction, continuing to ensure the superior breast is rolled laterally until the compression device replaces the anchor hand. The projection is labeled RCCRL or LCCRL (right craniocaudal rolled lateral or left craniocaudal rolled lateral).

Additional Observations of the Rolled Projection (RM, RL)

- Give thought to hand positions used for the direction of the rolled tissue. The technologist's hand that is in contact with the superior breast is the hand that is moved toward the technologist's body as compression is applied. This action ensures the hand continues to roll the breast in the labeled direction as it is removed from the field of view.

- Rolled view labeling follows the general description of the rolled direction of the tissue in contact with the compression device.
  ○ For CCRM, the superior tissue is in contact with the compression device and is rolled medially (Figure 7-192A).
  ○ For CCRL, the superior tissue is in contact with the compression device and is rolled laterally (Figure 7-192B).
  ○ For MLRI, the medial breast is in contact with the compression device and is rolled inferiorly (Figure 7-192C).
  ○ For MLRS, the medial breast is in contact with the compression device and is rolled superiorly (Figure 7-192D).

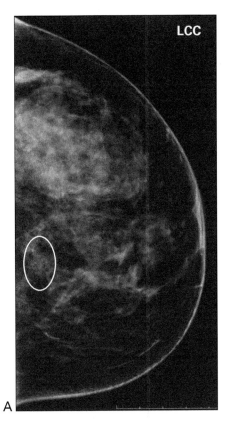
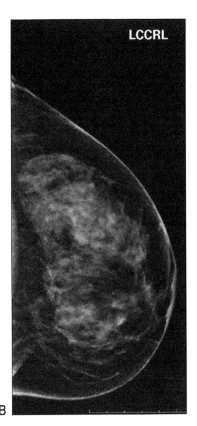

Figure 7-190
The use of rolled projections to define, confirm, or locate an abnormality is determined by radiologist guidance and/or protocol and may include the projection performed in both directions or a singular direction. **(A)** LCC projection demonstrating posterior ROI (*circle*), suspected superimposition of breast tissue. **(B)** LCCRL projection demonstrates separation of normal glandular tissue.

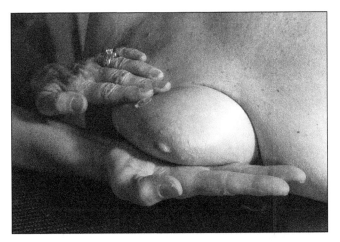

Figure 7-191
RCCRL projection demonstrating that the hand in contact with the inferior breast tissue withdraws in a medial direction as it relinquishes contact with the breast, leaving the hand securing the superior tissue to anchor the breast in the laterally rolled position.

From Below (FB) Projection (Caudocranial Projection)

Application

The FB projection uses an inferior to superior (caudocranial) x-ray beam direction, with the C-arm rotated 180° from the craniocaudal C-arm position. This projection is not commonly used as it can be challenging for the technologist and uncomfortable for the patient. The patient is required to straddle the tube housing in order to approach the unit. Although inverting the C-arm 180° positions the face shield to guard the abdomen from the field of view, it is challenging to ensure artifact-free images (Figure 7-193). The projection is used to evaluate abnormalities located in the superior breast as the area of interest is located closer to the detector, increasing sharpness due to reduced object-to-image receptor distance. The 180° rotation of the C-arm allows the compression device to

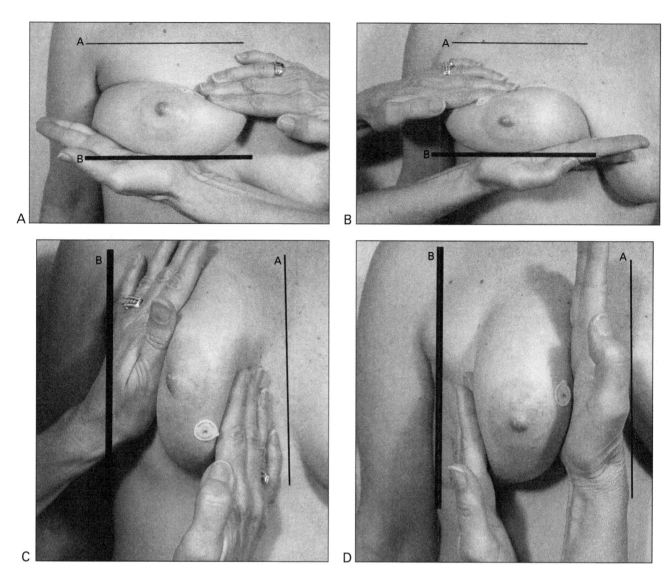

Figure 7-192
Rolled view labeling is determined by the rolled direction of the tissue in contact with the compression device. **(A–D)** the compression device (labeled *A*) and the image receptor (labeled *B*) assist in determining appropriate projection labeling; note the presence of a metallic marker to assist in visualizing the rolled tissue direction. **(A)** For CCRM, the superior tissue is in contact with the compression device and is rolled medially. **(B)** For CCRL, the superior tissue is in contact with the compression device and is rolled laterally. **(C)** For MLRI, the medial breast is in contact with the compression device and is rolled inferiorly. **(D)** For MLRS, the medial breast is in contact with the compression device and is rolled superiorly.

move the mobile inferior portion of the breast toward the fixed superior portion, providing a positioning benefit to patients with implanted medical devices and imaging the male breast. For some women with kyphosis, the FB projection may aid in capturing additional breast tissue; however, the same affect can be achieved by having the patient seated for the CC projection. Finally, the FB projection is used as the approach for presurgical needle localization or for core biopsy when the lesion is located in the inferior breast.

Case Study 7 Part **2-2**

1. Refer to Figures 7-193 and 7-194. Describe the use of the FB projection: when is it appropriate to use this projection; what are its advantages over the CC projection and its disadvantages; what is the acceptable angle of the IRSD; and why is it named FB rather than CC (caudocranial)?

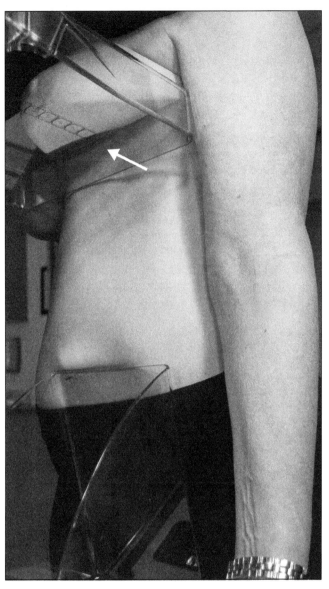

Figure 7-193
The FB projection uses an inferior to superior (caudocranial) x-ray beam direction, with the C-arm rotated 180° from the craniocaudal C-arm position. Although inverting the C-arm 180° positions the face shield to guard the abdomen from encroaching on the field of view, it is challenging to ensure artifact-free images; note the superimposition of the abdomen into the FOV (*arrow*) resulting in posterior artifact on the image.

From Below Projection Summary

1. The C-arm is rotated 180° with the image receptor and the compression device inverted from the CC position.
2. The patient faces the unit, straddling the tube housing. Adjust the height of the image receptor to a level allowing adequate visualization of the superior breast (or area of interest).
3. Elevate the IMF. With two flat hands, firmly sandwich the breast at the chestwall margin.

4. The patient leans forward, bringing the breast tissue onto the image receptor. Slide the hand in contact with the superior breast out following the path of the nipple.
5. To bring the superior breast tissue into closer proximity with the image receptor, and for additional patient comfort, place the patient's contralateral arm on the inverted undersurface of the image receptor and lay the patient's head on her arm (Figure 7-194).

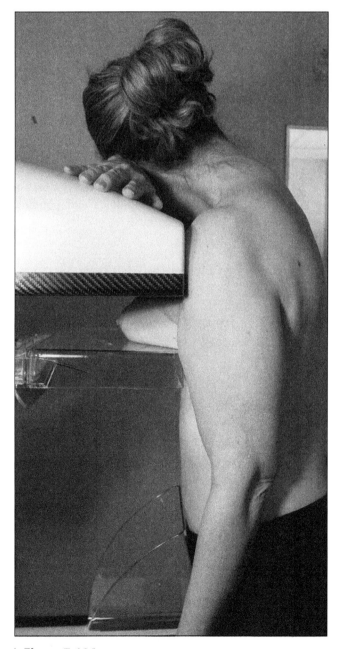

Figure 7-194
To bring the superior breast tissue into closer proximity with the image receptor, and for additional patient comfort, place the patient's contralateral arm on the inverted undersurface of the image receptor and rest the patient's head on her arm.

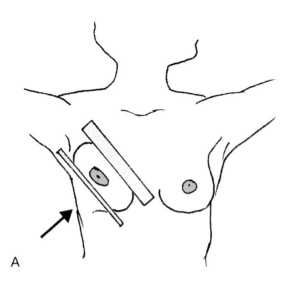

A

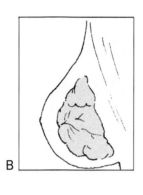

B

Figure 7-195
LMO projection. **(A)** Schematic illustrating the orientation of the C-arm for the LMO projection. **(B)** Schematic demonstrating the amount of the "glandular island" usually included with this view.

6. With the superior tissue in contact with the image receptor, anchor the breast to the image receptor with a flat hand against the inferior breast.
7. Apply compression, keeping the breast anchored to the image receptor until the compression device replaces the supporting hand in contact with the inferior breast.
8. Assess the breast tissue for skinfolds and potential patient artifacts prior to exposure.

Lateromedial Oblique (LMO) Projection

Application

The Lateromedial Oblique (LMO) projection (Figure 7-195) is a true reverse of the MLO projection, resulting in similar tissue demonstration as the MLO image.[8] The C-arm is rotated toward the ipsilateral breast, using an inferolateral to superomedial x-ray beam direction (lower outer quadrant to upper inner quadrant) (Figure 7-196). The LMO is effective as a replacement view for the MLO in patients who have an implanted medical device, history of open heart surgery, or other nonconforming situations. Using the principle of positioning, the inverted C-arm allows the compression device to move the mobile inferolateral tissue toward the fixed superomedial tissue, providing additional comfort to the patient by avoiding contact of the compression device with the superomedial region. The LMO also is used to further define lesion characteristics of abnormalities located in the superomedial aspect of the breast due to reduced object-to-image receptor distance.

Lateromedial Oblique Projection Summary

1. Rotate the C-arm to approximately 125° toward the ipsilateral breast. The position of the C-arm at this rotation is a true reverse from the C-arm position for

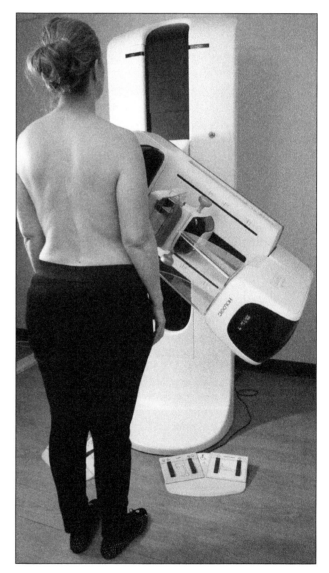

Figure 7-196
LMO projection. The C-arm is rotated toward the ipsilateral breast, using an inferolateral to superomedial x-ray beam direction (lower outer quadrant to upper inner quadrant).

the MLO projection. Further minor adjustment of the C-arm angle is necessary for each patient.

2. Determine the customized angle of the patient's pectoral muscle using method a or b:

   a. Because the C-arm for the LMO projection is inverted from the MLO position, it is advantageous to parallel the angle of the pectoral muscle to the inverted compression device rather than using the image receptor for this purpose.

   b. To determine the angle of C-arm rotation: 180° – angle of the MLO = angle for the LMO. For example, the MLO was done at 45°. The LMO angle is 180° – 45° = 135°; rotate the C-arm to 135°.

3. The patient stands facing the unit, midsternum slightly off center from the image receptor—toward the contralateral breast. This action ensures far medial tissue located at the sternum is included in the image. The medial aspect of the ipsilateral breast is in contact with the image receptor.

4. Adjust the height of the image receptor to the approximate level of the suprasternal notch. Additional minor adjustment may be necessary to ensure capture of superior and inferior margins of the breast for each patient.

5. Raise the patient's ipsilateral arm up and over, resting the arm on the image receptor (Figure 7-197).

6. Lean the patient onto the image receptor ensuring contact of the upper thorax and sternum.

7. Place a flat hand between the image receptor and the medial breast near the chestwall edge of the image receptor at the sternum, to gently pull and free any medial tissue caught under or behind the image receptor.

8. Using two hands, firmly capture and pull the breast tissue outward, approximately 90° from the chestwall.

9. Slide the hand in contact with the medial breast out following the path of the nipple.

10. With a flat hand, anchor the breast against the image receptor, supporting the lateral tissue in the outward and upward position to open the IMF as compression is applied; patient's feet and pelvis face the unit.

11. Lateral to medial projections allow additional rotation of the patient's thorax toward the image receptor as compression is applied for maximum capture of posterolateral tissue; completion of compression places the superior corner of the chestwall rise of the compression device just anterior to the latissimus dorsi muscle (Figure 7-198).

12. Ensure the IMF is open and free of skinfolds and airgaps by using fingers to sweep medial and lateral breast tissue downward.

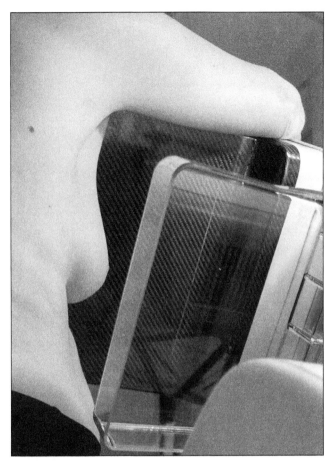

Figure 7-197
LMLO projection. The image receptor is adjusted to the approximate level of the suprasternal notch; the patient's ipsilateral arm is raised up and over, resting the upper humerus on the superior edge of the IRSD as she leans forward ensuring contact of the upper thorax and sternum to the chestwall edge of the image receptor.

Superolateral to Inferomedial Oblique (SIO) Projection

Application

The SIO projection utilizes an x-ray beam direction from superolateral to inferomedial (upper outer quadrant to lower inner quadrant). The C-arm is rotated to approximately 45° (Figure 7-199). Technologists easily recall this position of the image receptor by remembering the following simple concept: *the C-arm angle used to image the MLO for the right breast is the exact same C-arm angle used to image the SIO for the left breast, and vice versa* (Figure 7-200).

The SIO is useful in the following situations:

• The SIO projection best demonstrates the upper inner quadrant (UIQ) and lower outer quadrant (LOQ) of the breast free of superimposition of the upper outer and lower inner tissue.

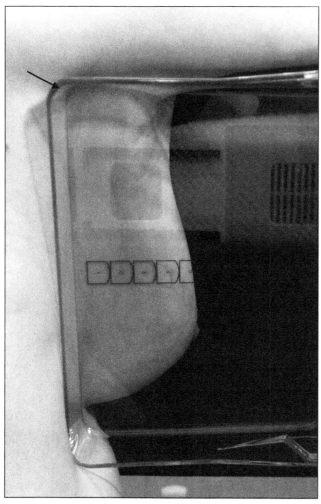

Figure 7-198
Lateral to medial projections allow additional rotation of the patient's thorax toward the image receptor as compression is applied for maximum capture of posterolateral tissue; completion of compression places the superior chestwall corner of the compression device just anterior to the latissimus dorsi muscle (*arrow*).

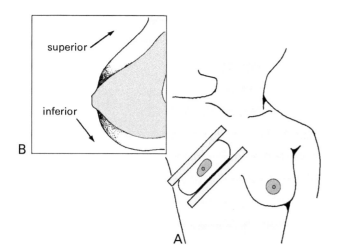

Figure 7-199
SIO projection. **(A)** Schematic of the orientation of the breast to the C-arm for the SIO projection. **(B)** Schematic demonstrating the amount of the "glandular island" usually included in this view.

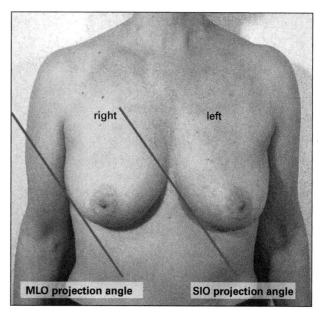

Figure 7-200
Technologists easily recall the position of the image receptor for the SIO projection by remembering the following simple concept: the C-arm angle, used to image the MLO for the right breast, is the exact same C-arm angle used to image the SIO for the left breast, and vice versa.

- For women with encapsulated breast implants, the 60° SIO may serve as an additional projection to visualize the UIQ and LOQ tissue hidden on the CC and the MLO views.
- A 45° SIO provides a perpendicular projection to the MLO and may be useful in distinguishing superimposition of breast tissue.
- For patients with chestwall anomalies, such as pectus excavatum, a 45° SIO can assist in capturing medial breast tissue not seen on the standard views.
- Finally, the SIO is an excellent complement to the MLO, visualizing the far posteroinferior breast in the IMF region. Using the superolateral to inferomedial x-ray beam direction while customizing the angle of the equipment to the IMF region of the patient allows for easier manipulation to include and open the IMF.

The SIO projection is sometimes mistaken for the reverse MLO projection, and technologists should have a detailed understanding of the x-ray beam directions and uses for these two very different projections.

Superolateral to Inferomedial Oblique Projection Summary

1. Rotate the C-arm approximately 45° in a superolateral to inferomedial x-ray beam direction.
2. The patient faces the unit, slightly off centering the sternum to the image receptor toward the contralateral breast. This action ensures the medial tissue attached to the sternum is included on the image (Figure 7-201).

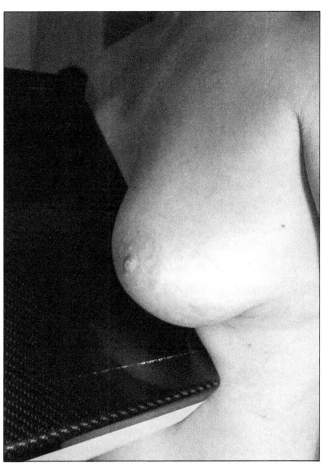

Figure 7-201
For the SIO projection, the patient faces the unit, slightly off centering the sternum to the image receptor toward the contralateral breast. This action ensures the medial tissue attached to the sternum is included on the image.

3. Bring the patient forward with the thorax and medial breast in contact with the image receptor.
4. Adjust the receptor height to approximately the suprasternal notch. Additional minor adjustment may be necessary to ensure capture of superior and inferior margins of the breast for each patient.
5. Raise the ipsilateral arm of the patient up and over the image receptor; rest the forearm, elbow flexed, on the superior edge of the receptor.
6. The patient leans toward the image receptor, with upper body supported by the mammography unit and sternum parallel to the receptor (Figure 7-202).
7. Adjust the C-arm to a customized angle for visualization of the IMF region and to enhance the patient's comfort.
8. Using a flat hand to capture the medial breast, place the fifth finger against the chestwall edge of the image receptor at the sternum, gently pulling and freeing any medial tissue caught under or behind the image receptor. Firmly, pull the breast tissue straight out away from the chestwall.

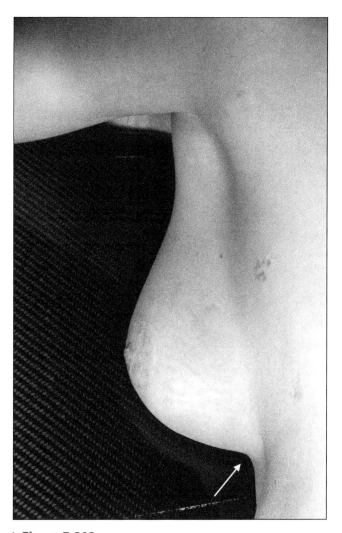

Figure 7-202
The image receptor height is adjusted to approximately the suprasternal notch. Raise the ipsilateral arm of the patient up and over the image receptor to rest the forearm, elbow flexed, on the superior edge of the IRSD. The patient leans toward the image receptor, with upper body supported by the mammography unit and sternum parallel to the receptor. Note the IMF presentation on the SIO projection (*arrow*).

9. The flat hand used to capture the medial tissue now rotates its position, coming in contact with the lateral breast, in order to capture and pull the lateral tissue outward, approximately 90° from the chestwall.
10. With a flat hand, anchor the breast against the image receptor, supporting the lateral tissue in the outward and upward position to open the IMF as compression is applied; patient's feet and pelvis face the unit.
11. Continue to lower the compression device along the posterior and lateral ribs, including as much lateral tissue as possible until the compression device replaces the anchoring hand (Figures 7-203 and 7-204).

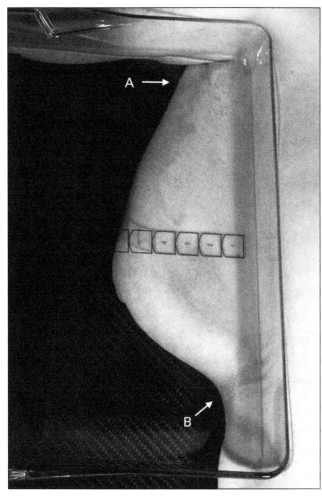

Figure 7-203
SIO projection. As compression is applied, the breast is anchored to the image receptor while the lateral breast is supported in an outward and upward position to open the IMF; the feet and pelvis face the unit. The compression device comes into contact with the posterior and lateral ribs, including as much lateral tissue as possible; note the decreased amount of superior tissue captured (*arrow A*) when compared to the MLO projection; and note the positioning benefit to the IMF region (*arrow B*) when using the SIO.

Techniques

Mammography technologists must be familiar with the specialized techniques described in Table 7-4. These techniques are used for problem solving in various breast imaging situations.

Spot Compression Technique

Spot compression is an invaluable technique used in mammography for further investigation of suspect findings identified on screening or diagnostic examinations. While the standard contact compression device uniformly compresses the entire breast, the true spot (7.5 cm) compression device provides focal compression to the ROI, separating overlapping tissue and reducing breast

thickness (Figure 7-205). This problem-solving technique allows better definition of lesion characteristics, assisting radiologists in determining the final BIRADS assessment for the patient, and their appropriate future care. This technique provides the following information:

- To confirm the presence of a lesion (is the lesion "real"?)
- To better evaluate the border of a mass lesion by minimizing overlapping tissue
- To capture and secure difficult-to-reach tissue
- Further definition of asymmetric tissue or architectural distortion

Case Study 7 Part 2-3

Refer to Figures 7-205 and 7-206.

1. List the reasons why a radiologist would request spot compression views.

2. Is spot compression done in conjunction with magnification or without?

3. Describe how the technologist transfers the area to be spot compressed from viewing the ROI on a computer monitor to placing this same area under the spot compression device on the mammography machine.

4. Will the use of DBT increase or decrease the need for spot compression images?

The technique of using the true spot compression device (7.5 cm) can be challenging to the technologist. The goal is to position the area of concern in the center of the spot compression device to achieve maximum compression advantage and to determine extent of disease (Figure 7-206). In reality, this goal is difficult to achieve, but the technologist can be reasonably successful by employing techniques using the transfer of careful measurements from the original image to the patient's breast, attempting to duplicate the original positioning using the spot compression device. The ACR describes the use of a three-point measurement technique[8] (Figure 7-207) using a ruler or the width of the technologist's fingers to target the lesion on the original image (Figure 7-208). Digital mammography equipment and PACS systems each are equipped with an electronic ruler for exact measurements of an ROI on the original image. The image used for measurement must be of "true size" proportion shown on the monitor for accurate information to be transferred to the patient's breast tissue. A CC image is used to provide an example of this measurement technique.

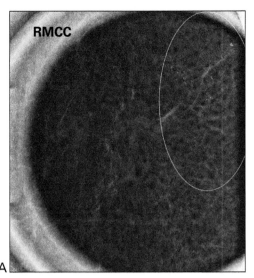
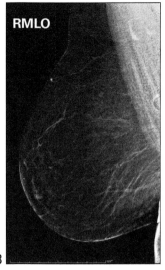
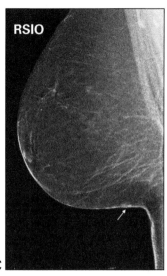

Figure 7-204
SIO positioning benefit for the IMF region. **(A)** RMCC demonstrates suspected dermal calcifications originally detected on the RCC (*circle*). **(B)** RMLO insufficiently visualizes IMF region. **(C)** SIO projection opens the IMF region for adequate evaluation of calcifications (*arrow*); subsequent magnified TAN projection proved dermal calcifications (see Figure 7-188A).

1. Measure from the skinline at the nipple to the ROI to find the depth of the lesion.
2. Draw an imaginary line from the nipple to the posterior margin of the image. Measure medially or laterally from the imaginary line to the ROI.
3. Measure from the ROI to the skinline edge.

Experienced technologists may rely on a two-measurement technique, omitting the third detail. The three-measurement technique offers an additional benefit as it addresses the potential of breast rotation differences between the original image and the spot compression image. Using a skin marker, place a very small mark on the skin indicating the target (Figure 7-209A). Carefully place the target point under the center of the spot compression device without introducing a change of position to the breast. Apply focal compression (Figure 7-209B). When the tissue is secured, but not yet fully compressed, make additional marks on the skin indicating the posterior edge of the compression device and two anterior points if desired. This "road map" is essential for repositioning when the ROI is not included on the image. Resourceful technologists have two colors of markers available for spot compression, using one color for the CC image and another color for the MLO image. When using a spot compression device, adequate breast compression cannot be evaluated by the same methods used with a standard contact compression device: tapping the skin for tautness. The spot compression device requires the technologist to evaluate compression individually for each patient and situation. Educating the patient using a teamwork approach, providing encouragement, and applying compression slowly yield a superior result. The measurement technique described for spot targeting in the CC projection is also commonly used for the MLO and Lateral projections. In addition to using the small spot compression device for defining lesion characteristics, it also may be used to capture and secure tissue in challenging circumstances. For larger area ROIs or for patients with very large breasts, the option of the 10-cm-size contact compression device may be useful.

Table 7-4 • This Table Provides a Quick Reference for Each of the Techniques Used in Mammography, Detailing Indications for Their Use and the Value They Contribute to Tissue Visualization

TECHNIQUE	ACR ID	TISSUE BEST VISUALIZED	APPLICATIONS
Spot Compression		ROI	Palpable abnormality, to visualize borders with better detail; often used in conjunction with magnification
Magnification	M	ROI	Improved resolution; better visualizes calcifications and borders of lesions
Triangulation		ROI	For further investigation when an abnormality is seen on only one standard image, to determine the location of an abnormality for biopsy
Implant Displaced	ID	Tissue anterior to implant	Patients with implants

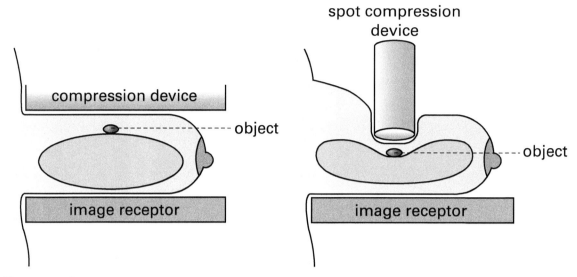

Figure 7-205
Spot compression, in either the contact or magnification mode, is used in mammography for further investigation of suspect findings. While the standard contact compression device uniformly compresses the entire breast, the true spot (7.5 cm) compression device provides focal compression to a ROI, separating overlapping tissue and reducing breast thickness. (Modified from Tabar L. *Diagnosis and In-Depth Differential Diagnosis of Breast Diseases.* Mammography Education, Inc.; 1990. Reprinted with permission of Mammography Education, Inc.)

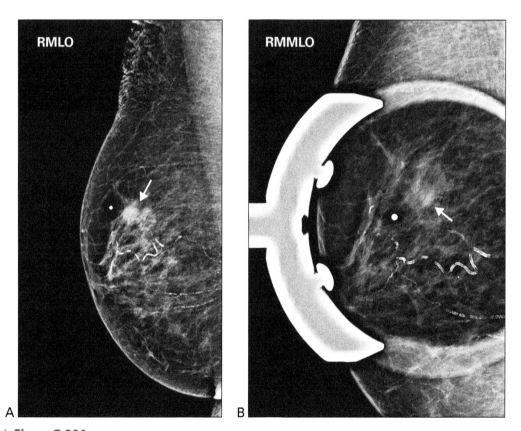

Figure 7-206
Spot compression technique. **(A)** Metallic marker placed on palpable lump in the RMLO projection demonstrates a lesion. **(B)** RMMLO with spot compression. Although it is challenging to position the area of concern in the center of the true spot compression device (7.5 cm), achieving this allows maximum compression over the ROI and better visualization of surrounding ROI tissue. Due to enhanced lesion characteristics demonstrated on the magnified spot compression image, a biopsy was recommended for this patient.

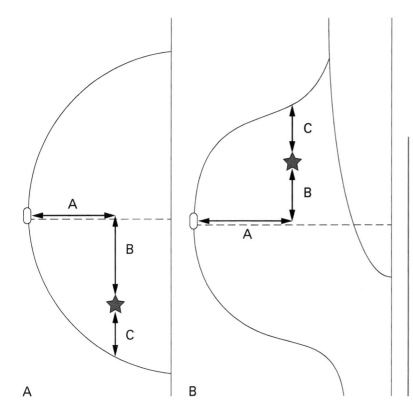

A   B

Figure 7-207
Positioning the lesion in the center of the 7.5-cm spot compression device can be accomplished using a three-point measurement technique. **(A)** CC projection: the depth of the lesion is measured (labeled *A*); the distance either medially or laterally from an imaginary line (indicated by *dotted line*) drawn from the nipple to the chestwall is measured (labeled *B*); the distance from the lesion to the skinline is measured (labeled *C*). **(B)** The same measuring concept is applied for the MLO or the Lateral projection; only "label *B*" is different; the distance either *superiorly* or *inferiorly* from an imaginary line (indicated by *dotted line*) drawn from the nipple to the chestwall. (Modified from American College of Radiology. *Mammography Quality Control Manual.* Reston VA: American College of Radiology Committee on Quality Assurance in Mammography; 1999.)

DBT may utilize the spot compression technique; however, it should be noted that the need to use additional imaging is reduced by approximately 40% with DBT.

Magnification Spot Compression Technique

When further evaluation of microcalcifications is needed or when trying to discern the border of a finite mass lesion detected on standard projection images, combining the technique of focal spot compression with the **magnification** mode enhances lesion definition because spatial resolution is increased (Figure 7-210). Combining these two problem-solving techniques (spot compression with magnification) assists radiologists in determining the final BIRADS assessment for the patient and their appropriate future care. The magnification

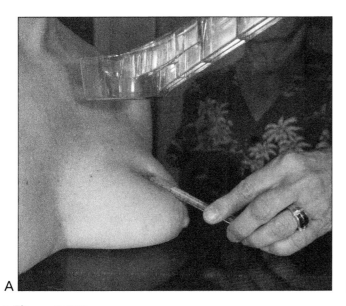

A

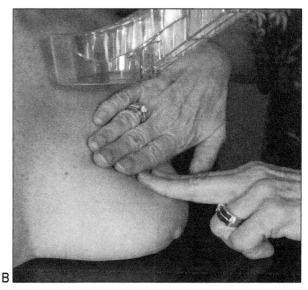

B

Figure 7-208
The ACR describes the use of a three-point measurement technique to target the lesion on the original image and to transfer these measurements to the patient's breast tissue. Employ either one of the following methods: **(A)** Use of a ruler: digital equipment uses an electronic ruler to measure the location of the lesion on the original image. **(B)** Use the width of the technologist's fingers as a ruler.

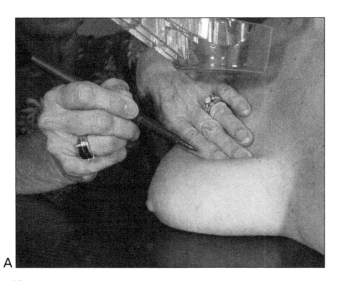
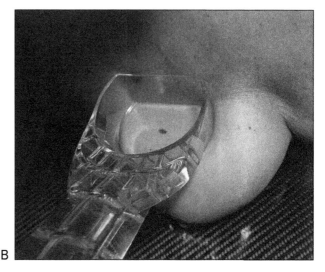

Figure 7-209
(A) To ensure the lesion is centered under the spot compression device, place a very small mark on the skin indicating the target. **(B)** Carefully, and mindful of minimizing rotation, move the breast placing the target point under the center of the spot compression device, and apply focal compression.

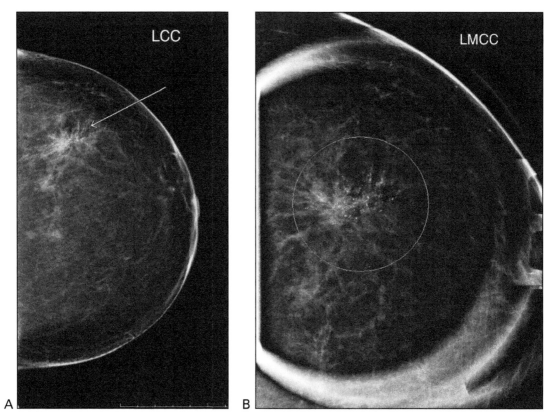

Figure 7-210
When trying to discern the border of a finite mass lesion or when further evaluation of microcalcifications is needed, combining the technique of focal spot compression with the magnification mode enhances lesion definition because spatial resolution is increased. **(A)** LCC standard projection demonstrating microcalcifications (*arrow*). **(B)** LMCC improves definition of lesion characteristics (*circle*) due to increased spatial resolution.

mode is not available in DBT due to the limited area of the detector surface used in magnification and the required sweep of the C-arm for tomosynthesis. Magnified spot compression for 2D FFDM imaging is valuable in determining:

- Additional mass information such as mass margins or the presence of microcalcifications
- Defining calcifications: size, shape, number, and distribution
- Confirming the presence of additional microcalcifications not visualized on the original screening image
- Evidence of additional masses
- Further definition of asymmetric tissue or areas of architectural distortion

Measurement techniques used in magnification spot compression are the same as those described for contact spot compression. The mag stand/tube housing configuration may be a limiting factor for some projections depending on where the area of concern is located within the breast.

Triangulation

Discussion of the triangulation technique is included in the Lateral projection discussed earlier in this chapter.

Implant Displaced (ID)-Modified Compression Technique for Augmented Breasts

Application

Imaging patients with breast implants due to breast augmentation can be challenging and requires specific training for technologists performing modified positioning/compression techniques. Implant imaging is addressed in the Mammography Quality Standards Act of 1992.[29] Under MQSA regulations, facilities are required to have procedures in place to identify patients with breast implants and to provide imaging projections for maximizing visualization of breast tissue. A typical examination for a woman with implants consists of images with the implant in place followed by images where the implant is excluded. The modified compression technique, recognized by the ACR as **implant displaced** (ID) views, used for imaging patients with breast augmentation offers an improvement in breast tissue visualization in 99% of patients[30] (Figure 7-211). This technique is appropriate for retromuscular (posterior to the pectoral muscle) or retroglandular (posterior to the glandular tissue, anterior to the pectoral muscle) implants, as long as the implant remains soft and free of encapsulation (Figure 7-212). This method allows capture and compression of breast tissue not visualized due to implant

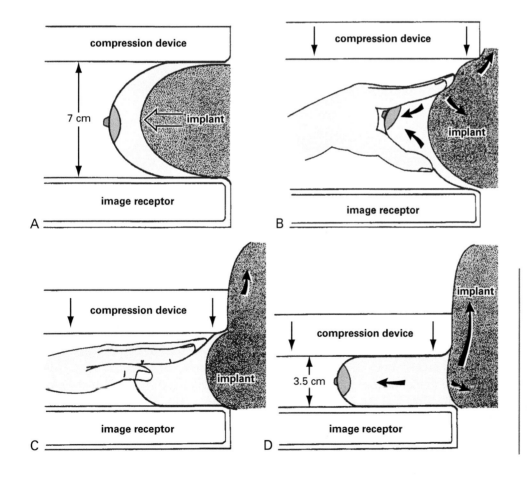

Figure 7-211
Modified compression technique. **(A)** Schematic of the breast with implants illustrating nondisplaced positioning and minimal compression. **(B–D)** Use of the *modified compression technique*, displacing the implant posteriorly and superiorly, to image the breast free of superimposition and with better compression. (Courtesy Dr. G. Eklund.)

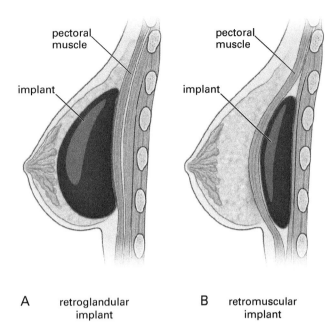

Figure 7-212
The modified compression technique, referred to as ID views, is appropriate for **(A)** retroglandular (posterior to the glandular tissue, anterior to the pectoral muscle) or **(B)** retromuscular (posterior to the pectoral muscle) implant placement.

superimposition on the nondisplaced images. The implant is manipulated posteriorly toward the chestwall ensuring its exclusion from capture and compression.[8,30] The portions of the breast anterior to the implant are brought forward onto the image receptor and held in position until compression is applied. The ID technique is performed in addition to the routine two-projection mammogram; it is not considered as a substitution because it does not include the most posterior margins of the breast (Figure 7-213). The mammography examination for women with implants includes the following projections for patients who present with soft, pliable implants. The total examination for both breasts includes eight images:

Routine Nondisplaced MLO and CC Projections (MLO and CC)
1. Routine nondisplaced MLO for the right and the left breast, labeled RMLO and LMLO
2. Routine nondisplaced CC for the right and the left breast, labeled RCC and LCC

Position the breast plus implant in the usual manner for the MLO and CC projections, with one very important difference: minimal compression, just enough to immobilize the breast, is used (Figure 7-214). Typically, a manual selection of exposure factors is used with the nondisplaced views; however, technologists should know the operating procedure for the digital system they are using.

Modified Compression MLO and CC Projections (MLOID) (CCID)
3. MLO with modified compression for the right and for the left breast, labeled RMLOID and LMLOID
4. CC with modified compression for the right and for the left breast, labeled RCCID and LCCID

Encapsulated Implants (Capsular Contracture)
The modified compression technique is performed easily on patients with soft, pliable implants. However, some patients develop a condition called capsular contracture, or **encapsulated** implants, making it difficult to manipulate the implant for the modified technique. This condition affects retroglandular implants more often than retromuscular implants. It may also be difficult to manipulate the implant of patients with very little natural breast tissue anterior to the implant. When ID views cannot be performed due to encapsulation, or difficulty in capturing tissue anterior to the implant in a small breasted woman, an additional nondisplaced Lateral projection is added to the routine nondisplaced CC and MLO views. This nondisplaced Lateral projection provides additional visibility of tissue superimposed by the implant on the nondisplaced CC and MLO projections (Figure 7-215).

Case Study 7 Part **2-4**

Refer to Figure 7-215.

1. When a woman with implants presents for imaging, what conditions prohibit manipulation of the implants to perform the ID technique?

2. When ID views cannot be performed, what is the geometric workaround to include all parts of the breast?

Implant Displaced Views

Craniocaudal (ID) Summary
1. The patient faces the technologist, bending forward at the waist, relaxed.
2. Using both hands, the technologist simultaneously "walks" the implant posteriorly toward the chestwall with her fingers, easing superior and inferior tissue forward to securely capture the natural breast tissue anterior to the implant (Figure 7-216).
3. While firmly holding the breast tissue anterior to the implant, instruct the patient to stand erect, facing the unit.

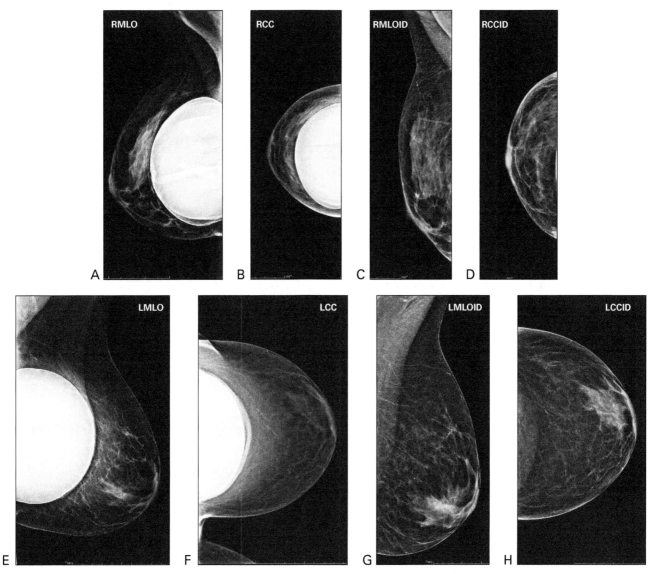

Figure 7-213
The modified compression technique allows capture and compression of breast tissue not visualized due to implant superimposition on the nondisplaced images. The ID technique is performed in addition to the routine two-projection mammogram; it is not considered as a substitution because ID views do not include the most posterior margins of the breast. Example: nondisplaced and ID projections of retroglandular placed implants, **(A)** RMLO, **(B)** RCC, **(C)** RMLOID, **(D)** RCCID and retromuscular placed implants, **(E)**LMLO, **(F)** LCC, **(G)** LMLOID, and **(H)** LCCID.

4. Place the patient's contralateral hand against her ribcage under the ipsilateral breast (Figure 7-217).
5. Adjust the height of the image receptor to the level of the breast tissue.
6. Using both hands, pull only the breast tissue anterior to the implant onto the image receptor.
7. The chestwall edge of the image receptor replaces the position of the fingers holding the inferior tissue (Figure 7-218A).
8. Continue to displace the implant on the superior aspect of the breast as compression is applied to the natural breast tissue (Figure 7-218B).

9. Use AEC if there is enough tissue to cover the AEC detector; if not, select a manual technique.

Mediolateral Oblique (ID) Summary
1. Customize the C-arm angle to the patient's natural pectoral muscle angle.
2. The patient faces the unit, slightly off center from the image receptor, ensuring the IMF region is engaged in front of the receptor.
3. Raise the patient's arm, placing the corner of the image receptor anterior to the latissimus dorsi muscle.

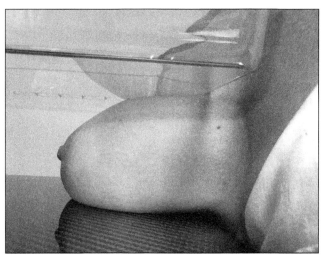

Figure 7-214
The mammography examination for women with implants includes a total of eight images. The four nondisplaced MLO and CC images include the breast plus the implant in the usual manner, with one very important difference: minimal compression, just enough to immobilize the breast, is used.

4. Slightly move the patient's thorax posteriorly, creating an airgap for the implant between the chestwall edge of the image receptor and the thorax.
5. Using both hands, the technologist simultaneously "walks" the implant posteriorly toward the chestwall

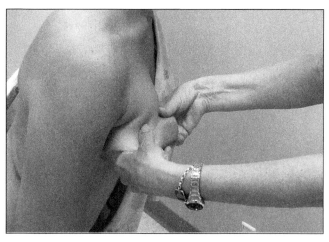

Figure 7-216
To perform the CCID view, the technologist uses both hands to simultaneously "walk" the implant posteriorly toward the chestwall with her fingers, easing superior and inferior tissue forward to securely capture the natural breast tissue anterior to the implant.

with her fingers, easing medial and lateral tissue forward to securely capture the natural breast tissue anterior to the implant.
6. With fingers securely holding the implant posteriorly, the edge of the technologist's fingers holding the implant at the lateral aspect of the breast is placed at the chest

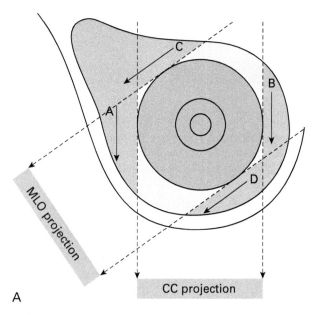

A

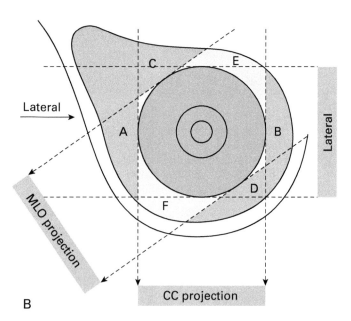

B

Figure 7-215
Imaging the patient with encapsulated breast implants: some patients develop encapsulated implants making it difficult to manipulate the implant for the modified implant technique. When ID views cannot be performed, a nondisplaced Lateral projection is included to visualize tissue not seen on the nondisplaced CC and MLO projections. When ID views cannot be performed, **(A)** labels *A* and *B* demonstrate tissue included on the CC projection; *arrows* indicate beam direction. Labels *C* and *D* demonstrate tissue included on the MLO projection; *arrows* indicate beam direction. *Light–gray* areas are not visualized using the routine nondisplaced projections. **(B)** An additional Lateral projection included in the exam increases tissue visualization of *light–gray* areas (labeled *E* and *F, arrow* indicates beam direction). (Modified from Eklund GW, Cardenosa G. The art of mammographic imaging. *Radiol Clin North Am.* 1992;30(1).)

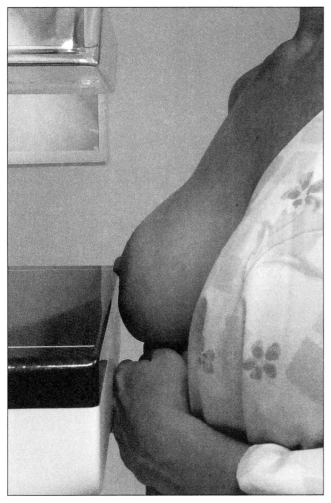

Figure 7-217
CCID views. To ensure the implant is posterior to the light field, a space is created between the chestwall edge of the image receptor and the patient's thorax. Place the patient's contralateral hand against her ribcage under the ipsilateral breast; the hand fills the space to ensure stability. Instruct the patient to stand erect, facing the unit.

wall edge of the image receptor; the implant should be positioned posterior to the receptor; the patient's thorax may need further adjustment during this maneuver to accommodate the implant size.

7. Continue to hold the implant posteriorly on the medial aspect of the breast as compression is applied to the natural breast tissue (Figure 7-219).

Additional Tip for Performing the MLOID Projection
- After walking the implant posteriorly toward the chestwall and placing the breast tissue anterior to the implant on the image receptor, while still holding the breast, instruct the patient to bend her ipsilateral knee and slouch. This action relaxes the thorax allowing easier

manipulation of the implant for the remainder of the positioning/compression maneuvers.
- MLOID views may exclude inferoposterior tissue. If necessary, the 10-cm-size contact compression device may be used to capture this tissue for further definition (Figure 7-220).

Additional Problem-Solving Projections

Sometimes, technologists need to "think outside the box," behaving more like a creative "portable" mammography technologist as opposed to rote performance of the standard projections on all patients. Technologists who think in terms of "What anatomy needs to be captured on the image?" and "How will the equipment work to achieve that capture with clarity?" move beyond the borders controlled by exact projection labels. Communication and consultation with the interpreting radiologist are necessary when stepping outside of the recognized boundaries of problem solving. Technologists familiar with standardized additional projections combined with equipment operation knowledge have the confidence to make innovative equipment modifications when confronted with challenging positioning/compression circumstances. Historical problem-solving projections exist that are not recognized in the ACR grouping of additional imaging projections, but remain invaluable for their contribution of mammographic problem solving. These tested projections have proved their reliability over time and are worthy of continued familiarity by technologists. These projections, illustrated in Table 7-5, are used in circumstances when suspected abnormalities are difficult to capture.

Medially Exaggerated Craniocaudal (XCCM) Projection

The medially exaggerated craniocaudal (XCCM) projection,[7] like the cleavage (CV) view, is another projection used to visualize the posteromedial aspect of the breast tissue (Figure 7-221). The CC projection emphasizes the inclusion of all medial tissue on the image due to the possible exclusion of this region on the MLO projection. However, for patients who have chestwall anomalies such as pectus excavatum or pectus carinatum, or for patients with posteromedial suspected abnormalities, the XCCM may be a valuable additional projection. It is performed by rotating the patient medially toward the image receptor, exaggerating the posteromedial tissue capture. The C-arm is positioned at 0° or customized to a shallower angle for each patient. Customizing this angle captures the natural attachment of the medial breast curvature to the thorax.

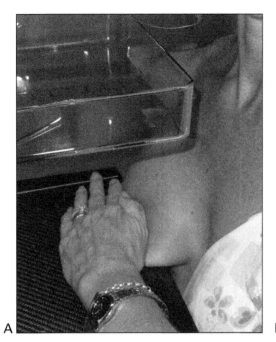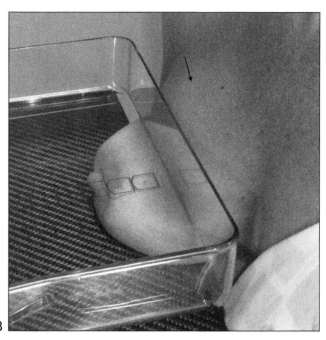

A   B

Figure 7-218
CCID views. The technologist uses both hands to pull the breast tissue forward, ensuring only breast tissue anterior to the implant is included on the image receptor. **(A)** As the natural tissue comes into contact with the IRSD, the chestwall edge of the image receptor replaces the work of the technologist's fingers that are in contact with the inferior breast tissue. **(B)** Compression is applied to the natural breast tissue anterior to the implant; note the "bulge" of the implant between the image receptor and the patient's thorax (*arrow*).

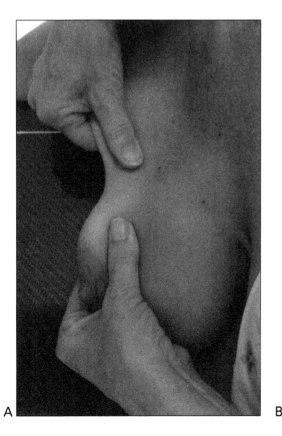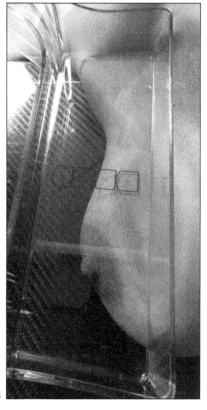

A   B

Figure 7-219
MLOID views: to accommodate the implant, a space is created between the chestwall edge of the image receptor and the thorax. **(A)** The technologist captures the natural breast tissue anterior to the implant by using both hands to simultaneously "walk" the implant posteriorly toward the chestwall while easing medial and lateral tissue forward. **(B)** The implant is secured in its "space" between the image receptor and the thorax as compression is applied to the natural breast tissue.

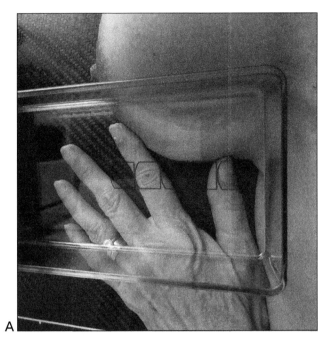
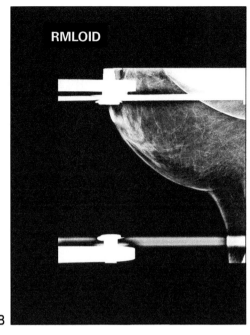

A   B

Figure 7-220
MLOID views may exclude inferoposterior tissue. **(A)** RMLOID view displaces the implant superiorly. **(B)** RMLOID demonstrates the IMF region using the 10-cm-size contact compression device; this projection is not included in established protocol for implant imaging, but can be added when warranted.

Table 7-5 • This Table Provides a Quick Reference for Additional Problem-Solving Projections Used in Mammography, Detailing Indications for Their Use and Tissue Best Visualized by Each View

PROJECTION	ID	C-ARM ANGLE	IMAGE RECEPTOR PLACEMENT	TISSUE BEST VISUALIZED	APPLICATIONS
Exaggerated Craniocaudal Medial	XCCM	0°–5°		Posteromedial	Capture of posteromedial region
Axilla	AX	70°–90°		Axillary content	Additional view for cancer patients on affected side, suspected inflammatory ca, lymphadenopathy, search for primary ca
20° MLO Mediolateral Oblique	20° MLO	20°		Entire glandular island, UOQ	Third projection for possible abnormality, patients with personal history of breast cancer
Elevated Craniocaudal or Pushed-Up CC	ECC	0°		Central and medial, high on the chestwall	Superior lesion not seen on CC

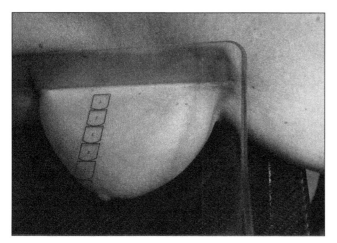

Figure 7-221
The XCCM projection, like the CV view, is an alternative projection used to visualize the extreme posteromedial aspect of the breast.

Medially Exaggerated Craniocaudal Projection Summary

1. Position the C-arm at 0° to 5°, with the x-ray beam directed superiorly to inferiorly.
2. Initially, the patient faces the unit. Rotate the medial aspect of the patient's body toward the image receptor. Patient's head is facing toward the ipsilateral side.
3. Adjust the level and angle of the image receptor to capture the natural curvature of the medial breast attachment to the thorax.
4. Place the contralateral arm on the side of the image receptor for stability.
5. Apply compression ensuring capture of posteromedial tissue.

Additional Tip for Performing the Exaggerated Craniocaudal Medial Projection Consider the use of the 10-cm (quad) contact compression device or 7.5-cm spot compression device for detected abnormalities difficult to capture.

Axilla (AX) Projection

Application

The axilla position, an anterior–posterior projection, visualizes the axillary region[6] (Figure 7-222). This projection assists in gathering information for patients who present with symptoms such as a lump high in the axillary region. An axillary projection can be considered as an additional view for breast cancer patients and for suspected inflammatory breast cancer. It may also be used for patients who present with lymphadenopathy (swollen lymph nodes) and when searching for primary cancer (after a diagnosis of unspecified cancer elsewhere in the body). Unilateral involvement of the lymph nodes is suggestive of an underlying occult breast cancer. Bilateral involvement indicates

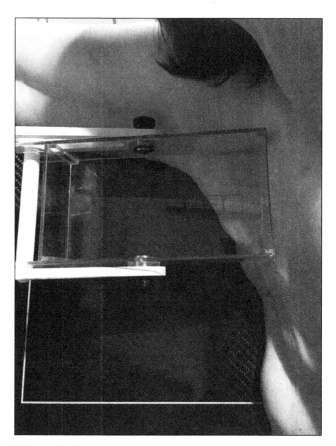

Figure 7-222
The axilla (AX) projection: completed axilla position utilizing the 10-cm-size contact compression device.

a systemic cause (e.g., infection, rheumatoid arthritis, lymphoma, and acquired immune deficiency syndrome).

Axilla Projection Projection Summary

1. Rotate the C-arm 70° to 90° and adjust the angle to best accommodate the patient's body.
2. The height of the image receptor allows visualization of the head of the humerus at the superior aspect of the image.
3. Begin with the patient standing with the posterior aspect of the shoulder in contact with the image receptor, anterior to posterior x-ray beam direction.
4. Rotate the patient approximately 15° toward the image receptor.
5. Lift the ipsilateral arm to shoulder level and extend laterally, with elbow flexed and arm resting on the C-arm.
6. The patient bends slightly forward at the waist, leaning laterally toward the unit, bringing the ribcage in contact with the image receptor.
7. The head of the humerus is at the superior aspect of the imaging field. The posterior aspect of the image receptor should include the glenoid fossa and possibly the ribs (Figure 7-223). Metastatic lymph nodes and recurrence can arise not only in the axilla but also inferior to the axilla and close to the ribcage.[6]

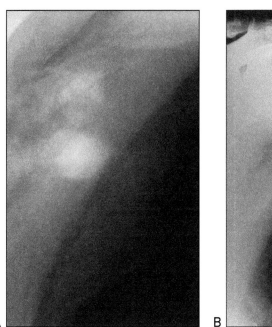
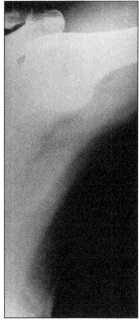

Figure 7-223
The axilla (AX) projection: variations of well-positioned axilla views. **(A)** Metastasized lymph nodes. **(B)** Image of complete axillary region.

8. Apply enough compression to minimize motion. If the patient has not had a mastectomy, it is sometimes necessary to bring a portion of the breast under compression.

20° Mediolateral Oblique Projection

Application

The 20° oblique (MLO) demonstrates the entire glandular island with less superimposition than the two-projection mammogram,[9] using a superomedial to inferolateral directed x-ray beam (Figure 7-224). This view is especially useful for visualizing the upper outer quadrant of the breast; however, it has many applications. The 20° oblique projection separates superimposed glandular structures by changing the angle and projection of tissue from the CC view. This is the same concept used to separate superimposed breast tissue when the rolled view technique is employed. It is useful as a third projection when seeking further evidence about a possible abnormality imaged on the MLO projection. The 20° oblique projection is also useful as a third view for both the unaffected and affected breasts in patients who have had breast cancer (see Chapter 10). These patients have an increased risk of either developing another carcinoma in the unaffected breast or of recurrence in the affected breast. A third projection gives the radiologist and patient an advantage in early diagnosis.

20° MLO Projection Summary

1. Rotate the C-arm approximately 20°, with the x-ray beam directed superomedial to inferolateral oblique.
2. The patient faces the unit (as for a CC projection), with thorax rotated slightly away from the image receptor, lateral aspect of the ipsilateral breast in contact with the unit.
3. The breast is placed on the image receptor. Turn the patient's head in either direction, whichever is most comfortable and facilitates acquisition of the lateral and posterior tissue.
4. The contralateral arm remains at the patient's side, with the ipsilateral hand placed at the lower aspect of the image receptor.
5. Elevate the IMF, adjusting the image receptor to the level of the IMF.

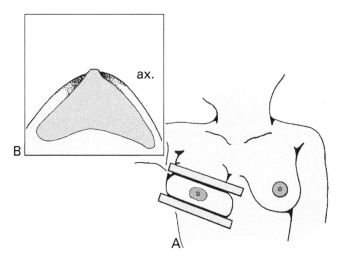

Figure 7-224
The 20° MLO. **(A)** Schematic of the orientation of the breast to the image receptor for the 20° MLO projection. **(B)** Schematic demonstrating the amount of the "glandular island" included with this view.

6. Using two hands, the technologist firmly captures the breast, gently pulling the breast tissue onto the image receptor with the patient's shoulders relaxed to better image the upper outer quadrant.

7. The patient should press forward, toward the unit, trying not to lean laterally toward the ipsilateral breast, which would result in the glandular tissue imitating that of the MLO projection.

8. Apply compression while continuing to gently pull the breast outward and forward (Figure 7-225).

Elevated Craniocaudal (ECC) Projection

Applications

The elevated craniocaudal (ECC) projection best visualizes central and medial abnormalities high on the chestwall[6] (Figure 7-226). This projection is an option when an abnormality presents in the superior aspect of the MLO and Lateral projections but is absent from the standard CC projection (Figure 7-227).

Elevated Craniocaudal Projection Summary

1. The C-arm is positioned at 0°, with the x-ray beam directed superiorly to inferiorly.

2. The patient faces the unit, placing distance between the patient and the image receptor to accommodate leaning excessively forward.

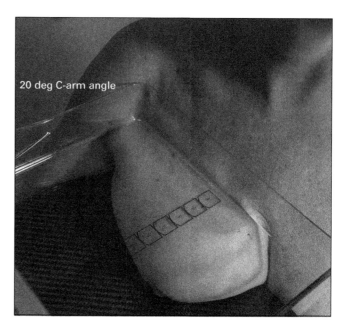

Figure 7-225
The 20° MLO demonstrates the entire glandular island with less superimposition than the two-projection mammogram. This view best visualizes the upper outer aspect of the breast.

3. Overelevate the breast, raising the image receptor above the IMF, taking advantage of the mobile inferior border. This allows access to tissue located high on the chestwall. Elevation of the IMF is dependent on the location of the suspected superior abnormality and is evaluated on each individual circumstance.

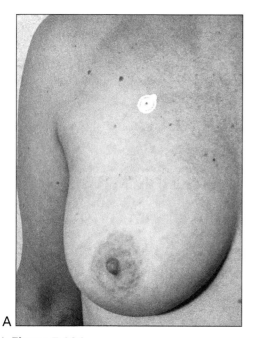
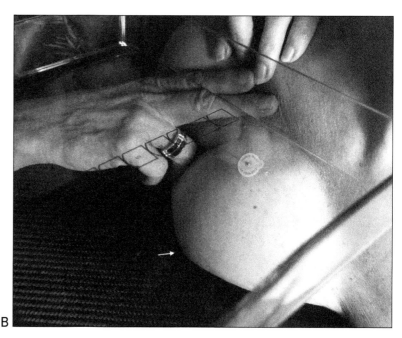

A   B

Figure 7-226
Elevated craniocaudal (ECC). **(A)** Abnormalities high on the chestwall, excluded from the CC projection, may be visualized with an ECC view. **(B)** To accomplish this view, overelevate the IMF, thus eliminating inferior breast tissue. Use minimal compression to maintain tissue visualization; note nipple rolled inferiorly (*arrow*).

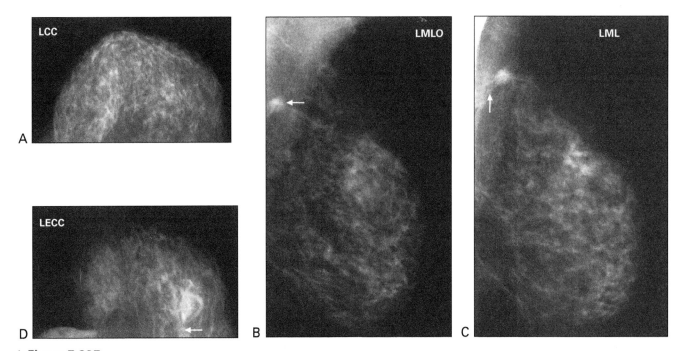

Figure 7-227
Elevated craniocaudal (ECC): routine screening exam (**A**—LCC and **B**—LMLO) reveals a speculated mass (*arrow*) on the LMLO. **(C)** An LML indicates the ROI location is medial, because it moves up from the LMLO (see Triangulation). **(D)** A LECC using minimal compression reveals the medial location of this proven carcinoma (*arrow*).

4. Using two flat hands, capture posterior tissue at the chestwall, and gently and firmly pull the breast outward and forward onto the image receptor.
5. Apply minimal compression to hold the breast in place. Vigorous compression may prohibit visualization.

Mammography Image Identification Requirements

Image Identification Labeling

Mammographic image identification, also known as "labeling," is defined by MQSA as recordkeeping data to ensure accuracy of several key identification points.[31] Each mammography image must include the following to comply with MQSA requirements (Figure 7-228):

- Name of the patient and an additional patient identifier
- Date of examination
- View and laterality
- Facility name and location (minimum facility information requires city, state, and zip code)
- Technologist identification
- Mammography unit identification (if there is more than one unit at the facility)

Image Laterality and Projection Labeling

The MQSA specifies the laterality and the projection identification is to be placed on the image in a location near the axilla, thereby indicating the position of the axilla on the image.[31] This is the only label that is permitted to be close to the breast, with all other labels placed far away so as not to be a distraction to the radiologist.

Mammography Infection Control

The MQSA requires facilities to establish policies and protocols for disinfecting mammography equipment in the case of contact with blood or other bodily fluids.[32] These MQSA requirements outline the facility's responsibility to comply with state or local regulations regarding infection control, to comply with manufacturer recommendations for disinfection of equipment, and to establish documentation methods demonstrating facility compliance. The image receptor, compression device(s), and face shield surfaces must be disinfected after coming into contact with bodily fluids; do not confuse disinfection measures with cleaning the machine surfaces in between patients. In between patients, the machine surfaces are cleaned with a solution recommended by the equipment manufacturer or by hospital cleaning protocols. By addressing hand sanitation and equipment disinfection prior to the mammography examination in front of the patient, the technologist provides additional reassurance that appropriate measures for infection control are maintained. Additional information on Infection Control requirements for mammography are provided in Chapter 15.

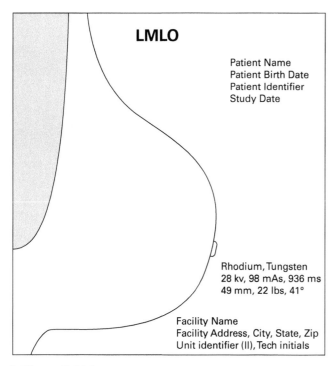

LMLO

Patient Name
Patient Birth Date
Patient Identifier
Study Date

Rhodium, Tungsten
28 kv, 98 mAs, 936 ms
49 mm, 22 lbs, 41°

Facility Name
Facility Address, City, State, Zip
Unit identifier (II), Tech initials

Figure 7-228
Mammographic image identification, also known as "labeling," is defined by MQSA. Each mammography image must include the following to comply with MQSA requirements: (1) name of the patient with additional identifier, (2) date of examination, (3) view and laterality, (4) facility name and location (minimum requirements include city, state, zip code), (4) technologist identification, and (5) mammography unit identification if applicable. The laterality and projection identification are placed near the axilla indicating the position of the axilla on the image. (Modified from American College of Radiology. *Mammography Quality Control Manual.* Reston, VA: American College of Radiology Committee on Quality Assurance in Mammography; 1999.)

Miscellaneous Examination Information

The following information has been gathered from technologists who have developed innovative problem-solving techniques through years of performing the mammography procedure. They have been collected and offered to the reader in our shared goal to improve image quality.

Positioning Assistance-Patient Feet Placement: CC and MLO Projections

The image quality of the CC and the MLO projections used for routine mammography can be positively or negatively affected by where the patient stands at the beginning of the positioning process. For this reason, many mammography facilities use a visual method of ensuring the patient's feet are appropriately placed in front of the image receptor prior to beginning the exam.

- Tape Method
  Tape is placed on the floor in front of the mammography unit in the shape of a "T." Using tape, the vertical line of the "T" is placed on the floor marking the exact center of the image receptor width. The horizontal line of the "T" is placed on the floor at approximately a hands-width distance from the chestwall edge of the image receptor (Figure 7-229A). When performing the RCC projection, the patient is asked to place her right foot on the vertical "T" line and toes behind the horizontal line of the "T." When performing the RMLO, the patient is asked to place her right foot on the left side of the vertical "T" line; however, her feet are forward to the horizontal line ensuring her abdomen is in contact with the image receptor. This process is reversed for the LCC and the LMLO.

- Footprint Method
  A footprint is placed on the floor in front of the mammography unit marking the exact center of the image receptor width. It is placed at a distance of an approximate hands width away from the chestwall edge of the image receptor (Figure 7-229B). To make the footprint, trace the sole of a shoe on cardstock. After cutting out the footprint, it can be laminated and taped to the floor. The footprint method functions the same as the tape method, replacing the vertical "T" line with the "footprint," with the "toe" edge of the "footprint" placed at an approximate hands-width distance from the image receptor.

Wearing Gloves

Wearing gloves while performing routine screening mammography is based on technologist preference. If the technologist chooses to wear gloves during the examination, it is beneficial to use tighter-fitting gloves similar to surgical gloves that conform to the hand rather than loose-fitting exam style gloves. Loose gloves may catch behind the image receptor at the chestwall edge, or between the patient's anatomy and the side edges of the image receptor, between the breast and the compression device, etc. When the patient presents with conditions indicating the presence of blood or bodily fluids, such as nipple discharge, open sores on the breast, or postcore biopsy clip images, safe infection control policies apply and gloves (either style) are always required.

Image Receptor Procedural Aids

The mammography procedure has long been acknowledged by physicians, technologists, and patients as an uncomfortable procedure. Technologists who work in this modality demonstrate empathy and compassion to patients as they strive to meet the standards of image quality while performing the examination. In addition to human empathy, two companies offer image receptor cover aids that provide

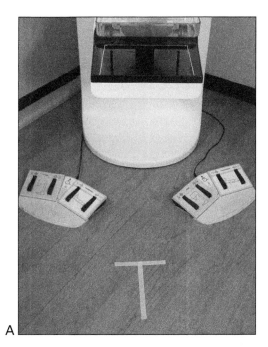
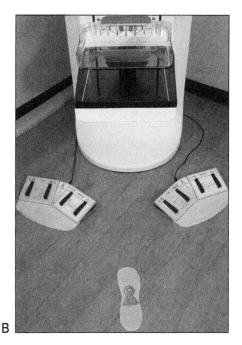

A

B

Figure 7-229
Positioning assistance: patient feet placement. The image quality of the CC and the MLO projections can be positively or negatively affected by where the patient stands in relation to the image receptor. Many facilities use a visual method to assist with verbal instructions when guiding the patient into position for the routine projections. **(A)** The tape method. **(B)** The footprint method.

options for further comfort to the patient. These receptor covers are single-use FDA-approved products that adhere to the image receptor providing a warmer surface for the patient. Additionally, it has been noted that these products may improve patient positioning through the grip enhancement of the material they are made of, which holds the breast tissue securely in place. At this time, these covers are not reimbursable through medical insurance. Facilities choosing to use these products must pay out of pocket for them or pass the cost on to the patient.

MammoPad Breast Cushion
MammoPad is a product offered by Hologic, Inc., Marlborough, MA. It provides a foam cushion surface to the image receptor promoting a warmer, softer approach to mammography with an additional benefit of enhanced grip during positioning (Figure 7-230A).

Bella Blankets
Bella Blankets, a product offered by the Beekley Medical Corp., Bristol, CT, is promoted as a protective coverlet. This product emphasizes its thin design and textured material to aid in positioning and infection control (Figure 7-230B).

The Card Trick

A common procedural aid used in mammography is the kitchen spatula. By design, its ultrathin flexible rubber rectangular shape provides an anchor to immobilize extremely thin tissue that would otherwise escape compression or assist the technologist in ID views.

A common problem experienced during the CC projection is the "extra" axillary tissue above the compressed breast that protrudes over the rise of the compression device and into the field of view. The spatula can be positioned horizontally between the chestwall rise of the compression device and the patient ensuring the tissue remains behind the compression device, out of the field of view. Another mammography aid easily used for the same purpose is a small plastic card (similar to a credit card or gift card) that technologists can carry in their pocket. When additional tissue protrudes into the field of view for the CC projection, the card is placed between the compression device and the patient ensuring the image is artifact free (Figure 7-231). As with any equipment used in mammography, these aids require cleaning between each patient use.

Wearing Jewelry: Technologist

Rings, watches, and bracelets that are thicker in diameter than extremely thin breasts at final compression pose a positioning challenge. Consistent problems with positioning and compression due to the interference of jewelry should be an indication to the technologist to reconsider wearing that particular article. Technologists who perform mammography and are required to wear medical alert jewelry should continue to do so.

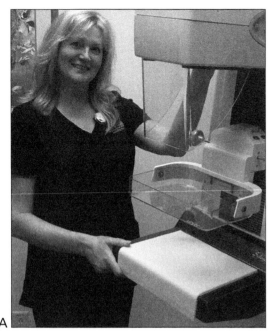

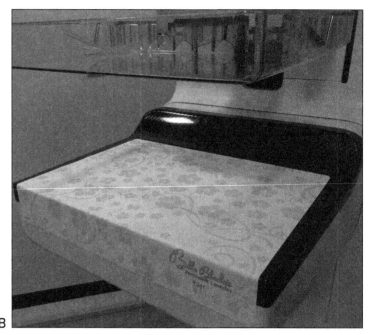

A   B

Figure 7-230
Two companies offer receptor covers that provide a more comfortable experience for the patient. These FDA-approved products are designed for single use and adhere to the image receptor providing a warmer surface for the patient. **(A)** The Mammo-Pad (Hologic, Inc., Marlborough, MA). **(B)** Bella Blankets (Beekley Medical Corp., Bristol, CT).

Artifact-Free Images: Jewelry, Accessories, and Hair

Ensuring that images are artifact free due to jewelry and accessories worn by the patient should be addressed by the technologist prior to taking the first exposure. Any article

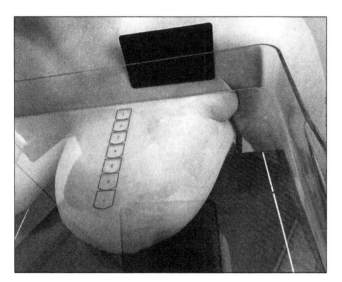

Figure 7-231
Mammography positioning aids may be used to prevent superior tissue from protruding into the FOV on the CC projection. A spatula or card (similar to credit card) placed between the compression device and the patient ensures the image is artifact free.

that can potentially be projected into the field of view should be removed prior to the exam to guard against unnecessary repeats to the patient. Patients who wear glasses pose not only a potential artifact concern for the image but also may impede adequate capture of posterior tissue. Patients who wear glasses during the CC projection subconsciously hold their head away from the face shield in an effort to protect the eye region from injury. This action results in posterior tissue being excluded from the image and creates difficulty for the patient to relax the muscles of her thorax and neck necessary for positioning. The removal of glasses is suggested to improve the positioning process for the CC projection, but the decision to comply with this request should be left up to the patient. For persons who have very poor eyesight, additional care should be taken to prevent potential injury:

- Wait until the patient has approached the unit and is familiar with her surroundings to remove her glasses.
- Remind her of the face shield location near her face.
- Return her glasses after the CC projections are completed.

Hair products pose potential artifacts on the mammography image. Disposable hairbands or pins used to secure hair from the field of view should be accessible to the patient.

Chapter 7, Parts 1 and 2 Summary

The artistic component and the scientific component of the mammography examination cannot be separated. The technologist performing this modality requires continued instruction, mentoring, and periodic refresher courses in positioning/compression techniques as surely as the mammography equipment requires its periodic inspections for reliability and safety. Positioning and compression are interdependent, requiring precision by the technologist to achieve established image criteria. Improving capture with clarity of mammographic features to meet established standards is most often accomplished using small intricate maneuvers that improve the image by millimeters or centimeters rather than inches. Although these image improvements may be small in measure, they may make the difference in detecting or not detecting cancer. During the last two decades, the landscape of breast imaging has changed offering additional imaging methods to optimize lesion identification and definition. The need for their additional use most often is gleaned from the screening mammogram. The technologist's understanding of basic techniques to position and compress the breast in order to provide an accurate representation of tissue for interpretation remains as important today as it was when mammography was the only radiographic modality available for the detection of breast cancer.

Review Questions, Chapter 7, Part 2

1. Explain the use of the LM projection or the ML projection to assist in determining triangulation of a lesion for core biopsy or needle localization.

2. Describe the use of the XCCL projection in a diagnostic setting versus a screening setting.

3. Describe the positioning used to obtain a tangential view for a lump found in the right breast at 2:00.

4. How is the labeling determined for the rolled views: RM, RL, RI, and RS?

5. What additional view best images the posteromedial tissue in close proximity to the sternum?

6. What are the requirements for mammographic image identification according to the MQSA?

References

1. Federal Register Department of Health and Human services/Food and Drug Administration. 21CFR Parts 16 and 900. Quality Mammography Standards; Final Rule.
2. Wentz G. *Mammography for Radiologic Technologists*. 2nd ed. St. Louis, MO: McGraw-Hill; 1997.
3. Cardenosa G. *Breast Imaging Companion*. 3rd ed. Philadelphia, PA: Wolters Kluwer; 2008.
4. FDA/MQSA/Guidance/Policy Guidance Help System/ Mammography Equipment Evaluation. Available at: https://www.accessdata.fda.gov/cdrh_docs/presentations/pghs/Polic_Guidance_Help_System.htm. Accessed February 23, 2017.
5. Logan WW, Norland QW. Screen-film mammography technique: compression and other factors. In: Logan WW, Muntz EP, eds. *Reduced Dose Mammography*. New York, NY: Masson; 1979.
6. Andolina VF, Lille S. *Mammographic Imaging: A Practical Guide*. 3rd ed. Philadelphia, PA: WK Lippincott Williams & Wilkins; 2011.
7. Kopans D. *Breast Imaging*. 3rd ed. Philadelphia, PA: Lippincott Williams & Wilkins; 2007.
8. American College of Radiology Committee on Quality Assurance in Mammography. *Mammography Quality Control Manual*. Reston, VA: American College of Radiology; 1999.
9. Andolina V. Chapter 23. Mammography. In: Frank ED, Long BW, Smith BJ, eds. *Volume 2, Merrill's Atlas of Radiographic Positioning and Procedures*. 11th ed. St. Louis, MO: Mosby Elsevier; 2007.
10. ACR practice parameter for the performance of screening and diagnostic mammography, Res. 11-2013. The American College of Radiology. Available at: https://www.acr.org/~/media/3484ca30845348359bad4684779d492d.pdf. Accessed February 23, 2017.
11. Lundgren B. The oblique view mammography. *Br J Radiol*. 1977;50:626–628.
12. Andersson I. Mammography in clinical practice. *Med Radiogr Photogr*. 1986;62(2).
13. Clinical Practice Guideline/Quality Determinants of Mammography/U.S. Department of Health and Human Services/Public Health Service/Agency for Health Care Policy and Research/Number 13/AHCPR Publication No. 95-0632; October 1994.
14. Majid A, de Paredes E, Doherty R, et al. Missed breast carcinoma pitfalls and pearls. *Radiographics*. 2003;23:881–895.
15. Sickles EA, D'Orsi CJ, Bassett LW, et al. ACR BI-RADS® mammography. In: *ACR BI-RADS® Atlas, Breast Imaging Reporting and Data System*. Reston, VA: American College of Radiology; 2013.
16. Eklund GW, Cardinosa G. The art of mammographic positioning. *Radiol Clin North Am*. 1992;30(1):21–53.
17. Eklund GW, Cardenosa G, Parsons W. Assessing adequacy of mammographic image quality. *Radiology*. 1994;190:297–307.
18. Bradley FM, Hoover HC Jr, Hulka CA, et al. The sternalis muscle: an unusual normal finding seen on mammography. *AJR Am J Roentgenol*. 1996;166(1).33–36.
19. Taplin SH, Rutter CM, Finder C, et al. Screening mammography: clinical image quality and the risk of interval breast cancer. *AJR Am J Roentgenol*. 2002;178:797–803.

20. MQSA Insights Articles. *Poor Positioning Responsible for Most clinical Image Deficiencies, Failures.* Available at: http://fda.gov/MQSA/MQSAInsightsArticles. Accessed February 23, 2017.

21. Keller BA, Evans KD. Fighting anxiety in order to improve the quality of breast imaging for women. eRADIMAGING.com. Available at: https://eradimaging.com/site/article.cfm?ID=758#.WdvXA1tSzIU. Published December 15, 2010. Accessed February 2017.

22. Deibel D, Heinlein R. Avoiding clinical image failure: a worksheet for clinical analysis. *Adv Admin Radiol Radiat Oncol.* 1998;8(4).

23. NCI-Funded Breast Cancer Surveillance Consortium (HHSN261201199931C). Breast Cancer Surveillance Consortium Web site: http://breastscreening.cancer.gov/statistics/benchmarks/screening/2009/table6.html. Accessed February 23, 2017.

24. Skaane P, Bandos A, Gullien R, et al. Comparison of digital mammography alone and digital mammography plus tomosynthesis in a population-based screening program. *Radiology.* 2013;267(1):47–56.

25. Genusaro G, Toledano A, DiMaggio C, et al. Digital breast tomosynthesis versus digital mammography: a clinical performance study. *Eur Radiol.* 2009;20:1545–1553.

26. Bick, et al. Tomosynthesis and the impact on patient management. EUSOBI March 2014. Vienna.

27. Butler RS, Crenshaw J, Kaira V, et al. How tomosynthesis optimizes patient workup, throughput, and resource utilization. *RSNA Annual Meeting.* Chicago, IL; 2013.

28. Ecklund GW. *Breast Imaging: Focus on Excellence (syllabus).* Sponsors: Medical College of Wisconsin, Medical Technology Management Institute; 1999.

29. FDA/MQSA/Guidance/Policy Guidance Help System/Breast Implants. Available at: https://www.accessdata.fda.gov/cdrh_docs/presentations/pghs/Polic_Guidance_Help_System.htm. Accessed February 23, 2017.

30. Eklund GW, Busby RC, Miller SH, et al. Improving imaging of the augmented breast. *AJR Am J Roentgenol.* 1988;151:469–473.

31. FDA/MQSA/Guidance/Policy Guidance Help System/Mammographic Image Identification. Available at: https://www.accessdata.fda.gov/cdrh_docs/presentations/pghs/Polic_Guidance_Help_System.htm. Accessed February 23, 2017.

32. FDA/MQSA/Guidance/Policy Guidance Help System/Quality Assurance-Equipment/Infection Control. Available at: https://www.accessdata.fda.gov/cdrh_docs/presentations/pghs/Polic_Guidance_Help_System.htm. Accessed February 23, 2017.

Special Imaging Applications

8

Objectives

- Gain an understanding of formulating creative solutions to achieve satisfactory image quality for individual patient situations when the use of standard projections is insufficient
- Understand alternative mammography projections that resolve issues of inadequate breast tissue capture with clarity
- Recognize the flexibility benefit of the mammography machine's C-arm design to enable creative problem-solving techniques that gain elevated image quality with increased comfort to the patient and with less exertion required of the technologist

---

Key Terms

- breast tissue margins
- complementary views
- exam management
- pectus carinatum
- pectus excavatum

INTRODUCTION

Under most circumstances, the 2-view mammogram, utilizing the standard CC and mediolateral oblique (MLO) projections of each breast, is sufficient to capture and display the breast tissue of patients who present for screening mammography.[1]

The two standard projections that comprise the screening mammogram are complementary; neither view adequately demonstrates all of the breast tissue. Each projection visualizes specific features of the breast adequately, while other features may not be sufficiently visualized or may be completely excluded from the image. The CC projection adequately demonstrates the anterior, central, medial, and posteromedial portions of the breast but is unreliable in visualizing the extreme lateral tissue. The MLO projection adequately demonstrates the extreme posterior margins and UOQ but may not visualize the medial and anterior tissue with equal clarity[2] (Figure 8-1). Most often, the mammography technologist has done her best to achieve satisfactory image quality that does not require additional exposure to the patient to complete the examination.

When a 2-view mammogram for screening purposes is completed, the technologist evaluates the four images contained in the study for adequate capture of breast tissue and for adequate visualization of tissue. To evaluate tissue capture, the technologist examines the images for anatomical structures and radiographic landmarks that confirm sufficient inclusion of breast margins (see Chapter 7). Evaluation of tissue visualization requires the technologist to examine all areas of the final image for verification of tissue clarity. Paying close attention to the positioning/compression execution of each projection and correlating this information to the image quality demonstrated on the radiograph(s) provides insight to the technologist in determining what factors may have contributed to any study inadequacies. These insights provide the technologist with immediate solutions customized for each examination circumstance allowing her to correct the suboptimal indications on the standard projections. As discussed in Chapter 7, this describes the proficiency of ***exam management***: *the technologist's ability to evaluate imaging compliance during the performance of the standard projections, whether the use of replacement or complementary projections will assist in achieving the goal of sufficient image quality, and the selection of specific projection(s) to accomplish the objective of adequate capture with clarity resulting in the least amount of dose to the patient.*

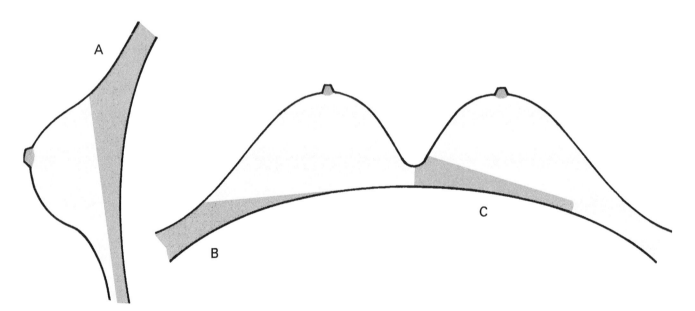

Figure 8-1
The "blind" areas of the standard mammography view. When the breast is compressed for the craniocaudal view, the superior–posterior portion of the breast is not imaged (*shaded area* in **A**). Furthermore, either a posteriomedial or a posteriolateral portion is not included, depending on how the patient is rotated (*shaded areas* in **B** and **C**). In the lateral view, the posteriolateral portion tends not to be imaged (**B**), whereas in the oblique view, the posteriomedial portion of the breast tends not to be imaged (**C**). The craniocaudal projection can be either laterally or medially oriented. Usually, it is obtained so that the lateral posterior portion is included rather than the medial posterior portion. This is logical only if two views are used, and the other view is the lateral, which tends to omit the posterior lateral portion. If, on the other hand, the oblique view is used together with the craniocaudal view as a two-view standard, it might be wise to obtain the craniocaudal in a more medially oriented fashion. This is recommended since the oblique projection tends to miss the juxtathoracic medial portion of the breast. (Reprinted with permission from Andersson I. Mammography in clinical practice. *Med Radiogr Photogr.* 1986;62:2. Copyright © 1986 Eastman Kodak Co.)

This chapter discusses special imaging situations that require the technologist to formulate solutions to adequately capture and display breast tissue when the CC and MLO projections are not sufficient due to individual patient attributes.

IMAGE QUALITY CRITERIA

The image quality criteria defined by the American College of Radiology (ACR) are thoroughly addressed in Chapter 7, along with established measurement practices to verify tissue capture. For convenience, the expected criteria for the CC and MLO projections are repeated in this chapter as a reminder to the reader of the important radiographic landmarks used to determine adequate tissue representation[3]:

Craniocaudal Projection Image Quality Criteria:

- Medial breast margin included on the image
- Desirable feature: reflection of the cleavage
- Desirable feature: presence of the contralateral breast
- Posterior nipple line (PNL) perpendicular to chest wall
- Pectoral muscle present 30% to 40% of the time
- Presentation of the retroglandular fat space
- As much lateral tissue as possible included on the image
- CC PNL measurement within 1 cm of MLO PNL measurement
- Adequate application of compression force

Mediolateral Oblique Projection Image Quality Criteria:

- Pectoral muscle presentation
  - Length to PNL (approximately 80% of the time)
  - Wide superior muscle
  - Anterior border of pectoral muscle convex in appearance
  - Gradual narrowing of pectoral muscle to inferior insertion point
- Inframammary fold (IMF) present and open
- Presentation of retroglandular fat space
- Posterior to anterior tissue adequately supported up and out
- Adequate application of compression force

In addition to evaluating the image criteria on the completed images, the technologist relies on her awareness of the positioning/compression process, noting any problematic areas of execution that may impact tissue capture and clarity. Only the technologist performing the positioning/compression maneuvers has the insight to evaluate the efficacy of her actions, as the effectiveness of the maneuvers are dependent on the cooperative ability of the patient and glandular distribution of the breast tissue.

During the evaluation of the images, the technologist draws on her awareness of the exam execution to discern reasons for observed suboptimal feature representation. This valuable information allows her to construct additional imaging solutions to improve features that may include one or more of the following problems:

- Breast tissue excluded from the image
- Inadequate compression
- Inadequate support and separation of tissue (MLO)
- Motion
- Artifacts
- Exposure

The technologist's expertise and efforts to ensure that as much breast tissue as possible is captured on the image and with adequate tissue clarity provide the opportunity for the interpreting radiologist to detect abnormalities.

WHEN SCREENING MAMMOGRAPHY REQUIRES PROBLEM-SOLVING PROJECTIONS

Even though the technologist has effectively executed a projection, visualizing all regions of the breast tissue on a single image is an unrealistic expectation (Figure 8-1). As mentioned earlier, the complementary nature of the standard projections used for screening mammography most often adequately completes the examination. Tissue missed on one view will most often be included on the opposing view.

Determining *if* additional imaging is warranted, and *how* to manage each mammography examination is dependent on individual patient and examination circumstances that the technologist encounters. The technologist familiar with mammography examination possibilities recognizes how significant her image quality expertise relates to each encounter. Let us take a close look at some mammography examination examples:

A. Most often performed. This screening mammography examination example successfully captures all margins of the breast tissue with clarity using the CC and the MLO projections; no additional imaging is warranted to complete the examination. Occasionally, example A will include the following scenario:
- The study demonstrates posterolateral tissue extending beyond the chestwall edge of the Image Receptor Support Device (IRSD) on the CC projection. The patient was positioned adequately by the technologist; the excluded tissue is satisfactorily visualized on the MLO projection (Figure 8-2).

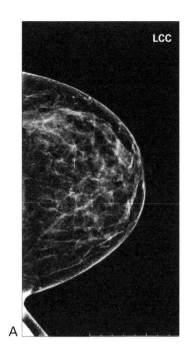
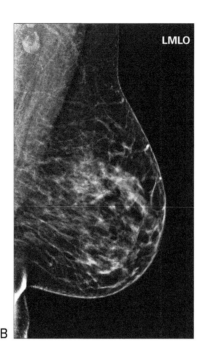

Figure 8-2
Screening study demonstrating adequate tissue coverage. LCC image with minimal posterolateral tissue excluded. **(A)** LMLO image visualizes posterolateral tissue excluded on CC image, adequately completing study **(B)**.

B. Occasionally performed. This screening mammography examination example does not capture all margins of the breast tissue with clarity using the CC and MLO projections; additional imaging is warranted to complete the examination. This examination is typified by the following example:

- The study demonstrates posterolateral tissue extending beyond the chestwall edge of the IRSD on both the CC and MLO projections. The patient was positioned adequately by the technologist, but the completed study results in nonvisualization of posterolateral tissue on both standard projections. Additional bilateral XCCLs improve the visualization of the excluded breast tissue, satisfactorily completing the screening mammography study (Figure 8-3).

The screening mammography examples described above require expert image evaluation skills by the technologist to determine if the standard projections have satisfactorily completed the imaging studies. Example B illustrates the technologist's combined expertise in recognizing inadequate image quality and in deciding which additional projections would best resolve the imaging problem.

Many examples exist of screening situations that require additional imaging to complete the examination due to individual patient attributes, even when the technologist has done her best to execute the standard projections. These imaging situations occur in approximately 15%, or 3 in 20 screening examinations.[4] Examples of these situations are described in greater detail in Chapter 7, Part 2, and in the Problem/Fix-It section of Chapter 7, Part 1.

C. Occasionally performed. This example uses problem-solving views to adequately capture breast tissue with clarity for the patient who presents with special imaging circumstances.

Case Study **8-1**

1. Refer to Figures 8-2 and 8-3. The patient in Figure 8-2 does not require an additional image to complete her screening examination, while the patient in Figure 8-3 requires an additional projection (XCCL). What is the difference between these examples?

Occasionally, the technologist encounters a patient who presents with physical, emotional, or psychological circumstances that impede the effectiveness of standardized imaging. These situations require the mammography procedure to be customized to the individual patient's specific situation. As with other radiographic procedures, the technologist performing the examination is challenged to formulate creative imaging solutions in order to achieve adequate image quality for each individual patient circumstance. Customizing the mammography examination for each patient's individual need may require the technologist to modify the procedure by:

- Using **complementary views** in addition to the CC and the MLO projections
- Replacing the CC or the MLO projection with problem-solving views.

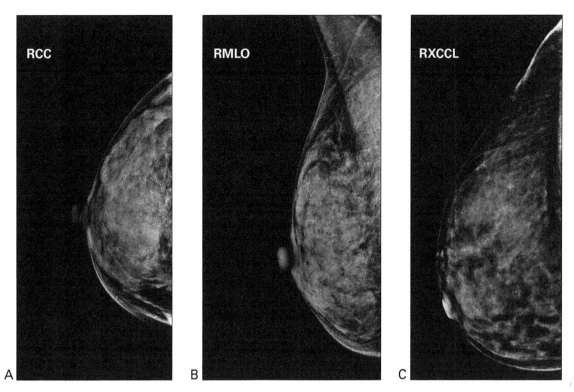

Figure 8-3
Screening study demonstrating posterior tissue excluded from both standard projections. RCC image excludes central and posterolateral tissue **(A)**. RMLO image excludes posterior tissue **(B)**. Complementary RXCCL image visualizes posterior central and posterolateral tissue **(C)**.

Imaging the small percentage of patients in which the standard projections do not adequately accommodate the examination may present a challenge for even the most experienced mammography technologist. The most significant factors in succeeding in the goal to provide a safe, efficient, and quality mammography examination for the patient in this setting requires the technologist to be proficient in the basic artistic components of mammography positioning/compression. These components, covered in more detail in Chapter 7, Part I, include the foundations of adequate breast capture with clarity in the mammography examination:

- Knowledge of **breast tissue margins** (Figure 8-4)
- Utilization of the positioning principle of mobile versus fixed breast margins (Figure 8-5)
- A comprehensive understanding of all problem-solving projections: their purpose and their execution
- A comprehensive understanding of mammography equipment operation: C-arm flexibility, appropriate selection of the compression device configuration, technique selection, etc.

When the technologist is confident in these basic positioning/compression skills, her proficiency in managing challenging situations to adequately capture breast tissue

with clarity, while ensuring patient comfort, is increased. These circumstances require the technologist to understand that the versatile design of the mammography equipment is intended to benefit her efforts to accommodate the patient's needs. This understanding, combined with a comprehensive knowledge of the problem-solving projections used in mammography, provide imaging solutions for a wide range of positioning impediments. In some instances, varying the angle of the C-arm in order to meet the positioning abilities of the patient may be an acceptable alternative to following exact projection definitions. There are numerous patient conditions that require an alternative approach to the 2-projection mammography examination. Additional projections for these patient situations are necessary to provide images that support the radiologist's ability to detect early indications of breast cancer should they be present. This requires the imaging solutions to manage the visualization of breast tissue through:

- Adequate capture
- Adequate tissue support for the MLO
- Adequate compression force
- Manage artifacts:
  ○ Motion artifacts
  ○ Patient artifacts
- Appropriate exposure

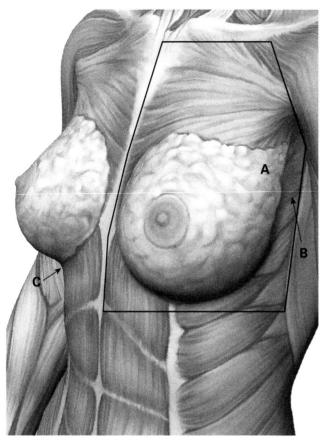

Figure 8-4
Superior to inferior and medial to lateral breast margins illustrated. Superior to inferior breast margins: 2nd or 3rd rib to 6th or 7th rib. Medial to lateral breast margins: sternum to latissimus dorsi muscle (midaxillary line). (Image from Shutterstock.)

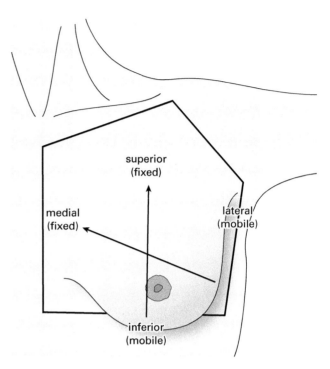

Figure 8-5
Positioning principle illustrated: mobile versus fixed breast tissue margins. Mobile margins: inferior and lateral. Fixed margins: superior and medial.

To better understand the concept of mammography exam management in situations where special imaging applications are necessary to better serve the patient, technologists should be familiar with basic examination principles that ensure a safe and positive patient experience.

BASIC MAMMOGRAPHY CONCEPTS FOR SPECIAL IMAGING CIRCUMSTANCES

Patient Safety

The subject of patient safety, specifically the radiologic technologist's responsibility to ensure the physical and psychological safety of the patient throughout all radiologic procedures, is recognized by the professional organizations associated with this health care field. The American Registry of Radiologic Technologists (ARRT) articulates these ideals in the ARRT Standard of Ethics.[5] The radiologic technologist is expected to "assess situations; exercise care, discretion, and judgment; assume responsibility for professional decisions; and act in the best interest of the patient"[5] as she provides care throughout the mammography procedure. Additionally, this subject is addressed in the American Society of Radiologic Technologists (ASRT) Mammography Curriculum. Included in its Clinical Practice objectives are the following requirements[6]:

- "Provide patient-centered, clinically effective care for all patients regardless of age, gender, disability, special needs, ethnicity, or culture."
- "Demonstrate competent assessment skills through effective management of the patient's physical and mental status."

Patient safety measures should be assessed for each individual patient and individual examination by the technologist. Depending on the specific needs of each individual patient, the technologist's responsibility for patient safety during the mammography procedure may include a wide range of safety considerations. These considerations are not limited to but may include implementing one or more of the following safety measures:

- The requirement of two technologists to safely execute the examination
- Seating the patient for the examination

- Securing wheelchair/equipment locks
- Securing the patient safely in the wheelchair
- Appropriate use of radiation protection

Patient Dignity

The subject of recognizing the dignity of each patient is also addressed in the ARRT Standard of Ethics. Within this Standard, the Code of Ethics #2 requires that the "radiologic technologist acts to advance the principal objective of the profession to provide services to humanity with full respect for the dignity of mankind."[5] Just as the technologist assesses the examination process to ensure the physical safety of the patient, she must also assess the potential to deliver the examination while ensuring patient dignity. The appearance of "struggling" to execute the examination should be minimized whenever possible. Behavior or indications by the technologist that imply a difficulty to execute the examination or problem solve may suggest that the patient is the cause of the problem. Providing two technologists for mammography procedures that are physically challenging for one technologist to perform due to strenuous examination execution requirements not only ensures the patient's safety and increases image quality but serves to preserves the dignity of the patient's experience.

Disability Etiquette

As in any radiologic procedure, the mammography patient may present with physical, emotional, or psychological conditions that require the technologist to provide special assistance during the examination. This encompasses a wide range of patient conditions, some of which may be classified as a disability. The Americans with Disabilities Act of 1990 was passed with the purpose to integrate people with disabilities into all aspects of life. According to the National Organization on Disability (NOD), more than 54 million Americans have a disability.[7] Understanding the approach that each patient desires, depending on their individual/specific need, can be difficult for the health care professional delivering their care. Sensitivity when interacting with people who have a disability supports the professional ethic of recognizing the dignity of humankind. The United Spinal Association has published a 35-page Disability Etiquette booklet entitled, "Tips On Interacting With People With Disabilities." This booklet contains valuable awareness information for a wide range of disabilities with tips that serve to create positive interactions (Figure 8-6). Technologists who are familiar and sensitive to specific disabilities are empowered to provide a positive experience

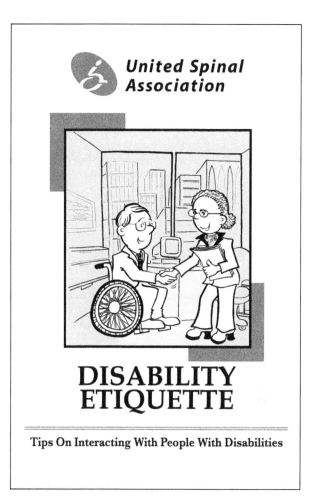

Figure 8-6
Disability Etiquette, Tips on Interacting With People With Disabilities booklet. Free publication from United Spinal Association provides awareness information for common disabilities and respectful interaction suggestions. (Accessible from United Spinal Association Website: unitedspinal.org. With permission from United Spinal Association.)

for the patient with a disability and to be comfortable while providing their care. To access more information on disability etiquette, visit the United Spinal Association Web site: unitedspinal.org.

Appropriate Documentation

An accurate account of examination specifics should be included in the documentation by the technologist in the designated location of the patient history form in the event that:

- Suboptimal images have been produced and accepted by the technologist due to positioning limitations of the patient
- Modifications to the mammography examination were made using replacement or complementary views to the standard projections due to positioning limitations of the patient

Patient Signature Date

To be filled out by the Technologist

Breast surface markings:
Moles
Scars
Pain
Lumps/Thickening
Nipple inversion

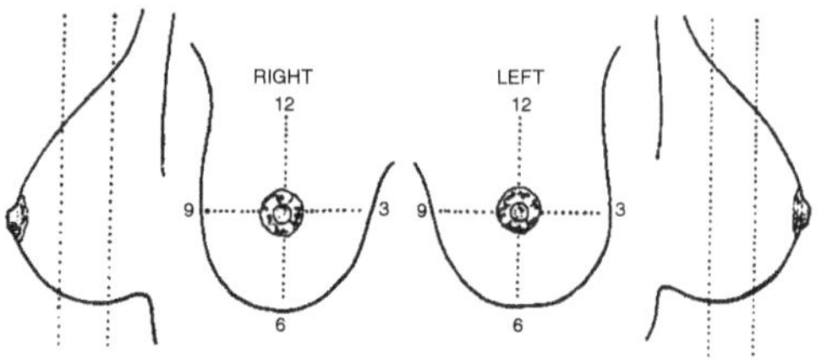

Technologist Comments:

Noted Exam Limitations:
Language Barrier: ☐ Physical Limitations: ☒ Body Habitus: ☐ Compression: ☐
Mammography examination performed with patient seated in wheelchair

Figure 8-7
An example of documenting patient positioning limitations in a designated location on the patient history form. This information alerts the interpreting physician to reasons for complementary projections or why substandard imaging is provided.

This critical documentation should accurately indicate to the interpreting radiologist the reasons for patient positioning limitations that would explain the imaging results accepted by the technologist for this particular study. It is important that the interpreting physician be informed of the medical condition of the patient and reasons for any substandard image that has been submitted for interpretation. Without this important documentation, the technologist is susceptible to speculation of poor imaging performance. Technologists should therefore follow the policies and procedures of individual mammography service practices in completing this documentation. An example of documenting patient positioning limitations in a designated location on the patient history form is provided in Figure 8-7.

GUIDANCE IN CHOOSING PROBLEM-SOLVING PROJECTIONS

When the mammographic examination is completed, the technologist evaluates the images to determine if the breast tissue is adequately visualized. When the complementary standard images of the right or the left breast demonstrate that the same area of breast tissue is excluded from both the CC and the MLO projections, the technologist must use problem-solving mammography views to capture and visualize the missing breast tissue. The ability to determine the area of breast tissue excluded from the completed study is essential in order to select the additional mammographic projection that serves to visualize the omitted area. Understanding the breast margins and landmarks combined with proficiency in image evaluation helps the technologist to determine which quadrant(s) of the breast are missing. Familiarization with the problem-solving projections provides the technologist with the insight necessary to choose the most suitable additional view(s) to complete the study. Understanding how the four quadrants of the breast are projected on the CC and the MLO images also provides a basis for choosing the appropriate problem-solving views (see Chapter 9). The significance of the technologist's ability to manage the mammography examination using her expertise in image evaluation and her perception of solving imaging problems using additional mammographic projections is appreciated in Figure 8-8.

The next section of this chapter provides an overview of patient conditions that may require the technologist to modify the mammography procedure in order to improve the quality of the examination while ensuring a safe and positive experience for the patient.

Image evaluation	Determining excluded breast tissue	Perform the problem solving projection that improves visualization of excluded tissue
A. Well positioned mammogram. The CC and MLO complement one another to form the complete study.	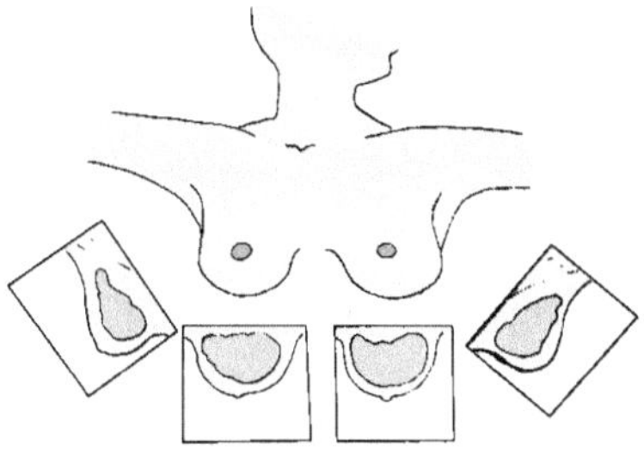	
B. The mammogram demonstrates medial tissue excluded from the CC projection; the central tissue excluded from the MLO corresponds to medial tissue. Review of breast margins confirm the posterior UIQ is excluded from the study.	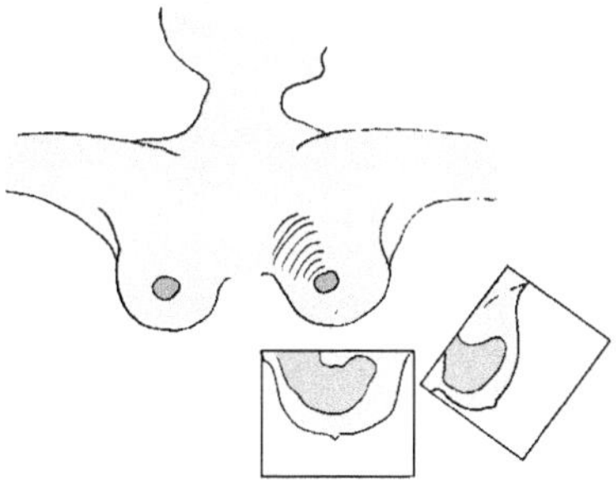	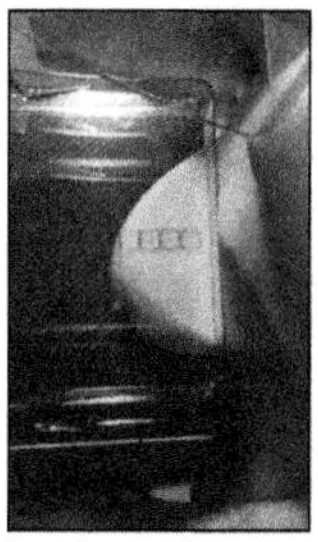 an SIO projection with the arm down
C. The mammogram demonstrates lateral tissue excluded from the CC projection; superior tissue excluded from the MLO. Review of breast margins confirms the posterior UOQ is excluded from the study.	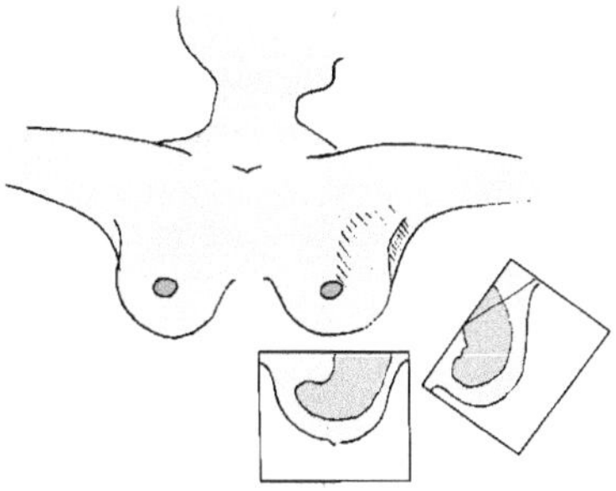	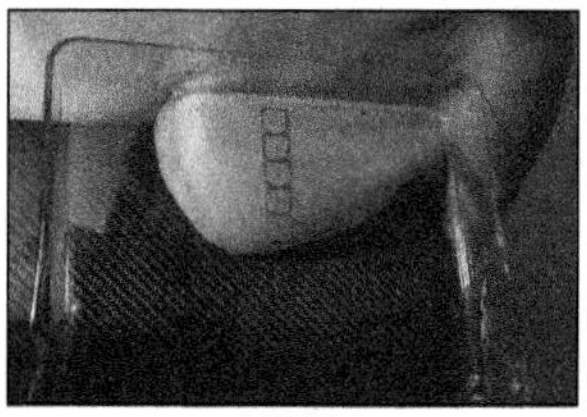 XCCL 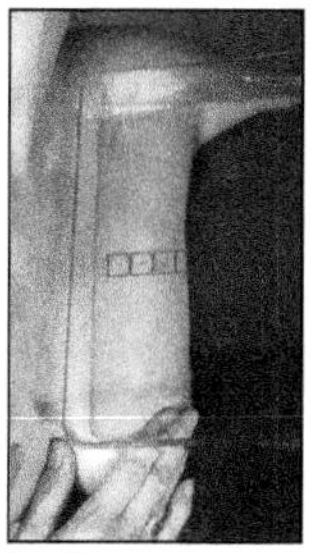 AT an XCCL and/or AT projection
D. The mammogram demonstrates lateral tissue excluded from the CC projection; inferior tissue excluded from the MLO. Review of breast margins confirms the LOQ is excluded from the study. (Note: the UOQ is well visualized on the MLO).	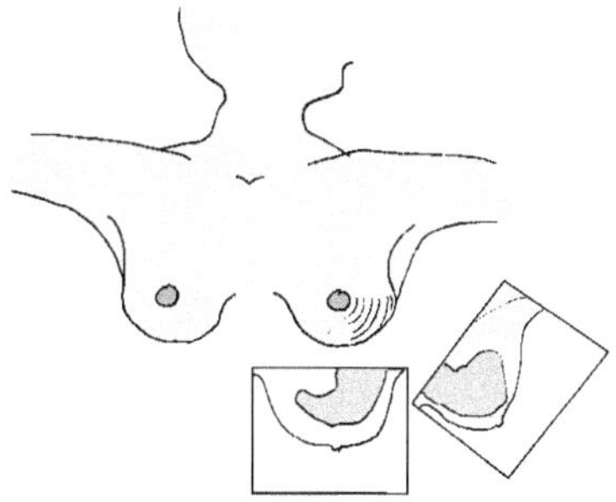	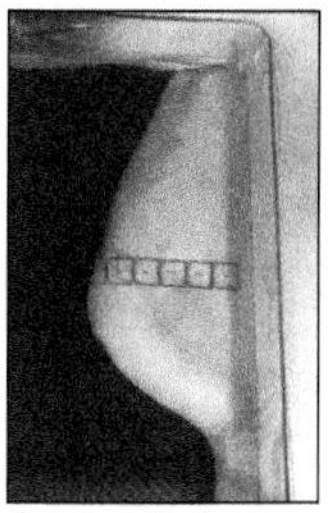 an SIO projection with the arm up and over (note the inclusion of the LOQ)
E. The mammogram demonstrates medial tissue excluded from the CC projection; inferior tissue excluded from the MLO. Review of breast margins confirms the LIQ is excluded from the study.	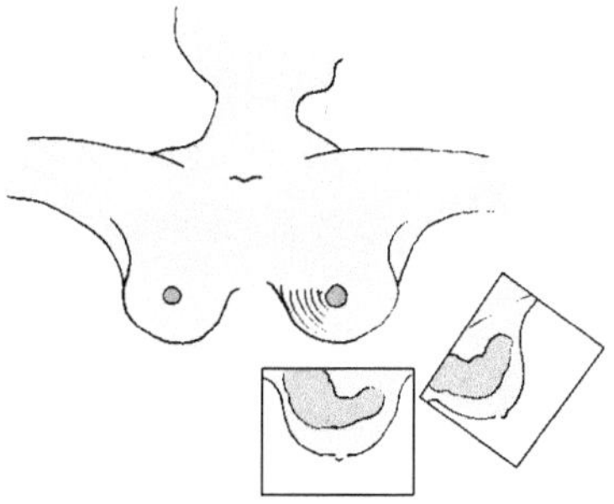	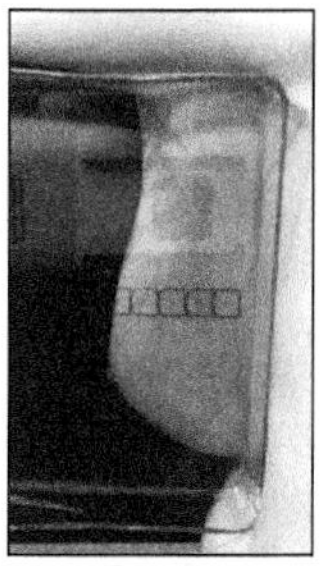 an LMO projection

Figure 8-8

Evaluating the mammogram and choosing complementary projections. Sample mammograms with tissue excluded from various quadrants and the additional views that demonstrate the excluded tissue. Select the one complementary view that demonstrates the area of excluded tissue whenever possible; however, some circumstances may require more than one extra view.

▌▌ SPECIAL PATIENT CONSIDERATIONS AND THE MAMMOGRAPHY PROCEDURE

Problem-Solving Projections

The most challenging breast tissue to capture on the standard projections used in the mammography examination is the posterior tissue. Even for the agile patient, the ability to be maneuvered into challenging positions for the procedure, while tolerating the compression required for the desired image quality results, can be demanding. As can be imagined, the goal to achieve adequate capture of breast tissue becomes a much more arduous examination process for the patient who presents with positioning/compression limitations. When the 2-view mammography examination must be modified to achieve desired image quality results, the technologist selects from various mammography problem-solving projections to customize the examination to the patient's specific needs. A complete list of problem-solving projections and their purpose are discussed in detail in Chapter 7, Part 2. The following additional imaging projections are recognized for their use in problem-solving applications for patients who have positioning limitations:

* Lateromedial projection (LM)
* Mediolateral projection (ML)
* Axillary tail (AT)
* Exaggerated craniocaudal lateral (XCCL)
* Exaggerated craniocaudal medial (XCCM)
* From below (FB)
* Axilla (AX)
* Superolateral to inferomedial Oblique (SIO)
* Cleavage view (CV)
* Lateromedial Oblique (LMO)

Depending on the examination circumstance and the patient's cooperative ability, the procedure may require the use of one or more problem-solving projections to complete the procedure. It should be noted that the technologist must assess each individual patient and her specific circumstance to determine the best examination approach. The technologist's ability to:

* Analyze the imaging situation
* Identify the obstacles affecting breast capture and adequate compression
* Identify the projections that resolve the problem

are key to providing effective patient care. The artistic component of the mammography examination plays an important role in creating the best imaging solutions for each situation. The technologist is advised to keep an open mind, using her knowledge and her creative abilities to develop strategies for these challenging situations. Table 8-1 provides the technologist with guidance and practical solutions to common imaging problems.

▌▌ SPECIAL IMAGING CIRCUMSTANCES

Familiarizing the mammography technologist with various patient conditions she may encounter prepares her to provide efficient, compassionate care that results in a satisfactory patient experience. This section describes special patient circumstances that require the technologist to modify the examination to the patient's specific need. The examples of patient conditions and the suggested resolutions described here are meant to prepare the technologist for imaging situations where she may be confronted with positioning limitations. Specifically, the problem-solving techniques describe solutions that increase the technologist's ability to control the thorax and breast in order to achieve successful positioning/compression goals. It should be noted that the following tips should be considered for the suggested examination modifications or problem-solving projections that are included for each patient circumstance described:

* The projections may or may not be useful when used with one another.
* Not all suggested strategies work in all scenarios.
* There is more than one way to solve a problem.

Table 8-2 provides quick reference imaging guidance for challenging patient conditions.

Imaging the Patient with Small Breasts

The extremely small-breasted patient may present imaging difficulties particularly if the breasts are also quite firm. The challenge for the technologist lies in the ability to:

* Capture the extreme posterior tissue
* Minimize skin folds
* Ensure breast tissue covers the automatic exposure control (AEC) (thus eliminating the need to set a manual technique)

Suggested Imaging Solutions

Resolving these issues requires the technologist to make specific adjustments in performing the mammography examination for smaller breasts:

1. Use the compression device designed especially for imaging the small breast or the male breast (sometimes referred to as the half paddle) (Figure 8-9). This smaller profile compression device enables the technologist to

Table 8-1 • This Quick Reference Table Provides Guidance and Practical Solutions to Some Common Positioning Problems

ANATOMICAL ANOMALY	PROBLEM	CAUSE	POSSIBLE SOLUTIONS
Small breast	Capture of extreme posterior tissue	Difficulty in positioning	Use compression device designed for imaging small breasts/males (half paddle) Ensure correct height of IR Use positioning techniques similar to implant imaging: grasp posterior tissue with fingers on superior aspect of breast, thumbs on inferior (or vice versa), to control tissue as patient is brought forward against IR Complementary XCCL often necessary Have patient exhale before quickly applying compression across ribcage as thorax "depresses"
	Minimizing skin folds	MLO: Insufficient axillary tissue introduces skin folds/air gaps	Increase C-arm angle to as much as 70° for MLO. Ensure correct height of IR.
	AEC tissue coverage	Breast tissue does not cover AEC	Acquire MLO view first; adjust resulting techniques for CC view
Pectus excavatum (depressed sternum)	Unable to visualize medial tissue on CC	Rib curvature does not allow IR and compression paddle access to medial tissue	Complementary view with attention to medial tissue: XCCM (5° angle) Replace CC with two views: XCCM and XCCL Use of 10-cm contact compression device
	Unable to visualize medial tissue on MLO Failure to image posteromedial tissue on MLO		Possible complementary LM/SIO views Possible replacement LMO for MLO
Pectus carinatum (pigeon breast)	Unable to visualize lateral tissue on CC	Rib curvature does not allow IR and compression paddle access to lateral tissue	Complementary XCCL view
	Unable to visualize lateral tissue on MLO		Replace MLO with LMO view Complementary SIO view
Kyphosis	Inhibited visualization of posterior tissue on CC	Curvature of spine does not allow access to IR without superimposition of head	Have patient sit in chair for CC Severe kyphosis: possible FB Complement to CC: XCCL
	Potential patient artifacts on image		Replacement for MLO: LMO Complement to MLO: LM/LMO
Frozen shoulder rotator cuff injury/surgery	Unable to visualize superior–posterior tissue on MLO	Shoulder immobility does not allow arm to be raised for superior posterior tissue capture	Begin MLO with IR in low position to accommodate patient's arm immobility. Slowly raise C-arm to patient tolerance. Slowly lower after image acquisition Replace MLO with LM. Patient's arm remains at side
Protruding abdomen	Prohibits visualization of posterior tissue on CC	Abdomen does not allow breast to fully access image receptor	CC: patient bends forward at the waist. Keeping patient's pelvis back from unit, guide patient's breast onto IR
	Prohibits visualization of posterior–inferior tissue on MLO		MLO/soft abdomen: no space between IR and patient abdomen. Before compression, tilt patient's pelvis down/back removing excess abdomen from FOV, opening IMF MLO firm abdomen: complementary LM/ML view to MLO
	Compromises IMF tissue	IMF tissue irritation	Use of positioning aid: MammoPad, Bella Blanket CC: slightly bend patient's knees
Large breast	Inadequate anterior compression; drooping breast	Nonuniform compression due to thick breast base, narrow apex Shoulder/axilla included under compression device	CC: use tilt compression device option if possible complementary CCAC view MLO: ensure correct IR height, axilla position; rotate triceps (underarm tissue) posteriorly, bending elbow Complementary MLOAC/MLAC MLO for breast mound with AT

(Continued)

Table 8-1 • This Quick Reference Table Provides Guidance and Practical Solutions to Some Common Positioning Problems *(Continued)*

ANATOMICAL ANOMALY	PROBLEM	CAUSE	POSSIBLE SOLUTIONS
	Drooping breast	Nonuniform compression/ gravity	Reduce C-arm angle to evenly distribute weight of breast on IR Complementary AC views
	Unable to visualize complete breast on CC projection	Breast size exceeds size of image receptor	Use larger size compression device CC: CC's to include lateral margins to medial tissue (possible small amount of medial cutoff) + CV, mosaic imaging (Figure 8-22B)
	Unable to visualize complete breast on MLO projection		MLO: mosaic imaging (Figure 8-22C) Complementary views: ML/LM for anterior tissue
Implanted medical device	Inadequate compression Compression device comes in contact with implanted medical device	Pacemaker, defibrillator, ports located in superior aspect of breast tissue Moving mobile margins of breast tissue to fixed while compressing fixed tissue is not feasible	CC: replace CC with FB MLO: replace MLO with LMO Pacemaker: CC image excluding pacemaker using adequate compression, MLO including pacemaker using only sufficient compression to stabilize breast, MLO excluding pacemaker using adequate compression

access the breast tissue more easily, thus controlling the amount of breast tissue secured beneath the compression device.

2. Ensure that the IRSD is raised to the height of the elevated IMF; positioning the IRSD too high or too low removes critical posterior tissue that is already challenging to secure.

3. Breast tissue may not completely cover the AEC sensors when performing the CC projection, requiring the technologist to set a manual exposure technique. To solve this problem, perform the MLO projection first. The MLO view images most of the breast tissue; inclusion of more breast tissue results in coverage of the AEC sensors, which permits phototiming the

Table 8-2 • This Quick Reference Table Provides Imaging Guidance for Challenging Patient Conditions

SPECIAL IMAGING APPLICATIONS	IMAGING REFERENCE GUIDE
#1 Small or male breasts	Note: use "half-paddle" compression device/spatula. CC + MLO (for males—possible FB in place of CC)
#2 Large breasts	CC anterior + CC middle + CC posterior/include medial + lateral margins MLO anterior + MLO middle + MLO posterior/include superior + inferior margins
#3 Implants	CC + MLO + CCID + MLOID If ID imaging cannot be performed + lateral image including implant
#4 Axillary tail tissue	CC + MLO + AT
#5 Obese body habitus	CC + MLO + ML/LM Rotate excessive upper arm posteriorly to rest behind detector
#6 IMF not imaged	Complementary ML/LM/SIO
#7 Protruding abdomen	CC: patient steps back and leans forward onto IR MLO: no space between abdomen and IR/patient's pelvis tilted down/back to open IMF
#8 Kyphosis	CC: performed with patient seated/possible FB/complementary XCCL MLO: replace with LMO/provide positioning aid if available (MammoPad, Bella Blanket)
#9 Pectus excavatum (depressed sternum)	CC + XCCM (5° angle) + LMO
#10 Pectus carinatum (pigeon chest)	XCCM + XCCL + LMO
#11 Frozen shoulder	CC + MLO: lower angled C-arm to accommodate immobile arm Replacement LM-arm at side
#12 Patient in wheelchair	CC + LM (if MLO not possible)
#13 Nipple not in profile (in both standard views)	Obtain complementary CCNP or MLONP/MLNP
#14 Skin folds	Obtain additional image with smoothed skin folds

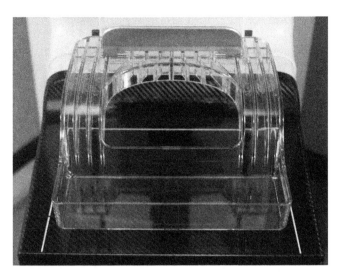

Figure 8-9
Small-breast compression device (sometimes referred to as the ½ paddle): this compression device is a modified version of the standard contact 18 × 24-cm compression device with a compression surface measuring only 9 cm from the chestwall edge. Advantageous when positioning small breasts, extremely thin breasts, males, and patients with implants because it allows the technologist increased access to the breast tissue.

exposure. Refer to the resulting technique provided on the phototimed MLO images to set the manual technique for the CC projections, making adjustments as necessary for any breast thickness changes.

4. The "two-handed pull" described in Chapter 7, Part 1, "positioning the CC projection" may not be effective with the extremely small breast. For better control, the technologist should use both hands to grasp the posterior breast tissue at the thorax, guiding the patient's upper body and breast tissue toward the image receptor, similar to the positioning methods of the implant patient.
5. Advise the patient to take in a breath and then exhale. As the patient exhales, the ribcage "collapses"; while the ribcage is collapsed, quickly move the compression device across the ribs.
6. The use of a rubber kitchen spatula to secure the breast tissue on the image receptor during the compression application may be beneficial.

Case Study **8-2**

1. Refer to Figures 8-9 and 8-10. When imaging a male patient or a small-breasted female, what positioning aids and techniques can help improve the amount of tissue included as well as improve the clarity of the image?

Imaging the Male Patient

Performing the male mammogram presents much the same positioning/compression challenges as the small, firm-breasted female. Additionally, hair on the chestwall causes the breast to slip out from under the compression device. This is more evident with the CC projection. It is critical that the nipple be imaged in profile on the male mammogram, as any pathology will be located directly posterior to the nipple (Figure 8-10A and B).

Suggested Imaging Solutions

1. Use the compression device designed especially for imaging the small breast or the male breast (sometimes referred to as the half paddle) (Figure 8-11) (see "Small-Breasted Patient" in this chapter).
2. Reduce amount of compression slightly.
3. Have the patient use the unit handrails to better secure the thorax to the chest wall edge of the IRSD.
4. Use of a positioning aid such as a mammography pad or liner (see Chapter 7) on the image receptor and compression device may help to increase the traction necessary to hold the breast tissue in place.
5. The use of a rubber kitchen spatula to secure the breast tissue on the image receptor during the compression application may be beneficial.
6. In imaging situations for the athletic male, who presents with a more developed and fixed pectoral muscle, the FB projection may be useful as a substitute for the CC view. Using the FB projection takes advantage of breast mobility, moving the inferior mobile tissue to the fixed superior breast tissue.

Imaging the Patient with Pectus Carinatum (Pigeon Breast)

Pectus carinatum is a condition in which the sternum protrudes outwardly (in varying degrees of severity) (Figure 8-12). Due to the shape of the thorax, the breast tissue is directed toward the lateral aspect of the anterior chestwall. Rarely is it possible to image the entire breast using the two standard projections.

Suggested Imaging Solutions

1. Perform the CC to image the medial tissue (the nipple will project laterally on the image).
2. Perform an XCCL to image posterolateral tissue excluded on the CC projection.
3. Perform the MLO projection to image posterolateral tissue and the upper outer quadrant of the breast. In most cases, the MLO view will not visualize posteromedial breast tissue.

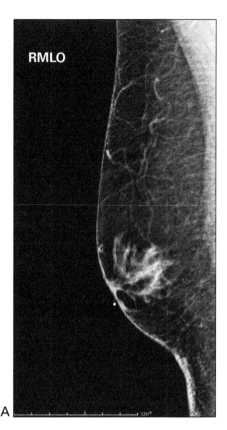 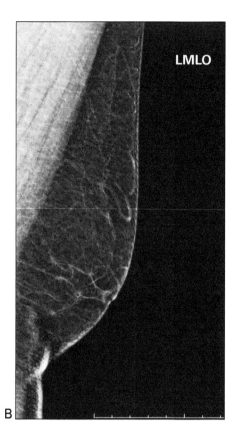

Figure 8-10
Male patient presenting with right breast subareolar lump. Mammography study confirms gynecomastia on RMLO image **(A)** and normal breast tissue LMLO **(B)**. Note metallic nipple marker on RMLO image and that the bilateral MLOs demonstrate the nipple in profile.

4. Consider using the LMO or the SIO projections to complement or replace to the MLO view.

Imaging the Patient with Pectus Excavatum (Depressed Sternum)

The sternum and ribs adjacent to the sternum are depressed inwardly (in varying degrees of severity) in this body habitus. Due to the sunken position of the posteromedial breast tissue, it is rarely possible to adequately visualize medial breast tissue using either of the standard projections (Figure 8-13).

Suggested Imaging Solutions

1. Perform the CC projection to image as much medial tissue as possible.
2. Depending on the severity of the **pectus excavatum**, consider replacing the single CC projection with both the XCCM and the XCCL projections, ensuring that central posterior tissue is adequately captured in at least one craniocaudal beam direction projection.
3. Perform the MLO to visualize posterolateral tissue.
4. Consider replacing the MLO with the LMO projection.
5. Depending on the severity of the pectus excavatum, consider supplementing the MLO/LMO with the SIO or the LM projection.
6. The lateral to medial beam direction can be painful due to the thorax positioned tightly against the imaging receptor chestwall edge. This discomfort can be relieved by using a positioning aid such as a mammography pad or liner.

Imaging the Patient with Kyphosis

Kyphosis describes a condition of an exaggerated rounding of the thoracic spine (Figure 8-14). It is a common presentation, in varying degrees of severity, in elderly women. Women who present for mammography with kyphosis may have an excessively hunched over appearance and difficulty straightening or moving their head and neck. Depending on the severity of the spinal curvature, the imaging challenges the technologist must solve for the patient with kyphosis include the following:

- Adequate breast tissue capture
- Manage patient artifacts (chin, ear, neck, etc.)
- Ensure safety and comfort during the examination

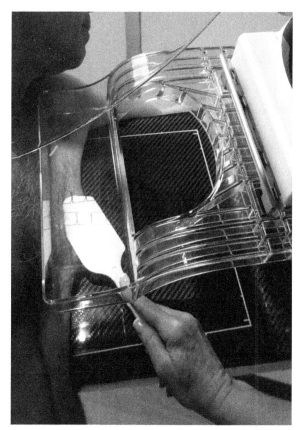

Figure 8-11
Illustration of male mammography MLO positioning techniques. Note the relaxed position of the patient, the use of the ½-paddle compression device and kitchen spatula to increase image quality outcome.

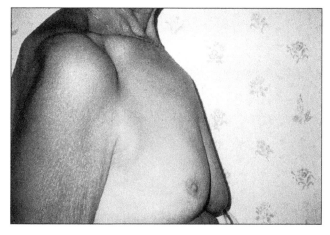

Figure 8-12
Pectus carinatum (pigeon chest). Pectus carinatum is characterized by an excessive protrusion of the sternum and ribcage. The standard projections used for screening mammography rarely complete the examination for patients with this condition.

Suggested Imaging Solutions

1. The patient should be seated for the CC projection. With the patient seated, her upper body can be positioned in an upright and vertical orientation to perform the CC view.

2. The FB view may be a useful replacement for patients who are unable to move their head and neck out of the field of view for the CC projection. When performing the FB view in these imaging situations, focus on capturing the medial and central breast tissue. If posterolateral tissue is excluded on the resulting image, an additional XCCL projection will be easily tolerated by this patient.

3. For the oblique projection, place the C-arm at any angle that best accommodates the positioning ability of the patient. The C-arm flexibility should be used to ensure minimum physical effort is expended by these patients.

4. The LMO may be a useful replacement for patients who are unable to move their head and neck out of the field of view for the MLO projection. The elderly woman with kyphosis may be thin, causing excessive discomfort when performing the LMO projection due to the position of the image receptor against the sternum. This discomfort may be reduced by using a positioning aid such as a mammography pad or liner placed on the image receptor.

5. The LM projection may be used as a complement to the oblique projection when necessary. This view provides an advantage of capturing either posterolateral or posteromedial tissue if it has been excluded on the oblique projection.

6. In the event that a lateral projection must replace the oblique view for the examination, the LM view provides an advantage over the ML view. The LM beam direction is preferred over the ML projection due to its ability to capture posteromedial tissue and the advantage it presents in capturing the extreme posterolateral breast tissue.

Imaging the Patient with a Frozen Shoulder/Rotator Cuff Injury

The CC positioning maneuvers are minimally affected when imaging the patient with shoulder immobility and may or may not require modifications to positioning techniques.

For patients who present with mobility limitations of the shoulder due to conditions such as a frozen shoulder or recent injury/surgery to the rotator cuff, positioning modifications are necessary in order to perform the MLO projection. Typical imaging for the MLO projection customizes the C-arm angle to the patient's pectoral muscle angle and the patient is asked to raise her arm up and over the image receptor, placing the point of the axilla just anterior to

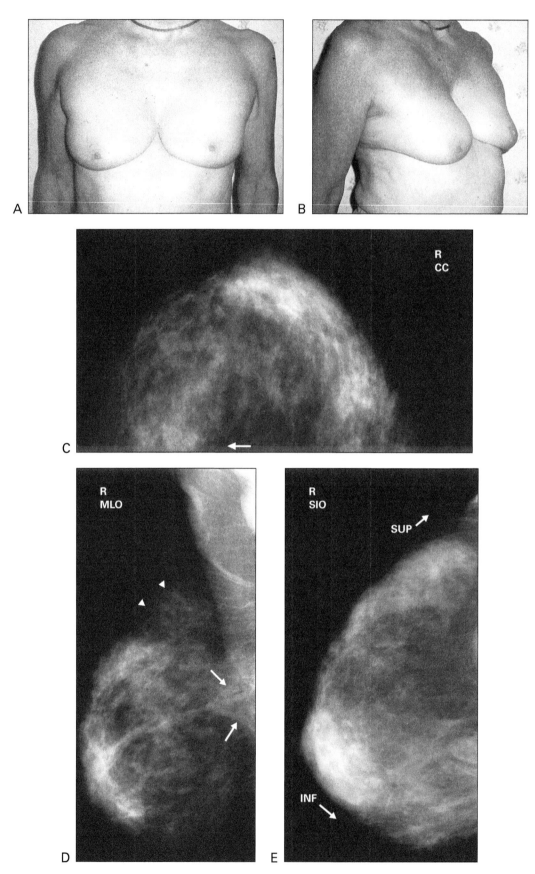

Figure 8-13
The patient with pectus excavatum **(A, B)** is characterized by a depressed sternum and adjacent ribs, prohibiting the visualization of all breast tissue in two standard projections. The CC **(C)** and MLO **(D)** of the patient with pectus excavatum demonstrates exclusion of the posteromedial tissue (*arrows*). Note the upper outer quadrant (*arrowheads*) is well visualized. An SIO view **(E)** allows capture of the nonvisualized posteromedial tissue.

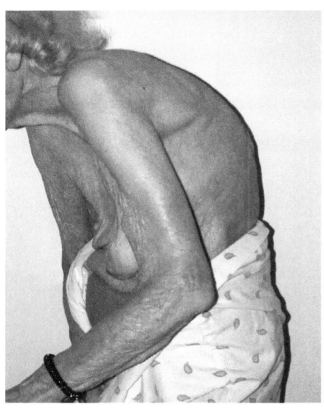

Figure 8-14
Patients with kyphosis may have an excessively hunched over appearance and difficulty straightening or moving their head and neck, requiring the technologist to use problem-solving projections for adequate tissue visualization.

the latissimus dorsi muscle on the IRSD corner. However, patients with conditions that affect shoulder mobility are unable to comply with this MLO positioning requirement that enables visualization of the superior posterior breast region (Figure 8-15).

For these situations, modifications of the MLO must be used to allow the affected shoulder to remain in a position that is tolerable to the patient throughout the procedure. When performing the MLO projection, the technologist should communicate with the patient explaining the following steps she is taking to minimize shoulder movement during MLO positioning.

Suggested Imaging Solutions

1. Lower the mammography image receptor so that the completed C-arm angle positions the superior edge of the image receptor well *below* the axilla of the affected shoulder.
2. Position the patient next to the image receptor with the superior proximal corner of the IRSD at the posterior edge of the breast margin at the approximate level of the nipple.
3. Never force the patient's shoulder from the position she is comfortable in.
4. Ask the patient to elevate the affected arm upward to a tolerable position, resting her arm on the image receptor (Figure 8-16).

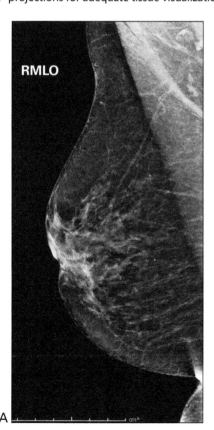

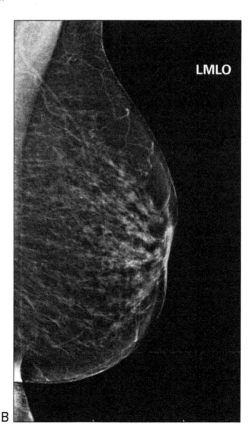

Figure 8-15
Example of comparison MLO images in patient presenting with left positioning limitations due to frozen shoulder. RMLO demonstrates expected radiographic landmarks that indicate adequate superior posterior tissue capture **(A)**. LMLO demonstrates decreased amount of superior posterior tissue visualization due to shoulder immobility **(B)**.

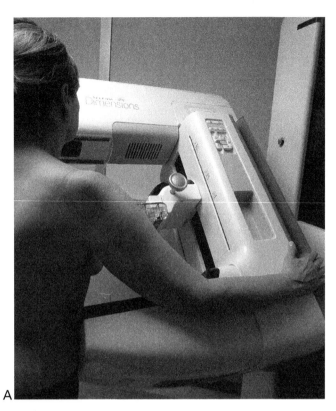
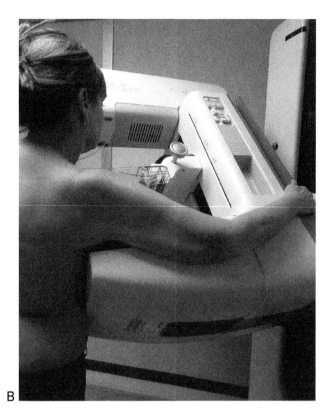

Figure 8-16
Patient comfort for shoulder immobility is addressed by lowering the angled C-arm for the MLO projection **(A)**, with gradual elevation as patient tolerance is monitored **(B)**. This technique allows for increased superior posterior breast tissue when positioning the MLO. The C-arm is lowered to accommodate the patient after image acquisition **(A)**.

5. Begin to slowly raise the image receptor as the IRSD corner makes contact with the axilla. Continue to raise the image receptor in small increments, one step at a time, while communicating with the patient after each small IRSD movement; monitor her discomfort as her arm continues to elevate.
6. Stop raising the image receptor when the patient states that her tolerance for elevating her arm has been reached.
7. After image acquisition, lower the mammography C-arm before removing the patient from position. This action reduces the need to lift the patient's arm as she is removed from the image receptor, thus ensuring her comfort.
8. Consider replacing the MLO with the LMO while keeping the patient's arm by her side, out of the field of view.
9. Consider using the LM as a complementary view to the MLO/LMO while keeping the patient's arm at her side, out of the field of view

Following these steps may benefit the patient who has minimal arm movement abilities. For the patient reporting for a screening mammography examination, consider consultation with her physician or the radiologist to verify the benefit of rescheduling the examination when improvement of tissue visualization is possible.

Imaging the Patient with a Protruding Abdomen

Patients who present for mammography with a large protruding abdomen thwart the ability of normal positioning techniques to capture inferior posterior breast tissue. This situation becomes more challenging if the abdomen is firm due to consequences of a patient in poor health. A protruding, firm abdomen not only impedes the capture of the IMF but also may compromise the ability to adequately compress the breast tissue (Figure 8-17).

Suggested Imaging Solutions

1. Adjusting the C-arm to a shallower angle for the MLO projection distributes the weight of the breast more evenly across the image receptor.
2. When additional imaging is necessary for further definition in the IMF region, an SIO projection may be beneficial for patients with a softer, pliable abdomen.
3. The LM projection included as a complement to the MLO view may improve the ability to capture and secure the IMF region due to the decreased thickness of tissue introduced between the image receptor and the compression device.

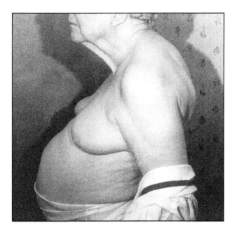

Figure 8-17
Patients with a large protruding abdomen challenge the ability to capture inferior posterior breast tissue. A firm abdomen due to consequences of poor patient health further complicates the ability for adequate compression in the MLO projection.

4. The abdomen should be tight against the chestwall edge of the image receptor when positioning the MLO projection. For the patient with a soft and protruding abdomen, have the patient tilt her pelvis in a downward motion. This action lowers the excess abdomen, positioning it toward the posterior margin of the image while opening the IMF region. This action is not as successful for the patient with a firm abdomen and, instead, may be resolved with the complementary ML projection.

Imaging the Patient with Compromised Balance

Assessing the physical, emotional, and psychological abilities of the patient begins when the technologist initially encounters the patient, greeting her for the examination. Walking with her to the changing room or the procedure room allows the technologist to assess the patient for any indications that may compromise patient safety during the procedure. One such indication is the observation that the patient's balance may be compromised and she is unsteady as she navigates her way to meet you. This may be observed when the patient gets up from her chair in the waiting room, walks to the changing room, or is asked to step up to the mammography machine. Imaging the patient for the mammography procedure requires the patient to be placed in somewhat challenging positions that require her to hold herself still for several seconds. Modern mammography suites further cause a problem for the patient whose balance may be compromised by using choices of flooring that can be easily cleaned for proper infection control. Although appropriate for proper infection control, these flooring choices also have the potential to be slippery if the patient should lose her balance during the imaging procedure.

When imaging patients with compromised balance, precautions should be taken to ensure their stability during the procedure.

Suggested Solutions: Compromised Balance

1. When the technologist has a concern that the patient's safety may be put at risk due to compromised balance, the mammography examination should be performed while the patient is seated.
2. Patients who present for mammography with walkers or canes that improve their balance should use these aids during the mammography procedure. The technologist should work around the stability aid so that the patient is secure while the examination is being performed.
3. For the MLO projection, the use of a steeper C-arm angle reduces the need for the patient to excessively lean onto the image receptor and away from their center of balance.
4. For the patient who is unsteady, the abrupt autocompression release option normally activated at the completion of the exposure may cause a "startle" reflex, which may affect patient stability. Deactivation of the autocompression release option during each exposure ensures patient stability until the technologist reaches the patient's side after the completion of the exposure. With the technologist providing additional assistance for stability to the patient, compression is released manually.

Additional note regarding an occasional positioning/compression challenge with the elderly patient:

Some women have breast tissue that compresses easily; their breast is extremely thin at the end of compression application. This has traditionally been described as the "pancake" breast. This type of breast includes specific challenges to the technologist in adequately securing the breast onto the image receptor and minimizing skin folds on the final image.

Suggested Solutions: Thin Breast

1. When possible, and if appropriate, use the half compression device (Figure 8-9) designed to allow the technologist better control over positioning/compression maneuvers.
2. The use of a rubber kitchen spatula to secure the breast tissue on the image receptor during the compression application may be beneficial.

Imaging the Patient in a Wheelchair

According to the United Spinal Association, Disability Etiquette, Tips on Interacting With People With Disabilities (Figure 8-6), people using wheelchairs have different disabilities with varying degrees of abilities. It may be possible for some people using wheelchairs to walk for short distances. Depending on the patient's condition, they may have use of their arms and hands, while others may not.[7] Successful imaging for mammography requires the image receptor to access all margins of the patient's breast and the ability of the patient to respond to positioning requirements. Modern mammography equipment is designed to enable capture of breast tissue using the flexibility of the C-arm to achieve this objective under various patient circumstances and abilities. As described for the patient with compromised balance, there may be situations when performing the mammography procedure with the patient seated may be the best choice to ensure patient safety. For patients seated in a chair, successful mammography imaging may be achieved, as the capture of posterior breast margins is not impeded by external interferences. In the case of performing the mammography procedure with a patient seated in a wheelchair, accessing the posterior breast margin is impeded due to the position of the wheelchair arm, obstructing the ability to achieve adequate breast tissue capture. There are multiple considerations when performing the mammography examination while the patient is seated in a wheelchair. Each examination should be assessed individually to achieve the highest image quality possible while ensuring patient safety, and each examination customized to the specific needs of the patient.

Suggested Solutions

1. The safety of the patient is of primary concern and should be addressed prior to conducting the examination. Address the *security* of the patient, assessing the need for wheelchair belts or other mechanisms that ensure patient safety as the procedure is performed. Ensure that wheelchair locks are adequately secured throughout the procedure.

2. Whenever possible, conduct the mammography procedure using the expertise of two technologists. Inevitably, the impediments to adequately capture and compress the breast tissue while ensuring patient safety may require more than one set of hands.

3. Conduct the medical intake interview seated next to the patient whenever possible (Figure 8-18). This courteous approach relieves the patient's need to strain her neck to make eye contact with the technologist. If that is not possible, standing at a slight distance from the patient also accomplishes this relief.

4. Communicate with the patient to ensure and verify that she can comply with what you are requesting of her.

5. If the patient uses a wheelchair belonging to the facility, it may be possible to detach the wheelchair arm on the side of the breast being imaged to better

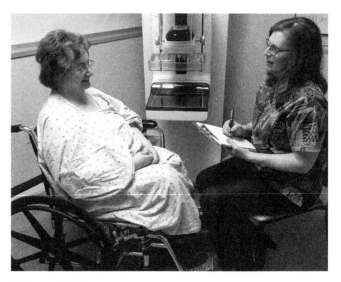

Figure 8-18
A courteous approach to conducting the medical intake interview. With the technologist seated, the patient does not need to strain her neck to make eye contact. If that is not possible, standing at a slight distance from the patient also accomplishes this relief.

access posterior tissue for the MLO or LM projection (Figure 8-19). If it is possible to detach the wheelchair arms, remove only one at a time in order to provide greater safety to the patient. Detach the right wheelchair arm when imaging the right breast, replacing the arm

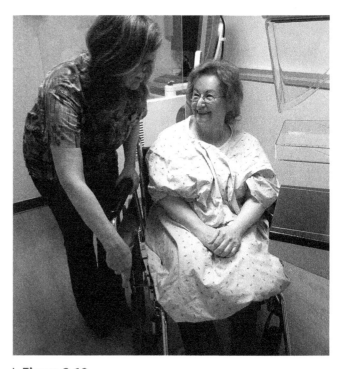

Figure 8-19
It may be possible to detach the wheelchair arm on the side of the breast being imaged to better access posterior tissue for the MLO or LM projection. For patient safety, detach and replace one arm from the wheelchair before progressing to the contralateral breast.

when imaging for the right breast has been completed. Repeat the same process for the left breast.

6. If the patient arrives in a personally owned powered wheelchair, consult with the patient before performing any modifications for the examination such as wheelchair arm detachment. According to the United Spinal Association, Disability Etiquette, Tips on Interacting With People With Disabilities, the wheelchair is part of the personal space of the person. Touching or pushing the wheelchair requires consultation with the patient.[7]

7. When the wheelchair arms are not able to be removed, an adult "booster seat" can be used to raise the patient higher in the wheelchair so that the breasts are now above the height of the wheelchair arms. The booster seat is easily made and is inexpensive: use a sturdy board, approximately 18 in. wide; wrap the board with padding, several inches thick; and cover with cloth. Place this on the seat of the wheelchair and have the patient sit down. The patient is still secure in the wheelchair; however, the extra height from the booster seat should elevate the patient so that the IRSD no longer contacts the wheelchair arms in the MLO projection.

8. When it is possible to detach the wheelchair arms, and the patient's safety can be ensured, it is possible to perform the standard projections for the patient seated in a wheelchair. When a replacement view is necessary for the MLO projection, the LM view is the preferred choice. The LM beam direction offers an advantage to the technologist and to the patient due to the following:
   - Removal of the face shield from the mammography equipment provides more space for the technologist as she positions the breast tissue, thus providing more control over breast tissue capture and compression.
   - The LM projection provides the ability of the technologist to gently rotate the patient toward the image receptor for slightly greater capture of the extreme posterolateral breast tissue as the compression is applied.

9. Placing a pillow between the back of the wheelchair and the thoracic spine of the patient may provide a stabilizing affect that assists the patient to remain in a forward position for greater capture of posterior breast tissue as she is positioned for the CC, MLO, or lateral projections.

10. Problem-solving for mammography imaging when the patient is seated in a wheelchair may require a combination of standard projections and complementary projections to complete the exam.

Performing the mammography examination for patients who are in a wheelchair requires the technologist to have comprehensive knowledge of these four imaging factors:

- Breast tissue margins
- Breast margin mobility
- Problem-solving projections
- Mammography equipment operation (including the purpose of specifically designed compression devices)

Often, the solutions arrived at to successfully achieve adequate breast tissue capture and compression will be a combination of one or more of the above suggested solutions and the technologist's ability to evaluate these four imaging factors.

Imaging the Patient with an Implanted Medical Device

Patients may present for mammography with implanted medical devices that require special imaging considerations when performing the mammography examination. Examples of these devices include pacemakers (Figure 8-20), defibrillators, and vascular access ports used

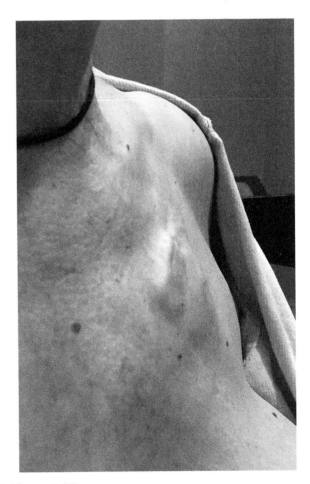

Figure 8-20
Illustration of pacemaker placement in the left superior breast region. This pacemaker location requires positioning/compression modifications to adequately capture and compress superior breast tissue.

to provide frequent medications and chemotherapy to the patient. Each imaging situation should be individually assessed by the technologist to determine what imaging approach should be considered to adequately capture and compress breast tissue. Generally, the unaffected breast may be managed by using the standard CC and MLO projections. The implanted medical device location is most often in the region of the superior or medial breast tissue margins, which describe fixed breast tissue margins. Standard projection positioning moves the mobile margins of the breast to the fixed tissue margin, applying the compression device across fixed tissue. For this reason, it may be necessary for the technologist to modify imaging of the affected breast by using replacement or complementary views to the standard projections. Modifications to the examination may include methods to avoid contact of the implanted medical device with the compression device as it moves across the fixed breast tissue margin:

1. Consider using the FB view in place of the CC projection.
2. Consider using the LMO projection in place of the MLO projection.
3. Consider using the LM projection as a complementary or replacement view to the MLO.
4. Consider a complementary view to the MLO using the 10-cm contact compression device to access and compress tissue surrounding the implanted device.

When imaging patients with pacemakers or defibrillators, it may be necessary to exclude the implanted device from the field of view to achieve adequate tissue compression. An example of a mammography study of a patient with a pacemaker is illustrated in Figure 8-21A–C. Figure 8-21A demonstrates adequate tissue compression in the CC projection with the pacemaker excluded from the image. Figure 8-21B demonstrates inclusion of the pacemaker on the MLO projection using enough compression force to adequately stabilize the breast tissue. Figure 8-21C demonstrates adequate tissue compression on the MLO projection with the pacemaker excluded from the image.

Imaging the Large-Breasted Patient

Patients who present for mammography with a larger breast size must be evaluated by the technologist for two separate imaging factors: adequate tissue inclusion and adequate compression application.

Adequate Tissue Inclusion

Occasionally, the active area of the 24 × 30-cm digital image detector is not sufficient to adequately include all margins of the breast due to breast size. In order for the CC image to include the entire breast from the medial margin to the lateral breast margin, and from the posterior margin

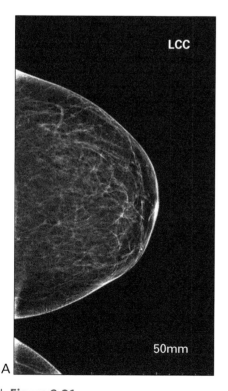
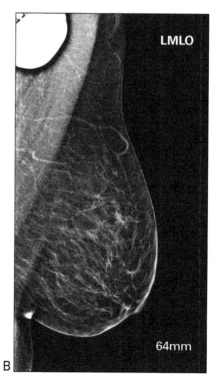
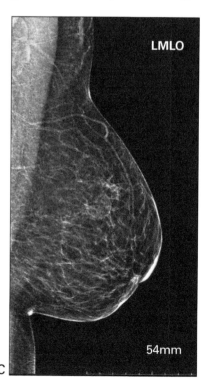

Figure 8-21
Mammography study of a patient with a pacemaker. LCC projection demonstrates adequate tissue compression; exclusion of pacemaker from the image **(A)**. LMLO projection demonstrates inclusion of the pacemaker with enough compression force to adequately stabilize the breast tissue **(B)**. Additional LMLO projection demonstrates adequate tissue compression; pacemaker excluded from the image **(C)**.

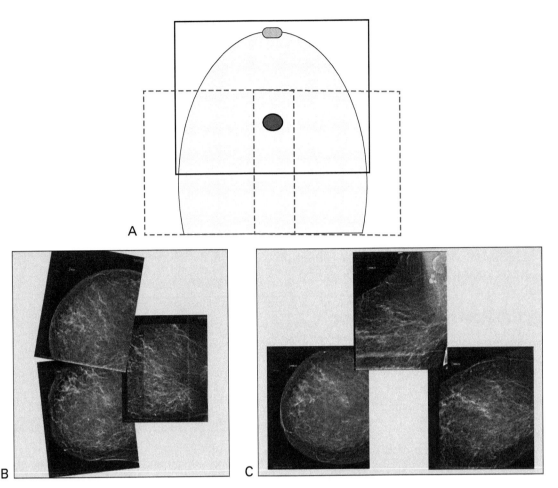

Figure 8-22
"Mosaic" or "tiling" imaging: overlapping images of the same projection allows visualization of the entire breast when the active area of the 24 × 30-cm digital image detector is not sufficient in size to adequately include all margins of the breast. Placement of a metallic marker centrally on the breast assists in providing image orientation for the interpreting radiologist **(A)**. Mosaic imaging of breast tissue in the CC projection demonstrating anteromedial, anterolateral, and posterior tissue **(B)**. Mosaic imaging of breast tissue in the MLO projection demonstrating inferior–posterior, anterior, and superior–posterior axillary tissue **(C)**.

to the anterior margin, it may be necessary to perform two or even three overlapping CC exposures. Likewise, for the MLO image to include the entire breast from the superior to inferior margin, and from the posterior to anterior margin, it may be necessary to perform two (or three) MLO exposures. The need for segmented exposures is determined by evaluating the width of the base of the breast for the CC projection, the length of the base of the breast for the MLO projection, and the distance from the base of the breast to apex. When imaging of the breast tissue requires overlapping images of the same projection to visualize all of the tissue due to breast size, it is referred to as "mosaic" or "tiling" imaging, as the tiles are fitted together to form a complete picture (Figure 8-22). Some technologists place a metallic marker on the center of the breast to accurately determine tissue inclusion and orientation on the completed radiographs (see Chapter 7).

Case Study **8-3**

1. Refer to Figure 8-21. When imaging a patient with an implanted device such as a pacemaker, infusaport, Port-A-Cath, etc., describe the special imaging techniques employed.

Case Study **8-4**

1. Refer to Figure 8-23. Describe the design feature of this compression device. When is it appropriate to use this design feature?

Adequate Compression Application

Patients presenting for mammography with a larger breast size may have a thicker (wide) breast base that tapers to a thinner (narrow) apex. For these patients, it is advantageous to use the tilt contact compression device. This unique compression device design provides a more uniform compression result from the thicker base of the breast to the thinner apex, especially when applying compression to a breast that is minimally compressible. The compression device conforms to the varying breast thickness as compression is applied, tilting toward the anterior breast when posterior compression has been achieved (Figure 8-23A and B). When the tilt compression device is not available, adequate tissue clarity may require an additional anterior compression view performed in the CC and MLO (or ML) projections (see Chapter 7).

Imaging the Postsurgical Patient

Reduction Mammoplasty

Patients with a history of reduction mammoplasty commonly present for the mammography procedure (Figure 8-24). Protocol for screening the patient with

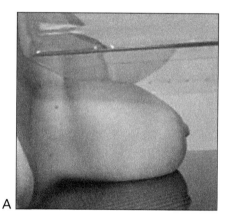

A

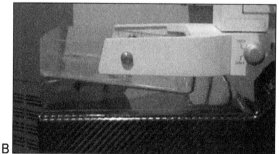

B

Figure 8-23
The tilt contact compression device design provides more uniform compression for patients with a thick breast base narrowing to a thinner apex **(A)**. The compression device conforms to the varying breast thickness as compression is applied, tilting toward the anterior breast when posterior compression has been achieved **(B)**.

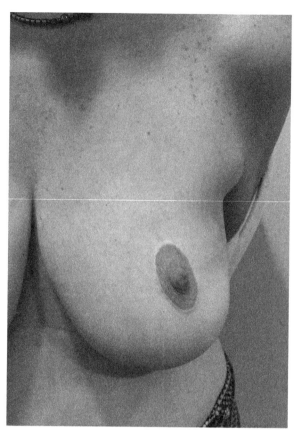

Figure 8-24
Patients with a history of reduction mammoplasty commonly present for the mammography procedure and do not typically require modifications for imaging. Note the higher nipple position on the breast after reduction mammoplasty is performed.

reduction mammoplasty includes the standard CC and MLO projections (Figure 8-25A and B) (see Chapter 10).

Breast Conservation Therapy (BCT) (Lumpectomy) Imaging

Chapter 10 provides an in-depth discussion of BCT and the imaging requirements associated with managing this patient. General guidelines suggest close mammographic surveillance at 6- or 12-month interval for 2 to 3 years. Some physicians recommend mammography of the affected breast after lumpectomy surgery (Figure 8-26), but before radiation therapy treatments begin to have a baseline study of the postoperative changes. The technologist should follow the facility protocols established for imaging the lumpectomy patient.

Suggested Solutions

1. Placing a scar marker on a BCT lumpectomy scar during screening and additional diagnostic imaging brings the area to the attention of the radiologist to facilitate the search for a new suspicious finding in and adjacent to the lumpectomy bed.

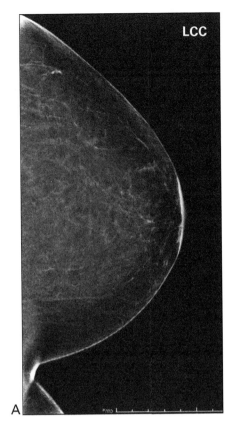
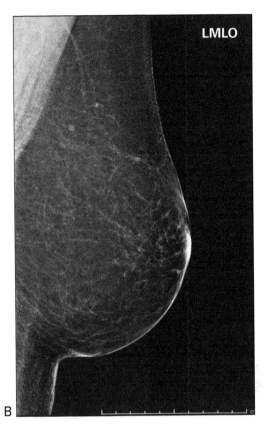

Figure 8-25
Mammography study example of reduction mammoplasty. LCC projection **(A)**, LMLO demonstrating slightly higher nipple position. Note the acceptable superior width of the pectoral muscle and the sufficient inclusion of the IMF, indicating adequate visualization of posterior breast tissue **(B)**. With reduction mammoplasty, the length of the pectoral muscle may not reach the PNL line on the MLO image; however, many other radiographic landmarks will be present.

2. Imaging protocols include the CC and the MLO projections.
3. Additional imaging may include the following contact or magnification projections:
   • ML + (MCC + MMLO of BCT site)
   • XCCL

Postmastectomy Imaging

Imaging of the postmastectomy chestwall (Figure 8-27) or following breast reconstruction is not routinely performed unless there is a new area of clinical concern. Figure 8-28A–C illustrates postmastectomy imaging projections, including the apex of the axilla, to detect recurrence of breast cancer. The technologist should follow the facility protocols established for imaging the postmastectomy patient. Imaging the postmastectomy patient may be requested after individual assessment of the patient by her oncologist and radiologist consult. The technologist may be asked to image the postmastectomy patient using the following:

• CC and MLO projections
• Spot magnification
• Imaging to include the axilla: AT and AX views

Irradiated Breast

Following radiation therapy, the breast may initially appear red or tan and edematous, and the patient may experience residual discomfort. In most cases, the breast will return to a more normal appearance with the passage of time (see Chapter 10). Imaging of the postirradiated breast requires the technologist to be sensitive to the discomfort of the patient. The breast must be gently handled during the positioning process. Communication with the patient during the compression application process will assist in ensuring the patient tolerates the procedure. When imaging the BCT patient who had radiation therapy treatments, review the previous images to discern the site of the original tumor, as periareolar incisions or excellent cosmesis can mask the surgical scar. The technologist should follow the facility protocols established for imaging the lumpectomy patient with radiation. The imaging study for this patient may include a tangential, magnified view of the tumor bed, obtained by positioning the surgical scar in tangent to the x-ray beam.

Managing the patient who has been diagnosed with breast cancer requires the technologist to be extra sensitive to the emotions she may be experiencing. Follow-up

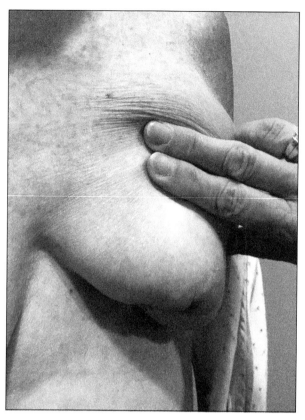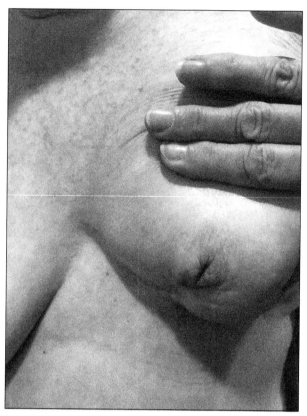

Figure 8-26
Patients with breast conservation therapy (BCT) (lumpectomy) surgical procedures commonly present for mammography. These patients may or may not have had radiation therapy treatments. Metallic scar markers indicate the surgical site. Gentle positioning techniques, slow application of compression, and a compassionate approach are essential for these patients.

care may produce feelings of great distress, anxiety, or sadness, often attributed to the fear of a possible recurrence.[8] Returning to the mammography suite may cause the patient to recall painful memories of her diagnosis and treatment. Many mammography services provide results to the diagnostic patient following the mammography procedure: this greatly reduces patient anxiety. Some mammography services, at the facility's discretion, allow the asymptomatic patient who has previously been treated for breast cancer to have a diagnostic mammogram or to return to screening mammography.[1] The technologist should demonstrate empathy and understanding to the breast cancer patient, validating her emotions while ensuring that the procedural process does not produce additional unnecessary anxiety. The following measures should be taken by the technologist and the facility to ensure that the emotions of the patient with a breast cancer diagnosis are respected:

- Gentle positioning/compression measures should be practiced.
- Additional imaging explained to the patient.
- Provide the imaging results as quickly as possible to the patient.

- Explain when and how the patient will receive her imaging results.

THE TECHNOLOGIST'S CONTRIBUTION

This chapter has provided several situations describing circumstances that challenge the mammography technologist's combined expertise in equipment operation and the artistic component of the mammography examination. These challenging imaging encounters are due to multiple situations that impede the capture and visualization of adequate breast tissue. Procedural impediments can be explained by various causes such as limitations in the patient's physical ability to cooperate with positioning requirements, inability to ensure the field of view is free of patient artifacts, or the limitation of space when imaging the patient in a wheelchair. Problem-solving for these situations depends heavily on the technologist's knowledge of additional mammography projections, the purpose of the additional projection, and her ability to correctly execute the necessary projection. Some of these challenging studies are infrequently encountered by the technologist, which further exacerbates the imaging situation due to the technologist's unfamiliarity of problem-solving projections, their purpose, and their execution. A simple solution to this problem is to periodically hold a positioning workshop for technologists to review the additional imaging projections and to allow each technologist to perform the view. These workshop solutions can be done through the voluntary assistance of a facility nurse or diagnostic technologist to act as the "patient." Staying current in the practice of all mammography projections and their intended purposes has the greatest impact in providing the technologist with the confidence necessary to creatively resolve difficult imaging situations.

▌▌ CHAPTER SUMMARY

Imaging the mammography patient who presents with a challenging situation requires additional time for the examination and for the technologist to demonstrate empathy and understanding to the patient. Respect for the patient includes allowing her to keep her gown on for the entire study unless it is the patient who decides it is a nuisance. Two technologists assigned to complete a challenging imaging study assures the patient a higher-quality examination with greater efficiency, increased safety, and less effort expended

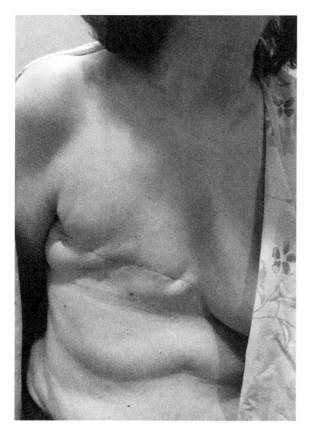

Figure 8-27
Imaging of the postmastectomy chestwall or of the breast mound after reconstruction surgery is not routinely performed unless there is a new area of clinical concern.

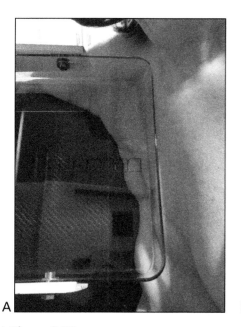 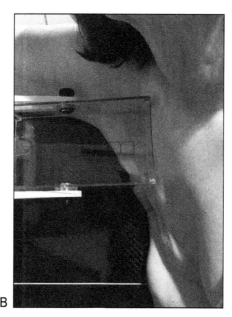 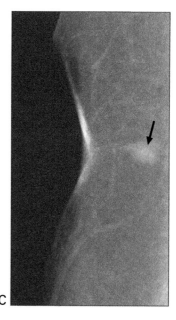

A B C

Figure 8-28
Postmastectomy imaging projections to detect breast cancer recurrence: tangential MLO projection over the surgical site **(A)**. Axillary projection (AX) using the 10-cm contact compression device to visualize the high apex of the axilla **(B)**. MLO image demonstrating recurrence of breast cancer **(C)**. Use of the magnification mode may also benefit postmastectomy imaging. The technologist should follow the facility protocols established for imaging the postmastectomy patient.

by the patient and by the technologist. The technologist who periodically reviews additional mammographic projections for problem-solving situations and updates her positioning/compression techniques by attending periodic positioning workshops is better equipped to manage a challenging imaging situation in the mammography setting.

Review Questions

1. Describe mosaic imaging and which patients would require this technique.

2. Describe problem-solving techniques that provide increased image quality and safety for the patient who is seated in a wheelchair.

3. Describe two examples of chestwall deformities that present imaging challenges in mammography, and why.

4. Describe the patient with kyphosis and what problem-solving techniques may be used when performing the mammographic study.

References

1. ACR Practice Parameter For the Performance of Screening and Diagnostic Mammography, Res. 11-2013. The American College of Radiology. Available at: https://www.acr.org/~/media/3484ca30845348359bad4684779d492d.pdf. Accessed February 12, 2017

2. Eklund GW, Cardenosa G. The art of mammographic positioning. *Radiol Clin North Am.* 1992;30(1):21–53.

3. American College of Radiology. *Mammography Quality Control Manual.* Reston, VA: American College of Radiology Committee on Quality Assurance in Mammography; 1999.

4. Majid A, et al. Missed breast carcinoma: pitfalls and pearls. *Radiographics.* 2003;23:881, 803–806.

5. The American Registry of Radiologic Technologists (ARRT) Standard of Ethics. Available at: https://www.arrt.org/docs/default-source/Governing-Documents/arrt-standards-of-ethics.pdf?sfvrsn=12. Accessed March 12, 2017

6. American Society of Radiologic Technologists (ASRT) Mammography Curriculum. Available at: https://www.asrt.org/docs/default-source/educators/curriculum/mammography/ed_curr_mammoadptd2013_20160606.pdf?sfvrsn=2. Accessed March 12, 2017

7. United Spinal Association. Free Publications, Disability Etiquette. Available at: https://www.unitedspinal.org/disability-publications/. Accessed March 10, 2017

8. Hartmann, Lynn C., et al. *Mayo Clinic Guide to Women's Cancers.* Mayo Clinic, 2007.

Thinking in Three Dimensions

9

Objectives

- Understand the descriptive terminology used to describe lesion location within the breast
- Determine the exact location of a lesion based on information obtained from mammogram images
- Determine the location of a lesion seen on only one standard mammographic projection

---

Key Terms

- central
- clock time
- lower inner quadrant (LIQ)
- lower outer quadrant (LOQ)
- periareolar
- subareolar
- upper inner quadrant (UIQ)
- upper outer quadrant (UOQ)

INTRODUCTION

The goal of this chapter is to encourage the technologist to think three-dimensionally. Each mammographic projection is a two-dimensional image of a three-dimensional organ; when combined, two projections can construct the three-dimensional breast. Each image is also a composite of numerous overlapping structures: medial structures overlap lateral structures, superior structures overlap inferior structures, and so on. The thicker the breast, the more structures there are to superimpose. Additionally, the tissue in the quadrants project differently from one view to another. Learning to think three-dimensionally helps the technologist accomplish the following:

• Evaluate the mammogram for missed breast tissue.
• Determine the location of a lesion in order to position the patient for a special view.
• Determine the location of a lesion in order to perform a correlative breast exam.
• Determine the location of a lesion in order to perform a stereotactic core biopsy procedure.
• Determine an optimal projection to view a lesion.
• Perform supplementary and special views with accuracy.

 CONSISTENT VIEWING

When viewing mammogram images, be consistent. Whether you view the images side by side or back-to-back, the technologist and radiologist must determine what format works best for them, and then, they need to stick with it. Routinely viewing images in the same manner familiarizes the technologist with breast tissue distribution—medial or lateral, superior or inferior, right or left, and so on. Additionally, an established format helps the technologist recognize patterns of pathology.

 DESCRIPTIVE TERMINOLOGY

Four quadrants divide the breast: **upper outer quadrant (UOQ)**, **upper inner quadrant (UIQ)**, **lower outer quadrant (LOQ)**, and **lower inner quadrant (LIQ)**. **Clock time** describes location within the breasts (Figure 9-1). Only 12:00 o'clock and 6:00 o'clock are the same location in both breasts. Note that 2:00 in the right breast represents the UIQ, whereas the same time in the left breast represents the UOQ. This opposite labeling is the same for all other clock times. Always describe the location of a lesion in terms of laterality, quadrant, and

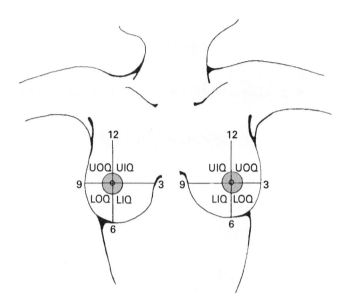

Figure 9-1
Clock time. Each breast is viewed as a clock and is divided into four quadrants, the upper outer quadrant (UOQ), the upper inner quadrant (UIQ), the lower outer quadrant (LOQ), and the lower inner quadrant (LIQ).

clock time (Figure 9-2). Also note the distance from the nipple, which is the only fixed point of reference in the breast. The terms **subareolar** and **periareolar** describe the area beneath the nipple and near (or around) the nipple area, respectively.

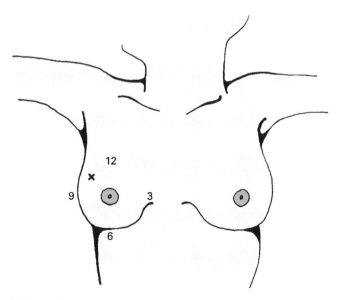

Figure 9-2
Descriptive terminology. Always describe a lesion in a consistent manner. For example, describe the lesion denoted by the "x" as "right breast UOQ at approximately the 10:30 position."

Case Study **9-1**

Refer to Figure 9-1. Describe how the clock time and quadrants differ between the left and right breasts.

MAMMOGRAPHIC SUPERIMPOSITION

Each mammographic image is a summation of tissue. It is possible to demonstrate areas of the breast free of superimposition of other glandular islands or one quadrant free of another. Figures 9-3 through 9-7 illustrate some of the common mammographic projections, the corresponding overlap, and the areas demonstrated free of superimposition.

Case Study **9-2**

Refer to Figures 9-3, 9-4, and 9-5. What tissue is superimposed in each of these three positions? Which positions provide true measurements of the ROI to the nipple?

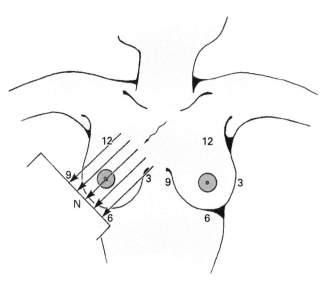

Figure 9-4
The MLO projection superimposes medial tissue over lateral tissue. Note:

1. The 12:00 to 1:00 area in the right breast (and 11:00 to 12:00 in the left) superimposes over the tissue in the UOQ.
2. A portion of the UIQ as it approaches 2:30 to 3:00 in the right breast (9:00 to 9:30 in the left) actually projects below the nipple.
3. The LOQ from 7:30 to 8:00 in the right and 4:30 to 5:00 in the left breast projects at the level of the nipple.
4. The LIQ of both breasts are demonstrated free of superimposition of other quadrants.

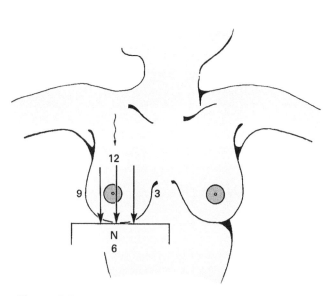

Figure 9-3
The CC projection superimposes superior over inferior tissue. This view is a true orientation of tissue to the nipple (i.e., measurement of a lesion's distance laterally or medially from the nipple is a true measurement).

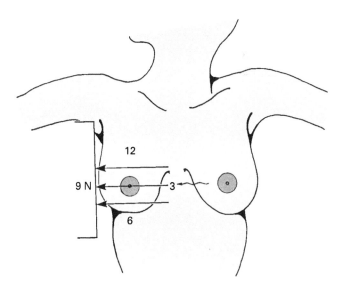

Figure 9-5
The Lateral projection superimposes medial over lateral tissue. This view is a true orientation of tissue to the nipple (i.e., measurement of a lesion's distance superior or inferior to the nipple is a true measurement). Note:

1. A 12:00 lesion is free of superimposition in this projection.
2. A 6:00 lesion is free of superimposition in this projection.

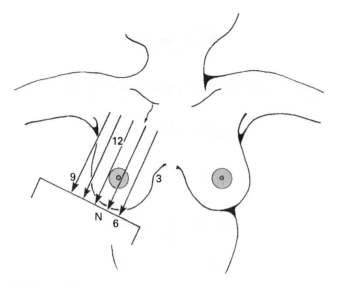

Figure 9-6
The 20° MLO projection superimposes superior over inferior tissue. Note:
1. 12:00 abnormalities will demonstrate lateral to the nipple.
2. The UOQ is free of superimposition in this projection.

▌ HOW ABNORMALITIES "MOVE" FROM PROJECTION TO PROJECTION

The nipple is the only fixed reference point in the breast. Except for centrally located lesions, which remain constant, a lesion's relationship to the nipple changes from one pro-

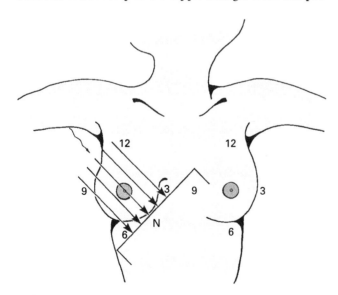

Figure 9-7
The superolateral to inferomedial oblique (SIO) projection superimposes lateral over medial tissue. Note:

1. The UOQ 10:30 area in the right breast (UOQ 2:30 area in the left) projects at nipple level.
2. The LIQ 3:30 to 4:30 area in the right breast (7:30 to 8:30 in the left) projects above or at the level of the nipple.
3. The UIQ and LOQ are projected free of superimposition.

jection to another. Understanding how a lesion "moves" in relationship to the nipple helps with localization, helps to demonstrate the area free of superimposition (if necessary), or facilitates with locating the lesion on a third view. Following a single lesion from projection to projection illustrates how it "moves" in relation to the nipple (Figure 9-8). Three rules hold true (barring any positional distortion of the mediolateral oblique [MLO] or Lateral):

1. When comparing the MLO projection to the Lateral projection, a lesion in the *medial* half of the breast *moves up* on the Lateral from its position on the MLO (Figure 9-9).
2. When comparing the MLO projection to the Lateral projection, a lesion in the *lateral* half of the breast *moves down* on the Lateral from its position on the MLO (Figure 9-10).
3. A **central** lesion has little to no movement from MLO to Lateral.

These rules are useful when a lesion is not seen with certainty on a craniocaudal (CC) projection and is only evident on the MLO projection. Comparing the height location of a lesion on the MLO projection to the height location on a Lateral (LM or ML) indicates where to search for the lesion on the CC image.

▌ APPROXIMATING LOCATION (FOR PALPATION AND/OR EXTRA VIEW)

Approximating a lesion's location (or at least its quadrant) guides the technologist in correlative palpation, in obtaining extra views, and in positioning for stereotactic core biopsy. Remember some basic concepts:

1. From the CC projection, we can determine whether a lesion is *medial* or *lateral* to the nipple and we can determine its distance from the nipple (Figure 9-11); superior and inferior cannot be determined from the CC image.
2. From the MLO and Lateral projections, we can determine whether a lesion is *superior* or *inferior* to the nipple and we can determine its distance from the nipple (Figure 9-12). Medial or lateral cannot be determined from the MLO or Lateral. A frequent mistake: a superior lesion is often assumed to be in the UOQ, when in fact a superior lesion could also lie in the UIQ. Remember to take into account the distortion of the MLO projection; that is, the MLO does not demonstrate a true relationship of structures to the nipple (refer to Figure 9-4) the way the Lateral does.
3. A centrally located lesion does not change its relationship to the nipple, regardless of the projection. However, if the nipple is excessively exaggerated in either projection, it may skew the nipple–lesion relationship.

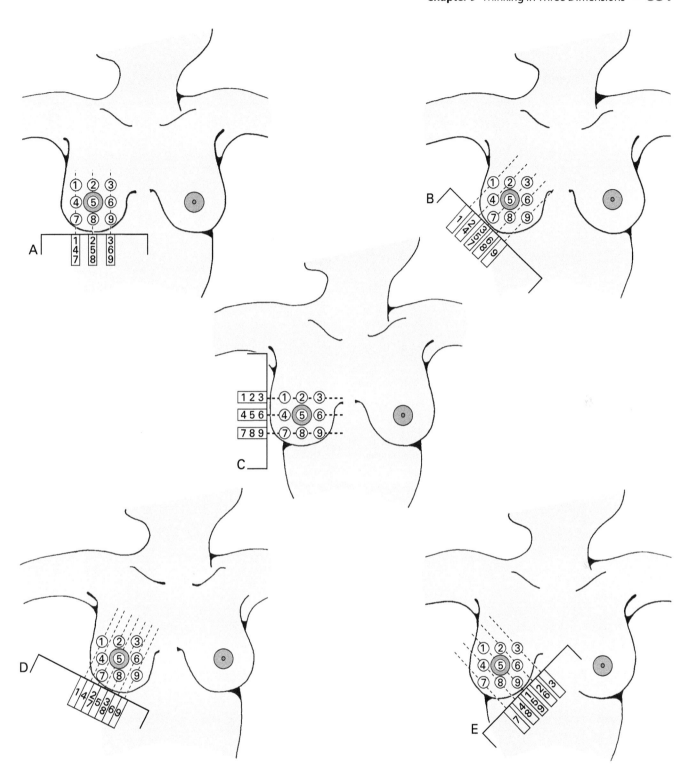

Figure 9-8
How abnormalities move. The schematics illustrate abnormalities in a grid array corresponding to superior, midbreast, and inferior and lateral, central, and medial locations. Numbers, corresponding to various placement of abnormalities, project on the image receptor outline. Follow any numbered lesion from projection to projection to gain an appreciation of how the lesion "moves" in relation to the nipple. In addition, these figures also illustrate which projection demonstrates a lesion free of superimposition of other quadrants. For example, lesion #3 is projected **(A)** medial to the nipple on the CC projection; **(B)** it is projected at the level of the nipple on the MLO view; **(C)** it is projected superior to the nipple on the Lateral view when compared to the MLO; this holds true for all abnormalities in the medial half of the breast. Note that the lesion moves up from the MLO view to the Lateral; this holds true for all medial abnormalities. **(D)** The lesion projects medial to the nipple (but in closer proximity to the nipple than on the CC view) on the 20° MLO view. **(E)** In the SIO position, lesion #3 is projected free of superimposition to other tissue. Therefore, the best view for imaging tissue in the UIQ of the breast is the SIO.

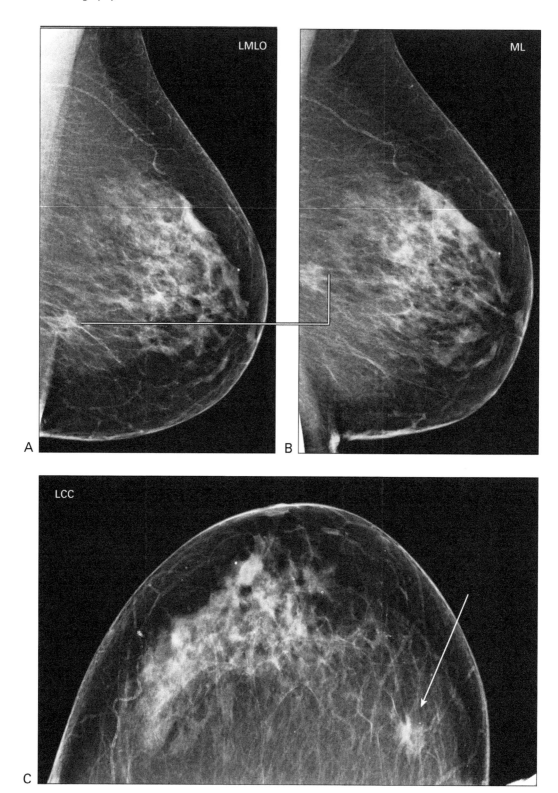

Figure 9-9
Medial lesion. Compare **(A)** the height of a lesion on the MLO projection to **(B)** the height on the Lateral projection. A lesion in the medial half of the breast is higher on the Lateral than its position on the MLO. **(C)** The CC view verifies the lesion lies medially (*arrow*).

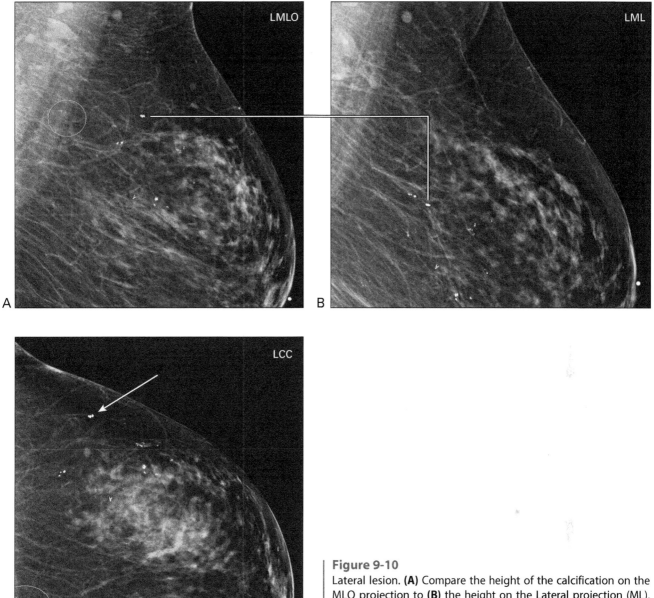

Figure 9-10
Lateral lesion. **(A)** Compare the height of the calcification on the MLO projection to **(B)** the height on the Lateral projection (ML). **(C)** A lesion in the lateral half of the breast (*arrow*) is lower on the Lateral than its position on the MLO. The CC view verifies the lesion lies laterally.

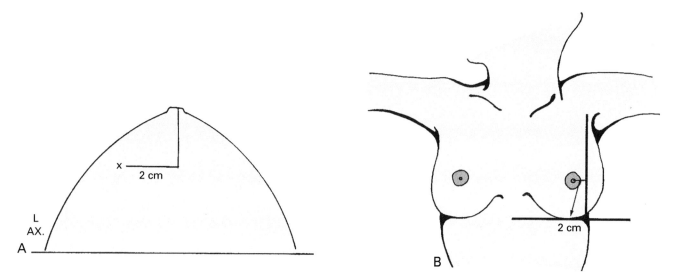

Figure 9-11
Medial or lateral. The CC projection **(A)** displays whether the lesion is medial or lateral and how far posterior from the nipple. **(B)** In this example, the lesion is 2 cm posterior to and 2 cm lateral to the nipple.

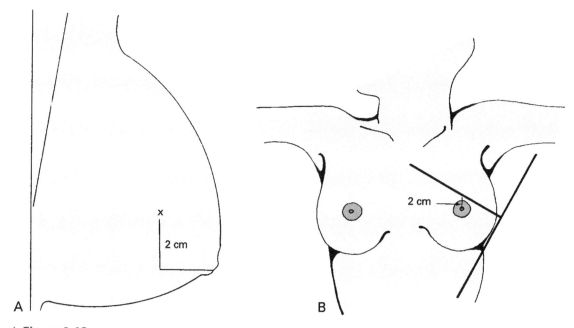

Figure 9-12
Superior or inferior. The Lateral (ML) projection **(A)** displays whether the lesion is superior or inferior to the nipple and how far posterior. **(B)** In this example, the lesion is 2 cm posterior to and 2 cm above the nipple.

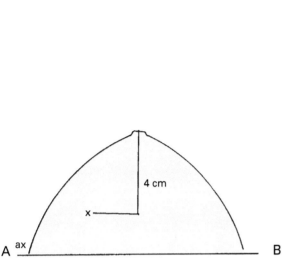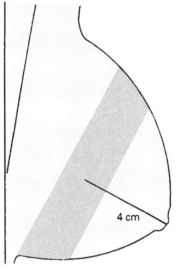

Figure 9-13
Lesion search. **(A)** A lesion evident on the CC projection is 4 cm posterior to the nipple. **(B)** To find the lesion on the complementary projection (in this case a MLO projection), measure a distance of 4 cm from the nipple; search a wider area to allow for nipple rotation to find the lesion.

Two projections are necessary to determine approximate location. When a lesion appears on one projection, determine its approximate distance from the nipple and examine the same plane in the complementary projection (allowing for rotation of the nipple) (Figure 9-13). If this search does not reveal the lesion, a third view will be necessary to determine whether the lesion is real or overlapped tissue. If real, it must be seen on a second projection to determine its location (see Chapter 10).

If the lesion is present on two projections, it is easy to approximate location. One method to locate a lesion, and by far the simplest, is to use one's own breast as a model (regardless of size relationship). Imagine in your own breast the possible location of the lesion on each of the views and correlate the findings to determine the lesion's approximate location (Figure 9-14).

Review Questions

1. What is the only fixed reference point in the breast?

2. Two projections are necessary to determine the approximate location of a lesion. Describe how to locate a lesion that is seen on only one of the standard (CC and MLO) views.

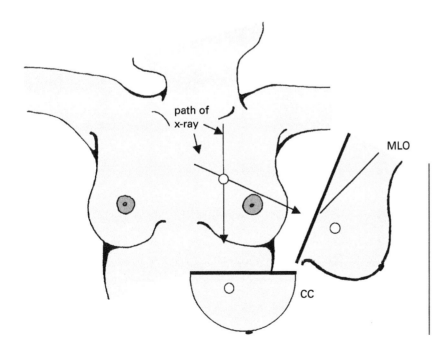

Figure 9-14
Locating a lesion: the quick method. This schematic illustrates another method to locate a lesion. The images are in the same relationship to the body, as they would be for the mammogram. The x-ray beam is always perpendicular to the image receptor. In order for the lesion to project medial to the nipple on the CC and superior to the nipple on the MLO, the lesion will have to lie along the perpendicular lines. Bisecting these lines reveals the approximate location of the lesion, left breast, UIQ at about 10:00.

Practical Applications in Problem-Solving

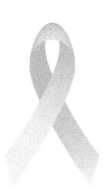

Detecting the suspected lesion is only half the job, proving the need for biopsy is quite another.

—Laszlo Tabar

Objectives

- Understand the steps necessary to establish a standardized protocol for working up findings found on the mammographic or clinical examination.
- Understand changes seen in the mammographic image due to surgical alterations.
- Understand the more common breast surgeries and how to best image these patients.

Key Terms

- Architectural distortion
- Asymmetry
- Calcifications
- Focal asymmetry
- Mass
- Superimposition

INTRODUCTION

This chapter illustrates the application of specific mammographic diagnostic protocols for specific breast problem-solving. Because each patient is unique, one approach may not address all problems. Yet, each problem identified, whether a clinical problem or a mammography finding, may have a standardized approach to problem-solving.

The mammogram as a tool of early breast cancer detection has a high sensitivity, finding most cancers. The false-negative rates of 5% to 25%[1,2] or higher may reflect cancers that are not evident on the mammogram, as well as cancer that is apparent on the mammogram, but perceived only retrospectively. Diagnostic errors by a radiologist are the chief alleged error associated with breast cancer malpractice. Many diagnostic errors by radiologists can be characterized as errors in either perception or interpretation.[3] This leaves room for improvement and no room for complacency.

Although the specificity of mammography is high in a screening population, it suffers low specificity in the diagnostic problem-solving imaging setting; the mammogram can suggest malignant or benign disease, but it is poor at distinguishing between the two. As a result, the average positive biopsy rate (PPV3) based on results of biopsies actually performed is 31.0% or one in three biopsies.[4] The widespread use of needle tests, such as fine needle aspiration cytology (FNAC) and large-gauge and vacuum-assisted needle core biopsy, has clearly impacted the diagnostic process, but these tests cannot replace an adequate and complete imaging workup of the patient. A full evaluation can improve both sensitivity and specificity of the mammogram.

The goal of this chapter is to improve both the sensitivity and specificity of mammography through problem-solving. The discussion begins with an overall approach to diagnostic problem-solving imaging and finishes with a section on imaging the surgically altered breast; these patients represent the majority of those undergoing diagnostic mammography.

ROLE OF THE TECHNOLOGIST

The technologist has a critical role in the problem-solving process. Technologists are the radiologist's eyes and ears in the screening and the diagnostic setting. Ensuring a complete and accurate breast health history from the patient, combined with good listening skills, is a critical attribute for a technologist to espouse. An accurate record of current clinical findings and personal history of risk factors, including prior invasive and noninvasive procedures, can impact the interpretation of the mammographic images and ultimately the course of action for the patient (Figure 10-1).

The technologist provides the radiologist with diagnostic images needed to make a definitive diagnosis. Knowledge of additional mammographic projections and their usefulness is essential. Appropriate high-quality diagnostic images combined with explanations written on the patient history form concerning additional images or additional diagnostic information from the technologist can make the difference in detecting a breast cancer, or canceling an unnecessary biopsy (Figure 10-2). Accurately correlating the referring provider's clinical exam or the patient's self-awareness findings and identifying the exact area in the

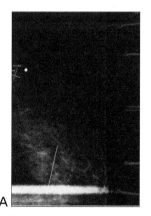 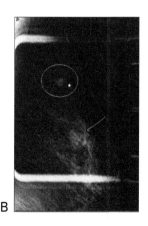 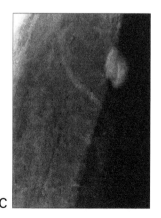 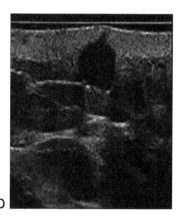

A B C D

Figure 10-1
Technologist input. A 51-year-old woman presents with a new palpable abnormality adjacent to a previous benign biopsy scar. The technologist placed a radiopaque marker (metallic BB) on the new palpable abnormality and a wire (*thin white line*) on the benign biopsy scar. Standardized diagnostic images obtained. **(A)** Spot compression CC and **(B)** spot compression MLO reveal a small well-defined superficial mass corresponding to the palpable abnormality—as indicated by the metallic BB. **(C)** Tangential image confirms the superficial location. **(D)** Ultrasound confirms a circumscribed mass with extension to the skin consistent with a benign sebaceous cyst.

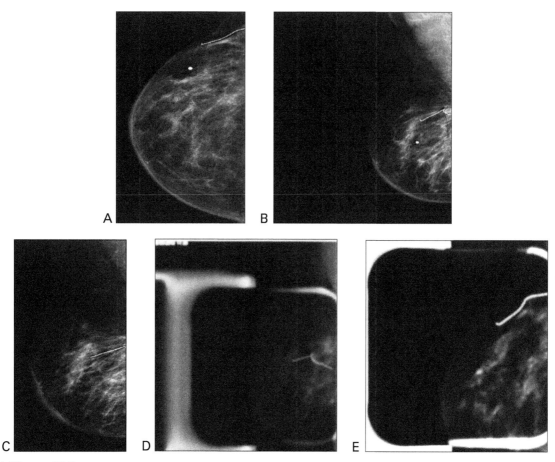

Figure 10-2
Biopsy cancelled. A 72-year-old woman referred for biopsy due to a new palpable abnormality adjacent to previous breast conservation therapy (BCT) site. Technologist placed a radiopaque marker (metallic BB) at the area of clinical concern and a wire (*thin white line*) at the previous BCT site. Technologist obtained standardized diagnostic images **(A)** CC, **(B)** MLO, **(C)** ML, **(D)** spot compression MLO, and **(E)** spot compression CC. Radiologist noted no mammographic abnormality at the area of clinical concern. Biopsy was cancelled, and further evaluation with ultrasound and/or MRI was recommended.

breast for the radiologist by placing a radiopaque BB on the area of clinical concern are essential.

Wende Logan-Young, MD, said, "We as mammographers are in a unique position to correlate what we see with what we feel." Take advantage of this.

INTRODUCTION TO STANDARDIZED IMAGING PROTOCOLS

Screening mammography requires at least two images of each breast. For the routine patient, these images have been standardized to CC and MLO projections of each breast, with or without additional 3D digital breast tomosynthesis (DBT) images. The addition of DBT to digital mammography (DM) has been shown to decrease recall rates and improve cancer detection rates.[5] Batch reading of screening exams can significantly reduce screening

mammography recall rates without affecting the cancer detection rate or the proportion of cancers diagnosed with favorable prognostic indicators.[6]

During diagnostic or problem-solving mammography, the exam is tailored to the patient's mammographic finding or sign or symptom of breast cancer. The lack of uniformity between radiologist's preferences of diagnostic images for specific breast problems can lead to inefficiencies in patient, technologist, radiologist, and facility time and resources. Different diagnostic imaging protocols may lead to distraction, fatigue, and potential medical errors.

There is growing evidence that distractions are increasing medical errors.[7] Distraction is the result of individuals interacting with their surroundings and technology and varies per individual differences, environmental disruptions, team awareness, and "rush mode"/time pressure.[8] This behavior can lead to error and affect patient safety and satisfaction. Radiologists may become distracted when they are interrupted by technologists who need to clarify which images are needed. Mammography technologists may become distracted trying to remember which set of images one radiologist prefers compared to another radiologist instead of focusing on patient care.

Radiologist fatigue has been a concern for years. Investigators have been studying its impact on diagnostic accuracy in image interpretation. Errors in medical image interpretation may be exacerbated by physician workload and multitasking. Medical error in medical image acquisition may be exacerbated by technologist workload and multitasking. Workload evaluation should consider all aspects involved in interpreting or acquiring images, especially in busy environments when administrative tasks and patient communication are integrated into clinical routines and distractions and interruptions occur regularly.[9]

Lean and Six Sigma Quality Improvement methodologies have been studied in their potential to reduce error and costs and improve quality within radiology. The measured outcomes studied have been organized into seven common aims: cost savings, reducing appointment wait time, reducing in-department wait time, increasing patient volume, reducing cycle time, reducing defects, and increasing staff and patient safety and satisfaction.[10] Each of these outcomes is critical in mammography.

The best the technologist can do are the following:

1. The radiology practice or facility should establish a standardized protocol for problem-solving or additional imaging per the problem indicated. The technologist must have a single specific standardized protocol for all patients with a specific clinical problem or screening mammography finding. This approach is not radiologist preference specific but rather clinical or mammography problem specific.
2. Become familiar with patterns of pathology, both clinically and mammographically.
3. Become comfortable viewing mammographic images and the areas of the breast best demonstrated on the image.
4. Understand mammography triangulation to localize a ROI using two-dimensional images of the breast and the distance from the nipple.

Establishing a Standardized Protocol

Each clinical or mammography finding should have specific additional imaging to determine the final recommendation for the patient: whether she can return to routine screening, or a short-interval follow-up is appropriate, or perhaps a biopsy for tissue diagnosis is required. Additional diagnostic imaging is highly advised in all incomplete or suspicious screening exams (BIRADS 0, 4, or 5). Without a complete diagnostic imaging workup, an assessment of probably benign (BIRADS 3) on a screening mammogram is discouraged. In fact, a probably benign assessment is included as a false-positive exam if, ultimately, breast cancer is not detected.

The following factors should be considered before a BIRADS final assessment category is assigned:

1. Clinical history
2. Patient history of risk factors including personal and family history of breast cancer
3. Prior mammography, breast ultrasound, or MRI findings

Each of these factors is critical for every patient. Tailoring the study to each patient's specific clinical or mammography finding is important to determine the BIRADS final assessment category and recommendation. A standardized protocol developed by the radiology facility will determine which images are needed for complete quality patient care (Tables 10-1 to 10-3).

Case Study **10-1**

1. Refer to Tables 10-1 to 10-3. Discuss the advantages to the radiologist, technologist, and the patient when standardized diagnostic protocols for specific breast problem-solving is implemented.

Patient Breast History Form

A breast history form (Figure 10-3) should be completed and signed by the patient, with the assistance of the

Table 10-1 • Standardized Protocols for BIRADS 0 Findings on Screening Mammogram

ADDITIONAL IMAGING NEEDED (BIRADS 0)	
#1 Calcifications	ML+ (MCC + MMLO of calcifications)
#2 Asymmetry on CC only	ML+ (SCC of asymmetry) + CCRM + CCRL
#3 Asymmetry on MLO only	ML+ (SMLO of asymmetry) + MLRS + MLRI
#4 Mass or focal asymmetry	ML+ (SCC + SMLO of mass)
#5 Architectural distortion	ML + (SCC + SMLO of architectural distortion)
#6 Skin lesion or calcifications	ML + (MCC + MMLO + TAN of calcifications)

Table 10-2 • Standardized Protocols for BIRADS 3 Findings on Previous Diagnostic Mammogram

SHORT-INTERVAL FOLLOW-UP (BIRADS 3)	
#7 Calcifications	CC + MLO + ML + (MCC + MMLO of calcifications)
#8 Mass or focal asymmetry	CC + MLO + ML + (SCC + SMLO of mass)
#9 Post-BCT	CC + MLO + ML + (MCC + MMLO of tumor bed)

Table 10-3 • Standardized Protocols for Findings on Clinical Exam

CLINICAL FINDING INDICATED	
#10 Palpable abnormality	CC + MLO + ML + (SCC + SMLO of palpable area) + US
#11 Nipple discharge	CC + MLO + ML + (MCC + MML of subareolar area) + US
#12 Focal pain	CC + MLO + ML + (SCC + SMLO of focal pain area) + US

Patient Label

Biopsy Date:

Biopsy Type:

Pathology: **Concordant** **Discordant**

Recommendation:

Screening Services

Type of Screening:

☐ Screening mammography: (completely without symptoms)

☐ Screening w/implants (please book two appointment slots)

Requested by:________________, M.D. Date:________

CBE

☐ Negative

☐ Positive (if checked, please complete diagnostic services section.)

Diagnostic Services

Diagnostic Evaluation:

☐ Clinical breast exam

☐ Imaging as needed (Mammo, U/S, MRI)

☐ Consultative Services (CBE, imaging and biopsy when indicated)

☐ Image-guided needle biopsy (ultrasound or stereotactic)

☐ Second Opinion Services

Requested by:________________, M.D. Date:________

Clinical Findings:

☐ Palpable lump

☐ Skin thickening

☐ Focal breast pain

☐ Abnormal nipple discharge

☐ Other: ________

Level of Suspicion

☐ Low

☐ Intermediate

☐ High

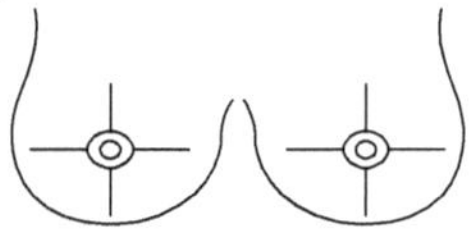

The patient was educated on this procedure taking into consideration the patient's learning needs.

Please have the patient complete this portion of the order form:

a. At the present time, have you or your doctor noticed any of the following changes or problems?

☐ Abnormal nipple discharge or change ☐ Palpable lump ☐ Dimpling

☐ Skin thickening ☐ New focal breast pain ☐ Other ________

b. Is this a follow-up from a recent abnormal mammogram within the last year? ☐ Yes ☐ No

c. Have you had a breast needle biopsy within the last two years? ☐ Yes ☐ No

d. Have you had a lumpectomy for breast cancer within the last three years? ☐ Yes ☐ No

CBC Office Use Only

By signing below, I have verified that my answers to the above questions are still accurate.

Name: ________________ Date: ________

Final BIRADS Assessment: B1 B2 B3 B4 B4a B4B B4C B5 B6 B0

Recommendation: Routine Short Interval F/U Biopsy Additional Imaging Other:

A

Figure 10-3

Sample patient history forms. **(A)** A simple patient history form that allows follow-up notes for biopsy if needed.

Patient History Form

For Technologist Notes Only:

Last Name:_____ First Name:_____ M.I._____

□ FTP

Birth date:_____ Phone:_____ Phone today if needed:_____

□ Cell phone

Health Care Provider to send reports to:_____

□ Results Called

1. Reason for Today's Exam: Annual Exam Follow-up New Symptoms or Clinical Finding

2. □ No □ Yes Do you have breast implants? □ Both □ Right □ Left

3. □ No □ Yes Are you still having menstrual periods? Date of last period:_____

   a. □ No □ Yes If you are still menstruating, beast feeding or possibly pregnant?

Known Clinical History

4. □ No □ Yes Have you ever been Diagnosed with Breast Cancer?
   If "Yes," please indicate which breast(s): □ Right □ Left

5. □ No □ Yes Have you ever been Treated for Breast Cancer?
   □ Mastectomy   □ Rt. Date:_____ □ Lt. Date:_____
   □ Lumpectomy   □ Rt. Date:_____ □ Lt. Date:_____
   □ Radiation   □ Rt. Date:_____ □ Lt. Date:_____
   □ Chemotherapy   Date:_____
   □ Chemoprevention Therapy Date:_____

6. □ No □ Yes Have you ever had Breast Surgery?
   □ Breast Reduction □ Rt. Date:_____ □ Lt. Date:_____
   □ Surgical Biopsy   □ Rt. Date:_____ □ Lt. Date:_____
   □ Needle Biopsy   □ Rt. Date:_____ □ Lt. Date:_____
   □ Other _____ □ Rt. Date:_____ □ Lt. Date:_____

Known Previous Breast Procedures

7. □ No □ Yes Have you had breast imaging studies at another facility? Facility _____
   □ Mammogram   □ Rt. Date:_____ □ Lt. Date:_____
   □ Breast Ultrasound □ Rt. Date:_____ □ Lt. Date:_____
   □ Breast MRI   □ Rt. Date:_____ □ Lt. Date:_____
   □ Other _____ □ Rt. Date:_____ □ Lt. Date:_____

Known Previous Breast Imaging

8. □ No □ Yes Are you currently using any hormone related treatments? If yes, what type?

Known Risk Factors

9. □ No □ Yes Have you ever given birth to a child? (Include all live births, still births, or cesarean sections. Do not include miscarriages or abortions.)
   If "Yes," your age at your first child's birth:_____

10. □ No □ Yes Do you have a history of breast cancer in your family? If yes, which relative(s)?
   □ Mother, age___ □ Sister, age___ □ Daughter, age___ □ Any males
   □ Other (please specify)

11. □ No □ Yes Do you have a history of ovarian cancer or BrCA in your family?

Known new Clinical Problems

12. □ No □ Yes Have you had a clinical breast exam by your health care provider? Date_____
   □ Within past 3 months □ 4 to 12 months ago □ Over 1 year ago □ Never

13. □ No □ Yes I or my Health Care Provider feel a new palpable lump or thickening. □ Rt. □ Lt.
14. □ No □ Yes I or my Health Care Provider noted new focal pain or tenderness. □ Rt. □ Lt.
15. □ No □ Yes I or my Health Care Provider noted new nipple discharge. □ Rt. □ Lt.
16. □ No □ Yes Other symptom: Please Specify: _____ □ Rt. □ Lt.

Known Previous Mammograms

Please mark the area in your breast where you or your Health Care Provider are concerned about.

18. Signature _____ Date _____

B

Figure 10-3 (*Continued*)
(B) A more complete patient history form that allows technologists to summarize important information in right hand column for radiologist to review. Either form can be scanned into PACS system for easy access.

technologist as needed. This form should include the following information:

1. Any clinical signs or symptoms of breast cancer detected by the referring provider or the patient, including any new palpable findings, breast thickening, nipple discharge, skin or nipple changes, or focal pain.
2. Personal history of breast cancer including surgical, radiation, and chemotherapy treatments. Draw all malignant biopsy scars on a diagram along with the date of the surgery.
3. Family history of breast cancer, including relationship (especially mother, sister, daughter, or any male family members) and age when diagnosed. Determination of premenopausal, perimenopausal, or postmenopausal status is helpful.
4. BrCA1 and BrCA2 status of any family members, if known.
5. History of prior benign biopsy. Draw biopsy scars on a diagram along with the date of the surgery.
6. History of recent nipple inversion, change, or nipple discharge—especially spontaneous, unilateral, bloody, or clear nipple discharge and the length of time the discharge has been present.
7. Presence of moles, birthmarks, or skin tattoos. Draw on the diagram.
8. History of hormonal replacement therapy or chemoprevention (i.e., tamoxifen).

9. Date of last menstrual period, including history of oophorectomy.
10. History of prior breast infections including mastitis or abscesses.
11. History of recent or remote breast trauma.
12. History of prior mammograms (date and location).

In addition to documenting the above information, it is critical that the technologist confidentially talk with the patient. The patient may exclude a symptom out of fear or because her physician said everything was fine on the/her clinical exam. The patient is most aware of any changes within her breast tissue. The technologist should ask the patient if she has any concerns about her breasts. The technologist can create an atmosphere that encourages the patient to discuss her concerns so that important information may not be overlooked (Figure 10-4).

Obtaining Prior Mammograms

Reviewing prior images for breast size and composition is helpful in determining the optimum technique for the mammogram. Preferably, at the time of the patient's appointment, prior mammograms are available. Although the availability of prior mammograms is helpful to identify new findings (Figure 10-5) and for reassurance of normal variation or stable findings, a patient should never be denied an appointment because of the lack of prior

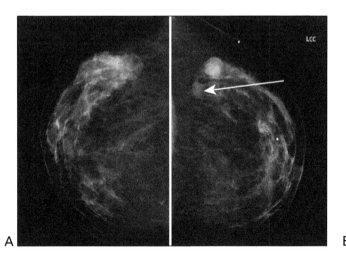
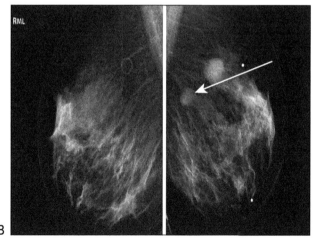

Figure 10-4
Accurate patient history. A 42-year-old woman presents for asymptomatic screening. After thoughtful questioning by the technologist, the patient confides she has two palpable lumps in her left breast that she did not reveal to her health care provider. The technologist marks the two masses with radiopaque markers (metallic BBs) and obtains standardized protocol diagnostic images for two left breast palpable abnormalities. Bilateral **(A)** CC and **(B)** MLO images reveal three masses in the left breast. The two palpable masses are marked with radiopaque markers (metallic BBs). The third mass (*arrows*) was felt by the technologist during positioning. Standardized diagnostic images, including CC, MLO, ML, and spot compression CC and spot compression MLO images, were obtained saving the patient, technologist, and radiologist time waiting for an additional imaging appointment. All three masses were biopsy-proven invasive ductal carcinoma.

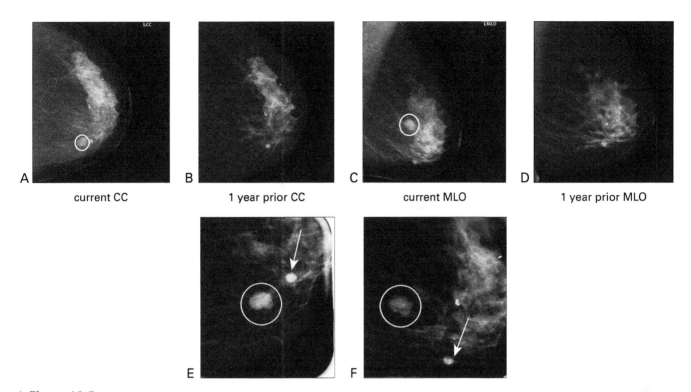

A   current CC   B   1 year prior CC   C   current MLO   D   1 year prior MLO

E   F

Figure 10-5
Comparison mammograms. A 47-year-old woman for screening mammogram. Having comparison mammograms available at time of the screening mammographic exam is critical for distinguishing new abnormalities. Both (**A and B**) CC and (**C and D**) MLO images demonstrate a new mass (*circle*) when compared to the previous mammogram acquired 1 year earlier. The patient needed to be recalled to complete the standardized diagnostic protocol for a mammographic mass. (**E**) Spot compression CC and (**F**) spot compression MLO images (*circle*) confirm the presence of a new circumscribed, oval high-density mass that retains its shape. Note the second high-density mass (*arrow*) not previously perceived. Both masses were biopsy-proven invasive ductal carcinoma.

mammogram access. The current mammogram may have an obvious suspicious finding that needs further evaluation that may or may not have been present on the prior mammogram. Although the previous mammogram may eliminate the need for further additional diagnostic imaging, any delay in identifying a suspicious finding may delay a breast cancer diagnosis and treatment.

Case Study **10-2**

1. Refer to Figure 10-5. Locating prior images on a patient who is new to a facility can be an enormous investment in time and effort. Discuss the advantages of having prior mammograms at the time of the patient's appointment.

Clinical Examination

The clinical examination is twofold and involves inspection and palpation.

Inspection

Before performing the mammogram, the technologist should document any suspicious skin or nipple changes or findings on the history sheet diagram (Figure 10-6). All skin lesions should be documented; skin moles and sebaceous cysts may appear as a breast mass on mammography. This documentation is especially important with 2D imaging; however, DBT has proven to be helpful in identifying skin

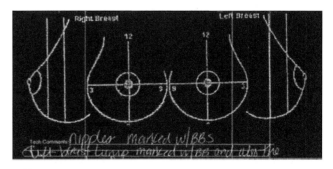

Figure 10-6
Documentation of visual breast inspection. Sample diagram with technologist notes.

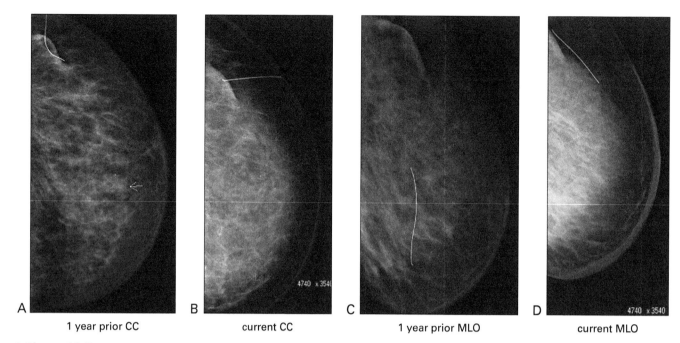

| 1 year prior CC | current CC | 1 year prior MLO | current MLO |

Figure 10-7

Physical inspection. **(A–D)** A 63-year-old woman with a surgical scar from prior breast conservation therapy (BCT). Metallic wire (*thin white lines*) clearly identifies the surgical scar and focal skin thickening from her recent surgery. Note the diffuse skin thickening, trabecular thickening, and increased breast tissue density on the current images; side effects from interval radiation therapy.

lesions and skin calcifications since these findings can be localized to the skin on stacked DBT images. Because many skin abnormalities can look suspicious on mammography and may not be immediately evident on initial inspection, a diagnostic mammogram with skin markers may be necessary to correlate with mammographic findings (Figures 10-7 and 10-8). A tangential image may be needed to document that the lesion is in the skin (Figure 10-9).

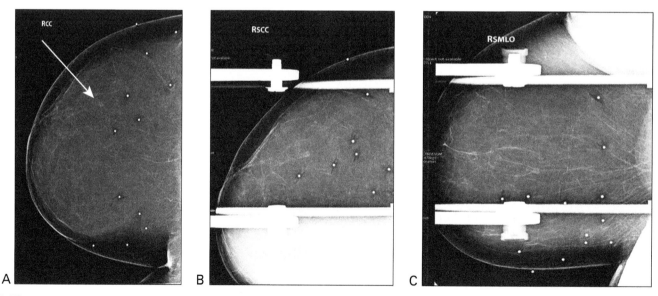

Figure 10-8

Skin markers. A 53-year-old woman recalled from screening for additional evaluation of a small mass in the right lateral breast (*arrow*). Radiopaque markers (metallic BBs) placed on multiple skin moles, which project as multiple masses on the mammogram. **(A)** CC, **(B)** spot compression CC, and **(C)** spot compression MLO images may be needed to determine if mammographic detected masses correspond to skin lesions. The small mass in the right breast lateral aspect does not correspond to any of the skin lesions. Mass was biopsy-proven invasive ductal carcinoma.

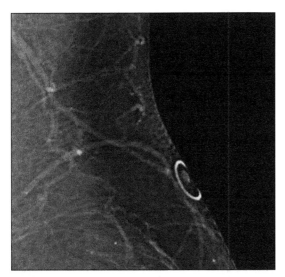

Figure 10-9
Skin lesion. A 49-year-old woman for screening mammography. Tangential image reveals a skin lesion marked with a radiopaque marker (*circle*). A tangential image may be helpful to document that a mammographic mass is actually located in the skin.

Palpation

It is not within the current scope of practice that mammography technologists are responsible to assess palpable clinical findings. Documentation and localization of any clinical findings on the patient history form and images by the technologist are critical to patient care. If a clinical finding is noted on a patient scheduled for screening mammography, the screening mammogram can be immediately converted to a diagnostic mammogram at the initial patient appointment and standardized protocol diagnostic images may be obtained (Figure 10-10).

Ultrasound

Breast ultrasound is complementary to mammography imaging. Since ultrasound utilizes a different diagnostic technology of ultrasonic sound waves, it complements mammography by detecting differences in tissue sound wave attenuation. The use of these two complementary modalities does not negate the suspicious findings of one modality versus the other. Yet, a negative ultrasound correlating to a possible resolved mammographic finding may boost the confidence of the radiologist that the exam is negative (Figure 10-11). Breast ultrasound is helpful in the evaluation of mammographic masses to determine their size, margin, and solid and cystic components (Figure 10-10). Ultrasound may also be helpful in determining if there is a solid or suspicious mass associated with focal asymmetries, architectural distortion, or calcifications.

Standardized Reporting

The ACR Atlas is designed to standardize breast imaging reporting and to reduce confusion in breast imaging

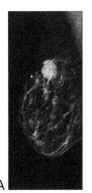 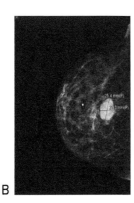 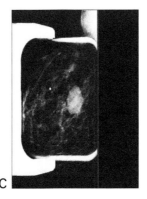 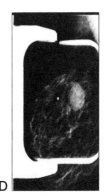 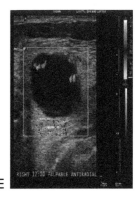

A　　B　　C　　D　　E

Figure 10-10
Palpation. A 61-year-old woman scheduled for a screening mammogram. A large palpable abnormality that was not reported by the patient or her health care provider was identified by the technologist. The screening exam was converted to a diagnostic exam at the patient's initial screening appointment. The technologist marked the new palpable abnormality with a radiopaque marker (metallic BB) and obtained standardized diagnostic images: **(A)** MLO, **(B)** CC, and **(C)** spot compression CC and **(D)** spot compression MLO. **(E)** Breast ultrasound performed on the same day reveals a vascular, suspicious solid mass. Biopsy confirmed invasive ductal carcinoma.

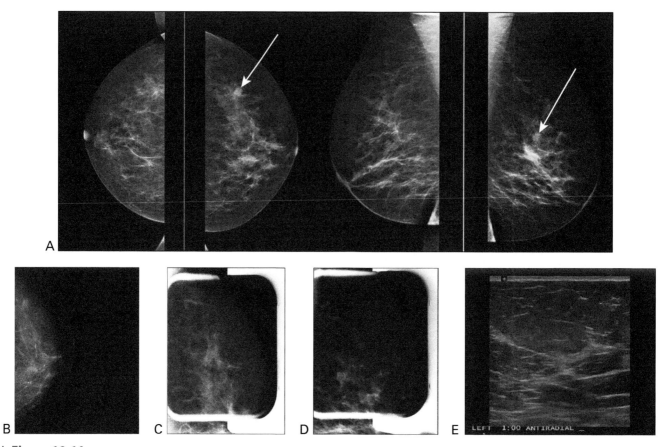

Figure 10-11

Superimposed breast tissue flattens with vigorous compression. A 66-year-old woman presents for a screening mammogram. **(A)** Bilateral CC and MLO images reveal a focal asymmetry (*arrows*) in the left breast. Further evaluation with standardized **(B)** ML and **(C)** spot compression CC and **(D)** MLO images reveal resolution of the focal asymmetry consistent with superimposed breast tissue. **(E)** Ultrasound evaluation of the 1 o'clock position reveals no ultrasound abnormality corresponding to the area of mammographic concern. Routine screening mammography recommended. BIRADS final assessment category 1: negative.

interpretation. It also facilitates outcome monitoring and quality assessment. The Atlas contains a lexicon for standardized terminology (descriptors) for mammography, breast US, and MRI. Standardized report organization and guidance include the following recommendations:

1. Describe the indication for the study: screening, diagnostic, or follow-up. Mention the patient's history.
2. Describe the breast composition.
3. Describe any significant finding using standardized terminology. Use the morphological descriptors: mass, asymmetry, architectural distortion, and calcifications. These findings may have associated features, like skin thickening, nipple retraction, calcifications, etc. Correlate these findings with any clinical information, mammography images, US exams, or MRI studies. Integrate mammography and US findings in a single report.
4. Compare to previous studies. Awaiting previous examinations for comparison should only take place if they are required to make a final assessment.
5. Conclude to a final assessment category. Use BIRADS categories 0 to 6 and the phrases associated with them.

If both mammography and US are performed, the overall assessment should be based on the most abnormal of the two breasts, based on the highest likelihood of malignancy.

6. Give management recommendations.
7. Communicate unexpected findings with the referring clinician. Verbal discussions between the radiologist, patient, and referring clinician should be documented in the report.

DIAGNOSTIC IMAGING OF INCOMPLETE SCREENING EXAM

(BIRADS 0: Incomplete—Needs Additional Imaging)

Imaging Calcifications

Lateral (ML or LM) plus magnified CC (MCC) and magnified MLO (MMLO)

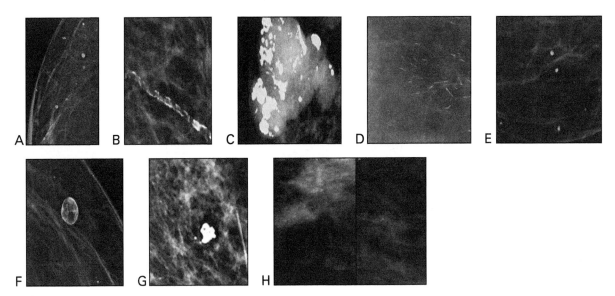

Figure 10-12
Magnification images of typically benign calcifications. Examples of benign calcifications. **(A)** Skin. **(B)** Vascular. **(C)** Coarse. **(D)** Large rod-like. **(E)** Round. **(F)** Rim. **(G)** Dystrophic. **(H)** Milk of calcium.

Breast **calcifications** are common. In fact, calcifications are the most common finding that undergoes breast biopsy. Most of these calcifications represent benign fibrocystic changes and do not signify carcinoma. The spatial resolution of routine screening mammography does not provide adequate visualization of calcifications to determine their morphology, number, and distribution; spatial resolution is critical to determining the need for biopsy.

Morphology

Many calcification morphologies determined as typically benign include skin, vascular, coarse, large rod-like, round, rim, dystrophic, and milk of calcium (Figure 10-12). These may not need diagnostic imaging for further evaluation. On the other hand, calcification morphologies classified as amorphous, course heterogeneous, fine pleomorphic, and

fine linear or fine-linear branching are considered suspicious and warrant further evaluation with biopsy for tissue diagnosis (Figure 10-13).

Amorphous (BIRADS 4B: moderate suspicion for malignancy) are small and/or hazy in appearance so that a more specific particle shape cannot be determined (Figure 10-13A).

Coarse heterogeneous (BIRADS 4B: moderate suspicion for malignancy) are irregular, conspicuous calcifications that are generally between 0.5 and 1 mm and tend to coalesce but are smaller than dystrophic calcifications (Figure 10-13B).

Fine pleomorphic (BIRADS 4C: high suspicion for malignancy) are usually more conspicuous than amorphous forms and are seen to have discrete shapes, without fine linear and linear branching forms, usually less than 0.5 mm (Figure 10-13C).

Fine linear or fine-linear branching (BIRADS 4C: high suspicion for malignancy) are thin, linear irregular calcifications

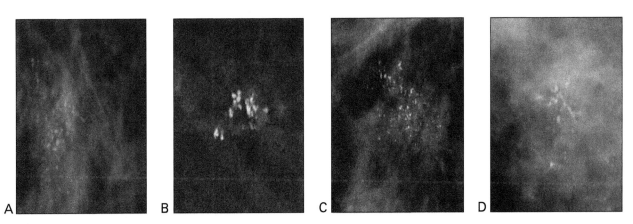

Figure 10-13
Magnification of suspicious calcification morphologies. Examples of suspicious-appearing calcifications. **(A)** Amorphous. **(B)** Coarse heterogeneous. **(C)** Fine pleomorphic. **(D)** Fine linear or fine-linear branching.

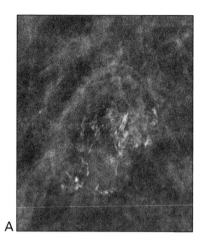 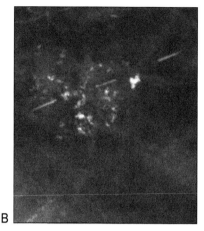 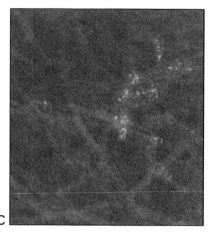

Figure 10-14
Early calcification morphologies may prove difficult to distinguish typically benign from suspicious. **(A)** Early fat necrosis. **(B)** Benign sclerosing adenosis. **(C)** Carcinoma.

that may be discontinuous; occasionally branching forms can be seen, usually less than 0.5 mm (Figure 10-13D).

It should be noted that the ACR BIRADS 5th edition no longer includes an indeterminate morphology calcification classification. Thus, short-interval follow-up of any calcification morphology is controversial. One exception is an isolated group of punctuate calcifications that is new, increasing, linear, or segmental in distribution or adjacent to a known cancer and can be assigned as probably benign or suspicious.

It can be difficult to determine the exact morphology of calcifications in their early stages of evolution. Many typically benign and suspicious calcifications look similar when they are very early in their development and not yet well formed. Perhaps some of these may undergo short-interval follow-up diagnostic imaging with the benefit that, given an additional 6 or 12 months of time, they may appear more typically benign; but this is done realizing the risk that instead they may appear more suspicious (Figure 10-14). A delay in diagnosis of carcinoma drives many early calcifications to undergo biopsy.

Distribution

Distribution of calcifications is at least as important as morphology in determining if they are benign or malignant. Distribution descriptors arranged according to the risk of malignancy (from least likely to most likely) include the following:

- Diffuse: distributed randomly throughout the breast
- Regional: occupying a large portion of breast tissue, with greater than 2 cm greatest dimension
- Grouped: few calcifications occupying a small portion of breast tissue; lower limit, five calcifications within 1 cm, and upper limit, a larger number of calcifications within 2 cm
- Linear: arranged in a line, which suggests deposits in a duct
- Segmental: suggests deposits in a duct or ducts and their branches

Diffuse calcifications, especially when they are widely scattered, are thought to be benign. Regional calcifications confined to one large area in the breast are also commonly considered benign. Grouped calcifications that occur in clusters of 5 or more in 1 cubic centimeter, especially if they are new or increasing, may require biopsy depending on their morphology. Calcifications with a linear or segmental distribution, following the pattern of the ductal system, are considered suspicious and warrant biopsy. These calcifications may represent carcinoma within the ductal system. Yet, it must be kept in mind that vascular calcifications occurring along the walls of blood vessels and large, rod-like calcifications occurring within ducts in plasma cell mastitis may also present in fine linear or fine-linear branching morphology—especially early in their development (Figure 10-15).

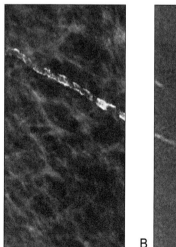 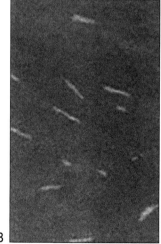

Figure 10-15
Benign calcifications. **(A)** Vascular calcifications line the walls of blood vessels; **(B)** plasma cell mastitis typically presents as large, rod-like calcifications occurring within the ducts. These benign processes can mimic fine linear or fine-linear branching morphology, especially early in their development.

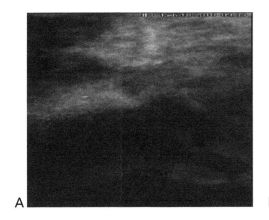
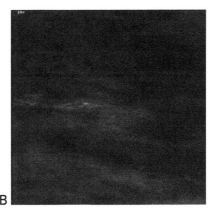

Figure 10-16
Milk of calcium. Calcium in microcysts that **(A)** layer on the Lateral image and **(B)** appear smudgy on the CC image.

Lateral Projection, Magnification, and Calcifications

A Lateral image, either ML or LM, is required for accurate localization in the breast. Choice of an ML or LM image is determined by the position of the calcifications within the lateral or medial breast. To minimize geometric unsharpness of the calcifications, the position that places the calcifications closest to the image receptor minimizes blur. Thus, calcifications in the lateral breast should be imaged in the ML projection, and calcifications in the medial breast should be imaged in the LM projection.

Additionally, a Lateral image, either ML or LM, allows identification of benign milk of calcium; this represents calcium in microcysts that appear smudgy on the CC image and layer on the Lateral image (Figure 10-16). MCC and MMLO images improve the spatial resolution of calcifications and facilitate the determination of benign, suspicious, or highly suspicious morphologies. Thus, additional evaluation and follow-up of calcifications require a Lateral and magnified CC and magnified MLO images (Figure 10-17).

Imaging Asymmetry

Asymmetries are findings that have different border contours than true masses and lack the conspicuity of masses.

Asymmetries appear like other discrete areas of fibroglandular tissue except that they are unilateral, with no mirror image correlate in the opposite breast. An **asymmetry** demonstrates concave outward borders and usually is interspersed with fat, whereas a mass demonstrates convex outward borders and appears denser in the center than at the periphery (Figure 10-18).

Types of Asymmetry

There are four types of mammographic asymmetries:

- Asymmetry as an area of fibroglandular tissue visible on only one mammographic projection, usually due to **superimposition** of normal fibroglandular tissue.
- **Focal asymmetry** visible on two projections, may represent superimposition of normal fibroglandular tissue or a true mass.
- Global asymmetry consists of a large asymmetry, over at least one quarter of the breast, and is composed of normal asymmetric fibroglandular tissue. Benign. No additional follow-up needed.
- Developing asymmetry is a new, larger, and more conspicuous asymmetry than was seen on a previous examination. This finding is highly suspicious for malignancy. Further evaluation with tissue diagnosis is needed.

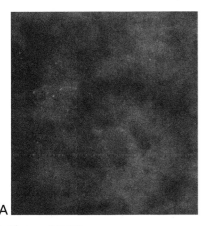
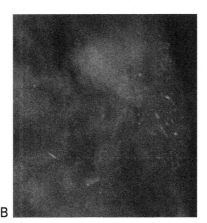
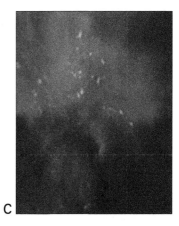

Figure 10-17
Additional evaluation and follow-up of calcifications require **(A)** Lateral, **(B)** magnified CC, and **(C)** magnified MLO images.

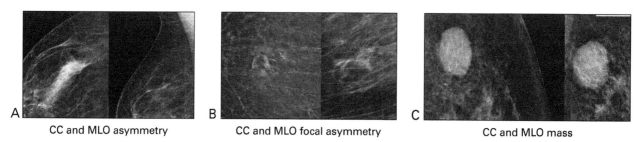

| CC and MLO asymmetry | CC and MLO focal asymmetry | CC and MLO mass |

Figure 10-18
Asymmetry and focal asymmetry versus mass. Asymmetries appear like other discrete areas of fibroglandular tissue except that they are unilateral, with no mirror image correlate in the opposite breast. **(A)** An asymmetry demonstrates concave outward borders and usually is interspersed with fat, **(B)** a focal asymmetry is identified on two images, whereas a **(C)** mass demonstrates convex outward borders and appears denser in the center than at the periphery.

Imaging Asymmetry Seen on One View Only

Lateral (ML or LM) plus CC Rolled Medial (CCRM) and
  CC Rolled Lateral (CCRL)
Or
Lateral (ML or LM) plus MLO Rolled Superior (MLORS)
  and MLO Rolled Inferior (MLORI)

A breast asymmetry is a non–mass-like area of fibroglandular density. Superimposition of normal fibroglandular tissue, Cooper ligaments, and blood vessels coursing through the breast all contribute to the mammographic finding of asymmetry seen on one image only. This finding accounts for many cases of BIRADS assessment category 0: incomplete—needs additional imaging. An asymmetry may be seen on either the CC or MLO screening mammogram image; the screening projection determines the diagnostic images that are needed. If identified on the CC image only, Lateral plus CC rolled medial (CCRM) and CC rolled lateral (CCRL) images should be obtained (Figures 10-19 and 10-20). If identified on the MLO image, a Lateral plus

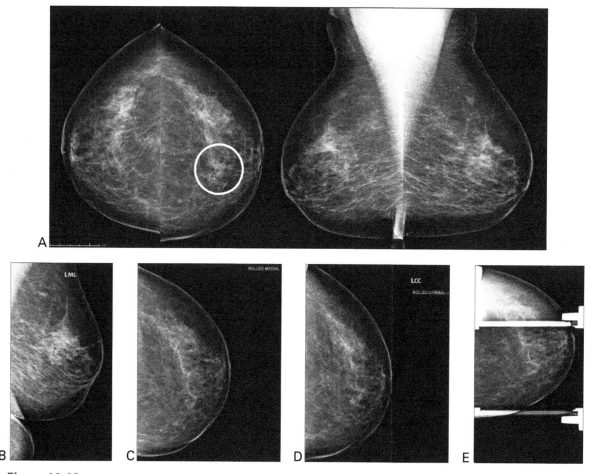

Figure 10-19
(A) Asymmetry identified only on LCC image (*circle*). **(B)** Lateral plus, **(C)** LCCRM, and **(D)** LCCRL images should be obtained. **(E)** Spot compression CC helps to confirm that there is no persistent abnormality.

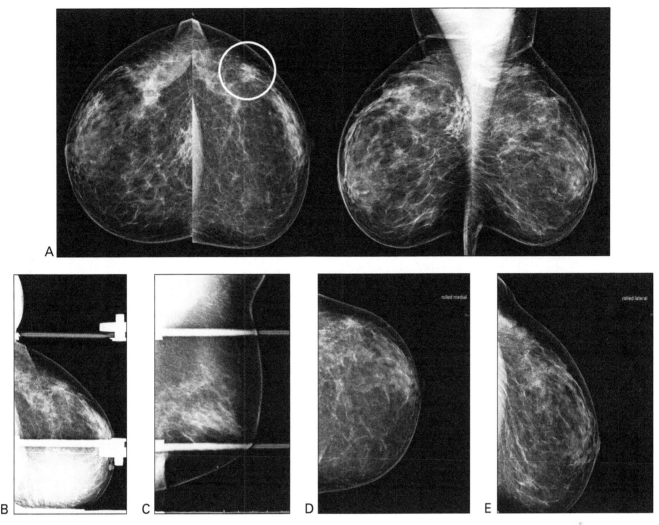

Figure 10-20
(A) Asymmetry identified only on LCC image (*circle*). **(B and C)** Two spot Laterals plus **(D)** LCCRM and **(E)** LCCRL images should be obtained.

MLO rolled superior (MLORS) and MLO rolled inferior (MLORI) should be obtained (Figure 10-21).

Imaging Focal Asymmetry

Lateral (ML or LM) and spot compression CC and spot compression MLO

A focal asymmetry is also a non–mass-like area of fibroglandular density. Unlike an asymmetry seen on one image only, a focal asymmetry is seen on both the CC and the MLO screening mammography images. If there are no associated findings such as architectural distortion or suspicious calcifications, a focal asymmetry typically represents superimposition of normal breast structures (Figure 10-22). This finding also accounts for many BIRADS assessment category 0: incomplete—needs additional imaging assessments. When identified on a baseline

screening exam, and after diagnostic imaging, a focal asymmetry may be assessed as a BIRADS assessment category 3: probably benign and undergo short-interval follow-up (Figure 10-23).

Diagnostic evaluation of this finding is different than that of an asymmetry seen on one image only. A Lateral plus spot compression CC (SCC) and spot compression MLO (SMLO) are required. A Lateral is required for accurate localization, while spot compression images are required to improve the compression on the suspicious area. Spot compression in the MLO projection instead of the Lateral projection is helpful to reproduce the same position as the original finding. Nonmagnified images are obtained to minimize technical changes of focal spot size and air gap that may confound image findings. Developing asymmetries identified on nonbaseline screening mammograms and that are persistent on diagnostic evaluation should have

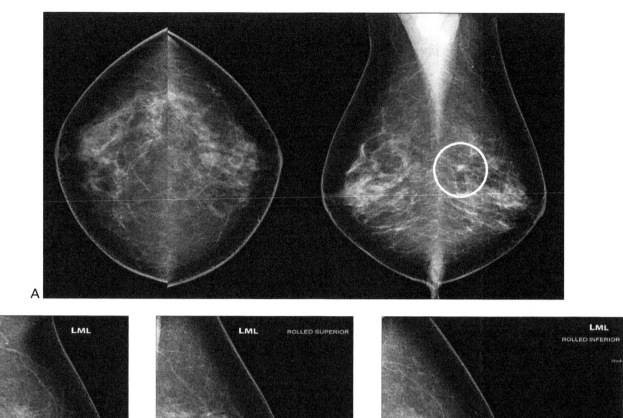

Figure 10-21
(A) Asymmetry identified only on the LMLO image (*circle*). **(B)** A Lateral plus **(C)** rolled superior and **(D)** rolled inferior images should be obtained. The asymmetry did not persist on the rolled images.

targeted ultrasound correlation. Recommendation of further evaluation with biopsy for tissue diagnosis is advised (Figure 10-24).

Asymmetry Summary

In summary, asymmetries are typically superimposition of normal fibroglandular tissue that spread out on spot compression images and appear similar to the surrounding normal fibroglandular tissue.

- A focal asymmetry will maintain its shape and density on spot compression. In fact, diagnostic imaging of a focal asymmetry may be categorized as an irregular, iso-, or high-density mass.

- Global asymmetries are large areas of normal fibroglandular tissue that do not require additional diagnostic imaging or follow-up.
- Asymmetries that are new, increasing in size, or more conspicuous are referred to as "developing asymmetries" and are highly suspicious for malignancy.
- Additional associated findings of architectural distortion or calcifications will further raise the level of suspicion.

Imaging a Nonpalpable Mass

Lateral (ML or LM) plus spot compression CC (SCC) and spot compression MLO (SMLO)

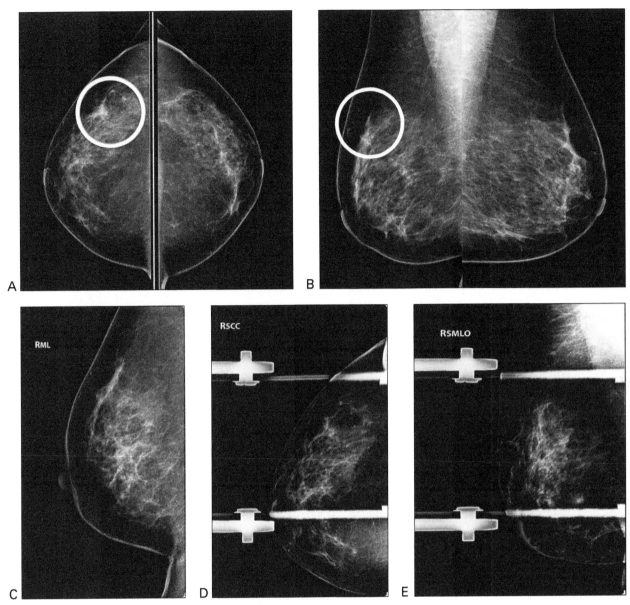

Figure 10-22
Focal asymmetry typically represents as superimposition of normal breast tissue. Bilateral **(A)** CC and **(B)** MLO images in an asymptomatic woman. There is a possible focal asymmetry in the right breast superolaterally (*circles*). **(C)** RML and **(D)** spot compression CC and **(E)** spot compression MLO images show resolution of the focal asymmetry. BIRADS 1: negative. Routine screening mammography recommended.

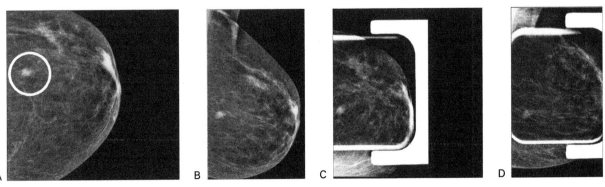

Figure 10-23
Baseline exam focal asymmetry. Even when a **(A)** focal asymmetry (*circle*) is present on two images, **(B)** Lateral and **(C and D)** spot compression images might be necessary for the radiologist to recommend a short-interval follow-up (BIRADS 3). Follow-up in 6 and 12 months were negative.

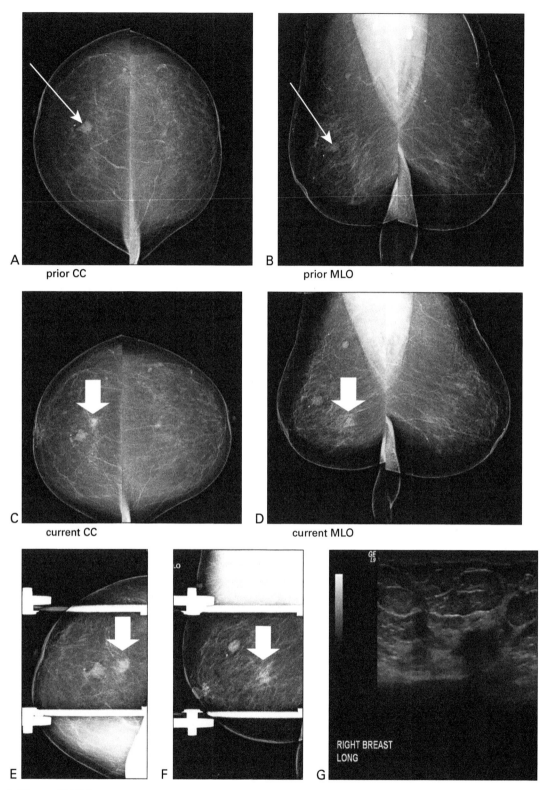

Figure 10-24

Developing asymmetry. A 47-year-old woman for a screening mammogram. Bilateral **(A)** CC and **(B)** MLO images reveal a central right breast biopsy-proven fibroadenoma (*arrow*). One year later, bilateral **(C)** CC and **(D)** MLO images show a developing asymmetry in the right breast central aspect posterior depth (*short arrow*). **(E)** Spot compression CC and **(F)** spot compression MLO reveal persistent focal asymmetry in the posterior breast. **(G)** Ultrasound confirms an irregular, hypoechoic mass. Asymmetries that are new, increasing in size, or more conspicuous are referred to as "developing asymmetries" and are highly suspicious for malignancy. Additional associated findings of architectural distortion or calcifications will further raise the level of suspicion. BIRADS 5—highly suspicious for malignancy. Biopsy-proven invasive ductal carcinoma.

A **mass** is a space-occupying three-dimensional lesion seen in two different projections. A mass is described by its:

- Shape: oval (may include 2 or 3 lobulations), round, or irregular
- Margins: circumscribed, obscured, microlobulated, indistinct, or spiculated
- Density: high, equal, low, or fat-containing.

All fat-containing lesions are typically benign and do not require diagnostic imaging or follow-up. Both solid and cystic masses typically retain their shape, margin, and density on spot compression images (Figure 10-25). A Lateral image is required for accurate localization, for ultrasound evaluation, and is required for all masses. SCC and SMLO images are required to further characterize mass features and to spread out adjacent normal fibroglandular tissue that can obscure identification of mass characteristics (Figures 10-26 and 10-27).

When multiple masses are present, each mass should be imaged. Multiple masses that have been present on previous mammograms and are increasing or decreasing in size do not need diagnostic imaging unless new suspicious associated findings are present (Figure 10-28).

Imaging Architectural Distortion

Lateral (ML or LM) plus spot compression CC (SCC) and spot compression MLO (SMLO)

Architectural distortion refers to distortion of normal breast structures with no definite mass visible (Figure 10-29). It has straight lines or spiculations radiating from a point and focal retraction, distortion, or straightening of the fibroglandular tissue (Figure 10-30). Architectural distortion can also be an associated feature. For example, a mass or calcifications may also have architectural distortion of surrounding fibroglandular tissue (Figure 10-31). Architectural distortion alone or as an associated finding, although

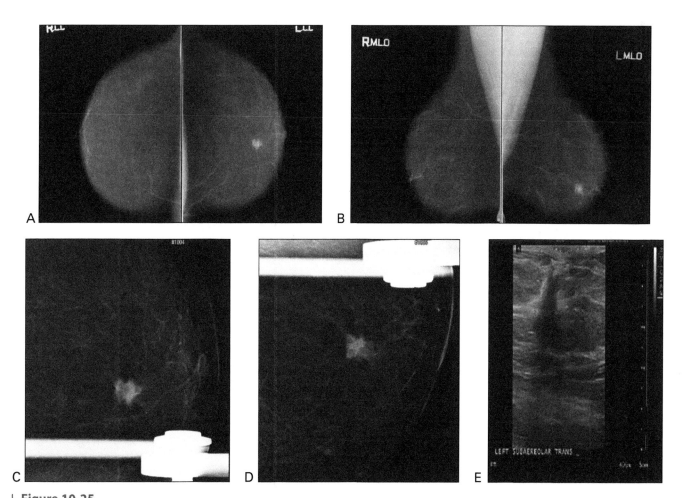

Figure 10-25
A 59-year-old woman for a screening mammogram. Spiculated, irregular, high-density mass noted on screening mammogram **(A)** CC and **(B)** MLO images. **(C)** Spot compression CC and **(D)** spot compression MLO images demonstrate that the mass retains its shape, margin, and density. **(E)** Ultrasound confirms a spiculated, irregular, hypoechoic mass. Biopsy-proven invasive ductal carcinoma.

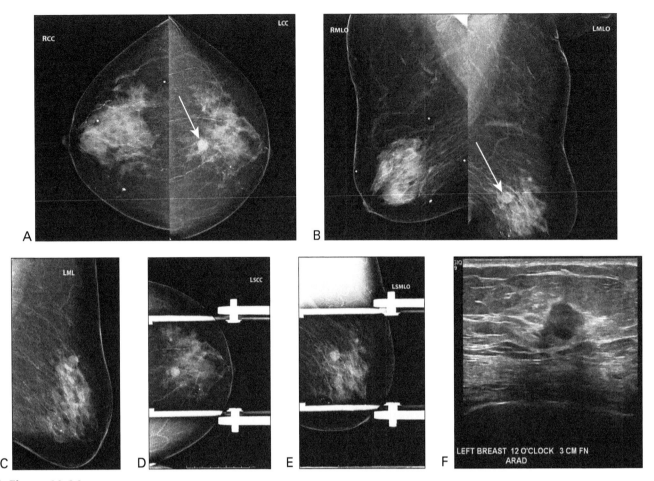

Figure 10-26

A 54-year-old woman for a screening mammogram. **(A and B)** A mass is noted in the posterior central aspect of the left breast (*arrows*). **(C)** Lateral and **(D)** spot compression CC and **(E)** spot compression MLO images are required to further characterize the mass features and for accurate localization for **(F)** ultrasound evaluation. Biopsy-proven invasive ductal carcinoma.

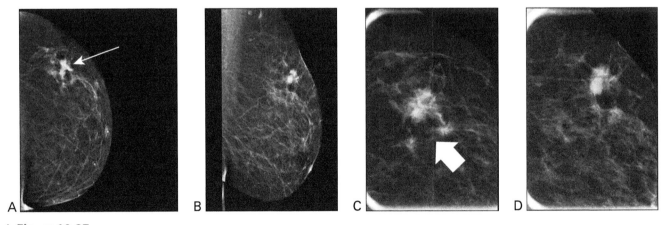

Figure 10-27

Value of Lateral and spot compression images. A 76-year-old woman for asymptomatic screening. **(A)** Left CC image reveals an irregular, high-density mass (*arrow*). **(B)** Lateral and **(C)** spot compression CC and **(D)** spot compression MLO images. Note that the shape of the mass persists and does not change upon vigorous compression. Spot compression images provide a dramatic example of cancer that does not spread out under compression. **(C)** Note that the normal superimposed tissue did spread out to reveal two additional irregular masses (*short arrow*) adjacent to initially detected mass. Biopsy-proved invasive lobular carcinoma with adjacent foci of carcinoma.

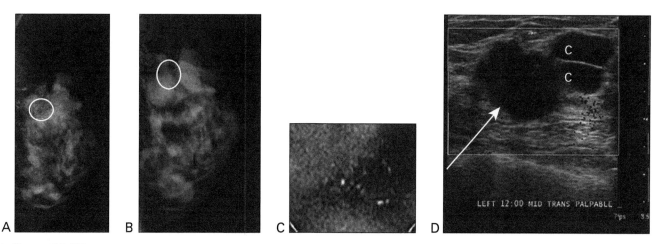

Figure 10-28
Multiple masses. A 56-year-old woman with a history of multiple cyst aspirations. Multiple masses that have been present on previous mammograms and are increasing or decreasing in size do not need diagnostic imaging unless new suspicious associated findings are present. **(A and B)** New grouped amorphous calcifications are noted (*circle*). **(C)** Magnification view of the calcifications. **(D)** Ultrasound reveals an irregular hypoechoic solid mass (*arrow*) with associated calcifications adjacent to multiple simple cysts (indicated by "*C*").

not commonly seen before the use of tomosynthesis, is a highly suspicious finding for malignancy (Figure 10-32). The differential diagnosis includes surgical scar, radial scar, and carcinoma (Figure 10-33).

Imaging Superficial Lesions and Calcifications

Grid localization with radiopaque marker plus TAN

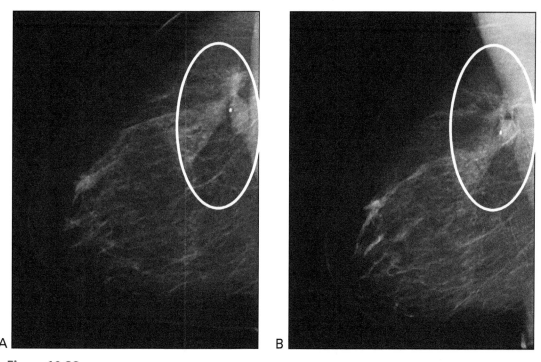

Figure 10-29
Architectural distortion. A 53-year-old woman for a screening mammogram. Right breast **(A)** CC and **(B)** MLO images reveal architectural distortion in the posterosuperior lateral breast. Architectural distortion (*circles*) results in straight lines or spiculations radiating from a point, and focal retraction, distortion or straightening of the fibroglandular tissue.

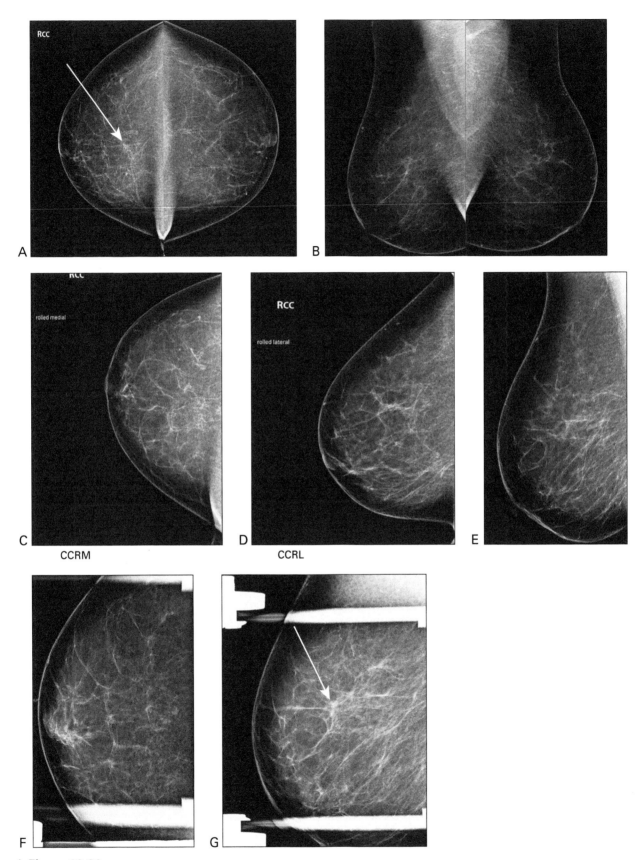

Figure 10-30

Architectural distortion. A 52-year-old woman for a screening mammogram. Bilateral **(A)** CC and **(B)** MLO images reveal possible architectural distortion noted in the right breast centrally; only seen on the CC image (*arrow*). **(C)** Rolled medial CC and **(D)** rolled lateral CC images were acquired and localized the architectural distortion to the superior breast. **(E)** Lateral and **(F)** spot compression CC and **(G)** spot compression MLO (*arrow*) confirm persistent architectural distortion. Biopsy-proven radial scar.

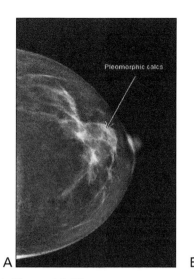
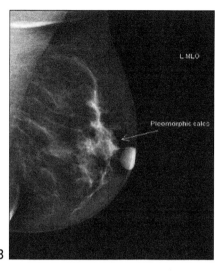
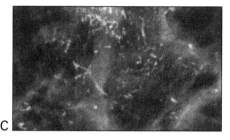

Figure 10-31
Architectural distortion as an associated feature. A 67-year-old woman for a screening mammogram. **(A)** CC, **(B)** MLO, and **(C)** magnification images reveal pleomorphic calcifications associated with architectural distortion. Together, these findings are highly suspicious of malignancy. BIRADS 5.

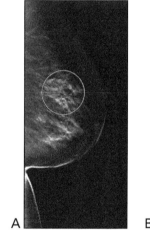
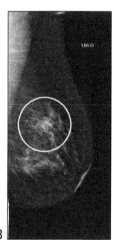
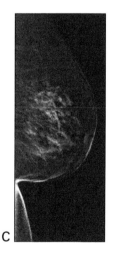
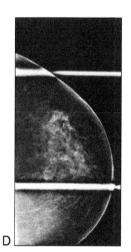
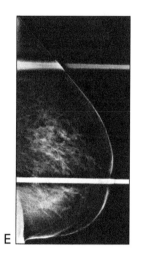

Figure 10-32
Architectural distortion on DBT. A 71-year-old woman for a screening mammogram. **(A)** Synthetic MLO and **(B)** 2D MLO images reveal architectural distortion in the superior lateral breast (*circles*). **(C)** DBT Lateral and **(D)** spot compression CC and **(E)** spot compression MLO confirm architectural distortion. Biopsy-proven invasive lobular carcinoma.

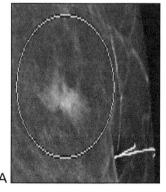
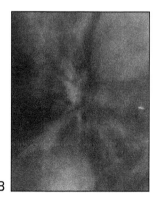
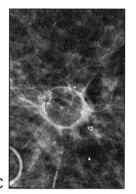
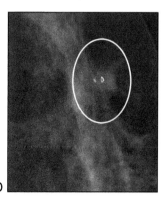

Figure 10-33
The differential diagnosis includes **(A)** surgical scar, **(B)** radial scar, **(C)** fat necrosis, and **(D)** carcinoma.

Skin lesions can project onto the mammogram and look as if they lie within the breast parenchyma. A tangential image better demarcates the borders of a superficial mass projecting into the subcutaneous fat. Magnification may enhance this projection, but when magnification is unavailable or unobtainable because of breast thickness or density, a tangential image may still offer the most information about a superficial mass or calcifications (Figure 10-34).

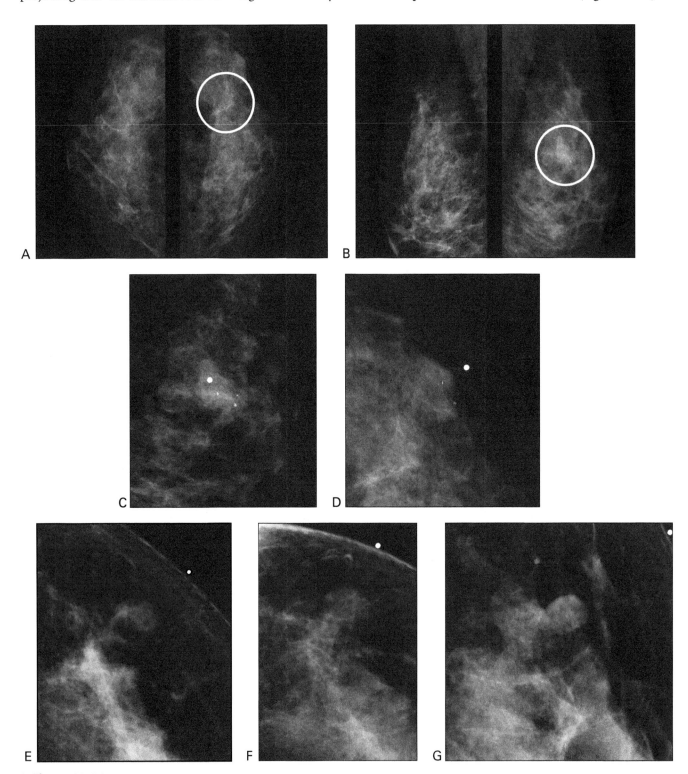

Figure 10-34
Superficial mass. A 47-year-old woman for a screening mammogram. Bilateral **(A)** CC and **(B)** MLO images reveal a superficial mass with associated calcification in the left lateral breast (*circles*). **(C)** Grid localization image with a radiopaque marker (metallic BB) placed on the mass and **(D)** tangential image confirm a superficial mass. Additional tangential images **(E–G)** better demarcate the borders of a superficial mass projecting into the subcutaneous fat. Biopsy-proven benign fibroadenoma.

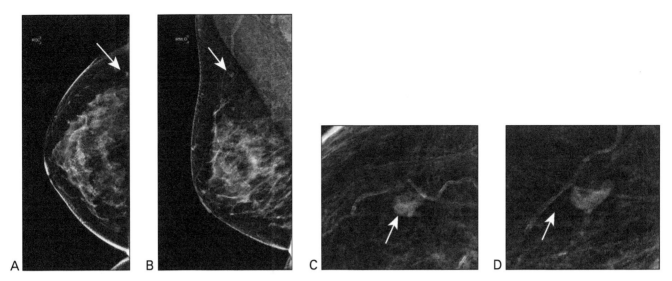

Figure 10-35
Imaging special cases. A 68-year-old woman for screening mammography. **(A)** CC, **(B)** MLO, **(C)** spot compression CC, and **(D)** spot compression MLO images of a well-defined mass with a fatty hilum. In the superior lateral breast adjacent to a blood vessel; consistent with a benign intramammary lymph node (*arrows*). Special cases are findings with features so typical that you do not need to describe them or describe them in detail on a screening mammogram report. No further diagnostic imaging is needed. Benign intramammary lymph node.

Imaging Special Cases

Special cases are findings with features so typical that you do not need to describe them or describe them in detail on a screening mammogram report. No further diagnostic imaging is needed. Examples of special cases include benign-appearing intramammary lymph nodes (Figure 10-35) and skin lesions.

Imaging Associated Findings

Associated findings include skin or nipple retraction (Figure 10-36), skin or trabecular thickening, axillary lymphadenopathy, architectural distortion, and calcifications. These play a role in the final assessment of a primary finding such as a focal asymmetry or mass. For example, a BIRADS 4 suspicious for malignancy mass could become

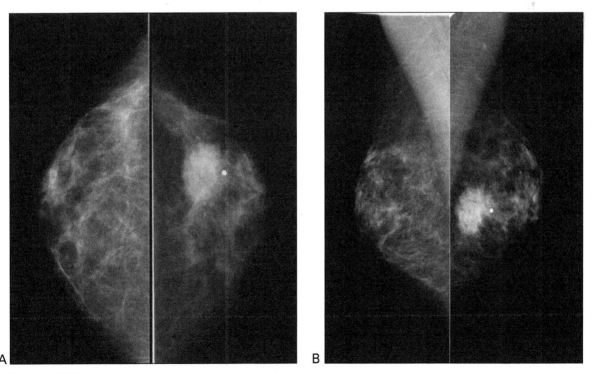

Figure 10-36
Associated findings: skin retraction. A 75-year-old woman with a new palpable mass and skin retraction. Bilateral **(A)** CC and **(B)** MLO images. A radiopaque marker (metallic BB) was placed at the location of the palpable abnormality and skin retraction.

BIRADS 5 highly suggestive of malignancy assessment if seen in association with nipple retraction.

DIAGNOSTIC IMAGING OF SHORT-INTERVAL FOLLOW-UP EXAMINATION; BIRADS 3: PROBABLY BENIGN

Short-interval follow-up, at 6 or 12 months, of probably benign mammographic findings require routine CC and MLO images of the entire breast and diagnostic images of the specific mammographic finding. Refer to the standardized protocols specific for the mammographic finding as noted above in Diagnostic Imaging of the Incomplete Screening Mammogram. Direct comparison with the prior screening and diagnostic images is mandatory. Although any changes from the prior mammogram should be evaluated with suspicion, stability of any suspicious findings should also be re-evaluated for a recommendation of biopsy for tissue diagnosis. In addition, routine screening CC and MLO images of the contralateral breast may be indicated.

Imaging Calcifications

CC and MLO plus Lateral (ML or LM) plus magnified CC (MCC) and magnified MLO (MMLO)

Imaging Focal Asymmetry or Mass

CC and MLO plus Lateral (ML or LM) plus spot compression CC (SCC) and spot compression MLO (SMLO)

DIAGNOSTIC IMAGING OF CLINICAL EXAMINATION FINDINGS

Imaging Palpable Abnormality or Thickening

CC and MLO plus Lateral (ML or LM) plus spot compression CC (SCC) and spot compression MLO (SMLO) (Figure 10-37). Radiopaque marker placed on skin at area of palpable abnormality (Figure 10-38).

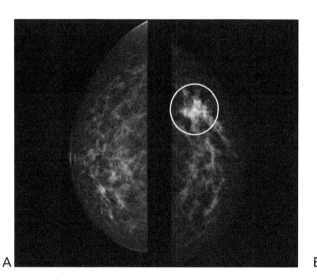

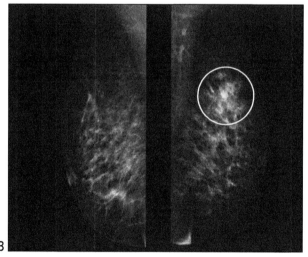

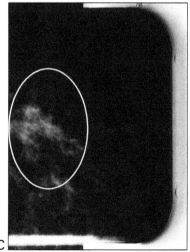

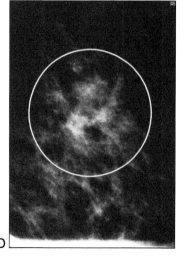

Figure 10-37
Imaging palpable thickening. A 53-year-old woman with palpable thickening without a discrete mass. In the left superior lateral breast, as noted by her health care provider. No radiopaque marker placed due to inability of the patient and technologist to identify this area of thickening. Thickening was noted on the patient history form. Bilateral **(A)** CC and **(B)** MLO plus Lateral (not shown) and **(C)** spot compression CC and **(D)** spot compression MLO images reveal focal asymmetry with associated architectural distortion in the left superior lateral breast (*circles*). Biopsy-proven invasive lobular carcinoma.

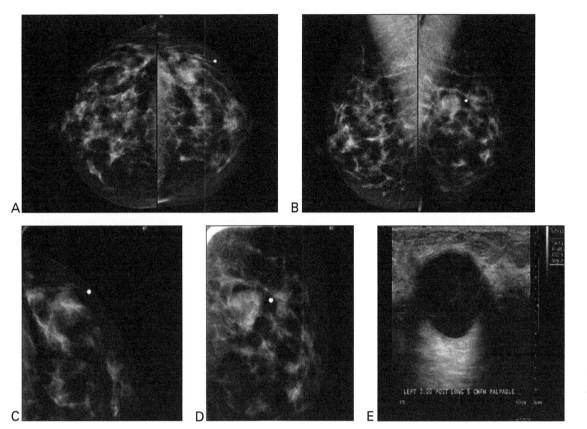

Figure 10-38
Imaging palpable abnormality or thickening. A 48-year-old woman with a new palpable abnormality. Radiopaque marker (metallic BB) placed on the skin at the area of palpable abnormality. **(A)** Bilateral CC and **(B)** MLO plus Lateral (not shown) plus **(C)** spot compression CC and **(D)** spot compression MLO reveal an obscured, round isodense mass. **(E)** US confirms a complex solid and cystic mass. Biopsy-proven invasive papillary carcinoma.

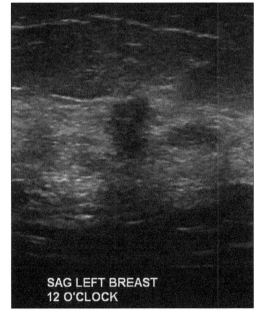

Figure 10-39
Imaging palpable abnormality or thickening. A 46-year-old woman with a palpable abnormality and extremely dense tissue on the mammogram. A mammographically occult suspicious irregular hypoechoic mass on ultrasound. Biopsy-proven invasive ductal carcinoma.

Discrete masses have a level of suspicion on clinical exam, but the clinical exam alone cannot be a reliable tool to exclude malignancy. Ultrasound of the palpable abnormality or thickening should be obtained to evaluate for a possible mammographically occult abnormality, especially in dense breast tissue (Figure 10-39).

Imaging Nipple Discharge

CC and MLO plus Lateral (ML or LM) plus retroareolar spot compression CC (SCC) and retroareolar spot compression MLO (SMLO)

Nipple discharge that is unilateral, single duct, spontaneous, clear, or bloody is suspicious for malignancy. Although these nipple discharges are more commonly caused by benign fibrocystic changes, it is critical to evaluate for an underlying retroareolar mass. Ultrasound of the retroareolar area may be helpful to locate an intraductal nodule or dilated duct associated with a benign papilloma (Figure 10-40). Surgical duct excision of a papilloma provides symptomatic relief of problematic nipple discharge. An underlying malignancy may also cause nipple discharge that may be spontaneous and not elicited by

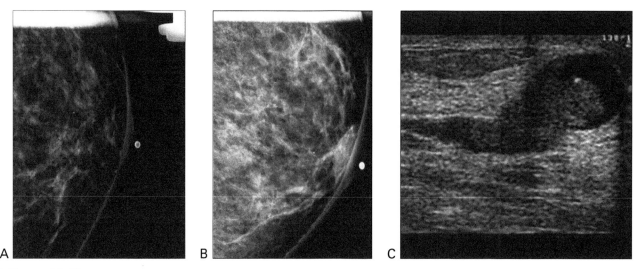

Figure 10-40
Imaging nipple discharge. A 37-year-old woman with single duct, spontaneous bloody nipple discharge. Retroareolar spot compression **(A)** CC and **(B)** MLO images reveal no mammographic abnormality corresponding to the nipple discharge. **(C)** Ultrasound of the retroareolar breast confirmed an intraductal mass. BIRADS 4a. Low suspicion of malignancy. Biopsy-proven benign papilloma.

manipulating the nipple or mammographic compression. Nipple discharge suspicious for malignancy tends to be clear or bloody. Nipple discharge caused by fibrocystic change tends to be milky white, green, brown, or black in color.

Imaging Focal Pain

CC and MLO plus Lateral (ML or LM) plus spot compression CC (SCC) and spot compression MLO (SMLO). Radiopaque marker placed on skin at area of focal pain (Figures 10-41 and 10-42).

Breast pain is any discomfort, tenderness, or pain in the breast or underarm region, and it may occur for sev-

eral reasons. All or part of one or both breasts may be affected differently. Diffuse breast pain tends to not be worrisome. Fibrocystic breast changes are a common cause of breast pain. Pain may be cyclical or noncyclical. Cyclic breast pain appears to have a strong link to hormones and the menstrual cycle. Cyclic breast pain often decreases or disappears with pregnancy or menopause. Fibrocystic breast tissue can contain lumps or cysts that tend to be more tender just before menstruation. An imbalance of fatty acids within the breast cells may affect the sensitivity of breast tissue to circulating hormones. Certain hormonal medications may also cause noncyclic breast pain, including some infertility treatments and oral birth control pills. Also, breast tenderness is a possible

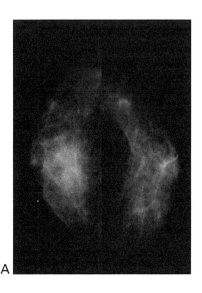

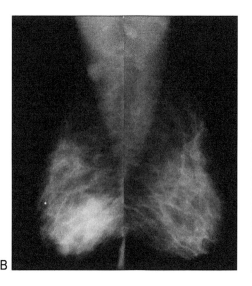

Figure 10-41
Imaging focal pain. A 58-year-old woman with focal pain in the right breast for 1 week. A radiopaque marker (metallic BB) was placed on the area of focal pain. Bilateral **(A)** CC and **(B)** MLO plus **(C)** Lateral images reveal global asymmetry directly beneath the radiopaque marker. Spot compression images could not be obtained due to the patient's complaint of pain upon compression.

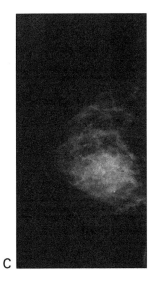
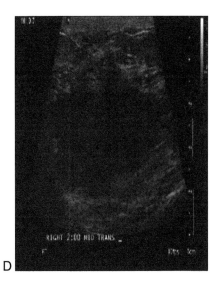

C   D

Figure 10-41 (*Continued*)
(D) Ultrasound confirms an irregular hypoechoic solid mass. Biopsy-proven acute, chronic and granulomatous inflammation, and abscess formation.

side effect of estrogen and progesterone hormone therapies that are used after menopause. Breast pain may be associated with certain antidepressants, including selective serotonin reuptake inhibitor (SSRI) antidepressants. Women with large breasts may have noncyclic breast pain related to the size of their breasts. Neck, shoulder, and back pain may accompany breast pain due to large breasts. Breast pain associated with breast surgery and scar formation can sometimes linger long after incisions have healed.

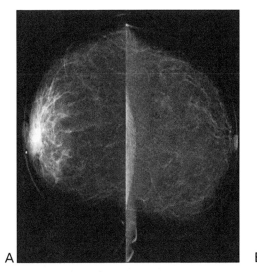
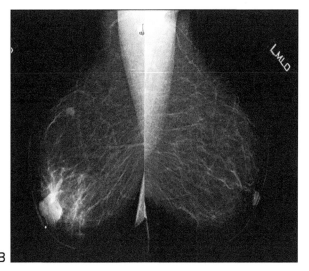

A   B

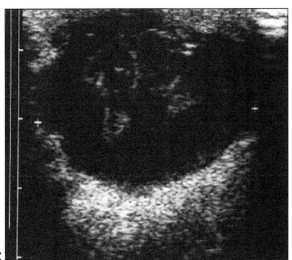

C

Figure 10-42
Imaging focal pain. A 39-year-old woman with focal pain after breast-feeding. Bilateral **(A)** CC and **(B)** MLO images. Lateral and spot compression CC and spot compression MLO projections were not obtained due to patient's complaint of pain. A radiopaque marker (metallic BB) was placed on the skin in the area of focal pain. An indistinct mass with associated skin and trabeculae thickening is seen in this area. **(C)** Ultrasound confirms a complex solid and cystic mass. Biopsy-proven abscess.

DIAGNOSTIC IMAGING OF SURGICALLY ALTERED BREAST

Any invasive breast surgery, whether for diagnosis, prophylaxis, therapy, or cosmetic purposes, may alter the physical and mammographic appearance of the breast, complicating the diagnostic evaluation and occasionally necessitating additional imaging evaluation.

A basic understanding of the procedures and implications for imaging women with surgically altered breasts is justified due to the volume of breast surgery attributed to:

- Open surgical biopsies
- Reduction mammoplasty
- 2+ million women with breast implants who are now of screening age[11]
- The number of women opting for breast conservation therapy (BCT; lumpectomy with or without radiation)[6] and breast reconstruction
- BrCA1 and BrCA2 gene–positive women who opt for prophylactic mastectomy

In addition to questioning the patient about prior surgeries, the technologist, especially in the screening situation, must pay attention to the clinical signs of postoperative change. The patient's breast history form should include a diagram of this physical inspection and should also include the following information:

- Surgical intervention: type and approximate date.
- Location of scars.

- Keloid formation.
- Skin retraction at site of tissue removal—This may be the only evidence of surgical intervention with excellent cosmetic results in a barely perceptible periareolar incision. Alternatively, skin retraction may be a sign of tumor recurrence.
- Marked asymmetry in size or shape between breasts.

Mammographic Changes due to Surgery

Any of the following mammographic changes may appear secondary to surgical intervention:

- Architectural distortion (Figure 10-43)
- Asymmetry, focal asymmetry, or masses (Figures 10-44 and 10-45)
- Calcification: especially course heterogeneous, rim, or round calcifications of fat necrosis (Figure 10-46)
- Diffuse or focal trabecular thickening or edema (Figure 10-47)
- Skin thickening or nipple retraction (Figure 10-48)

Asymmetry or Focal Asymmetry

Mammographic changes can resolve and new changes emerge simultaneously because of surgical intervention. Typically, the density and size of benign postoperative changes decrease rapidly in the first few months and may resolve entirely. When postoperative changes do not resolve completely, any residual changes may remain stable indefinitely.

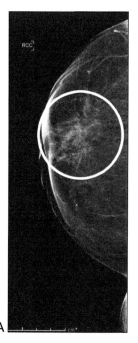 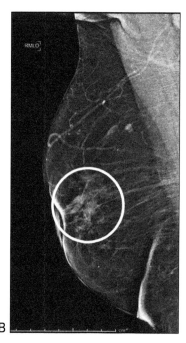 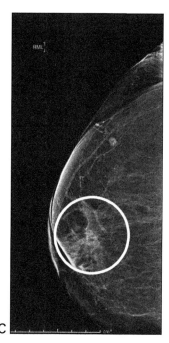

Figure 10-43
Benign postoperative architectural distortion. **(A)** CC, **(B)** MLO, and **(C)** ML images reveal benign postoperative architectural distortion at the BCT site (*circles*).

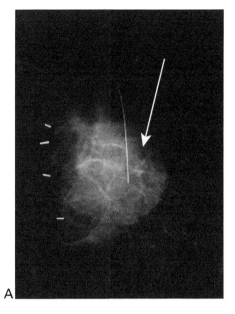
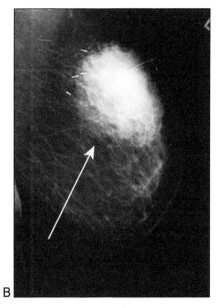

Figure 10-44
Benign postoperative mass. A 62-year-old woman with recent BCT surgery postoperative hematoma. A skin marker (*thin white line*) is placed along the surgical scar. An indistinct, high-density mass is noted in the tumor bed consistent with postoperative hematoma/seroma. The well-defined mass evident on the **(A)** CC and **(B)** MLO images (*arrows*) proved to be hematoma/seroma.

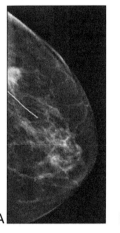
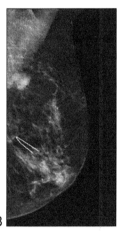
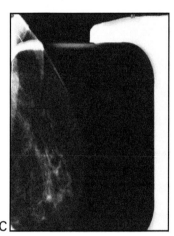
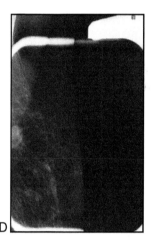

Figure 10-45
Benign postoperative stable mass. A 62-year-old woman with a history of left breast invasive ductal carcinoma and lumpectomy; this is her third year follow-up mammogram. **(A)** CC, **(B)** MLO, and **(C)** magnified CC and **(D)** magnified MLO images reveal a benign postoperative mass at the BCT site consistent with chronic hematoma/seroma.

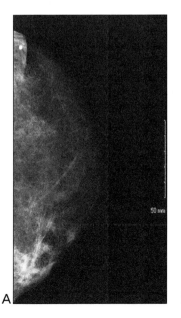
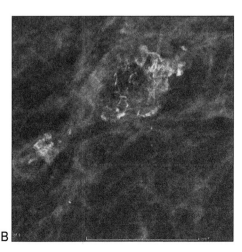

Figure 10-46
Benign postoperative calcifications. A 47-year-old woman with a history of left breast invasive lobular carcinoma and BCT. Two-year follow-up mammogram **(A)** CC and **(B)** magnified CC reveals postoperative developing calcifications at the medial BCT site consistent with fat necrosis.

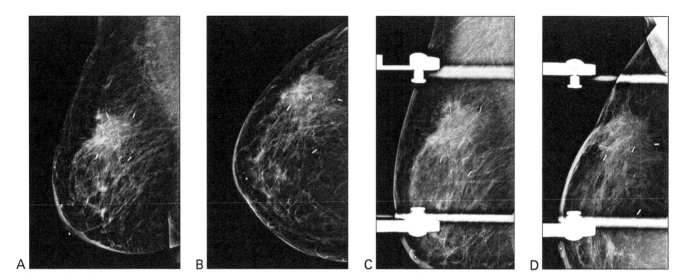

Figure 10-47
Benign postoperative trabecular thickening or edema. A 78-year-old woman with a history of right breast invasive ducal carcinoma and BCT. One-month follow-up mammogram **(A)** MLO, **(B)** CC, **(C)** spot compression MLO, and **(D)** spot compression CC images reveal postoperative trabecular thickening at the BCT site consistent with focal edema.

However, benign calcifications of fat necrosis may increase over time and some asymmetries or focal asymmetries will continue to coalesce, becoming denser and more spiculated, but smaller, before eventually stabilizing. A complete and accurate patient history form is especially important in the latter cases (Figure 10-49). Once postoperative changes stabilize over two successive mammograms, subsequent changes at the surgical site may warrant further investigation (Figures 10-50 to 10-52).

Architectural Distortion

One of the most common and problematic postoperative changes is architectural distortion. This change can mimic

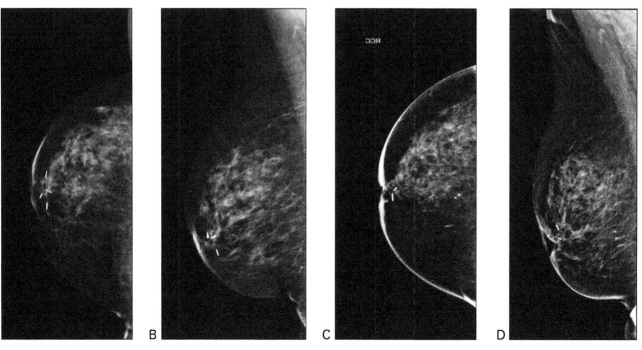

Figure 10-48
Benign postoperative skin thickening and nipple retraction. A 61-year-old woman with a history of right breast invasive ducal carcinoma and BCT. Six-month **(A)** CC, **(B)** MLO, and 18-month follow-up mammogram **(C & D)** after radiation therapy. **(C)** CC and **(D)** MLO images reveal postoperative skin thickening and nipple retraction consistent with postoperative and radiation change.

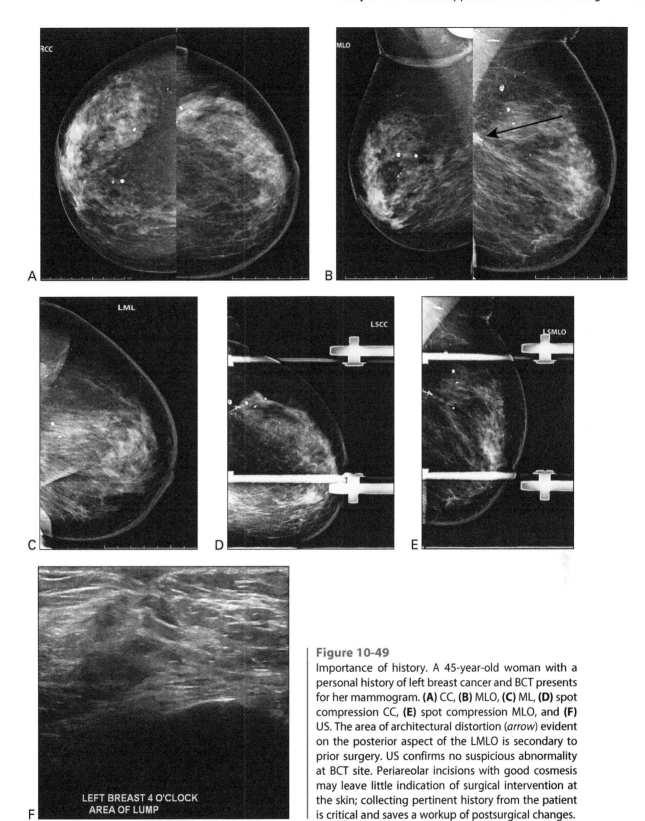

Figure 10-49
Importance of history. A 45-year-old woman with a personal history of left breast cancer and BCT presents for her mammogram. **(A)** CC, **(B)** MLO, **(C)** ML, **(D)** spot compression CC, **(E)** spot compression MLO, and **(F)** US. The area of architectural distortion (*arrow*) evident on the posterior aspect of the LMLO is secondary to prior surgery. US confirms no suspicious abnormality at BCT site. Periareolar incisions with good cosmesis may leave little indication of surgical intervention at the skin; collecting pertinent history from the patient is critical and saves a workup of postsurgical changes.

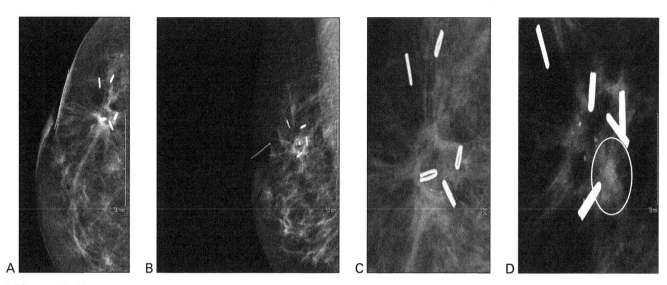

Figure 10-50
Post-BCT change. A 47-year-old woman with a personal history of breast cancer and BCT 4 years prior. **(A)** Prior CC, **(B)** prior MLO, and **(C)** prior spot compression CC reveal stable post-BCT change. **(D)** One year later, spot compression MLO reveals a new small mass at the BCT site (*circle*). Biopsy-proven recurrent invasive ductal carcinoma.

a suspicious, spiculated mass (Figure 10-53). The following features of postoperative scarring, plus the history of surgical intervention at the site, can resolve the need for a diagnostic and/or additional imaging evaluation: surgical scars may change in appearance on multiple views (Figure 10-54), whereas cancer tends to maintain its shape. Cancer will most often have lines radiating from a central mass; the surgical scar presents as lines radiating from either a lucent center or multiple lucent centers or will exhibit no apparent mass-like center (Figures 10-55 and 10-56).

Imaging Reduction Mammoplasty

CC and MLO

Breast-reduction mammoplasty is one of the top five cosmetic surgeries performed in the United States.[11] The typical breast-reduction procedure involves making a keyhole incision around the nipple, extending it to the 6 o'clock region of the breast, and vertically down to the breast crease. A wedge of breast tissue is excised and the edges of the exposed tissue are brought together and sutured closed. Thus, a band of tissue distortion is often noted in the inferior or lateral breast where the tissue was brought back together (Figure 10-57). The nipple and areola are transposed or transplanted to a higher area on the breast and a portion of the inferior breast is resected, thus decreasing the size of the breast (Figure 10-58). Preoperative screening mammography is indicated to

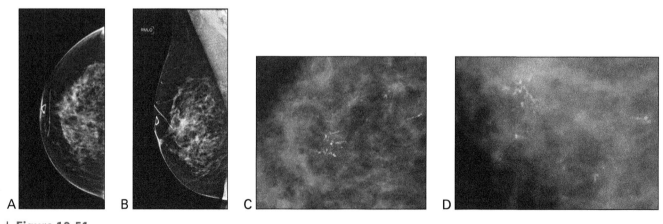

Figure 10-51
Post-BCT change. A 63-year-old woman with a personal history of breast cancer and BCT 7 years prior. **(A)** CC, **(B)** MLO and **(C)** magnified CC, and **(D)** magnified MLO reveal new grouped fine pleomorphic calcifications adjacent to the BCT site. Biopsy-proven recurrent invasive ductal carcinoma.

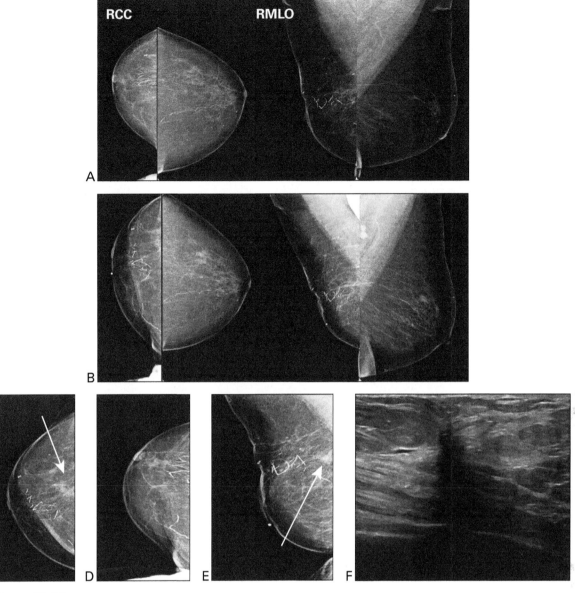

Figure 10-52
A 62-year-old woman with a personal history of right breast cancer; status post partial mastectomy. **(A)** Note asymmetry of breast size and development of calcifications on the right partial mastectomy site. **(B)** One year later, complaint of a palpable abnormality in the right central breast. **(C)** CC demonstrates posterolateral asymmetry *(arrow)*. **(D)** CC rolled lateral image demonstrates posterolateral asymmetry. Note that the asymmetry moves medially, localizing the abnormality to the inferior breast. **(E)** MLO shows the abnormality *(arrow)*. **(F)** Targeted ultrasound reveals a spiculated mass along the chestwall. This mass was biopsy-proven invasive ductal carcinoma.

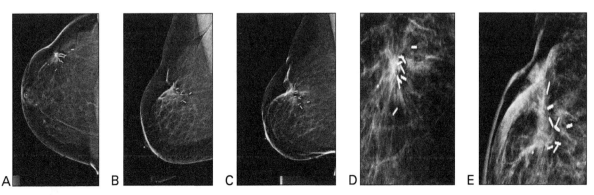

Figure 10-53
Postoperative architectural distortion. A 71-year-old woman with postoperative BCT; scarring mimics a spiculated mass. **(A)** CC, **(B)** MLO, **(C)** ML, and **(D)** spot compression CC and **(E)** spot compression MLO. Surgical scars may change in appearance on multiple images.

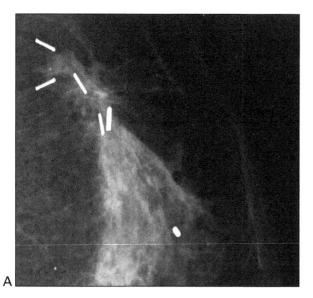
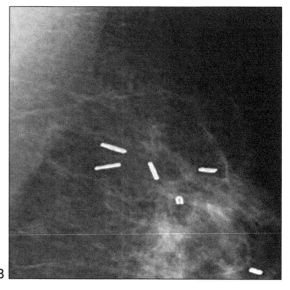

Figure 10-54
Typical scar. A 58-year-old woman with a personal history of breast cancer and BCT. **(A)** Magnified CC and **(B)** magnified MLO images reveal a typical surgical scar. The architectural distortion does not appear to originate from a dense center as with carcinoma. This area opens and spreads out on the magnified MLO image. Changes in appearance on different images is the hallmark of benign surgical scar.

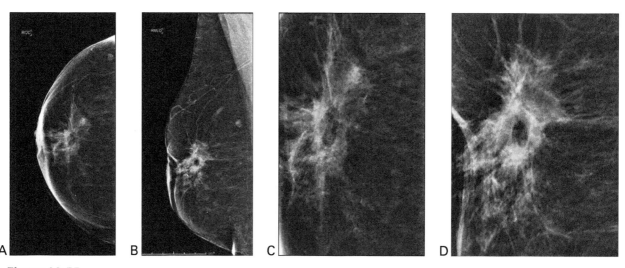

Figure 10-55
Typical scar. A 69-year-old woman with a personal history of breast cancer and BCT. **(A)** CC, **(B)** MLO, **(C)** magnified CC, and **(D)** magnified MLO images reveal lines radiating from a lucent center with no apparent mass.

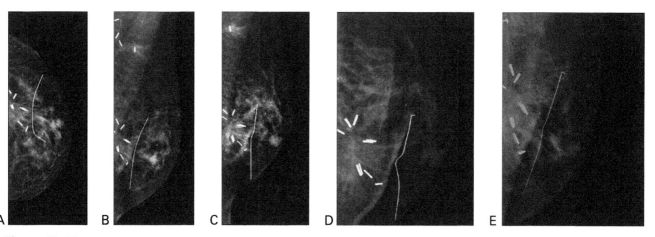

Figure 10-56
Typical scar. A 73-year-old woman with a personal history of breast cancer and BCT. **(A)** CC, **(B)** MLO, **(C)** ML, **(D)** magnified CC, and **(E)** magnified MLO images reveal the surgical scar presents as lines radiating from no apparent mass-like center.

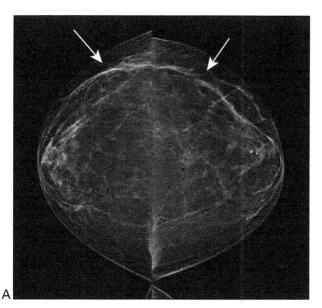 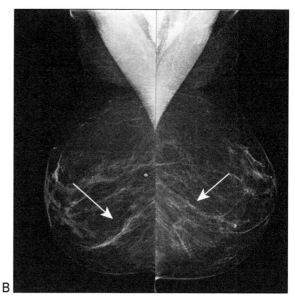

Figure 10-57
Post breast-reduction mammoplasty changes. A 58-year-old woman status post breast-reduction mammoplasty. Bilateral **(A)** CC and **(B)** MLO images. Note the distortion of breast tissue along the inferior and lateral breast where the surgical excision is closed (*arrows*). The typical breast-reduction procedure involves making a keyhole incision around the nipple, extending it to the 6 o'clock region of the breast, and vertically down to the breast crease.

evaluate for a suspicious mammography finding suggestive of malignancy.

Mammographic characteristics of reduction mammoplasty may include any or all of the following (Table 10-4):

• As with any surgery, hematoma, seroma, architectural distortion, fat necrosis with oil cysts, and calcifications can occur.

Imaging of Breast Implants

CC + MLO + CCID + MLOID

Breast implants are used for cosmetic augmentation, correction of congenital anomalies, and reconstruction after mastectomy. However, approximately 80% of breast augmentation surgery is for cosmetic purposes.[12] Past and current

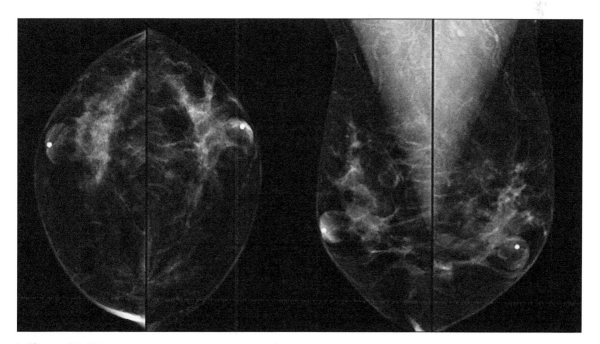

Figure 10-58
Post breast-reduction mammoplasty changes. A 45-year-old woman status post reduction mammoplasty. High-lying nipples are marked with radiopaque markers (metallic BB). The nipple and areola are transposed or transplanted to a higher area on the breast and a portion of the inferior breast is resected, thus decreasing the size of the breast.

Table 10-4 • Mammographic Characteristics of Reduction Mammoplasty May Include Any or All of the Following

Skin thickening
Architectural distortion and fibroglandular redistribution to the inferior breast
High nipple position
Nipple tilt
Retroareolar band
Areolar thickening
Postsurgical fat necrosis calcifications

implant design goals include minimization of immunological reaction from the patient, decreased implant migration and rupture, and increased implant radiolucency while maintaining good cosmetic results and patient satisfaction.

The density and position of saline or silicone implants interfere with the mammographic study regardless of the implant type. Additionally, benign side effects of implantation can both mask and mimic cancer. In addition to the recommended routine views, described in Chapter 7, the mammographic study may include the following:

- Tangential views of lumps or areas of asymmetry
- Magnification views to evaluate early capsular calcifications
- Axilla views to evaluate silicone spread into the lymph nodes
- Additional projections to assure visualization of the entire breast

Imaging is useful to evaluate implant integrity, to determine the amount and location of free silicone, and to detect residual silicone after implant removal. Although magnetic resonance imaging is superior to mammography and ultrasonography in detecting implant rupture, it is not as good at detecting free or residual silicone. Mammography is limited to the immediate breast and axilla and is not useful to image the chestwall.

The technologist should be aware that the patient with implants might have pain due to implant contracture or free silicone. These issues and the substantial number of sensational media reports about the potential link to systemic disease can produce anxiety for the patient who may already be concerned about the effects or effectiveness of mammography. Use caution when compressing the implanted breast, allowing the patient to control the examination.

The technologist should be aware of the following physical attributes associated with implants and include any pertinent and accurate information on the patient history form:

- Hardened implant
- Sudden softening of a hardened implant
- Lump
- Breast pain or tenderness
- Neck and shoulder pain
- Chestwall pain
- Change in breast size
- Sudden change in appearance
- Breast asymmetry

Implants may have a single or double lumen filled with silicone, saline, or a combination of both. Solid silicone of some type provides the shell, usually a silicone elastomer, which may vary in thickness and texture or have attached fastening "tabs" to prevent host reaction and migration, respectively. The shell may have a valve for filling, which is evident on the mammogram. A single implant or "stacked" implants may provide augmentation.

Currently, placement of the implant behind the pectoral major muscle (retro or subpectoral) is common (Figure 10-59), but earlier placed implants may lie anterior

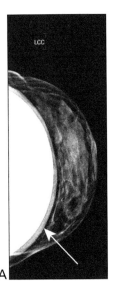 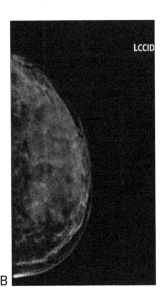 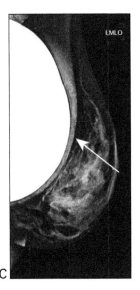 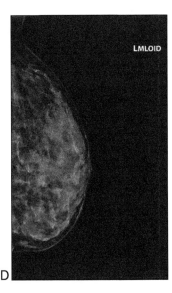

Figure 10-59
(A–D) Retropectoral silicone implant. A 56-year-old woman with left breast retropectoral implant. The implant lies behind the pectoral muscle (*arrow*). No valve is present because this is a silicone implant.

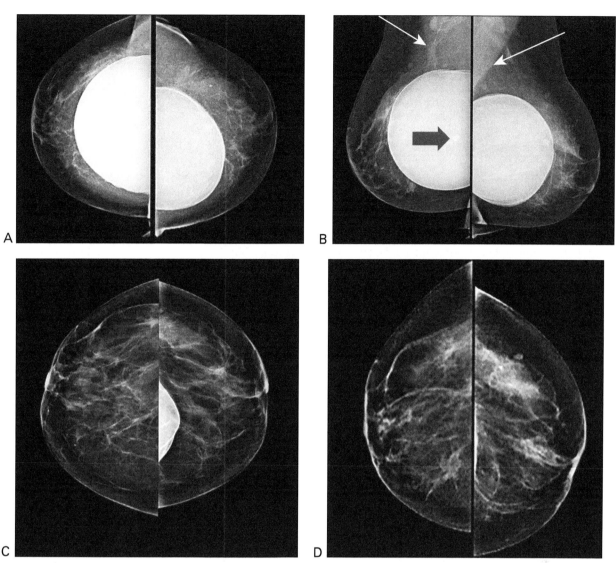

Figure 10-60
A 49-year-old woman with bilateral subglandular implants. Bilateral **(A)** CC, **(B)** MLO, and bilateral **(C)** CC implant-displaced and **(D)** MLO implant-displaced images. The implant is placed in front of the pectoral muscle (*long arrows*). A valve (*short arrow*) is present and most visible on the right MLO image.

to the pectoral muscle (subglandular) (Figure 10-60). Placement of the implant, either subpectoral or subglandular, is dependent on multiple factors, including the cosmetic effect within the breast and cost considerations (Table 10-5). Subglandular implants improve the contour of an otherwise flaccid breast. Subpectoral implants require a native breast with adequate fullness and provide increased protection of the implant from trauma but are costlier. The placement is usually evident on the mammogram. The presence of a valve in saline implants (Figure 10-61) versus no valve in silicone implants may be helpful to differentiate implant type.

Complications

Early complications from implantation are confined to the previously mentioned surgical possibilities. Later difficulties mostly affect the locoregional area.[13] Silicone implants or implants of any other material have not been proven to cause breast cancer; however, some literature[14,15] report a higher percentage of invasive cancer, a higher percentage of metastatic axillary lymph nodes, and diseases in more advanced stages in women with implants. Suggested reasons for this advanced stage of detection may be because it is difficult to access and image the breast tissue, difficulty

Table 10-5 • Submuscular and Subglandular Implants

SUBMUSCULAR IMPLANTS (PLACED BETWEEN THE PECTORALIS MAJOR AND MINOR MUSCLES)		SUBGLANDULAR IMPLANTS (PLACED BEHIND THE BREAST TISSUE AND ANTERIOR TO THE PECTORALIS MUSCLE	
ADVANTAGES	DISADVANTAGES	ADVANTAGES	DISADVANTAGES
Lesser degree of capsular contracture	Possible weakening of pectoral muscle	Can be placed with local anesthesia	Increased frequency of capsular contracture
Skin ripples due to folds in the implant shell are less evident	More susceptible to wear and tear due to exercise	Greater augmentation	Skin ripples due to folds in the implant shell are more evident
Implant is less palpable	Implant may move during exercise	Muscular activities have less effect on the implant's wear and tear	Implant is more palpable

in imaging due to the radiodensity of the implant, the host reaction to the implants, or silicone that can obscure (and mimic) cancer (Figure 10-62).

Capsular Contracture

Implants can be problematic. Many implant difficulties occur because of the periprosthetic capsule or fibrous scar tissue that develops around the implant. Whether the implant is subpectoral or subglandular, the foreign body reaction forms a fibrous capsule around the implant and creates a fibrous scar encompassing the implant (Figure 10-63). This is a natural reaction and, in fact, the developers of implants relied on this mechanism to protect the implant from rupture into the breast tissue.

The fibrous capsule may remain soft with much postoperative care, including massage, to keep this capsule pliable. But often, the fibrous capsule hardens and may calcify over time (Figure 10-61). A classification system, Baker's scale[16], labels the degree of hardening or eventual contracture or shrinkage of the capsule (Table 10-6). Severe breast implant contracture can cause deformity of the breast, displacement or migration of the implant, and discomfort for the patient. It can also make imaging the breast more difficult due to the incompressibility and immobility of the implant, especially on implant-displaced images. Asymmetric contracture from one breast to the other is prevalent. Other common deformities of implants include:

• Focal herniation or bulges where the implant remains intact but pushes through or focally deforms the fibrous capsule. Upon clinical examination, the patient may exhibit a focal mass.

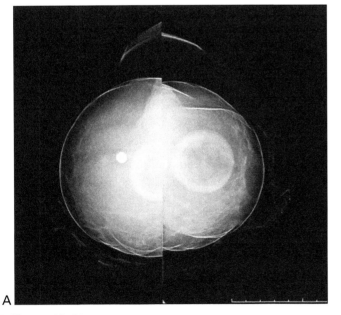
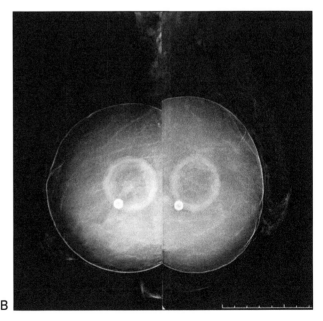

A   B

Figure 10-61
Saline implant valve. A 65-year-old woman with bilateral subglandular saline implants. Bilateral **(A)** CC and **(B)** MLO images. The visible valve identifies that these are saline implants. Implant displacement images could not be obtained due to the inflexibility of these encapsulated implants. Most of the breast tissue is hidden by the implant.

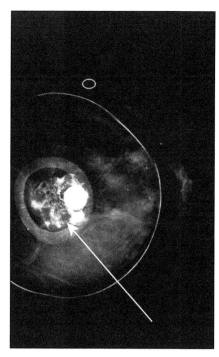

Figure 10-62
Capsular calcification at the valve. A 57-year-old woman with left subglandular saline implant. Dense calcification of the implant capsule in the region of the valve (*arrow*) may mimic cancer or make mammographic interpretation difficult.

- Folds in the elastomer shell can occur with both subglandular and subpectoral implant types but may be more apparent both clinically and mammographically with the subglandular type due to the better imaging of the implant contour in the subglandular position.

Implant Rupture and Bleed

Implant rupture is uncommon; however, this complication is more likely to occur as the implant ages; more than 60% are not intact after 12 years.[17] This is a very different understanding from patients that were told that their implant would have minimal risk of rupture. Interestingly, an early advertisement of silicone implants in the 1960s demonstrated that a car could run over an implant without it rupturing. All silicone implants, even if well intact, eventually bleed or diffuse silicone through the elastomer shell.[12,13] Regardless of a rupture or tear in the capsule, leaks are either intracapsular, where the silicone remains within the fibrous capsule or scar, or extracapsular, where the silicone escapes the fibrous capsule or scar. The following summarizes the potential results of rupture or bleed:

- Distortion of implant or breast
- Change in size of implant or breast

- Collapse of implant in the case of saline implants. The saline is quickly reabsorbed in the body leaving only a collapsed shell in place
- Migration of silicone to the following:
  - Fascial planes
  - Breast tissue
  - Axillary lymph nodes and channels
  - Ducts
  - Surrounding muscle
  - Abdominal wall
  - Ipsilateral arm
  - Rare instances of distant migration of silicone to any place in the body
  - Siliconomas or granulomas
  - Fibrosis
  - Locoregional pain or tenderness

Although intracapsular leak is less worrisome, a ruptured silicone implant should be detected as soon as possible to prevent leakage of extracapsular silicone into the body and the resulting possible problems. Early detection of implant rupture allows for the least complicated removal, if indicated.

Implant Removal

Patients may choose to remove or replace an implant for many reasons including severe contracture, deflation, or proven leak. Removal or explantation should include removal of the fibrous capsule to better evaluate the integrity of the implant. The surgeon removes as much of the free silicone as possible, but it is not unusual for residual silicone to remain in the breast.

Imaging Breast Conservation Therapy Patient

CC + MLO + ML + MCC + MMLO of BCT site with a radiopaque marker on the scar.

The purpose of mammography in the conservatively treated breast is to:

1. Confirm removal of the tumor
2. Identify postoperative fluid collection
3. Detect residual and recurrent tumor
4. Screen the contralateral breast for cancer
5. Screen the ipsilateral breast for a new primary cancer

Some physicians recommend mammography of the affected breast after lumpectomy surgery but before radiation therapy treatments begin to have a baseline study of the postoperative changes. The side effects of radiation

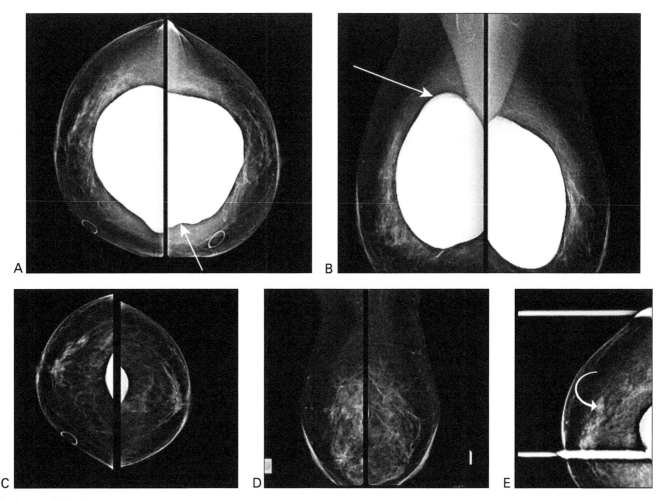

Figure 10-63
A 73-year-old woman with bilateral subglandular silicone implants. Bilateral **(A)** CC, **(B)** MLO, and **(C)** CC implant-displaced and **(D)** MLO implant-displaced and **(E)** spot compression CC implant-displaced images. Focal herniations (*short arrow*) and bulges (*long arrow*) through the fibrous capsule can occur over time causing distortions to the implant contour. The density and position of saline or silicone implant interfere with the mammographic study regardless of the implant type. Benign effects of implantation can both mask and mimic cancer, such as this small breast mass (*curved arrow*).

therapy can exacerbate these changes (and create new ones) and complicate the mammographic picture.

The technologist should prudently adapt the standardized protocols for an optimal mammographic examination when imaging the BCT patient. Information such as the

Table 10-6 • Baker's Grading of Capsular Contracture

GRADE	PHYSICAL FINDINGS
Grade I	Breast is soft with natural appearance
Grade II	Implant can be palpated; less soft; natural appearance
Grade III	Breast is firm with implant visible, some distortion
Grade IV	Breast is hard; obvious spherical distortion; may be cold and painful

tumor location and mammographic manifestation, that is, mass, calcification, etc., of the original tumor is required to provide the most adequate follow-up studies. Please note that the original mammography findings of a malignancy do not predict the findings of a recurrent malignancy. For example, calcifications originally detected and confirmed as malignant may recur as calcifications or a mass and vice versa. It is the current standard of care that the surgeon marks the edges of the surgical bed with surgical clips.

After BCT surgery, close mammographic surveillance is common. Typically, the patient is imaged at 6- or 12-month intervals for 2 to 3 years. Postsurgical and irradiation changes can both mimic and mask recurrence. However, these BCT changes follow sequential phases before eventually stabilizing. Any change after stabilization (stability is deemed as no change over two consecutive mammograms) is a strong indication for recurrence. Stability in surgical and radiation changes is reached at about 2 years when recurrences may begin to become evident. The following are frequent mammographic findings in the conservatively treated breast (see earlier discussion for explanation and regression of these changes) that can signal recurrence in the tumor bed:

- New or increasing asymmetries, focal asymmetries, or masses
- New or increasing diffuse accentuation of the glandular tissue density
- New or increasing skin thickening
- New or increasing architectural distortion
- New or increasing suspicious calcifications

Marking a BCT Lumpectomy Scar

Placing a scar marker on a BCT lumpectomy scar during screening and additional diagnostic imaging is beneficial for the radiologist. This brings the area to the attention of the radiologist and facilitates the search for a new suspicious finding in and adjacent to the lumpectomy bed. Positioning a lumpectomy scar tangential to the x-ray beam allows the radiologist to determine if the suspicious area is a scar or a new finding in the breast. The technologist can use the magnification technique and place a radiopaque wire to mark the scar for optimal results. Jewelry wire or even a small staple with tape can be cost-effective in marking the skin at the site of the lumpectomy scar.

Hematoma, Seroma, and Abscess

Hematoma, seroma, and abscess may present as a focal asymmetry or mass on the mammogram. A hematoma is a collection of blood, and a seroma is a collection of serous (clear proteinaceous) fluid. The patient may present with a firm palpable abnormality after surgery; however, mammography may be the first indication of a residual hematoma or seroma. Hematoma or seroma presents in early stages as a circumscribed, high-, or isodense mass on the mammogram.

In some cases, the hematoma or seroma will resolve entirely. In other cases, the mass will become smaller but quite dense and may even develop a spiculated margin, possibly creating difficulty for the interpreting radiologist. Eventually, this mass will stabilize. An accurate surgical history is critical in these cases, especially in the absence of a prior mammographic study.

Additional evaluation with targeted ultrasound is necessary to prove the mass is cystic. A hematoma may appear solid on ultrasound, secondary to the coagulation of blood; aspiration may or may not be possible depending on the thick consistency of the fluid. Image-guided aspiration or core biopsy may be necessary to distinguish between a hematoma and residual or recurrent carcinoma.

Short-interval mammography to follow the hematoma until it resolves or stabilizes may be useful.

Fat Necrosis

Fat necrosis is the death and necrosis/liquefaction of fat interspersed in breast tissue, caused by tissue trauma. Mammographic changes secondary to fat necrosis include architectural distortion and coarse heterogeneous, rim, or round calcifications. Architectural distortion is caused by possible fibrosis and scarring in the tissue. An oil cyst, created by organized, liquefied fat, may calcify along its wall creating rim calcifications that are typically larger than 2 to 3 mm in diameter. An oil cyst may be palpable. Rim calcifications may progress into round, smooth calcifications as the oil cyst continues to calcify. Suspicious course heterogeneous calcifications may also occur as smaller areas of tissue are traumatized. Even highly suspicious fine pleomorphic calcifications may occur in fat necrosis and can be difficult to distinguish from true malignant calcifications.

Calcifications

Postoperative fat necrosis calcifications may increase as other surgical changes resolve and, in some cases, may be the only residual evidence of previous surgical intervention within the breast. Distinguishing postoperative fat necrosis calcifications from residual or recurrent malignant calcifications can be difficult. It is thought that benign fat necrosis calcifications may increase for up to 2 years and then stabilize. Postoperative fat necrosis usually presents as coarse, round, or rim calcifications when associated with a hematoma, seroma, or oil cyst. Grouped fine-linear or branching calcifications are suspicious for residual or recurrent carcinoma. After a period of stabilization (usually two successive mammograms), an increase in calcifications in the lumpectomy bed are suspicious for malignancy.

Breast Tissue Edema

Edema from breast tissue inflammation and the disruption of lymphatic flow most often occurs after radiation treatment in the conservatively treated breast. Edema appears as a diffuse or focal increased density of the fibroglandular tissue and trabecular thickening and is worse in the first year after radiation treatment and then gradually decreases and stabilizes over the next 2 years. After a period of stabilization, any increase in breast tissue density is considered suspicious for malignancy.

Skin Thickening

Skin thickening may occur secondary to edema or may occur at any site of surgical incision and scar formation.

Skin thickening may completely resolve or will reduce and stabilize over time.

Imaging the Postmastectomy Patient

Imaging of the postmastectomy chestwall or following breast reconstruction is not routinely performed unless there is a new area of clinical concern. Ultrasound or MRI may be needed for any new palpable abnormalities. Mammography of the reconstructed breast is controversial. However, mammographic detection of a clinically occult recurrence in the reconstructed breast justifies this type of evaluation.[18] Long-term survival of the cancer patient is affected by local recurrence[19]; therefore, the earliest detection provides the best prognosis.

Reconstruction after Mastectomy

Saline or silicone implants are used for reconstruction after mastectomy and create similar issues as implants for augmentation, including the difficulty of mammographic technical factors for adequate imaging. Autologous myocutaneous flaps, however, provide a radiolucent reconstruction and are gaining popularity. Predictable surgical scars for each type of reconstruction are evident.

Autologous reconstruction typically has an adipose replaced appearance and some isodense fibroglandular tissue that represents the muscle component of the flap. This procedure involves transplanting tissue such as from the anterior abdominal wall rectus muscle (transverse rectus abdominis myocutaneous [TRAM] flaps) to the chestwall area to create a breast mound. During the procedure, the vascular supply to the transposed tissue must be maintained. Subsequent tattooing or surgical construction can create a nipple and areola complex.

Autologous implants may use one of three muscles: rectus abdominis, latissimus dorsi, and gluteus maximus, with the most popular being the TRAM flap.

Review Questions

1. Discuss the information necessary for an accurate patient clinical history and ways that it can affect the mammographic examination.

2. Discuss asymmetries—what they are and how they can be imaged.

3. Discuss some of the physical changes caused by surgery of the breast.

References

1. Kerlikowske K, Grady D, Rubin SM, et al. Efficacy of screening mammography. A meta-analysis. *JAMA*. 1995;273(2):149–154.
2. Bird RE, Wallace TW, Yankaskas BC. Analysis of cancers missed at screening mammography. *Radiology*. 1992; 184(3):613–617.
3. Logan-Young W, Dawson AE, Wilbur DC, et al. The cost-effectiveness of fine-needle aspiration cytology and 14-gauge core needle biopsy compared with open surgical biopsy in the diagnosis of breast carcinoma. *Cancer*. 1998; 82(10):1867–1873.
4. Available at: http://breastscreening.cancer.gov/data/benchmarks/screening/.
5. Haas BM, Kalra V, Geisel J, et al. Comparison of tomosynthesis plus digital mammography and digital mammography alone for breast cancer screening. *Radiology*. 2013;269(3):694–700.
6. Burnside E, Park J, Fine J, et al. The use of batch reading to improve the performance of screening mammography. *AJR Am J Roentgenol*. 2005;185(3):790–796.
7. Freeman R, McKee S, Lee-Lehner B, et al. Reducing interruptions to improve medication safety. *J Nurs Care Qual*. 2013;28(2):176–185. doi:10.1097/NCQ.0b013e318275ac3e.
8. D'Esmond L. Distracted practice and patient safety: the healthcare team experience. *Nurs Forum*. 2017;52(3):149–164. doi:10.1111/nuf.12173.
9. Fiske S, Krupinski E. Improving patient care through medical image perception research. *Policy Insights Behav Brain Sci*. 2015;2(1):74–80.
10. Amaratunga T, Dobranowski J. Systematic review of the application of Lean and Six Sigma Quality Improvement methodologies in radiology. *J Am Coll Radiol*. 2016;13(9):1088. e7–1095.e7. doi:10.1016/j.jacr.2016.02.033.
11. Available at: http://www.thebreastsite.com/breast-surgery/breast-reduction-statistics.aspx. Accessed October, 2009.
12. Newman J. Mammographic evaluation of the augmented breast. *Radiol Technol*. 1998;69(4):319–338.
13. Caskey CI, Berg WA, Hamper UM, et al. Imaging spectrum of extracapsular silicone: correlation of US, MR imaging, mammographic, and histopathologic findings. *Radiographics*. 1999;19:S39–S51.
14. Silverstein MJ, Handel N, Gamagami P, et al. Breast cancer in women after augmentation mammoplasty. *Arch Surg*. 1988; 123(6):681–685.
15. Dershaw DD, Chaglassian TA. Mammography after prosthesis placement for augmentation or reconstructive mammoplasty. *Radiology*. 1989;170:69–74.
16. Baker JL. Classification of spherical contractures. Presented at the Aesthetic Breast Symposium, Scottsdale, AZ; 1975.
17. Cohen BE, Biggs TM, Cronin ED, et al. Assessment and longevity of the silicone gel breast implant. *Plast Reconstr Surg*. 1997;99(6):1597–1601.
18. Hogge JP, Zuurbier RA, de Paredes ES. Mammography of autologous myocutaneous flaps. *Radiographics*. 1999;19: S63–S72.
19. Overgaard M, Hansen PS, Overgaard J, et al. Postoperative radiotherapy in high-risk premenopausal women with breast cancer who receive adjuvant chemotherapy. Danish Breast Cancer Cooperative Group 82b Trial. *N Engl J Med*. 1997;337(14):949–955.

Bibliography

ACR BI-RADS Atlas Breast Imaging Reporting and Data System. 5th ed. Reston, VA: American College of Radiology; 2013.

Harvey J, March DE. *Making the Diagnosis: A Practical Guide to Breast Imaging Expert Consult—Online and Print.* Philadelphia, PA: Elsevier Saunders; 2013.

Monsees BS, Destouet JM. Mammography in aesthetic and reconstructive breast surgery. *Perspect Plast Surg.* 1991;5(1):103–119.

Leibman AJ, Styblo TM, Bostwick J III. Mammography of the post construction breast. *Plast Reconstr Surg.* 1997;99(3):698–704.

Digital Mammography

Mammography Machines

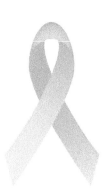

The consummate professional, in any profession, is the person who not only knows all the 'bits and pieces', but also understands how they fit together. He or she can analyze ideas, situations, and problems and offer intelligent guidance. We can all think of several people who fit this description, and most often aspire to emulate them. In my opinion, a professional technologist is someone who can do more than produce a quality diagnostic image; he or she is the person who understands the many factors involved in creating that image and controlling its quality. —**McKinney**[1]

Objectives

- Identify the various components of the mammography machine: the purpose and function for each.
- Discuss the special features and benefits for mammography x-ray tube designs.
- Describe the special requirements for proficient use of the mammography machine's phototimer.
- Discuss the design and rationale for the digital detector.

Key Terms

- automatic exposure control (AEC)
- computer-aided detection (CAD)
- constant potential generation
- exposure status index
- soft grid

- heel effect
- Mammography Accreditation Program (MAP)
- photoelectric effect
- ripple

INTRODUCTION

Mammographic image production begins long before breast manipulation during positioning in an attempt to capture as much breast tissue as possible on that image. Positioning the breast, initiating the x-ray exposure, and processing the image are the *final* steps in the imaging process. The "professional technologist" also understands how to maximize the inherent strengths in the design features of the mammography machine while minimizing the weaknesses.

Although some patients attempt to position their own breasts during the mammogram, it is the technologist who should position the breast. The technologist also needs to control the mammography machine.

A new era of mammography began in the United States in the late 1960s with the sale of the first dedicated mammography machine from the CGR Company. The new era continued to develop in the early 1970s with the introduction of the first single-emulsion, single-screen recording system from the DuPont Company. The 1970s focused on reducing x-ray dosage. Film imaging evolved into lower-dose screen-film systems; in direct response, xeroradiography was forced to modify its methods to lower its radiation dose to compete with the changes in screen-film mammography.

The 1980s phased out the use of general x-ray machines and xeroradiography techniques and replaced them with dedicated screen-film mammography machines to improve the quality of images at lower x-ray doses. Although the benefits of mammography were apparent, the results of screening trials showed the need for additional improvements in imaging.

The 1985 Nationwide Evaluation of X-ray Trends (NEXT-85)[2] evaluated dose and image quality at 232 sites in the United States and found disturbing results (Table 11-1). Only 64% of facilities had acceptable processing conditions. In 1986, Galkin et al. of Philadelphia surveyed 29 dedicated mammography facilities and found processing conditions varied tremendously; 41% demonstrated an unacceptable variation in processor performance over a 15-day period. Radiation doses ranged from 26 to 260 millirads per view.[3]

During the 1980s, the ACS implemented the National Breast Cancer Awareness Screening Program. The ACS was concerned about recommending women have routine mammograms because many were not high-quality exams. The ACS contacted the American College of Radiology (ACR). By 1986, the ACR designed and began pilot testing a **Mammography Accreditation Program (MAP)** to ensure image quality. This *voluntary* program was implemented in 1987. The first years of MAP showed great variability in the tested components. "We conclude from the ACR accreditation data and other surveys that image quality and dose vary widely, and that quality control practices are well below recommended standards ... There is a quality crisis in mammography."[3]

The 1990s was an era of improving image quality, equipment performance, and interpretive skills: quality images, quality control, and quality assurance. When the Women's Health Equity Act was passed in 1991, MQSA became a reality in 1992. MQSA regulates four areas: (a) site survey questionnaire, (b) phantom image, (c) clinical image, and (d) equipment performance. The Secretary of the Department of Health and Human Services designated the FDA to oversee MQSA.

The 2000s were a turbulent era. It began with great promise: January 2, 2000, digital mammography is approved by the FDA; February 11, 2011, digital breast tomosynthesis (DBT) is approved. The technology used to create the image keeps improving. But in October 2015, the mammography community is stunned by new ACS guidelines that reduce the customary annual mammogram exam to biannual (every other year). Current practice had reached a point where we could find stage 0 (DCIS) disease, and suddenly, the guidelines for mammography changed. See Table 11-2.

Table 11-1 • NEXT[a]

YEAR OF STUDY	SITES WITH ACCEPTABLE PROCESSING CONDITIONS (%)
1985	64
1988	81
1992	86

[a]Nationwide Evaluation X-ray Trends Summary of NEXT results.

Table 11-2 • Four Decades of Developments

1970s Dose reduction
• Dedicated machines
• Single-emulsion film
• Intensifying screen
1980s Equipment
• Xeromammography dies
• Dedicated mammography:
  ◦ Machines
  ◦ Films
  ◦ Processors
1990s Quality assurance
• 1985 NEXT
• 1987 Voluntary MAP
• 1991 Women's Health Equity Act
• 1992 MQSA
2000s Technological advancements
• 2000 2D digital mammography
• 2011 digital breast tomosynthesis

Each decade of modern-day mammography has had a theme: 1970s, dose reduction; 1980s, dedicated mammography equipment; 1990s, quality assurance; 2000s, technological advancements.

▌▌ THE MAMMOGRAPHY MACHINE

The mammography machine has but one purpose: to detect subtle changes in normal healthy breast tissue and image the tissue with the greatest clarity possible. Physicians depend on these images to detect abnormal diseased tissues at their earliest stage when intervention produces its best results. The perfect mammography machine—one that does everything for everybody all the time, does not exist; trade-offs must be accepted.

Various technologies for breast cancer detection are in clinical use: x-ray (mammography), ultrasound, nuclear medicine, CT, PET, and magnetic resonance (MR), each with their own specialized machines. Some are considered alternative methods and techniques to x-ray machines, which are considered the gold standard for mammography. Chapters 20 and 21 address other modalities and their applications. This chapter helps you understand the critical operating and design features of an x-ray mammographic machine and its relationship to the digital imaging process.

In 1986, the National Council on Radiation Protection and Measurements (NCRP) established guidelines that required use of dedicated equipment when performing screen-film mammography.[4] A dedicated mammographic machine is the only type of equipment that is specifically designed to adequately visualize the parts of the breast from which cancer develops. A variety of digital equipment is currently available, ranging from low-cost mammographic machines with few features to high-cost machines with many built-in features. Many machines offer optional peripheral add-on accessories.

Although the objective of all dedicated mammography machines is to produce clinically useful information on the computer monitor, manufacturers may choose to engineer and design their equipment with slight differences to accommodate the unique technical demands of digital mammography.

Every manufacturer attempts to accommodate several factors that influence the mammogram: such as the choice of digital detectors, differences in technologists' skills and knowledge of mammography, and most importantly, patients of all ages, shapes, and sizes, each possessing a unique temperament. Some equipment may offer automated features; other machines may require adjustments to accommodate key operating variables. Each facility must select the equipment that best meets its needs and budget. What factors should be considered when selecting a mammographic machine?

Performance

This chapter focuses on the technical factors in equipment design that affect production of an image. The most important ability the technologist can develop is to understand and master these factors to produce consistent, high-quality, diagnostic images. While "ergonomics" or "human engineering" features such as color, style, and number and location of controls are of value, they are not discussed in detail. However, these are equipment features to consider even though they do not directly affect image production. Equipment selection is a trade-off between the equipment features and your budget. Price should not be the only factor when selecting equipment. The basic considerations for equipment should include the following:

Space

The examination room should accommodate the gantry and acquisition workstation and provide enough space for the technologist to move around and assist the patient for proper positioning. Additional space may be needed to accommodate women in wheelchairs and for storing some supplies and/or equipment accessories in the examination room.

Electrical Requirements

Provide proper dedicated electric power for the mammography machine. Some machines plug into wall outlets, while others require three-phase or 220 wiring to be installed. In every case, a dedicated line is recommended.

Ergonomics

The machine should be user friendly to both the patient and the operator. The basic components of a standard mammography machine are shown in Figure 11-1.

Case Study **11-1**

Refer to Figure 11-1 and the text and respond to the following questions:

1. Name as many parts of the mammography machine C-arm as you can and describe the function(s) for each.

2. Name as many parts of the acquisition workstation as you can and describe the function(s) for each.

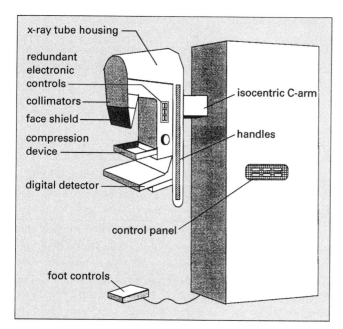

Figure 11-1
Dedicated mammographic unit.

The labels in the figure read: x-ray tube housing, redundant electronic controls, collimators, face shield, compression device, digital detector, isocentric C-arm, handles, control panel, foot controls.

The C-Arm

The C-arm's range of vertical movement should accommodate both tall women (approximately 6 ft) and those who need to sit; the minimum range of travel is 66 cm to 140 cm above the floor. The space beneath the image receptor support device (IRSD) should be open and free of encumbrances so that the patient can sit, if she needs to, for the examination.

The C-arm should rotate at least 180°. The point at which the C-arm connects to the tower (collar) should be isocentrically designed so that when moving from the CC projection to the MLO projection, the height does not need to be adjusted. Currently, the C-arm on most machines needs to be lowered several inches when changing from the CC to the MLO projection.

Electronic Controls

Electronic controls on both sides of the C-arm provide easy access for the technologist to adjust the height of the C-arm and raise and lower the compression device while the patient is being positioned. Grips or handles should be available to the patient to maintain a difficult or awkward position. Patient handles should be different from the technologist's handles, which contain the switches for operating the C-arm movements.

Compression Device-to-Receptor Distance

This distance (with the compression device raised as far away from the IRSD as possible) should allow adequate

space when positioning an obese woman for an MLO projection, when magnifying an area in a large breast, when raising the compression device over the needle during preoperative localizations, or when performing upright stereotactic core biopsies. The minimum measurement should be approximately 20 cm.

Tube Housing and Face Shield

This area of the unit should remain as small as possible to facilitate positioning of the patient's head for the CC projection in the contact and magnification modes. With DBT machines, the wider face shield should mount on the stationary C-arm, not on the moving tube housing; this reduces "patient collisions" with the tube housing and face shield.

Foot Controls

Remote foot controls for vertical movement of the C-arm and the compression device free the hands of the technologist while positioning. The amount of compression exerted by the foot pedal control should be minimal; final compression of the breast should always be done using a hand-controlled device. The hand-controlled device provides feedback to the technologist so that she feels the resistance the breast offers. The foot on the foot pedal on the floor cannot feel the resistance the breast offers.

Image Receptor Support Device

The IRSD is a fixed size, measuring approximately 24 cm × 30 cm. Gone are the days of two different size Buckies (18 cm × 24 cm and 24 cm × 30 cm) available with analog machines. In digital imaging, the IRSD is one size.

The size of the compression device now controls the size of the x-ray exposure field. The 18-cm × 24-cm compression device is used with the smaller breast and the (approximately) 24 cm × 30 cm is used with larger breasts.

Transmission of x-rays to the undersurface of the image receptor should be limited to no more than 0.1 mR/exposure. This shields the patient's abdomen from receiving x-ray exposure during the CC projection, plus this prevents x-rays from passing through the IRSD into adjacent walls when the C-arm is angled for an oblique or a Lateral projection; one reason why lead is not required in the walls of mammography rooms.

Acquisition Workstation

The acquisition workstation is the part of the mammography machine where the x-ray exposure controls are located. It is "command central" for the technologist because this component of the mammography system is where commands are given to the computer to acquire and process the images:

- The computer software should be easy to read and to adjust.
- The monitor should be 3MP to allow visualization of microcalcifications, the irregular borders of a mass, to perform interventional procedures, and to evaluate an image for motion.
- All machines must have automatic exposure control (AEC). When the exposure is completed, the workstation should indicate the technical factors used.
- An auxillary compression release device must be located on this panel. The unit must be able to disengage this release device during needle localizations or core biopsies.

Technical Capabilities

Density Selection

This leftover feature from the analog era has, in essence, no function in digital imaging. With digital imaging, density selection instructs the AEC to deliver more or less x-ray dose to the patient.

Kilovoltage

Molybdenum target tubes should have a range of at least 24 to 35 kVp in no greater than 1 kVp increments. Lower settings may be used in specimen radiography and higher settings for special views. Rhodium and tungsten target tubes should have a range of at least 28 to 45 kVp in no greater than 1 kVp increments.

Milliamperage Selection

Milliamperage (mA) selection may be fixed or variable. If the mA value automatically decreases while increasing the kVp, it should occur outside the range of settings routinely used for mammography: the 25 to 35 kVp range.

Time Selection

What is the range of time (from shortest to longest) allowed for an exposure? With short exposures when imaging a thin adipose-replaced breast, be certain the exposure time is long enough so grid lines are not visible.

Source-Image Detector Distance

The minimum source-image detector distance (SID) is 55 cm or more for contact imaging and 60 cm or more for magnification. Most mammography machines today have an SID in the range of 65 cm to 70 cm.

Collimators

Collimator blades are located inside the tube housing. They automatically open or close depending on the size of the compression device that is installed.

The x-ray field may extend beyond the IRSD at the chestwall edge, but only by a maximum of 2% of the SID.

Field Light

The brightness of the light source should be 160 LUX or higher. Misalignment of the x-ray/light field can be a maximum of 2% of the SID.

Unlike general x-ray procedures where we collimate the x-ray exposure field to match the size of the body part being imaged, when we perform the CC and MLO projections, no collimation is permitted. Since we are not allowed to collimate, turning on the field light is done only to check if an extraneous part of the patient's body encroaches in the light field:

- CC projection—the shoulder on the lateral margin of the breast; the chin on the medial border
- MLO projection—the opposite breast

Breast Thickness Scale

The compression thickness scale should be accurate to within 0.5 cm. The AEC takes into account the composition of the breast as well as the compression thickness.

Alignment

The focal spot, compression device, and image receptor must align perfectly at the chestwall edge to ensure that all posterior breast tissue is included.

Automatic Technique Selection

Machines must have a postexposure display that indicates the technical factors used: kVp, mAs, target material, filter, focal spot size, compression device size, and whether or not a grid was employed. The benefit of this feature is to produce an image using an acceptable length of exposure time to reduce motion blurring and/or patient dose, but without compromising the image quality.

Exposure Control

Typically, the machine manufacturer has two exposure buttons or levers, or the technologist must step on a foot pedal at the AWS. This feature ensures the operator can make an exposure only when completely outside of the x-ray field.

Radiation Shield

A radiation shield for the operator is required. "Equivalent attenuation to at least 0.08 mm of lead at 35 kVp or the maximum kVp, if less, and extend from ≤15 cm above the floor to a height of at least 1.85 m and sufficiently wide (at least 0.6 m) to intercept x-rays scattered from the breast and the unit which might otherwise expose the operator. To limit operator exposure to well below 0.1 mSv/wk based on 40 patients/d, 5 days/week. If shield is moveable it must interlock to prevent exposure if not in place properly."[5]

Filtration

X-ray tube filtration eliminates the soft end of the x-ray spectrum; photons that are not strong enough to penetrate the breast so they contribute nothing to the image, they simply increase the dose to the patient. Filtration also reduces the harder end of the x-ray spectrum; higher energy photons are lower in contrast. Filtration produces monochromatic characteristic wavelengths.

If multiple filters, the machine must clearly display which filter is in place when the exposure is made.

Backup Timer

The backup timer terminates the exposure with a sound or visual indicator. The suggested limits are 250 mAs minimum to 600 mAs maximum. Magnification mode requirements will be different.

Automatic Exposure Control

This device must maintain a consistent exposure regardless of the kVp setting used, thickness of the compressed breast, and/or ratio of glandular-to-adipose components.

The AEC should be able to determine if the time on the backup timer will be exceeded and, if so, should be able to terminate exposure to the patient within 50 milliseconds or 5 mAs.

Needle Localization Capability

The compression device for needle localization either has a series of concentric holes or a large rectangular cutout. See Chapter 17. The concentric-hole compression device holds the breast in place as the needle is inserted, but use caution when raising the device over the hub of the needle. With the cutout system, the breast *pillows* through the opening and is less stable during needle placement; adequate compression for visualizing small or low-density lesions cannot be achieved; however, raising the compression device over the hub of the needle should not present a problem.

Image Production Factors

The ability to produce a quality image is the most important consideration in selecting and using equipment. Even though the space that a mammography unit occupies, the ease with which one can exchange imaging accessories, and the availability of redundant electronic controls may be important considerations, none of these have a direct influence in producing the image. A summary of the six most important design/imaging features in the production of a good image are presented in Table 11-3. Each feature is discussed more thoroughly in this chapter. An understanding of the interrelationships between these six features enables the technologist to maximize a machine's strengths and to minimize its deficiencies.

Electrical Requirements and Efficiency

X-ray tubes require an efficient use of electrical power. Two methods for delivering power are alternating current (AC) and direct current (DC). Electronic circuits require DC, and state-of-the-art dedicated mammography machines require a smooth, ripple-free delivery of DC electrical power.

The method by which electrical power is generated in a dedicated mammography machine influences several important operating features: efficiency, x-ray intensity, exposure time duration, and dose yield. The output of a mammographic x-ray tube should be at least 800 mR/sec at 28 kVp, when measured 4 cm from the chestwall edge, centered laterally, and 4.5 cm above the image receptor plane. The unit should be able to sustain this exposure for a minimum of 3 seconds. The compression device is left in place during measurement of the output. Insufficient output creates longer (above 3.5 seconds) exposure times or requires higher kVp settings.[5] A short discussion of basic electricity is presented here to aid the reader in understanding the key role of electrical power in producing a useful clinical image.

Alternating voltage or current is usually defined as voltage or current that changes its strength according to a sine curve. Alternating voltage reverses its polarity on each alternation, and an AC reverses its direction of flow on each alternation. The point of maximum voltage, also called the crest voltage or peak voltage of the sine curve, occurs at 90° (Figure 11-2). Effective voltage (the beginning and ending portion of the usable waveform during the production of x-rays) starts at 45° and continues to 135° (Figure 11-3).

The frequency of the alternating voltage or current is the number of cycles (completed sine waves) per second (c/sec). In the United States, the standard is 60 c/sec or 60 Hz.

Table 11-3 • Equipment Design Factors in Producing a Digital Image[a]

DESIGN FEATURE	AFFECTS	DESIGN FEATURE	AFFECTS
Electrical requirements and efficiency	Exposure time SID Contrast Scatter Filtration Space requirements kVp + mAs selection	Magnification	kVp + mAs selection Exposure time Dose Radiographic sharpness SID Contrast Scatter
	Dose HVL[b] Ripple	X-ray tubes	Filtration Magnification
Grids	Exposure time Contrast Scatter Dose kVp + mAs selection		Dose Collimation kVp + mAs selection Exposure time Radiographic sharpness Contrast Scatter Heel effect
Compression and compression devices	Exposure time Scatter Radiographic sharpness kVp + mAs selection Dose Contrast		HVL SID Focal spot size
		Automatic exposure control	Exposure time Dose kVp + mAs selection

[a]Each equipment design feature influences several imaging factors; for example, x-ray dose is influenced by all six design features, while the HVL will be influenced only by two. If the manufacturers were to change any one of the six features listed here, the impact of this modification would be felt in other areas as well.
[b]HVL, half-value layer.

However, electronic circuits require direct current (DC power). The effective voltage component of the AC waveform is equal to the DC power. Half-wave rectification changes AC to DC by using only the positive (+) alternation (from 0° to 180°) of the input voltage, thus effectively cutting off the alternating waveform (Figure 11-4). This causes the DC voltage to fluctuate with the same frequency as the AC input. This is extremely inefficient because the output power is much less than the input. Full-wave rectification is more efficient. This reverses the polarity of one alternation of the input sine wave. Thus, DC voltage fluctuates with a frequency two times that of the input sine wave (Figure 11-5). This delivers an average or effective voltage twice as large as

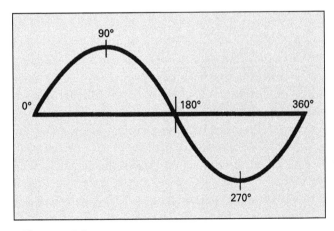

Figure 11-2
The highest portion of the sine wave occurs at 90°. An electrical measurement taken here indicates the peak voltage being supplied.

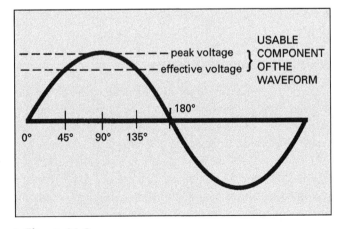

Figure 11-3
During the production of x-rays, the useful portion of a sine wave is from the effective voltage up to the peak voltage and down to the effective voltage. The rest of the waveform is unused.

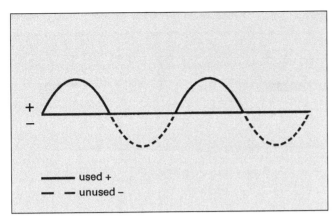

Figure 11-4
Half-wave rectification is an inexpensive means of converting AC to DC; however, it is very inefficient (50%). Use of half-wave rectification would result in exposure times twice that of full-wave rectification, or almost three times the exposure of a constant potential unit.

that of half-wave rectification; however, the peak output voltage remains the same.

A filtered circuit smooths the fluctuating DC output so that the equipment will operate even though the output voltage is not completely smooth. These small fluctuations are known as **ripple**, which is measured by frequency and amplitude. A filtered circuit is used to compress the peaks of the individually fluctuating DC pulses and to fill the valleys between the pulses. Capacitors store energy and then release this energy between the pulses (into the valleys) to smooth out the ripple. Tremendously large capacitors (so large, they're impractical) would have to be used to achieve near-DC power for mammography machines operated at a 60-Hz line frequency. *Thus, when operating a mammography machine, one has always had to account for the effects of ripple* (Figure 11-6).

One method of achieving pure DC power (0% ripple) is to use a battery. However, considering the kVp values needed for mammography, this is impractical. The battery would have to be larger than the capacitors needed for smoothing the waveform at 60 Hz to produce DC in a

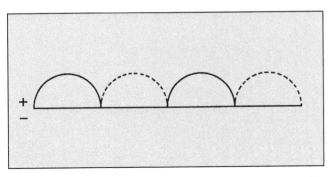

Figure 11-5
Full-wave rectification is twice as efficient as half-wave, but 30% less time efficient than power produced by constant potential.

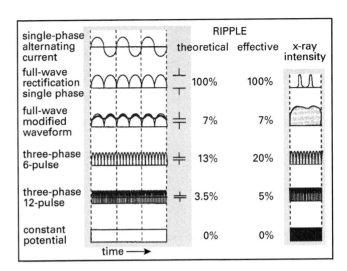

Figure 11-6
Tube current and x-ray intensity diagrams. Alternating voltage output from the x-ray transformer is converted into DC by means of full-wave rectification. Single phase, single phase with modified waveform, three phase/6 pulse, three phase/12 pulse, and constant potential circuits show progressively less variation with time of the voltage curve (decreased "ripple effect"). Short pulses of x-ray intensity are produced by the single-phase generator, whereas steady x-ray intensity results from the constant potential system. (Published in Feig SA. Mammography equipment: principles, features, selection. *Radiol Clin North Am.* 1987;25(5):897–911; Copyright Elsevier 2018.)

filtered circuit. Another method called **constant potential generation** is practical and is used by all manufacturers in currently available mammography machines. This method produces this efficient and desirable energy state by turning the waveform on and off rapidly and using only the peaks of each waveform. By using a microprocessor to control the on–off action, power is delivered efficiently.

All manufacturers produce mammography machines using high-frequency inverter technology (meaning over 10,000 Hz) with constant potential output (meaning less than 13.5% ripple). However, a further distinction must be made: the most efficient constant potential machines will have 2% ripple; the less efficient machines between 5% and 13% ripple. The amount of ripple should remain essentially equal for small and large focal spot operation.

The significant point of this discussion is that *mammography machines operate differently and should be used according to their ripple content.* Because of the varying ripple, different mammography machines require the use of different keV or kVp settings. Without proper keV or kVp settings, the exposure times might become prohibitively long. Table 11-4 lists the proper settings when comparing dedicated mammography machines to the varying ripple.

High-frequency/constant potential machines have several advantages. Weigl[6] compared a conventional single-phase generator with a high-frequency/constant potential generator

Table 11-4 • Power Variations in Mammography Machines[a]

GENERATOR SETTING (kVp)		CONSTANT POTENTIAL GENERATOR RIPPLE (kV)		3-PHASE, 6-PULSE GENERATOR, 20% RIPPLE (kV)	SINGLE-PHASE GENERATOR (FILTERED), 25%+ RIPPLE (kV)
		5%	13%		
25	=	24.4	23.4	22.5	21.9
28	=	27.3	26.2	25.2	24.5
32	=	31.2	29.6	28.8	28.0

[a]Discussion of kilovoltage (kV) rather than kilovolt peak (kVp) settings is more appropriate when making comparisons between machines. Kilovoltage factors in the inefficiency (or ripple content) of a machine. The average (or effective) kilovoltage equals kilovolt peak minus one-half ripple.

(a multipulse generator) also supplied by a single-phase line. He noted the following primary differences:

1. Dose yield and exposure times. We have already seen that dose yield of a three-phase generator is approximately 60% higher than the dose yield of a single-phase generator. This means that a multipulse generator (high-frequency/constant potential) also has a higher dose yield than a conventional single-phase generator.
2. Skin dose. Comparative depth dose measurements illustrate that the skin dose for the same film dose is considerably less from a high-frequency generator than the skin dose from a conventional single-phase generator, due to the different high-voltage wave shapes.
3. Space requirements. A further advantage of high-frequency technology is the reduced size. The generator does not consume much space, and it consists only of the control desk and the single tank tube unit; no additional high-tension transformer or electronics cabinets are necessary.[6]

High-frequency/constant potential machines have the following advantages:

1. The ability to use lower kV settings; thus, contrast is increased.
2. The increase in mR/s means x-ray production is more efficient; greater efficiency results in shorter exposure times.
3. Less patient motion is likely with shorter exposure times.
4. The patient receives a lower x-ray dose.
5. X-ray tube should last longer because output is higher.
6. Decrease in unit size. Smaller components are used when building a machine; therefore, the machines are compact and consume less space.

The radiation output waveform should have less than 5% kVp ripple (≤10% exposure ripple). Rise time (time until kVp is accurate and regulated) and the time to terminate an exposure should be less than 16 milliseconds.

kV Selection

In 1992, the General Electric Company introduced the first serious contender to the molybdenum target tube, at least for selected cases (Figure 11-7). This tube has a target with two different materials: molybdenum/vanadium and rhodium. The melting point of rhodium, 1,966°C, versus molybdenum's 2,610°C, requires lower mA stations to compensate for the lower thermal loading capacity.

"The subject contrast ... decreases with increasing thickness (for a fixed kVp) and increasing kVp (for a given phantom thickness), regardless of the incident spectrum [Mo/Mo; Mo/Rh; Rh/Rh] ... Subject contrast is greatest

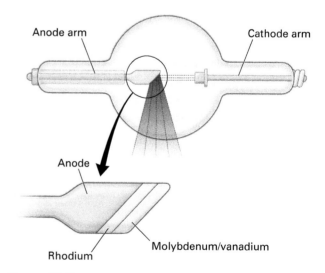

Figure 11-7
Dual track x-ray tube: rhodium and molybdenum/vanadium. Large and small focal spot sizes for each track. Rhodium is used for thick, glandular breasts; molybdenum for all the rest.

for Mo/Mo and least for Rh/Rh at lower kilovolt peaks. As kilovoltage increases, the Mo/Mo contrast decreases more rapidly than Mo/Rh or Rh/Rh, and for some combinations of breast composition and thickness, the Mo/ Mo combination produces less subject contrast than Mo/Rh or Rh/Rh. This crossover occurs at progressively lower kilovolt peaks as the breast attenuation (i.e., thickness or glandular content) increases"[7].

X-rays are produced using two methods: the Compton effect (Figure 11-8) and the **photoelectric effect** (Figure 11-9). In analog mammography, the photoelectric effect produced the special high-contrast x-ray spectrum necessary to find a (white) cancer hidden in (white) fibroglandular tissue.

The photoelectric effect depends on the atomic number of the substance (the target material) that is bombarded. Elements with atomic numbers between 40 and 45 give off characteristic radiation in the 15- to 30-keV (kilo-electron volt) range; the photoelectric effect dominates in this range.

- Molybdenum, with an atomic number of 42, produces K-edge characteristic peaks at 17.4 and 19.6 keV; the K-absorption edge is 20 keV. A 0.03 mm molybdenum filter is used with a molybdenum target to absorb anything produced below 17 keV or above 20 keV, resulting in a very narrow band of monochromatic radiation (Figure 11-10). This is optimal for adipose breasts and smaller to average size breasts of any composition; but the thicker, more glandular breast attenuates the x-ray beam so that it is only the higher energy (read "lower in

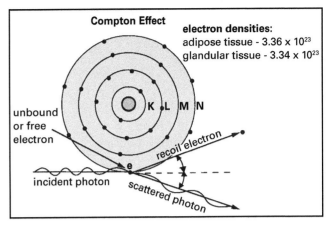

Figure 11-8
The Compton effect releases an outer-shell electron. The radiation emitted is the difference between the incoming x-ray photon's energy level and the amount of energy required to remove the loosely held outer-shell electron. Because only a portion of the incoming photon's energy is transferred in this interaction, the photon continues to travel, but with less energy. This photon may have more collisions and give up more of its energy, always at a different quality of radiation. (Adapted from Johns HE. *The Physics of Radiology*. Springfield, IL: Charles C Thomas; 1964.)

contrast") photons that exit out the bottom of the breast plus scatter that create the image. Molybdenum becomes ineffective at approximately 32 kVp. Breasts requiring the use of kVps in this range will be better served by switching to an alternative target material.

- Rhodium, having a higher average energy of x-ray photons, penetrates thick and/or glandular breasts and should be used with breasts that compress to 6 cm or

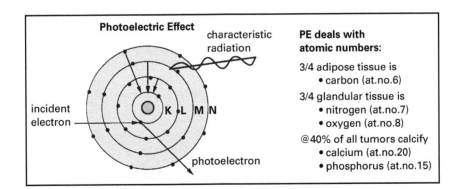

Figure 11-9
In the photoelectric effect, an electron from the cathode of the x-ray tube strikes the target and removes a tightly bound inner-shell electron, a photoelectron. The original x-ray photon then disappears because it expended all of its energy. The hole created by the ejected photoelectron is then filled by an electron from an outer orbit. Characteristic radiation is emitted as the outer-shell electron gives up some of its energy in moving closer to the nucleus. (Adapted from Johns HE. *The Physics of Radiology*. Springfield, IL: Charles C Thomas; 1964.)

Mammographic X-ray Spectra

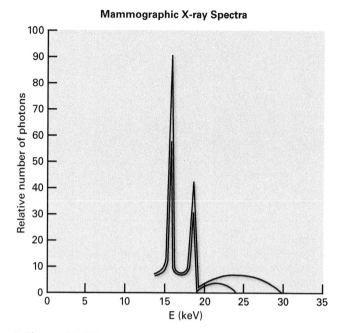

Figure 11-10

Typical x-ray emission spectra (normalized to unit area) used in mammography. A 0.03-mm molybdenum filter is used for the molybdenum target, and the spectra from 24 and 30 kV settings are shown. (Image courtesy of Eureka X-ray Tube, Inc.)

greater. [7–11] This has proven useful for approximately 15% of women.[9] With the "new anode/filter combinations there will be a decrease in dose without a loss of contrast if used appropriately. If inappropriate, then contrast will be significantly reduced with only a minimal reduction of dose".[12] See Table 11-5.

Rhodium, with an atomic number of 45, produces K-edge characteristic peaks at 20.1 and 22.7 keV; the K-absorption edge is 23.2 keV. A 0.03 mm rhodium filter is used with a rhodium target to absorb anything produced below 20 keV or above 23 keV, resulting in a very narrow band of monochromatic radiation.

Table 11-5 • Comparison of Molybdenum and Rhodium Characteristics

	Mo	Rh
Atomic no.	42	45
Melting point C	2,610	1,966
K-edge keV	17.4	20.1
	19.6	22.7
K-absorption keV	20.0	23.2

• Tungsten, with an atomic number of 74, produces characteristic peaks at 57.98 and 59.32 keV. Tungsten target tubes are used predominately with digital imaging. Various filters are used with a tungsten target.

The photoelectric effect deals with atomic numbers. In examining the composition of the breast, the atomic numbers of the two major components of breast tissue are closely grouped. Three-quarters of the mass of adipose tissue is composed of carbon atoms (atomic number 6). Three-quarters of the mass of glandular tissue is composed of nitrogen (atomic number 7) and oxygen (atomic number 8). Approximately 40% of breast cancers present with microcalcifications; calcium (atomic number 20) is also composed of phosphorus (atomic number 15).

The objective then is to produce contrast that will distinguish among atomic numbers 6, 7, 8, 15, and 20. This is a formidable task for any system to accomplish and the reason why it is crucial to keep the factors that degrade contrast to a minimum.

The Compton effect deals with electron densities. The electron density of fat is 3.36×10^{23} electrons/g, whereas that of glandular tissue is 3.34×10^{23} electrons/g. There is *no contrast differentiation here*; thus, every effort should be made to avoid Compton scatter.

"According to Johns and Cunningham, in soft tissue at 20 keV there is a 70% likelihood of photoelectric absorption and a 30% chance of Compton interaction.... At 26 keV, there is an equal chance of either interaction".[13] As noted by Feig, "a low kV beam is essential to maximize the number of photoelectric interactions. Below 20 kV, the Photoelectric Effect predominates in all soft tissue. From 20 kV to 28 kV, most absorption in fat is due to the Photoelectric Effect, whereas most absorption in fibroglandular tissue results from the Compton Effect. Above 28 kV, Compton scattering accounts for most interactions within those tissues. These relationships occur because the Photoelectric Effect increases more rapidly with a decrease in energy than does the Compton Effect. Therefore, contrast between fat and fibroglandular tissue increases with a reduction in kV. To achieve the highest contrast practically attainable, settings of 25 kV to 27 kV should be used in **screen/film mammography**".[14] (emphasis added) "Settings of 26–27 kV may be useful when performing magnification or grid studies, and settings in the low 20s can be used with specimen radiography".[15]

Settings of 25 kV with a molybdenum target tube create the highest possible image contrast while maintaining an acceptable radiation dose for the patient. This was the premise for analog imaging. However, digital image production is quite different from film-based imaging.

Traditionally, kVp controls contrast and mAs controls density; this concept is transformed with digital imaging. In digital imaging, contrast is equivalent to grayscale and density is equivalent to brightness. kVp and mAs do not affect grayscale and brightness; in digital imaging, grayscale and brightness are controlled by computer processing algorithms and by window width and window level functions. kVp controls penetrance of the x-ray photons. Digital imaging can use higher kVp settings because kVp no longer controls grayscale display. Instead, grayscale levels are controlled by the window/level adjustments. Increased kVp settings result in decreased mAs settings.

Tungsten target tubes were unacceptable to use with analog imaging because the atomic number and characteristic peaks of tungsten are well outside the preferred 15- to 30-keV range in which the photoelectric effect predominates. But with the uncoupling of kVp and contrast, most digital mammography machine manufacturers have switched from molybdenum/rhodium target tubes to tungsten. They match their digital detector design to the x-ray spectrum emitted by the tube.

The intended use of an alternate filter and/or target material is to produce images at a lower dose without reducing image quality (Figure 11-11). With digital mammography machines, the exposure indicator alerts the technologist to the quality of the exposure.

X-Ray Tube

The x-tube is the heart of the x-ray machine. On the outside, the x-ray tube designed for mammography may resemble other medical x-ray tubes, but the interior design dramatically affects the operating characteristics and performance features necessary to produce a mammogram. A basic understanding of the problems mammography poses to x-ray tube engineers, and their solutions to these unique problems, permits further critical evaluation of a mammography machine.

Measured Output Rate

"Because of varying design characteristics of x-ray tubes, SID, window construction, and ripple performance of different generators ... specification of tube current can be misleading in predicting x-ray output. Measured output exposure data are much more useful."[16] The output of the mammographic unit should be at least 800 mR/sec at 28 kV, measured 4 cm from the chestwall edge, centered laterally, and 4.5 cm above the image receptor plane. The unit should be able to sustain this exposure for a minimum of 3 seconds. The compression device is left in place when measuring the output. Insufficient output means longer (above 3.5 seconds) exposure times or requires higher kilovolt peak settings.[5]

Filtration

Molybdenum target tubes use molybdenum and rhodium filters, usually 0.03 mm thick, to provide an almost monochromatic beam by filtering out the energy levels above 20 keV and below 17 keV. Do not substitute aluminum filtration for molybdenum filtration when using a molybdenum target tube; this will shorten the exposure time while severely compromising the contrast of the radiograph. Rhodium target tubes use rhodium filters; tungsten target tubes employ various filters, including aluminum filters for DBT. If overfiltration of the x-ray beam occurs, a built-in microswitch should prohibit exposure.

Glass windows are used in general x-ray machine tubes; mammography x-ray tubes should have a beryllium window rather than glass. Glass acts as a filter when dealing with the soft end of the x-ray spectrum, and it filters out photons that would provide contrast in mammography.

Half-Value Layer

The half-value layer (HVL) affects radiographic contrast and dose. The HVL is measured 4 cm in front of the edge of the image receptor, centered laterally, with the compression device left in place.

For a molybdenum target/molybdenum filter tube the HVL should be equivalent to the value of the kilovolt peak/100 + 0.03 in machines of high-purity aluminum, with an upper limit not to exceed kilovolt peak/100 + 0.12 in machines of aluminum. The HVL should not decrease by more than 20% after removal of all material between the x-ray filter and the breast—that is, minimum filtration should come from the K-edge filter and not from the beryllium window, the mirror, or the compression device.[5]

Stationary Versus Rotating Anode

An advantage of a rotating anode is a higher tube loading capability; therefore, the mA can be higher and exposure times can be reduced. The disadvantage is that

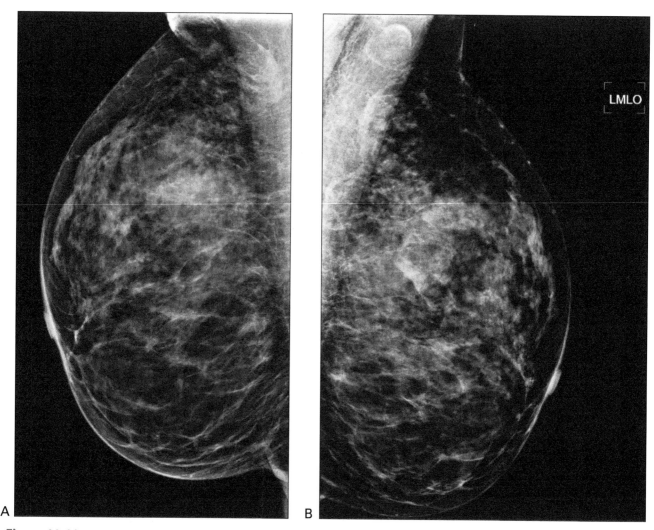

Figure 11-11
Molybdenum versus rhodium radiographic images of the breast. **(A)** Rhodium: 4.5 cm compressed thickness. **(B)** Molybdenum: 4.5 cm.

there is more off-focus radiation produced with a rotating system. "This ... may comprise from 5% to 25% of the total radiation output. Like scatter radiation, off-focus radiation adds an overall haze to the image, reducing the image contrast."[17] Much of the off-focus radiation can be removed by inserting a diaphragm inside the tube housing; however, make sure that an unacceptable increase in the HVL has not occurred as a result. Stationary tubes produce less off-focus radiation, but have lower tube rating capabilities.

Heel Effect and Anode Angle

Because x-rays are produced 8 μm inside the target material, the angled target absorbs some of the x-rays it just produced—hence the **heel effect** (Figure 11-12).

Diagnostic x-ray tubes exhibit the heel effect in a left-to-right pattern; the intensity of the x-rays is strongest at the cathode side of the tube and diminishes in strength toward the anode side. Mammography x-ray tubes exhibit the heel effect just as diagnostic tubes do, except the pattern is turned 90° so that the strongest x-rays are at the chestwall, diminishing outward toward the nipple (the cathode side of the tube is closest to the patient's chestwall, while the anode side of the tube is toward the nipple).

Production of the x-ray beam requires a flow of electrons from the filament (cathode) of the tube to the surface of the anode. This electron stream is driven or forced to flow by the kV level, while the amount of electron flow is controlled by the mA. If the controlling factors (either kV or mA) increase, the heat load to the anode increases. Tube

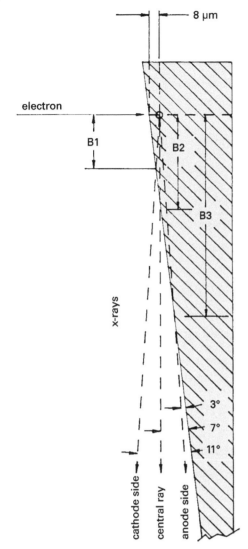

Figure 11-12
Illustration of the heel effect—self-absorption of x-rays in the upper target layer. X-ray production occurs 8 µm *inside* (**at circle**) the target (**shaded area**). Because the target is angled, the differences in exit lengths (**B1 through B3**) result in a falloff of radiation from chestwall (**cathode side**) to nipple (**anode side**), known as the heel effect. (Image courtesy of Eureka X-ray Tube, Inc.)

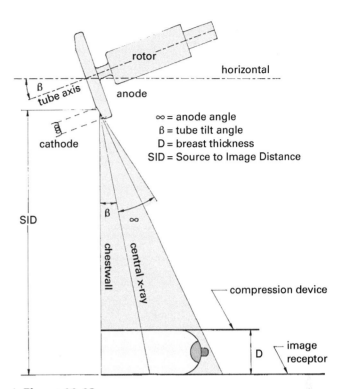

Figure 11-13
Tube angle relationships. X-ray tubes produce a diverging x-ray field. Mammography tubes use only one-half of this diverging beam—that from the chestwall out. If the other half were used, posterosuperior tissue along the chestwall would not be visualized because of the divergence of the beam. The x-ray unit must provide the proper target angle plus tube tilt to assure a perpendicular ray through the chestwall and yet still provide coverage for the large imaging format (approximately 24 × 30 cm). This combined angle (target angle plus tube tilt) is a function of the SID of the machine. (Image courtesy of Eureka X-ray Tube, Inc.)

manufacturers angle the anode surface to distribute the heat better; thus, a larger stream of electrons can be used to yield higher mA values, and the angle also results in a smaller effective focal spot for better resolution. The disadvantage is a more pronounced heel effect: a reduction in beam intensity as viewed from the chestwall to the nipple. Newer tube designs provide a balance between tube angle and focal spot size and the resulting optical density falloff, or heel effect.

The heel effect, exposure level, and the size of field coverage depend on the angle of the x-ray tube's target, the amount of tube tilt, and the SID (Figure 11-13). Trade-offs in this facet of x-ray tube design are common because these three factors (heel effect, exposure level, and field coverage) are closely interrelated. The steeper the anode angle (the closer to 0°), the more heat units the tube can withstand; but the heel effect will be greater. The greater the heel effect, the lower the intensity of the x-ray beam at the anode (nipple) side. The lower the x-ray intensity at the nipple side of the IRSD, the less field coverage available for the "24" dimension of a 24-cm × 30-cm image receptor.

Effective focal spot sizes from many different mammography machines can be identical, regardless of the anode angle (Figure 11-14). The factors affected by the anode's

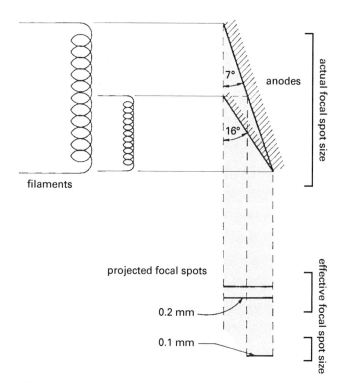

Figure 11-14
Projected focal spot sizes versus anode angle. Using a steeper anode angle with respect to the image plane (on this diagram it is the 7° angle), the actual focal spot (area on target's surface that the electrons strike) will be larger, while the projected focal spot (effective focal spot at image plane) will be the *same size* as that produced by a more angled target (the 16° angle). The advantage of a 7° anode angle is that the system will withstand more heat units because the target face is almost twice the length of that achieved with the other angle. This is known as the line focus principle. The disadvantages are that the heel effect on the 7° anode will be far greater, there will be a larger variation in the flux or photon energy (see Figure 11-15), and size of field coverage will be less. (Image courtesy of Eureka X-ray Tube, Inc.)

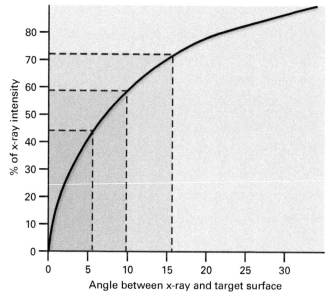

Figure 11-15
The heel effect produced by a 7° angled target will be greater than that from a 16° angled tube. The intensity of the x-rays provided by the steeper target (7°) will be 45%, whereas that from the 16° target will be 72%. (Image courtesy of Eureka X-ray Tube, Inc.)

angle are (a) the actual focal spot size, (b) the amount of heat units the target can withstand, (c) the heel effect, and (d) variations in the flux rate (intensity of the x-rays) (Figure 11-15). Because effective focal spots are measured at the half-angle axis, the longer the SID the smaller the half-angle. Hence, the larger the actual focal spot will be. The positive effect of this design permits a higher mA loading of the tube; however, there is an adverse effect with this design also. The inverse square law states that the intensity of radiation varies inversely as the square of the distance; that is, as the tube is moved farther away from the digital detector, the x-ray intensity reaching the digital detector diminishes. In practical terms, to go from a 60 cm SID to a 65 cm SID, the mAs must be increased by 20% to maintain the same exposure on the image. A 10 cm increase in the SID requires a 36% increase in mAs.

Focal Spot Projection

Mammography machine focal spots are much smaller than general x-ray machines. Mammography exams are primarily done for screening purposes; thus, we are searching for the earliest signs of breast cancer. In order to detect early disease, the image must contain exquisite detail. Resolution depends on a small focal spot size as well as small pixel size. The large focal spot of the typical mammography machine measures 0.3 mm, while the small focal spot is 0.1 mm. These focal spots are so small that they cannot withstand many heat units, but they do produce excellent resolution.

The projection of the focal spot as a function of the central ray is another factor that relates to tube design. "It is extremely important that the unit be designed such that the [chestwall] ray projects parallel to the chestwall. If the [chestwall] ray from the tube (the ray that is perpendicular to the IRSD) is toward the center of the image receptor ... a few mm of tissue close to the chestwall is not imaged unless the compression device is moved in or out"[16] (Figures 11-13 and 11-16).

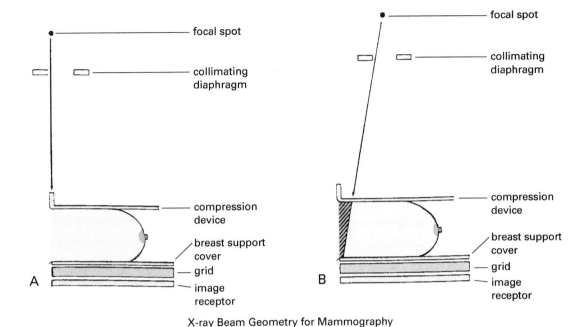

X-ray Beam Geometry for Mammography

Figure 11-16
(A) The correct alignment of the focal spot over the edge of the IRSD. Posterior and/or superior breast tissue is not lost. **(B)** Incorrect alignment causes a loss of tissue. (Reprinted with permission from AAPM Report No. 29 "Equipment Requirements and Quality Control for Mammography", Report of Task Group No. 7 Diagnostic X-Ray Imaging, August 1990.)

The resolution toward the nipple edge of the IRSD can be three or four times sharper than at the chestwall edge of the image (Figure 11-17). This factor becomes critical during magnification (Figure 11-18). Using the small 2-inch diameter spot compression device for magnification restricts imaging to the area that aligns at the chestwall edge (Figure 11-19). Ideally, the area of the breast under clinical suspicion should be placed away from the chestwall edge of the breast support so that the tissue is under the part of the x-ray tube that provides the best resolution.

The "Sweet Spot"

A mammographic unit that uses an x-ray tube with a biangular design (large and small focal spots use separate angles on the target for production of x-rays) has a "sweet spot" that is approximately 4 cm from the chestwall for each focal spot. With all other mammography x-ray tube configurations, this area of high resolution will range from 4 to 8 cm from the chestwall edge out toward the nipple edge. Although the biangular design has a decided advantage when performing magnification views, the current angle of the target produces a dramatic optical density falloff because of its heel effect. Tilting the beam filter at the opposite angle of the target can reduce falloff.

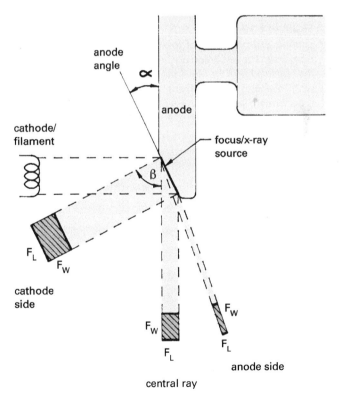

Figure 11-17
Projection of focal spot size as a function of the central ray. Resolution contains two dimensions: width and length. Only the length resolution (F_L) is two times worse at the chestwall; the width resolution (F_W) is unchanged. The apparent (effective) resolution is approximately the ratio of the orthogonal dimensions. (Image courtesy of Eureka X-ray Tube, Inc.)

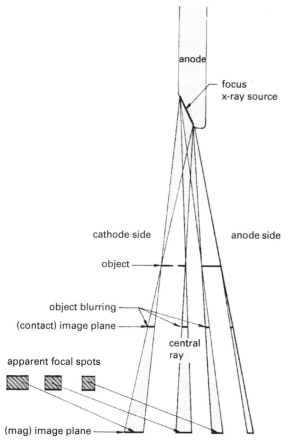

Figure 11-18
Blurring and projection of focal spot size as a function of the central ray. The resolution on the anode side of the tube (toward the nipple edge of the IRSD) will be better than that at the chest-wall. This holds true whether magnification or contact imaging is performed. (Image courtesy of Eureka X-ray Tube, Inc.)

Case Study **11-2**

Refer to Figure 11-17 and the text and respond to the following questions.

1. Why do we have a focal spot width versus a focal spot length?

2. What is the "sweet spot" of the x-ray tube? Where is it located?

X-Ray Tubes and Filters

In the 1980s, mammography was the hot topic among the radiology community. Sales of mammography machines escalated and mammography conferences

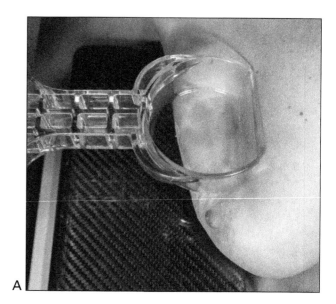

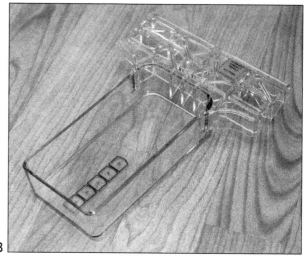

Figure 11-19
(A) The 2-inch round spot compression device requires precise positioning and restricts the imaged area close to the edge of the IRSD. **(B)** The 4-inch rectangular spot compression device allows visualization of a larger area of breast tissue.

proliferated exponentially. By the mid 1980s, it became apparent that there was a need for standardization in education and equipment. Diverging opinions among educators and also among mammography equipment designers caused dissent within the ranks of mammographers.

In 1990, the Centers for Disease Control granted funding to the ACR to "identify aspects of mammography amenable to improvement through education, research, and the implementation of quality assurance procedures and to develop educational materials, courses, and recommendations to assist in improving quality assurance in mammography. The expected outcome of this work was a higher, more uniform standard of quality in mammography."[18]

One component of this cooperative agreement project culminated in the 1995 ACR publication of a white paper *Recommended Specifications for New Mammography Equipment: Screen-Film X-ray Systems, Image Receptors, and Film Processors.* The avalanche of sales of mammography machines in the 1980s contributed to the manufacture of machines that were not designed well. To capture market share and keep abreast of every innovation created by their competitors, various assortments of machines were quickly designed, fabricated, and sold. Some machines contained good features, while other designs were ill equipped for the complex work involved in screening mammography. A classic example of this flawed thinking was that less expensive machines were built expressly to screen asymptomatic women; the more expensive (read "higher-quality") machines were the diagnostic machines. Typically, the screening machines were underpowered, had larger focal spots, high HVL, and fewer accessories. The manufacturers had it wrong; screening machines must be of *high* quality to image the small lesions. When screening the asymptomatic population, we search for the earliest signs of breast cancer, to detect very small lesions. Here is where one should use the best machines.

The consensus of *Specifications for New Mammography Equipment* was to stop manufacturing machines that would not produce good images. However, the authors of this paper did not want to dissuade future innovations in imaging (i.e., digital mammography). Although the paper declares that the ideal analog mammography unit consists of a molybdenum target tube, a beryllium window, and a molybdenum filter that meets the criteria of minimum HVL, an alternative combination of target material, window, and filter can be used if it provides comparable contrast and detail to the above combination at an equal or reduced dose to the breast.[19] Figure 11-20 is a graphic depiction of various target materials and filters, various kVp settings, and the contrast they produce.

Automatic Exposure Control

"The discovery of AEC dates back to Russell H. Morgan in 1942. Morgan used a theory developed by Heinrich Franke, who recognized that on every radiograph there is a dominant area, the darkening of which is proportional to the average darkening and general

Contrast/Dose

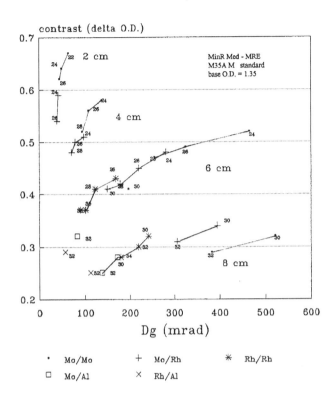

contrast: 1 cm gland–lipid   DR Jacobson

Figure 11-20

This is a composite plot of dose and contrast as a function of anode/filter/kilovolt peak for simulated breast thicknesses of 2, 4, 6, and 8 cm. (Image courtesy of Dr. Jacobson, PhD., Medical College of Wisconsin.)

appearance of the entire image. This theory has formed the basis on which every AEC device operates. Radiation that is transmitted through an object is converted into an electronic signal, which terminates the exposure when the predetermined level of radiation has been reached."[20]

Automatic exposure control (AEC) has been a standard feature on most diagnostic x-ray equipment for many years, but has been incorporated in mammography machines only since the early 1970s. Phototimer designs have only recently been adapted as effective for mammography. The unique problems associated with breast imaging required waiting for the development of "smart" phototimers that relied on more advanced electronic technology to reproduce accurate densities on the image. Before the development of the smart phototimer, most skilled technologists used manual techniques.

To understand the unique phototiming problems that the breast presents, we must first look at the anatomy of the breast (Figure 11-21). The side view of the breast reveals the skinline at the outer edge, the subcutaneous fat layer immediately beneath the skin, the ductal structures and functional glandular tissue, the retroglandular adipose tissue, the pectoral muscle to which the breast is attached and that extends down to the level of the nipple, and finally the ribcage. Breast cancer does not develop in the skin or in adipose tissue; it originates within the ductal structures or the functional glandular tissue. Therefore, this tissue must be adequately visualized.

Adipose tissue appears dark on the image because the soft x-ray photons used for mammography are strong enough to penetrate the fatty component of the breast; thus, many photons exit the bottom of the breast and interact with the digital detector. The glandular tissue, however, is very dense and absorbs more of the soft x-ray photons; therefore, only a few exiting photons strike the digital detector. Thus, the glandular tissue appears white on the image.

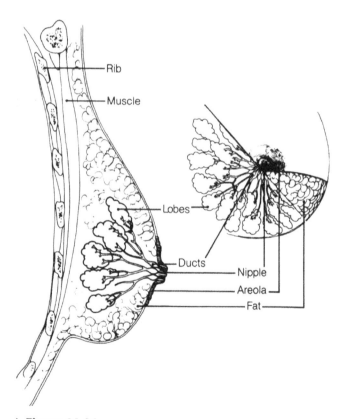

Figure 11-21
The breast structure: rib, muscle, lobes, ducts, nipple, areola, fat. (From: National Cancer Institute - Visuals Online, Susan Spangler, illustrator.)

Smart Phototimer

The AEC with a digital mammography machine is dose dependent. The field service engineer programs the dose to be delivered to the patient into the mammography machine's computer. This method of phototiming is more stable than its predecessor—the ion chamber. Rarely do we over or under expose the image.

The smart phototimer consists of a series of photocells rather than a single pickup. These multiple detectors are connected in parallel to provide better consistency in exposure level from one view and one patient to another. For example, when imaging a glandular breast that has one area of adipose tissue, if one of the photocells is placed under that tissue while the others are positioned under glandular tissue, this phototimer averages the signals of both areas. The image should not be overexposed nor should it be underexposed. This is only one feature that makes the newer phototimers more reliable.

Smart phototimers "remember" and "repeat" kV settings; thus, they can respond to varying kV settings. Earlier ion chamber models were unable to respond to different settings; when the kVp setting changed, an adjustment had to be made to the density setting. Smart phototimers do not need additional adjustments to the density setting. Once the desired exposure level is established, and the "0" or "normal" density setting is programmed, the density setting will rarely need to be changed. With today's digital mammography machines, the density setting instructs the machine to deliver more or less dose to the patient; it no longer controls the density of an image because of the window-leveling feature available with digital imaging.

Smart phototimers also respond to varying breast tissue thickness. Most breasts tend to be thicker in the oblique position than in the CC position. The density setting on a single-pickup ion chamber phototimer usually needed to be increased when a woman was in the oblique position. Smart phototimers recognize and compensate for breast thickness as the positions change.

The phototimer should be able to do the following:

1. Track (maintain the same exposure level) from one kVp setting to another
2. Compensate for differences in breast thickness
3. Obtain an adequate exposure level for varying breast tissue compositions
4. Provide a kVp and mAs readout after the exposure terminates
5. Reproduce accurate exposure levels on each image (reproducibility)

AEC Reproducibility

The AEC device should produce images that do not vary more than 0.12 optical density units from the mean optical density for breast thicknesses of 2 to 6 cm of PMMA and kVps that are appropriate for those thicknesses. The mean optical density is where performance is evaluated at an optical density above 1.20 and with an imaging system average gradient of 3.0. Note that if an average gradient other than 3.0 is used, the value of 0.12 should be scaled linearly with the film gradient (i.e., the higher the film gradient, the higher the allowed optical density variation), so that the specification is based strictly on the performance of the x-ray equipment.[5]

A suboptimally exposed image is virtually impossible to take with a smart AEC device. Figure 11-22 illustrates the range of technical factors for varying tissue composition and thickness. A "potential disadvantage of phototiming is that it might encourage a radiologist to employ an inexperienced technologist to do mammography, or assign infrequent mammography rotations to many technologists instead of forming a small cadre of highly skilled ones. It must be remembered that selection of exposure parameters is a relatively simple task whereas proper positioning and compression of the breast truly defines the success of the technologist, and thereby, of the images she produces. Phototiming must not serve as an excuse for slipshod technical performance; the result may well be correctly exposed yet poor quality mammograms."[21]

Automatic Technical Factor Selection

The automatic technical factor selection on mammography machines has several options. Depending on the machine manufacturer's definition and terminology, this phototiming function can be as simple as allowing the machine to select everything: the target and filter combination, as well as the kVp and mAs settings, or a semiautomatic phototiming option could be used instead, where the technologist selects the target and filter, while the phototimer selects the kVp and mAs. Or it may be that the technologist selects the phototiming option that provides images with the highest contrast index, or perhaps she selects the dose option to intentionally reduce the contrast in the image in order to reduce the dose to the patient. Manufacturers provide differing options.

Reciprocity Law Failure

The RLF of a film used with an intensifying screen states that as the length of exposure time increases, there is no

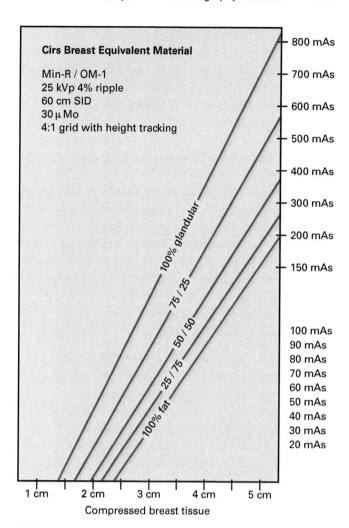

Figure 11-22
Milliamperage seconds as a function of type of breast tissue and thickness of breast with compression. The constant factor is the kVp setting. The variables include (1) the ratio of adipose to glandular tissue (ranging from 100% glandular to 100% adipose tissue) and (2) the thickness of the breast, which ranges from 1.5 to 5 cm. A 4.5-cm thick, 100% glandular breast would require approximately a threefold increase in mAs to obtain an optical density equivalent to that of its 100% adipose counterpart. A 3-cm thick glandular breast would require only a twofold increase in mAs. (Image courtesy of Transworld Radiographic X-Ray Systems.)

linear increase in the density on the film. For example, if two identical films were to be exposed, one for a period of time and the other for twice that amount of time, the second film would not be twice as dark in its density measurement as the first.

Digital machine phototimers respond linearly, so unlike analog phototimers, they do not have to be programmed to compensate for RLF. In digital imaging, making exposures longer than necessary results in an undesirable increase in dose to the patient, the possibility of patient motion, and can result in more noise on the image.

In digital imaging, the kV is increased as the breast thickness, and/or amount of glandular tissue increases in order to keep the dose to the patient reasonable. The kV setting is matched with the breast thickness/composition to optimize the contrast/noise ratio. With use of higher kV, the contrast in the raw image is lower, but image processing restores the contrast. With digital systems, at a fixed patient dose, using low kV results in a high contrast but noisy image; use of higher kV results in lower contrast but a smoother image. Somewhere in the middle is a sweet spot that is the best compromise between contrast and noise. Image processing then adjusts the contrast to display the high-contrast image the radiologist is used to seeing.

Image Acquisition and Quality

Mammography uses a digital detector to measure and convert the signal that passes through the breast. This signal is recorded, digitized, and quantified into a grayscale display that represents the amount of signal deposited in each pixel. Postprocessing software organizes this data into a meaningful display on the acquisition monitor.

Digital systems are designed to automatically optimize the image, regardless of the accuracy of the phototimed exposure. The acquisition workstation computer compares the received signal with that of an ideal image and applies specific algorithms (i.e., thickness compensation, conspicuity) to "fix" the image so that it is acceptable; this is one reason why there are few technical repeat images, because the computer fixes our images for us.

The purpose of this automatic optimization function is to reduce repeated exposures to the patient due to technical errors, but an unintended consequence has been a failure by the technologist to select correct technical factors. With the uncoupling of image contrast and brightness to the dose delivered to the patient, it is possible to slightly reduce the dose and then window/level the image to make the image look acceptable. However, if the dose to the patient is too low, the image will be noisy. If the technique is too high, the image is acceptable, but the dose to the patient is higher than necessary to produce an acceptable image. The technologist needs a method to visually assess whether a correct technique was used to produce the image. In analog mammography, this was done by examining the film on the viewbox for over- or underexposure; the digital mammography technologist does this assessment by checking the exposure status indicator.

Exposure Status Indicator The **exposure status indicator** has a few aliases, depending on the equipment manufacturer: EI number, DEI number, S value. This is a numerical indicator of exposure data to (a) monitor the dose to the patient and (b) alert us to acceptable image quality by monitoring that adequate x-ray exposure has reached the detector. The readout of the exposure status indicator depends on the x-ray tube target material, filtration, SID, collimation, and image processing algorithms.

Attempts are underway to standardize the exposure status indicator among the various equipment manufacturers. Not only does the name vary between manufacturers, the acceptable/unacceptable range varies, while some manufacturers do not even make this feature available to the technologist. In 2009, the AAPM, the Medical Imaging Alliance, and the International Electrotechnical Commission developed a method to standardize the exposure status indicator for all digital equipment.

The exposure status indicator should display immediately after the exposure terminates to let the technologist know if the level of exposure is okay. The deviation index (DI) should be zero. If the image is underexposed, a negative DI displays; if overexposed, a positive DI displays. A posted technique chart and use of a phototimer helps prevent dose creep.

Magnification

Magnification should produce quality images—images that are sharp and that are produced with an acceptable radiation dose. Magnification increases the radiation dose to the patient because her breast is placed on the magnification stand breast platform, so it is much closer to the x-ray tube.

The equipment should allow compression and collimation to only the area of the breast that is of concern and should also allow full-field magnification imaging; some radiologists prefer collimation to just the ROI, while others want the entire field imaged so they can see associated landmarks (i.e., the nipple or the skinline).

Magnification factors range from 1.4× to 2×. When compared with routine breast imaging, the magnification ranges are as follows:

$$1.4 \times \text{mag} \begin{cases} \text{nongrid technique} & 1.9 \times \text{increase in dose} \\ \text{grid technique} & 0.9 \times \text{increase in dose} \end{cases}$$

$$2 \times \text{mag} \begin{cases} \text{nongrid technique} & 4 \times \text{increase in dose} \\ \text{grid technique} & 1.7 \times \text{increase in dose} \end{cases}$$

To maintain acceptable doses and exposure times, "grids are not recommended for use with magnification since both the air gap … and the small field size reduce scattered radiation…. The use of a grid increases patient exposure, increases tube loading and increases motion artifacts due to the prolonged exposure time."[16]

Aside from the increase in dose as the magnification factor increases, another problem is introduced: maintaining radiographic sharpness. To maintain a sharp image as the magnification factor increases, the focal spot must either be significantly reduced (it cannot because this is an internal part of the equipment's design) or the thickness of the body part being radiographed must be decreased. "While some machines are equipped to provide 2× magnification geometry, most focal spots perform better at 1.5× magnification. Images at lower magnification are usually sharper due to the finite size of the focal spot."[16] For 1.5× magnification, the optimal "equivalent" focal spot size is about 0.2 mm, while for 2× magnification, the optimal equivalent focal spot is about 0.1 mm. A nominal focal spot measurement is not a reliable indicator of the resolving capability of a mammographic unit. The actual size of the focal spot is allowed to be +50%. The focal spot resolution test provides specific data for the calculation of resolution in line pairs per millimeter (lp/mm).[14]

Magnification Factor Versus Focal Spot Size

Screen-film mammography systems are able to resolve approximately 20 to 22 lp/mm. 2D FFDM machines resolve 9 to 10 lp/mm. However the contrast resolution of digital imaging more than offsets its limited spatial resolution. DQE is the preferred method to evaluate resolution.

A brief discussion of basic imaging concepts demonstrates how improved imaging technology influences magnification. Figure 11-23 shows a mammographic x-ray machine and the geometric resolution (line pairs per millimeter) for two focal spot sizes. Note how the smaller focal spot improves resolution.

With magnification, regardless of the magnification factor, the recording system is still limited to resolving the current 20 to 22 lp/mm, while 2D FFDM has spatial resolution of 9 to 10 lp/mm. With the parameters set in Figure 11-24 (unknown SID, unknown breast thickness, 0.15 mm measured focal spot), using a 1.5× magnification factor allows visualization of 13 lp/mm at midbreast, whereas with 2× magnification, this is reduced to 7 lp/mm. Because the focal spot cannot be reduced to give more line pairs of resolution, the thickness of the radiographed object must be altered. Furthermore, the higher the magnification factor, the thinner the object needs to be. The

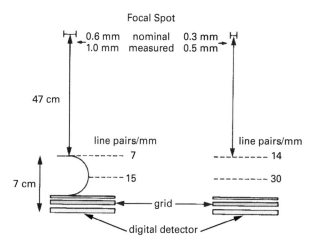

Figure 11-23
Example of the use of a grid in routine imaging of the breast. The distance from the top of the breast to the film measures 7 cm. The smaller of the two measured focal spots would therefore obtain good resolution on the resulting radiograph. The very top of the breast induces a bit of geometric unsharpness (the 14 lp/mm produced by the equipment is worse than the 21 lp/mm current recording systems can visualize), but by the time midbreast is reached, the radiographic resolution is being limited by the recording system (the equipment is now able to produce 30 lp/mm although the recording system is unable to "see" more than 21 lp/mm). Remember that the part of the object closest to the film always has the best resolution, while the part farthest from the film has the worst. With the larger of the two focal spots, only the bottom half of the breast, closest to the film, would have good resolution. (Reprinted from Haus AG. Recent advances in screen/film mammography. *Radiol Clin North Am.* 1987;25(5): 913–928. Copyright © 1987 Elsevier. With permission.)

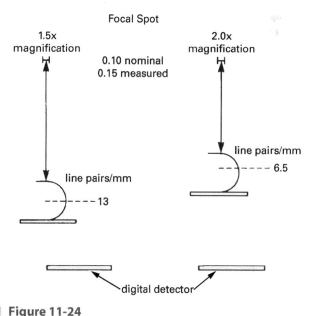

Figure 11-24
Compares mammographic x-ray unit geometric resolution (line pairs/millimeter) for 1.5× and 2.0× magnifications. (Reprinted from Haus AG. Recent advances in screen/film mammography. *Radiol Clin North Am.* 1987;25(5):913–928. Copyright © 1987 Elsevier. With permission.)

Table 11-6 • Line Pair Resolution in Magnification[a]

FOCAL SPOT SIZE (MM)	MAGNIFICATION FACTOR							
	1.5	1.6	1.7	1.8	1.9	2.0	2.1	2.2
10	20.00	16.67	14.29	12.50	11.11	10.00	9.09	8.33
11	18.18	15.15	12.99	11.36	10.10	9.09	8.26	7.58
12	16.67	13.89	11.90	10.42	9.26	8.33	7.58	6.94
13	15.38	12.82	10.99	9.62	8.55	7.69	6.99	6.41
14	14.29	11.90	10.20	8.93	7.94	7.14	6.49	5.95
15	13.33	11.11	9.52	8.33	7.41	6.67	6.06	5.56
16	12.50	10.42	8.93	7.81	6.94	6.25	5.68	5.21
17	11.76	9.80	8.40	7.35	6.54	5.88	5.35	4.90
18	11.11	9.26	7.94	6.94	6.17	5.56	5.05	4.63
19	10.23	8.77	7.52	6.58	5.85	5.26	4.78	4.39
20	10.00	8.33	7.14	6.25	5.56	5.00	4.55	4.17

[a]These numbers represent the resolving ability *at the surface the breast rests on* (the magnification platform). To figure the actual number of line pairs per millimeter (lp/mm), one would need to factor in how high above this surface the lesion lies in the breast using the following formula: where 1.1 is a constant, FOD is the focal spot-object distance (in centimeters), FS is the focal spot size (millimeters), and OFD is the object-film distance (in centimeters).
Source: Courtesy of Transworld Radiographic X-ray Systems.

number of line pairs per millimeter that can be resolved at various magnification factors and focal spot sizes are given in Table 11-6. Chapter 7 provides a further description of positioning in relation to magnification.

The focal spot resolution test requires a high-contrast resolution bar pattern. This bar is placed parallel to the image receptor at a distance of 4.5 cm above the breast support surface and within 1 cm of the chestwall edge of the IRSD and centered laterally. To pass the resolution test, the mammography machine must meet the minimum criteria: identify 11 lp/mm with the pattern oriented perpendicular to the anode–cathode axis and 13 lp/mm when parallel to the A–C axis. The bars must appear separated over at least 50% of their length when viewed with a 1× (or higher) magnifier.[5]

Do not use the focal spot size measurement test; it is not as precise. The x-ray tube manufacturers did not standardize the reference angle specification, which made measuring the focal spot size an unreliable indicator of resolving capacity. Using the line pair resolution test measures the system performance and is the preferred method to evaluate a system.

Grids

Contrast is important in mammography. Anything that contributes to contrast degradation is undesirable, and one should attempt to avoid or reduce such contributing factors. Maintaining high contrast is difficult because the breast has minimal inherent subject contrast; in addition, the "soft" x-ray spectrum used is easily attenuated.

Scatter production is the primary cause of contrast degradation. Scatter adds to the overall exposure of the image, so it detracts from contrast (Figure 11-25). Two methods to combat scatter are (a) use of specially constructed soft grids for mammography and (b) vigorous compression of the breast. The latter method is discussed in the next section of this chapter.

Case Study 11-3

Refer to Figures 11-25, 11-26, 11-29, and 11-30 and respond to the following questions.

1. Why do we want to reduce scatter?

2. What are the two primary methods used to reduce scatter?

3. What are the two styles of grids used in mammography?

Grids improve contrast by allowing primary x-rays to pass through their interspace material, while the lead strips absorb the secondary scatter (Figure 11-26). Consequently, this method to increase contrast increases the x-ray dose to the patient by as much as three times that of a study performed without a grid.

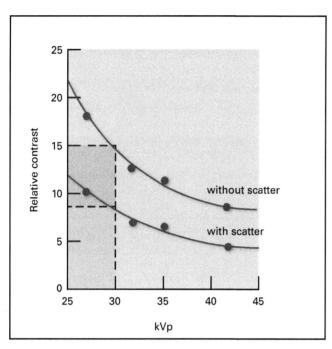

Figure 11-25
Variation of subject contrast with x-ray energy, with and without the effect of scatter. Contrast increases dramatically as x-ray energy is decreased and scatter is eliminated. At 30 kVp, contrast is roughly doubled when scatter is eliminated. (Reprinted with permission of Anderson Publishing Ltd. from Zammenhof RG, Homer MJ. Mammography part 1. Physical principles. Appl Radiol. 1984;13(5):86. Copyright © Anderson Publishing Ltd.)

Moving grids have been in existence since 1978 when the Philips Medical Company introduced the **soft grid** for mammography. Moving grid ratios are usually 5:1. As the grid ratio increases, the cleanup of the scattered radiation also increases, but a corresponding increase in radiation dose to the patient results as well. Various types of fibrous interspace material (carbon fiber, pressed cardboard, or wood) instead of aluminum interspace material (as is common with diagnostic x-ray grids) allow the Bucky factor to remain low—between 2 and 2.5. The pressed carbon fiber surface of the IRSD breast platform, which is separate from the actual grid, acts as a protective cover for this fragile grid, especially when the grid is subjected to the forces used in compressing the breast. Pressed carbon is strong yet attenuates very little of the x-ray beam.

The IRSD platform should be rigid enough so that the motion of the grid is not impeded when the breast is firmly compressed. The breast support surface should be strong enough so that when a 5-cm diameter, 0.5-cm thick disk is placed on the breast support, above the center of the image receptor, and compressed using the full pressure of the compression device, the motion of the grid is not impeded.[5]

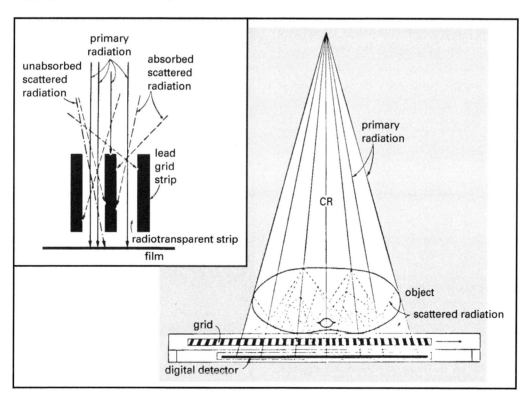

Figure 11-26
Location and function of a grid (inset: detail of a grid). Note how a large portion of the scattered radiation is absorbed, but image-forming radiation passes through. (From "Controlling Scattered Radiation," in Cahoon's Formulating X-Ray Techniques, 9th ed., Thomas T. Thompson (John Cahoon), pp. 83–109, Fig 4.10, page 94. Copyright, 1979, Duke University Press. All rights reserved. Republished by permission of the copyright holder. www.dukeupress.edu.)

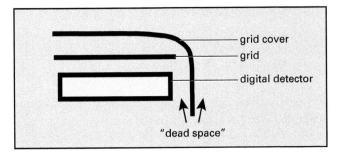

Figure 11-27
Side view of an IRSD. The space between the edge of the digital detector and grid and the grid cover that contacts the patient's skin must be minimized. Breast tissue that rests on top of this area will not be visualized.

When examining the IRSD platform, make sure the chestwall bend of the surface that covers and protects the grid is not too thick. The edge of the grid should be as close to the edge of the cover as possible; there should be just enough extra space for the grid to move freely. The important point is to minimize the "dead space"—any area of the IRSD on which breast tissue rests but will not be visualized (Figure 11-27). This nonvisualized area affects all standard views. In addition to minimizing the dead space, the area on either side of the active imaging field must be kept as small as possible to avoid lateral edge dead space (Figure 11-28). This nonvisualized area affects any view in which the corner of the IRSD is placed in the axilla. A certain amount of dead space is necessary to allow the grid to reach operating speed before the x-ray exposure begins; the grid lines will then be blurred out during the exposure. Accommodating this space becomes critical when performing the oblique

view, in which visualization of the upper portion of the tail of Spence is essential.

In 1995, a revolutionary new grid was introduced, the high-transmission cellular (HTC) grid. The conventional grid is linear, whereas the HTC grid is a honeycomb-shaped structure that can absorb more scatter x-rays while allowing the through transmission of more primary x-rays. As a result, a higher-contrast image is produced at a dose comparable to that of a 5:1 linear grid. The cellular/honeycomb pattern is self-supporting so interspace material is eliminated (Figure 11-29).

Compression and Compression Device

Vigorous breast compression has an important role in mammography. Sickles'[21] summary of Logan and Norlund's[22] reasons for compression includes the following:

• Decreased motion unsharpness (vigorous compression effectively immobilizes the breast, even for exposures as long as 3 to 4 seconds)

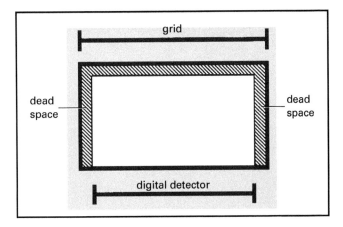

Figure 11-28
A moving grid will always be larger than the digital detector. Lateral edge dead space must be kept to a minimum because breast tissue that rests atop this area will not be visualized on an MLO or Lateral view.

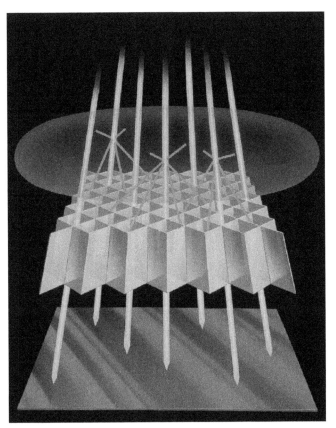

Figure 11-29
HTC grid. Crosshatch grid design uses air as interspace material. Removes more scatter than a conventional mammography grid yet the radiation dose is equal to or less than a linear grid. (Image courtesy of Hologic, Inc., and affiliates.)

- Decreased geometric unsharpness (compression brings intramammary abnormalities closer to the image receptor)
- Increased contrast (compression reduces the amount of scattered radiation by decreasing thickness)
- Separation of superimposed areas of glandular tissue (vigorous compression spreads apart overlapping islands of dense breast tissue, thereby reducing confusion caused by superimposition shadows and facilitating the visualization of the borders of mass lesions)
- Reduced radiation dose (by decreasing breast thickness, fewer photons are needed to expose the image receptor)
- More uniform density (vigorous compression flattens the base of the breast to the same degree as the more anterior regions, permitting optimal exposure of the entire breast in one image)
- More useful assessment of the apparent density of masses (cysts and benign glandular tissue usually flattened more easily with vigorous compression than carcinomas; therefore, they appear to be of lower density because, size for size, their decreased thickness stops fewer x-rays)

The only negative aspect of compression is the varying degree of discomfort each woman experiences. Every woman has her own level of tolerance for compression.

Figure 11-30 depicts how much compression can increase contrast on an image; examples of adequate compression versus inadequate compression can be found in Chapter 7. Although good compression is a necessity, a statement concerning overcompression of the breast is warranted. "Compression forces in the range of 160–250 N (36–56 lbs.) should be obtainable. A minimum of 200 N should be generated by the compression systems in order to sufficiently compress large, dense breasts. Compression forces higher than 250 N may be harmful and should not be obtainable."[23]

Compression Device Design

Manufacturers have dramatically improved the design of compression devices from that of earlier versions. The design and fabrication of the compression device is extremely important to allow visualization of posterior breast tissue and to maintain contrast on the image. A compression device:

- Should be made of thin transparent plastic
- Must have a straight chestwall edge, that is, no "cutout" for the ribs

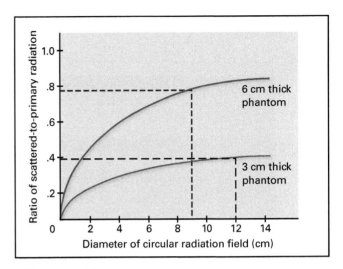

Figure 11-30
With a 6-cm thick, minimally compressed breast that measures 9 cm in diameter, 80% of the film density results from scatter. If that same breast were reduced to 3 cm in thickness with good compression, with an increase in diameter to 12 cm, scatter would contribute to only 40% of the density. Thus, there would be a twofold increase in contrast. (Adapted from Barnes GT, Brezovich IA. Intensity of scattered radiation in mammography. *Radiology.* 1978;126:243.)

- Must have sufficient height and angulation of the chest-wall edge
- Must have a squared off rather than a rounded chestwall edge
- Must remain parallel to the IRSD when compression is applied
- Must have perfect vertical alignment between its chest-wall edge and that of the IRSD
- Must be controlled by hand during final compression, although the initial positioning and compression should be aided by a motor-driven assembly

Thin Plastic Composition The use of fire-retardant polycarbonate plastic is recommended. This plastic attenuates little of the x-ray beam compared with Plexiglass, which is used by many manufacturers. The thicker the plastic, the more rigid the compression device, but also the greater the attenuation factor. Although the attenuation from the compression device will not cause the radiologist to miss a carcinoma, this minor design feature does affect the clinical image. The use of 1.5- to 2-mm thick polycarbonate is preferred.

Straight Chestwall Edge The compression device should have a straight chestwall edge. Since 1987, all manufacturers have produced the straight-edge design (Figure 11-31).

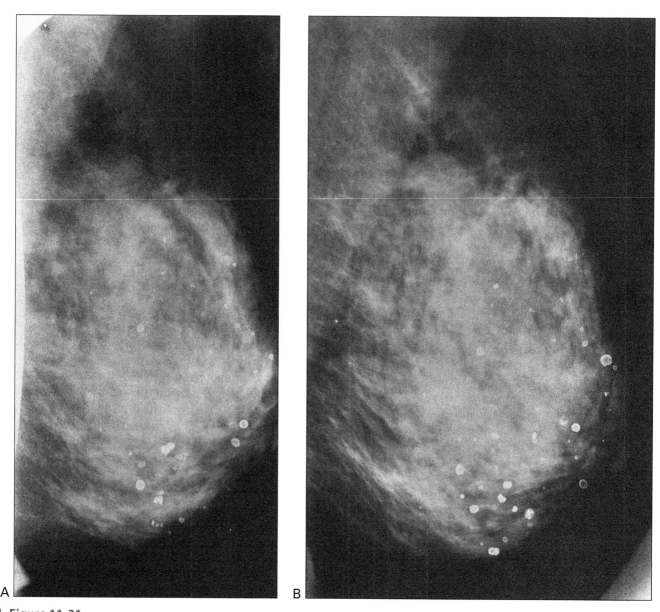

A   B

Figure 11-31
(A) An oblique view mammogram performed with a curved compression device causes loss of visualization of tissue at the chestwall. **(B)** An oblique view of the same patient performed with a straight-edged compression device visualizes much more posterior tissue.

Height and Angulation of Chestwall Edge   The chestwall rise of the compression device should extend upward approximately 2 in. in height and form an 85° angle with the horizontal edge (Figures 11-32 and 11-33). The 2-inch height in this design helps to prevent the axillary fold from superimposing itself over the posterolateral aspect of the breast while performing the CC projection. A compression device with a short chestwall rise requires the patient to sublux her shoulder, which pulls some of her lateral breast tissue off the IRSD.

Additionally, the 2-in. height helps avoid shearing fractures of a thin plastic compression device when vigorously

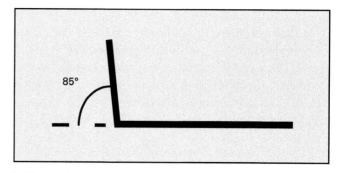

Figure 11-32
Side view of a compression device.

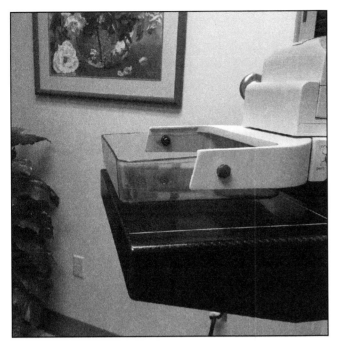

Figure 11-33
The chestwall rise of the compression device should extend upward approximately 2 in. and should angle slightly toward the patient. Note that the edge is squared rather than rounded at the chestwall. Also, the compression device must be parallel to the IRSD.

compressing the breast. With compression devices made of thinner plastic, an 85° angle near the patient's ribcage permits enough forward displacement of the plastic as she leans into the machine while being positioned to avoid superimposing the ribs and plastic over the central posterior aspect of the breast.

Squared-Off Chestwall Edge The chestwall edge or bend of the compression device should be squared off with a small radius rather than rounded (Figure 11-34). The

sharper edge allows the compression device to grip the tissue closer to the ribs than a curved edge would. Curved edges allow some of the breast tissue closest to the ribs to "roll" backward and not be compressed.

Parallel Alignment with Image Receptor The compression device should remain perfectly parallel to the image receptor during final compression of the breast. The breast must be compressed to a flat, even thickness over its entire surface. Any inclination of the compression device will usually result in less compression of the thickest portion of the breast, exactly the area that requires the most. Figure 11-35 illustrates the correct and incorrect relationship of the compression device to the IRSD. More than a 1-cm difference in measurement from the chestwall edge to the nipple edge is unacceptable.[5] A specialty compression device that does not remain parallel to the image receptor, a tilting compression device, should be used when the breast is noncompressible. The tilting compression device has been specifically designed to distribute compression evenly across a noncompressible breast.

Vertical Alignment with Image Receptor The chestwall edge of the image receptor and the chestwall rise of the compression device must be in perfect vertical alignment along the full length of the image receptor. Figure 11-36 illustrates proper alignment. Posterior breast tissue will not be imaged if the IRSD and compression device are not properly aligned. The compression device can extend up to 2 mm beyond the chestwall edge of the image receptor.[5]

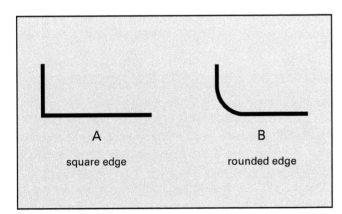

Figure 11-34
Side views of a (*A*) square-edged versus a (*B*) rounded-edged compression device.

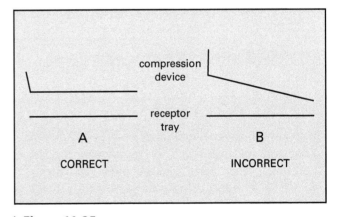

Figure 11-35
(**A**) The correct relationship between the compression device and IRSD. (**B**) Incorrect sloping of the compression device. This sloping arrangement is allowed with *specially designed* tilting compression devices.

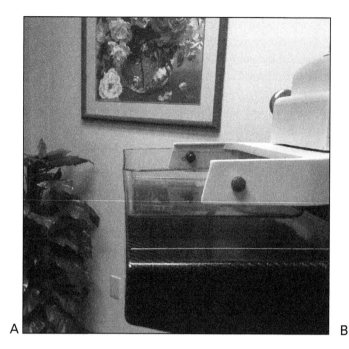

A

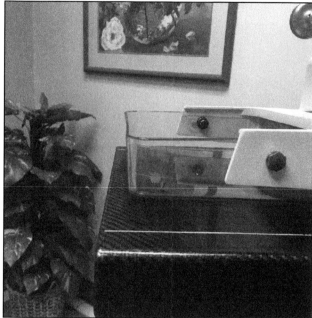

B

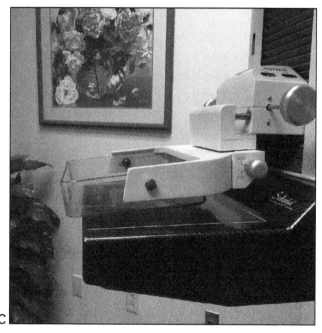

C

Figure 11-36
The chestwall edge of the compression device must have a straight edge. This straight edge must align perfectly with the edge of the IRSD, as shown in **(A)**. The alignment of the compression devices shown in **(B)** and **(C)** will miss posterior tissue.

Initial and Final Compression

There are two controls for breast compression: motorized (automatic) and manual. While positioning the breast, apply initial compression with the motorized device activated by a foot pedal. This foot pedal device should be preset to an amount sufficient to "hold the breast in position" but yet not enough force to adequately compress the average breast. Without reservation, the force the foot pedal applies should never be enough to overcompress the

breast. Final compression should be applied manually and should be controlled by the technologist.[5]

The technologist uses a hand-controlled compression device for two reasons: (a) the patient needs reassurance that a person, not a machine, controls the compression amount that will be applied to her breast, and (b) the technologist can feel the resistance increase when turning the handwheel and receives feedback when the breast is adequately compressed. The compression device should not slip back after final compression.

An automatic or technologist-directed release mechanism immediately removes compression after the x-ray exposure has ended. An override feature is essential to disengage the automatic release function when necessary (e.g., preoperative wire localization or for a patient whose balance is unsteady). If a power failure occurs, there must be an emergency release mechanism.

Spot Compression Device and Quadrant Paddles

The "spot" or "coned-down" compression device included with many mammography machines is small, perhaps 2 inches in diameter. These devices are adequate to use with patients who have a nonpalpable area in a small breast, or they can be used on any breast size that has a palpable lesion. However, they are of limited value in attempting to obtain an extra view of a nonpalpable lesion in a large breast. If the technologist cannot locate a suspicious nonpalpable area during the first attempt with this small compression device, the patient will typically allow a second try with some resistance. Additional attempts will not be tolerated. A quadrant paddle should be available and used. Quadrant paddles are approximately 3 to 4 in. wide. This paddle usually allows the nipple to be visualized as a point of reference when performing special views of the breast (Figure 11-19).

▌ COMPUTER-AIDED DETECTION

Introduction

Computer-aided detection (CAD) in mammography is a valuable technique to aid in improving the sensitivity of screening mammography. The concept is simple: use a computer's strengths (rapid processing of complex data, consistency, programmed attention to repetitive tasks without distractions or fatigue) to aid in the repetitive task of searching for the signs of breast cancer in screening mammograms. When CAD is used in mammography, there is a synergy, a combination of human strengths of the physician and the computational strengths of the computer that lead to improved sensitivity—better results. CAD is like a powerful spell checker, a valuable tool, to aid the physician in the detection of breast disease.

Many factors contribute to making the interpretation of a screening mammogram difficult:

- The differences between malignant and benign tissue are sometimes small, with careful attention needed to find suspicious microcalcifications and masses.

- Another difficulty is that the number of women with breast cancer in a screening population is low, typically 3 to 10 per 1,000 women screened,[24,25] with the majority of those cases being normal.

- Most mammography facilities have a large number of patients and therefore a large number of mammograms to interpret, sometimes with a relatively short amount of time per case.

- There can be many distractions for the interpreting radiologist in busy settings.

All of these factors combine to cause false-negative screening mammograms because of oversights: a mammogram interpreted as normal that shows clear signs of breast cancer. Studies have shown that the false-negative rate for screening mammography ranges from 20% to 40%.[26–30]

Facilities tried "double reading" to help solve this problem. Using two radiologists to independently review the mammograms increases the sensitivity of screening mammography by 5% to 15%.[31,32] However, depending on the method used to combine the two interpretations of the radiologists, there can be a corresponding decrease in the specificity.[33] In addition, many facilities have logistical and financial difficulty in implementing a double-reading method.

This leads to the alternative discussed here—using a computer to help the radiologist visually analyze the mammogram to detect the abnormalities associated with the presence of breast cancer. The goal of the system is not to replace the radiologist, but to provide extra information to ensure that the radiologist has looked at all of the suspicious locations on the mammogram. The interpretation of the suspicious locations remains the decision of the radiologist. The use of computers for detection is different from computer-aided diagnosis, in that computer analysis gives more guidance as to the degree of malignancy of a particular location. Currently, there is no commercially available system in the United States that provides computer-aided diagnosis in mammography. The FDA-approved CAD for analog mammography in 1998, digital mammography approval in 2001, and DBT CAD for Hologic's C-view in 2013.

How CAD Works

The first step to enable CAD to work in a mammography facility is to obtain an image of the mammogram in a digital version for the computer to analyze. The mammogram is formatted into a grid of rows and columns, and each small square is called a pixel. Digital mammography automatically captures an image in this digital format.

After the digital image is captured the CAD computer analysis begins. The different algorithms (an "algorithm" is a method of applying mathematical or logical tools to a task, in this case by a computer) are usually built around well-known techniques based on computer vision or image analysis from other fields. What the programmers try to do is to use these techniques to search for the same pattern recognition features as the radiologist. Most algorithms are separately developed for the detection of microcalcifications and masses (or subsets of masses, such as spiculated masses), because the features of those abnormalities are so different. This is analogous to the fact that radiologists use different visual techniques to see microcalcifications compared with mass lesions.

In a simple sense, the computer algorithms are searching for either clusters of bright spots (microcalcifications) or large white areas (masses). Just as a radiologist is taught by looking at many known examples of both normal and malignant cases, the programmers use large databases of biopsy-proven cases to develop new ways for the computer to examine the image. An important development of the analysis is to learn to recognize the known abnormalities while endeavoring not to point out normal structures or artifacts in the image (again, mimicking the process used by radiologists). Most algorithms work by assigning some sort of "probability" to a suspicious region. Then regions that have a probability higher than a certain threshold will make it to the final list.

Once the analysis has determined the locations to point out, this information must then be conveyed to the radiologist. The marked areas are viewed on the radiologist's monitors. The CAD marks can be displayed by simply depressing the CAD button. Figure 11-37 shows examples of screening mammograms with markers superimposed.

The cardinal rule with using this technology is that the radiologist is the person making the final interpretation of the mammogram. The radiologist is instructed to view the mammogram without the CAD results displayed to determine their own ROI and then activate the CAD results before making the final decision. This process allows the radiologist to act as his or her own "second reader."

Integration of CAD into a Clinical Environment

The CAD systems available today are designed as an aid to screening mammography; therefore, only standard views are processed. Integration of CAD into the digital environment is virtually seamless. The digitally acquired images are automatically routed through the CAD computer (Figure 11-38). The results are displayed at the radiologist's workstation.

Measuring the Performance of a CAD System

The heart of the CAD system is the quality of the algorithm and its accuracy. Considerable research has been done to develop and measure that aspect.[25,34–36]

Marker Accuracy

The output of a CAD system is markers at locations found by the algorithm to have suspicious features. To evaluate how well the CAD algorithm works, determine the accuracy of the markers—how often are the markers at locations known to be cancer and how frequently are noncancer locations marked. The two quantities used to capture this are (a) the sensitivity of the system and (b) the average number of marks per four-view case. The sensitivity is defined as the number of cancer cases correctly marked by the CAD system divided by the total number of cancer cases. The average number of marks per case is the total number of marks shown divided by the total number of cases. No CAD system has 100% sensitivity, underscoring the importance of having the radiologist read the cases carefully themselves (Figure 11-39).

Cases Used for the Evaluation

To be able to evaluate the performance numbers presented, it is important to know the types of cases used for the measurement. The cancer cases must be chosen in an unbiased way and must represent all types of cancer that would be encountered in a clinical setting. This allows the radiologist to evaluate how well the system will mark the abnormalities commonly seen in the clinic. Although one can measure the average number of marks per case for the cancer cases, it is more illustrative to use normal cases, because those cases are more typical of the cases seen in a screening environment (where typically 95% of the cases are read as normal).

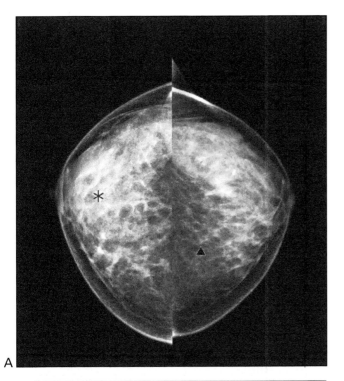

A

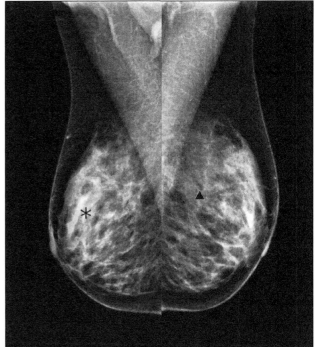

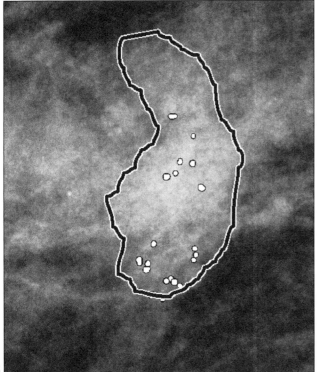

B

Figure 11-37
(A) CAD display of ROIs marked for review by the radiologist. The radiologist may agree with the computer that the finding is significant, or she/he can disagree with the computer's finding. **(B)** The radiologist can prompt the display unit to identify the *specific* areas the computer deemed significant. (Image courtesy of Hologic, Inc., and affiliates.)

Workflow

Integration of CAD into the workflow is straightforward. Digitally acquired images flow from the technologist's workstation through the CAD computer to the radiologist's monitor(s) for display of the results.

Clinical Studies with CAD

The introduction of CAD into the mammography facility depended on several technological advances happening together: improvements in the quality of mammograms, progress in image analysis techniques, advancements in

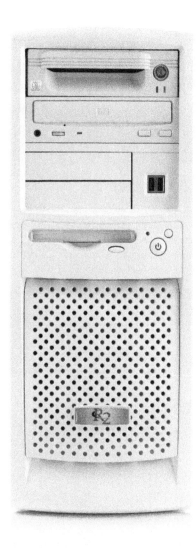

computers that allowed fast processing and lots of storage space, and enhancements in the quality of film digitizers. As these advances occurred, many research groups working on prototype components were publishing their results.

Many of the first studies documented the ability of CAD algorithms to correctly mark the location of known cancer on mammograms. As measured on a database of 1,083 consecutive biopsy-proven cancer cases, work from the first company to obtain FDA approval showed a sensitivity of 98% (399/406) for detecting microcalcifications and 86% (580/677) for masses while placing an average of 2 marks per four-film case. Other early studies[37,38] measured radiologists' performance reading mammograms with and without CAD; they showed improved sensitivity and specificity when they read cases with CAD in a controlled test setting. A multicenter study[30] not only measured the false-negative rate of screening mammography (number of mammograms called negative when they really showed signs of breast cancer) but measured the ability of a CAD system to correctly mark the missed cancers. The authors reported a false-negative rate of 21% and that the CAD system marked 77% of the missed cancers (Figure 11-40). All of these retrospective studies[34,35,39–45] demonstrate the potential of CAD to aid the radiologist with the task of finding those few cancers in the screening population.

However, an important step is to use CAD systems on a daily basis in screening facilities (prospective trials). One of the first prospective trials to investigate the feasibility of using CAD for screening mammography was started at the University of Chicago in April of 1995.[46] Another prospective study analyzed the effect of using a CAD system on the number of women recalled for additional views or workup.[30] The results showed that the radiologists did not recall more patients after the CAD system was installed compared with before installation. Commercial CAD

Figure 11-38
A digital CAD computer. (Image courtesy of Hologic, Inc., and affiliates.)

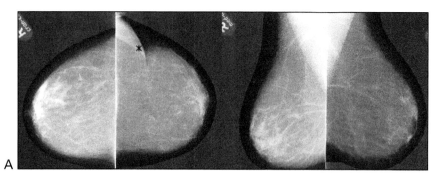
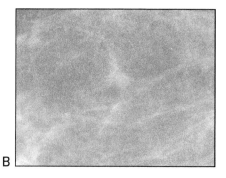

Figure 11-39
(A) Example of a cancer not marked by CAD. The one asterisk is on a skinfold on the LCC view. There is a small, low-contrast spiculated mass in the right breast upper outer quadrant that was not marked by the CAD system. **(B)** A digitally enhanced version of the RCC view of the mass. (Image courtesy of Hologic, Inc., and affiliates.)

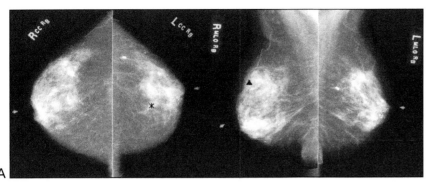
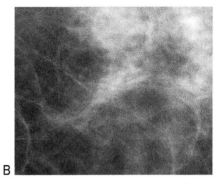

Figure 11-40
An example case drawn from the clinical studies on missed cancer. The mammogram shown was read as negative, with the cancer being detected on the subsequent screening mammogram 13 months later. **(A)** The CAD system marks the spiculated mass only on the LCC view. **(B)** A digitally enhanced version of the spiculated mass from the LCC view. (Image courtesy Hologic, Inc., and affiliates.)

systems, in use for two decades, have improved their algorithms and refined the resulting marks to make them easier to use, "more intuitive," for the radiologist.[47]

Future Directions

The evolution of CAD algorithms in the last few years has focused on a steady increase in sensitivity and an accompanying decrease in the number of marks per case. At some point, the accuracy of the computer algorithms may approach that of a radiologist, in which case the partnership will be redefined. Some future applications of more developed algorithms could be a flag to alert technologists to take extra views before the patient has left the facility, to show the radiologist enhanced or magnified views of the suspicious areas, and to use CAD as a "first screener" that would classify some mammograms as normal to allow radiologists to concentrate their efforts on the difficult mammograms.

Much of the research currently underway at academic institutions is to develop computer tools that help the radiologist not with the detection of abnormalities, but tools to help the radiologist distinguish benign versus malignant locations (interpretation). It will be the development of these tools that will move CAD into the realm of computer-aided diagnosis, redefining the role that computers play in finding breast cancer at its earliest stages.

Summary

A competent mammography technologist must have a thorough understanding and mastery of the relationship and interdependence between the mammography machine components, accessories, processing environment, and patient positioning techniques.

This chapter presented the following points:

- The ergonomic features that make mammography machines easier to operate
- The electromechanical features of mammography machines that are critical to producing a clinically useful image of the breast
- The basic considerations and the underlying physics of mammography that are important in selecting and using equipment to ensure that high-quality images are produced
- The entwined relationship between the mammography machine, the recording system, and the processing environment
- An introduction to CAD and its integration into a clinical environment with x-ray mammography machines

The trend in equipment design is to automate digital mammography with improved machines and useful peripheral equipment. However, producing a good clinical image is still based on the technologist's understanding of how the equipment produces a high-quality image. The objective of the professional technologist is to be in full control of all the factors that produce a high-quality image. A woman's life depends on it.

Review Questions

1. The mammography x-ray tube is "special" due to the focal spot size and target materials used. A brief explanation please.

2. The mammography grid is unique. Describe some of its attributes.

3. What is the difference between computer-aided detection versus computer-aided diagnosis? Which is used in mammography?

References

1. McKinney W. Sensitometry. The professional's test tool. *Radiol Technol.* 1996;67(6):477–478.

2. Hendrick RE. Quality assurance in mammography. *Radiol Clin North Am.* 1992;30(1):243–255.

3. Barnes D. Mammographers face crisis in QC. *Diagn Imaging.* 1991;13(12):73–78.

4. *Mammography-A User's Guide.* NCRP Report No. 85. Bethesda, MD: National Council on Radiation Protection and Measurements; 1986.

5. Recommended Specifications for New Mammography Equipment. Screen-Film Systems, Image Receptors, and Film Processors. ACR 1995.

6. Weigl W. A new high-frequency controlled x-ray generator system with multi-pulse wave shape. *I Radiol Eng.* 1983;1(1):7.

7. Gingold E, Wu X, Barnes G. Contrast and dose with Mo/Mo, Mo/Rh, Rh/Rh target-filter combinations in mammography. *Radiology.* 1995;195:639–644.

8. Tobin M, Bednarek D, Rudin S. Dependence of contrast and dose on variations in mammographic parameters. AAPM, 1995.

9. Kimme-Smith C, Wang J, DeBruhl N, et al. Mammograms obtained with rhodium vs. molybdenum anodes: contrast and dose differences. *Am J Roentgenol.* 1994;162:1313–1317.

10. Heidsieck R. Dual target (Molybdenum/Rhodium) x-ray tubes for mammographic applications: dose reduction with image quality equivalents to standard mammographic tubes. *Radiology.* 1991;181:311.

11. Kimme-Smith CM, Sayre JW, McCombs MM, et al. Breast calcification and mass detection with mammographic anode-filter combinations of molybdenum, tungsten, and rhodium. *Radiology.* 1997;203:679–683.

12. Jacobson D. *Mammographic dose and contrast as a function of anode and filter material.* Presented at AAPM July, 1994.

13. Stears JG, Gray JE, Frank ED, eds. Radiologic exchange. *Radiol Technol* 1990;61(3):221.

14. Feig S. Fundamental considerations in xeromammography and screen/film mammography. Syllabus for the Categorical Course on Mammography. *J Am Coll Radiol.* 1984.

15. Tabar L, Dean P. Optimum mammography technique. *Adm Radiol.* 1989;54–56.

16. *Diagnostic X-ray Imaging Task Group No. 7: Equipment Requirements and Quality Control for Mammography.* AAPM Report No.29. American Institute of Physics, 1990.

17. Ranallo FN. Physics of screen-film mammography. In: Peters ME, Voegeli DR, Scanlan KA, eds. *Handbook of Breast Imaging.* New York: Churchill Livingstone; 1989.

18. *The National Strategic Plan for the Early Detection and Control of Breast and Cervical Cancers.* U.S. Department of Health and Human Services, 1990.

19. Yaffe M. Recommended specifications for new mammography equipment: report of the ACR-CDC focus group on mammography equipment. *Radiology.* 1995;197:19–26.

20. Sterling S. Automatic exposure control: a primer. *Radiol Technol.* 1988;59(5):421.

21. Sickles EA. Dedicated equipment. Syllabus for the Categorical Course on Mammography. *J Am Coll Radiol.* 1984.

22. Logan WW, Norlund AW. Screen-film mammography technique: compression and other factors. In: Logan WW, Muntz EP, eds. *Reduced Dose Mammography.* New York: Masson; 1979.

23. ECRI: mammography machines. *Health Devices.* 1989; 18(1):41.

24. Sickles EA. Quality Assurance: how to audit your own mammography practice. *Radiol Clin North Am.* 1992;30: 265–275.

25. Ellis RL, Meade AA, Mathiason MA, et al. Evaluation of computer-aided detection systems in the detection of small invasive breast carcinoma. *Radiology.* 2007;245(1):88–94.

26. Bird RE, Wallace TW, Yankaskas BC. Analysis of cancers missed at screening mammography. *Radiology.* 1992;184: 613–617.

27. Harvey JA, Fajardo LL, Innis CA. Previous mammograms in patients with impalpable breast carcinoma: retrospective vs blinded interpretation. *Am J Roentgenol.* 1993;161: 1167–1172.

28. Beam C, Layde P, Sullivan D. Variability in the interpretation of screening mammograms by US radiologists–findings from a national sample. *Arch Intern Med.* 1996;156: 209–213.

29. Elmore J, Wells C, Lee C, et al. Variability in radiologists' interpretations of mammograms. *N Engl J Med.* 1994;331: 1493–1499.

30. Warren-Burhenne LJ, Wood SA, D'Orsi CJ, et al. Potential contribution of computer aided detection (CAD) to the sensitivity of screening mammography. *Radiology.* 2000;215: 554–562.

31. Antinnen I, Pamilo M, Soiva M, et al. Double reading of mammography screening films—one radiologist or two? *Clin Radiol.* 1993;48:414–421.

32. Thurfjell E, Lernevall K, Raube A. Benefit of independent double reading in a population-based mammography screening program. *Radiology.* 1994;191:241–244.

33. Taplin SH, Rutter CM, Elmore JG, et al. Accuracy of screening mammography using single versus independent double interpretation. *Am J Roentgenol.* 2000;174:1257–1262.

34. Ko JM, Nicholas MJ, Mendel JB, et al. Prospective assessment of computer –aided detection in interpretation of screening mammography. *Am J Roentgenol.* 2006;187(6):1483–1491.

35. Jiang Y, Nishikawa RM, Schmidt RA, et al. Potential of computer-aided diagnosis to reduce variability in radiologist's interpretations of mammograms depicting micro calcifications. *Radiology.* 2001;220:787–794.

36. Skaane P, Kshirsagar A, Stapleton S, et al. Effects of computer-aided detection on independent double-reading of paired screen-film and full-field digital screening mammograms. *Am J Roentgenol.* 2007;188:377–384.

37. Kegelmeyer WP, Pruneda JM, Bourland PD, et al. Computer-aided mammographic screening for spiculated lesions. *Radiology.* 1994;191:331–337.

38. Chan HP, Doi K, Vyborny CJ, et al. Improvement in radiologists' detection of clustered microcalcifications on mammograms: the potential of computer-aided diagnosis. *Invest Radiol.* 1990;25:1102–1110.

39. Taplin SH, Rutter CM, Lehman CD. Testing the effect of computer-assisted detection on interpretive performance in screening mammography. *Am J Roentgenol.* 2006;187(6): 1475–1482.

40. Freer TW, Ulissey MJ. Screening mammography with computer-aided detection: prospective study of 12,860 patients in a community breast center. *Radiology.* 2004;220: 781–786.

41. Birdwell RL, Bandodkar P, Ikeda DM. Computer-aided detection with screening mammography in a university hospital setting. *Radiology.* 2005;236:451–457.

42. Morton MJ, Whaley DH, Brandt KR, et al. Screening mammograms: interpretation with computer-aided detection—a prospective evaluation. *Radiology.* 2006;239:375–383.

43. Cupples TE, Cunningham JE, Reynolds JC. Impact of computer-aided detection in a regional screening mammography program. *Am J Roentgenol.* 2005;185:944–950.

44. Gilbert FJ, Astley SM, McGee MA, et al. Single reading with computer-aided detection and double reading of screening mammograms in the United Kingdom National Breast Screening Program. *Radiology.* 2006;241:47–53.

45. Dean JC, Ilvento CC. Improved cancer detection using computer-aided detection with diagnostic and screening mammography: prospective study of 104 cancers. *Am J Roentgenol.* 2006;187:20–28.

46. Nishikawa RM, Giger ML, Wolverton DE, et al. *Prospective Testing of a Clinical Mammography Workstation for CAD: Analysis of the First 10,000 Cases. Digital Mammography.* Dordrecht, Netherlands: Kluwer Academic Publishers; 1998.

47. Ikeda DM, Birdwell RL, OShaughnessy KF, et al. Computer-aided detection output on 172 subtle findings on normal mammograms previously obtained in women with breast cancer detected at follow-up screening mammography. *Radiology.* 2004;230:811–819.

Creating the Digital Image

12

Objectives

- List the key factors that made mammography the last x-ray procedure to convert to digital imaging.
- Explain the impact the ACRIN/DMIST study had on the acceptance of digital technology for mammography.
- Identify the components of a digital mammography system.
- Describe two methods of digital image production.
- Describe how a digital image is created and processed.
- Sequence the steps of image production and evaluation of the digital image.
- Explain the postprocessing features available to the radiologist at the reviewstation.
- Define the terminology for digital image creation, storage, transmission, and retrieval.

Key Terms

- algorithms
- American College of Radiology Imaging Network/Digital Mammographic Imaging Screening Trial (ACRIN/DMIST)
- bit depth
- detective quantum efficiency (DQE)
- digital array
- Digital Imaging and Communications in Medicine (DICOM)
- direct conversion
- dynamic range
- flat panel detector
- hospital information system (HIS)
- indirect conversion
- Integrating the Healthcare Enterprise (IHE)
- matrix
- modality worklist (MWL)
- modulation transfer function (MTF)
- noise
- Picture Archival Communication System (PACS)
- pixel
- postprocessing refinements
- radiology information system (RIS)
- signal-to-noise ratio (SNR)
- window center
- window width

INTRODUCTION

Mammography is usually one of the last imaging modalities to benefit from technological advances because of its special demands and unique requirements. It is a screening examination; few medical imaging modalities place an emphasis on screening the asymptomatic population. People do not voluntarily schedule themselves for an annual total body x-ray to see if a bone is fractured or if plaque is accumulating in a coronary artery. Only when symptoms are present do people seek medical relief and physicians to order the appropriate diagnostic imaging examination(s).

The mammography technologist, on the other hand, routinely images seemingly healthy women looking for early developing breast disease. It is this quest to find small breast cancer that makes us unique and requires that we wait until technology advances so that it can visualize the early development and subtle differences of abnormal changes in breast tissue. Mammography is very demanding, requiring sophisticated technology and skillful professionals who pay attention to detail.

General diagnostic x-ray procedures look for gross anatomical disruptions: broken bones that are out of alignment, 2-cm × 3-cm lung masses, blood clots that diminish the flow of blood. When digital imaging first appeared in the radiology department in the early 1980s, even though it was in its infancy, it could visualize these larger structures. Mammography had to wait patiently until the technology advanced to enable visualization of structures as small as a grain of sand (microcalcifications) or as faint as a low-density mass whose borders exhibit fine spiculation and is hidden within glandular tissue.

IN THE BEGINNING

The start of the new century began a spectacular shift from screen–film (analog) mammography to digital mammography. Hospital radiology departments and free-standing diagnostic imaging facilities were already well underway toward an all-digital interchange of diagnostic images and medical records in the rest of the x-ray disciplines: total paperless and filmless imaging. Beginning in January 2000, digital technology applied to mammography became the focus for medical equipment manufacturers, medical researchers, and clinical practitioners. Mammography finally joins the digital age. See Table 12-1.

An Odd Couple

At first glance, it appears unlikely that an agency concerned with warfare [Ballistic Missile Defense Organization (BMDO)] and a community concerned with healing would have a single feature in common.[1]

Table 12-1 • Digital Mammography Begins

DIGITAL MACHINE	FDA APPROVAL
GE 2000D	1/28/2000
Fischer SenoScan	9/25/2001
LoRad CCD	3/15/2002
Hologic Selenia	10/2/2002
GE Senograph DS	2/19/2004
Siemens Novation DR	8/20/2004
GE Essential	4/11/2006
Fuji CR	7/10/2006

The BMDO is committed to the development of innovative technologies for our national defense. Medical imaging is the fortunate recipient of advanced technology from many research and development (R&D) projects funded by BMDO; military defense technologies are nearly a decade ahead of medical technology. Technological advancements from the military have had a profound influence on the medical field:

- From the military's nuclear energy technologies, the medical imaging field benefited from the development of linear and particle accelerators for use in PET.
- Lasers, used in everything from tissue ablation to permanent hair removal, had their origin in military radar-related projects.
- From the missile defense program, where jet fighter pilots have just a few seconds to identify missiles or the shape of incoming planes, the radiology community now uses pattern recognition software to detect the shape of breast cancer: CAD, or computer-aided detection, evolved from MAD, missile-aided detection.
- Digital imaging benefited from silicon pixel development and from computer enhancement capabilities.
- Computed radiography's (CR) imaging plate technology was developed, in part, from a government contract to develop light-trapping materials that, when exposed to infrared light, give off an intensity that corresponds to the initial x-ray exposure.
- The CCD technology initially used in stereotactic machines and in LoRad's initial FDA submission for full-field digital mammography (FFDM) approval originally was developed by Thermotrex Corporation for the Strategic Defense Initiative.
- The "stitching" together of the 12 CCDs used in the full breast platform to yield a seamless image of the entire breast was technology developed by the National Aeronautical and Space Administration (NASA) for the panoramic images from the Voyager spacecraft.

During the 1960s, the heydays of the race to the moon, capital investment money flowed freely into the electronics and advanced technologies fields. Today, however, we live in a very different economic climate. With shrinking budgets for government R&D projects, those that are approved tend to be multipurpose projects with many potential uses for defense and for commercial venues.

In both military and medical terms, it is far better to recognize an event in its earliest stages than to cope with an all out conflict ... often, an abnormal cell differs from its normal counterpart in only the subtlest change of architecture or even one mismatch in the genetic code. By the time a collection of cells is sufficiently different from its background to enable detection, the cancer has often metastasized.[1]

Looking Forward to Digital Mammography

In 1991, the NCI convened a group of experts to review the current methods of breast cancer detection and to identify new and effective technologies. The workshop was called "Breast Imaging: State of the Art and Technologies of the Future." The attendees promoted formation of the National Digital Mammography Group. This focus group encouraged and made recommendations for funding research of digital mammography and related technologies. One of the stellar highlights promoted by this workshop was the seedling foundation of the **American College of Radiology Imaging Network/Digital Mammographic Imaging Screening Trial (ACRIN/DMIST)**. ACRIN/DMIST investigated the efficacy of digital versus analog imaging.

The first prototype digital mammography machine was introduced at the 1995 Radiological Society of North America (RSNA). The FDA approval process for digital mammography machines was slow and exacting. FDA considered these machines to be a significant risk device, thus the protracted approval process. Digital mammography units were considered a higher-risk device than general diagnostic x-ray digital equipment, which was accorded FDA approval in a routine process. The FDA did not want to find out, after granting approval, that digital machines in use for many years missed breast cancers during the screening process. So the FDA was rigorous in its scrutiny of this specialized application of digital technology. At a minimum, digital mammography had to be equivalent to screen–film mammography, the existing gold standard for breast cancer detection.

Early Comparisons of Analog Versus Digital Imaging

ACRIN/DMIST

The ACRIN/DMIST study involved a long time frame to complete its comparison of the effectiveness between analog and digital machines. In the interim, modest studies involving fledgling digital machines answered the burning question: Is digital better? One of the first clinical studies, published in 2002, reported that analog imaging found 33 cancers and missed 9; digital found 25 and missed 17; 18 cancers were found by both technologies.[2]

Digital mammography, even in its formative years, showed a statistically significant difference in recall rates: analog 14.9% and digital 11.8%.[2]

Although these initial studies comparing analog and digital techniques showed digital imaging as equivalent to analog imaging, digital sales were tepid at best. Digital equipment was 1.5 to 4 times more expensive than analog equipment. With the lower medical insurance reimbursement rates associated with mammography, most facilities delayed purchase of digital equipment until the September 2005 release of the preliminary ACRIN/DMIST results. These results showed digital surpassed analog imaging when imaging a glandular breast, and the results were equal when dealing with an adipose breast. By mid-2006, digital mammography equipment sales were "red hot"[3] (Table 12-2). Mammography facilities that had delayed purchase now had proof the new equipment was worth the additional expense.

ACRIN/DMIST was the impetus for digital equipment sales because it validated the benefits of digital imaging:

- Improved image quality, especially with the glandular breast
- Decreased radiation dose
- Increased productivity for mammography technologists
- Postprocessing enhancements of the image at the radiologist's reviewstation
- Faster and more efficient interventional procedures.

Table 12-2 • FFDM Moves into Mammography Facilities

	FFDM UNITS	# FACILITIES WITH FFDM
Jan 2004	451	345
Jan 2005	778	556
Jan 2006	1,160	832
Jan 2007	2,090	1,453
Jan 2008	3,945	2,627
Jan 2009	6,181	4,086
Jan 2010	7,755	5,246

Source: U.S. Food and Drug Administration. *MQSA National Statistics.* Silver Spring, MD: FDA; 2010. Available at: http://www.fda.gov/Radiation-EmittingProducts/MammographyQualityStandardsActandProgram/FacilityScorecard/ucm113858.htm

ACRIN/DMIST: American College of Radiology Imaging Network/ Digital Mammographic Imaging Screening Trial

ACRIN/DMIST was funded by a $26.3 million grant from NCI. Imaging began in September 2001 and continued through 2004. It involved 49,528 women who had an analog mammogram and a digital mammogram done the same day; 33 mammography facilities in the United States and Canada participated in the study, and all examinations were independently interpreted by two radiologists. ACRIN/DMIST answered the question—How does digital mammography compare with screen–film mammography, the accepted gold standard in breast cancer detection? The results:

Digital mammography is significantly better in imaging women who fit *any* of the following criteria[4]:

1. Under age 50; independent of breast tissue density
2. Women of any age with heterogeneously (very dense) or extremely dense breast tissue
3. Pre- or perimenopausal women of any age, or women who had their last menstrual period within 12 months of their mammogram

There is no apparent benefit of digital over analog imaging for women who fit *all* of the following three criteria[4]:

1. Over age 50
2. Those who do not have heterogeneously or dense breast tissue
3. Those no longer menstruating

Up to 28% more cancers were found with digital mammography than screen–film mammography in women age 50 and younger, pre- and perimenopausal women, and in women of any age who have radiographically dense breast tissue. The ACRIN/DMIST sensitivity results for women with dense breast tissue were 55% for analog imaging and 70% for digital imaging.

▮▮ THE DIGITAL IMAGE

Static Versus Dynamic Image

Photographs, drawings, and paintings are all static images; digital images are dynamic—an interactive image that can be explored in greater detail, seen in various lighting, stored in its original form, and modified to serve many purposes. It is this ability to manipulate the image that makes digital attractive, but the underlying true value of a digital image is that it can more accurately display a structure and its relationship to its surroundings. In medical imaging,

where physicians need to see a structure and understand the exact relationship or change in that structure from normal to abnormal, the dynamic manipulation of a digital image can be a gift of life for many women.

Digital Imaging Advantages

Health information typically moves at the pace of the receptionist at your doctor's office; fast-moving electrons flowing through wires win the race against paper reports. A radiology department with digital imaging services looks more like a business office than a medical office. Darkrooms have been replaced by computers; darkroom aides have been replaced by IT/Picture Archival Communication System (PACS) personnel; viewboxes have been replaced by computer monitors; and conversations about computers dominate. General diagnostic x-rays (i.e., chest x-rays, knees, and feet) have been digital for almost five decades; mammography was the last to go digital. The time finally arrived for mammography to benefit from the advantages of digital imaging.

1. *ACRIN/DMIST results.* This study was the definitive work to demonstrate digital's superior imaging of the glandular breast. ACRIN/DMIST was conducted with the early formulation of digital imaging; digital imaging technology has improved in the 20 years since the trial began.
2. *Dynamic range.* The dynamic range afforded by digital mammography (16,000:1) is far superior to analog imaging (100:1). The optical densities (ODs) displayed on film are limited to 100 shades of gray, not all of which can be displayed at any one time because the OD of the film is limited and fixed and is determined by the x-ray exposure technique. The digital image, on the other hand, is dynamic due to the computer's window/level attribute. Through the magic of the central processing unit (CPU), the radiologist can manipulate a digital image through 16,000 shades of white–gray–black. Because of a linear rather than sigmoidal response curve and the radiologist's postprocessing window/level feature, the toe section of the OD range can be thoroughly explored, one shade of gray at a time. With digital imaging, the electronic signal output is directly proportional to the transmitted x-ray intensity.
3. *Productivity.* Digital allows for four improvements to productivity.
   • First, for the technologist: by using digital equipment she can perform more mammograms per hour than she could with analog equipment. Darkroom and film processing chores are eliminated. The time saved is used to complete two to three more examinations per hour.
   • Second, interventional procedures are faster: primarily preoperative wire localizations and stereotactic

core biopsies. Compare and contrast the digital display of an image on the monitor within 10 seconds of the exposure, to the technologist leaving the room to process a film through a 90-second processor to see an image produced with an analog unit.

- A third and important boost in administrative productivity occurs because the digital image is transferred quickly and easily within the radiology department to the radiologist's monitors, to network connected sister sites, and within the hospital or the healthcare system if so desired. A click of the mouse and the electrons that comprise the digital image are on their way through a network. Film courier services, messengers, and mail delivery of analog images are replaced by digital technology just as e-mail messages have greatly reduced "snail mail" volume.

- Finally, the goal of sending medical information (images and associated reports) to many locations simultaneously is achieved with digital mammography. Images are available to radiologists and referring physicians for timely consultation; associated reports, from scheduling through billing, flow through hospital networks and web-based PACS systems for more efficient administration. The central theme is viewing images and medical records simultaneously at different locations.

4. *Efficiency.* There are at least three ways in which digital imaging improves efficiency.

- There are fewer radiologist requests for additional views with digital systems. The radiologist can manipulate the original image (resize, magnify, invert, make the image lighter or darker) to examine a region of interest (ROI) without destroying or losing the original image or the need to recall the patient for a diagnostic workup.

- A second efficiency is again the consequence of the postprocessing features available to the radiologist reading digital images. Fewer patients are recalled for repeat views because of underexposed or overexposed images. The ACRIN/DMIST study demonstrated a significant reduction in the patient recall rate using digital imaging.

- A third benefit is the ability to access images at any time. Digital images are stored in PACS. Images are viewed on computer monitors connected to the facility's network. If a referring physician is not connected to the network, perhaps the images could be viewed via the Internet. The digital examination can be downloaded to a CD. If none of these options is available, then an image can be printed on film and sent to the referring physician. Unlike film, where we make a copy of the original image and send the copy to a referring physician, all printed digital images are originals.

5. *Fewer employees.* With digital imaging, one technologist is now able to perform almost twice the number of screening mammograms per day compared with analog systems. Facilities can reduce the number of technologists; however, a word of caution: highly trained, skilled, and experienced mammography technologists are difficult to find and retain. Holding a technologist to a regimented routine to image one patient every 15 minutes 5 days a week for 50 weeks a year will result in "burnout" rather quickly, as dedicated as she may be. Other staffing also can be reduced. Support staff, darkroom personnel, couriers, and film librarians all go the way of the Pony Express because of digital technology's advancements. When the patient appears for her digital mammogram, PACS catalogs and stores the information.

6. *Added workspace.* After converting to digital mammography, facilities reclaim workspace formerly occupied by the darkroom, film library, and mammography rooms into increased space for office, storage, patient dressing rooms, or larger waiting rooms. Mammography machine manufacturers state that one digital mammography machine can replace 2.5 analog machines; theoretically, two digital units can replace five analog rooms.

7. *Technological improvements.* Digital technology offers advanced platforms in imaging; analog systems cannot. Digital breast tomosynthesis, contrast enhanced mammography, and 3D reconstruction all require digitally captured information; all have demonstrated some specialized applications in mammography. Other technological improvements are in the postprocessing functions. For example, digital mammography's dynamic range permits equal visualization from the skinline to the chestwall.

    Telemammography, sending images from one facility to another via satellite or high-speed transmission line, is possible with digitally encrypted images.

8. *Patients demand digital mammograms.* In the 5 years before the ACRIN/DMIST results were published, a total of 700 digital mammography machines were sold and operational in the United States. One year after the results were published, the number of digital units almost doubled; and doubled again the year after that. Reports of the ACRIN/DMIST study appeared in newspapers, on television, and in popular women's magazines. When women called a facility to schedule their mammography appointment, they asked if the facility had a digital unit. If the facility said no, they phoned a different center. Although most women didn't know the difference between analog and digital imaging, they were influenced by marketing campaigns and requested

a digital mammogram because they were told "it's a clearer picture." They wanted to be the beneficiary of this exciting new technology.

Every improvement, while it has advantages, also has some disadvantages.

Digital Imaging Disadvantages

Some disadvantages appear in the early stages of newer technologies and are transitory; these are considered part of the growing pains and soon disappear. These are largely resolved once the machines are operational and in the marketplace. Other disadvantages are more complex and difficult to resolve quickly, or they can be an unexpected event that requires immediate attention and fast resolution.[5,6]

Resolved Issues

1. *Cost effectiveness.* Initially all facilities had to replace their analog machines with digital machines, replace film libraries with PACS, install PACS monitors throughout the work area, and invest in broadband. This was expensive.
2. *Dual operation.* When facilities had multiple mammography machines, typically, they could not afford to replace all of their older analog technology machines with the more expensive new digital units. They operated using both and maintained darkrooms and film libraries that coexisted with PACS.

Ongoing Issues

3. *Increased operating cost.* Yearly service and maintenance contracts for digital mammography machines, radiologist reviewstations, and PACS made mammography services more costly to operate. Operating without service contracts is like not purchasing health insurance; one major "illness" can deplete a bank account.
4. *Spatial resolution.* This is perhaps an outmoded concept. We are accustomed to the 20 to 22 lp/mm resolution of screen–film mammography. A first and erroneous impression is that the 9 to 10 lp/mm of digital mammography is inadequate. It is, however, the contrast resolution and the dynamic range in digital imaging that makes digital imaging surpass the performance offered by analog systems. So what appears to be a negative is mitigated by digital imaging's strengths.
5. *Consolidation.* Movement toward digital mammography had an unwanted side effect. Digital mammography, with its higher equipment costs and required higher patient volume, could not be financially justified in many smaller and rural facilities. What were their alternatives? Some facilities were forced out of the mammography business, whereas others combined efforts and/or networked with regional hospitals and larger

imaging practices to continue offering mammography services. All consolidation options required patients to travel farther for a mammogram, wait longer for an appointment, or both.

6. *Increased time for radiologists.* It takes a radiologist longer to read a digital mammogram than to read an analog examination. The productivity of a radiologist was cut in half; the time required to interpret a digital mammogram is approximately 60% longer than reading an analog examination.[6–8]
7. *Image Receptor Support Device (IRSD).* The IRSD on the digital machine is one size. There are no interchangeable Buckys (18 cm × 24 cm and 24 cm × 30 cm) as with analog machines. The digital platform is permanently fixed to the x-ray C-arm. The digital mammography technologist uses the same size breast platform for imaging a 28AA or a 44DD breast. Imaging smaller breasts is more challenging.
8. *Digital image standardization.* Efforts to standardize digital imaging and integrate connections for digital imaging compatibility with equipment from different manufacturers continue. **Digital Imaging and Communications in Medicine (DICOM)** is the universal standard used to transfer images and data among PACS devices.[9] DICOM was created by the National Electrical Manufacturers Association (NEMA) to view and transmit digital medical images with the use of DICOM tags.

   DICOM Part 10 describes a file format for the distribution of images. This data is the foundation on the DICOM header of the digital image. Examples of DICOM tags:
   - (0008,0020) study date
   - (0010,0020) patient ID
   - (0020,0062) image laterality
   - (0054,0220) view code sequence
   - (0018,1114) estimated radiographic magnification factor

   There will always be display issues between the older and newer equipment. The **Integrating the Healthcare Enterprise (IHE)** mammography subcommittee is the group charged with improving connectivity issues. By creating the IHE Mammo Standard, a facility will be able to use multiple vendor equipment to produce, process, display, store, send, query, retrieve, and print images. Until all digital manufacturers adhere to this standard, the radiologist spends additional time clicking, dragging, and flipping images in order to read the examination. In addition, the current and prior images may be of different sizes (scaling), and the window/level settings are different.
9. *Monitor resolution.* The resolution on the 5-megapixel (MP) monitors radiologists use to read mammograms is much sharper than for those used in reading general

diagnostic x-ray examinations. However, the mammography monitors, good as they are, cannot display the same sharp pixel-by-pixel resolution captured by the digital array of the mammography machine. Monitors are the weakest link in the imaging chain.

End of the Road for Analog

Our past experience with technology is that with continued use it is either refined, applied to other endeavors, or replaced by even better technology. Photographs evolved from early tin types through paper–film photography to Polaroid to digital photography, music from magnetic coil rolls through reel-to-reel tapes to eight-track cassettes, while digital mp3 and iPods are the current rage. Most of this older technology is now resigned to dusty attics and flea markets; the classic best to museums and private collections.

Every technological advancement impacts the equipment used; its assigned space in the house, office, or factory; and storage associated with the technology. Computers hold the record for the fastest evolution; experienced computer users understand Moore's principle that every 18 months, there will be some significant improvement. From supercomputer to home PCs to laptops, from floppies to CDs to flash drives, and from KB experimental kits to off-the-shelf terabyte processors are but a few examples. This scenario of rapid development in technology is all around us; it influences our lives with new materials, robots, and new ways to live and work.

Early adopters of new technology immediately replace their older technology mammography machines with the new models. Some mammography facilities wait to replace their perfectly functional older machines until they can no longer be properly maintained and serviced, while others will wait for government regulations to place a sunset date on the old technology, just as they did in 2009 with analog TV broadcasting being phased out in favor of high-definition digital programming. Beginning in 2017, health insurance companies began a reduction in payment to mammography facilities that continue to use analog equipment as well as those who perform digital mammography using CR technology. Stay tuned.

▊▊ HOW IS AN IMAGE CREATED IN FFDM?

What Does Digital Mean?

Digital is a different and more precise way to display information using electric signals, such as voltage, to represent arithmetic numbers. For example, how *exact* should the

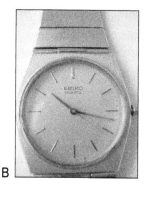

Figure 12-1
(A) Example of digital time. Time can be measured as precisely as one wishes. **(B)** Example of analog time measured in hours, minutes, and seconds.

measurement of time be? You can be casual: it's morning about 10 AM; or a bit more formal: it's 10:17 AM; or if the occasion (such as a sports race) calls for exact precision, you may present time to include a fraction of a fraction of a second as 10:17:21:36 (Figure 12-1).

Digital precision is also useful in determining measurements such as weight, temperature, and distance. Digital methods exist to measure the flow of liquids in pipes, assess temperatures for processing a wide range of manufactured goods (from baby food, to steel, and plastics), and detect the speed of cars on a highway, along with many more practical purposes that contribute to our lives. Inherent in all these digital applications is the use of numbers and the decimal system.

With analog mammography, creation of an image depended on a system converting x-rays into a light source, specialized film, and processing equipment to visualize structures within the breast. It was a meld of chemistry, physics, and mechanics that progressed wonderfully over the years, enabling clinicians to visualize structures as small and faint as microcalcifications and as subtle as distortion associated with a very small mass. It got the job done well enough to become the "gold standard" for all future development. Yet, further development and improvement in imaging only occurs with the ability to see smaller changes that occur earlier in the development of breast disease. Analog mammography machines, like the analog watch with a second hand, are not capable of displaying more refined measurements.

Four Basic Functions

The four basic functions in x-ray image production are as follows:

1. Acquisition
2. Processing
3. Display
4. Storage

With analog imaging, the *film* was common to all four functions; it followed a set production chain with few variables possible in each function. A latent image was captured on a film; that film was then taken into a darkroom where chemistry and the mechanics of rolling the film through a processor dropped the processed film out of the dryer section. Next, the film was placed on a viewbox for physician review and interpretation. And finally, the film was stored away in a medical film library. The design and use of film always involved making trade-offs because the film performed all four functions; optimization of one factor came at the expense of another. Changes to any function irretrievably impacted the image in the subsequent stages.

Digital mammography is filmless. Yet all four functions occur and produce the desired results as surely as a digital watch with no hands tells time (Figure 12-1). Digital imaging uncouples the four functions so each can be more exacting and expert and not be at the mercy of the other three functions. Digital imaging can push the limits of any function independently to get better results.

With digital imaging, a latent image is created in the digital array to visualize x-ray photons that passed through a breast. There is no film to handle, no specialized processing chamber to take this array to, and no extra equipment or chemicals that physically form, shape, or fashion an image we can see. Instead, we rely on fast-moving electrons invisible to the naked eye to acquire the shape and form of the structures within the breast as surely as those physical/anatomical structures are captured on x-ray film. So how does FFDM do this magic?

Fashioning an Invisible Cloak

After completing the x-ray exposure, we do not remove the exposed digital array from the C-arm of the mammography machine and carry it to the darkroom. Instead, the latent image in the digital array is processed by a different piece of equipment—the computer. After the computer processes the latent image, we do not hang the computer on the viewbox to look at the image; instead, we look on a computer monitor that displays the image. When we are finished viewing the image on the computer monitor, we do not place the monitor into a patient's x-ray jacket and send it to the monitor library for storage; instead, we send the digital image electrons to a different piece of equipment in the digital mammography system—the PACS archive center. At the core of digital mammography is the computer, a digital marvel in its own right that keeps everything in a common code so the digital images can be easily transferred from one part of the system to another; it maintains communications between the digital mammography machine, the computer, the viewing monitors, and then to PACS.

From the patient's perspective, the digital mammogram examination is virtually identical to the analog examination.

The room is the same, the machines look alike, positioning is the same, compression is the same, and x-rays are still used to create the images. The only difference she notices is that the technologist never leaves the room to process the films because the images now appear on a monitor in the room several seconds after the x-ray is taken.

The digital mammogram, from the technologist's viewpoint, is easier and faster than the analog examination with one notable exception—fixing an electronic mistake. One quickly learns to avoid misspelling the patient's name and to make certain the view is labeled correctly. These digital mistakes cannot be as easily fixed as in analog imaging with a paper label and pen. When a technologist is finished positioning the patient and dismisses her, in essence she has completed the digital examination. She does not walk to the reading room to hang films; the images are automatically routed to the monitor at the radiologist's reviewstation.

The digital mammogram, from the radiologist's perspective, has changed with definite advantages and disadvantages. Digital images are available within seconds, detailed and exquisite, particularly images of the glandular breast; however, review and interpretation require more time, especially when postprocessing enhancements of the digital images are necessary.[4–8,10,11]

What Exactly Is a Digital Image?

What exactly is a digital image? The short answer: electronic signals processed into assigned shades of gray. We understand the art of analog imaging because we have a film we can touch. We see the results of our work when a film drops out of the film processor, and we make judgments about how to further handle an underexposed or overexposed film. However, we are not able to hold a digital image in our hands so the digital imaging process is somewhat of a mystery. Filmless imaging is a major departure from the past, with significant benefits for medical imaging.

The relationship of radiation to the breast and its ability to pass photons through living tissue is the same for analog and digital mammography systems. The difference between the approaches begins with *how* the x-ray photons are collected, processed, displayed, and stored. The digital camera you take with you on vacation can collect, process, and display light passing though its optics (lenses). Digital mammography systems collect, process, and display x-ray photons without use of an optic system; yet the two digital imaging concepts are much the same. The digital mammography machine's computer converts signal strengths from x-rays that pass through the breast tissue into numbers; computers "like" numbers. The computer rapidly constructs an image based on the signal strength numbers, each with an assigned value for lightness or darkness.[12]

We Have an Image

X-rays that pass through the breast are collected, measured, and stored in the digital imaging system as an electronic "signal" as surely as light is collected, measured, and processed by chemicals to display light and dark shadows on a photographic film. Signal equates to measurable or detectable information and, in our case, is represented as voltage or current. The amount of voltage or current is assigned a numeric value. Computers and their software instructions, called **algorithms**, process the numbers into meaningful data.

The amount of voltage is what determines the shade of gray at each specific location. In digital mammography, more x-ray photons collected in an area on the detector produce a "high signal" and areas with few x-ray photons recorded produce "low signal" (Figure 12-2). More x-rays pass through adipose tissue in the breast; this area of the digital detector is struck by more x-ray photons (high signal). Glandular tissue attenuates many of the x-ray photons so fewer x-rays pass through the breast and strike the digital detector (low signal). Every place on the surface of the

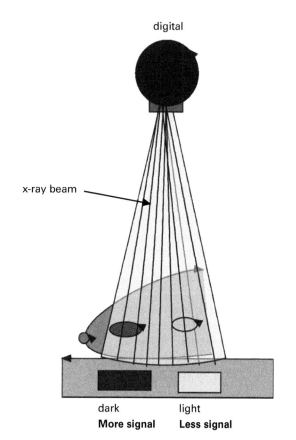

Figure 12-2
X-rays readily pass through adipose tissue and strike the digital detector, causing an increase in photons as measured by the pixels. This area of the image displays increased signal, which corresponds to darker shades of gray. Objects that attenuate x-ray photons result in lower signal, thus lighter shades of gray.[8,9]

digital detector, as small as the period at the end of this sentence, can receive a signal. Further, these small dot-like spaces (called **pixels**) are arranged in ordered rows and columns; there are millions of pixels in the array. Electronic wires connected to the array send a readout of how much radiation reached each specific location.[12,13]

Each pixel records shades of gray, depending on how many photons struck the pixel. The range of grays is quantified as bits. The number of bits (**bit depth**) represents the maximum number of pixel values, or shades of gray. Mammography flat panel digital detectors typically use 14 bits; 2^{14} = 16,384 shades of gray. The 16,384 shades of gray comprise the vast **dynamic range** of digital imaging (Figure 12-3).

Digital mammography images are displayed on high-resolution monitors. These are no ordinary general diagnostic x-ray monitors; they present extra fine detailed images for radiologists to display and interpret mammograms. MQSA recommends mammography monitors be 5-MP monitors as compared with the 2- to 3-MP PACS monitors used to display general diagnostic x-ray images, although it is permissible to interpret mammograms from the less resolute monitors.

While reviewing the digital image on the monitor, the radiologist has various **postprocessing refinements** (additional computer algorithms) that allow better visualization of structures in the breast.[12–14] These include window/leveling, zoom, and inverting an image.

When the radiologist completes a review of images on the high-resolution monitor, the images are stored in the facility's PACS system. A PACS network is a central server that acts as a database storing images from all digital modalities. A physician interpreting an examination can call up prior patient examinations from PACS and display these images on a high-resolution monitor; a referring physician with a standard computer monitor can access PACS to simply display images for reference. While the referring physician's monitor does not have the resolution of the radiologist's monitors, it is only the radiologist who is interpreting the examination and thus requires sharp resolution.[12,13,15]

How Do We Create a Digital Image?

Production of the digital image begins at the gantry of the mammography machine (Figure 12-4). The gantry is the C-arm structure that consists of the x-ray tube, collimator, faceshield, compression device, grid, and digital array. The x-rays that exit out of the bottom of the breast strike the digital array.

The digital array is either a direct detector or an indirect detector; but for preliminary discussion, both are treated as the same. A separate discussion of the two approaches and their differences appears later in this chapter.

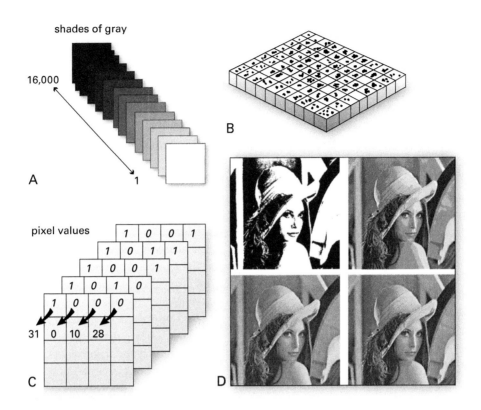

Figure 12-3
(A) The 16,000 shades of gray the digital array can detect. **(B)** The shade of gray for each pixel is determined by the number of photons that interact with the pixel. **(C)** Digital detectors are typically 14-bit registers, which means each pixel can record 2^{14} different shades of gray. **(D)** The number of bits in an image determines the number of gray levels. As the number of gray levels increases, more detail can be portrayed. Illustrated here is this effect for an image with 1, 3, 5, and 7 bits (2, 8, 32, and 128 gray levels). (**B** and **C** images courtesy of Dr. Don Jacobson, PhD., Medical College of Wisconsin.)

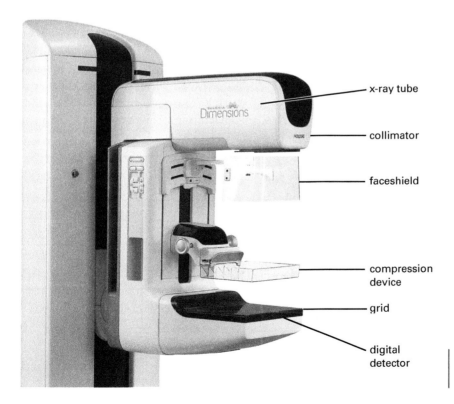

x-ray tube

collimator

faceshield

compression device

grid

digital detector

Figure 12-4
Production of the digital image begins at the gantry.

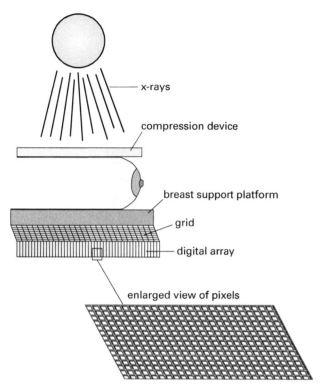

Figure 12-5
The digital array. Millions of individual pixels comprise the matrix of the digital detector.

The Digital Array

The x-ray photons that pass through the breast continue on to strike the **digital array**. The array is like a two-dimensional sheet of graph paper with thousands of columns and rows. Each small square within this graph is known as a pixel. There are 10 to 25 million pixels in a typical digital array; the collection of pixels is also called a **matrix**[12,13,15] (Figure 12-5).

Think of the digital array as a "waffle-like plate" with a series of tiny bins (pixels) in a grid pattern; each bin can store electrical charges. At the beginning of the x-ray exposure, all

Table 12-3 • Comparison of Imaging Modalities and Matrix Size

DIGITAL IMAGING MODALITY	MATRIX SIZE
Nuclear medicine	128 × 128
MRI	256 × 256
CT	512 × 512
CR	2,048 × 2,048
DR	2,048 × 2,048
Digital mammography	5,000 × 6,000

the bins are empty. When the x-ray exposure is terminated, each bin holds different amounts of x-ray photons (small electrical charges). Each pixel is assigned a numeric value based on the number of photons that were deposited in the pixel. This discrete value represents a brightness level (Figure 12-6).

There are several conflicting requirements for determining the optimal size of a pixel in digital mammography. Make the pixels too large and one cannot visualize the small structures necessary for diagnosis. Make them too small and they individually don't receive enough x-rays and are noisy; in addition, the file storage requirements become enormous.

Your family's digital camera is based on the same principle and has greatly improved picture detail and sharpness from the early 3-MP cameras to today's 20-MP cameras. More pixels translate into sharper images because more information about the image is available (Table 12-3). However, more pixels also means memory storage fills up faster. Millions of bits of information require more time to readout and display an image. A sufficiently large memory to accept data and readout the large amounts of information (detail) is a crucial element in all digital imaging endeavors, whether using your family camera or a digital mammography machine.

As pixels become smaller, the resolution increases (Figure 12-7); however, it becomes more difficult to manufacture the array. These newer arrays require more sophisticated manufacturing techniques at greater expense

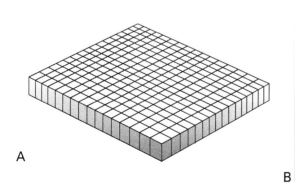

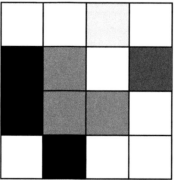

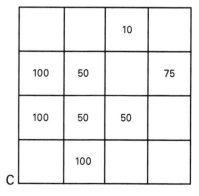

Figure 12-6
(A) Before the x-ray exposure, all the pixels are empty. **(B)** After the exposure, the pixels record the number of photons that interacted with each pixel. They display this as a shade of gray. **(C)** How the digital detector "sees" the number of photon interactions.

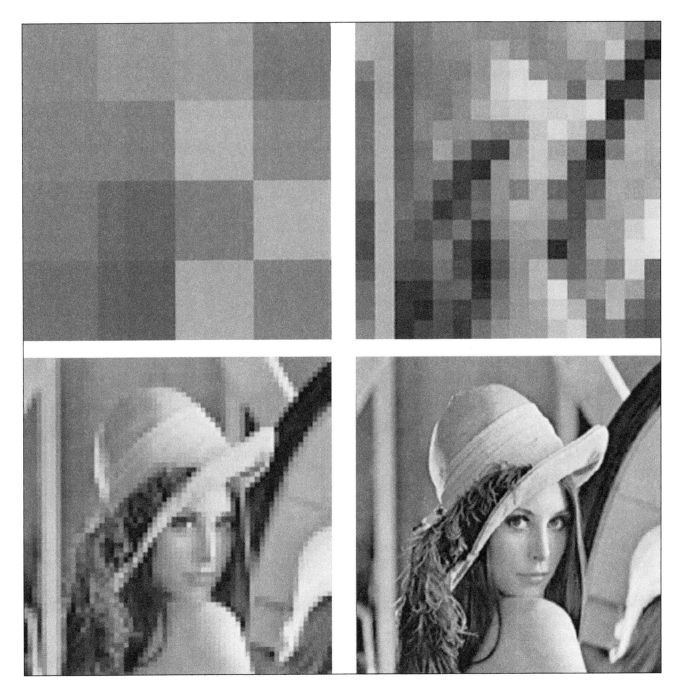

Figure 12-7
The number of pixels in an image determines the spatial resolution of an imaging system. This determines how fine a structure can be portrayed. Illustrated here is an image with 4, 16, 64, and 256 pixels in each direction. Note that as the number of pixels increases, finer details can be displayed.

to assure quality control. Continued improvements to digital imaging systems consider an optimal balance of: pixel size, resolution, manufacture cost, time to display an image created from millions of these smaller pixel size data bits, and the total amount of data these small pixels create that must now be stored in picture archive and communications systems (PACS).[16–18]

In digital mammography, the size of a lowly microcalcification determines the size of pixels in the array. Pixels must be smaller than the calcium in order to display them.

We visualize microcalcifications that are 0.1 to 0.2 mm, which is the equivalent of 0.004 to 0.008 in., the width of a human hair (Figure 12-8). It is humbling to consider that this basic requirement pushed digital imaging to its limits in order to perform digital mammography. As pixels are made smaller, fewer x-rays will strike each individual pixel; some pixels will not receive an adequate signal to include in the construction of the digital image. Without an adequate signal from these pixels, the image appears "noisy"—a visual kind of electronic static.[12,13,15]

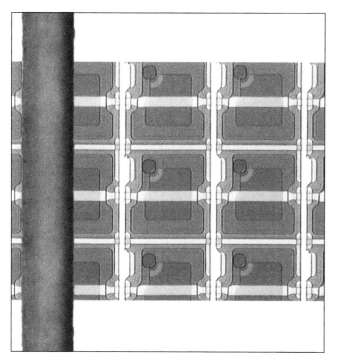

Figure 12-8
Compare the size of a human hair and a series of pixels. (Image courtesy of Hologic, Inc. and affiliates.)

A Mag-View of a Pixel

The millions of pixels each contain a transistor connected to a series of wires; this combination is called a thin-film transistor, or TFT.[19] When the digital array is struck by x-rays, the varying x-ray intensities are captured as very small electrical voltages that are stored in the transistors; each pixel registers a unique voltage (signal) (Figure 12-9). The readout electronics measure these voltages (signals). Reading each pixel empties the pixel of its charge.

The first step in this readout process is to identify which pixel is to be read. This is accomplished by electronically turning on and off a switch connected to that specific pixel. The voltage signal represents the number of x-ray photons absorbed by that pixel; the voltage signal per pixel is so small that it must be amplified so that it can be processed. The amplified signal passes into a circuit called "sample and hold." This circuit stores the voltages and measures the strength of the signal. The sample-and-hold circuit creates an analog signal; this analog signal must be converted into a digital signal in order to be processed by and stored in a computer.

Analog-to-digital converters (ADCs) convert the analog signal to a digital signal; they do this for each individual pixel. The greater the ADC signal, the more x-ray photons struck that individual pixel.[12,15]

The ADC sends the digital raw image to the technologist's workstation (acquisition workstation—AWS) where the computer applies image-correcting algorithms that visually enhance the appearance of the image on the monitor (Figure 12-10).

Preview Image Processing

Once the preview image arrives at the AWS, the computer automatically applies several image-correcting or image-enhancing software functions. These algorithms improve visualization of detail by correcting minor mechanical defects (such as dead pixels) and enhancing visual perception (e.g., window/level).

1. The digital array's matrix is composed of millions of pixels. Odds are very good that some of these pixels will not work, that is, they no longer readout the correct voltage signal in response to the number of x-ray photons that

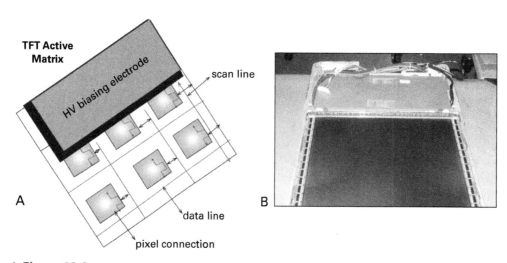

Figure 12-9
(A) An enlarged view of a TFT. Each pixel contains one TFT. **(B)** Wires located on three sides of the digital array readout the electric charge deposited in each pixel by interaction of x-ray photons with the pixel. Reading empties the pixel of signal. (Image courtesy of Hologic, Inc. and affiliates.)

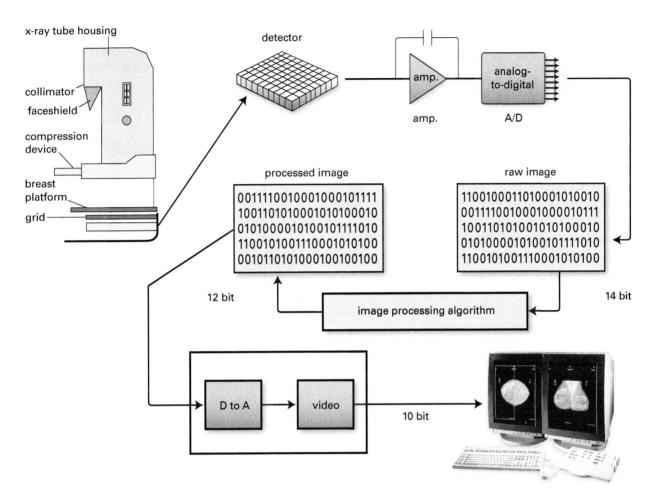

Figure 12-10
From acquisition to display of a digital image. (Courtesy of Dr. Don Jacobson, PhD., Medical College of Wisconsin.)

interacted with the pixel. These nonworking pixels are known as "dead pixels." The pixel is stuck in the "0" (open position) or in the "1" (closed position) so that it always reads the same voltage output regardless of the number of x-ray photons that struck it. Dead pixels appear as either a white or a black dot. The dead pixel is brought back to life by the service engineer. Service "maps" the location of this errant pixel from its exact location in the rows and columns of the matrix; this location is programmed into the AWS computer. On all subsequent exposures, the AWS computer applies a correction factor to each dead pixel. This correction factor is an averaging of the signal values from the dead pixel's neighboring pixels.

2. Another algorithm automatically applied to the preview image is a field of uniformity correction. The concept is if all the pixels were exposed to a uniform x-ray field, the voltage signal in all pixels would be equal. However, during the manufacturing process, not all of the pixels are created equal; that is, if neighboring pixels are exposed to the same number of x-ray photons, the voltage output will be similar but not identical. The field uniformity algorithm multiplies the signal from each

pixel by a correction value to compensate for pixel-to-pixel variations and render the image more uniform.

3. The digital array can record thousands of distinct pixel values, or shades of gray, while the computer monitor can display only 256 to 1,024 shades of gray at a time. Another automatic background image-processing algorithm contracts the 14 bit or 16,384 shades of gray into a more manageable range so that our eyes can distinguish structures in the breast. This algorithm reduces the data to 4,096 (12 bit) shades of gray for storage in PACS. This is further reduced to 8 to 10 bits (256 to 1,024 shades of gray), the number of gray tones suitable for computer monitor display. At first blush, it might seem that we are throwing away a lot of information, reducing each pixel's number of shades of gray from 16,000 to 256; however, the human eye cannot see more shades of gray so nothing perceptible is lost.

4. We can adjust the grayscale and brightness levels of the image on the monitor; this function is called windowing. The window postprocessing feature is one of the wonderful benefits of digital imaging; however, when the image is first displayed, the person viewing the image does not

want to spend time manipulating the image so that it is not too light or too dark. The computer optimizes the display of the image on the monitor so the technologist and radiologist will typically not have to apply window/leveling to their initial review of the image.

5. When the x-ray exposure terminates, the preview image appears on the technologist's monitor. Computer algorithms are applied to the image to optimize the display. In the digital world each radiologic examination, whether imaging a chest, a breast, or a bone, has a typical histogram stored in the computer for comparison. The computer uses a look-up table (LUT) for image processing; it compares your image to what it "should be." If your image is "off," the computer uses the LUT to correct density and contrast for display.[12,15]

6. Another algorithm, known as peripheral equalization, allows us to visualize from the skinline to the pectoral muscle. The overexposed subcutaneous adipose tissue plus the burned-out skinline are made brighter by the computer to match the appearance of the tissue in the center of the breast. At the same time, this algorithm darkens the area under the pectoral muscle so that it too matches the appearance of the tissue in the center of the breast[20,21] (Figure 12-11).

7. Lesion conspicuity algorithms enhance the contours and shapes of structures in the breast. This is accomplished by contrast and edge enhancement, by spatial and frequency filtering, and by suppressing electronic **noise**. Edge enhancement makes calcifications and spiculation more visible; however, there is a concomitant increase in noise. Smoothing makes large, low-contrast structures such as cysts, lymph nodes, and masses easier to perceive.[10,21]

Window/Level

The AWS is linked with the facility's information system, or network. The AWS has a hard drive that temporarily stores the image while long-term storage takes place in

PACS. PACS stores and distributes the images to workstations, printers, etc., via the network. PACS also supplies the **modality worklist (MWL)** to the AWS.

When the technologist accepts the images she just acquired, the images are automatically routed to various destinations electronically: for example, to PACS, CAD, and the radiologist's reviewstation. The primary duty of the radiologist is to review the images on a monitor. Part of this review process involves windowing: interactive processing of the image that adjusts the grayscale and brightness levels. Windowing involves **window width** and **window center**[12,15] (Figure 12-12).

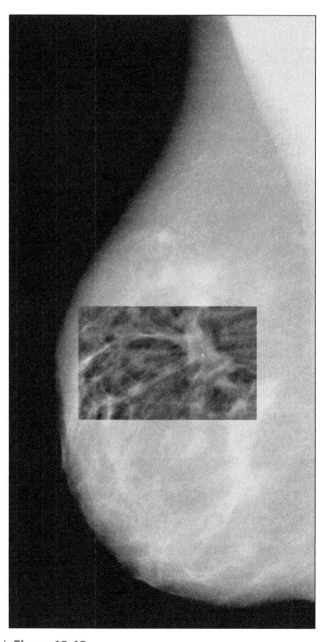

Figure 12-12
An example of image processing applied to an image. In this instance, a small region of the mammogram has been modified to enhance the contrast (conspicuity) of a cancer.

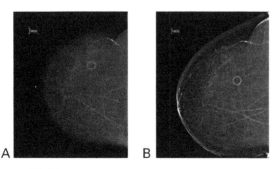

Figure 12-11
(A) This is the preview image that first appears after the x-ray exposure terminates. **(B)** Shortly thereafter the final image, with numerous algorithms applied to enhance the image, takes its place.

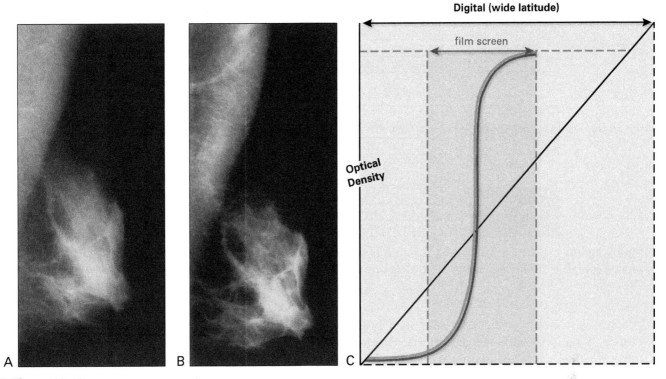

Figure 12-13
(A) A low-contrast image. **(B)** A high-contrast image. **(C)** Film–screen imaging produces high-contrast images; however, the narrow latitude captures only 100 shades of gray. The wider latitude offered by digital imaging provides us with high contrast, low contrast, and all levels in between.

1. *Window width* computer manipulation is like making contrast adjustments on your television set. This determines the range of pixel values displayed within the grayscale on the monitor. Since the monitor is capable of displaying only 256 shades of gray at a time while the image stored in PACS typically has 4,096 shades of gray, the radiologists could conceivably spend a great deal of time "windowing" if they wanted to visualize all 4,096 shades of gray.

   The computer displays only those pixels whose values fall inside the specified range of 256 shades of gray.

If the value in the pixel is lower than this range, the pixel will display black; if the value in the pixel is above the specified range, the pixel will display white. Increasing the window width results in a broader range of pixel values; this is less contrast. Decreasing the window width results in a narrow range of pixel values; this is high contrast (Figure 12-13).

2. *Window center* computer manipulation adjusts brightness. This function sets the center pixel value around which the window width is positioned (Figure 12-14). Increasing the window center results in a darker image;

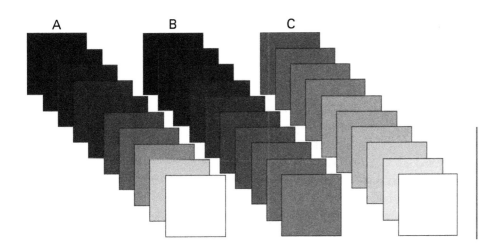

Figure 12-14
(A) The digital array captures 16,384 shades of gray. This is contracted to 4,096 shades in PACS. **(B)** By adjusting the window center to higher values, darker shades of gray display on the monitor. **(C)** Decreasing the window center results in lighter shades of gray.

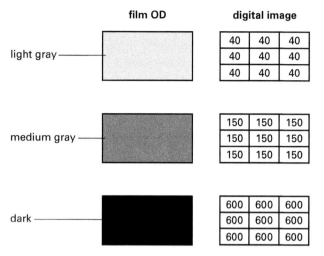

Figure 12-15
Varying optical densities of film versus how the digital system interprets optical densities.

decreasing the window center results in a brighter image. A high window center setting makes the image darker because more tissues with high image pixel values are within the displayed grayscale.

The pixel value determines the shade of gray displayed on the monitor; if the pixel was struck by many x-ray photons, the pixel displays a black image; white if struck by few photons; and shades of gray if an intermediate number of interactions (Figure 12-15). A typical digital mammography image stored in PACS contains 4,096 pixel values (2^{12} bits). This mammographic dynamic range far exceeds what our eyes can perceive, but by windowing the radiologist can manipulate the image to better visualize structures in the breast.

QUALITY OF THE IMAGE

Flat-fielding

The digital detector is composed of millions of pixels. If they were all struck by the same number of x-rays, some pixels would produce a larger signal, while others will produce a slightly lower signal. Accurate detection of signal intensity, the strength of the voltage striking each pixel, is crucial to producing quality images. Sensitivity of digital detectors to signal intensity can change over time; thus, digital systems require strict adherence to QC procedures. Generally, requirements include weekly updating of field uniformity of the array. This calibration procedure uses a uniform phantom to bring the system back to optimal settings. The quality of the digital image depends on maintaining the millions of pixels in the array so that they all respond equally to uniform radiation exposure.

The procedure called flat-fielding consists of two parts: (a) calibration and (b) correction. (a) The calibration component of flat-fielding is one of the QC tests a technologist performs. The technologist x-rays a uniform phantom, making multiple exposures. The computer averages the multiple images to determine the average response to x-rays for each pixel. This data is now used to correct all subsequent images. (b) The correction component of flat-fielding is done automatically as an image is acquired; the computer applies algorithm processing to smooth the appearance of the image. Because this variation in signal intensity (mottle) always occurs at the same place in the digital detector and with the same intensity, the corrections determined during the calibration step are performed to bring the pixels back to optimal efficiency.

A well-designed digital system balances contrast, spatial resolution, and dose efficiency; in digital terminology, these are determined by the dynamic range, **signal-to-noise ratio (SNR)**, contrast-to-noise ratio (CNR), small pixel size, **modulation transfer function (MTF)**, and **detective quantum efficiency (DQE)**. From a physics perspective, digital imaging is expected to improve clinical performance relative to film imaging due to the following:

1. A lower x-ray dose to the patient because the digital array is more efficient in detecting incident x-ray photons.
2. Better visualization of microcalcifications due to the superior dose performance for the smallest objects.
3. An improved display of breast structures from the nipple all the way to the densest chestwall region, resulting from the linear response throughout the vast dynamic range, and the ability of digital image processing to equalize image quality throughout the range of densities in a breast.

Factors that Affect Image Quality

The physics principles involved with applying radiation to the breast demonstrates analog and digital imaging have much in common. The advantage for digital mammography comes from the fundamental differences in how the x-ray energy that passes through the breast is collected, processed, displayed, and stored.

With analog mammography, the film assumes all four roles: image collection, image processing, image display, and image storage. Once a film is exposed, the quality and appearance of the image is determined. In contrast, digital mammography separates these four roles. Image collection is done by the digital image array. Image storage is handled by the facility's PACS. Image display is handled by the radiologist's computer reviewstation. Image processing: the digital image can be manipulated by the computer to optimize the signal at each pixel and for each region of the breast under review. This is facilitated by the wide dynamic range of digital detectors.[12,15]

Contrast is extremely important for both analog and digital imaging. Contrast is the ability to differentiate the x-ray attenuation coefficiencies for all breast structures and types of tissue; for example, adipose tissue is a dark shade of gray, while glandular tissue is a light shade of gray, Cooper's ligaments are white, and so on. In general, tumors appear white similarly to glandular components, and this is why cancer detection is so difficult in mammography. Contrast is essential so small differences in x-ray attenuation, or observed white in the mammogram, are visible and allow the detection of cancer among the clutter of normal breast tissue.

In analog imaging, contrast is primarily controlled by the x-ray tube target material and the kVp used; digital imaging uses image processing, which is essentially windowing the image differently. Digital imaging relies on wide dynamic range detectors to effectively perform this windowing throughout the range of breast tissue, allowing optimal visualization from adipose tissue to glandular tissue.[22]

Resolution is the ability to visualize very small structures. Analog imaging relies on the size of the focal spot and the line pairs of resolution offered by the screen–film recording media. Spatial resolution in digital is less than half as good as analog imaging, and yet comparison of phantom images between the two methods shows digital "sees" more clearly.[12,15,21] The ACR phantom minimum requirements for analog imaging are four fibers, three spec groups, and three masses. Yet digital imaging using the same phantom "sees" more fibers, spec groups, and masses. Clearly, there is something more to resolution than line pairs/mm.

Noise, in any form, is the #1 enemy of resolution; it obscures detail by making the image "grainy." Noise is signal that does *not* originate from the object; it is fluctuations in intensities. If you x-ray a homogenous phantom, you will see slight variations of density throughout the image. All x-ray images exhibit this noise or mottle. Sources of noise for analog imaging come from the light of the intensifying screen (line spread function), the film emulsion, the film processing cycle, and x-ray quanta. Digital imaging also has sources of noise—the primary cause being the x-ray quanta, with others including electronic noise in the digital array and imperfect QC calibration procedures or system drifts. In general, for the same amount of x-ray radiation striking the patient, the noise is lower in a digital image than in a film image. This is especially important for imaging the smallest objects and for the lowest contrast objects and manifests itself in the generally superior ACR phantom scores, for example. Even though film mammography can image more line pairs/mm than digital, in a real breast imaged with clinical x-ray doses, the noise of film is sufficiently higher than digital images. This difference gives digital imaging superior performance.

Evaluating the Digital Image

Different technologies require different measuring tools to evaluate the quality of an image. Digital imaging uses tools appropriate for evaluation of electronic signals: SNR, MTF, and DQE.[12,15,21,22]

1. SNR: Signal-to-Noise Ratio. SNR measures the quality of information in the image and is determined by the number of x-ray photons absorbed by the digital detector. Signal is the difference in intensity of two areas in the breast, for example, cancer and the adjacent normal issue. The digital imaging chain optimizes the image according to the SNR. Digital imaging utilizes higher kVp settings and tungsten target tubes to enrich the number of photons that exit the breast to strike the array, thus ensuring a higher SNR. The use of higher kVp and harder metal targets/filters results in lower contrast. However, the dynamic range of more than 16,000 shades of gray and the ability to manipulate the image to improve the contrast between structures and the background clearly offset the loss of contrast (Figure 12-16) (also refer to Figure 12-20).

2. MTF: Modulation Transfer Function. MTF evaluates the overall system resolution. It measures the signal transfer over a range of spatial frequencies. This evaluates how well the imaging system transfers shapes or

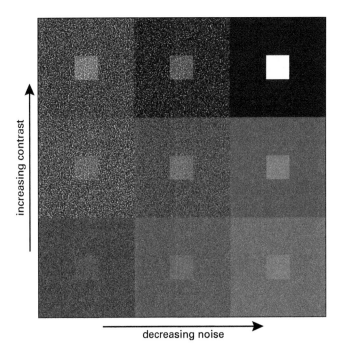

Figure 12-16
SNR and contrast. Although digital image contrast can be manipulated, this capability cannot overcome a high noise level. Nor can a low noise level compensate entirely for poor contrast performance. As a result, when viewed in isolation, neither parameter alone is enough to quantify digital image quality.

structures from the incident to the output x-ray pattern. The individual MTF of each subsystem in the imaging chain (e.g., pixel size, focal spot size, line spread function, magnification) is taken into account. MTF is measured under perfect laboratory conditions using a bar pattern with 100% contrast under noiseless conditions—not clinically relevant conditions. You can have a very high MTF value but yet not be able to visualize a lesion due to the pixilation of the image (Figure 12-17).

3. DQE: Detective Quantum Efficiency. DQE is a measure of the combined effects of noise and contrast expressed as a function of object detail; DQE also compares dose (Figure 12-18).

   An ideal image would have a DQE of 100%; this is visualization of all the line pairs of the physicist's line pair phantom. However, no system can image all the line pairs because of noise. DQE is the best method to measure detector performance of both contrast and

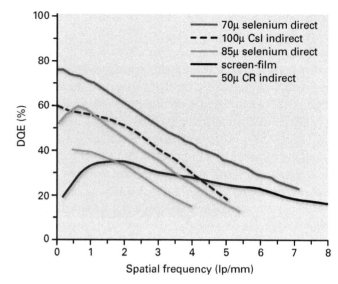

Figure 12-18
Dose efficiency as shown by the detective quantum efficiency for various types of imaging methods. (Image courtesy of Dr. Andrew Smith, Hologic, Bedford, MA.)

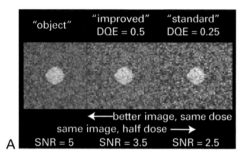

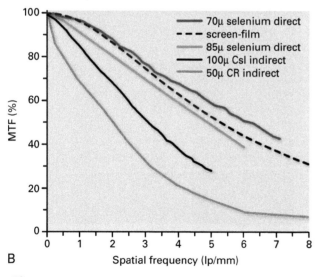

Figure 12-17
(A) The SNR = 2.5 image is too resolute in that each pixel is clearly identifiable; it is difficult to tell which are background pixels and which belong to the periphery of the mass. The SNR = 5 image is not as resolute but it is easier to identify the boundaries of the mass. **(B)** Resolution performance as shown by the modulation transfer function comparing various types of imaging methods. (Image courtesy of Dr. Andrew Smith, Hologic, Bedford, MA.)

noise. It measures the percent of x-rays that strike the detector and are absorbed. A quantum efficient system produces higher-quality images at a lower dose.

$$DQE = \frac{SNR^2 \text{ at Detector Output}}{SNR^2 \text{ at Detector Input}}$$

DQE relates to detectability of objects and is a great single measure for image quality. You control DQE by:

1. Increasing the number of x-rays that reach the detector
2. The efficient detection of x-rays by use of an efficient scintillator and high-pixel fill factor
3. An efficient coupling of scintillator and photodetector
4. Low electronic noise

Maximize the SNR to achieve a high DQE; increased signal and decreased noise provides greater visibility of small structures.

Case Study 12-1

Refer to Figure 12-16 and the text and respond to the following questions.

1. What is contrast?

2. What is noise?

3. In mammography why do we want high contrast and low noise?

◾◾ DIGITAL MAMMOGRAPHY DEPARTMENT

Parts of the Whole

The digital mammography department finally caught up with the other medical imaging services—using sophisticated systems to capture images and send and store those images and related information electronically (Figure 12-19).

1. Gantry—This is the section of the mammography machine that houses the x-ray tube, digital array, the breast positioning and compression mechanism, and paddles. Patients are most familiar with the gantry because this is where they are positioned and compressed.
2. AWS—Acquisition workstation. This is the computer and monitor interface between the gantry and the technologist.

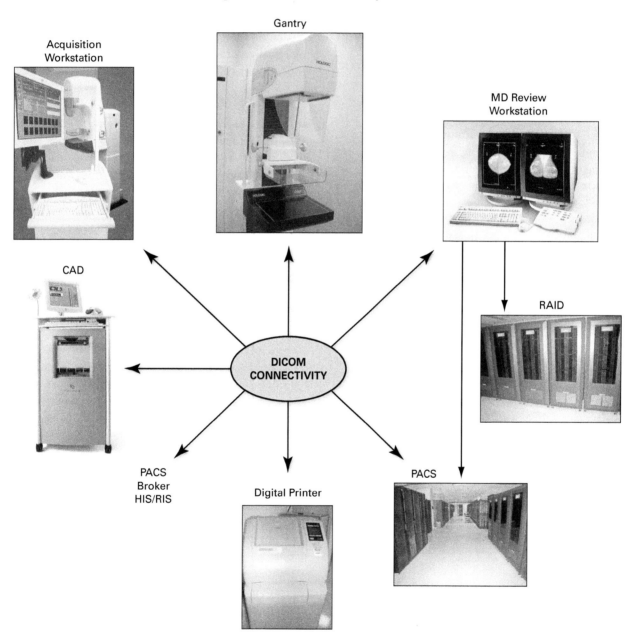

Image Archive & Connectivity

Acquisition Workstation

Gantry

MD Review Workstation

CAD

RAID

DICOM CONNECTIVITY

PACS Broker HIS/RIS

Digital Printer

PACS

Figure 12-19
Wilhelm Roentgen would be amazed if he visited a radiology department today. Everything familiar is gone: darkrooms replaced by a room full of computers, electronic image processors, and monitors; glass plates, chemicals, and film replaced by digital arrays; and cables that connect everything for instant image display.

Case Study 12-2

Refer to Figure 12-19 and the text and respond to the following questions.

1. Which component contains the digital array?

2. Which component(s) does the technologist utilize?

3. Where is PACS physically located?

4. Why do all the components interact with "DICOM connectivity"?

3. MDRS—Physician reviewstation. After the technologist acquires the digital image, the AWS computer sends the images to the output devices, one of which is the MDRS. The physician interprets the softcopy images at this workstation.

4. **PACS—Picture archival communication system.** A vast computer network for long-term storage of all digital images. An output destination.

5. CAD—Computer-aided detection. CAD is a "second reader" that assists the radiologist in detecting regions of interest in the image. This is a computer on the network containing software that analyzes digital mammograms and identifies areas of potential concern to avoid being overlooked by the radiologist. In facilities that use CAD, the computer is accessed as an output destination.

6. Printer—An output destination. Typical is a laser printer similar to the kind used to print CT and MRI examinations, with a mammography software upgrade. In November 2015, the FDA permits facilities that no longer print images to discontinue use and QC of this device.

Digital Mammography Room

The digital mammography room contains the gantry and AWS. This machine has a permanently mounted digital array. The array is one size and one size only; there is no exchange of Bucky sizes as in analog imaging. Even though the digital detector is only one size, systems utilize different size compression devices to match the breast size. Digital examinations do not take as long for the technologist to perform so more examinations can be done on the unit each day. Additionally, fewer repeat images are required, which again increases the productivity of the new machine.

Acquisition Workstation

The gantry and C-arm components of digital machines are similar from manufacturer to manufacturer so the technologist quickly feels comfortable positioning the patient using different manufacturer's machines. Learning computer commands at the technologist's console is usually the difficult part; technologists learn a new skill and vocabulary to operate a digital mammography machine.

Paperwork Be Gone

Well almost. An organized computer-based information system links the patient information between the mammography facility, radiology services, billing, and the required reporting to government and insurance agencies; it also facilitates appointment scheduling, delivery of the physician's report, delivery of radiographic images, and finally storage of all data in an information base. What took 59 steps to accomplish in the analog world requires just 9 steps with digital.[19] Learning the alphabet soup of computer networking systems involved can be somewhat disorienting. But with experience and practice DICOM, **hospital information system (HIS)**, **radiology information system (RIS)**, HL7, and others involved in coordinating the paperwork and images to flow smoothly, you'll appreciate the digital system.

The paperless process begins when the patient phones the mammography center to schedule her appointment. The centralized scheduler enters the woman's personal information into the computer; the language used by the computer is HL7 (health level seven). The computer operates using a RIS program or HIS: this is a database that stores, manipulates, and distributes patient data.

When the patient arrives at the mammography center, the receptionist selects the woman's name from the MWL, a list of patients scheduled for that day generated by RIS/HIS. Use of the MWL ensures the patient data are entered consistently and correctly from one year to the next. The technologist should always verify the spelling of the name, and that the appropriate procedure (screening, diagnostic, wire localization, etc.) was entered correctly by the receptionist at the time of registration *before pressing the x-ray button to begin the examination*. The "almost" from the section title refers to the avoidable hassle of having to fix incorrect data after the examination is started and incorrect information is accepted by the computer. This paperless system does not come with erasers or whiteout. So, with that cautionary note and a newly enforced discipline of reading carefully before acting, you will enjoy one of the benefits of digital mammography.

Before the examination begins, the technologist selects the woman's name from the MWL at the AWS. The technologist then positions the patient and compresses the breast the same way she did with the analog machine. The IRSD of the digital machine is one size, not two interchangeable sizes as with the analog machine. The complex electronics and expense to replace the digital platform, should it be "mishandled," necessitated design of the digital machine with a permanently mounted one-size IRSD.

The x-ray tube on the digital machine can be either molybdenum (Mo) and/or rhodium (Rh) or the digital machine may use tungsten (W). Digital detectors offer their best performance with harder beams, and that is responsible for the increasing popularity of Rh and especially W anodes (Figure 12-20). The technologist can phototime the digital examination, having the system select the appropriate target, filter, kVp, and mAs. The AEC electronics are capable of selecting the combination of exposure factors that yield the best dose versus the best quality image.

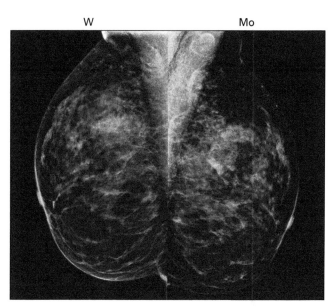

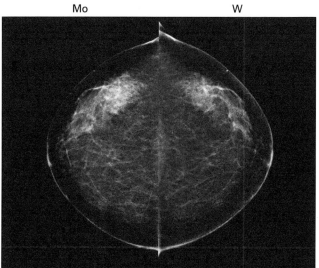

Figure 12-20
An example of tungsten (W) images versus molybdenum (Mo) images. (Image courtesy of Hologic, Inc. and affiliates.)

AEC: Phototiming the Image

We are familiar with the analog method of placing the photocell(s) under the glandular tissue to achieve the proper amount of OD darkening. The photosensors are located in the IRSD, beneath the Bucky and the cassette.

Phototiming with digital is different. With digital imaging, we cannot have photosensors located "under the cassette" because there is no cassette. One cannot position the photosensors under the electronic-rich digital array because the electronics would be in the way of the photons as they exit the breast and no signal would strike the photosensors.

Nor can the digital machine have a phototimer device on the top surface of the digital array. The exquisite imaging performance of the digital array would show the phototimer as an artifact superimposed in the breast.

How then does the digital phototimer work when it cannot be placed on top or under the array? The answer—the array itself acts as the photosensor. At the initiation of the exposure, a short (0.05 second or so) low-dose x-ray pulse is sent through the breast. The digital array is quickly sampled by the computer, which searches for the densest areas (Figure 12-21), and calculates the optimal final exposure techniques so as to generate a high-quality image. The main x-ray exposure then continues. This all happens automatically and efficiently behind the scenes with minimal technologist input.

In the digital world, we rarely have underexposed or overexposed images. This is partially because the automatic exposure control is very accurate and also because postprocessing with the window/level feature uses all the information about the photons captured in the detector array. Its wide dynamic range with over 16,000 shades of gray allows for accurate "reconstruction" of structures.

So, how do we ascertain whether or not we have an acceptable digital image since we cannot use the too light/too dark criteria used with film? The answer is the exposure number. Computers and digital imaging are all about making numbers do wonderful things for us.

S#, EI, DEI, REX, …

When the digital machine phototimer terminates the exposure, a number displays on the AWS monitor along with the image. This number should fall within an acceptable range, as stated by the equipment manufacturer. The acceptable range is a numerical index that indicates the exposure range, which ensures a diagnostic image is produced with an appropriate radiation dose.[12,15]

If the exposure number is too low, the image looks noisy because the signal to the matrix is not sufficient to overcome the noise inherent in the imaging process. If the

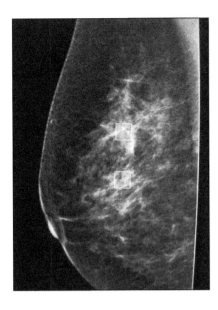
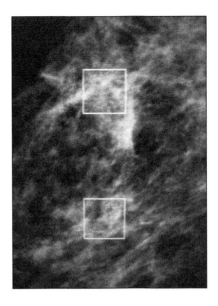

Figure 12-21
The two areas the AEC selected to calculate the final exposure technique.

exposure number is higher than the ideal range, the digital image looks good; however, the patient receives more radiation than required to produce the image. If the exposure number is significantly higher than the optimal range, the pixels are saturated; they receive so much signal that they cannot distinguish between different tissue types. It is possible, due to the window/level function, to produce an image that is technically "bad" and yet on the monitor looks good.

With most digital machines the AWS computer is programmed to automatically window/level the image to preordained (calculated) values so the technologist and radiologist do not have to perform this function. Other equipment manufacturers have the technologist establish the window/level display for each exposure to look good to them. Close monitoring of the QC tests that track the exposure number reliability/reproducibility are important to ensure the production of a good image with an acceptable dose.

Accept or Reject?

On termination of the x-ray exposure, the image displays on the AWS monitor in the mammography room (Figure 12-22).

The preview image appears approximately 10 seconds after the technologist releases the x-ray exposure button. The preview image is a partial readout of the signal that accumulated in the 25 million pixels; no image-correcting algorithms have been applied. The technologist immediately begins assessment of the preview image: is the positioning adequate? Radiographic landmarks visible? Skin wrinkles? Correct electronic view marker (e.g., RCC, LCC)?

Shortly after the preview image appears, the finished image takes its place. Now, the technologist examines the details: exposure number okay? Motion? Since the AWS

monitor is not the same resolution quality as the radiologist's monitors, the technologist may activate the full resolution box or enlarge the entire image to check for motion. If the technologist is performing diagnostic imaging of an ROI, she has many of the same postprocessing features on her AWS as are available to the radiologist.

If the technologist rejects the image, the computer prompts her to select a category for the reject reason. This feature makes the dreaded reject/repeat QC test at least tolerable. If she accepts the image, she continues on with the next projection. Should the technologist change her mind and choose to unreject a previously rejected image, a mechanism is in place to permit this. If, on the other hand, she changes her mind and wants to reject a previously accepted image, depending on the configuration setup of

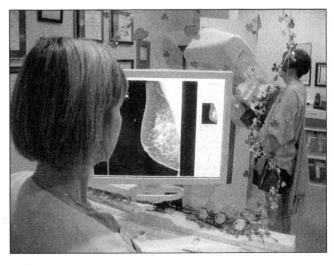

Figure 12-22
The technologist stays in the room for the entire digital examination since it is no longer necessary to leave to develop films in a darkroom.

the acceptance feature, this can be done quite easily or it can be a very time consuming activity.

Outputs

After accepting the image(s), the digital image is automatically routed to the predetermined outputs: PACS, CAD, RT workstation, MD reviewstation, and printer. If for whatever reason the images do not reach some of the selected destinations, the technologist is able to resend the images.[12,15,23]

PHYSICIAN REVIEWSTATION

Softcopy review of the digital mammogram images takes place at the radiologist's reviewstation (Figure 12-23). Generally, this consists of two 5-MP monitors on which to review the images, a 3-MP multimodality monitor on which to view breast ultrasound and/or MRI examinations, and a keypad for efficient postprocessing commands.[23] Mammography reviewstations are more comprehensively designed with advanced postprocessing features for faster review of mammography examinations.

The special high-resolution monitors can be a component of the digital imaging system designed by a mammography machine company, or they may be monitors manufactured by a PACS company. It is permissible to read from monitors even if they are not 5 MP; however, virtually, all radiologists use 5-MP monitors. The early cancers discovered today on screening mammograms are so small that use of lower-resolution monitors, while permissible, is foolhardy.

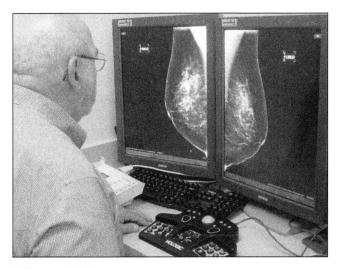

Figure 12-23
A radiologist at his reviewstation.

The digital reading room is dark. The suggested ambient room light for reading analog images is 50 lux or less, while digital is 20 lux or less. If a film viewbox is in the reading room, the digital monitors should be positioned at right angles to minimize the spectral reflection.

Previous Digital Examinations

When a facility has previous digital examinations to compare with the current digital examination, the previous cases must be retrieved from PACS storage. This retrieval process occurs in one of three ways:

1. *Manual*—An employee of the facility retrieves prior examinations from PACS before the patient's mammogram appointment. Previous examinations are now on the radiologist's reviewstation for comparison with the current examination.
2. *Prefetch*—This retrieval method requires a broker connected to the facility's HIS/RIS system. When the patient's mammogram appointment is entered into the computer, the study order triggers the retrieval of prior examinations; this usually occurs automatically in the middle of the night when PACS is not busy.
3. *Autofetch*—This automatic retrieval method is set into motion when the first image from the current examination arrives in PACS or at the radiologist's reviewstation. If multiple AWS and/or radiologist reviewstations are located at a facility, they need to "talk" to one another. A workflow manager (server) will direct the routing, auto- or prefetching, and the archiving of images.

Hanging Protocols

Digital mammography is flexible and responsive to radiologists' preferences when they review an examination. The various scenarios for constructing the hanging protocols in digital far exceed the options in analog. The following examples illustrate only a few hanging protocols from all the possible combinations available to radiologists (Figure 12-24).

A computer can be programmed to display images whichever way the radiologist wants to read them.[12,15,16] The actual choices are dependent on the mammography software provided by the equipment vendor. Dedicated digital imaging systems offer more sophisticated programs. A PACS vendor will generally have only basic reading functions; their mammography software is considered a works in progress for many companies trying to become all things for all systems. While PACS vendors are responsible for all imaging modalities, mammography

Dr. A

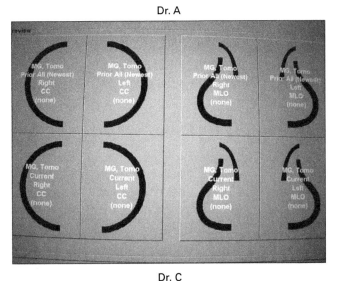

Dr. B

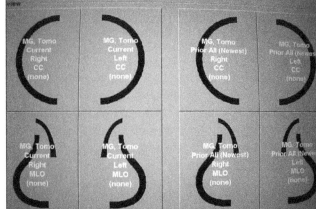

Dr. C

Dr. D

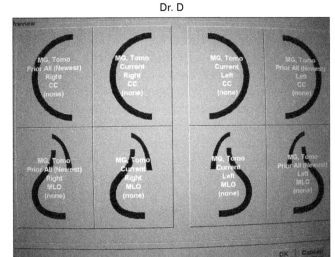

Figure 12-24
Examples of radiologist's hanging protocols.

equipment manufacturers specialize because they cater to only one modality.

Postprocessing Image Enhancements

A radiologist has many "tools" available for viewing and enhancing mammogram images. While all the tools are designed to improve visualization, not every tool is used by every radiologist; they have their favorites and specific conditions for applying them. A radiologist may spend little time using these tools to read the basic four-image screening examination of an adipose replaced breast. Yet may spend more time and use more postprocessing tools when reading diagnostic examinations or when dealing with a predominately glandular breast. It does take longer for a radiologist to read digital examinations than to read analog examinations; studies cite up to 60% longer.[11,23]

Paradoxically, it is the fantastic "tools" available to the radiologist for postprocessing an image that increases their workload.[6,7,10,12,15,16] Some of the tools include the following:

1. Window/level: the computer records, pixel by pixel, how much electronic signal was captured. Radiologists can manipulate this data very easily to view areas of the image as light or as dark as they wish and as high in contrast or low in contrast as they choose (Figure 12-25).

2. Full resolution box: a radiologist can activate the full resolution box and move it throughout the image (Figure 12-26). The image inside the box is the highest resolution display offered by the digital array. Use of the full resolution box should not be confused with a mag-view. A magnified view is created on the mammography machine using a small focal spot and a magnification imaging platform.

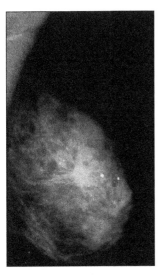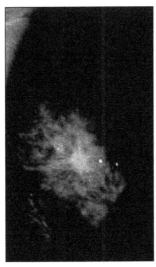

Figure 12-25
In analog imaging two separate x-ray exposures would be required to obtain these differing contrast and optical density images. Contrast and brightness levels are dynamic with digital imaging. Only one x-ray exposure was required; computer manipulation supplies the rest. (Image courtesy of GE Healthcare. Milwaukee, WI.)

3. Zoom: the entire image displays in full resolution. The breast cannot be zoomed and displayed in its entirety since the image is too large to fit on the monitor; the radiologist pans the image (moves superior–inferior, anterior–posterior) until it has been viewed in its entirety (Figure 12-27).
4. Inversion: what is white on the image now shows up black, and what was black is now white (Figure 12-28). The technique is especially useful when looking for calcifications.
5. Measurement: calipers opened on an area are dragged across the image and closed. The distance between the two points displays in millimeters (mm) (Figure 12-29).
6. Rotation: useful for making back-to-back comparisons of images (Figure 12-30).
7. CAD: toggle a keypad button to display the CAD marks (Figure 12-31).

Case Study **12-3**

Refer to Figure 12-25 and the text and respond to the following questions.

1. If these are analog films, what is the difference between them, and how was this accomplished?

2. If these are digital images, what is the difference between them, and how was this accomplished?

3. What other digital postprocessing tools are available to the radiologist?

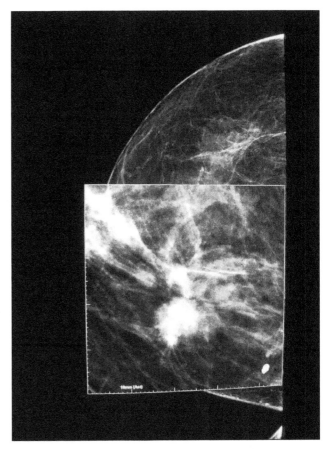

Figure 12-26
The portion of the breast inside the box displays at full resolution. The full resolution box can be positioned anywhere on the image.

It is possible to activate multiple postprocessing features at the same time.[12,15,21,22,24] For example, you can zoom, invert, and window/level all at the same time. The postprocessing features are conveniently located on a keypad for the radiologist (Figure 12-32). This keeps the functions confined to a space-saving location to minimize moving a mouse across a mouse pad. Use of the keypad facilitates the interpretation process for the radiologist.

Electronic Wax Pencil

When radiologists read analog images, they marked an ROI on the film using a China marker or wax pencil. In the digital world, the radiologist marks with an electronic wax pencil (Figure 12-33).

After placing a mark around the ROI, a radiologist may/may not attach an electronic message (annotation). A radiologist may elect to save the markings and annotations in PACS, which can be useful when sending images to the referring physician. Saving markings and annotations depends on the capabilities of the PACS system; some may or may not support this function. Some PACS systems can support GSPS (grayscale presentation state).

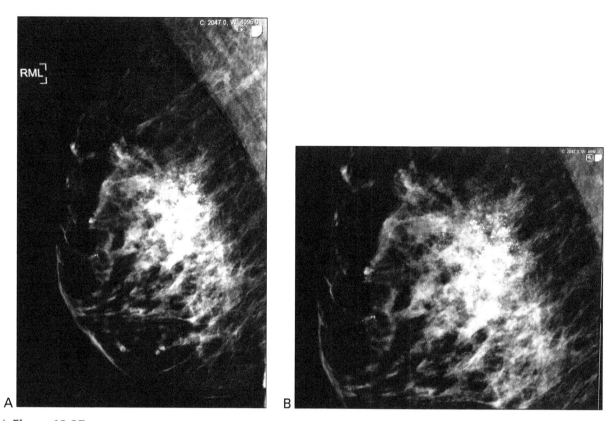

Figure 12-27
(A) Decreased resolution is required to visualize the entire breast on a monitor. **(B)** One step in the radiologist's hanging protocol displays the image at full resolution, where the breast is now larger than the monitor. In order to inspect the breast, the radiologist must move the zoomed image on the monitor.

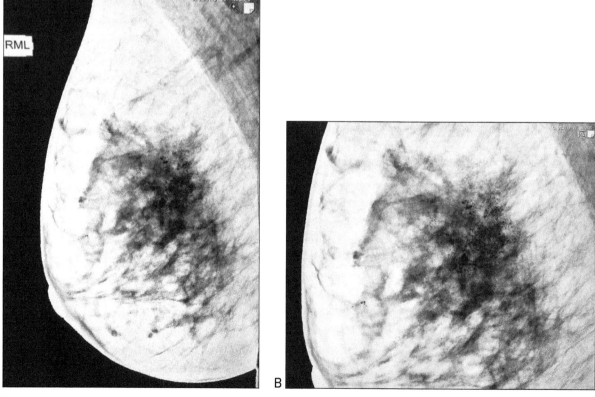

Figure 12-28
Inversion. **(A)** What was black is now white, and what was white is now black. **(B)** Inversion plus zoom. This technique is especially valuable in visualizing calcifications.

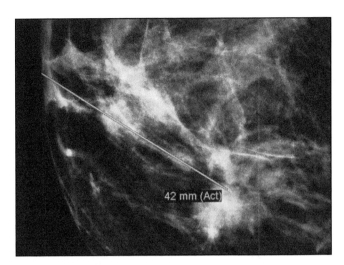

Figure 12-29
Example of an electronic ruler.

With GSPS, the markings are stored in PACS as an overlay. If the PACS system cannot support GSPS, then the markings may be saved as secondary capture (SC). With SC, the markings are saved by creating a copy of the image with the marks attached. The result: if you took four images and the radiologist made a mark on one of them, there will now be five images stored in PACS. The SC image has less resolution than the GSPS because it is an electronic copy, but it serves the purpose to identify the location of a marking.

The Weakest Link

The weakest link in analog imaging was human eyesight; in digital imaging, it is the radiologist's monitors. The monitors can only display a fraction of the information captured by the digital array; in fact, the digital image resolution must be reduced to display on the monitor.[12,15,25]

The typical home PC computer monitor has approximately 1,000 × 1,000 pixels; the 5-MP mammography monitors are 2,000 × 2,500 pixels for a total of 5 million pixels; yet the digital array totals nearly 25 million pixels. Use of the full resolution box or the zoom postprocessing enhancement brings us closer to the individual pixel display resolution; however, with this expansion of the image, the breast is now too large to display on the monitor. The radiologist must move the image superior–inferior–anterior and posterior to inspect all of the breast tissue, one section at a time (Figure 12-27). This movement adds time to the evaluation process.

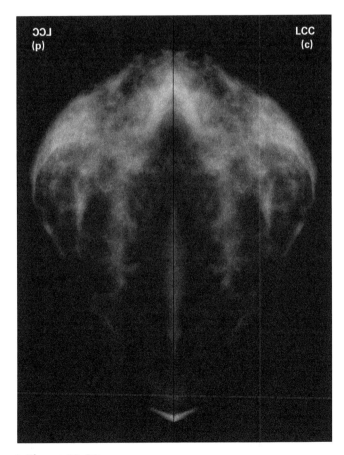
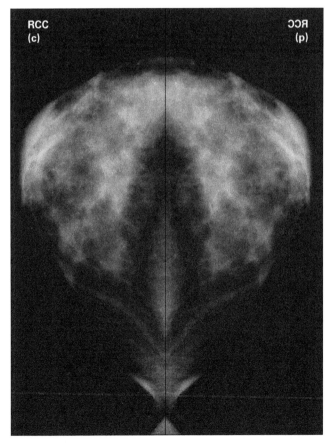

Figure 12-30
Radiologists often compare current (c) and prior (p) images oriented back-to-back to evaluate symmetry/asymmetry.

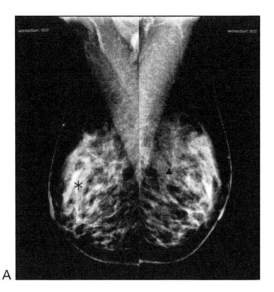
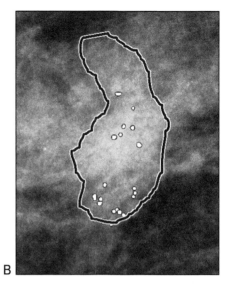

Figure 12-31
(A) CAD indicates a ROI to the radiologist by placing symbols on the image. **(B)** The monitor refines the display to depict the specific structures the computer deemed significant. (Images courtesy of Hologic, Inc. and affiliates.)

When digital mammography first became commercially available, the monitors were of the cathode ray tube (CRT) vintage, much like our old home TV sets. Large glass vacuum tubes were coated with a phosphor that gave off light when electrons struck the tube. Its strong suit was that black is the darkest black. CRT tubes quickly gave way to the liquid crystal display (LCD) technology used today in laptop computers and flat screen TVs. The strength of the LCD technology is that its light source is placed behind the LCD and displays the entire color range of white. Mammographers are interested in "white" (Figure 12-34).

PRODUCING THE DIGITAL IMAGE: VARIATIONS ON THE THEME

Direct and Indirect Conversion

There are several methods for producing digital images[26] (Table 12-4). They can be most clearly characterized in terms of *how* the electronic image is generated: direct-to-digital imaging and nondirect imaging. Direct-to-digital systems automatically generate signal and send the image to the controlling computer. In nondirect, the

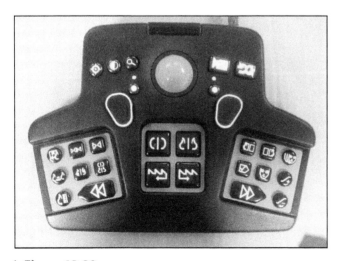

Figure 12-32
The keypad contains the most frequently used postprocessing tools and functions available to the radiologist.

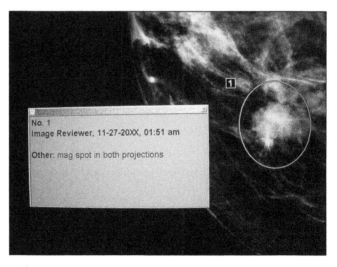

Figure 12-33
An electronic wax pencil mark with accompanying annotation for the technologist.

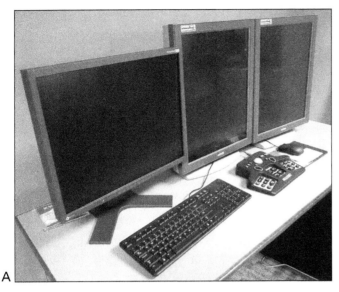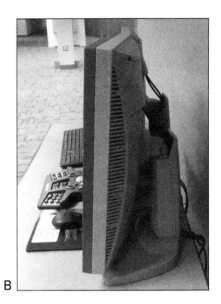

Figure 12-34
(A) An example of LCD monitors. **(B)** Profile of an LCD monitor.

technologist must intervene. CR is an example of nondirect. The technologist must remove the exposed CR plate and transport it to an image plate reader in order to generate the image.

The direct-to-digital systems have two conversion methods: (1) indirect and (2) direct conversion. Each has advantages and disadvantages.

1. **Indirect conversion** methods are similar in behavior to screen–film imaging: x-rays produce light to form a light image, which is then detected by some sort of light-sensitive system. Film was the first method using indirect conversion, but of course, this is not digital technology. The indirect digital conversion methods are CR mammography and a system that uses cesium iodide (CsI).
2. There is only one type of **direct conversion** digital imaging. With this method, x-rays directly produce the image. Amorphous selenium (a-Se) detectors are used in direct conversion systems.

CR mammography is being phased out of use in the United States. In 2017, health insurance companies began reducing payment schedules to facilities that use this digital technology. CR mammography is no longer included in this edition of the textbook.

Table 12-4 • Digital Imaging Methods

DIRECT TO DIGITAL	NONDIRECT DIGITAL
Indirect conversion (CsI)	Indirect conversion (CR)
Direct conversion (a-Se)	

Direct-to-Digital Detectors

Flat Panel Detectors

Flat panel detectors refer to detectors that are built as large assemblies that automatically generate images when exposed to x-rays. As we learned, these can use either direct or indirect conversion methods of absorbing the radiation.

Both direct and indirect flat panel detectors are used in FFDM. The indirect method, similar to capturing a screen–film image, is a two-step process: (a) convert the x-rays to light and (b) record the light on the digital array. The direct method uses a single step process: x-rays are (directly) converted into an image. No intermediary step is involved.

Indirect Flat Panel Conversion Detector

The indirect flat panel detector produces an image in much the same manner as screen–film imaging (Figure 12-35). The x-ray photons that pass through the breast strike the scintillator material, which is made of cesium iodide. The scintillator material converts x-rays into light. The light is detected by photodiodes and converted into electrons. The electrons form the digital image. As with screen–film imaging, it is the diffusion of light in the scintillator that results in a less resolute image (blur).

The Indirect Imaging Process

The scintillator is composed of cesium iodide (CsI); it is a phosphor screen, similar in function to the intensifying screen in the screen–film cassette. The CsI screen emits light when struck by x-ray photons. The CsI material then channels the light to a layer of photodiodes that converts

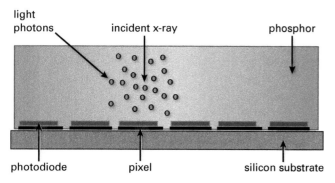

Figure 12-35
Indirect conversion detectors work by absorbing x-rays, which give off light scintillations that are detected by photodiodes. (Image courtesy of Dr. Andrew Smith, Hologic, Bedford, MA.)

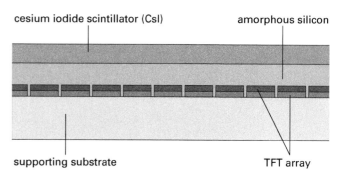

Figure 12-36
Top layer: CsI scintillator. Middle layer: amorphous silicon. Bottom layer: TFT array.

light into electrical signals. The photodiodes are mounted on a substrate of amorphous silicon (a-Si) that houses the array of electronic switches and signal lines that sit atop the pixels. Each light-sensitive diode element is connected by TFTs to a control and a data line. This results in a collection of digital data that describes precisely the x-ray intensity that strikes each pixel (Figure 12-36).

A close bonding process intimately joins the CsI scintillator material and the a-Si photodetector to reduce the loss of light as it is transferred from one layer to the other. If you make the CsI layer thinner to reduce the light spread, the thinness now adversely affects the absorption quantum efficiency. The CsI crystals are grown as needle-like columnar structures to channel the light to the photodiode surface. This columnar structure is conducive to minimizing the loss of light during the transfer process; however, there is still some degree of light spread that degrades the resolution. Light diffusion is a source of less resolution as up to 3 pixels away from the source (about 50 pixels in all) receive signal from one incoming x-ray.

Indirect Conversion Resolution

The resolution of the indirect detector is 100 μm (0.1 mm). This is the distance between two transistors. If the pixels were made smaller, would this improve the spatial resolution? The inherent resolution of this digital system is determined by light spread, not by pixel size; therefore, making pixels smaller will not make the image sharper.

Another factor that causes reduced resolution is the location of the portion of the digital array that actually "captures" the image. In screen–film imaging, the film is placed at the top surface of the intensifying screen. The film is in intimate contact with the intensifying screen, and it responds to the light emitted by the screen. The TFT array, where the digital image is captured, is at the bottom of the digital array and is not in contact with the scintillator layer. The light from the scintillator is channeled down to the TFTs; light spread occurs during the "channeling," thus a reduction in spatial resolution (Figure 12-37).

If the scintillator were made thinner to reduce the distance the light diffuses, thus creating a sharper image, the array would become less efficient in absorbing x-ray photons and the SNR would suffer.

Direct Flat Panel Conversion Detector

The direct flat panel detector produces an image in much the same manner as xeromammography did. The x-ray photons that pass through the breast strike the photoconductor, which is made of amorphous selenium (a-Se) (Figure 12-38). This interaction produces an electrostatic

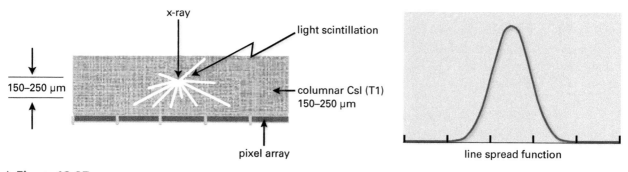

Figure 12-37
Indirect conversion detectors utilize a scintillating layer to absorb the x-ray and generate light photons, which are detected by a photodiode array. (Image courtesy of Dr. Andrew Smith, Hologic, Bedford, MA.)

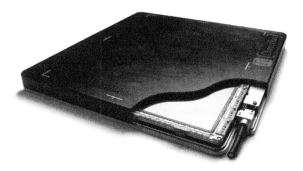

Figure 12-38
The direct detector is made of amorphous selenium. This converts x-rays directly into an electrical charge. (Image courtesy of Hologic, Inc. and affiliates.)

image with high spatial resolution. The flat panel plate is uniformly charged. The x-ray exposure causes the plate to discharge, with the degree of discharge proportional to the amount of radiation striking the plate.

The Direct Imaging Process

X-rays strike the amorphous selenium photoconductor surface; electron-hole pairs (+ and − ions) are created by knocking electrons off the selenium atoms. A high-voltage electric field is applied across the selenium layer; positive and negative electrodes are placed on the upper and lower surfaces, and an electric field is applied. This voltage differential propels the electrons in one direction and electron holes in the other. Ions travel in a straight line to the TFTs because of the voltage differential; lateral light spread is minimal, on the order of 1 μm. Therefore, the spatial resolution is not affected (Figure 12-39).

Direct Conversion Resolution

a-Se is ideal for use in mammography; it is a very good detector of x-rays in the mammographic energy range. Selenium was used in the 1970s to 1980s with xeromammography so the manufacturing process is well understood. It has high x-ray absorption efficiency with excellent intrinsic resolution. The x-ray absorption capability (quantum efficiency) of the direct process is 95%; analog imaging is 50% to 70%; and CsI scintillators are 50% to 80% (Figure 12-40).

The a-Se photoconductor layer can be made thicker to absorb more x-rays, thus making data collection more efficient. With a thickness of 250 μm, this detector stops 95% of the incident x-rays. If this layer is made thicker, it does not create increased light blur, as it would with the indirect method.

Direct detectors do not have light spread, so the spatial resolution is limited only by the pixel size. Depending on the equipment manufacturer, 70 to 85 μm pixel sizes are typical. As monitor technology advances, future efforts will be directed toward reducing the direct detector pixel size to provide better resolution. The indirect method cannot be improved because its limiting factor is light spread (blur), not pixel size.

In all detectors, there is an inherent lower limit in the size of the pixel. If pixels are made too small, while the resolution may improve, the overall system may not. Very small pixels receive too few x-rays to generate an image, and the image is noisy. In addition, smaller pixels make large data sets that are challenging to transmit, store, and display.

Direct Conversion Weaknesses

All technology has advantages and disadvantages. The resolution of the direct conversion array is limited only by the

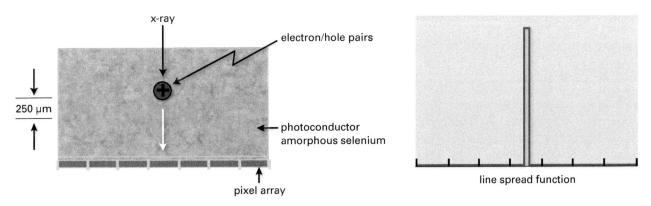

Figure 12-39
Opposite electric charges are applied at the top and bottom surfaces of the a-Se layer. When x-rays strike the a-Se layer, the ions travel in a straight line to the TFTs. Spatial resolution is sharp because there is virtually no lateral light diffusion. The transistor array absorbs the electrical charge and measures the charge from the ions. The measurement of the charge is converted into a digital image. (Image courtesy of Dr. Andrew Smith, Hologic, Bedford, MA.)

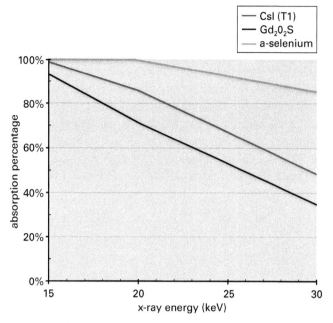

Figure 12-40
Percent absorption of incident x-rays for materials used in screen–film, Gd_2O_2S 34 mg/cm²; indirect conversion CsI(Tl), 73 mg/cm²; and second-generation selenium, 250 µm thick. (Image courtesy of Dr. Andrew Smith, Hologic, Bedford, MA.)

size of the pixels. As pixels are made smaller, the amount of data in an image rapidly increases. This results in a longer wait time for the image to be read out by the TFTs and displayed on the technologist's monitor; additionally, with more information acquired with each image, more storage space is required in PACS.

Another disadvantage is drifting of the dark signal, aka "ghosting." The direct digital array produces an electronic signal even in the absence of an actual radiation exposure. The array is constantly "cleaned" to empty the TFTs of this dark signal.

Summary

Digital imaging is more than the sum of new technology, science, and mathematics; it is a shift in our thinking, concepts, and language. It is all about how we think, see, and express our questions and answers. Invisible electrons move with the speed of light, sometimes through wires, sometimes through the air; they are shaped by digital technology to capture lifesaving images and our words about them for our medical decision-makers in ways not available to them a mere decade ago.

As our minds decide what we want to see, and how we want to see it, we turn to digital technology for solutions to these present needs and our future hopes.

Review Questions

1. Why was mammography the last of the imaging modalities to go digital?

2. What conclusions came out of the ACRIN/DMIST study?

3. List the advantages of digital mammography.

4. The IHE Mammography Subcommittee is charged with improving connectivity issues between multiple vendor equipment. Why is this necessary?

5. What is the difference between the matrix, a pixel, and a TFT?

6. What function does flat-fielding provide?

7. Compare and contrast the indirect and direct-to-digital methods.

References

1. Zimmermann J. *BMDO Technology Applications in Biomedicine.* Washington, DC: National Technology Transfer Center, Washington Operations for the Ballistic Missile Defense Organization; 1997.

2. Lewin JM, et al. Clinical comparison of full field digital mammography and screen-film mammography for detection of breast cancer. *Am J Roentgenol.* 2002;179:671–677.

3. Frost & Sullivan. North American X-ray mammography market. February 6, 2006, Internet article. Available at: www.frost.com/prod/servlet/report-toc.pag?ctxixplink=fcmctx3searchquery=north+american+x-ray+mammography+market&repid=f793-01-00-00-00&bdata=ahrocdovl3d3dy5mcm98dc5jb20vc3jac9jyxrhbg9nlxniyxjjac5kb89xbwvevriehq9b-m9ydg6ryw1lcljyw4rec1yyxkrbwftbw9ncmfwahkrbwfya-2voqh5au2vhcm-noifjl3vsdhnafkaxmjc3mdy1ntayotlx&ctxixplabel=fcmctx4

4. Pisano ED, et al. Diagnostic performance of digital versus film mammography for breast cancer screening. *N Engl J Med.* 2005;353(17):1773–1783.

5. Yee KM. Managing the transition to digital mammography. Aunt Minnie.com; 2007. Available at: www.auntminnie.com/index.aspx?sec=spt&sub=tir&pag=dis&ltemld=74564

6. Mullaney R, Burbage D, Evantash A, et al. Making the transition to digital mammography. *Comm Oncol.* 2007;4(11):678–680.

7. Berns EA, Hendrick RE, Solari M, et al. Digital and screen-film mammography: comparison of image acquisition and interpretation times. *Am J Roentgenol.* 2006;187:38–41.

8. Digital mammo takes longer to interpret than screen-film. *Advance Magazine*; June 14, 2004:18.

9. Massat MB. *A Clinical Perspective of Digital Mammography: Evaluating Choices in Mammography Displays.* Crystal Lake, IL: Massat Media, LLC.

10. Miner HT, Wang J, Neely AE, et al. Timed efficiency of interpretation of digital and film-screen screening mammograms. *Am J Roentgenol.* 2009;192:216–220.

11. Undrill PE, O'Kane AD, Gilbert FJ. A comparison of digital with screen-film mammography for cancer detection: results of 4,945 paired examinations. *Radiology.* 2001;218(93):873–880.

12. Pisano E, Yaffe M, Kuzniak C. *Digital Mammography.* Baltimore, MD: Lippincott Williams & Wilkins; 2004.

13. Indrajit IK, Verma BS. Digital imaging in radiology practice: an introduction to few fundamental concepts. *Indian J Radiol Imaging.* 2007;17(4):230–236.

14. Goldstraw EJ, Castellano I, Ashley S, et al. The effect of premium view post-processing software on digital mammographic reporting. *Br J Radiol.* 2009;10:1259.

15. Mahesh M. AAPM/RSNA physics tutorial for residents. Digital mammography: an overview. *Radiographics.* 2004;24: 1747–1760.

16. Reiner B, Siegel E, Carrino J. Workflow optimization: current trends and future directions. *J Digit Imaging.* 2002;15:141–152.

17. Pisaro W, Zuley M, Baum J, et al. Issues to consider in converting to digital mammography. *Radiol Clin North Am.* 2007;45(5):813–830.

18. Smith, AP. *Fundamentals of Digital Mammography: Physics, Technology, and Practical Considerations.* Bedford, MA: Hologic, Inc.; 2005.

19. Sudharsanan R. *Thin Film CdZnTe Detector Arrays for Digital Mammography.* Bedford, MA: Spire Corporation; 1999.

20. Cole EB, Pisano ED, Kistner EO, et al. Diagnostic accuracy of digital mammography in patients with dense breasts who underwent problem-solving mammography: effects of image processing and lesion type. *Radiology.* 2002;223: 845–852.

21. Pisano ED, Cole EB, Hemminger BM, et al. Image processing algorithms for digital mammography: a pictorial essay. *Radiographics.* 2000;20:1479–1491.

22. Pisasno ED, Gatsonis CJ, Hendrick E, et al. Diagnostic performance of digital versus film mammography for breast cancer screening. *N Engl J Med.* 2005;353(17): 1773–1783.

23. Trambert M. *Digital Mammography Integrated with PACS: Real World Issues, Considerations, Workflow Solutions, and Reading Paradigms.* Santa Barbara, CA: Department of Radiology, Santa Barbara Cottage Hospital.

24. Provost V, Pauwels H, Marchai G, et al. Evaluation of clinical image processing algorithms used in digital mammography. *Med Phys.* 2009;36(3):765–775.

25. Weiser J. LCD monitors beyond radiology. *Imaging Economics.* July 2004.

26. Monnin P, Gutierrez D, Bulling S, et al. A comparison of the performance of digital mammography systems. *Med Phys.* 2007;34(3):906–914.

Nonimaging Components of the FFDM Network

13

Objectives

- Understand the unique requirements of mammography within a digital radiology department
- Become familiar with the additional networking and hardware components needed before digital mammography imaging is performed
- Become familiar with the terminology used to describe the systems and requirements of these components
- Understand the development of an efficient workflow within the digital mammography environment

---

Key Terms

- bandwidth
- data compression
- digital imaging and communication in medicine (DICOM)
- firewall
- fit to film
- hanging protocols
- health level 7 (HL7)
- hospital information system (HIS)
- information technology (IT)
- Kaizen
- lookup tables (LUT)
- magneto-optical disks (MOD)
- mammography information system (MIS)
- migrate
- modality worklist
- network area storage (NAS)
- network backbone
- PACS administrator

- picture archiving and communication system (PACS)
- pixel to pixel
- productivity
- radiology information system (RIS)
- redundant array of independent disks (RAID)
- request for proposal (RFP)
- router
- server
- storage area network (SAN)
- switch
- teleradiology
- true size
- virtual private network (VPN)
- window center
- window level
- window width
- workflow
- workstations

INTRODUCTION

Due to the inception of digital imaging in 1981, hospital radiology departments and private radiology facilities are more advanced in computerization than the average medical office. However, mammography was the last of the radiology disciplines to convert to digital imaging. This was due in part to the technical demands necessary to produce and to store high-quality digital mammography images and also in part to Federal regulations that made the process of developing the complete full-field digital mammography (FFDM) imaging systems more complicated for the manufacturers and more challenging to incorporate into an existing digital imaging network.

The majority of technologists are health care workers, not computer scientists. So when computer terms and acronyms enter the conversation, we tend to feel overwhelmed. The goal of this chapter is to make a little more sense of the alphabet soup and how it affects what the mammography technologist does on a day-to-day basis.

Advantages and Disadvantages of FFDM

Technologists are efficient when working in a digital environment. The technologist spends as much time in the mammography room with each patient as she did when she worked with analog equipment, but much of the background work, such as film processing and paperwork, is eliminated. Therefore, she is able to image more patients within the same timeframe, possibly doubling the number of examinations per unit.[1] The increased **productivity** of the technologist results in increased income for the facility.

Although the digital technologist is more productive, this advantage can also be considered a limitation. As the technologist spends more time in the mammography room imaging almost twice the number of patients, she has less face-to-face interaction with the radiologist. This means that considerable care must be taken to avoid mistakes when relaying patient histories or other pertinent information. Another limitation of the increased time spent isolated in the mammography room is that technologists have less opportunity to consult with coworkers on the technical aspects of a case; therefore, each technologist must be secure and have confidence in her skills.

For the radiologist, the conversion from analog imaging to digital imaging may in some ways seem counterproductive. Studies show that it takes almost twice as long for a radiologist to read a digital mammography exam than to read an analog exam.[2,3] Reasons for this loss in productivity are as follows:

• The radiologist can electronically manipulate the images; this adds time to the interpretation process.

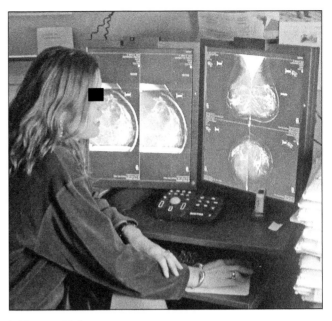

Figure 13-1
The radiologist reads FFDM images at the softcopy review workstation utilizing tools such as window and level, zoom, and pan to glean even more information from a single image. CAD markings are also available to the radiologist as she scrolls through the examination in hanging protocols that are personalized for each physician.

• Having to scroll through files to see current and prior images (hanging protocols).
• Learning curve to become familiar with the software at the reviewstation and computer, including PACS.
• Time delay if images were not prefetched from PACS.
• Network speed.

However, there are reasons why FFDM is attractive to the radiologist (Figure 13-1; Table 13-1). Of course, this infers that the FFDM system and picture archiving and communication system (PACS) are working in sync.

• **More tools at their disposal to electronically manipulate images.** These tools allow the radiologist to more easily find areas of suspicion. The radiologist can electronically change the look of the image to suit his/her personal preference; this can result in a greater positive predictive value (PPV) and fewer false negatives (FN). This electronic image manipulation also takes pressure off the technologist because the technique factors for acquisition of FFDM images are broader ranged, resulting in fewer repeated images.
• **Images cannot be lost.** There is no longer a need to worry about films that have been sent out to referring physicians not being returned; the digital image is always available on PACS. This saves time for the file room staff and eliminates frustration on the part of the radiologist.

Table 13-1 • Advantages and Disadvantages of FFDM

ADVANTAGES	DISADVANTAGES
Improved contrast resolution, which benefits patients with dense tissue	Cost of equipment
Reduction in cost of consumables (film, processing chemicals, etc.)	Cost of additional hardware (infrastructure, PACS, workstations, laser printers, archiving, etc.)
Fewer repeated images for technical factors (too dark, too light)	Possible increase in support staff for techs and radiologists
Increased technologist efficiency. Less technologist time needed per examination	Less technologist/radiologist interaction
Possible increase of PPV— radiologist has more tools and is able to manipulate images to optimize visualization.	More time needed for radiologist to read examination

- **Easy to pull up images if a referring doctor or surgeon calls to discuss a patient.** It takes much less time for the radiologist to electronically recall an exam from PACS than for the radiologist to contact a film librarian to locate the film jacket and deliver it to the reading room while the caller waits on the phone.

CHOOSING EQUIPMENT THAT IS BEST FOR YOUR FACILITY

Cost

FFDM is expensive. The FFDM machine itself is only part of the expense. Depending on the infrastructure that may already be in place, other financial considerations include the radiologist reviewstation, computer-aided detection (CAD), breast density measurement, PACS, radiology information system (RIS), networking, archiving, IT/PACS department personnel, and architectural and physical changes that may be necessary to accommodate the digital equipment. Evaluating the assets you already have helps you to determine your plan for the digital system. Almost always, this begins with the budget.

Determining Need and Making Decisions

It is important to obtain as much knowledge and information about FFDM as possible before jumping into a purchase that might not be the right fit for your facility.

Half the battle is learning the language that comes along with digital imaging. Chapters 11 and 12 will help you get started with understanding the process.

Most likely a single vendor will not be able to solve all of your equipment needs, which may include not only the mammography machine but also the RIS functions such as scheduling and reporting and modality worklist and PACS-type functions that include acquisition, display distribution, workstations, archiving, and disaster recovery. In addition, peripheral equipment is required: CAD, printers, and CD burners. The best place to start is to consider your current environment and discuss the goals of your facility.

The first step toward choosing new equipment is to inventory the existing equipment and determine your current status.

- Is your facility already digital? Do you already have an existing laser printer, PACS, RIS, network connectivity, and IT/PACS support personnel?
- Are other imaging departments in your facility already using digital imaging? Is it CR, direct radiography (DR), or a combination?
- What is the geography of your mammography department? Are you an independent single site, or part of a multisite facility? If multisite, what resources are available at the other sites? Are screening and diagnostic mammograms performed at the same site? Is the mammography department separate or contiguous with a general imaging department?
- Where will the mammography images be interpreted?
- Where will the FFDM equipment be placed?
- Is there a wired network in place that can support the bandwidth required for mammography imaging?
- Is there an information system in place: HIS or RIS?

Keep connectivity and compatibility in mind when considering the purchase of any equipment. A current PACS system and network may not be compatible with a new FFDM system. Transfer, display, and storage of FFDM images may be more rigorous than an older PACS system can handle.

RFPs: Choosing a Vendor, Site Visits

When making any large purchase for a facility, it is always wise to use an RFP—**request for proposal**—process. This can help you focus on your needs and reduce your susceptibility to smooth sales pitches by helping you weed out unsuitable choices and allow for more accurate comparisons between products and services. Provide as much specific detail as possible about your practice and your needs within the RFP to avoid vague inferences from the vendor as to what you will be purchasing. There are templates available online to help design an RFP around your specific needs.

The best RFP proposals include information about the size of the practice, the location of the facility and the types of services that are offered, potential growth expectations, a profile of the facility's managed care payers, information about the employees and system users, details about other systems that will need to be integrated with the equipment you are purchasing, and data storage requirements.

In addition to providing information about your own facility, request information about the vendor to get a better idea of their qualifications to provide you with the services you need. This could include information regarding the company's history, longevity, and future plans, whether it is a private or publicly traded company, the location of the company and its service center, HIPAA compliance and how it is accomplished, system audit features, disaster support plans, company representation following the sale, and participation in the Integrating the Healthcare Enterprise (IHE) mammography profiles. IHE participation assures you that the vendor is working with the rest of the mammography community to overcome compatibility issues between their equipment and other vendors' equipment.

Once the RFP is developed, an identical packet can be submitted to each vendor bidding on your proposal. The cover letter should give an overview of the project and specifications of the technology or service you are in need of. It should also advise vendors of due dates for proposals and estimates for dates when decisions will be made. To avoid confusion, let the vendors know if you will accept electronic submissions or if you expect all proposals to be submitted in a specific format.

Once the responses come in, you can compare and eliminate the unqualified candidates and then schedule meetings with the finalists. Plan site visits to view each of the finalist's equipment and question current users. The people within your facility who will use the new equipment or supply service should be included on these visits; they will be able to help determine the equipment that will work best for your individual situation.

THE NETWORK INFRASTRUCTURE

Image Storage, Archiving, Transfer, and Retrieval

Invisible Electrons

To most mammography technologists, the "network" is represented by a cable from the acquisition workstation that plugs into the wall. Beyond the wall is a pipeline that moves data and images from one place to another throughout a facility, or even beyond. The infrastructure consists of servers, switches, firewalls, more cabling, and possibly even wireless routers. This area is the domain of **information technology (IT)** personnel and the PACS administrator.

So, what are these things on the other side of the wall?

- A **server** is defined as a multiuser computer that provides a service (e.g., database access, file transfer, remote access) or resources (e.g., file space) over a network connection.
- A **firewall** is a dedicated piece of equipment, or it can be software running on another computer, which inspects network traffic passing through it, and denies or permits passage on the basis of a set of rules. Its basic task is to regulate the flow of traffic between computer networks. It is used to prevent intrusion into a private network from a public access network.
- A **switch** is a device that connects segments of the network and directs the information to its proper destination.
- A **router** is a device that forwards information to designated recipients.

The **network backbone** is this collection of equipment and the direct connection from one piece to the next piece that enables communications across the network. This is usually the fastest part of the network, or the "interstate freeway" of the information highway. All the other roads converge here to get their destination faster.

Each link within the network chain, and the manner in which they are connected, has an impact on the speed with which information is transported and to where it can be transported. The network can be very simple or very complex, depending on the functions it performs and the number of devices on the network. There is no set blueprint of how a network should be set up. Each network is unique to the facility that designs and uses it.

Network Bandwidth

Bandwidth is the maximum rate that data may be transferred across a network. It is measured in bits per second. It is the size of your "information highway." Because digital mammography images are quite large, they need a higher bandwidth—a wider road—to travel quickly throughout the network without causing a "traffic jam" (Figure 13-2).

How much bandwidth you have determines how quickly files are moved within the network and how quickly they can be called up on a workstation. The number of images moving through the network at one time is also a factor in how fast they move—the more cars on the highway, the slower the traffic is likely to be. Adequate bandwidth is necessary so that your radiologists aren't sitting around waiting to look at studies that are caught in traffic.

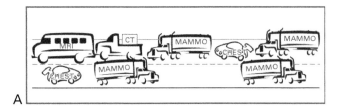

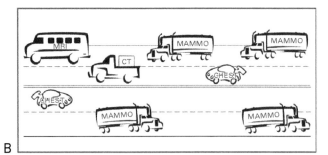

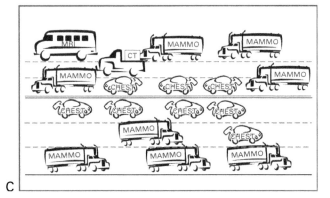

Figure 13-2
The information highway bandwidth determines how fast images can travel through the PACS network. Speed is determined by the size of the image and the volume of the traffic. The larger the bandwidth, the faster images can travel, even with a higher volume of large images and traffic. **(A)** A narrow bandwidth allows images to travel, but the speed may be slow, depending on traffic within the network. **(B)** A broader bandwidth allows the same traffic to travel a bit more smoothly. **(C)** A minimum 1 GB bandwidth will allow larger images, and more of them, to travel faster through the network.

Of course, the broader the bandwidth, the more costly the service; but cost needs to be assessed in relation to the productivity of the radiologist and the patient volume. Currently, a bandwidth of 1 gigabyte (GB) is usually recommended for mammography applications. However, bandwidth is not the only factor that can limit the throughput of the network. The speed of the servers and storage networks also plays a part.

Communication and Languages

In order for the many different components of an imaging system to work together and communicate effectively, they need to speak the same language. That is the mission of the IHE (Integrating the Healthcare Enterprise) initiative. Devised by leaders in health care imaging and health care industries, IHE works to improve the way computer systems in health care share information. Systems developed in accordance with IHE communicate with one another better, are easier to implement, and enable health care providers to use information more effectively.

IHE promotes the use of established standard computer languages such as **health level 7 (HL7)** and **digital imaging and communication in medicine (DICOM)** to address specific clinical needs. HL7 is the language used by the RIS to store a database of patient demographics, usually in the form of text.

DICOM is a very specific standard language for PACS. It moves images and image information around the system using query, retrieve, and send commands. A piece of equipment that is said to be "DICOM compatible" means that the equipment uses the DICOM language and should be able to communicate and interact with other pieces of DICOM-compatible equipment. For instance, an FFDM machine from manufacturer A should communicate with a hardcopy film laser printer from manufacturer B.

The DICOM header is a behind-the-scenes attachment to each image that contains tagged files to convey patient demographics (name, date of examination, DOB, etc.), imaging information (view, laterality, kilovolt peak [kVp], compression thickness, degree of obliquity, etc.), and display parameters for the image.

Unfortunately, as in any language, sometimes, there are disparities in the interpretation, and information can be lost in translation—in this case from one manufacturer to another, within the DICOM header. This can interfere with archiving or display. This possible lack of communication is almost as frustrating and vexing to the manufacturers as it is to the users of the equipment. Improvement in equipment communications was the driving force behind the establishment of the IHE, as vendors worked to produce equipment that could be used in conjunction with equipment from other vendors.

HIS, RIS, and MIS

Before we begin imaging a patient, we need some basic information: her name, date of birth, home address, phone number, insurance information, patient ID number, etc. This is considered the patient demographic information—information that identifies her as a specific individual within the patient population. This is the information that is contained within a **radiology information system (RIS)**, a **hospital information system (HIS)**, or a **mammography information system (MIS)**. Correct data entry of initial patient demographics in the information system is critical to successful patient identification.[4] The demographics entered in the information system will be linked to all future data related to this specific patient, including billing and images.

HIS is a database of demographic information used throughout an entire hospital or health care system by all departments; RIS is a database of the information used within a radiology department; and MIS is the information used solely within the mammography department. It often can be an integral part of transcription and recall, as well as the medical outcomes audit. Depending on the size of a facility and how the information in the database is used, a facility may use all of these systems in a cooperative network to store and supply demographic information, or it may use these systems independently of each other. To simplify the rest of the chapter, from now on when we refer to RIS, it simply suggests the information system.

The accepted standard computer language used in information systems is called HL7. This is not a language that a receptionist or scheduler needs to know to be able to input patient information; it is the universal language that allows RIS to communicate with PACS and with other RIS systems. HL7 is a protocol that can take the patient information that has been typed into a patient scheduling and billing software program and encode it in a format that can be accepted by PACS. It can be thought of as a translation tool rather than a language.

Modality Worklist

As simple as it may seem, consistent adequate labeling of all images is the single most important aspect of storage and retrieval in an electronic environment.[5] This is typically managed through a **modality worklist** that is generated by RIS or HIS. This allows all patient demographics to be imported into the image file consistently—on all images and for all examinations that the patient has performed, linking them to each other as part of the patient's electronic medical file. Without a modality worklist, images may be irretrievable or at the very least may take many personnel hours to find and retrieve.

A modality worklist prevents manual entry of patient demographic data by the technologist, which can be inconsistent; the difference in input from using all uppercase letters one year to lowercase the next year could prevent the images from linking together in one electronic patient file. If the patient data ever changes, it is changed globally through RIS, not on an individual examination or image.

RIS works with PACS to create a modality worklist for each digital modality within the facility. The worklist, with the demographic data of each patient, is sent to the acquisition workstation where the patient is scheduled to be imaged (Figure 13-3).

Case Study **13-1**

1. Refer to Figure 13-3B. Explain the electronic steps that take place from the time the patient arrives at the mammography facility until her report of the results of the examination are delivered to her referring physician.

The worklist can be programmed to display not only the complete listing of all current examinations, but it should also be able to sort into lists relevant only to the individuals who currently need the information. There could be a specific list for Mammo Room #1, a list for Mammo Room #2, a list for Dr. Jones, and so on; workers in those areas would need to choose only from the list of patients that they need to image or whose charts they need access to. This can also work as a means of enforcing HIPAA regulations by limiting employee access to patient records.

When ready to begin a patient examination, the technologist needs only to select the correct patient name from the worklist at the acquisition workstation. The patient information, name, ID number, age, etc., is automatically attached to all the images acquired on that patient as part of the DICOM header. The acquisition device and PACS have been set up with a list of studies that have been predetermined according to the facility. The study defines specific views, or images, that must be taken to complete the study. For instance, if the technologist selects "screening mammogram," the acquisition device and PACS have been set up to anticipate four images: RCC, LCC, RMLO, and LMLO. These images are sent or pushed to PACS from the acquisition workstation after being reviewed for completeness by the technologist.

PACS

There is no way around it—once you begin producing digital images, you must have a method to store and transfer them. Typically, **PACS** consists of an archive device, diagnostic review workstations for the radiologists, clinical review workstations for the technologists, servers to distribute the images throughout the network, and software to manage the database and workflow.

PACS is the component of the imaging network where everything comes together. The images can be viewed,

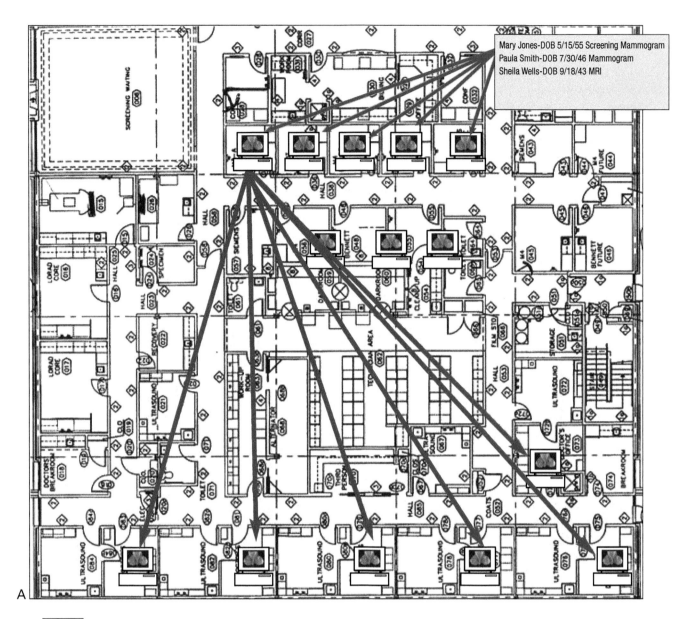

Mary Jones-DOB 5/15/55 Screening Mammogram
Paula Smith-DOB 7/30/46 Mammogram
Sheila Wells-DOB 9/18/43 MRI

A

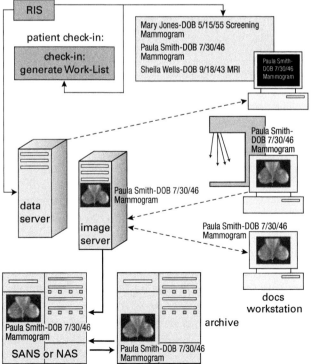

RIS

patient check-in:

check-in:
generate Work-List

Mary Jones-DOB 5/15/55 Screening Mammogram
Paula Smith-DOB 7/30/46 Mammogram
Sheila Wells-DOB 9/18/43 MRI

Paula Smith-DOB 7/30/46 Mammogram

Paula Smith-DOB 7/30/46 Mammogram

Paula Smith-DOB 7/30/46 Mammogram

Paula Smith-DOB 7/30/46 Mammogram

data server

image server

Paula Smith-DOB 7/30/46 Mammogram

docs workstation

Paula Smith-DOB 7/30/46 Mammogram

archive

SANS or NAS

B

Figure 13-3

The basic network. **(A)** Within the network, each modality is assigned a worklist of patients scheduled to have an examination. Once the technologist completes the examination, images can be seen by any radiologist within the department. **(B)** The patient's demographics are stored in RIS. Once the patient arrives at the facility, her information is sent to a modality worklist, which tells the technologist at the modality (mammography machine acquisition workstation) that the patient is ready for her examination. The digital images are taken and linked with the patient's demographic information. All of this digital data is sent to the short-term image server, where it can be accessed instantly by the radiologist at the softcopy review workstation. After a predetermined length of time, the images may be stored in a near-line server or in long-term archiving. These images are still available to the radiologist at any time, but may take longer to bring up on a workstation.

interpreted, and then stored, forever connected with the patient data from RIS, so that these images can be retrieved and viewed as needed. The goal is a completely electronic environment where images and cases can be brought up on a computer workstation anywhere, anytime, and quickly. Depending on the size of the facility, this may, or may not, be a hugely complicated expense. If a facility already has PACS in place, keep in mind that mammography is relatively new to the digital imaging world and connectivity and compatibility issues still exist.

Electronic Storage: Image Size

Electronic storage can be managed on-site or off-site, by PACS servers, or stored on removable media such as CD, DVD, or tape. Whichever media type is considered, be aware of technology obsolescence; you should ensure that data can be migrated from one system to another as technology advances so that the data will always be retrievable. In addition, you need to assure that you have an adequate network, with enough bandwidth to move the data from archive to workstation. Bandwidth controls the speed with which the data can be moved and the amount of data that can be moved at one time.

Digital image storage space is measured in megabytes (MB). FFDM images have the dubious honor of being some of the largest digital images in the radiology department. A single FFDM image is approximately 50 MB; multiply that by four views per patient, and the average 2D digital mammogram requires approximately 200 MB of storage space in PACS. The size of a DBT exam is approximately 1,229 MB. By comparison, a single-view chest x-ray uses only about 1 MB. Table 13-2 gives several comparisons for digital image sizes and text file sizes. In addition, it can help calculate and plan the amount of storage space your facility will need, based on the number and type of digital examinations you perform. When estimating how much storage space you will need, think ahead; storage needs for mammography are very large compared with most other examinations.

Image Compression

Digital images are large data packets; these large packets present storage and display challenges for PACS. One way to reduce the size of a digital image, thus reducing the challenge to PACS, is through compression of the data packet. Electronic **data compression** allows data to be stored in a smaller packet, thus requiring less space; space is money. A smaller packet also improves transmission performance, allowing images to travel faster over the network. There are two ways to compress data: *lossy compression*, where some of the information on the image is lost forever, and *lossless compression*, where all of the information is retained.

Lossy compression allows a greater degree of compression, requiring much less storage space, and allows images to be transferred much faster. This can be performed at ratios of up to 30:1. However, when an image is compressed this much, some data are lost and the image quality can never be fully recovered. Therefore, at this time, lossy compression can**not** be used to archive FFDM images or to recreate an image for final interpretation. This may change as imaging technology advances.

Lossy compression is accomplished by averaging the pixel data and removing information within a tolerable level so that when the image is brought out from storage, some of the information will be gone. The tolerable level depends on the examination and the relevance of contrast and resolution to its interpretation.

Because of the importance of contrast and resolution in the interpretation of mammograms, lossless compression is recommended. The ratio of compression with lossless is about 2:1. Even though this sounds insignificant, it is important when you realize that a 200-MB examination can now fit in an area of only 100 MB, actually doubling the storage capacity. Currently, the FDA recommends that mammography facilities use only lossless compression when storing the data from FFDM examinations.

Storage and Image Archiving

Once digital images have been obtained, they need to be stored and archived on some type of medium. In analog imaging, the film, which is also a part of the imaging chain, is stored. Today, the film would be called a hardcopy image. However, in the digital world, there is limited need for a hardcopy image, and in reality, a hardcopy image is counterproductive to the cost-saving benefits of digital imaging. The money saved due to removing film and printing costs is instead placed into the electronic storage of the images.

Storage needs to be evaluated from several different aspects:

* Storage for the studies that you need instant access to (online)
* Storage for studies that you need occasional access to (near-line)
* Long-term storage for archiving (offline)

There are no set standards for information storage; each facility needs to determine what combination will work best for their patient volume and workflow.

Online storage is used for daily work. It needs to be fast, and it is the most expensive type of storage; an analogy, this is like short-term parking at the airport—closest parking to the terminal, shortest time to get to the terminal, but the most expensive fee to park your car so close to the building.

Table 13-2 • Visualizing Data and Storage Space[a]

ABBREVIATION		BIT	NIBBLE	BYTE	KILOBIT	KILOBYTE	MEGABIT	MEGABYTES	GIGABYTE	TERABYTE
b	Bits in a	1	4	8	1,024	8,192	1,048,576	8,388,608	8,589,934,592	8,796,093,022,208
	Nibbles in a		1	2	512	2,048	262,144	2,097,152	2,147,483,648	2,199,023,255,552
B	Bytes in a			1	128	1,024	131,072	1,048,576	1,073,741,824	1,099,511,627,776
Kb	Kilobits in a				1	8	1,024	8,192	8,388,608	8,589,934,592
KB	Kilobytes in a					1	128	1,024	1,048,576	1,073,741,824
Mb	Megabits in a						1	8	8,192	8,388,608
MB	Megabytes in a							1	1,048,576	1,073,741,824
GB	Gigabytes in a								1	1,048,576
TB	Terabytes									1
PB	Petabytes									
EB	Exabytes									
ZB	Zettabytes									

Approximate size of several digital radiography examinations
- 1 MB = one view chest x-ray
- 5 MB = one view cervical spine
- 10 MB = one view lumbar spine examination
- 50 MB = one view of a digital mammogram

Some useful comparisons
- 5 bytes = the average English word
- 2 kilobytes = one typewritten page
- 5 megabytes = complete works of Shakespeare, 1 typical mp3 song, 30 seconds of broadcast—quality video
- 100 megabytes = 8 minutes of broadcast video, 20 King James Bibles
- 3 gigabytes = 200,000 telephone book pages

[a]The chart above represents data sizes in true binary values, but it should be noted that most hard disk manufacturers use a decimal value to calculate storage. For example, a 100-GB drive is actually only 1,000,000,000 bytes, or 100 GiB (gibibytes), which is really only 940 GB.
Source: Information extracted from http://www.asimweb.org and "How Much Information?" UC Berkeley School of Information Management and Systems, 2003.

This is where the current images taken by technologist at the acquisition workstation are sent, as are prior studies that have been retrieved for comparison by the radiologist. The length of time that a patient's study remains "online" is dictated by the needs of the facility; patients with a diagnosed cancer or who will be recalled for additional testing often stay online for up to 6 months or more, as they will likely be reviewed during that time. A screening mammogram that has been interpreted as negative may remain online only for a limited time, perhaps a week or a month. Because it is more expensive to keep patient records here, the object is to clear out studies that will not need to be reviewed again for quite a while to make room for incoming studies.

Near-line storage is somewhat slower than online but is also less expensive; an analogy, this is like long-term parking at the airport—a little farther walk to get to the terminal takes a little longer to get there, but moderate in price. Images of patients who are likely to have additional exams within a year are often stored here, such as breast cancer patients undergoing radiation therapy. The images are easier to access than if they were offline, but it is less expensive than taking up space in the online storage.

Offline storage, or deep archive, is the slowest and the least expensive type of storage; an analogy, this is like off-site parking at the airport—the farthest away from the terminal takes the longest amount of time to get to/from, but is the least expensive parking fee. This may include PACS servers, DVD, CD, and tape storage media. This storage is for studies of patients whose examinations are completed, and it is not likely that they will be returning for at least another year. When the patient does schedule an appointment, RIS will send a message to PACS to retrieve the prior images from the offline storage; the prior images will then go online, waiting to be accessed when the patient comes in. Retrieval of the information is transparent, meaning that an order is automatically sent from RIS when an appointment is scheduled; thus, no additional step needs to be performed by the scheduler.

In addition to these storage options, a redundant disaster archive, typically located off-site, is necessary. In the event of a natural disaster, such as a flood, studies that are stored at a location physically separate from the facility will be saved and are available for restoration, even if the facility does not survive. Generally, this is accomplished through a third-party service provider.

Storage Hardware

Once you have an idea of how many examinations you will be storing in each of these "virtual waiting rooms," you can make a decision about how nice the waiting room will be (space and speed) on the basis of your budget. The bigger the storage space and the faster it can deliver your images, the more expensive it will be. On the positive side, technology improves constantly; comparable space will probably decrease in price from year to year.

Redundant array of independent [or inexpensive] disks (RAID) is a fast and relatively inexpensive type of image storage using multiple hard drives for sharing or replicating data among the drives. It is the most commonly used short-term storage technology. A RAID consists of several magnetic storage disks, whereby the data are spread over multiple devices to improve performance and increase reliability. In case of a single disk failure, information can be regenerated using redundant information (called "checksums") stored on another disk within the device. Storage appliances that use RAID technology are configured in one of two manners: as a SAN or a NAS.

Storage area network (SAN) is the most expensive type of RAID. These are high-performance, high-availability storage networks with the ability to cross great distances using fiber channel components and fiberoptic interfaces. SANs are accessible by multiple host computers. All images are online all the time, so retrieval is immediate. This is also referred to as a "spinning disk RAID."

A **network area storage (NAS)** server is generally used as an archive and for prefetching images. A stand-alone solution that attaches directly to a network, it can also easily integrate into Microsoft Windows, Novell NetWare, Unix/Linux, and Macintosh networks. Multiple NAS servers can be used within a network to increase storage capacity. These storage devices usually are combined on a very fast network using a high-speed dedicated communications channel for image transfer.

Magneto-optical disks (MOD) are similar to a CD or DVD, with each disk holding 5 GB or more of data. They often are used within a "jukebox," a storage device that utilizes a number of MOD or DVDs. Accessing saved images from a MOD can take up to a minute, so these are generally used for long-term storage, and they can be rather expensive.

Tape libraries are the most cost-effective method of storage, but are not as reliable as optical media, access is slower, and there is a chance that obsolescence of the technology may be imminent.

Data Migration

As we all know, nothing ever stays the same. Technology continues to change and advance at a rapid pace, and as it does, older technology becomes obsolete. However, the images and data that we have acquired need to remain accessible even as we upgrade our equipment.

In our everyday lives, we can see how this has happened when we want to watch a movie in our home. BETA videotapes gave way to VHS, which in turn were overcome by DVD, and more recently, NetFlix. Many of us have family video from the 1980s that we despair of ever seeing again because we no longer have the hardware to play the tapes on. If only we'd had the foresight to **migrate** that data to a newer technology, it would still be accessible.

The same threat of obsolescence is also true as images are stored within PACS. However, Federal and state regulations require you be able to access those images for at least 7 to 10 years. When purchasing new equipment, make certain that the vendor guarantees that all the data you currently have will be accessible or is able to be migrated into the new technology where it will be accessible.

▌▌▌ WORKSTATION

Workstations within a PACS network are not all the same (Figure 13-4). A diagnostic reviewstation is specifically used for the softcopy interpretation of images by the radiologist. The key feature of this type of workstation is the monitor; it must have very high resolution to enable the radiologist to see every detail on the image. For mammography, it is suggested that at minimum a 5-megapixel monitor be used for diagnosis. In addition to the high-resolution monitor, these reviewstations usually have specialized keypads to enhance the functions used most often by radiologists, making it faster and easier for them to maneuver through each case.

A QA workstation is often used by clinicians within a PACS network and by technologists as they perform a final review of each case before it is sent on to the radiologist to be read. These generally have monitors that are not as high in resolution as those in a diagnostic reviewstation, but are slightly higher in resolution than those at the acquisition workstation. QA workstations are usually about 3 megapixel; acquisition workstations usually have 2 megapixel monitors. Acquisition workstations can be upgraded to 3 megapixel monitors.

Viewing Functions and Hanging Protocols

Although these are covered in more detail in Chapter 12, Creating the Digital Image, they are a function of PACS. These include, but may not be limited to, image and information management, basic display features, image manipulation, image metrics, advanced functions, and modality-specific features.

Image and information management deals with anything needed to retrieve the correct images and the corresponding information. This would include the worklist, thumbnail images, clinical information, and importing and exporting images.

Some *display features* that are commonly used for mammography include image ordering, hanging protocols, landscape/portrait display, and pixel and screen-size matching. Cine display, image linking, stereo display, and reference lines are additional display features.

- Image ordering is the sequence of image display—what views of the study the radiologist wants to see first, then second, and so on.
- **Hanging protocols** go one step beyond image ordering by arranging the images on the reviewstation exactly as they would be hung on a viewbox or film alternator.

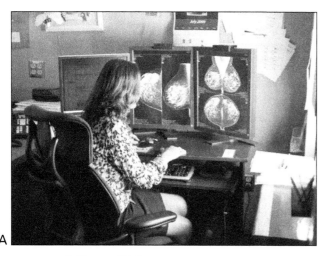

A

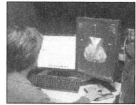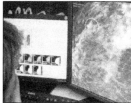
Technologist reviews requested views before performing exam

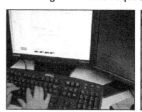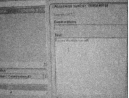
B Technologist adds notes about exam

Figure 13-4
PACS workstations allow the radiologist **(A)** and the technologist **(B)** to communicate with each other.

Each radiologist has a preferred way of looking at the images in a study, particularly in mammography. Therefore, hanging protocols and image order should be configurable dependent on the user.

Image manipulation features allow changes to the presentation of individual images. These include the following:

- Rotating or flipping the image
- Inverting the image to create a "negative" image where black appears white or white appears black
- Zooming to increase the size of the image
- Panning to move the center point of the image
- A loupe to enlarge only a small area of the image
- Window width and window center

Window width and **window center** also manipulate the image; this is oftentimes referred to as **window/leveling**. Window width is mapping of the range of information (shades of gray) within the image, while the window center identifies the center value of the information. DICOM data typically include more information than can be displayed at one time on a computer monitor. Individual image points may be stored in PACS using 4,096 (or more) intensity levels, but are represented on the computer monitor with only 256 levels of gray. All medical imaging workstations provide a way for the source data to be mapped to the display, and this is what is known as windowing. Adjusting the window center and width allows different tissue types to be visualized.

Lookup tables (LUT) are often included in the DICOM header to display the image with a certain "look" that is the radiologist's preference. This is a predetermined manipulation of the image, but different LUT can be applied to an image to change the look.

Presentation state storage allows a manipulated image to be saved and stored and then retrieved at a later date in the same state.

Image metrics are the numeric measurements taken of the image. Most common is the measurement function used to determine the size or location of pathology seen on an image. A region of interest (ROI) can also be measured using a histogram, a graph showing the distribution of pixel values and their frequency within the area. This demonstrates the characteristics of a certain area within the image and can be helpful in determining distinguishing aspects of a tumor or mass, particularly in CT or MR.

Advanced functions are more often used for CT and MR. They include multiplanar reconstruction, 3D, and image fusion where images from different modalities can be fused into one image.

Modality-specific functions include applications such as sound for ultrasonography and spectroscopy for MR images.

Computer-Aided Detection

CAD is another available link within the PACS network chain for FFDM images. CAD has become a standard of care for many mammography practices and is utilized with digitally acquired studies. The CAD equipment must be compatible with PACS, with the image acquisition equipment, and must be approved by FDA for use with both.

More information on CAD can be found in Chapter 11, Mammography Machine.

Telemammography

Teleradiology is the electronic transmission of radiological patient images from one location to another for the purposes of interpretation and/or consultation. Through teleradiology, images can be sent to another physical location within a practice or to other locations around the world. Growth in telemammography has not been as rapid as in other fields of radiology due to several factors, the most significant being the technical demands and the need for specialized equipment to transmit and display mammograms. Compatibility with client sites is a constant concern for practices that read images from other sites. A **virtual private network (VPN)** between a client site and a telemammographer is one method of overcoming the obstacles; however, most teleradiology companies have inevitably had some integration issues. Most employ a full-time information technology expert to anticipate, intercept, and resolve compatibility issues.

Adequate bandwidth to transmit large mammography files from the acquisition site to the reading rooms is another obstacle. Because of the extraordinarily high resolution of mammography images, FFDM files can exceed 100 MB per study and are difficult to transfer efficiently.

Easy, rapid access to prior studies is another problem faced by telemammographers. Unavailability of prior images necessarily slows the process since final reports cannot be produced until comparison studies are considered.

Credentialing is another major obstacle. Mammographers, like all radiologists, must be licensed in the state where the study originates, not merely in the state where it is read. Currently, state regulations vary widely, but to be on the safe side, many teleradiology companies opt to be licensed in every state. This can be a financial burden, especially on smaller telemammography operations.

Breast imaging is generally associated with a higher liability for radiologists than nonbreast imaging, so malpractice insurance is a major concern for telemammography groups. In spite of the financial and technical challenges and liability risks, some mammography experts believe the future of mammography lies in telemammography due to the lack of fellowship trained breast imaging specialists throughout the country.

Laser Printer

Although one of the strengths of digital imaging is the ability to make a radiology department "filmless," there may still be times when hardcopy images must be printed from PACS or from the acquisition workstation.

- Currently, accrediting bodies for FFDM, including the ACR, allow clinical images to be submitted in either a printed format or an electronic format; in the future, the printed film option will undoubtedly be discontinued and only electronic filing allowed.
- Not all referring physicians and surgeons are able to access imaging networks or have imaging workstations available for their use. The patient's exam may need to be printed for physicians outside the facility's network.
- When prior images, taken at a different facility, are uploaded into PACS, compatibility issues may arise. If unable to upload the prior exam, a request for printed film images is made.

If a facility chooses to maintain the ability to print films, they are required to have access to a high-resolution laser printer, whether it is located off-site or on the premises (Figure 13-5). According to the FDA, the printed image must be comparable in quality with the image seen on the softcopy review workstation.

When printing FFDM images, there are variables to be aware of:

- **Fit to film**—For convenience and economy, this is the print format of choice. Large and small breasts all fit neatly on an 8- × 10-in. film. However, this can be a prob-

lem when the images are being sent to a surgeon or used as reference during core biopsy because the location of the area of interest is difficult, if not impossible, to measure accurately.
- 1:1—**Pixel to pixel**—The image is printed at 100% of the pixel count at acquisition. Depending on the pixel count, or resolution, of the printer, this can give an image so large that more than one film is required to print each view of the breast. For example, an image acquired on a 70-μm pixel size detector and then printed from a laser printer with a resolution of 40 μm will require approximately twice as much area on the film.
- **True size**—When performing an analog mammogram, the resulting image is a replica of the true size of the patient's breast. The reference points for measurement (nipple and lesion) will be true to scale, so that if a lesion measures 3 cm from the nipple on the film, in reality, it will be 3 cm from the nipple in the breast tissue. Printing a digital image at the true size setting assures that films being used for surgical reference will not confuse the surgeon and cause a biopsy to be performed in the wrong area of the breast. However, just as with analog imaging, the correct size of the hardcopy needs to be chosen in order for all the breast tissue to be included.

WORKING IN THE DIGITAL ENVIRONMENT

FFDM can be overwhelming for physicians, technologists, and support staff. Digital imaging is a heavily computerized paradigm that may seem impossible to learn, especially for the staff that is unfamiliar even with home computing. Physicians, technologists, and administrators need to understand digital technology and to overhaul workflow patterns because of the investment in time to learn this technology and the associated costs of the equipment.

In-house meetings and seminars on FFDM and PACS technology can help a great deal toward staff compliance and enthusiasm. Allow all staff members to contribute ideas regarding workflow—they understand in detail how the facility functions, and their input is invaluable. Always keep them updated on issues, problems, and changes. Technical changes with equipment can happen so quickly that keeping the staff apprised of what is happening can often be overlooked, so make an effort to update communications on a regular basis. When you do receive feedback from the staff, take any relevant information to the vendor. The vendors can use this relevant information to improve their product, and it may help resolve problems with your own equipment.

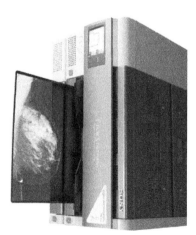

Figure 13-5
The Sony UPDF750 laser printer has the higher resolution necessary for producing hardcopy mammography images but takes up very little space.

Staff Training

Keep in mind that staff members all have varying levels of skill when it comes to using computer equipment. Regardless of their computer literacy when they begin, all will become proficient on the equipment if given adequate training and time to practice. Equipment vendors are a great resource for on-site training. Often, the training is included with the vendor agreement when the equipment is purchased. Additional training can be costly—be sure to negotiate enough training time in your contract to accommodate your facility and all of the technologists and radiologists who need to be trained. It is often wise to negotiate a few revisits from application specialists. This allows the staff time to use the equipment and then have any specific questions or problems addressed.

Ergonomics

Technology also brings about changes in the way we work. For the technologist, there may be less footwork and paperwork involved with digital imaging, but more time is spent using a computer and standing in one room. Depending on the facility, the mammography room may hold not only the x-ray unit and acquisition workstation but possibly also a PACS workstation and a "dashboard" to follow the progress of each patient (Figure 13-6).

Computer workstations need to be fitted to a height that is easy for all of the technologists to use—the short and the tall—and they need to be placed in a location that is easily accessible to the technologist as she works. Common complaints by technologists in the digital mammography world include back pain and sore feet (because they are doing less walking and more standing in one place), carpel tunnel problems (due not only to the repeated wrist movement used for compression but also due to computer typing and mouse clicking), and headache (attributed to concentration on computer monitors).

Similarly, the way the radiologist works has also changed. Rather than using viewboxes, the radiologist now has a panorama of computer screens. The radiologist may continue to have a viewbox adjacent to the computer workstation for reviewing hardcopy images. Important ergonomic considerations for the radiologist's reading area include placement of this equipment to reduce glare on the computer monitors and to reduce neck strain as the radiologist looks at images from one modality and then shifts to the other. Computer screens should be tilted forward slightly to provide depth and perspective to the image. Ambient light should come from behind the monitors. The chair needs to be comfortable for the physician to accommodate his/her height and reduce back strain.

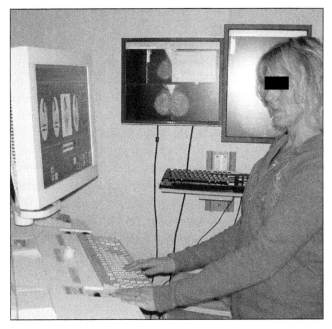

Figure 13-6
The acquisition workstation area can be an ergonomic nightmare for the technologist. Multiple computer monitors for acquisition, PACS access, and patient management are all important tools in the digital environment, but it can be difficult to fit everything into the small spaces usually allotted for mammography.

Establishing a New Workflow

One of the draws of FFDM is being able to image the same number of patients using fewer staff and equipment. Efficiency is the goal; thus, new **workflow** processes are developed.

To optimize the efficiency that FFDM can achieve, changes must be made in the workflow and in the way processes are performed. The best way to avoid any delays or financial pitfalls is to plan for these changes before you face them. First, understand what your current processes are, then figure out how to make those processes more efficient, and, finally, diagram how those can be transitioned to a workflow that will work within the digital technology.

Efficiency: Kaizen

Kaizen is a Japanese philosophy that focuses on continuous improvement throughout all aspects of life. When applied to the workplace, Kaizen activities continually improve all functions of a business, from manufacturing to management and from the CEO to the assembly line workers.[6] By improving standardized activities and processes, Kaizen aims to eliminate waste. Kaizen was first implemented in several Japanese businesses, including Toyota, during the country's recovery after World War II and has since spread to businesses across the world.[7]

The Kaizen philosophy can be applied to any type of business, including health care. Kaizen is a daily activity, the purpose of which goes beyond simple productivity improvement. It is also a process that, when done correctly, humanizes the workplace, eliminates overly hard work, and teaches people how to learn to spot and eliminate waste in business processes. People at all levels of an organization can participate in Kaizen, from the CEO down.

A Kaizen event is a meeting that representatives involved in each part of the process attend, to make improvements that are actually within the participants' ability to change. The event can be held for improvement across the enterprise, a department, or a specific process within a department. Kaizen events are often facilitated by consultants from outside the business who specialize in workflow optimization.

Charting your current workflow gives you perspective to streamline your process. Start from the moment the patient calls to make an appointment, all the way through her visit, how the billing takes place, to the moment the report is sent out to the referring physician. Each step within the entire patient visit should be charted, no matter how menial it might seem (Figure 13-7). Then look at who is performing each task, and how you can make it more efficient. Even the most efficient-appearing facility will find ways to eliminate steps using this process.

Case Study 13-2

1. Refer to Figure 13-7. All businesses must be efficient and productive in order to maintain a margin of profitability. The Kaizen method is one such attempt to streamline workflow efficiency. List some actions that make the mammography service more streamlined.

Creating New Positions

After you chart which employee is doing each job within the process, you will be better able to define how the technology affects each position. Some positions may be phased out, new positions may be created, and other positions will evolve to compensate for the process changes (Figure 13-8).

Choosing a PACS Administrator

Selecting a **PACS administrator** is one of the more important decisions that a facility makes. This person is responsible for making certain that all the images are stored in the PACS correctly and are retrievable, that all the different components within the imaging chain (acquisition, CAD, laser printers, workstations, etc.) work together and are compatible, that archiving and disaster recovery is adequate, and that image production and the flow of the image within the network is accurate and timely.

The PACS administrator is responsible for the operational administration and network management of all PACS servers and workstations. This includes the following functions and activities:

* Daily system monitoring
* Storage media management
* User management
* Network management
* Quality control and performance monitoring
* Study monitoring and patient information management
* Training for new and ongoing users
* Troubleshooting and problem-solving
* Security, including development and monitoring of policies and procedures
* Providing proactive technical administration, planning, coordination, and documentation[8]

Hanging protocols, DICOM compatibility, and importing RIS data—the PACS administrator must be someone who is not only computer literate but knows the processes, workflow, and preferences of the department and its physicians (Figure 13-9).

There are many schools of thought as to what skill level a PACS administrator is required to have to perform the job effectively. There are job description guidelines, but the requirements are primarily up to the PACS administrator's employer. Many PACS administrators have an IT background, but most do not. Many are employees who were promoted to PACS administrator because they exhibited the aptitude and desire to perform these tasks. Some are technologists, but this also is not a prerequisite for the position in most facilities.

There are several PACS certification examinations developed by organizations to help prepare PACS administrators for their new roles. These organizations include PACS Administrators Registry and Certification Association (PARCA) and the Society for Imaging Informatics in Medicine (SIIM).

In addition to the PACS administrator, there is also a need for several PACS "super-users." These employees have enhanced access to the PACS system, though not as much as the administrator. Super-users can set up files within PACS or change settings as needed, on a limited scale. Generally, these users are supervisors within the department.

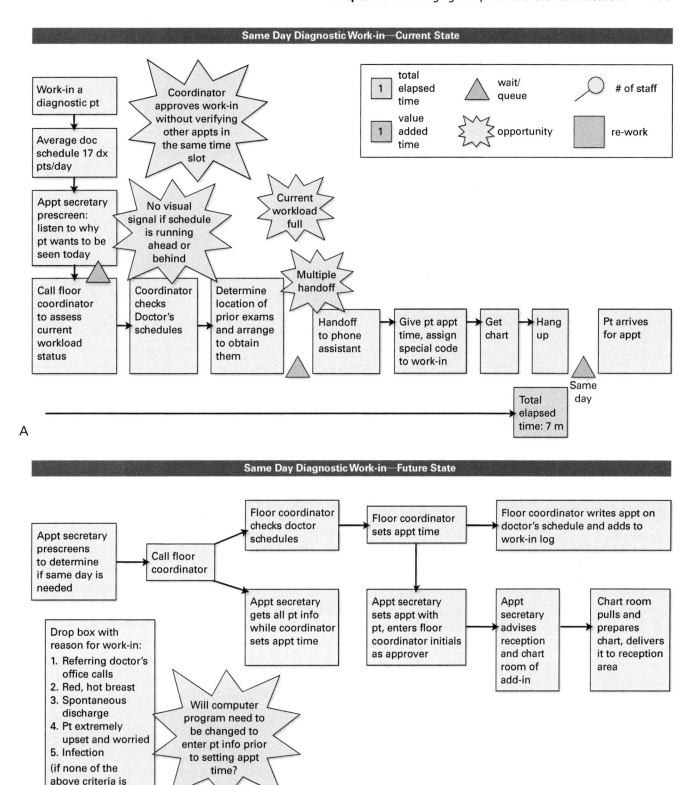

Figure 13-7
An example of charting workflow during a Kaizen event. This event was held to improve the process of working a diagnostic patient into the schedule. Chart A shows the current workflow and areas where time is wasted or the process could be improved. Chart B shows the workflow after the Kaizen team came up with suggestions and solutions to improve the flow.

FFDM (DIGITAL)

APPOINTMENT IS MADE	Patient information put into RIS
	RIS sends information to PACS
PATIENT CHART IS PULLED	PACS prefetches patient EMR and prior digital images from archives, brings them to SAN or NAS server
PATIENT CHECKS IN AT RECEPTION DESK	Patient information added to worklist, making patient EMR available to tech for review
PATIENT TAKEN TO CHANGING ROOM	Updated worklist seen at modality, indicating to tech that patient is ready to be imaged
	Tech reviews prior images and requisition at workstation
IMAGE IS OBTAINED	Tech reviews patient history and takes appropriate images
IMAGE IS PROCESSED	Images are reviewed by tech at acquisition
PATIENT IS RELEASED	Tech sends images to PACS and CAD (if part of facility protocol) from acquisition workstation
IMAGES ARE INTERPRETED	Radiologist pulls up patient file from worklist on diagnostic workstation includes new and prior films
	Report is dictated or entered in computer by MD
CATEGORY ASSIGNED	Recall generated if necessary
REPORT IS SENT	Report is transcribed and sent electronically to radiologist for electronic signature
	Report is automatically faxed, emailed or printed and mailed to referring MDs. Copy is saved in patient EMR
PATIENT CHART IS RE-FILED	Patient name removed from all worklists, patient data sent to archives.

Figure 13-8
Workflow chart comparing steps taken during an FFDM examination.

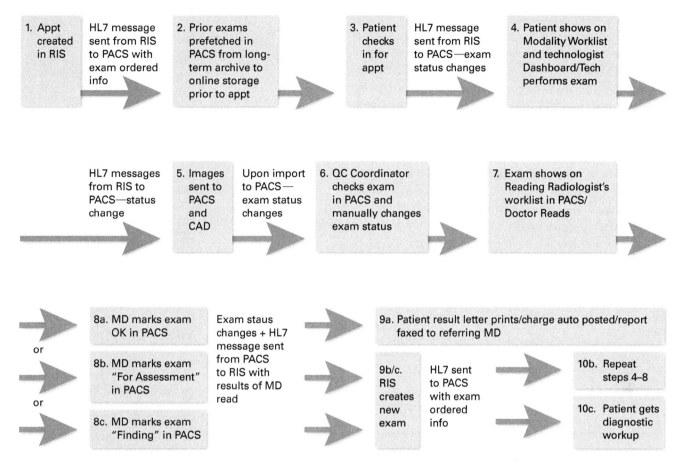

Figure 13-9
Representation of the RIS–PACS workflow that is the responsibility of the PACS administrator.

▌▌▌ DOWNTIME ISSUES AND TROUBLESHOOTING

At some point, service issues will arise. FFDM technology is relatively new, and the issues that occur are sometimes unprecedented and unfamiliar to technologists and service personnel. As the technology matures, these issues arise less frequently, but are still not uncommon.

When looking at your digital workflow, be sure to take into account potential problems that may come up. When a mammography machine is first installed, there are usually a few difficulties that need to be resolved. Networking problems, DICOM compatibility issues, licensing issues, software problems, and electronic component glitches are just some of the many surprises that can be waiting around the corner. The more complicated the machinery and electronics, the more things there are likely to go wrong. At this point, most FFDM machine manufacturers have worked out the major bugs in their equipment so installation problems are less likely to occur. Purchasing equipment that is suited to the facility's networking, PACS, and the infrastructure that is already in place

will make a difference to the ease of installation. Be sure to specify these items in your RFP before purchasing equipment.

As the staff becomes familiar with the equipment, downtime becomes less of an issue. Be aware that initially productivity will not be as much as the vendor promised; there is always a learning curve as technologists and radiologists familiarize themselves with the full potential of the new equipment. As with any equipment, there will be error codes to deal with and occasions when the operator's manual isn't enough to solve an issue.

Most vendors provide a "help desk" phone number that connects you with service personnel who can answer your questions and talk you through an equipment problem. Often, this is all that is needed to correct a problem and get the machine operational again. Some manufacturers offer a service where they can connect into your equipment online and perform some service operations through this remote access. If this fails, they may need to send a service engineer to your facility, especially if the issue is related to hardware, such as a defect in the grid, detector, or x-ray tube.

The resources vendors offer vary greatly, as can differing levels of service contracts within the same vendor's options. Be sure to consider the service options carefully when purchasing FFDM equipment. Also, be aware that some vendors offer better help desks than others. Ask the vendor how their service and help is structured, because you will probably rely on it a lot, especially during the first year with the new equipment. Find out if you are connected to a live person when you call or if you must leave a message and wait for them to call you back. Find out the origin of the service; if you are located on the East coast, will you need to wait until 11:00 AM for a service representative from the West coast to call you back?

Equipment service is an important issue that should be addressed before the equipment is installed. Installation itself may be a factor to consider:

* Is there a need for architectural changes to the department or the room where the machine will be placed?
* Are the necessary electrical requirements already in place?
* Is there a need to make changes to the existing HV/AC system to accommodate the heat load given off by the FFDM machine or the radiologist's reviewstation?

Consider these issues before the machine is delivered to avoid downtime from postponement of installation.

Service

Once FFDM equipment is purchased, it must be properly maintained in order to consistently produce quality images. New equipment comes with a warranty, but after that first year of free service, the equipment must continue to be maintained. A service contract for FFDM equipment is costly. Without a service contract, repairs can be difficult and expensive. Without a service contract, noncovered equipment will be last on the list for a service call, and when service engineers arrive, it is more expensive to pay by the hour, and parts are more expensive. Additionally, downtime means loss of revenue; it is important to keep the equipment working so that patients continue to be imaged without interruption.

The cost of replacement parts for FFDM machines is very expensive; to replace a defective digital detector could cost more than $45,000. Additionally, when you purchase a service contract from the manufacturer, you can be sure that your software will be upgraded as new versions become available. Service calls are answered promptly and often can be handled online, with the service personnel accessing your equipment and fixing problems without even stepping into your facility.

Review Questions

1. Workstations used by radiologists and technologists vary. Discuss how the function of each workstation might affect the workflow and image quality.

2. Discuss the differences between online, near-line, and offline storage.

3. Discuss how bandwidth can affect workflow within a facility.

References

1. Rush B. *The Impact of New Technologies, Imaging Economics*. Available at: http://www.imagingeconomics.com/issues/articles/2003-10_17.asp. Accessed October 17, 2003.
2. Ishiyama M, et al. Comparison of reading time between screen-film mammography and soft-copied, full-field digital mammography. *Breast Cancer*. 2009;16(1).
3. D'Orsi CJ. 1–26 Follow-up and final results of the Oslo I study comparing screen-film mammography and full-field digital mammography with soft-copy reading. *Breast Dis*. 2007;18(1):56–57.
4. Oosterwijk H. *PACS Fundamentals*. Dallas, Texas: OTech, Inc.; 2004.
5. Andolina V, Wade T. *Digital Mammography—A How-To Manual for Seamless Implementation*. Marblehead, MA: HCPro, Inc.; 2006:49.
6. Imai M. *Kaizen: The Key to Japan's Competitive Success*. New York: Random House; 1986.
7. Europe Japan Centre. In: Colenso M, ed. *Kaizen Strategies for Improving Team Performance*. London, UK: Pearson Education Limited; 2000.
8. Radiology PACS Administrators Website. Available at: http://www.pacsadminforum.com/Job%20Description/Pacs_Admin_Job_Desc.html. Accessed November 29, 2016.

Bibliography

Dreyer K, et al. *PACS: A Guide to the Digital Revolution*. 2nd ed. New York: Springer; 2006.

FDA. *MQSA Final Regulations, Policy Guidance Help System*. Silver Spring, MD: FDA; 2014.

Oosterwijk H. *PACS Fundamentals*. Dallas, TX: OTech, Inc.; 2004.

Orenstein BW. Eight keys to digital mammography success. *Radiol Today*. 2007;7(19):30.

Page D. Teleradiologists tap neglected long-distance breast imaging; December 2007. Available at http://www.diagnosticimaging.com/display/article/113619/1189067

Trambert M. Digital mammography integrated with PACS: real world issues, considerations, workflow solutions, and reading paradigms. *Semin Breast Dis*. 2006;9:75–81.

Digital Breast Tomosynthesis (DBT)

14

Objectives

- To compare DBT to earlier methods of imaging using 2D mammography
- To understand how DBT imaging is performed
- To examine the benefits of 3D imaging for mammography
- To review current requirements for DBT

Key Terms

- 2D
- 3D
- combo mode
- lossless compression
- modality-specific training

- projection
- reconstruction
- synthesized 2D image
- superimposition
- tomosynthesis

▮▮ INTRODUCTION

The transition from analog imaging to digital imaging in mammography took approximately 17 years: 2000 to 2016 (Table 14-1). This 17-year sojourn gave us our first hint of the future: using the digital platform to perform **3D** imaging of the breast. Digital breast **tomosynthesis** (DBT), also known as 3D mammography, is remarkable technology.

Breast imaging began in 1924 as grainy, low-contrast, gray-scale **2D** film images; a mere 87 years later, we have this phenomenal quasi-3D imaging capability. Although in its infancy, having gained FDA approval in 2011, DBT already leads to further technological progression: functional-based imaging techniques using the tomosynthesis platform. Future disease detection possibilities seem endless. We are excited and grateful for every imaging improvement along the way and see even more progress in the future.

The authors fantasize about what breast disease detection methods will encompass when we reach the end of our working careers; our crystal ball shows us using radiation combined with a contrast agent to create some type of image, perhaps incorporating breast restraint versus breast compression. The authors are grateful to the visionaries who relentlessly pursue new technologies that prove effective for discovery of disease:

- at an earlier stage of development
- when treatments are more effective and more tolerable for the patient
- and that increase long-term survival

DBT in a Nutshell

During acquisition of the DBT scan, the x-ray tube moves in an arc across the breast. The mammography machine acquires x-ray exposures, known as projections, at multiple angles throughout the arc of travel; the projection exposures are then reconstructed into a series of cross-sectional images that can be displayed rapidly, similar to a cine' movie. The computer reconstructs an image of the breast in height planes, much the same way a CT or MRI scan does. The DBT scan helps discern if an ROI is truly a significant finding.

DBT is a screening tool and a diagnostic device and is also used to perform interventional procedures. By far, its greatest impact is in the screening environment where improved sensitivity combined with a reduction in recalls of patients for additional views is a remarkable combination.[1–4] The use of DBT is shown to increase lesion and margin visibility and yield a 10% to 54% increase in invasive cancer detection, an 18% decrease in stage diagnosis from stage 2–4 to stage 1, and a reduction of 15% to 37% in false-positive findings that lead to recalling patients for additional imaging.[5,6] Skaane et al.[7] studied a mixture of breast densities to compare 2D FFDM versus DBT. This study reports a 40% increase in invasive cancer detection with DBT and a 27% increase in overall cancer detection, yet the false-positive rate decreased by 15%.

Several studies evaluate the ability of DBT to find invasive versus noninvasive cancers:

- Skaane et al.[7] report a 40% increase with invasive cancers and no increase with noninvasive.
- Ciatto et al.[8] report a 50% increase with invasive cancers and no increase with noninvasive.
- Rose et al.[9] report a 53% increase with invasive cancers and no increase with noninvasive cancers.

Although the studies do not show an increase in detection of noninvasive cancers, they do demonstrate a 40% to 53% increase in invasive cancers detected with DBT over 2D FFDM. Cancers not identified on a 2D FFDM exam will continue to grow, with treatment of this disease at a more

Table 14-1 • Transition from Analog to FFDM: Difference

YEAR	TOTAL	ANALOG	FFDM	DIFFERENCE
2003	13,645	13,189	465	291
2004	13,659	12,903	756	364
2005	13,635	12,515	1,120	843
2006	13,601	11,638	1,963	1,842
2007	13,608	9,803	3,805	2,247
2008	13,293	7,241	6,052	1,592
2009	12,727	5,083	7,644	1,313
2010	12,412	3,455	8,957	1,160
2011	12,287	2,170	10,117	952
2012	12,471	1,402	11,069	1,126
2013	13,109	914	12,195	1,069
2014	13,844	580	13,264	1,734
2015	15,357	359	14,998	1,736
2016	16,959	225	16,734	

The gradual replacement of analog mammography machines with 2D FFDM machines. By the end of 2016, virtually all mammography machines are digital, whether 2D or 3D.

advanced state placing a heavier burden for recovery on the patient. 3D offers the potential to find invasive cancers earlier. Earlier is always better.

Detection of our nemesis, invasive lobular carcinoma (ILC), has been reported with DBT. Detection of ILC is significantly higher with DBT, especially in the glandular breast. 2D FFDM is more than twice as likely to miss ILC in a glandular breast than when imaged with DBT.[10]

TRANSITION

History repeats itself: out with the old, in with the new. Our transition from film to screen-film, from screen-film to 2D FFDM, and from 2D FFDM to DBT all follow the same pathway.

Technologist Transition

For the 2D FFDM technologist, the transition to DBT is quite simple.

1. Mammography machine
   Companies that manufacture 2D FFDM machines also manufacture DBT machines. In fact one manufacturer (GE) currently attaches an accessory package onto their 2D FFDM machine to convert it into a DBT machine; this configuration will likely be phased out as dedicated DBT units proliferate and 2D FFDM machines are phased out of production. History repeats itself: the ceiling-mounted x-ray tube and x-ray table (1924) gave way to a dedicated analog mammography machine; the analog machine (1965) is replaced by 2D FFDM equipment; and now 2D FFDM (2000) is being replaced by a DBT machine (2011) (Figure 14-1).

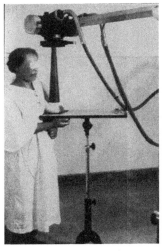

ceiling mounted
x-ray machine (1924)

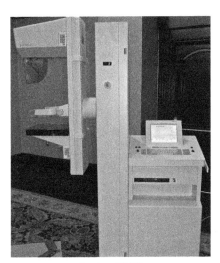

Analog (1965)

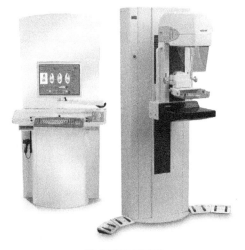

2D FFDM (2000)

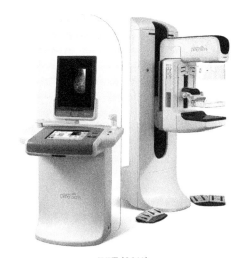

DBT (2011)

Figure 14-1
Mammography begins in 1924 with the one and only ceiling-mounted x-ray machine. In 1965, the first dedicated mammography machine is manufactured; direct exposure film is initially used as a recording system but is replaced in 1972 with a screen-film cassette. 2D FFDM arrives on the scene in January 2000, closely followed by DBT in February 2011.

Due to using these similarly designed machines for decades, technologists are familiar with operation of the control functions of the equipment: foot pedals to raise/lower the C-arm and compression device, hand control features, exposure buttons or levers, etc. However, there are differences between the earlier machines and DBT machines; operation of the AWS software is the "new" part of the equipment technologists have to learn. The DBT acquisition workstation monitor display is a modification of the 2D FFDM version, so it retains many familiar operational practices, but there are new features (Figure 14-2).

2. Positioning and compression

Positioning and applying compression to the breast in DBT is currently the same application as in 2D FFDM. Refer to the section later in this chapter on compression for a more comprehensive discussion about this controversial topic. For now, it is safe to say that compression remains the same whether acquiring a 2D FFDM or a DBT image.

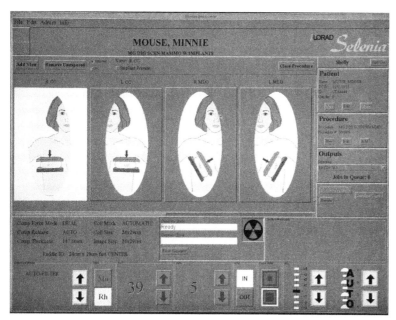

2D FFDM

DBT

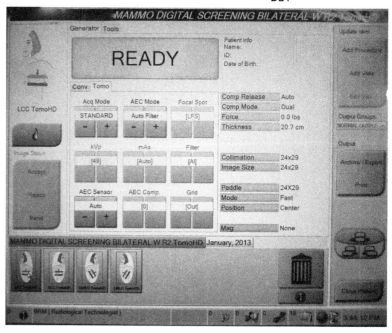

Figure 14-2

The digital mammography machine is computer operated and controlled. The technologist who operates a 2D FFDM machine transitions easily to a DBT machine. Basic computer functions are inherent to all computers.

3. X-ray exposure

Initiation of the x-ray exposure remains the same for 2D FFDM and DBT. X-ray tube target and filtration combinations may have changed, but we continue to photo-time, which allows the computer to select appropriate target and filter combinations, kVp settings, and mAs values (Figure 14-3).

4. Image processing

Upon termination of the x-ray exposure, 2D FFDM and DBT technologist behavior remains the same: critique the image for radiographic landmarks associated with proper positioning and compression, and examine the image for motion artifact. 2D FFDM and DBT post-exposure image processing by the mammography machine computer is inherently different; however, this function does not involve the technologist. Each mammography machine computer performs its own unique image processing task: 2D FFDM generates a 2D image, while DBT creates a 3D set of cross-sectional images.

5. Image display

Technologists utilize the AWS computer monitor to assess the quality of the image for proper positioning, compression, and motion. When the image is considered acceptable, it is sent to PACS for permanent storage and to the radiologist for interpretation. This function is the same for 2D FFDM and DBT.

For the mammography technologist, the change from 2D FFDM to DBT is simple and straightforward:

• The C-arm and its operation remains the same.
• Become familiar with new computer software functions at the AWS in order to acquire the DBT scan.

Modality-Specific Training

MQSA mandates technologists must have 8 hours of **modality-specific training** in DBT, although we (the authors) are hard-pressed to find enough material to fill an

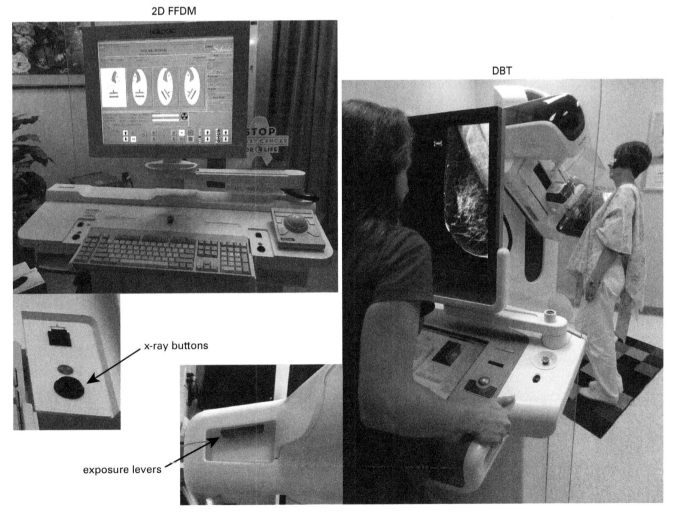

Figure 14-3
2D FFDM and DBT machines share a common legacy. C-arm functions, patient positioning and compression, initiating the phototimed exposure, and evaluation of the resulting image are very similar whether performing 2D FFDM or DBT exams.

8-hour seminar syllabus because there are not many changes for the technologist who transitions from 2D FFDM to DBT imaging.

When MQSA took effect in 1994, the technologist had to have 8 hours of modality-specific training in screen/film imaging. In January 2000, FDA granted approval to GE for the first 2D FFDM system; FDA mandated technologists must have 8 hours of modality-specific training in 2D FFDM before they can independently perform exams. The same 8-hour requirement holds for DBT. History repeats itself.

Years of Transition: 2D FFDM to DBT

When FDA approved the first 2D FFDM system in January 2000, the death knell for analog imaging and the darkroom sounded. It took approximately 17 years for the United States to complete the transition from analog to digital imaging. A major contributing factor for the long period to change was cost. Change is expensive. Every facility, large or small, has to consider a major impact to their budget to update their mammography service operations. Mammography services of every size need to purchase a new 2D FFDM machine, dismantle the darkroom, replace the film library with PACS, increase broadband access, and make other physical changes related to introduction of the new digital machine: PACS workstations for the technologists, scanners to import paperwork into PACS; purchase a CD burner and laser film printer; and repaint the mammography room.

Our patients become the driving force for change. This part of personal life had already changed for them in the 1990s: digital cameras replaced their old roll of film cameras. Vacations, parties, and family gatherings are no longer captured on rolls of film and stored in photograph albums; instead, these precious and valuable personal memories are now captured by a filmless camera and the digital images are stored in the cloud. Either old photographs are packed into a box destined for a closet or attic or they are converted and saved in a digital format. The patients understand the benefits derived from new technology; they either read or hear about the new filmless technology for mammograms. They have their imaging done at mammography facilities that offer the new and improved digital service.

A New Reality: Things Change

With the results of the ACRIN/DMIST study published in September 2005, the technical and clinical advantages of the newer 2D FFDM technology versus the older analog technology are settled; mammography facilities must provide the new preferred clinical service or withdraw from that marketplace. Once the first 2D FFDM machine is installed in a facility in a city, competitor facilities are under financial pressure to follow suit or lose patients to that facility.

Women seek and use more medical services than do men; they drive the economics for a medical facility's well-being: when family members need radiology services, they go to the same facility where Mom has her mammogram. When new and significant improvements associated with breast imaging occur, women prefer and demand these updated services. The new reality is that mammography services have shorter time frames to update in order for the facility to stay competitive.

- 1924, the first mammogram performed
- 1965, the first dedicated mammography machine
- 1972, screen-film mammography introduced
- 2000, 2D FFDM approved by FDA
- 2011, DBT approved by FDA

Many in the mammography community have hope we will go directly from analog imaging to DBT, but this transition takes longer than expected. 2D FFDM is initially considered "a stepping stone, a bridge to cross over" from analog mammography to DBT. We did not expect it would take 11 years (2000 to 2011) to cross the bridge.

The replacement of analog mammography machines with the five to six times more expensive 2D FFDM counterpart happens slowly. Two landmark events cause this delay.

1. ACRIN/DMIST
   2D FFDM is approved in January 2000. Many mammography facilities delay replacement of their analog machines until the ACRIN/DMIST results are published, or they delay replacement with the expectation FDA approval of DBT is immanent. Why replace an analog machine with an expensive 2D FFDM machine, only to soon replace it with a more expensive DBT machine?

   Until the results of ACRIN/DMIST are published in September 2005, only 100 2D FFDM machines per year are sold in the United States. Prudent business managers delay replacement of their analog machine, hoping to replace it with a DBT machine. As time marches on, with no approval for DBT by the FDA, facilities trying to be fiscally prudent delay the purchase of new equipment until forced into action by a competitor facility that is the first in their marketplace to offer services.

2. The Great Recession
   In December 2007, the economy suddenly contracts; recession immobilizes the nation. For the first time ever, The Fed "breaks the buck," reminiscent of the great economic depression in the 1930s. A run on the

Table 14-2 • Transition from Analog to FFDM

YEAR	TOTAL	ANALOG	FFDM
2003	13,645	13,189	465
2004	13,659	12,903	756
2005	13,635	12,515	1,120
2006	13,601	11,638	1,963
2007	13,608	9,803	3,805
2008	13,293	7,241	6,052
2009	12,727	5,083	7,644
2010	12,412	3,455	8,957
2011	12,287	2,170	10,117
2012	12,471	1,402	11,069
2013	13,109	914	12,195
2014	13,844	580	13,264
2015	15,357	359	14,998
2016	16,959	225	16,734

The Great Recession wreaks havoc in all aspects of the economy, right down to purchase of a mammography machine. Sales of digital mammography machines climb steadily until the Recession of 2008. 2011 is the low point with fewer than 1,000 digital machines sold that year. As the economy slowly improves, so do sales of mammography machines.

banks, companies shed employees, mortgage lending grinds to a near halt, and everyone cinches their belt tightly. Economic rebound does not happen until 2014. Tightly controlled government policies tend to favor and preserve a slower and steadily improving economy.

Speculation: If the economy had not experienced such a sudden and violent contraction, would the acceptance of DBT as a replacement of analog imaging and 2D FFDM have occurred sooner? See Table 14-2.

In February 2011, FDA finally approves DBT. At this time, the new mammography machine is two to three times more expensive than 2D FFDM; upgrades to PACS are required; broadband capacity must expand; unless the facility has a radiologist reviewstation made by the DBT manufacturer, purchase or lease of a compatible computer system is required; and radiologists must learn a new set of skills: how to interpret the DBT scan.

Between 2011 and 2014, sales for the more expensive DBT units progress on a slow upward trajectory. By mid-2014, clinical acceptance and demand skyrocket for the newer technology. Manufacturers must ramp up quickly to keep pace with the increased demand from the medical community and from patients.

Patient Selection and Management

The transition from older technology to new takes time. The transition years, when facilities exchange their 2D FFDM machines for DBT machines, follow the same historical pathway as when we transitioned from analog machines to 2D FFDM machines. For example, a facility has five older technology machines. They cannot afford to

replace all five machines at once so the new machines are phased in, one at a time.

Until all the older technology mammography machines at a facility are replaced with the newer DBT machines, a process must be in place to determine which patients are taken into the 2D FFDM room and which are selected for the DBT room. When all the 2D FFDM machines are replaced by DBT machines, patient triage is no longer necessary.

Factors to consider for patient triage into either a 2D FFDM room or a DBT room:

- Greatest benefit
  ○ DBT's greatest benefit is in the screening environment. Patient throughput in the screening environment results in a larger volume of patient exams. With an approximate 40% reduction in recalls for additional views of a ROI, DBT reduces the number of diagnostic exams. Diagnostic exams require a longer appointment time; reducing the number of diagnostic exams frees up more time for screening appointments.
- Dense breast
  ○ DBT is more effective in finding disease in the glandular breast. Women with dense breast tissue benefit the most from a DBT exam.[7,8,11–15]

When there are more patients scheduled than can be accommodated on a DBT machine, an additional triage system must be in place to determine who is imaged in the new DBT room and which patients are imaged in the 2D FFDM room.

- Next available
  ○ As a technologist escorts her patient toward the mammography room, if the DBT room is not in use, she directs the patient into this room.
- Schedule DBT exam time
  ○ If a patient specifically requests a DBT exam, a scheduled appointment time ensures she is imaged in that room.
- Triage patients
  ○ Patients with adipose breast tissue (BIRADS A and B) are imaged in the 2D FFDM room. Patients with heterogeneously dense or radiographically dense breast tissue (BIRADS C and D) are imaged in the DBT room.

▮▮ DBT: WHO, WHAT, WHERE, WHEN

Concept: 2D versus 3D

From 1924 to 2011, the three-dimensional breast is imaged with two-dimensional x-ray images, thus the need to perform multiple projections of each breast. Film,

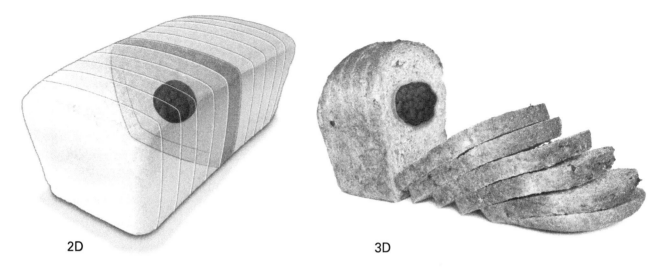

2D   3D

Figure 14-4
A comparison is made between a loaf of bread and a breast. A cancer is in the geographic center of the bread/breast. 2D: bread/breast tissue completely surrounds the cancer. It does not matter how we position the loaf of bread/breast, superimposition always impedes visualization of the cancer. (Modified from Shutterstock.) 3D: slice the loaf of bread and examine each slice individually. The cancer is readily apparent when the one slice of bread containing the cancer is examined. DBT permits visualization of individual height planes (slices) of tissue. (Modified from Shutterstock, Inc.)

xeromammography, screen-film imaging, and 2D FFDM all require multiple projections for a complete clinical exam.

3D imaging does not have the same constraints as 2D. Refer to Figure 14-4. Consider the loaf of bread is a "breast." If a cancer is placed in the exact geographic center of the loaf (top to bottom, end to end, and side to side), it is difficult to visualize the cancer with two-dimensional imaging due to **superimposition** of the "bread/tissue" that surrounds it. It does not matter whether we image the loaf in the CC projection, MLO, FB, Lateral—the image always has the issue of superimposition. The thicker the breast (or loaf of bread) surrounding the cancer, the greater the likelihood for superimposed structures.

Let us "slice" the loaf of bread; in essence, this is what DBT imaging does to the breast. We now examine each individual slice of our loaf of bread, one at a time. Eventually, we arrive at the one slice in which the cancer is located. We

can readily view the cancer because now there is no bread on top of, beneath, or on either side (Figure 14-5).

In 2D imaging, the thicker the breast, the more tissue there is to superimpose on the cancer, making it more difficult to see. With 3D imaging, since we examine each height plane individually (look at each slice of the loaf of bread, one at a time), the thickness of the compressed breast is immaterial (Figure 14-6).

Case Study **14-2**

Refer to Figure 14-5. How do 3D images differ from 2D images?

Case Study **14-3**

Refer to Figure 14-6. What are projection images? Reconstructed images?

Case Study **14-1**

Refer to Figure 14-4. Describe DBT in a nutshell: how does the mammography machine acquire x-ray images; how are x-ray exposures processed and displayed; what are appropriate uses for DBT (e.g., screening/diagnostic/interventional procedures) and which provides the greatest benefit?

Our breasts are three dimensional, while images such as photographs and x-rays are two-dimensional representations. Refer to Figure 14-7. In the CC projection, the implants appear to be normal. The MLO projection demonstrates a vertical herniation of the implant. If the woman has a 3D exam, the herniation is evident on the scan in the CC projection.

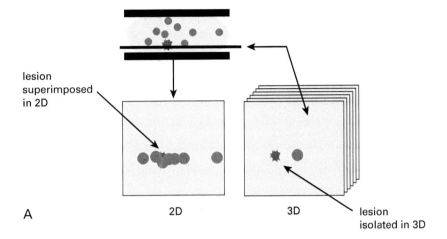

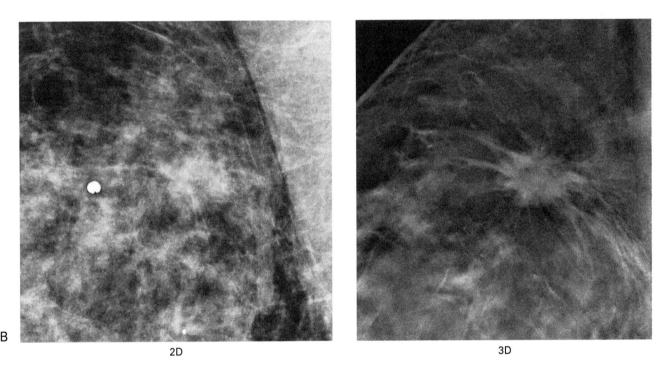

Figure 14-5
Tomosynthesis is a three-dimensional mammographic examination that can minimize the effects of structure overlap within the breast. **(A)** 2D imaging visualizes all height planes on top of as well as underneath one another, while 3D views one height plane at a time. Only the structures located at that height plane are visible; structures located in other height planes misregister or are blurred out. (Adapted from Hologic, Inc., and affiliates.) **(B)** An example of the clarity of 3D imaging. (Images courtesy of Hologic, Inc. and affiliates.)

What Is DBT?

What is DBT? There are three answers; all are related and intertwined because DBT relies on a different mechanical device and image presentation to provide a 3D anatomical view of the breast for medical diagnosis.

1. DBT is currently one of the best ways to view, detect, and determine the exact location of cancer in breast tissue.
2. The x-ray tube moves in an arc to capture a series of sequential images. The information displays in individual height planes (like slices in a loaf of bread).

3. For medical physicists and technologists, the transition into DBT is quick and simple. It is the radiologist who encounters a learning curve with this new technology. Basic tenets of 2D interpretation may/may not hold true in 3D imaging. It takes several months for the radiologist to become accustomed to the presentation of a 3D image.

In 2D FFDM imaging, the x-ray tube remains stationary, positioned directly above the breast. In DBT, the x-ray tube sweeps in an arc across the breast (Figure 14-8): from side to side in the CC projection and from superior

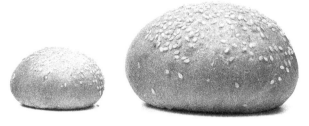

Figure 14-6
Slice both the loaf of bread and a roll into 1-mm-thick slices; the thicker loaf of bread is composed of more individual slices than is the thinner roll. There is more tissue to superimpose with a thicker breast imaged with 2D. 3D is not impacted by a thicker or thinner breast because each height plane (slice) is viewed individually. (Image from Shutterstock, Inc.)

to inferior in the angled projection. As the x-ray tube travels along the arc, a series of exposures (**projection** images) are taken. A computer then reconstructs the multiple exposures into images that are viewed as individual height planes or, more likely, scanned as a set of images similar to a cine' movie (**reconstruction** images).

While movement of the DBT x-ray tube is reminiscent of a kidney IVP tomogram, the kidney images are low resolution, while the DBT images are high-resolution images

that surpass the quality of CT and MRI scans. All DBT equipment manufacturers currently move the x-ray tube in an arc across the breast. This does not preclude future designs from scanning in different patterns.

Is There a Need for DBT?

In 2D imaging, there will always be tissue overlap of normal structures. These structures (e.g., fibroglandular elements, blood vessels, suspensory ligaments) are scatted throughout the breast and at differing height planes. The thicker breast has more tissue in which superimposition can occur (Figure 14-9).

It is easy for cancers, large or small, to become "invisible" among the structure noise in a 2D FFDM image (Figures 14-10 and 14-11). Conversely, tissue overlap can produce the opposite effect: instead of a cancer hiding in normal tissue, making it more difficult to see, overlap of normal breast structures can appear to be a cancer. Frequently, when a woman returns for additional imaging, the subsequent exam demonstrates what appears to be a cancer is due to fortuitous superimposition of structures[16] (Figure 14-12).

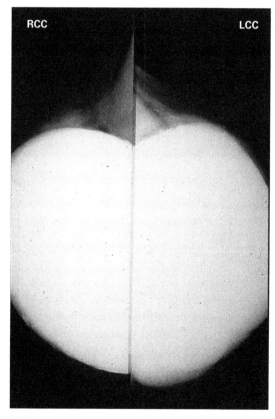
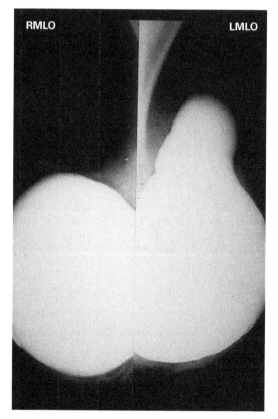

Figure 14-7
The left breast implant has a large herniation visible in the MLO projection. Even in retrospect, the herniation is not readily apparent on the CC projection. If 3D imaging were done, the herniation will be appreciated in the CC projection.

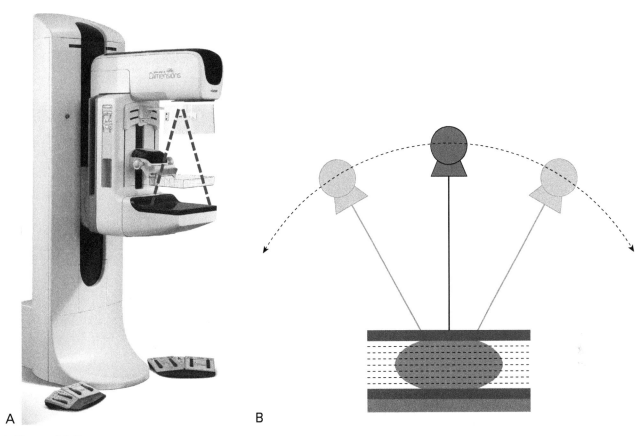

Figure 14-8
2D geometry versus 3D acquisition. **(A)** A single x-ray exposure captures a single image of the breast with 2D imaging. The x-ray tube remains stationary, in a neutral position. **(B)** 3D image acquisition occurs as the x-ray tube moves in an arc across the breast. Multiple exposures are made as the tube travels throughout the angular range.

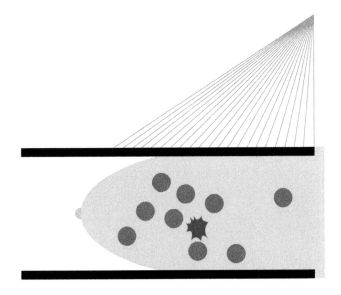

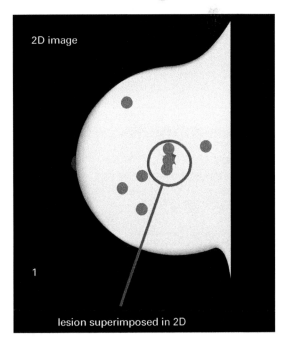

Figure 14-9
With 2D imaging, cancers can "hide" among the anatomic structure noise inherent in breast tissue. The thicker the breast, the more tissue there is to superimpose on top of or underneath a cancer, obscuring visibility. Conversely, normal structures can easily summate and look like a cancer. (Adapted from Hologic, Inc., and affiliates.)

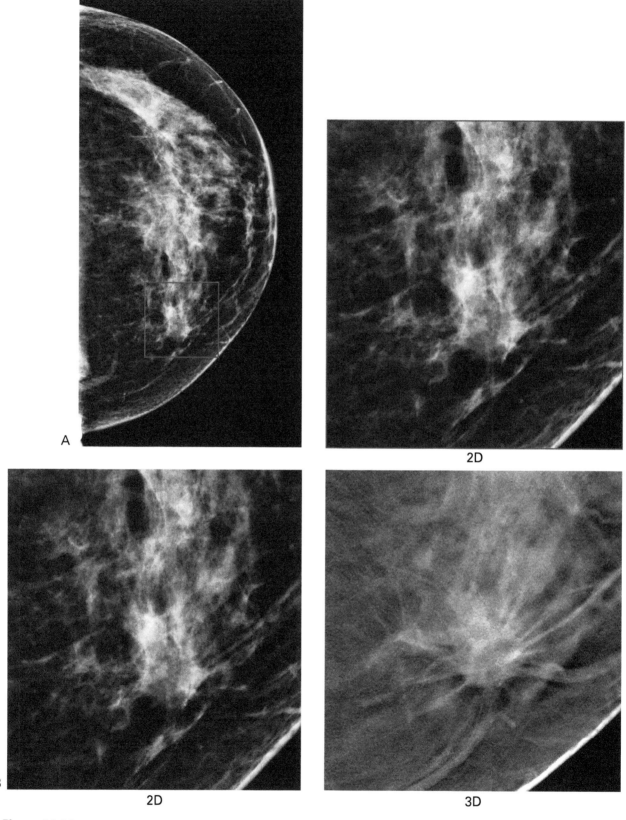

Figure 14-10
2D versus 3D visualization. **(A)** A cancer viewed in 2D, with normal structures slightly obscuring the cancer. (Images courtesy of Hologic, Inc. and affiliates.) **(B)** The cancer is clearly seen on the 3D image. Viewing a single height plane negates superimposition. (Images courtesy of Hologic, Inc. and affiliates.)

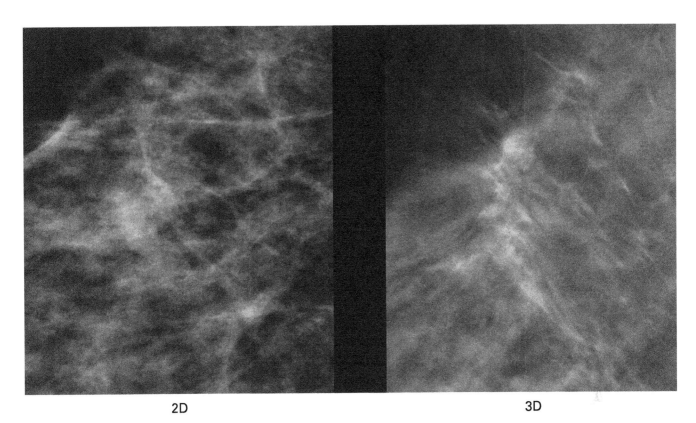

2D   3D

Figure 14-11
An example of the clarity of a cancer with architectural distortion imaged in 3D compared to 2D. (Image courtesy of Hologic, Inc. and affiliates.)

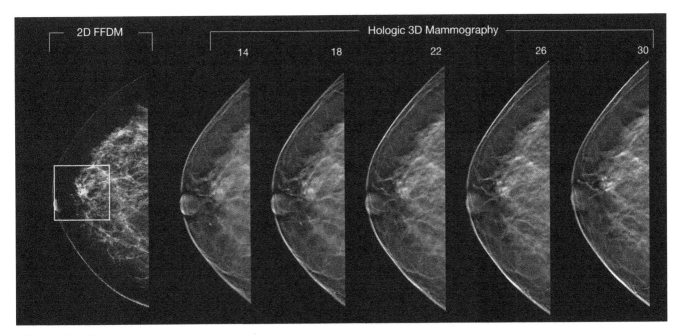

Figure 14-12
Structures converge in the retroareolar region, making this part of the breast prone to summation artifact. Eighty percent of additional images are done for benign summation of structures. (Image courtesy of Hologic, Inc. and affiliates.)

A study by Haas et al.[14] screened 13,000 patients, comparing 2D FFDM with DBT. This study shows a decrease in recall rates for all breast density groups with DBT imaging:

- Fatty: 31% reduction
- Scattered fibroglandular: 25% reduction
- Heterogeneously dense: 39% reduction
- Extremely dense: 57% reduction.

DBT decreases the need for diagnostic exams, thereby allowing these longer appointment slots to convert to screening time slots. In addition, radiologists are faster interpreting screening exams than diagnostic; a reduction in diagnostic exams and an increase in screening exams increases their productivity.

DBT Strengths

Breast cancers typically present one of two ways: approximately 40% exhibit microcalcifications, while the majority present as a mass with or without architectural distortion. Both microcalcification and mass cancers appear white on a mammogram. Finding a "white" cancer in a breast with fibroglandular tissue, which displays white on a mammogram, is challenging. Statistics report missed cancers in the radiographically dense breast range between 52% and 76%; this study utilized analog imaging.[17]

The results of the ACRIN/DMIST study proved digital mammography, with a dynamic range of 16,384 shades of gray, is significantly better than analog imaging, with 100 shades of gray, at imaging the breast containing fibroglandular tissue. 2D FFDM and DBT utilize this wide dynamic range; 16,384 shades of gray provide greater contrast resolution. The ACRIN/DMIST study proved 2D FFDM is better at imaging the breast containing fibroglandular tissue; however, this study did not report an increase in the detection of cancers; analog and 2D FFDM both miss 15% of cancers. The ability to find more cancers happened when FDA approved DBT. The combination of the vast dynamic range of digital mammography plus viewing individual height planes of tissue free of superimposition is a technologic advancement in breast cancer detection.

It has long been recognized that DBT improves detection of mass lesions. Viewing a single height plane of breast tissue at a time cancels out structural noise; the result is improved visualization of lesions. This is especially true when viewing a radiographically dense breast where the fibroglandular tissue displays white on the mammogram, and breast cancers also image as white. The ability of DBT to scroll through the breast in 0.5 or 1 mm height plane thicknesses negates the problem of structure superimposition. Mass cancers tend to be taller than wide; radiologists look for vertical structures. A study by Rafferty et al.[18] reports a 2× to 3× increase in cancer detection in the dense breast. This study compares 2D FFDM versus the combo mode of DBT. Fifty-four percent of cancers found with DBT have dense breast tissue versus 21% of cancers found with 2D FFDM only.[19]

Unexpected Benefit

During the transition years, many decisions are made about triage for patients into either a 2D FFDM room or the room with the new DBT machine. When DBT cannot be offered to all patients, initial decisions are made based on which patients benefit most from a DBT exam. The popular consensus is that radiographically dense breasts benefit most. Thus, fatty replaced breasts are generally assigned to the 2D FFDM room.

As DBT machines completely replace 2D FFDM machines, DBT becomes the standard of care for all patients; thus fatty replaced breasts now routinely undergo DBT. Interpreting radiologists are shocked to discover DBT finds unsuspected cancers in breasts where cancer "can't hide"[1,12,13] (Figure 14-13).

DBT is very good at finding noncalcified breast cancer in scattered and heterogeneously dense breast tissue. Seventy percent of cancers in these tissue types are seen only or better with DBT. Patients with fatty and those with extremely dense tissue have cancers seen slightly better[1] or seen equally well with DBT.[13]

Can DBT Find Cancers that Calcify?

Question: Can DBT find cancers that calcify? Answer: yes, but DBT technology employs minor adjustments to view calcifying lesions.

The radiologist interprets calcifications based on:

1. Morphology: the shape of calcifications
2. Distribution: diffuse, clustered, regional, or linear pattern
3. Time: stability or change over time

Both 2D FFDM and DBT are able to evaluate the morphology and stability of calcifications. DBT's dilemma is with distribution. 2D imaging readily permits the evaluation of calcifications based on their distribution;

2D provides the radiologist with the ability to evaluate a volume of tissue to ascertain whether calcifications are tightly grouped or clustered and to view the ominous linear pattern. DBT, on the other hand, makes the evaluation of clustered and linear calcifications more difficult (Figure 14-14).

Whether viewing the DBT cine' movie or viewing each height plane individually, the evaluation of calcifications as a cluster or in a linear pattern is difficult due to the thinness of the individual height planes. When calcifications are identified on a DBT exam, the radiologist either corroborates with the 2D image or (s)he views several DBT height planes simultaneously; this process is called "slabbing" (Figure 14-15).

The slabbing technique takes several adjacent individual height plane reconstructions and adds them together: if a single piece of bread equals a single height plane, slabbing is like a piece of Texas toast. This thicker "slab" provides the radiologist with the ability to evaluate calcifications as a cluster or to identify the linear distribution due to the added

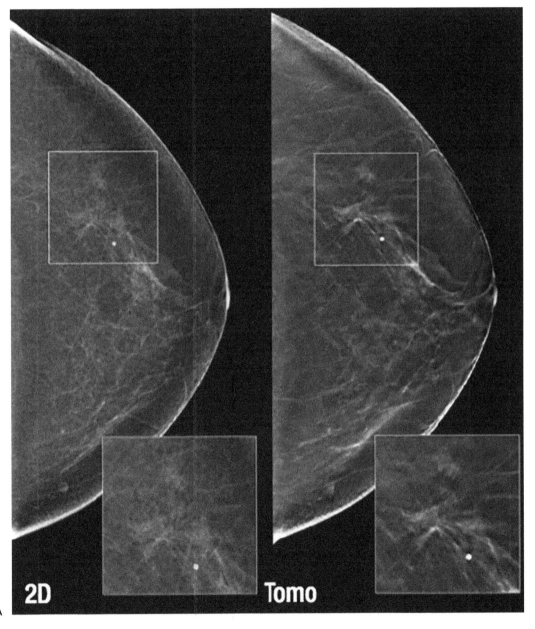

Figure 14-13
Unexpected benefit of 3D imaging of the adipose breast. **(A)** Cancer is better visualized on the 3D exam. (Image courtesy of Hologic, Inc. and affiliates.)

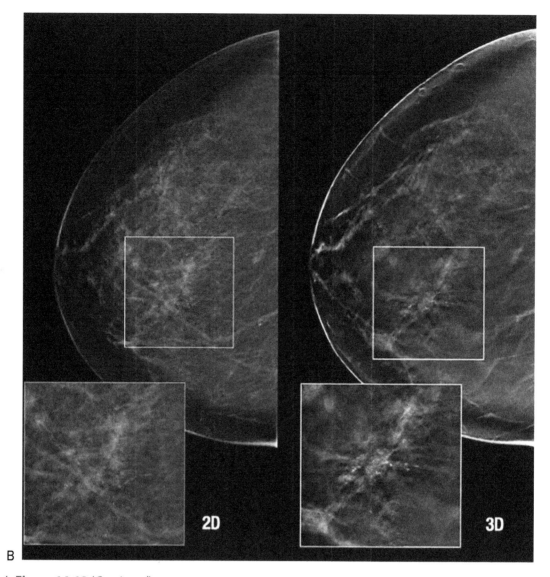

Figure 14-13 (*Continued*)
(B) Another example of the benefit of 3D imaging with an adipose breast. (Image courtesy of Hologic, Inc. and affiliates.)

thickness of the slabbed tissue. Typically, reconstructed images (the single slice of toast) are viewed at 1 mm thick height planes, while slabs (Texas toast) are approximately 15 to 20 mm thick. With a 15- to 20-mm-thick volume of tissue, the radiologist is able to judge if the calcifications are tightly clustered versus dispersed and can appreciate the linear pattern and extent.

Slabbing averages several adjacent reconstruction planes to suppress low-contrast, low-frequency artifacts that arise from pixel sharing of digital image data. Slabbing reduces high-frequency noise and reduces artifacts from out-of-plane objects.

THE COMBO MODE

Radiologists have interpreted 2D mammograms since 1924. Between 1924 and January 2011, exams were film, xeromammography, screen-film, or 2D FFDM. For 87 years, radiologists have viewed 2D images; they are comfortable with 2D interpretation.

On February 11, 2011, FDA grants Hologic approval for DBT imaging. To provide assistance to radiologists through the learning curve associated with interpretation using the new DBT technology, Hologic suggests acquiring images in the "combo mode":

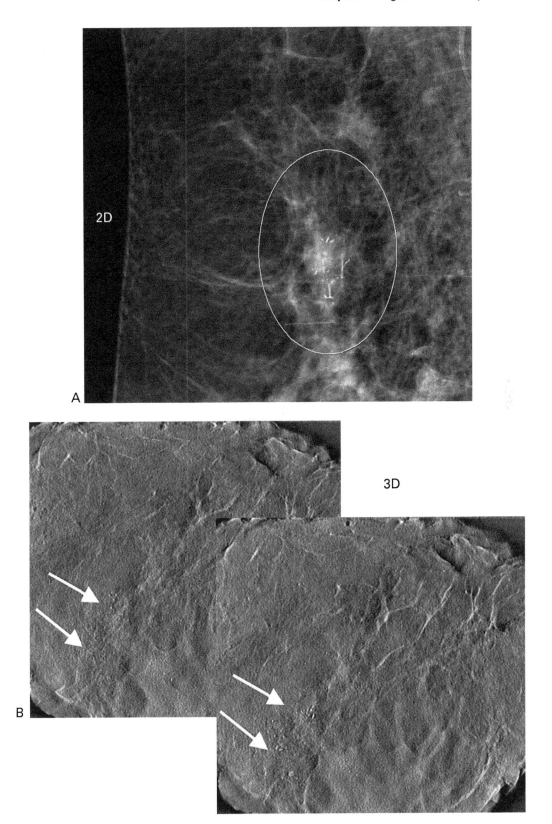

Figure 14-14
Viewing microcalcifications. **(A)** 2D depiction of microcalcifications. It is easy to evaluate these as a cluster due to the thickness of the volume of breast tissue. **(B)** Microcalcifications are clearly visualized on 3D images; however, it is very difficult to ascertain if the calcifications are clustered due to the thinness of each height plane. (Image courtesy of Hologic, Inc. and affiliates.)

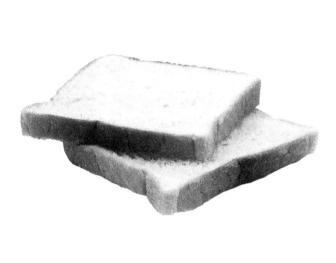

regular toast   Texas toast

Figure 14-15
When calcifications are discovered on a 3D exam, the radiologist expands the thickness of the viewed tissue, known as "slabbing." Slabbing is like Texas toast versus a regular, thinner slice of bread. The thicker slab of tissue permits evaluation of a volume of tissue to determine clustering and distribution of the calcifications. (Images from Shutterstock, Inc.)

Combo mode

The patient is positioned and compressed. The technologist acquires both 2D and 3D images. Only then is the patient released from compression. One advantage for the radiologist is that the 2D and 3D images are coregistered.

If a technologist were to position a patient for the 2D images, and later bring the patient back into the mammography room to acquire 3D images, even though it is the same technologist positioning the same patient in the same projection, the 2D FFDM image will be similar, but not identical, to the DBT image because both images were not acquired under the same compression. Coregistration only applies when the patient is positioned, compressed, exposed for the 2D image, and then exposed for the 3D image; only then is compression released.

Coregistration helps the radiologist along the learning curve during the transition from the familiar appearance of the 2D FFDM image to the new DBT scan. As the radiologist reviews the 3D cine' movie and identifies a ROI, they can simultaneously view the familiar 2D FFDM image (Figure 14-16).

Single-View DBT?

During the radiologists' transition from 2D FFDM to DBT, they quickly realize it requires a longer time to

interpret a combo mode exam because they must evaluate both 2D (RCC, LCC, RMLO, LMLO) and 3D (RCC, LCC, RMLO, LMLO) image sets. They wonder: can we acquire a single 2D FFDM projection (RCC and LCC) and then perform a single DBT scan of each breast (RMLO and LMLO)? The MLO projection is considered the single view of choice because it images more breast tissue compared to the CC projection. Viewing only one 2D FFDM and one DBT projection rather than two 2D FFDM and two DBT projections of each breast requires less time for interpretation.

Studies have been and are conducted to evaluate this approach.[20–24] A study by Beck et al.[25] concludes about half of lesions are equally well seen on both CC and MLO projections, but 34% are better or only seen on the CC projection and 7% are only seen on one view. Rafferty et al.[26] reports 15% are better seen on the CC projection, 12% are better seen on the MLO, and 9% are visualized only on the CC projection. Therefore, if only a 3D CC projection and a 2D MLO projection were done, cancers that are best or only visualized on a 3D MLO could be missed; or if a 2D CC projection and a 3D MLO projection were done, cancers that are best or only visualized on a 3D CC could be missed.

So the popular consensus is "no," we need to acquire bilateral DBT scans. There are no published single-view DBT studies that show increased sensitivity and specificity compared to 2D FFDM. There are several reasons for this:

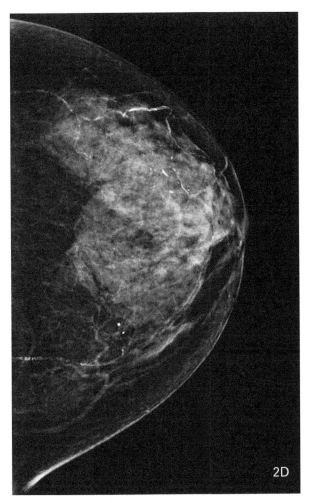 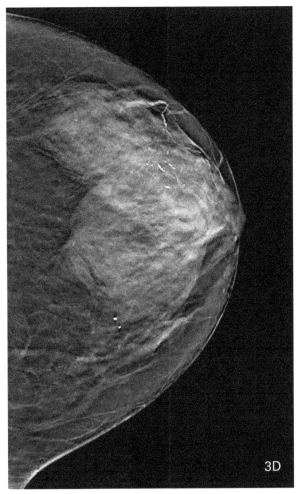

Figure 14-16
Coregistration permits the radiologist to view the 2D and 3D images side by side. The patient is in the exact same position. (Images courtesy of Hologic, Inc. and affiliates.)

- Screening trials to prove the efficacy of mammography began in the 1970s. Many of the very early trials incorporated a single 2D MLO projection. The investigators quickly learned the limitations of a single view; subsequent trials consisted of two-view mammography.[27]
- Neither the CC nor the MLO projection captures all of the breast tissue.
- Some cancers are discovered easily on one projection and are not well visualized on the other.
- CT and MRI image the body in a 360° angular range. Due to the 360° collection of data, CT and MRI perform true orthogonal multiplanar reconstructions: sagittal, coronal, and transverse. In DBT the angular range varies between 15° to 50°, depending on the manufacturer. DBT computers perform "computer magic" to reconstruct the cine' movie from images acquired within a limited angular range; this is sometimes called "pseudotomographic imaging" or "quasi-3D imaging."
- FDA approval for the GE Senoclaire DBT machine is based on documentation as "noninferior" (equal) to 2D FFDM; reader studies were conducted with a single 2D FFDM CC projection in combination with a single DBT MLO projection.[28] DBT manufacturers who conduct reader studies incorporating the combo mode are awarded FDA approval based on documentation as "superior" to 2D FFDM.
- CC DBT scans find substantially more cancers than do DBT MLO scans.[29]

When the radiologist becomes comfortable interpreting DBT exams, it is their personal decision whether or not to continue acquiring 2D FFDM images. Caveat* GE's FDA approval states a 2D FFDM CC projection **must always** be done.[28]

Combo-Mode Benefits

To gain FDA approval, DBT manufacturers must complete reader studies. Radiologists are invited to participate, interpreting exams done in various combinations. Hologic, the first company to gain DBT approval from FDA, conducts two reader studies; refer to Figure 14-17.

FDA grants Hologic permission to make the statements listed in Box 14-1. None of these statements can be made for the transition from analog to 2D FFDM; however, they are valid for the transition from 2D FFDM to DBT.

The transition from analog to 2D FFDM makes the darkroom obsolete and improves imaging of the glandular breast. 2D FFDM does not improve the ability to detect cancers, yet it is widely embraced because it leads to advanced imaging capabilities. DBT is the first of the improved platforms, with a reported 30% increase in breast cancer detection.

Radiologist Reading Time

Compared to analog interpretation, radiologists are less productive when it comes to interpreting digital mammograms:

- Average time to interpret an analog mammogram: 127 seconds
- Average time to interpret a 2D FFDM mammogram: 240 seconds[30]

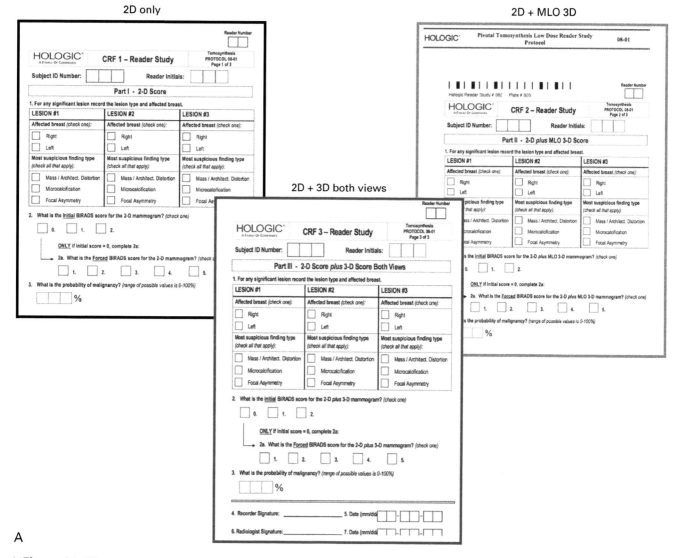

Figure 14-17

Hologic reader studies. **(A)** Reader studies compare (1) 2D FFDM versus (2) 2D FFDM plus a single DBT image versus (3) the combo mode. (Image courtesy of Hologic, Inc. and affiliates.)

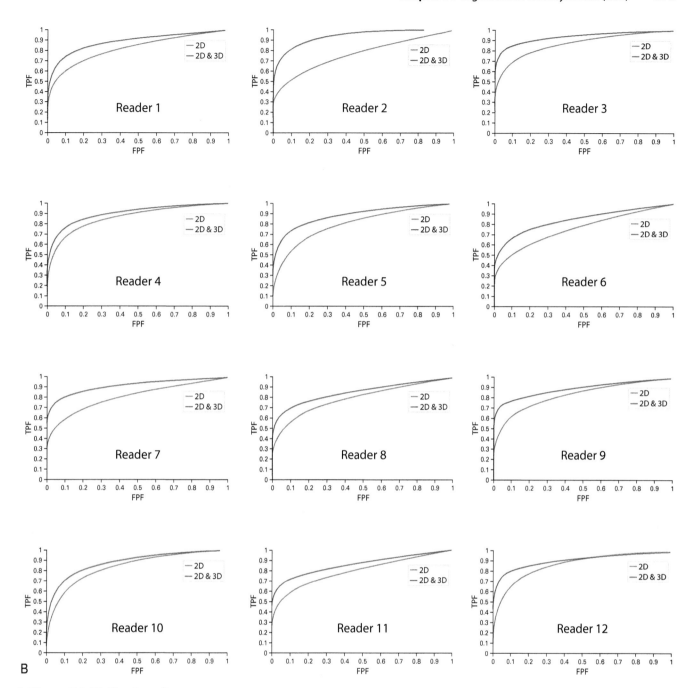

Figure 14-17 (*Continued*)
(B) Reader studies show an increase in sensitivity and specificity with the combo mode. (Source: FDA Executive Summary. Meeting of the Radiological Devices Advisory Panel. September 24, 2010. Gaithersburg, MD; 2010.)

A paper by Zuley et al.[31] reports:

- 1.8 minutes to interpret a 2D FFDM exam
- 2.16 minutes to interpret a combo-mode DBT exam

A paper by Skaane et al.[12] reports:

- 49 seconds to interpret a 2D FFDM exam
- 92 seconds to interpret a combo-mode exam

Others say DBT reading time is 50% longer than 2D FFDM.[32]

As with anything new, a learning curve ensues. After reading 2,000 DBT exams, Dang et al.[33] report a 40% reduction in interpretation time—to 60 seconds.

DBT increases reading time when interpreting a combo-mode exam. However, much of this loss of productivity by the radiologist will be recovered because DBT reduces the number of exams in which the radiologist recalls the patient for additional views; this is reported to be approximately 40%. Diagnostic exams require a longer deliberation time by the radiologist; screening exam interpretation is much faster. So although a screening combo-mode DBT exam requires more time to interpret than a 2D FFDM screening exam, this additional time requirement is partially offset by an approximate 40% reduction in diagnostic exams.

A further reduction in time to interpret a combo-mode exam is proposed by Dustler et al.[34,35] This group is exploring the possibility of viewing 2-mm-thick height planes rather than the current 0.5 or 1 mm. The thicker height planes shorten the length of the cine' movie.

GE's FDA submission included a CC projection in 2D and a 3D MLO projection as a way to reduce the reading time required by the radiologist. However, this did not show a separation in the ROC curves for sensitivity and specificity the way that a combo-mode exam does.

Combo-Mode Dose

The radiation dose for either a 2D or a 3D exam is approximately equal. However, when *both* a 2D and 3D exam are performed, the combo-mode dose is twice that of either a 2D or a 3D exam. Some feel the benefits from a combo-mode exam outweigh the increased radiation risk:

- Combo-mode total dose is less than the MQSA maximum permissible dose.
- Combo-mode dose is less than the yearly background radiation from living on earth.
- Combo-mode exam reduces the need for additional views by approximately 40%.
- Combo mode shows a 30% increase in breast cancer detection.

Further comparisons of radiation dose delivered to the average 4.5 cm, 50% glandular/50% adipose breast under various scenarios:

- 2D tungsten target tube dose: 1.2 mGy
- 2D molybdenum target tube dose: 1.6 mGy
- Combo-mode dose when acquired with a tungsten target tube: 2.65 mGy
- MQSA maximum permissible dose per view: 3 mGy

The combo-mode dose is less than the maximum permissible dose established by MQSA. An approximate dose for analog imaging, as reported in the ACRIN/DMIST study, is 2.0 mGy. The combo-mode dose of 2.65 mGy is slightly higher than the dose in screen-film mammography.

Reduced Dose Solution

Part of the process of developing new technology is to plan ahead: how to overcome an obstacle that new technology creates. The dose doubling attributed to the combo mode is an example of one such obstacle; the patient receives the dose from a 2D FFDM exam as well as from the DBT exam—twice the dose.

DBT manufacturers came up with a solution. Rather than acquire a 2D FFDM exam by exposing the patient to radiation, DBT manufacturers program the computer to synthesize this exam instead. The computer creates these images by collapsing data from the reconstructed DBT images (Figure 14-18).

Hologic refers to this computer process as C-View; GE as V-Preview; and Siemens named this process Insight. DBT was first approved in February 2011; C-View approval was granted in May 2013. For 2 years, Hologic had to contend with this dose controversy. Note: this feature is an option available for a facility to purchase.

Studies are done to compare the efficacy of 2D FFDM versus the combo mode versus DBT in conjunction with the synthetic view.[36,37] The most extensive review of the ability of a synthetic view to replace a 2D FFDM image is conducted by Skaane et al.[38]; more cancers are detected with a DBT scan and C-View image than with 2D FFDM alone.

The **synthesized 2D image**:

- Reduces the dose to the patient
- Reduces the time the patient is compressed
- Reduces exam time
- Extends the life of the x-ray tube and the digital detector
- May aid the radiologist's determination if calcifications are clustered or in a linear pattern
- Facilitates review between current and prior exams

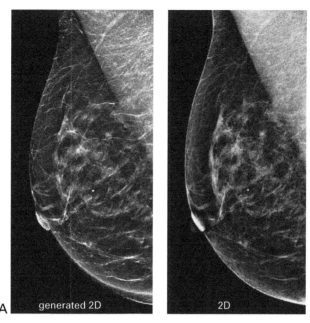

A generated 2D   2D

RCC—image comparison

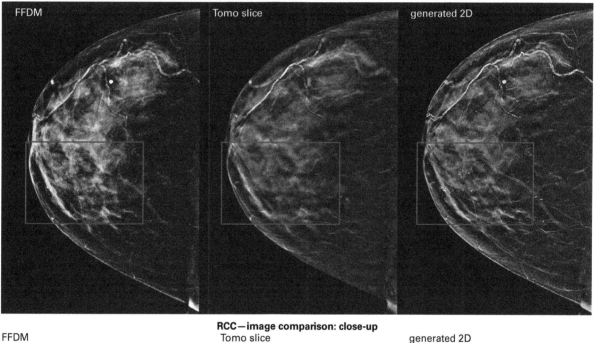

FFDM   Tomo slice   generated 2D

RCC—image comparison: close-up

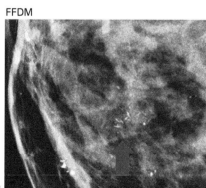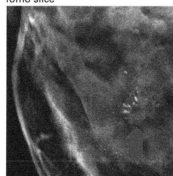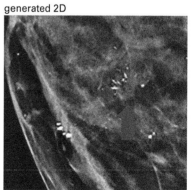

FFDM   Tomo slice   generated 2D

B

Figure 14-18

(A) When imaged in the combo mode, the patient receives twice the x-ray dose because the patient is imaged with both 2D and 3D acquisitions. The solution to reduce the dose is to replace the actual 2D acquisition with a computer synthesis instead. The information used by the computer to synthesize the image is gathered from the 3D acquisition. (Images courtesy of Hologic, Inc. and affiliates.) **(B)** A comparison of 2D FFDM, DBT, and the synthesized image. (Images courtesy of Hologic, Inc. and affiliates.)

Currently, as part of a 2D + 3D tomosynthesis screening exam, the Hologic C-View image and the Siemens Insight image are FDA approved as a substitute for the 2D FFDM images; GE, as part of its FDA application, requires a 2D FFDM CC projection must always be acquired. The Hologic C-View, the GE V-Preview, and the Siemens Insight computer synthesized images are not approved as a stand-alone exam; they always accompany the 3D exam.

PHYSICS PRINCIPLES

Physics Principle Trade-Offs

Digital imaging ventures into the radiology department in 1981 when Fuji introduces CR technology for use with general x-ray exams: chest, knees, feet, etc. In 2000, mammography belatedly enters the digital world. The immediate advantages for 2D FFDM are primarily logistical:

* Storage
  PACS rather than a film library
* Portability
  Original images can be viewed simultaneously in different locations
* Contrast control
  Electronic images can be manipulated postacquisition: window/level, zoom, invert, etc.
* Improved Detector Quantum Efficiency (DQE)
  Detectors absorb more x-rays allowing better image quality and higher dose or the same image quality with lower dose.

The transition from analog imaging to 2D FFDM is a lateral move (Table 14-3). While 2D FFDM improved diagnostic confidence and improved control of diagnostic image quality, it still missed the same percentage of cancers as analog imaging. The transition from 2D FFDM to DBT is a leap forward in detection (Figure 14-19). DBT's ability

Table 14-3 • Similar Technologies

ANALOG MAMMOGRAPHY	2D FFDM
• 1924–1999	• 2000–2011
• Gold standard	• Gold standard
• Low dose	• Low dose
• Grayscale Images	• Grayscale images
○ Black = adipose tissue	○ Black = adipose tissue
○ White = glandular tissue and cancer	○ White = glandular tissue and cancer
○ Gray = everything else	○ Gray = everything else
• 2D	• 2D
○ Multiple views CC, MLO, ML, LM, etc.	○ Multiple views CC, MLO, ML, LM, etc.

A comparison of analog and 2D FFDM mammography. Only the time frame is different.

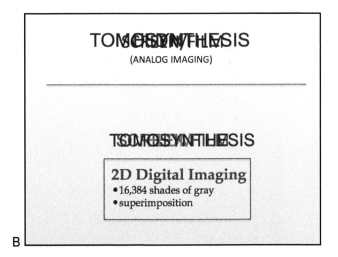

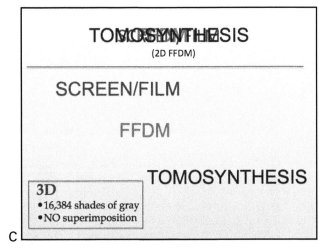

Figure 14-19
(A) Analog imaging. Words are superimposed on top of and underneath one another in this 2D depiction. With a limited dynamic range of only 100 shades of gray, it is difficult to determine how many words there are, nor can we discern what the words are. **(B)** 2D FFDM has a dynamic range of 16,384 shades of gray; thus, we recognize there are three words. Due to superimposition, it is not clear what the words are. **(C)** 3D imaging incorporates the vast dynamic range of 16,384 shades of gray, and it unsuperimposes the words. The words are readily apparent.

to view breast tissue in height planes free of superimposition is a tremendous technological advancement. However, if we evaluate DBT from a purely "physics" viewpoint, one might be led to believe this imaging technique is inferior to 2D FFDM:

- Resolution is reduced—affects all manufacturers
  - Analog spatial resolution is 20 lp/mm; 2D FFDM is 9 lp/mm; DBT is between 3 and 6 lp/mm.
- Binning—by some manufacturers
  - Combining 2 vertical pixels with 2 horizontal pixels (Hologic) reduces the 25 million pixels in the digital detector to approximately 6 million; the reason for reduced resolution. Binning results in increased SNR but decreased MTF in the binned direction, parallel to the detector. GE and Siemens do not bin.
- Use of a grid—by some manufacturers
  - A grid cleans up scattered radiation. Nongrid images are not as "contrasty," thus a loss of contrast resolution. GE uses a grid; Hologic and Siemens do not use grids; however, Hologic is working on a prototype grid. Siemens PRIME is a computer algorithm to cancel out the effects of scatter on their DBT images in place of a grid. The computer subtracts the scattered radiation signal and uses the primary signal to reconstruct the cine' movie. This is a challenging approach requiring robust computer calculations. This scatter correction software is not yet FDA approved; it is a future enhancement.
- Tungsten target x-ray tube—by most manufacturers
  - Tungsten has a higher atomic number than molybdenum, the target material used in analog imaging. The characteristic energy of tungsten is 59 keV, while molybdenum is 17.9 and 19.5 keV. Higher-energy photons produce lower-contrast images. All DBT manufacturers, except for one, use tungsten target tubes with various filter combinations. GE continues use of molybdenum/rhodium target tubes, with rhodium being the preferred target material used with DBT scans.
- Filtration
  - Analog imaging employs use of a molybdenum filter with a molybdenum target to enrich the characteristic photons that produce contrast in an image. Filters such as aluminum are used by some DBT manufacturers to make the beam harder, thus more penetrating.
- High kVp
  - kVp controls contrast; the lower the kVp, the higher the contrast. Analog imaging typically uses molybdenum at 25 kVp. Most DBT manufacturers use tungsten at higher kVp settings for increased penetration.

- Compression
  - Breast restraint as opposed to breast compression leaves the breast thicker due to less compression force. A thicker breast creates more scattered radiation; scatter reduces contrast.

When we perform DBT imaging, some manufacturers purposely employ trade-offs that render the image less contrasty and less resolute. Theoretically, it should be more difficult to visualize a cancer, yet the opposite happens. The cancer is easier to see due to reduced superimposition of structures.

Breast Compression

In theory, the force for DBT compression should be minimal: breast restraint rather than breast compression.

In 2D FFDM, applying "adequate" compression to a breast is a skill each mammography technologist learns. Technologists learn by doing. What is too much compression? Too little compression? Every technologist has to practice this positioning skill on many patients to determine a force of compression that is tolerable to the patient yet produces a quality image for the radiologist.

The seven reasons for compression, as stated in Table 14-4, are all valid and necessary for 2D FFDM to successfully find a small (white) mass cancer or (white) microcalcifications inside (white) glandular breast tissue. However, in DBT, not all seven reasons for compression are valid.

An analogy helps here. If we think of the breast as a loaf of bread, do we want to compress the loaf so that each slice becomes indistinguishable from one another (Figure 14-20)? Of course not. So, in theory, DBT wants the bread/breast in its natural (uncompressed) state to retain the separate height planes in order to identify internal structures.

Two of the seven reasons for compression (less motion and reduced patient dose) continue to be valid reasons for compression in DBT. Currently, we compress the breast in DBT to the same degree we do with 2D FFDM. However, when functional-based imaging techniques are combined

Table 14-4 • Compression

	2D	3D
Reduces thickness of breast	Yes	No
Uniform penetration	Yes	No
Separate glandular tissue	Yes	No
Reduce geometric unsharpness	Yes	No
Improve contrast	Yes	No
Less motion	Yes	Yes
Reduce patient dose	Yes	Yes

The reasons for breast compression. All seven reasons are valid with 2D imaging; only two reasons are valid with 3D imaging.

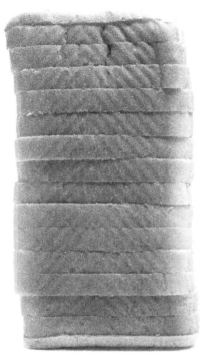
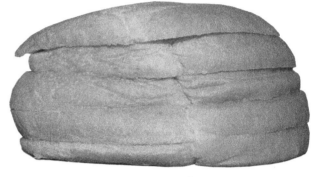

uncompressed   compressed

Figure 14-20
3D imaging views the breast in individual height planes, like viewing one slice of bread at a time. We do not want to take the loaf of bread and compress it so that the slices are indistinguishable from one another. Breast compression takes structures at many different height planes and compacts them into fewer height planes. This negates the beneficial effects of DBT. (Uncompressed image from Shutterstock, Inc.)

with DBT, we must reduce the force of compression. Compression stops blood flow in and out of the breast. Functional–based imaging techniques require normal blood flow to see if areas enhance.

Investigators research the effects of reduced compression. Saunders et al.[39] found no significant difference in the conspicuity of mass and/or calcifying lesions with a 12% reduction in compression force when the dose is constant for varying breast tissue composition and thickness. Fornvik et al.[40] studied full compression followed by a 50% reduction in compression force, with the same acquisition parameters used for both exams. Results: three subject reviewers found no evident difference in image quality between the two compression forces.

More research needs to be done in this aspect of breast restraint versus breast compression.

Motion

If we are ultimately able to reduce the force applied to the breast, what affect will this have on image quality, specifically resolution?

Motion unsharpness is the most common patient-related artifact.[41] Motion can be all-encompassing (the entire breast) or it can be region specific (one area of the breast). Motion can range from subtle to gross. Repeating images due to patient motion increases the radiation dose to the patient. Motion has the potential to cause a cancer to be missed due to degradation of the image (Figure 14-21).

It has always been the responsibility of the technologist to evaluate each image for motion. This responsibility assumes a more important role in DBT. In 2D imaging, whether analog or 2D FFDM, if the technologist does not detect motion on an image, the radiologist will be quick to see it. This happens because the technologist and radiologist evaluate the same image. In DBT, the radiologist and the technologist do not view the same image; motion in DBT is identified on projection images, it is not readily apparent on reconstructed images. Rarely will a radiologist look at projection images; they view reconstructed images.

One DBT manufacturer (Hologic) bins pixels for faster acquisition of multiple exposures during tube movement;

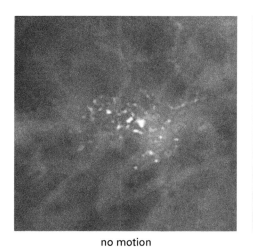 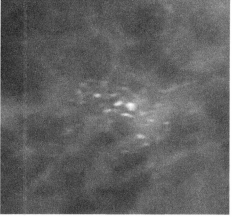

no motion   motion

Figure 14-21
Motion is a potential problem when we ease the force of compression. It has always been the responsibility of the technologist to review an image for motion artifact. This is more important in DBT. (Images courtesy of Hologic, Inc. and affiliates.)

they trade off a loss of resolution due to binning for faster tube travel and less likelihood of patient motion due to less time under compression. Binning reduces spatial resolution; this diminished resolution makes it difficult for the radiologist to see motion. DBT manufacturers who do not bin have slightly higher spatial resolution; however, the length of time to acquire the scan is longer. With a longer scan time, patient motion is more likely to occur.

Spatial Resolution

Spatial resolution, reported in line pairs per millimeter (lp/mm), evaluates sharpness of an image. Analog imaging has the best spatial resolution: 20 to 22 lp/mm, followed by 2D FFDM, and finally DBT (Figure 14-22).

The human "spatial resolution" test is the Snellen eye chart, which measures the ability of the eye to resolve shapes or letters. The 20 to 22 lp/mm resolution of an

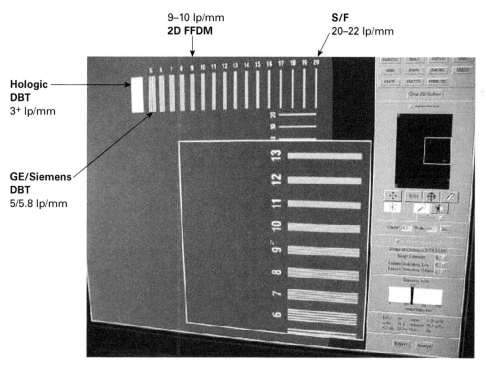

Figure 14-22
A comparison of spatial resolution. DQE is a better predictor of digital image quality. Most of the time, it is a reduction in spatial resolution, not patient motion, that results in DBT images looking less resolute than 2D images.

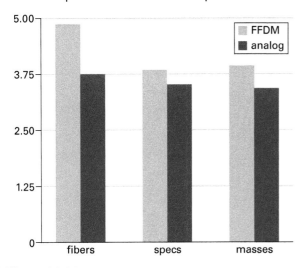

Comparison of ACR accreditation phantom scores

Figure 14-23
3D imaging, with reduced spatial resolution, visualizes more fibers, spec groups, and masses than analog imaging due to the increased contrast resolution of digital imaging.

analog system is equivalent to 20/20 vision on the eye chart; 9 to 10 lp/mm of 2D FFDM is like 20/400 vision; and 3 to 6 lp/mm of DBT is the equivalent of a human without eyes!

How can DBT's poor spatial resolution depict a cancer better than a 2D FFDM or analog image with better resolution? DBT has better contrast resolution (16,384 shades of gray) than analog imaging (100 shades of gray) plus it eliminates superimposition of structures, which 2D FFDM cannot do. Contrast resolution and unsuperimposition of structures more than offset a reduction in spatial resolution (Figure 14-23).

▌▌ IMAGE QUALITY

Manufacturers of DBT machines all design their equipment with slightly different technical features (Table 14-5).

Manufacturers optimize the image produced by their machine by incorporating various technical specifications: SID, angular range, reconstruction method, x-ray tube target and filtration material, etc. Because DBT is a new breast imaging technology, we do not have precedent machine designs to compare to see which approach produces the best image.

Design Features

Many design features impact the quality of an image. Some features are visible, for example: tube motion, angular range, SID, scan time in seconds, etc. Others are not visible, yet also are important; for example: tube target material, filtration, reconstruction method, etc. Let's consider several of these features in greater detail.

1. X-ray tube target material

   All manufacturers except for one have moved away from molybdenum/rhodium target tubes to tungsten. A variety of filters, depending on the machine manufacturer, are incorporated with a tungsten target tube. Molybdenum target tubes produce high-contrast images; in digital imaging, with 16,384 shades of gray available through window/leveling, we can electronically manipulate a tungsten target image until there are comparable contrast indices to molybdenum (Figure 14-24).

   Manufacturers always balance a series of trade-offs they are willing to accept for each technical

Table 14-5 • DBT Machine Design Characteristics

	HOLOGIC 2.11.11	GE 8.26.14	SIEMENS 4.21.15	PHILIPS	PLANMED	FUJI 1.23.17	GIOTTO
Pixel size (μm)	70	100	85	50	83	50	85
X-ray tube target	W	Mo Rh	W	W	W	W	W
Tube motion	Continuous	Step and shoot	Continuous	Continuous	Continuous	Continuous	Step and shoot
Angular range (°)	15	25	50	NA	30	15 or 40	40
Number projection exposures	15	9	25	21	15	15	15
Scan time (seconds)	4	7–10	25	3–10	20	4	4/9
Reconstruction method	FBP	Iterative	FBP	Iterative	Iterative	Modified FBP	Iterative with total variation

DBT is brand new technology; no precedent equipment designs are available to deduce which design features produce the best image. Manufacturers all design their machines with different characteristics and features.

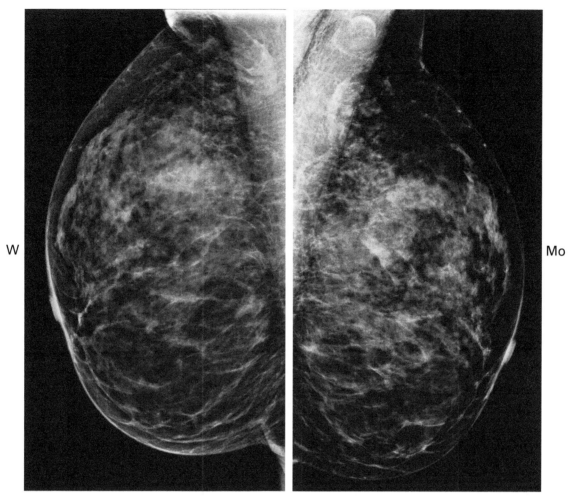

Figure 14-24
A tungsten target x-ray tube was used to produce the image on the left; molybdenum was used for the image on the right. Before the 16,384 shades of gray available with digital imaging, mammograms produced by tungsten target tubes were unacceptable. Today with the vast dynamic range of digital imaging, window/level the tungsten image until the contrast index is similar to that of a molybdenum image.

specification, for example, in DBT, the use of a rhodium target versus a tungsten target x-ray tube. The a-Se digital detector is matched with the tungsten target x-ray tube to produce an optimal image. Tungsten permits higher mA output and the use of higher kVp to minimize focal spot blur from the continuous motion design feature.

Impact of tungsten target tubes:

- Dose
  - Lowers dose to the patient because photons are more penetrating.
- Optimal exposure
  - DBT manufacturers optimize exposure to the patient. The signal difference-to-noise ratio (SDNR) increases with an increase in patient dose, up to

a certain point before it levels off. Increasing the dose beyond this point does not result in increased image quality due to an increase in anatomic noise. This is reminiscent of reciprocity law failure (RLF) in analog imaging.[42,43]

- Higher mA stations
  - The harder target material can withstand more heat units. mA stations increase, typically from 100 mA with molybdenum target tubes to 200 mA with tungsten. Higher mA stations permit a shorter exposure time.
- Higher kVp settings
  - A slightly higher energy spectra results in increased SNR. The use of higher kVp settings also reduces the dose to the patient. Additionally, the use of higher kVp settings shortens exposure time.

- Shorter exposure time
  - Shorter exposure times minimize the likelihood of patient motion and focal spot blurring during short x-ray pulses used with the continuous motion DBT sweep.
- Contrast
  - There is reduced contrast information in the signal when using a tungsten target tube.

2. Tube motion

There are two styles of tube motion: step-and-shoot and continuous motion.

The step-and-shoot design is mechanically challenging. The tube moves in the standard arc, but it stops at set degrees throughout the arc to make an exposure. The step-and-shoot motion: tube moves, stops to make an exposure, moves another few degrees, and stops to make an exposure. The mechanical challenge is for the tube to come to a complete stop when the exposure is made so there is no focal spot blur.

The continuous motion design has its own challenges. Exposures are made as the tube travels throughout the arc resulting in focal spot blur, which produces unsharpness in the DBT images. This necessitates a very short pulse width to reduce this blur. This is one reason for the transition away from molybdenum target tubes to tungsten with higher kVp settings, higher mA stations, and higher heat unit tolerance.

3. Angular range, number of projection exposures, and scan time

Angular range, number of projection exposures, and scan time are all interrelated. Angular range is the number of degrees the x-ray tube moves during travel along the arc. Manufacturers have varying opinions as to this design feature; it ranges from a low of 15° to 50°.

Angular range and the number of projection exposures are key to a system's ability to decrease the impact of overlapping tissue (Figure 14-25). Angular range directly affects depth resolution. A wider angular range results in better out-of-plane resolution, with worse in-plane resolution; out-of-plane artifacts are reduced because they are spread over a wider range in the considered plane. The wider arc angle yields better separation of structures at different heights due to the decreased width of a physical slice, thus tissue overlap is reduced. This is better for separation of structures at different height planes, but it results in less sharpness with calcifications. The longer arc requires a longer scan time; pay particular attention for patient motion.

A narrow angular range yields a rapid scan time; however, it does not reduce overlapping structures as much as a wider scan angle. The smaller angle is better for microcalcifications as this provides better in-plane resolution due to the increased depth of field, with worse out-of-plane resolution.

In theory, DBT manufacturers want to maximize the number of projections as well as maximize the distance the x-ray tube travels as this yields the highest image quality. However, the number of projections must be tempered by the dose delivered to the patient. Divide the dose to the patient by the number of projections, with the result being the amount of signal provided to the computer to generate an image. Too many projections decrease the signal to a point where electronic noise is more dominant than the amount of signal.

As the angular range increases, exposures made at the extremes of the arc result in shallow incident angles that result in degradation of spatial resolution.

Manufacturers research distribution of x-ray exposures throughout travel of the tube along the angular range. Should projections be evenly spaced throughout the arc, or should they occur in an irregular distribution (Figure 14-26)?

Nishikawa et al.[44] examined nonuniform distribution: half the total exposure dose is delivered at 0° (the central projection), while the remaining dose is divided equally among the remaining projections. Das et al.[45] evaluated uniform versus nonuniform distribution. The conclusion: uniform distribution results in better image quality.

Each manufacturer designs their machine to produce what they believe is optimal image quality.

4. Reconstruction algorithm

The series of projections are processed by a computer reconstruction algorithm: filtered back projection (FBP) or a modification of the iterative method. The reconstruction method uses the different locations of the same tissue, depending on the angle in the arc of travel at which the x-ray exposure is acquired, to compute the vertical position of the tissue. The computer algorithm estimates the 3D distribution of the tissue into planes parallel to the detector.

Due to the limited distance the tube travels, DBT displays anisotropic spatial resolution (ASR) (Figure 14-27). ASR displays high resolution in planes parallel to the

	Hologic 2.11.11	GE 8.26.14	Siemens 4.21.15	Philips	Planmed	Fuji 1.23.17	Giotto
pixel size (um)	70	100	85	50	83	50	85
x-ray tube target	W	Mo Rh	W	W	W	W	W
tube motion	continuous	step and shoot	continuous	continuous	continuous	continuous	step and shoot
angular range (degree)	15	25	50	NA	30	15 or 40	40
number projection exposures	15	9	25	21	15	15	13
scan time (seconds)	4	7 - 10	25	3 - 10	20	4/9	2
reconstruction method	FBP	iterative	FBP	iterative	iterative	modified FBP	iterative with total variation

A

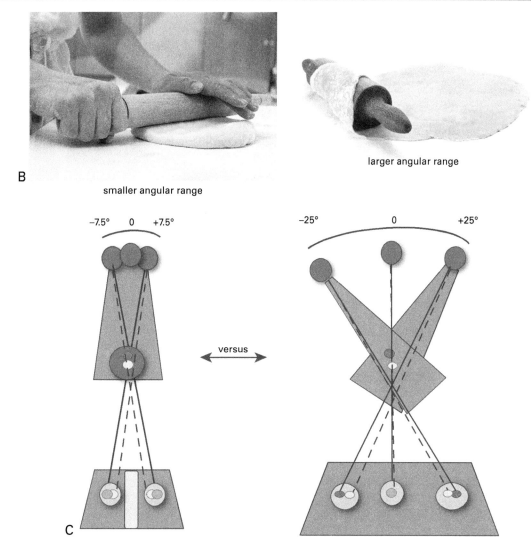

B   smaller angular range

larger angular range

versus

C

Figure 14-25
Angular range is the distance the DBT x-ray tube moves during acquisition of the projection images. **(A)** Each DBT machine manufacturer determines the optimal distance the tube moves based on their design specifications. **(B)** This ranges from a low of 15° to a high of 50°. The smaller angle is better for visualization of microcalcifications, while it is worse for determining superimposition of structures. (Image from Shutterstock, Inc.) **(C)** The wider angular range separates structures at different height planes more completely; however, it is worse for imaging microcalcifications. The narrow angular range is better for visualizing microcalcifications; however, it is worse at separating overlapping structures.

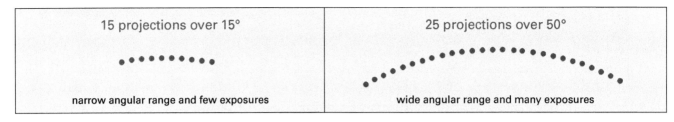

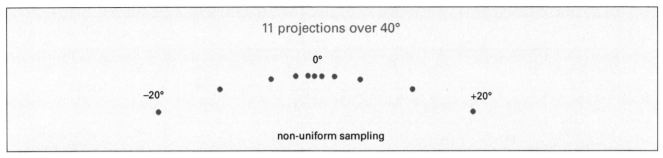

Figure 14-26
DBT is new technology. Each design feature is scrutinized by engineers and physicists, who hope their design specifications produce the best image quality. One such design feature is distribution of x-ray exposures as the tube travels throughout the angular range.

detector; spatial resolution in the perpendicular direction is considerably lower. However, even resolution in the perpendicular plane is adequate to minimize tissue superimposition.

Manufacturers use the FBP technique or an iterative method.

The FBP algorithm had its origins during the 1960s with CT. It is a mathematical technique that gives an idea of

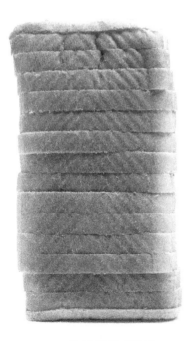
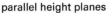

parallel height planes

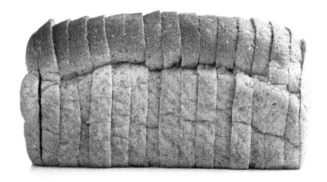

perpendicular height planes

Figure 14-27
All DBT manufacturers display the 3D scan with ASR (anisotropic spatial resolution). When the computer reconstructs the projection images, the height planes are viewed parallel to the digital detector; this provides the best resolution. Resolution in the perpendicular plane, while reduced, is adequate to evaluate whether tissue is superimposed or is a significant lesion. (Images from Shutterstock, Inc.)

spatial distribution in height planes parallel to the plane of the detector. By shifting the single projection views according to the height of a specific feature, the information of that feature is summed up, while the information of features from other heights are misregistered. A problem associated with back-projection reconstruction is geometric blurring. The optimal way to eliminate the patterns of blur is to use a ramp filter.

There are variations of iterative reconstruction techniques. This reconstruction method derives from the early days of CT. It is a repetitive process where the reconstructed image is estimated and then improved by comparing the structure detail to the measured projection data and minimizing differences. This is repeated many times to optimize the image. The technique reduces noise and dose while improving both spatial and contrast resolution. It is computer intensive.

PACS STORAGE

2D FFDM files are large because high resolution images are necessary for a mammogram (Figure 14-28). DBT scans are much larger than the large 2D FFDM file. The large DBT data file presents a challenge for storage in PACS.

2D FFDM:	uncompressed 88 MB
	compressed 22 MB
DBT:	uncompressed 1.2 GB
	compressed 320 MB
Combo mode:	uncompressed 1,317 MB
	compressed 342 MB

Because a DBT scan is so large, compression is employed. There are two types of compression for digital

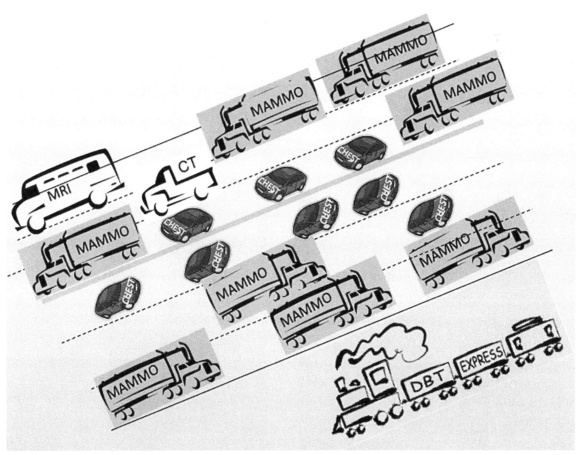

Figure 14-28
Data file size of digital x-ray images are large:
A chest x-ray is like a sports car.
A CT scan is like a pickup truck.
An MRI scan is like a school bus.
A four-view 2D FFDM exam is like an 18-wheeler.
A DBT scan is like a railroad train.

x-ray images: lossy compression and **lossless compression**. Mammograms are not allowed to be lossy compressed, they can only be lossless compressed. Other types of x-ray images, for example, chest x-rays, knees, feet, can be lossy compressed (Figure 14-29). Compressed images take up less storage space in PACS.

When a medical event is over (e.g., a broken leg has healed), the x-ray images can be lossy compressed for

lossy compression

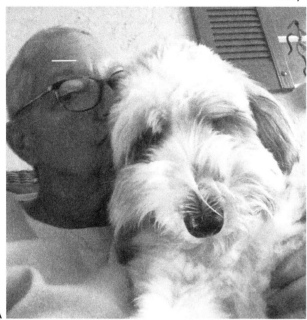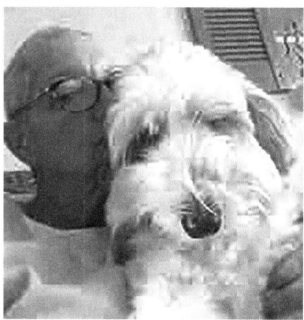

A

lossless compression

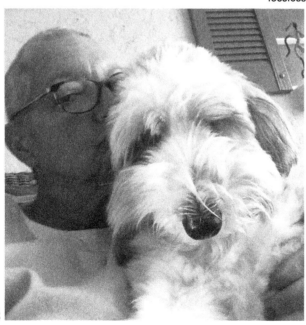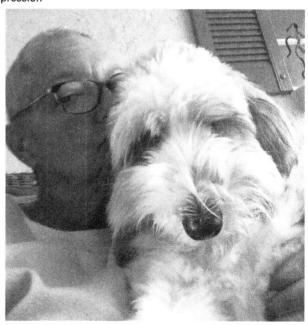

B

Figure 14-29
Digital x-ray data file size is very large. Compression is used to reduce storage size demands. There are two types of data compression: lossy and lossless. **(A)** Lossy compression is acceptable in general x-ray exams. It is not allowed for use in the storage of mammography images. (Courtesy of the Goddard family.) **(B)** Lossless compression is on the order of 4:1. This minimal compression is acceptable for the long-term retention of mammogram images.

storage purposes. The likelihood these images will be viewed again is low, so the trade-off of loss of resolution for a smaller amount of storage space is acceptable. The loss of resolution that occurs with lossy compression cannot be undone.

On the other hand, mammograms are allowed only a slight reduction in resolution; mammograms can only be lossless compressed, typically 4:1. This slight degradation of resolution is deemed acceptable. Radiologists always compare current mammogram images to priors so the resolution needs to remain sharp.

The data file size of the DBT exam is quite large: 1.2 GB. When lossless compressed, it is still large: 320 MB. Hologic, the first manufacturer to gain FDA approval for DBT, was faced with the task to reduce the data file size even further. Hologic took the 1.2 GB size and created a storage standard, Secondary Capture Tomo Object, to reduce this to 136 MB. This 136 MB file cannot be further compressed.

Compressing image data relies on the ability to decompress the same data in order to view the DBT scan on a reviewstation. In this early stage of DBT entrance into the mammography marketplace, the individual manufacturer's DBT scans either display only or best on their brand reviewstation. If the radiologist wishes to use a PACS system to display the DBT scan, the PACS companies must support display of the DICOM Breast Tomosynthesis Object; PACS companies are in the early stages of deciphering and displaying this information. As each newly FDA-approved DBT manufacturer enters the marketplace, PACS manufacturers must adapt.

The display of the DBT scan is challenging for the DBT manufacturer as well as a PACS company wanting to allow their reviewstation to display the scan. Items that present a challenge:

- Correct image orientation
- Display current and prior exams
- Synchronize same size/comparing current to prior images
- Hanging protocols
- Annotation: marking tools plus display
- Comparable size: true size, actual size
- Measurement tools
- Correct gray-scale display
- Accommodate both cine' and manual scroll viewing
- Smoothly scroll at a rapid frame rate without skipping frames, through all planes and all views

For now, a DBT exam is best viewed on a reviewstation made by the manufacturer of the AWS.

Summary

Without curious people who have a vision of a different way to image the breast, we would still be using a ceiling-mounted x-ray tube and x-ray table to produce images circa 1924. Through the dogged efforts of Dr. Daniel Kopans and research engineers L.T. and L.E. Niklason, breast tomosynthesis is the latest tested and proven advancement in breast cancer detection. We owe much gratitude to those with the conviction and fortitude to follow another pathway.

Review Questions

1. 2D imaging has always had to contend with superimposition of tissue; the thicker the breast, the greater the impact of this negative factor of imaging a 3D object in a 2D imaging format. What is superimposition?

2. The benefits of DBT are legion. Provide a short explanation of each benefit.

   - Increased lesion/margin visibility
   - Increased detection of invasive cancers
   - A decrease in stage detection
   - A decrease in false-positive findings

3. Refer to Figure 14-21. Which image does the technologist use to evaluate motion?

4. Anisotropic spatial resolution displays high-resolution images in which plane?

5. Which exam has the largest data file?

References

1. Skaane P, et al. Comparison of digital mammography alone and digital mammography plus tomosynthesis in a population-based screening program. *Radiology*. 2013;267(1): 47–56.
2. Genusaro G, et al. Digital breast tomosynthesis versus digital mammography: a clinical performance study. *Eur Radiol*. 2009;20:1545–1553.
3. Bick U, et al. Tomosynthesis and the impact on patient management. *EUSOBI March 2014*, Vienna; March 2014.
4. Butler RS, et al. How tomosynthesis optimizes patient workup, throughput, and resource utilization. *RSNA Annual Meeting*, Chicago, IL; 2013.
5. Zuley ML, et al. Digital breast tomosynthesis versus supplemental diagnostic mammographic images for evaluation of non-calcified breast lesions. *Radiology*. 2013;266(1):89–95.

6. Bonafede M, et al. Value analysis of digital breast tomosynthesis for breast cancer screening in a commercially insured US population. *Clinicoecon Outcomes Res.* 2015;7: 53–63.

7. Skaane P, et al. Prospective trial comparing full field digital mammography (FFDM) versus combined FFDM and tomosynthesis in a population based screening programme using independent double reading with arbitration. *Eur Radiol.* 2013;23(8):2061–2071.

8. Ciatto S, et al. Integration of 3D digital mammography with tomosynthesis for population breast cancer screening (STORM): a prospective comparison study. *Lancet Oncol.* 2013;14(7):583–589.

9. Rose SL, et al. Implementation of breast tomosynthesis in a routine screening practice: an observational study. *AJR Am J Roentgenol.* 2013;200(6):1401–1408.

10. Gandini G, et al. Comparative study with digital mammography (DM) combined with digital breast tomosynthesis (DBT) for detection of invasive lobular carcinoma (ILC). *RSNA Annual Meeting*, Chicago, IL; 2013.

11. Uchiyama N, et al. Diagnostic impact of adjunction of digital breast tomosynthesis (DBT) to full field digital mammography (FFDM) and in comparison with full field digital mammography (FFDM) breast imaging. *11th International Workshop on Digital Mamography (IWDM 2012)*, Philadelphia, PA; July 2012.

12. Skaane P, et al. Comparison of digital mammography (FFDM) and FFDM plus DBT in mammography screening for cancer detection according to breast parenchyma density. *RSNA Annual Meeting*, Chicago, IL; 2014.

13. Philpotts LE, et al. Tomosynthesis in breast cancer visualization as a function of mammographic density. *RSNA Annual Meeting*, Chicago, IL; 2013.

14. Haas BM, et al. Comparison of tomosynthesis plus digital mammography and digital mammography alone for breast cancer screening. *Radiology.* 2013;269(3):694–700.

15. Destounis SV, Morgan R, Arieno A. Screening for dense breasts: digital breast tomosynthesis. *AJR Am J Roentgenol.* 2015; 204(2):261–264.

16. Sickles EA. *SBI Forum Post*, Orlando, FL; January 2012.

17. Kolb TM, Lichy J, Newhouse JH. Comparison of the performance of screening mammography, physical examination, and breast ultrasound, and evaluation of factors that influence them: analysis of 27,825 patients. *Radiology.* 2002;225:165–175.

18. Rafferty EA, Niklason L, Smith A. Comparison of FFDM with breast tomosynthesis to FFDM alone: performance in fatty and dense breasts. *Tomosynthesis Imaging Symposium*, Duke University; 2009.

19. Geisel J, Raghu M, Durand M, Haas B, Lapia K, Hooley R, Butler R, Philpotts, L. Cancer Detection rates on screening 2D versus combined 2D + Tomosynthesis Imaging. *American Roentgen Ray Society (ARRS) Annual Meeting*, Washington, DC; April 2013.

20. Rafferty EA, Niklason LT, Jameson-Meehan LA. Breast tomosynthesis: 1 view or 2? *Radiol Soc N Am.* 2006:SS601–SS604.

21. Baker JA, Lo JY. Breast tomosynthesis: state-of-the-art and review of the literature. *Radiology.* 2011;18(10):1298–1310.

22. American Roentgen Ray Society (ARRS) Annual Meeting, Washington DC; April 2013.

23. Zackrisson S, et al. Performance of one-view breast tomosynthesis versus two-view mammography in breast cancer screening—first results from the Malmo breast tomosynthesis screening trial. *ECR 2014*, Vienna, Austria; March 2014.

24. Wallis MG, et al. 2 view and single view tomosynthesis versus full field digital mammography: high resolution x-ray imaging observer study. *Radiology.* 2012;262(3):788–796.

25. Beck N, et al. One-view vs 2-view tomosynthesis: a comparison of breast cancer visibility in the MLO and CC views. *ARRS Annual Meeting*, Washington, DC; April 2013.

26. Rafferty E, Niklason L, Jameson-Meehan L. Breast tomosynthesis: one view or two? *RSNA Annual Meeting*, Chicago, IL; 2006.

27. Tabar L, et al. Swedish two county trial: impact of mammographic screening on breast cancer mortality during 3 decades. *Radiology.* 2011;260(3):658–663.

28. GE Senoclaire Summary of Safety and Effectiveness. 26 August 2014. http://www.accessdata.fda.gov/cdrh_docs/pdf13/p130020b.pdf

29. Zuley ML, et al. Analysis of cancers missed on digital breast tomosynthesis. *RSNA Annual Meeting*, Chicago, IL; 2014.

30. Haygood TM, et al. Timed efficiency of interpretation of digital and film-screen screening mammograms. *AJR Am J Roentgenol.* 2009;192:216–220.

31. Zuley ML, et al. Time to diagnosis and performance levels during repeat interpretations of digital breast tomosynthesis: preliminary observations. *Acad Radiol.* 2010;17(4):450–455.

32. Sonnenschein M. The use of breast tomosynthesis with C-view images and tomosynthesis guided biopsy in daily practice: our experience in Switzerland. *Symposium S423, European College of Radiology Annual Meeting*, Vienna, Austria; 2014.

33. Dang PA, et al. Addition of tomosynthesis to conventional digital mammography: effect on image interpretation time of screening examinations. *Radiology.* 2014;270(1):49–56.

34. Dustler M, et al. Image quality of thick average intensity pixel slabs using statistical artifact reduction in breast tomosynthesis. *12th International Workshop on Digital Mammography (IWDM 2014)*, Gifu City, Japan; June–July 2014.

35. Dustler M, et al. A study of the feasibility of using slabbing to reduce tomosynthesis review time. Medical Imaging 2013: Image Perception, Observer Performance, and Technology Assessment 867311 March 26, 2013. *Proc SPIE.* 2013;8673:83761L.

36. Zuley M, et al. Comparison of 2 dimensional synthesized mammograms versus original digital mammogram alone and in combination with tomosynthesis images. *Radiology.* 2014;271(3):664–671.

37. Wallis MG, et al. Two view and single view tomosynthesis versus full field digital mammography: high resolution x-ray imaging observer study. *Radiology.* 2012;262(3):788–796.

38. Skaane P, et al. 2 view digital breast tomosynthesis screening with synthetically reconstructed projection images: comparison with digital breast tomosynthesis with full field digital mammographic images. *Radiology.* 2014;271(3):655–663.

39. Saunders RS, et al. Can compression be reduced for breast tomosynthesis? Monte Carlo study on mass and microcalcification cancer conspicuity in tomosynthesis. *Radiology.* 2009;251:673–682.

40. Fornvik D, et al. The effect of reduced breast compression in breast tomosynthesis: human observer study using clinical cases. *Radiat Prot Dosimetry.* 2010;139;118–123.
41. Geiser WR, et al. Challenges in mammography: part 1. Artifacts in digital mammography. *AJR Am J Roentgenol.* 2011;197(960):1023–1030.
42. Kempston M, Mainprize J, Yaffe M. Evaluating the effect of dose on reconstructed image quality in digital tomosynthesis. *Proceedings of the 8th International Workshop on Digital Mammography*, Springer Berlin Heidelberg, Manchester; 2006:490–497.
43. Timberg P, et al. Impact of dose on observer performance in breast tomosynthesis using breast specimens. *Proc SPIE.* 2008;6913:69134J.
44. Nishikawa RM, et al. A new approach to digital breast tomosynthesis for breast cancer screening. *Proc SPIE.* 2007;6510:65103-C–65108-C.
45. Das M, et al. Evaluation of a variable dose acquisition technique for microcalcification and mass detection in digital breast tomosynthesis. *Med Phys.* 2009;36:1976–1984.

Quality Assurance in Mammography

15

Objectives

- Understand current and historical regulatory compliance for facilities that deliver mammography services.
- Understand the purpose and scope of a quality assurance program for mammography services.
- Understand the quality control component of the quality assurance program.
- Understand the regulatory personnel requirements for the delivery of mammography services.
- Understand the regulatory equipment requirements for mammography.
- Understand the responsibilities of the radiologist, medical physicist, and radiologic technologist in the QA/QC program.
- Gain an understanding of the medical outcomes audit required by the MQSA regulations.

Key Terms

- American College of Radiology (ACR)
- Food and Drug Administration (FDA)
- Mammography Accreditation Program (MAP)
- Mammography Quality Standards Act (MQSA)
- quality assurance (QA)
- quality control (QC)
- Policy Guidance Help System (PGHS)
- MQSA (FDA) Annual Inspection

SAFEGUARDING PATIENT CARE AND IMAGE QUALITY

Since the 1930s, medical imaging departments have historically participated in programs to increase the quality of patient care and to control costs by monitoring equipment performance and procedures.[1] Today's health care environment, including medical imaging modalities, requires strict adherence to regulations established by the U.S. Government; additional requirements may be imposed by individual states, health care accrediting agencies, local governments, and individual health care organizations with the intent to improve patient care. Continuous quality improvement (CQI) has become a familiar language to medical professionals in the health care industry; CQI is involved across all aspects of patient care.

Breast imaging, the most regulated of all imaging modalities, requires superior image quality due to the soft tissue nature of the anatomy and the similar appearance of normal versus abnormal tissue. Therefore, the mammographic detection of early breast cancer is dependent on the performance of the mammography equipment, the technologist procuring the image, and the radiologist who interprets the image. These three critical components of mammography services affect image quality and outcome accuracy, which ultimately impact patient safety, care, and satisfaction. To assure that these processes consistently perform according to the rules and regulations of the Mammography Quality Standards Act (MQSA), quality management that includes a robust quality assurance program to monitor all components that contribute to patient safety, employee safety, and image quality is required.

HISTORY OF QUALITY ASSURANCE IN MAMMOGRAPHY

In 1987, in an effort to standardize the quality of mammography in the United States, the **American College of Radiology (ACR)** implemented a voluntary accreditation program for mammography facilities. The ACR **Mammography Accreditation Program (MAP)**[2] gave facilities the opportunity to prove the delivery of superior mammography services by meeting established ACR standards for equipment, personnel, quality assurance, image quality, and dose. This program was positively received by facilities offering mammography services to their customers, and by 1991, half of the 10,000 mammography units in the United States had applied for accreditation. The voluntary ACR Mammography Accreditation Program was available from 1987 to 1991; 70% of the units that applied for accreditation were successful on their first attempt.[3] From 2001 to 2003, almost a decade after the implementation of the MQSA, statistics clearly demonstrated its effect on improving mammography quality and services; the first attempt pass rate rose to 86%.[2] The latest (2012) statistics from the ACR Web site cite first attempt pass rates of 93.8%.[4]

Prior to 1992, the responsibility to ensure mammography quality across the United States fell to individual states or the motivation of individual facilities. During that year, the Senate Committee on Labor and Human Resources determined that mammography services across the country were fraught with problems ranging from the use of substandard equipment, inadequately trained radiologic technologists and interpreting physicians, insufficient quality assurance programs, and lack of government oversight.[5] The quality variance of mammography services offered across the country was evident. The ACR had begun a successful process of ensuring quality services and imaging for patients through a voluntary program, but not all facilities complied. The time had come to standardize care, ensuring quality for all women having mammography.

MAMMOGRAPHY QUALITY STANDARDS ACT OF 1992

In response to the hearings conducted by the Senate Committee on Labor and Human Resources exposing the inconsistent quality of mammography services in the United States, **the Mammography Quality Standards Act (MQSA)** was passed into law by Congress on October 27, 1992. The purpose of MQSA was to "guarantee sufficient oversight of mammography facilities to ensure that all women nationwide receive adequate quality mammography services."[5] Mammography facilities under the auspices of the Department of Veterans Affairs are exempt from MQSA, but to their credit follow their own program for mammography services that is equal to the standards established in the MQSA. Under MQSA, in order to legally perform mammography after October 1, 1994, facilities would be required to become accredited by an approved accreditation body (AB) and certified by the Secretary of Health and Human Services. The Secretary delegated the authority to approve accrediting bodies and to certify facilities to the FDA. Due to the volume of facilities (approximately 10,000) that required certification, the FDA implemented the law in stages, which allowed continued access to mammography services to patients as facilities underwent the certification process; this staged implementation also reduced the workload burden on the accrediting bodies. The first stage implemented by the FDA, The Interim

Rule, went into effect on February 22, 1994. This document, published in the *Federal Register*, defined requirements for facilities to follow that were adapted from standards already developed by the ACR, the Health Care Finance Administration, and by individual states. The Interim Rule secured acceptable quality practices for facilities to meet as they prepared for the increased standards that would be implemented under the Quality Mammography Standards: Final Rule that took effect on April 28, 1999. Among additional regulations, the Final Rule addressed standards that would further define requirements for personnel, equipment, and communication of results to the patient. The MQSA was extended by the Mammography Quality Standards Reauthorization Acts (MQSRA) of 1998 and 2004.

THE SCOPE OF MQSA AND MQSRA

Understanding the scope of MQSA and MQSRA is essential for facilities that offer mammography services to their customers. According to the Code of the Federal Register (CFR 21), "FDA believes that high quality mammography extends from the production of high quality mammographic images to the communication of results to the patient."[5] Every facet of mammography service that impacts the quality of patient care and accuracy of results, including the management of appropriate follow-up care for the patient, has been addressed by the FDA. The requirements established under the MQSA are understood to be the minimum requirements, and facilities are expected to know and carry out what is contained within the law. The FDA/MQSA Web site includes an extensive "Guidance" portal that uses lay terminology to describe how facilities can best comply with the MQSA. The **"Policy Guidance Help System" (PGHS)** is designed for easy navigation of the MQSA standards, allowing the reader to familiarize themselves with every facet of the law. The PGHS supplies much of the material covered in this chapter. At times, it was necessary to borrow direct verbiage from the PGHS in order to ensure accuracy when describing a regulation. The following topics contained within the MQSA require meeting specific standards for facilities that produce, process, or interpret mammograms:

- Facility accreditation and certification
- Equipment
- Personnel
- Medical records and mammography reporting
- Quality assurance—general
- Quality assurance—equipment
- Quality assurance—medical outcomes audit

- Imaging patients with breast implants
- Consumer complaint mechanism
- Clinical image quality
- Annual on-site inspection by an MQSA inspector

FACILITY ACCREDITATION AND CERTIFICATION PROCESS

To lawfully provide mammography services in the United States, facilities must be certified by the **Food and Drug Administration (FDA)** or an FDA-approved State Certifying Agency (SCA). Currently, the FDA has approved the states of Illinois, Iowa, South Carolina, and Texas to be State Certifying Agencies. State Certifying Agencies certify facilities that are located within their own state borders. Prior to becoming certified, a facility must first go through an accreditation process. Certification and accreditation are two separate processes that must be successfully completed prior to the delivery of mammography services. Facilities who successfully satisfy these requirements are designated as an MQSA-certified Mammography Facility and are sent a certificate from the FDA or SCA that must be placed in a prominent area where it may be easily viewed by patients (Figure 15-1). Every facility is required to hold (*physically have in their possession*) an FDA or SCA certificate prior to performing mammography.

Case Study 15-1

Refer to Figures 15-1 and 15-2. Explain the differences between the accreditation process and the certification process. What agencies administer these processes?

The process for accreditation is initiated by contacting an FDA-approved AB to apply for accreditation. The FDA has approved the American College of Radiology (ACR) and the states of Arkansas, Iowa, and Texas as accreditation bodies. Since 2013, the ACR has provided an online process for submission of the information required for the accreditation application. When the initial paperwork for the application process is deemed acceptable, the facility receives further testing information needed to complete the accreditation process. The material that is collected and sent for review by the AB must be submitted within the time frame defined by the AB. This review verifies that the facility has met the established standards for:

- Mammography equipment
- Personnel qualifications
- Clinical image quality

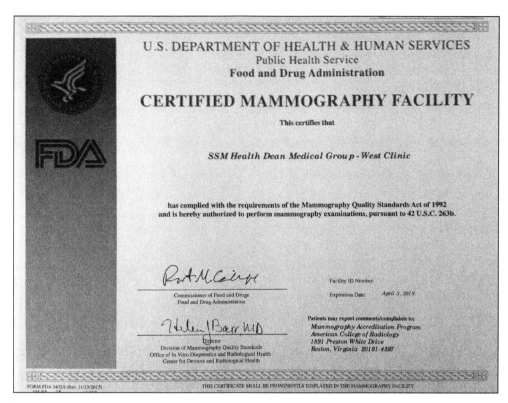

Figure 15-1
Only facilities that are recognized as an FDA Certified Mammography Facility may offer mammography services in the United States. (Source: Photo courtesy of SSM Health, Dean Medical Group.)

- Quality assurance
- Quality control
- Phantom image quality

Most, if not all, of the standards included on this list, are covered under the subject of quality assurance or quality control and are included in Chapters 15 and 16, with the exception of the submission process of required material for clinical image quality to the AB. Although every detail of the submission process is not completely explained in the MQSA, the process is covered in detail on the ACR Web site under "Mammography Accreditation Program Requirements."[6] When submitting clinical images to the AB for evaluation, the facility's images go through the following process:

- Clinical image evaluation is performed by at least two qualified reviewers (radiologists) every 3 years during the accreditation or reaccreditation process.
- Facilities must submit two separate patient examinations consisting of CC and MLO images for each mammography unit; the images must be performed within a specified time frame as defined by the AB. The submitted images include examinations that:
  ◦ Demonstrate predominantly adipose tissue (Category A or B in the BI-RADS)[7]
  ◦ Demonstrate predominantly glandular tissue (Category C or D in the BI-RADS)[7] (refer to Figure 7-21).

- The examinations submitted are required to be interpreted as "negative" (BI-RADS-1). Under certain conditions, accrediting bodies may grant a facility the option to send a "benign" assessment (BI-RADS-2) when submitting images. Facilities should follow the instructions and processes of the AB when submitting images for accreditation and reaccreditation.
- The submitted images should be considered the facility's "best work" and should be approved by the Lead Interpreting Physician (LIP).
- In November 2015, the ACR began accepting electronic submission of images for the Clinical Image Evaluation Accreditation process.
- Two qualified reviewing physicians independently evaluate eight separate attributes of the submitted images[5]:
  ◦ Positioning: Sufficient breast tissue imaged to ensure the detection of disease (and to ensure that cancers are not missed due to inadequate positioning).
  ◦ Compression: Adequate compression applied to the breast that promotes the separation of overlapping breast structures and decreases motion.
  ◦ Exposure: The use of appropriate exposure levels that adequately demonstrate breast structures without overexposure or underexposure to the image.
  ◦ Contrast: Subtle soft tissue variances of the breast visualized through adequate contrast evident on the image.

○ Sharpness: Breast structures demonstrate distinct margins without blur.

○ Noise: Noise should not obscure breast structures, nor should it mimic structures that are not actually present.

○ Artifacts: Artifacts induced by the equipment or process or from external sources should not be apparent on the image.

○ Exam Identification: Image identification requirements include specific patient and exam information. Please refer to Figure 7-228 for the complete list and an illustration of exam identification.

• The eight exam attributes are evaluated separately using a one through five scoring system, with number one correlating to the poorest demonstration of the attribute and number five correlating to the best demonstration of the attribute. Image quality is considered deficient when a one or a two is given in any attribute category or when the Posterior Nipple Line measurement fails (indicating posterior tissue has been excluded).[6]

Documentation of the clinical image review is provided to the facility. The documentation is required to include reasons for assigned scoring should deficiencies be noted in the attribute categories along with information for improvement.

Facilities who lawfully offer mammography services and currently hold a MQSA certificate reapply to the AB for renewal every 3 years. Upon successful verification and review of materials submitted to the AB from the facility, the AB sends the facility appropriate verification documents of accreditation (Figure 15-2), and the AB notifies the FDA or SCA, who in turn issues the facility a new MQSA certificate to permit the continued delivery of mammography services. Certification must be renewed by the facility prior to its expiration date to remain in compliance with the MQSA. The certificate renewal process is cyclical, repeating the steps necessary to become accredited, resulting in a new FDA certificate allowing another 3 years of compliance for the facility.

First-time applicants to the MQSA certification process are granted an FDA/SCA 6-month provisional certificate, which provides time to collect the necessary data and clinical images required for the AB review. Upon successful verification and review of criteria submitted by the facility to the AB, the AB notifies the FDA or SCA, who in turn issues the facility a full (3-year) MQSA certificate permitting the continued delivery of mammography services. Facilities that satisfy the accreditation process and are designated as an MQSA-certified Facility are also advised, prior to performing mammography services, to ascertain if there are individual State and/or local laws pertaining to this service.

In addition to the mandatory accreditation process for mammography services, the ACR also offers voluntary accreditation for stereotactic breast biopsy (SBBAP), breast ultrasound (BUAP), and breast MRI. When a facility

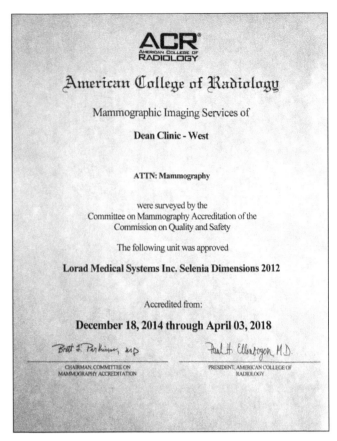

Figure 15-2
Prior to becoming a Certified Mammography Facility, each facility must pass the FDA accreditation process which includes criteria for each individual mammography unit. (Source: Photo courtesy of SSM Health, Dean Medical Group.)

becomes accredited in all of these modalities, they are awarded the distinction of being a Breast Imaging Center of Excellence (BICOE).

CLINICAL IMAGE QUALITY

The quality of clinical images produced at a facility and the relationship to accurate interpretation directly correlates to the potential to detect breast cancer and is appropriately addressed at the very beginning of the CFR21. Because deficient image quality impacts the need for additional image evaluation and impacts the ability of the interpreting physician to detect breast cancer, the MQSA explicitly includes "clinical image quality" as a separate standard, stating "Clinical images produced by any certified facility must continue to comply with the standards for clinical image quality established by that facility's accreditation body."[5] Separately including this standard in the MQSA directly informs the facility producing mammography images that image quality should be maintained continually and not isolated to the accreditation process. The intention to ensure that quality mammography is provided to every patient is addressed by two processes in the MQSA:

1. The accreditation and reaccreditation process requires the submission of clinical images for evaluation ensuring image quality standards are achieved.
2. The annual AB process of conducting onsite visits and random clinical image reviews evaluates the clinical image quality of selected mammography services throughout the United States to further verify that facilities appropriately address and maintain clinical image quality through quality assurance.

The 1999 ACR Mammography Quality Control Manual includes a thorough explanation of the eight attributes evaluated on the clinical images submitted for the accreditation process in a section titled "Clinical Image Evaluation." This section of the manual was excluded in the 2016 ACR Digital Mammography Quality Control Manual; however, the section was added to the ACR Web site in 2016. The Clinical Image Evaluation portion of the 1999 ACR Mammography Quality Control Manual may be accessed using the following web address: acraccreditation.org.[8]

In September 2016, the FDA announced its EQUIP (Enhancing Quality Using the Inspection Program) initiative. EQUIP adds three questions to the inspection process; one question emphasizes the responsibility of the LIP to provide oversight of the QA/QC program discussed later in this chapter under QA/AC Quarterly Review. The remaining EQUIP questions pertain to the following MQSA standards that address image quality[9]:

- *900.12(i): Clinical image quality. Clinical images produced by any certified facility must continue to comply with the standards for clinical image quality established by that facility's accreditation body.*
- *900.12(d)(1)(i),(ii)(A)(B):*
  - *(ii) Interpreting physicians. All interpreting physicians interpreting mammograms for the facility shall:*
  - *(A) Follow the facility procedures for corrective action when the images they are asked to interpret are of poor quality, and*
  - *(B) Participate in the facility's medical outcomes audit program.*

Implementation of the initiative, which strengthens the process to ensure that the Interpreting Physician (IP) addresses images of inferior quality that are submitted for interpretation, began in January 2017. The EQUIP program incorporates the following questions posed to facilities during the annual MQSA inspection process regarding the facility's actions to safeguard image quality[10]:

- Does the facility have procedures for corrective action (CA) when clinical images are of poor quality? (Yes/No)
  - Do the procedures include a mechanism for providing ongoing IP feedback on image quality to RTs or other designated facility personnel? (Yes/No)
  - Do the procedures include a mechanism for documenting any needed corrective actions and documenting the effectiveness of any corrective actions taken? (Yes/No)
- Does the facility have procedures to ensure that clinical images continue to comply with the clinical image quality standards established by its accreditation body? (Yes/No)
  - Do the procedures include a mechanism for regular reviews of image quality attributes of a sample of mammograms performed by each active RT and a sample of mammograms accepted for interpretation by each active IP? (Yes/No)
- Is there documentation of such review since the last inspection? (Yes/No)

The plan to launch the EQUIP program over a 3-year period allows the inspection process to educate and inform facilities about the expectations of EQUIP during the first year. During the second year of implementation, facilities that do not demonstrate compliance of the EQUIP program will receive a Level 2 citation, requiring corrective action. During the third year, a repeat Level 2 citation will be issued to the facility for noncompliance, requiring a written response to the FDA within 15 days and will be referred to its AB for evaluation of clinical images.[10]

According to information published on the FDA Web site regarding EQUIP, documentation that could satisfy the EQUIP requirements for image quality review include the following examples:

- Summary report
- Clinical image review records
- LIP signed statement that a review was performed
- Documentation of memos to mammography technologists and to IPs

PERSONNEL REQUIREMENTS

The MQSA ensures that personnel involved in the production, processing, and interpretation of mammography are initially qualified to perform their responsibilities and that they maintain the expertise necessary to support their application to mammography. These requirements apply to the interpreting physicians, medical physicists, and radiologic technologists who all contribute in some way to the mammography services and image quality delivered by the facility. These requirements also apply to any mammography personnel performing quality assurance responsibilities related to the program. In order to meet the MQSA standards for personnel, three categories of compliance must be met:

- Initial qualifications
- Continuing education
- Continuing experience

These three categories of personnel compliance for the MQSA are further defined in Table 15-1 for interpreting physicians, Table 15-2 for medical hysicists, and Table 15-3 for radiologic technologists. Especially useful to the radiologic technologist is the form found on the FDA Web site in the Policy Guidance Help System (PGHS) titled "Radiologic Technologist Qualification Worksheet" (Figure 15-3) that clearly describes requirements the technologist must complete prior to performing mammography examinations and the requirements she must complete to continue performing mammography according to the MQSA.

Table 15-1 • Acceptable Documents for Interpreting Physicians (PGHS)

REQUIREMENT	OBTAINED PRIOR TO 10/1/94	OBTAINED 10/1/94 TO 4/28/99	OBTAINED AFTER 4/28/99
State license	1. State license/copy with expiration date 2. Confirming letter from State licensing board 3. Pocket card/copy of license	1. State license/copy with expiration date 2. Confirming letter from State licensing board 3. Pocket card/copy of license	1. State license/copy with expiration date 2. Confirming letter from State licensing board 3. Pocket card/copy of license
Board certification (ABR, AOBR, or RCPSC)	1. Original/copy of certificate 2. Confirming letter from certifying board 3. Confirming letter from ACR 4. Listing in ABMS directory	1. Original/copy of certificate 2. Confirming letter from certifying board 3. Confirming letter from ACR 4. Listing in ABMS directory	1. Original/copy of certificate 2. Confirming letter from certifying board 3. Confirming letter from ACR 4. Listing in ABMS directory
Formal training (2 months—interim regs) (3 months—final regs)	1. Letters or other documents from US or Canadian residency programs 2. Documentation of formal mammography training courses 3. Category I CME certificates	1. Letters or other documents from US or Canadian residency programs 2. Documentation of formal mammography training courses 3. Category I CME certificates	1. Letters or other documents from US or Canadian residency programs 2. Documentation of formal mammography training courses 3. Category I CME certificates
Initial medical education (40 hours—interim regs) (60 hours/15 in last 3 years—final regs)	1. Attestation 2. Letter from residency program 3. CME certificates 4. Letter or other document confirming in-house or formal training	1. Letter from residency program 2. CME certificates 3. Letter or other document confirming in-house or formal training	1. Letter from residency program 2. Category I CME certificates 3. Letter or other document confirming in-house or formal training (Category I)
Initial experience (240) (any 6-month period—interim regs) (last 6 months vs. 6 months in last 2 years of residency—final regs)	1. Attestation 2. Letter or other document from residency or training program or mammography facility	1. Letter or other document from residency or training program or mammography facility—done under direct supervision	1. Letter or other document from residency or training program or mammography facility—done under direct supervision
Initial Mammographic Modality Specific Training—8 hours—final regs	1. Attestation for training or experience with investigational units 2. Mammography Modality Specific CME certificates (Category I or II) 3. CME certificates (Category I or II) plus agenda, course outline or syllabus 4. Confirming letters from CME granting organizations 5. Letters, certificates or other documents from manufacturers' or other formal training courses 6. Letter from facility where experience was obtained documenting experience in the new mammographic modality	1. Attestation for experience with investigational units 2. Mammography Modality Specific CME certificates (Category I or II) 3. CME certificates (Category I or II) plus agenda, course outline or syllabus 4. Confirming letters from CME granting organizations 5. Letters, certificates or other documents from manufacturers' or other formal training courses 6. Letter from facility where experience was obtained documenting experience in the new mammographic modality	1. Attestation for experience with investigational units 2. Mammography Modality Specific CME certificates (Category I or II) 3. CME certificates (Category I or II) plus agenda, course outline or syllabus 4. Confirming letters from CME granting organizations 5. Letters, certificates or other documents from manufacturers' or other formal training courses
Continuing experience (960/24 months)	N/A	N/A	1. Letter, table, facility logs or other documentation from residency or training program or mammography facility

Table 15-1 • Acceptable Documents for Interpreting Physicians (PGHS) (*Continued*)

REQUIREMENT	OBTAINED PRIOR TO 10/1/94	OBTAINED 10/1/94 TO 4/28/99	OBTAINED AFTER 4/28/99
Continuing Education (15 CME/36 months—interim regs) (15 Category I CME/36 months—final regs)	N/A	N/A	1. CME certificates (Category I) 2. Confirming letters from CME granting organizations
Continuing Mammographic Modality Specific Education—final regs (enforcement delayed indefinitely)	N/A	N/A	1. Mammography Modality Specific CME certificates (Category I) 2. CME certificates (Category I) plus agenda, course outline or syllabus 3. Confirming letters from CME granting organizations
Requalification–experience–done under direct supervision	N/A	N/A	1. Letter, table, facility logs or other documentation from residency or training program or mammography facility
Requalification–education	N/A	N/A	1. CME certificates (Category I) 2. Confirming letters from CME granting organizations

The table summarizes the types of documentation that interpreting physicians may use to document their initial qualifications, as well as their continuing requirements and requalification requirements, prior to MQSA and under the interim and final regulations.
Source: FDA/MQSA Web site: Home/Radiation Emitting Products/Mammography Quality Standards Act and Program/Guidance (MQSA)/Policy Guidance Help System/Personnel/Interpreting Physician/Acceptable Documents for Interpreting Physician (www.fda.gov). Accessed October 10, 2016.

Table 15-2 • Acceptable Documents for Medical Physicists (PGHS)

REQUIREMENT	OBTAINED PRIOR TO 10/1/94	OBTAINED 10/1/94 TO 4/28/99	OBTAINED AFTER 4/28/99
State license or approval	1. Original/copy of State license or approval/copy with expiration dated 2. Confirming letter from State licensing board	1. Original/copy of State license or approval/copy with expiration date 2. Confirming letter from State licensing board	1. Original/copy of State license or approval/copy with expiration date 2. Confirming letter from State licensing board
Board certification (ABR, AOBR, or RCPSC)	1. Original/copy of certificate 2. Confirming letter from certifying board 3. Pocket card/copy of certificate 4. Confirming letter from ACR	1. Original/copy of certificate 2. Confirming letter from certifying board 3. Pocket card/copy of certificate 4. Confirming letter from ACR	1. Original/copy of certificate 2. Confirming letter from certifying board 3. Pocket card/copy of certificate 4. Confirming letter from ACR
Degree in a physical science–final regs (Master's pathway) (Bachelor's pathway)	1. Original/copy of diploma 2. Confirming letter from college or university 3. FDA approval letter	1. Original/copy of diploma 2. Confirming letter from college or university 3. FDA approval letter	1. Original/copy of diploma 2. Confirming letter from college or university 3. FDA approval letter
Initial physics education—final regs (20 semester hours—Master) (10 semester hours—Bachelors)	1. College or university transcripts 2. Confirming letter from college or university 3. Master or Bachelor degree specifically in physics 4. FDA approval letter	1. College or university transcripts 2. Confirming letter from college or university 3. Master or Bachelor degree specifically in physics 4. FDA approval letter	1. College or university transcript 2. Confirming letter from college or university 3. Master degree specifically in physics 4. FDA approval letter
Survey training—final regs (20 contact hours—Master) (40 contact hours—Bachelors)	1. Attestation 2. Letter or other document from training program 3. CME/CEU certificates 4. Letter or other document confirming in-house or formal training 5. Training gained performing surveys 6. FDA approval letter	1. Letter or other document from training program 2. CME/CEU certificates 3. Letter or other document confirming in-house or formal training 4. Training gained performing surveys 5. FDA approval letter	1. Letter or other document from training program 2. CME/CEU certificates 3. Letter or other document confirming in-house or formal training 4. Training gained performing surveys 5. FDA approval letter

(*Continued*)

Table 15-2 • Acceptable Documents for Medical Physicists (PGHS) (*Continued*)

REQUIREMENT	OBTAINED PRIOR TO 10/1/94	OBTAINED 10/1/94 TO 4/28/99	OBTAINED AFTER 4/28/99
Initial experience—final regs (1 facility—10 units—Master) (1 facility—20 units—Bachelor)	1. Attestation 2. Copy or coversheet of survey 3. Letter from facility or listing from company providing the physics survey services documenting performance of survey done 4. FDA approval letter	1. Copy or coversheet of survey 2. Letter from facility or listing from company providing the physics survey services documenting performance of survey done 3. FDA approval letter	1. Copy or coversheet of survey done under direct supervision 2. Letter from facility or listing from company providing the physics survey services documenting performance of survey done under direct supervision 3. FDA approval letter
Initial mammography modality-specific training—8 hours—final regs	1. Attestation for training or experience with investigational units 2. Mammography modality-specific CME/CEU certificates 3. CME/CEU certificates plus agenda, course outline, or syllabus 4. Confirming letters from CME/CEU granting organizations 5. Letters, certificates, or other documents from manufacturers' or other formal training courses 6. Letter from facility where experience was obtained documenting experience in the new mammographic modality	1. Attestation for experience with investigational units 2. Mammography modality-specific CME/CEU certificates 3. CME/CEU certificates plus agenda, course outline, or syllabus 4. Confirming letters from CME/CEU granting organizations 5. Letters, certificates, or other documents from manufacturers' or other formal training courses 6. Letter from facility where experience was obtained documenting experience in the new mammographic modality	1. Attestation for experience with investigational units 2. Mammography modality-specific CME/CEU certificates 3. CME/CEU certificates plus agenda, course outline, or syllabus 4. Confirming letters from CME/CEU granting organizations 5. Letters, certificates, or other documents from manufacturers' or other formal training courses
Continue experience (2 facilities—6 units/24 months—final regs)	N/A	N/A	1. Copy or coversheet of survey 2. Letter from facility or listing from company providing the physics survey services documenting performance of survey done
Continuing mammographic modality-specific education—final regs (enforcement delayed indefinitely)	N/A	N/A	1. Mammography modality-specific CME/CEU certificates 2. CME/CEU certificates (plus agenda, course outline or syllabus 3. Confirming letters from CME/CEU granting organizations
Requalification experience—final regs—done under direct supervision	N/A	N/A	1. Copy or coversheet of survey done under direct supervision 2. Letter from facility or listing from company providing the physics survey services documenting performance of survey done under direct supervision
Requalification education	N/A	N/A	1. CME/CEU certificates 2. Confirming letters from CME/CEU granting organizations 3. Letters, certificates or other documents from manufacturers' or other formal training courses

The table summarizes the types of documentation that medical physicists may use to document their initial qualifications, as well as their continuing requirements and requalification requirements, prior to MQSA and under the interim and final regulations.
Source: FDA/MQSA Web site: Home/Radiation Emitting Products/Mammography Quality Standards Act and Program/Guidance (MQSA)/Policy Guidance Help System/Personnel/Medical Physicist/Acceptable Documents for Medical Physicists (www.fda.gov). Accessed October 10, 2016.

Table 15-3 • Acceptable Documents for Radiologic Technologists (PGHS)

REQUIREMENT	OBTAINED PRIOR TO 10/1/94	OBTAINED 10/1/94 TO 4/28/99	OBTAINED AFTER 4/28/99
State License	1. State license/copy with expiration date 2. Confirming letter from State licensing board 3. Pocket card/copy of license	1. State license/copy with expiration date 2. Confirming letter from State licensing board 3. Pocket card/copy of license	1. State license/copy with expiration date 2. Confirming letter from State licensing board 3. Pocket card/copy of license
Board certification (ARRT or ARCRT)	1. Original/copy of current certificate 2. Confirming letter from certifying board 3. Pocket card/copy of certificate	1. Original/copy of current certificate 2. Confirming letter from certifying board 3. Pocket card/copy of certificate	1. Original/copy of current certificate 2. Confirming letter from certifying board 3. Pocket card/copy of certificate
Initial training (~40 hours–interim regs) (40 hours–25 supervised exams–final regs)	1. Attestation 2. Letter or other document from training program 3. CEU certificates 4. Letter or other document confirming in-house or formal training 5. ARRT(M) Mammography certificate 6. California Mammography certificate 7. Arizona Mammography certificate 8. Nevada Mammography certificate	1. Letter or other document from training program 2. CEU certificates 3. Letter or other document confirming in-house or formal training 4. Approved RT training courses 5. California Mammography certificate 6. Arizona Mammography certificate 7. Nevada Mammography certificate	1. Letter or other document from training program 2. CEU certificates 3. Letter or other document confirming in-house or formal training 4. ARRT(M) Mammography certificate but only if issued after 1/1/01 5. Certain State issued Mammography certificate(s)-facilities need to check with their State inspectors
Initial mammography modality-specific training—8 hours—final regs	1. Attestation for training or experience with investigational units 2. Mammography modality -specific CEU certificates 3. CEU certificates plus agenda, course outline or syllabus 4. Confirming letters from CEU granting organizations 5. Letters, certificates, or other documents from manufacturers' or other formal training courses 6. Letter from facility where experience was obtained documenting experience in the new mammographic modality	1. Attestation for experience with investigational units 2. Mammography modality-specific CEU certificates 3. CEU certificates plus agenda, course outline or syllabus 4. Confirming letters from CEU granting organizations 5. Letters, certificates, or other documents from manufacturers' or other formal training courses 6. Letter from facility where experience was obtained documenting experience in the new mammographic modality	1. Attestation for experience with investigational units 2. Mammography modality-specific CEU certificates 3. CEU certificates plus agenda, course outline or syllabus 4. Confirming letters from CEU granting organizations 5. Letters, certificates, or other documents from manufacturers' or other formal training courses
Continuing experience (200/24 months—final regs)	N/A	N/A	1. Letter, table, facility logs, or other documentation from training program or mammography facility
Continuing mammographic modality-specific education—final regs	N/A	N/A	1. Mammography modality-specific CEU certificates 2. CEU certificates (plus agenda, course outline or syllabus 3. Confirming letters from CEU granting organizations 4. Letters, certificates, or other documents from manufacturers' or other formal training courses
Requalification—experience—final regs—done under direct supervision	N/A	N/A	1. Letter, table, facility logs, or other documentation from training program or mammography facility (done under direct supervision)

(Continued)

Table 15-3 • Acceptable Documents for Radiologic Technologists (PGHS) (*Continued*)

REQUIREMENT	OBTAINED PRIOR TO 10/1/94	OBTAINED 10/1/94 TO 4/28/99	OBTAINED AFTER 4/28/99
Requalification education	N/A	N/A	1. CEU certificates 2. Confirming letters from CEU granting organizations 3. Letter or other document confirming in-house or formal training 4. Letters, certificates, or other documents from manufacturers' or other formal training courses

The table summarizes the types of documentation that radiologic technologists may use to document their initial qualifications, as well as their continuing requirements and requalification requirements, prior to MQSA and under the interim and final regulations.
Source: FDA/MQSA Web site: Home/Radiation Emitting Products/Mammography Quality Standards Act and Program/Guidance (MQSA)/Policy Guidance Help System/Personnel/Radiologic Technologist/Acceptable Documents for Radiologic Technologist (www.fda.gov). Accessed October 10, 2016.

Radiologic Technologist Qualification Worksheet
This worksheet may be used by facilities to help ensure that their personnel meet all applicable requirements prior to providing mammography services.

Initial Qualifications Met Before 4/28/99 (INTERIM)	Initial Qualifications Met After 4/28/99(FINAL)
Need one of the following:	Need one of the following:
___ General radiography license (any State)	___ General radiography license (any State)
___ General certification (ARRT or ARCRT)	___ General certification (ARRT)
Need one of the following:	Need all of the following:
___ 40 hours of mammography training ___ ARRT (M) ___ CA Mammography Certification ___ AZ Mammography Certification ___ NV Mammography Certification ___ Completion of prior FDA accepted course or training	___ 40 hours of mammography training including the following subjects: ___ Breast Anatomy ___ Physiology ___ Positioning/Compression ___ QA/QC ___ Breast Implants
(attestation allowed if training completed prior to 10/1/94)	___ 25 supervised patient exams (generally up to 12.5 hours can be counted toward the 40 hours, but must be documented)

START DATE _____
(The later of 10/1/94 or date the last initial qualification was completed)

___ 8 hours initial training in additional mammographic modality used (if applicable)
DATE COMPLETED _____

Continuing Qualifications

All of the following:

___ 200 patient exams in the 24 months prior to the current date
(applicable 24 months after start date)

___ 15 CMEs in the 36 months prior to the current date
(applicable 36 months after start date)

Figure 15-3
Radiologic Technologist Qualification Worksheet (PGHS). (Source: FDA/MQSA Web site: Home/Radiation Emitting Products/ Mammography Quality Standards Act and Program/Guidance (MQSA)/Policy Guidance Help System/Personnel/Radiologic Technologist/Radiologic Technologist Overview [www.fda.gov]. Accessed October 10, 2016.)

Additional personnel qualifications and credentialing may be fulfilled through professional association with the following organizations:

- ACR (American College of Radiology): Professional medical association—members include radiologists and medical physicists (www.acr.org).
- AAPM (American Association of Physicists in Medicine): Professional organization—members include medical physicists (www.aapm.org).
- ASRT (American Society of Radiologic Technologists): Professional association—members include medical imaging and radiation therapy technologists (www.asrt.org).
- ARRT (American Registry of Radiologic Technologists): Credentialing organization for medical imaging, interventional procedures, and radiation therapy technologists (www.arrt.org).
- ARMRIT (American Registry of Magnetic Resonance Imaging Technologists): Registry and certifying organization for MRI technologists (www.armrit.org).
- ARDMS (American Registry for Diagnostic Medical Sonography): Governing organization of ultrasound professionals (www.ardms.org).

EQUIPMENT REQUIREMENTS

Only equipment specifically designed for the purpose of imaging the breast can be used to perform mammography under the MQSA (Figure 15-4). Today's landscape of digital mammography units complies with strict equipment requirements established in the interim regulations of

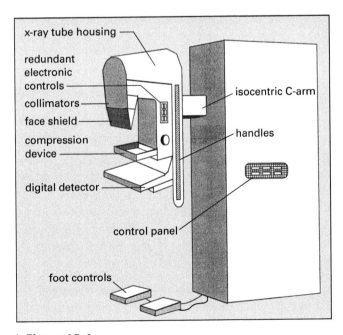

Figure 15-4
Dedicated FFDM DR mammography unit.

x-ray tube housing

redundant electronic controls

collimators

face shield

compression device

digital detector

isocentric C-arm

handles

control panel

foot controls

the MQSA and later more stringent equipment component requirements effective October 28, 2002 that were addressed in the Final Rule. Only mammography equipment approved for use by the FDA may be used to produce mammography images. Table 15-4 provides a list of manufacturers and their mammography units currently approved by the FDA. Prior to clinical use, mammography equipment must be evaluated by a medical physicist. This is required for a new equipment purchase, equipment that has been disassembled and reassembled (i.e., moving a unit within the same organization), or if major components of the equipment have been changed or repaired.[9] In these cases, a Mammography Equipment Evaluation (MEE) is performed by a medical physicist verifying that all components of the unit have met the standards established by the FDA for that unit manufacturer. Due to the number of approved FFDM/DBT, units utilized for mammography in the United States, including a complete list of all manufacturers MEEs in this chapter is not possible. For the purpose of providing an example of what is included in an MEE, the equipment components included in an MEE for three manufacturers are illustrated in Figure 15-5A–C.[11] A complete list of MEE equipment requirements for each manufacturer can be found on the FDA Web site and the ACR Web site listed in this chapter under "Where to Find Help With Compliance". Equipment requiring evaluation by the medical physicist includes all equipment that is used in the entire mammography imaging chain. For FFDM, this applies to the mammography unit, the radiologist's workstation/monitors (soft copy image display), and the laser printer (if applicable). Medical physicists are also required to perform annual surveys on mammography equipment previously installed and accredited. The results of the medical physicist's evaluation must be sent to the facility within 30 days of the date of the survey.[9] Physicist MEEs or annual surveys are reviewed during the MQSA inspection and at the request of the AB. Further discussions explaining the components mandated for mammography units and the required quality control for dedicated FFDM mammography units can be found in Chapters 11 and 16, respectively.

MEDICAL RECORDS AND MAMMOGRAPHY REPORTING

Required Contents and Terminology of the Mammography Report

The report generated by the IP for each mammography examination provides important information to the patient and her referring physician. To ensure this communication is consistent and understood across all medical practices,

Table 15-4 • FDA Approved FFDM and DBT Systems (PGHS)

Siemens Mammomat Fusion	09/14/15
Siemens Mammomat Inspiration with Tomosynthesis Option (DBT) System	4/21/15
GE SenoClaire Digital Breast Tomosynthesis (DBT) System	8/26/14
Fuji Aspire Cristalle Full-Field Digital Mammography (FFDM) System	03/25/14
Siemens Mammomat Inspiration Prime Full-Field Digital Mammography (FFDM) System	06/11/13
iCRco 3600M Mammography Computed Radiography (CR) System	04/26/13
Philips MicroDose SI Model L50 Full-Field Digital Mammography (FFDM) System	02/01/13
Fuji Aspire HD Plus Full-Field Digital Mammography (FFDM) System	09/21/12
Fuji Aspire HD-s Full-Field Digital Mammography (FFDM) System	09/21/12
Konica Minolta Xpress Digital Mammography Computed Radiography (CR) System	12/23/11
Agfa Computed Radiography (CR) Mammography System	12/22/11
Fuji Aspire Computed Radiography for Mammography (CRM) System	12/8/11
Giotto Image 3D-3DL Full-Field Digital Mammography (FFDM) System	10/27/11
Fuji Aspire HD Full-Field Digital Mammography (FFDM) System	9/1/11
GE Senographe Care Full-Field Digital Mammography (FFDM) System	10/7/11
Planmed Nuance Excel Full-Field Digital Mammography (FFDM) System	9/23/11
Planmed Nuance Full-Field Digital Mammography (FFDM) System	9/23/11
Siemens Mammomat Inspiration Pure Full-Field Digital Mammography (FFDM) System	8/16/11
Hologic Selenia Encore Full-Field Digital Mammography (FFDM) System	6/15/11
Philips (Sectra) MicroDose L30 Full-Field Digital Mammography (FFDM) System	4/28/11
Hologic Selenia Dimensions Digital Breast Tomosynthesis (DBT) System	2/11/11
Siemens Mammomat Inspiration Full-Field Digital Mammography (FFDM) System	2/11/11
Carestream Directview Computed Radiography (CR) Mammography System	11/3/10
Hologic Selenia Dimensions 2D Full-Field Digital Mammography (FFDM) System	2/11/09
Hologic Selenia S Full-Field Digital Mammography (FFDM) System	2/11/09
Siemens Mammomat Novation S Full-Field Digital Mammography (FFDM) System	2/11/09
Hologic Selenia Full-Field Digital Mammography (FFDM) System with a Tungsten (W) target	11/2007
Fuji Computed Radiography Mammography Suite (FCRMS)	07/10/06
GE Senographe Essential Full-Field Digital Mammography (FFDM) System	04/11/06
Siemens Mammomat Novation DR Full-Field Digital Mammography (FFDM) System	08/20/04
GE Senographe DS Full-Field Digital Mammography (FFDM) System	02/19/04
Lorad/Hologic Selenia Full-Field Digital Mammography (FFDM) System	10/2/02
Lorad Digital Breast Imager Full-Field Digital Mammography (FFDM) System	03/15/02
Fischer Imaging SenoScan Full-Field Digital Mammography (FFDM) System	09/25/01
GE Senographe 2000D Full-Field Digital Mammography (FFDM) System	01/28/00

The following FFDM and DBT units have been approved for use in mammography facilities by the FDA since January 2000.
Source: FDA/MQSA Web site: Home/Radiation Emitting Products/Mammography Quality Standards Act and Program/Facility Certification and Inspection/Digital Accreditation (www.fda.gov). Accessed October 10, 2016.

the MQSA stipulates the content and terminology used in the report. To satisfy MQSA requirements, the report must include the name of the patient and an additional identifier, the date of the examination, and the name of the physician who interpreted the mammogram. Additionally, the report must contain an overall final assessment assigned by the IP. The MQSA separates these final assessments into categories.[9] The final assessment categories were developed for the Breast Imaging and Reporting Data System (BI-RADS) by the ACR,[7] with minor changes noted in the MQSA final assessments.[5] The decision to use these final assessment categories was based upon the established use and familiarity of the ACR BI-RADS final assessment categories in the medical community prior to the enactment of the MQSA. Table 15-5 lists the assessment categories required by the MQSA to be incorporated in the mammography report. The words in quotations under the left column of the table are required to be included in the report for the designated assessment category or when no assessment category can be assigned. The verbiage under the right column of the table is provided to explain the categories and may be used by the IP if desired. In addition to the final assessment category, the MQSA regulation also requires the report to include recommendations to the provider and patient for further action, should it be necessary. The FDA PGHS (discussed later in this chapter) addresses additional assessment categories included in the Approved Alternative Standards[9] (also discussed later in this chapter) for their specific application in mammography:

• Postprocedure mammograms for marker placement.
• Known biopsy-proven malignancy: appropriate action should be taken.
• Separate assessment of findings for each breast.

MEDICAL PHYSICIST'S MAMMOGRAPHY QC TEST SUMMARY
Full-Field Digital—Siemens

Site Name		**Report Date**	
Address		**Survey Date**	
Medical Physicist's Name		**Signature**	
X-Ray Unit Manufacturer	Siemens	**Model**	
Date of Installation		**Room ID**	

QC Manual Version # _____ *(use version applicable to unit tested; contact mfr if questions)*

Accessory Equipment

	Manufacturer	Model	Location	QC Manual Version #
Review Workstation*			☐ On-site ☐ Off-site	
Film Printer*			☐ On-site ☐ Off-site	

FDA recommends that only monitors and printers specifically cleared for FFDM use by FDA's Office of Device Evaluation (ODE) be used. See FDA's Policy Guidance Help System www.fda.gov/CDRH/MAMMOGRAPHY/robohelp/START.HTM.

Survey Type (☐ Mammo Eqpt Evaluation of new unit (include MQSA Rqmts for Mammo Eqpt checklist))   (☐ Annual Survey)

Medical Physicist's QC Tests
("Pass" means all components of the test passes; indicate "Fail" if any component fails. Tests must be done for both on and off-site equipment.)

PASS/FAIL

1. **Site Audit/Evaluation of Technologist QC Program**
2. **Mechanical Inspection**
3. **Acquisition Workstation Monitor Check**
4. **Detector Uniformity**
5. **Artifact Detection**
6. **Collimation, Dead Space & Compression Paddle Position**
7. **AEC Thickness Tracking**
8. **Spatial Resolution**
9. **SNR, CNR and AEC Repeatability**
   Measured values: SNR _____   CNR _____
   CV for mAs and entrance air kerma ≤5%
   Max deviation of mean pixel values and SNR within ±15% of mean for measurements
10. **Image Quality**
    Largest 5 fibers, 4 speck groups and 4 masses visible*
    *(*largest 4 fibers, 3 speck groups and 3 masses acceptable if spatial resolution and CNR pass)*
    Phantom image scores: Fibers _____   Specks _____   Masses _____
11. **Radiation Dose**
    Average glandular dose for average breast is ≤3 mGy (300 mrad)   _____ mrad
12. **HVL and Radiation Output**
13. **Tube Voltage Measurement & Reproducibility**
14. **Film Printer Check**
15. **Review Workstation (RWS) Tests** *(for all RWS, even if located offsite; NA if only hardcopy read)*

*** YOUR MEDICAL PHYSICIST MUST SUMMARIZE HIS/HER RESULTS ON THIS FORM ***

A

Figure 15-5
(A) Example #1 of Medical Physicist MEE, Manufacturer Specific. (Source: ACR Web site: www.acraccreditation.org Quality Control and Equipment Evaluation Forms/Medical Physicist Evaluation Forms/Medical Physicist Mammography QC Test Summary-Manufacturer Specific.)

MEDICAL PHYSICIST'S MAMMOGRAPHY QC TEST SUMMARY
Full-Field Digital—General Electric

Site Name	**Report Date**
Address	**Survey Date**
Medical Physicist's Name	**Signature**
X-Ray Unit Manufacturer General Electric	**Model**
Date of Installation	**Room ID**

QC Manual Version # *(use version applicable to unit tested; contact mfr if questions)*

Accessory Equipment

	Manufacturer	Model	Location	QC Manual Version #
Review Workstation*			☐ On-site ☐ Off-site	
Film Printer*			☐ On-site ☐ Off-site	

FDA recommends that only monitors and printers specifically cleared for FFDM use by FDA's Office of Device Evaluation (ODE) be used. See FDA's Policy Guidance Help System www.fda.gov/CDRH/MAMMOGRAPHY/robohelp/START.HTM.

Survey Type ☐ Mammo Eqpt Evaluation of new unit (include MQSA Rqmts for Mammo Eqpt checklist)   ☐ Annual Survey

Medical Physicist's QC Tests

("Pass" means all components of the test passes; indicate "Fail" if any component fails. Tests must be done for both on and off-site equipment.)

PASS/FAIL

1. **Flat Field**
2. **Phantom Image Quality**

	Fibers	Specks	Masses
Phantom IQ Test on AWS			
Phantom IQ Test on Printer			

3. **CNR Measurement** *(NA for DS, Essential or Care if Sub-System MTF test done)*

   CNR [____] *(Required for both new unit Mammography Equipment Evaluations and Annual Surveys)*

   Change in CNR ≤0.2 *(NA for Mammography Equipment Evaluations)*
4. **MTF Measurement** *(NA for 2000D, DS, Essential or Care if Sub-System MTF test done)*
5. **AOP Mode and SNR**
6. **Collimation Assessment**

	Mammo Equipment Evaluation			Annual Survey		
	Ess/Care	DS	2000D	Ess/Care	DS	2000D
24 cm x 30.7 cm	x	NA	NA	x	NA	NA
19 cm x 23 cm tests	x	x	x	NA	x	x

7. **Evaluation of Focal Spot Performance** *(NA for 2000D, DS, Essential or Care if Sub-System MTF test done)*
8. **Sub-System (MTF)** *(NA for 2000D if MTF and Focal Spot Performance tests done; NA for DS, Essential or Care if CNR, MTF and Focal Spot Performance tests done)*
9. **Breast Entrance Exposure, Average Glandular Dose and Reproducibility**

   Average glandular dose for average breast is ≤3 mGy (300 mrad) [____] mrad

   Exposure reproducibility (CV) for air kerma (R) and mAs is ≤0.05
10. **Artifact Evaluation and Flat Field Uniformity**
11. **kVp Accuracy and Reproducibility**
12. **Beam Quality Assessment (Half-Value Layer Measurement**
13. **Radiation Output**

    Radiation output is ≥800 mR/s [____] mR/s
14. **Mammographic Unit Assembly Evaluation**

    Meets requirements for motion of tube-image receptor assembly

    Meets requirements for compression paddle decompression
15. **Review Workstation (RWS) Tests** *(for all RWS, even if located offsite; NA if only hardcopy read)*

*** YOUR MEDICAL PHYSICIST MUST SUMMARIZE HIS/HER RESULTS ON THIS FORM ***

B

Figure 15-5 *(Continued)*
(B) Example #2 of Medical Physicist MEE, Manufacturer Specific. (Source: ACR Web site: www.acraccreditation.org Quality Control and Equipment Evaluation Forms/Medical Physicist Evaluation Forms/Medical Physicist Mammography QC Test Summary-Manufacturer Specific.)

MEDICAL PHYSICIST'S MAMMOGRAPHY QC TEST SUMMARY
Full-Field Digital—Lorad

Site Name		**Report Date**
Address		**Survey Date**
Medical Physicist's Name		**Signature**
X-Ray Unit Manufacturer	Lorad/Hologic	**Model**
Date of Installation		**Room ID**

QC Manual Version # _(use version applicable to unit tested; contact mfr if questions)_

Accessory Equipment

	Manufacturer	Model	Location	QC Manual Version #
Review Workstation*			☐ On-site ☐ Off-site	
Film Printer*			☐ On-site ☐ Off-site	

*FDA recommends that only monitors and printers specifically cleared for FFDM use by FDA's Office of Device Evaluation (ODE) be used. See FDA's Policy Guidance Help System www.fda.gov/CDRH/MAMMOGRAPHY/robohelp/START.HTM.

Survey Type ☐ Mammo Eqpt Evaluation of new unit (include MQSA Rqmts for Mammo Eqpt checklist)   ☐ Annual Survey

Medical Physicist's QC Tests
("Pass" means all components of the test passes; indicate "Fail" if any component fails. Tests must be done for both on and off-site equipment.)

PASS/FAIL

1. **Mammographic Unit Assembly Evaluation**
2. **Collimation Assessment**
3. **Artifact Evaluation**
4. **kVp Accuracy and Reproducibility**
5. **Beam Quality Assessment—HVL Measurement**
6. **Evaluation of System Resolution**
7. **Automatic Exposure Control (AEC) Function Performance** _(NA for systems without AEC)_
8. **Breast Entrance Exposure, AEC Reproducibility and Average Glandular Dose**
   Average glandular dose for average breast is ≤3 mGy (300 mrad) [_____] mrad
9. **Radiation Output Rate**
10. **Phantom Image Quality Evaluation**
    Phantom image scores: Fibers [_____] Specks [_____] Masses [_____]
11. **Signal-To-Noise Ratio and Contrast-To-Noise Ration Measurements** _(values required for all tests)_
    SNR _(value)_ [_____]
    CNR _(value)_ [_____] _(Required for both new unit Mammography Equipment Evaluations and Annual Surveys)_
    CNR should not vary by more than ±15% _(NA for Equipment Evaluation)_
12. **Diagnostic Review Workstation (RWS) QC** _(for all RWS, even if located offsite; NA if only hardcopy read)_
13. **DICOM Printer QC** _(Mammography Equipment Evaluations only)_
14. **Detector Flat Field Calibration** _(Mammography Equipment Evaluations only)_
15. **Compression Thickness Indicator** _(Mammography Equipment Evaluations only)_
16. **Compression** _(Mammography Equipment Evaluations only)_

*** YOUR MEDICAL PHYSICIST MUST SUMMARIZE HIS/HER RESULTS ON THIS FORM ***

C

Figure 15-5 _(Continued)_
(C) Example #3 of Medical Physicist MEE, Manufacturer Specific. (Source: ACR Web site: www.acraccreditation.org Quality Control and Equipment Evaluation Forms/Medical Physicist Evaluation Forms/Medical Physicist Mammography QC Test Summary-Manufacturer Specific.)

Table 15-5 • Modifications In the Assessment Categories Used In Medical Reports

(A) "Negative"	Nothing to comment upon (if the interpreting physician is aware of clinical findings or symptoms, despite the negative assessment, these shall be explained)
(B) "Benign Finding(s)"	Also a negative assessment
(C) "Probably Benign Finding(s)"	Initial short-interval follow-up suggested. Finding(s) has a high probability of being benign
(D) "Suspicious Abnormality"	Biopsy should be considered. Finding(s) without all the characteristic morphology of breast cancer but indicating a definite probability of being malignant
(E) "Highly suggestive of malignancy"	Appropriate action should be taken. Finding(s) has a high probability of being malignant
(F) "Known Biopsy-Proven Malignancy"	Appropriate action should be taken
(v) "Incomplete: Need additional imaging evaluation and/or prior mammograms for comparison" (In cases where no final assessment category can be assigned due to incomplete workup)	Shall be assigned as an assessment and reasons why no assessment can be made shall be stated by the interpreting physician

Source: FDA/MQSA Web site: Home/Radiation Emitting Products/Mammography Quality Standards Act and Program/Guidance (MQSA)/Policy Guidance Help System/Approved Alternative Standard Requirements/#11 Modifications In the Assessment Categories Used in Medical Reports (www.fda.gov). Accessed October 10, 2016.

Separate from the reporting requirements of the MQSA for mammography, the Breast Imaging and Reporting Data System (BI-RADS) was initiated in the 1980s by the ACR to address the variance of reporting practices among radiologists as well as to address the need for making appropriate recommendations for management of patient care to the healthcare provider. Participation from a wide range of professional, governmental, and medical organizations such as the American Medical Association, the National Cancer Institute, the Centers for Disease Control and Prevention, the FDA, the American College of Surgeons, and the College of American Pathologists ensured the success and acceptance of the system.[12] The ACR BI-RADS encompasses a complete reporting mechanism that defines the reporting structure for radiologists to use, a "lexicon" or "dictionary" to describe benign and malignant processes, requires decision making for appropriate patient care, and communicates the report clearly to other physicians and the patient. The assessment categories correlate to an assessment category code that has a significant purpose. These codes assist in facilitating a system of quality improvement for interpreting physicians, an integral aspect of the ACR BI-RADS. Table 15-6 includes the assessment categories and correlative codes used in the ACR BI-RADS.

Throughout its development the BI-RADS was intended to adapt and change according to new technologies introduced to improve breast care.[12] In keeping with that logic,

Table 15-6 • ACR BI-RADS® Assessment Categories

ASSESSMENT	MANAGEMENT	LIKELIHOOD OF CANCER
Category 0: Incomplete—Need Additional Imaging Evaluation and/or Prior Mammograms for Comparison	Recall for additional imaging and/or comparison with prior examination(s)	N/A
Category 1: Negative	Routine mammography screening	Essentially 0% likelihood of malignancy
Category 2: Benign	Routine mammography screening	Essentially 0% likelihood of malignancy
Category 3: Probably Benign	Short-interval (6-month) follow-up or continued surveillance mammography	>0% but ≤2% likelihood of malignancy
Category 4: Suspicious	Tissue diagnosis	>2% but <95% likelihood of malignancy
Category 4A: *Low suspicion* for malignancy		>2% to ≤10% likelihood of malignancy
Category 4B: *Moderate suspicion* for malignancy		>10% to ≤50% likelihood of malignancy
Category 4C: *High suspicion* for malignancy		>50% to <95% likelihood of malignancy
Category 5: Highly Suggestive of Malignancy	Tissue diagnosis	≥95% likelihood of malignancy
Category 6: Known Biopsy-Proven Malignancy	Surgical excision when clinically appropriate	N/A

Source: Sickles EA, D'Orsi CJ, Bassett LW, et al. ACR BI-RADS® Mammography. In: ACR BI-RADS® Atlas, Breast Imaging Reporting and Data System. Reston, VA: American College of Radiology; 2013.

since its first publication in 1993, the ACR has expanded the BI-RADS to include breast ultrasound and breast MRI, although only mammography requirements are included under the MQSA.

Case Study 15-2

Refer to Table 15-6. Describe the BI-RADS assessment categories. Explain why a BI-RADS classification has relevance to a referring physician but not to a patient.

Communication of Mammography Results to the Patient

The early detection of breast cancer increases the likelihood of survival of the patient and increases the potential for conservative treatment options. Treatment plans initiated in a timely manner from the time of diagnosis are dependent on the organized dissemination of reporting to the patient and primary physician. To ensure that the patient receives the mammography report and to ensure that the patient understands the information contained within the report, the facility is required to send every mammography patient a written summary of the report, in lay terms, within 30 days of the examination. Additionally, when "suspicious" or "highly suggestive of malignancy" is assigned for the assessment category, the facility must demonstrate that communication to the patient takes place "as soon as possible." FDA guidance further defines "as soon as possible" as 3 to 5 days after the *interpretation date* of the exam rather than the date the study was performed.[9] Additionally, when the report contains the category assessment, "incomplete-need additional imaging evaluation," communication with the patient is recommended as soon as possible.

Conveying the report using computerized methods such as patient portal access through the facility's network is acceptable to the FDA; however, the facility must be able to demonstrate their established electronic system of communication to the patient if asked to do so during an MQSA inspection. When electronic communication is not possible for patients, communication using paper form is required.

For patients who receive mammography services but do not identify a health care provider, facilities are required to include a final report along with the lay summary to the patient.

RECORD KEEPING

Obtaining and comparing previous mammography images to the current examination demonstrates improved reporting accuracy. Radiologists who compare current images to previous studies are able to evaluate subtle changes in breast tissue and better determine stability. Following this practice demonstrates decreased false positive recalls by 40% to 60% and improves earlier breast cancer detection by 25%.[13–22] The ACR Practice Parameters for Screening and Diagnostic Mammography includes this topic. The American Cancer Society, the National Cancer Institute, Office of Women's Health, U.S. Department of Health, and Human Services all mention on their Web sites that in preparation for a mammogram, patients should make previous mammography examinations available to the facility where they intend to have their next mammogram.

The importance of this practice is widely recognized. The potential impact to the patient when previous studies are not available for comparison can translate to additional image evaluation, delayed cancer detection, increased medical costs, and increased anxiety. For these reasons, the FDA places requirements on facilities to ensure that patients have access to their previous mammography studies and upon request these images are sent to facilities conducting current examinations for comparison purposes.

Image Retention (Storage)

Facilities are required to maintain mammography reports and images for a period of not less than 5 years. If the patient does not return to the facility for additional mammograms, the facility is required to maintain the images and reports for a period of 10 years. MQSA has regulations regarding long term storage of digital mammograms. Mammograms can only be lossless compressed. Lossless compression describes a method of data storage that enables the image to retain data information equal to the original image when regenerated. Examples of lossless versus lossy compression storage are included in Chapter 13 and illustrated in Figure 14-30. Laws concerning patient medical records may also be imposed by State and local government; facilities should be aware of and observe these additional regulations.

Image Transfer

A patient's access to his or her imaging records is also assured through specific FDA regulations that prohibit facilities from inflating costs when patients request the transfer of images. Facilities are only allowed to pass on to the patient the associated cost of performing this service. Individual states and local laws may also affect the process of image transfer.

QUALITY ASSURANCE— GENERAL

In the beginning of this chapter, we discussed the role of quality assurance and its focus to improve patient care. The MQSA describes essential requirements for equipment, personnel, and processes that must comply with established standards of quality. To safeguard these broad objectives, **quality assurance (QA)**, a management program, is used to ensure that **all** components contributing to patient care and image quality must be established for the mammography service to demonstrate that it consistently achieves the standards of MQSA through the systematic monitoring and maintenance of its practice. The FDA gives specific direction for facilities to encompass the "safety, reliability, clarity, and accuracy" of mammography services when establishing a QA program[5] (Box 15-1). The QA scope for mammography services essentially evaluates the application of the MQSA standards for each individual facility. Facilities are required to demonstrate a system that ensures that the personnel standards, equipment standards, and policies affecting the patient throughout the entire imaging service are such that they meet the requirements of the MQSA. To demonstrate that the QA program is effectively carried out, personnel in charge of the program, or who provide equipment and QA oversight, or who provide the routine management of QC within the QA program, must have appropriate training and be qualified for these responsibilities. Facilities are required to:

1. Assign responsibility of the QA program and each of its processes to individuals with appropriate qualifications to perform their assigned responsibilities

---

BOX 15-1

Quality Assurance Program

Citation:

900.12(d): Quality Assurance—general. Each facility shall establish and maintain a quality assurance program to ensure the safety, reliability, clarity, and accuracy of mammography services performed at the facility.

MQSA Regulation addressing Quality Assurance as stated in the Policy Guidance Help System (PGHS).
Source: fda.gov/Mammography Quality Standards Act and Program/ Guidance/PGHS/Quality Assurance. Accessed December 9, 2016.

---

2. Establish a records system which can demonstrate the organized collection of all information defined for the QA program, which includes policies, quality control records, corrective action, and equipment service/ repair of the mammography service operation

Assignment of Responsible Individuals

Lead Interpreting Physician

The facility must identify a "lead interpreting physician." This individual has the general responsibility of ensuring that the quality assurance program meets the requirements of the MQSA and of ensuring that only qualified personnel are assigned to quality assurance responsibilities and the performance of quality assurance tasks.

Medical Physicist

Facilities are required to engage the services of a qualified medical physicist. This individual is responsible for conducting Mammography Equipment Evaluations (MEE) when necessary and the required facility annual survey. During these equipment inspections, the medical physicist evaluates the equipment safety and reliability by performing and analyzing the quality control tests, the phantom image quality, and dose. Additionally, during the annual survey, the quality control tests performed by the QC technologist and the QA/QC program records are reviewed by the medical physicist for verification and to recommend improvement if necessary. The medical physicist is required to submit a report to the facility of the completed evaluations within 30 days of the survey. Appropriate credentials of the medical physicist should be retained by the facility for accreditation, certification, and annual FDA inspection purposes.

Quality Control Technologist

The facility must identify a quality control technologist. This individual is responsible for the performance of the quality assurance tasks that are not assigned to the lead interpreting physician or the medical physicist. The designated QC technologist must be an individual that has the qualifications to perform mammography. Other individuals may be permitted to perform the required QC tasks; however, appropriate documentation of training is necessary ensuring their abilities to properly perform and evaluate the QC tests. When other qualified personnel step in to assist the QC technologist with testing procedures, the QC technologist retains supervisory responsibility, ensuring that the testing performance by other individuals meet the MQSA standards.

Quality Assurance Records

To verify that a facility delivers mammography services that meet the requirements of the MQSA, the lead interpreting physician, the medical physicist, and the QC technologist are required to ensure that records of the mammography service operation are updated and secured. These records should be well organized and include documentation that address:

- The safety and protection of the patient and personnel
- Mammography procedures and technique charts
- The qualifications of personnel performing quality assurance responsibilities
- Quality control testing (see Quality Assurance—Equipment)

Records related to quality control testing are required to include performance results analysis and documentation. When testing results fall outside of acceptable parameters for any component in the imaging chain, it is necessary to follow a corrective action process. The corrective action process, along with the results of retesting the component, must be documented and included in the records for quality control. Facilities are required to retain all QA records until their next annual (FDA) inspection has been completed or until the test has been performed two additional times at the required frequency, whichever is longer.[9] In addition, the medical physicist needs to review all QC records since his/her previous evaluation. Facilities should also be aware of and observe State and local laws governing quality assurance records. One easy and effective means of judging which QC records need to be in the QC manual is to simply retain all QC records from the current and previous calendar years. Any older QC records can be safely discarded. In September 2016, the FDA introduced the EQUIP initiative to address existing MQSA standards that pertain to image quality and quality assurance. The image quality component of EQUIP is addressed in this chapter under clinical image quality. The MQSA standard addressed by the EQUIP initiative pertaining to quality assurance reminds facilities that the responsibility of the QA/QC program to ensure that "records concerning employee qualifications to meet assigned quality assurance tasks, mammography technique and procedures, quality control (including monitoring data, problems detected by analysis of those data, corrective actions, and the effectiveness of the corrective actions), safety, protection and employee qualifications to meet assigned quality assurance tasks are properly maintained and updated" falls to the LIP. Beginning January 2018, facilities must show compliance of adhering to this MQSA standard.[10]

Quality Assurance—Equipment

An effective quality assurance program for mammography should be established and then maintained. This program should ensure that all the components that contribute to the quality, safety, reliability, and accuracy of the service are consistently addressed in order to meet the current required standards. Within this framework, equipment performance, a major component of image quality is addressed through its quality control program. **Quality control** is the part of the quality assurance program that focuses on equipment performance (technical performance) and reliability to ensure quality, safety, and accuracy to the patient and to the mammographic image. To ensure that established regulatory equipment standards are met upon installation, and consistently achieved for daily operation, quality control testing and evaluation are required to be performed by qualified personnel. Medical physicists perform Mammography Equipment Evaluations (MEE) when new equipment has been installed; when major changes take place to the equipment, such as major repairs or major component replacements (this includes the disassembly or reassembly of equipment within the same facility); or when yearly equipment inspections are due. Required annual medical physicist inspection of equipment typically requires the same testing as the MEE but is considered an "annual survey" rather than an MEE. Periodic quality control is performed by the QC Technologist to ensure the equipment continues to meet established standards of safety and quality that have been determined through the medical physicist's testing procedures. A more in-depth discussion of this process is included in Chapter 16. Quality control establishes standards (parameters) for equipment operation, periodically tests equipment components for performance verification, and analyzes testing data in an effort to detect problems that may negatively impact image quality prior to being observed on the mammographic image. Additionally, quality control practices include required "corrective action" when acceptable testing standards are not met. All manufacturers of mammography equipment are required to comply with the established equipment standards defined by the MQSA. A complete discussion of equipment standards and quality control is included in Chapters 11 and 16.

Quality Assurance—Medical Outcomes Audit

The scope of quality assurance for the mammography service includes a method to measure the effectiveness of the program as well as the program's ability to identify the opportunity for improvement. The FDA addresses these aspects by requiring facilities to establish a system that can "ensure the reliability, clarity, and accuracy of the interpretation of mammograms."[9] This regulation is satisfied through the implementation of a medical audit that requires the collection of information including pertinent patient data, mammography reporting data, and biopsy/pathology data, in order to calculate aggregate performance outcomes for the practice as a whole and for each individual interpreting physician. To comply with the MQSA, the following minimum requirements are included in the medical audit:

- A method to track all mammography examinations performed at the facility.
- A method to track positive assessments ("suspicious" and "highly suggestive of malignancy") and to correlate the biopsy pathology report with the radiologist's mammography report.
- A method of gathering pathology reports when a biopsy is recommended, and if the biopsy was performed, at a minimum to learn whether the result was benign or malignant.
- A method to identify patients imaged at a facility and subsequently discovered by the facility that the patient was diagnosed with breast cancer. The facility is required to demonstrate a procedure of obtaining (or attempting to obtain) the pathology report and to review the prior examination.
- The identification of the auditing interpreting physician if different than the lead interpreting physician. The auditing interpreting physician is responsible for the review and documentation of the medical audit results at least every 12 months. This process requires the auditing interpreting physician to analyze the information contained in the medical audit and to disseminate the aggregate results as well as the individual outcome results to each interpreting physician.[9]

Expanded Medical Audits

Facilities may choose to go beyond the minimum requirements of the MQSA medical audit to include a greater scope of performance outcomes for the aggregate practice and each interpreting physician. Conducting a meaningful medical audit and analyzing the information contained in it are demanding and complex. For the purposes of ensuring that mammography technologists are familiar with the process and terminology commonly used in the basic medical audit by mammography practices,

information from the ACR BI-RADS Basic Clinically Relevant Audit and from other audit resources is included in this section. The purpose of the medical audit analysis is to measure the quality of the mammography practice and to address the three major goals of screening mammography[23–26]:

1. The goal to find a high percentage of cancers that exist in a screening population. Sensitivity and cancer detection rate (number of cancers found per 1,000 women screened) can measure this percentage.
2. The goal to maintain acceptably low biopsy recommendations and additional imaging evaluation requests of screening cases while finding cancer. The recall rate and the positive predictive value are used in finding this rate.
3. The goal to find cancers that are small and confined to the breast. Calculate the rate of minimal (invasive cancer ≤1 cm or in situ ductal carcinoma) and node-negative cancers found.

Often the responsibility of preparing the medical audit for the lead interpreting physician or the Auditing Interpreting Physician falls to the manager, lead mammography technologist, or quality control technologist. The process of entering the audit data and preparing the audit allows the technologist to become familiar with audit terminology used in the data collection process and to describe performance outcomes. Understanding the terminology used in the medical audit is helpful for appreciating the potential benefits gained from conducting the medical audit and its implications for quality improvement.

Medical Audit Process and Calculations Overview

The process of conducting a medical audit begins with the collection of raw data from the patient's electronic medical record (EMR) and from referring physician offices outside of the facility. Pertinent data extracted from these sources include patient information, mammography final assessments and information contained in the pathology reports from performed biopsy procedures. This information can sometimes be difficult to collect due to a transient population and the difficulty in accessing patient records outside of the facility. Consequently, diligent efforts to obtain data are necessary to demonstrate meaningful performance outcome results. Fortunately, computer systems and software designed to analyze the data exist to accomplish the steps in the audit process. When data have been gathered from the information contained in the EMR and patient reports, it is possible to extract additional data for the audit including[23–26]

- Raw data:
  - ○ Dates included in the audit period
  - ○ Number of screening examinations performed
  - ○ Number of diagnostic examinations performed
  - ○ Number of additional imaging evaluations requested
  - ○ Number of recommendations for surgical consultations or biopsies
  - ○ Biopsy results
    - ▪ Benign or malignant
    - ▪ Separate fine needle aspiration cytology (FNAC's) and core biopsy cases
  - ○ Tumor staging
    - ▪ Size
    - ▪ Nodal status
    - ▪ Histologic type: in situ (ductal) or invasive (ductal or lobular)
    - ▪ Grade

The end result of the medical audit is to quantify practice accuracy for the three areas that impact screening mammography. (Diagnostic mammography performance outcomes may also be separately calculated.) Before the desired performance outcomes can be calculated, the raw data must be converted to derived data. Before this conversion can be accomplished, all mammography examinations must first be categorized into one of the following four groups[23-26]:

- True positive (TP)
- True negative (TN)
- False negative (FN)
- False positive (FP)

Figure 15-6 provides a visual example of the process that categorizes each screening examination into a positive or negative group.

Women who are screened for breast cancer:

- with a mammography report indicating a positive result are placed in the top half of the graph (positive)
- with a mammography report indicating a normal result are placed in the bottom half of the graph (negative)

Both of these groups are further categorized using the results of the biopsies that have been performed and results provided to the facility. The biopsy results are assigned to one of four groups from (Figure 15-6): positive examinations in the left column, negative in the right column:

- True positive (TP): Tissue diagnosis of cancer within 1 year after a positive examination (BI-RADS® Category 0, 4, or 5 for screening examination)
- Negative (TN): No known tissue diagnosis of cancer within 1 year of a negative examination (BI-RADS® Category 1 or 2 for screening examination)

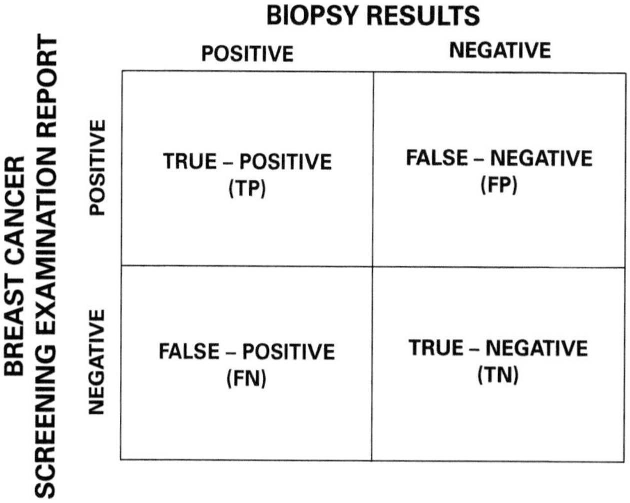

Figure 15-6
A chart used to visually explain the process of categorizing the screening examination: first chart position is determined by positive or negative interpretation result and second chart position is based on positive or negative biopsy result. (Source: Linver MN, et al. The mammography audit: a primer for the Mammography Quality Standards Act (MQSA). *Am J Roentgenol.* 1995;165:19–25.)

- False positive (FP): The false positive category is further separated into three definitions[23]:
  - ○ FP_1: No known tissue diagnosis of cancer within 1 year of a positive screening examination (BI-RADS® Category 0, 4, or 5)
  - ○ FP_2: No known tissue diagnosis of cancer within 1 year after *recommendation* for biopsy or surgical consultation on the basis of a positive examination (BI-RADS® Category 4 or 5)
  - ○ FP_3: Benign tissue diagnosis within 1 year after recommendation for biopsy on the basis of a positive examination (BI-RADS® Category 4 or 5)
- False negative (FN): Tissue diagnosis of cancer within 1 year of a negative examination (BI-RADS® Category 1 or 2 for screening examinations)[23,24]

Using the raw data and the information gained from categorizing the mammography examinations, derived data

Case Study 15-3

Refer to Figure 15-6. The medical outcomes audit is a mechanism to evaluate the interpretation capabilities of the radiologist. Describe the four biopsy classifications that categorize the biopsies into a positive or a negative group.

BOX 15-2

The Basic Clinically Relevant Audit

A. **Data to Be Collected**
1. Modality or modalities.
2. Dates of audit period and total number of examinations in that period.
3. Number of screening examinations; number of diagnostic examinations (separate audit statistics should be maintained for each).
4. Number of recommendations for additional imaging evaluation (recalls) (ACR BI-RADS® Category 0—"Need Additional Imaging Evaluation").
5. Number of recommendations for short-interval follow-up (ACR BI-RADS® Category 3—"Probably Benign").
6. Number of recommendations for tissue diagnosis (ACR BI-RADS® Category 4—"Suspicious" and Category 5—"Highly Suggestive of Malignancy").
7. Tissue diagnosis results: malignant or benign, for all ACR BI RADS® Category 0, 3,4 and 5 assessments (ACR suggests that you keep separate data for fine needle aspiration/core biopsy cases and for surgical biopsy cases). MQSA Final Rule requires that an attempt is made to collect tissue diagnosis results for those mammography examinations for which tissue diagnosis is recommended.[2]
8. Cancer staging: histologic type, invasive cancer size, nodal status, and tumor grade.
9. MQSA Final Rule also requires analysis of any **known** false-negative mammography examinations by attempting to obtain surgical and/or pathology results and by review of negative mammography examinations.[2]

B. **Derived Data to Be Calculated**
1. True positives (TP)
2. False positives (FP_1, FP_2, FP_3)
3. Positive predictive value (PPV_1, PPV_2, PPV_3)
   a. In a screening/diagnostic facility, PPV may be obtained in one or more of three ways:
      i. PPV_1—based on positive cases at screening examination, which includes recommendation for anything other than routine screening (BI-RADS® Categories 0, 3, 4, 5)
      ii. PPV_2—based on recommendation for tissue diagnosis (BI-RADS® Categories 4, 5)
      iii. PPV_3—based on results of biopsies actually performed (otherwise known as biopsy yield of malignancy or positive biopsy rate [PBR])
   b. If screening exclusively, obtain in only one way:
      i. PPV_1—based on "positive" cases at screening examination, which includes recommendation for anything other than routine screening (BI-RADS® Categories 0, 3, 4, 5)
4. Cancer detection rate
5. Percentage of invasive cancers that are node negative
6. Percentage of cancers that are "minimal" (minimal cancer is defined as invasive cancer ≤ 1 cm, or ductal carcinoma in situ [DCIS] of any size)
7. Percentage of cancers that are stage 0 or 1
8. Abnormal interpretation (recall) rate for screening examinations

Source: Sickles EA, D'Orsi CJ, Bassett LW, et al. ACR BI-RADS® Mammography. In: ACR BI-RADS® Atlas, Breast Imaging Reporting and Data System. Reston, VA: American College of Radiology; 2013.

can be calculated to demonstrate important performance proficiencies of the mammography program to detect breast cancer and to demonstrate the abilities of each interpreting physician. Box 15-2 provides an example of raw and derived data for an ACR Basic Clinically Relevant Audit.

The information in the medical audit provides a further benefit to interpreting physicians because they can compare their statistics to published benchmarks of performance. Table 15-7 provides the current information regarding Analysis of Medical Audit Data published on the Breast Cancer Surveillance Consortium (BCSC) Web site: http://www.bcsc-research.org. These data are derived from large numbers of screening mammography examinations. Additional information for diagnostic performance outcomes is also available on the BCSC Web site. Although the

definitions and analysis included in the medical audit are complex, they are included in this chapter for the purpose of ensuring that the technologist understands the scope of the medical audit and that she understands its correlation to evaluate and improve the quality of the mammography program at her facility.

Sensitivity

Sensitivity: the probability of finding a cancer when cancer exists, or the percentage of all patients found to have breast cancer within 1 year of screening who were correctly diagnosed by screening (Sensitivity = TP/TP + FN).[24] Sensitivity describes how often disease is detected when it is actually present.[27]

Table 15-7 • Analysis of Medical Audit Data: BCSC Mammography Screening Benchmarks[a]

Cancer detection rate (per 1,000 examinations)	4.7
Median size of invasive cancers (in mm)	14.0
Percentage node negative of invasive cancers	77.3%
Percentage minimal cancer[b]	52.6%
Percentage stage 0 or 1 cancer	74.8%
Abnormal interpretation (recall) rate	10.6%
PPV$_1$ (abnormal interpretation)	4.4%
PPV$_2$ (recommendation for tissue diagnosis)	25.4%
PPV$_3$ (biopsy performed)	31.0%
Sensitivity (if measurable)[c]	79.0%
Specificity (if measurable)[c]	89.8%

[a]Original article describes methodology in detail.[3] BCSC data are updated periodically and reported at http://breastscreening.cancer.gov/data/benchmarks/screening/. Updated data are presented in this table, comprising 4,032,556 screening mammography examinations, 1996–2005, collected from 152 mammography facilities and 803 interpreting physicians that serve a geographically and ethnically representative sample of the United States population. Average data are presented here, but the source material also includes data on ranges and percentiles of performance.
[b]Minimal cancer is invasive cancer ≤ 1 cm or ductal carcinoma in situ.
[c]Sensitivity and specificity are measured with reasonable accuracy only if outcomes data are linked to breast cancer data in a regional tumor registry.
Source: BIRADS Atlas Follow up section: Sickles EA, D'Orsi CJ. ACR BI-RADS® Follow-up and Outcome Monitoring. In: ACR BI-RADS® Atlas, Breast Imaging Reporting and Data System. Reston, VA, American College of Radiology; 2013.

Positive Predictive Value

Positive predictive value (PPV) is defined as the number of cancers proven by biopsy divided by the number of examinations interpreted as positive.[28] There are three separate definitions of PPV that may be used for calculation depending on the practice setting and based upon the three definitions of a false positive.

- PPV$_1$: (abnormal findings at screening): The percent of all positive screening examinations (BI-RADS® categories 1, 4, or 5) that result in a tissue diagnosis of cancer within 1 year. An initial screening assessment of Category 4 or 5 is unusual, but possible.[28]
- PPV$_2$: (biopsy recommended). The percent of all examinations recommended for biopsy or surgical consultation as a result of screening that resulted in the diagnosis of cancer (BI-RADS® Category 4 or 5).[7,25]
- PPV$_3$: (biopsy performed). The percent of all biopsies actually done as a result of screening that resulted in the diagnosis of cancer. This is also known as the biopsy yield of malignancy or the positive biopsy rate (BI-RADS® Categories 4, or 5).[23,26]

Knowing which PPV definition is applied for calculations is important when comparing facility audit data to published data.

- For practices that perform only screening mammography, only PPV$_1$ is used in evaluating the data.
- For practices that perform both screening and diagnostic mammography, all three definitions may be used to evaluate the data.

Specificity

The probability of interpreting an examination as negative when cancer does not exist; or the percentage of all patients not diagnosed with breast cancer within 1 year of screening whose screening examinations were correctly identified as normal.[23,24] Specificity describes how often patients who are disease-free are found to be cancer-free.

Cancer Detection Rate

Defined as the number of cancers detected per 1,000 women screened by mammography. The cancer detection rate provides the greatest value when calculating screening examinations only, describing those women who are asymptomatic and represent the true screening population. When sufficient raw data have been collected, the following cancer detection rates can also be calculated[24]:

- Separate calculations for
  - Prevalent cancer rate (cancers detected at first-time screening examinations)
  - Incident cancer rate (cancers detected in return screening examinations
- Cancer detection rates in diagnostic examinations
- Cancer detection rates in various age groups

Prognostic Factors for Breast Disease

- Tumor Size
  Mortality rates from breast cancer are directly related to tumor size. Therefore, when tumors are small and confined to the breast, the disease prognosis is better. Tumor size will vary depending on the percentage of screening versus diagnostic examinations performed, with larger tumors found in symptomatic patients than tumors found in the screening population. Documentation of tumor size is provided in the pathology report.[24]

- Node Positivity
  Mortality rates from breast cancer are directly related to prevalence and extent of nodal metastasis. Therefore, the lower the rate of lymph node involvement, the better the disease prognosis. The ratio of positive nodes to the total number of removed nodes is contained in the pathology report. The node positivity rate is the number of patients who have positive nodes compared with the total number of cancer patients. These data are converted into a percentage.[24]

Recall Rates

Recall rates deal with the percentage of screening exam patients for whom "need additional evaluation" (ACR BI-RADS "0") is recommended. Additional evaluation may consist of compression views, magnification, ultrasound, etc. The recall rate is evaluated to ensure that it is not too high, indicating that unnecessary examinations are being performed. Unnecessary exams negatively affect the cost effectiveness and integrity of the screening program. The recall rate can also be used in the calculations for FP_1 and PPV_1 in a facility that performs only screening examinations. Published reports note that the recall rate may decrease as the interpreting physician gains in experience.[24]

The Medical Audit Illustrated

A helpful exercise to illustrate the medical audit was devised by Gale Sisney, MD, a Breast Imaging Specialist and an instructor for radiologists and technologists through Global Radiology Outreach. To demonstrate the cancer detection rate, 1,000 playing cards are used to symbolize 1,000 screening examinations interpreted by a radiology practice in 1 week; the practice consists of ten radiologists. The cards are selected from 25 decks of playing cards, with an appropriate number of cards removed for the exercise. Playing cards are given to each interpreting radiologist, symbolizing the examinations they interpreted for the week.

1. Set out 25 decks of playing cards = 1,300 cards total.
2. Take out all Aces, Kings, and 2's = 1,000 cards total.
3. Take out one 3 of clubs, one 3 of diamonds, one 3 of spades, and two 3 of hearts = 995 cards total.
4. Add back 5 King of hearts = 1,000 cards total.
5. Shuffle the cards and give out 100 cards to each of the 10 radiologists.
6. Look at their individual and aggregate numbers.

Kings = True positive cancer diagnosis (TP).
Queens and Jacks: Exams that may look like a king, but are benign tissue (FP).
Number cards: Exams that are benign (TN).

Perfect interpretation accuracy for each individual radiologist and for the practice as a whole, occurs if the cards are correctly identified as follows:

- All King of hearts will be identified as cancer (TP).
- Each Jack and Queen will be recognized as a recall, but will be benign (FP).
- Each number card will be recognized as benign (TN).

Statistically:

$$\text{Sensitivity} = (TP/TP + FN) \frac{\begin{array}{c}\text{Number of kings assessed} \\ \text{as Category 0, 3, 4, 5}\end{array}}{\begin{array}{c}\text{Total number} \\ \text{of kings (5)}\end{array}}$$

$$\text{Specificity} = (TN/TN + FP) \frac{\begin{array}{c}\text{Number of cards assessed} \\ \text{as Category 1, 2}\end{array}}{\begin{array}{c}\text{Total number of cards that} \\ \text{are not kings (995)}\end{array}}$$

$$\text{Recall rate} = \frac{\text{All cards assessed as Category 0, 3, 4, 5}}{\text{Total number of cards (1,000)}}$$

$$PPV_1 = \frac{TP}{\text{Number of positive screening exams}}$$
$$\frac{\text{Number of kings assessed as Category 0, 3, 4, 5}}{\text{Number of cards assessed as Category 0, 3, 4, 5}}$$

$$PPV_2 = \frac{TP}{\begin{array}{c}\text{Number of screening or diagnostic exams} \\ \text{recommended for tissue diagnosis}\end{array}}$$
$$\frac{\text{Number of cards assessed as Category 4, 5}}{\begin{array}{c}\text{Number of cards diagnosed with cancer} \\ \text{within 1 year}\end{array}}$$

$$PPV_3 = \frac{TP}{\text{Number of biopsies performed}}$$
$$\frac{\begin{array}{c}\text{Number of biopsies with tissue} \\ \text{diagnosis of cancer within 1 year}\end{array}}{\text{Number of biopsies performed}}$$

$$\text{Cancer detection rate} = \frac{\begin{array}{c}\text{Number of kings with tissue} \\ \text{diagnosis as cancer}\end{array}}{\text{Total number of cards}}$$

$$\text{Minimal Cancer Rate} = \frac{\begin{array}{c}\text{Number of kings diagnosed} \\ \text{with cancer} \leq 1 \text{ cm or DCIS}\end{array}}{\begin{array}{c}\text{Total number of kings} \\ \text{diagnosed with cancer}\end{array}}$$

This exercise helps to visualize the outcome performance for each interpreting radiologist and the practice as a whole as well as to illustrate the random nature of when actual cancers may be present in a practice for detection.

Using this exercise, multiply the number of examinations interpreted by 4 to symbolize a practice that interprets 4,000 examinations in a month, etc. With only 5 cancers expected to be identified in 1,000 screening examinations per interpreting physician, the illustration assists in demonstrating the random nature of the medical audit.

Analysis of Data

Calculation of individual and collective interpreting abilities permits comparison of performance between interpreting physicians as well as to published acceptable parameters of performance. This knowledge provides opportunities for improvement that ultimately increase the quality of the entire mammography program.

Quality Assurance "Policies and Compliance"

Quality standards that assure all aspects of image production, interpretation, and communication of results are addressed in the rules and regulations of MQSA. Within these statutes are patient care specifics that address the following:

• Safe infection control practices
• Appropriate imaging for patients with breast implants
• A means for patients to express concerns regarding mammography service and potential noncompliance of MQSA.

Because these areas are specifically addressed in the MQSA regulations, facilities must document that they follow the requirements as stated in the law. Facility compliance is corroborated by developing policies that delineate specific procedures used to adhere to the stated regulation. Accompanying logs or records may be necessary to document compliance or when corrective action is taken.

Infection Control

Ensuring that patients are not exposed to contaminated equipment is a common requirement of all radiology modalities and is addressed in mammography services by disinfecting the image receptor, face shield, and compression device between each patient. MQSA further stipulates facilities establish an infection control process that addresses proper methods to clean and disinfect mammography equipment after exposure to blood or other infectious materials. The procedures used for proper disinfection of equipment must also comply with regulations imposed by Federal, State, or local stipulations. Further MQSA requirements specify that the facility should follow the equipment manufacturer's recommendation for disinfection, and if they are unavailable, to use generally acceptable practices

of infection control until they are made available. Logs or records of compliance should be maintained by the facility for quality assurance and inspection purposes.

Patients with Breast Implants

To ensure that the maximum amount of breast tissue is visualized when performing mammography on patients with breast implants (for augmentation), the ACR describes the Implant Displacement (ID) views to be included in the examination. This technique, when combined with the nondisplaced images, provides the greatest opportunity to visualize the natural breast tissue of the patient. For these reasons, MQSA addresses this subject, assuring women who have breast implants that appropriate techniques to obtain images will be used during their procedure. MQSA lists two directives regarding breast implants:

1. The facility must establish a method to identify women who have breast implants prior to the actual mammographic examination. Facilities may opt to *not* image patients with implants. Identification of patients with implants prior to their scheduled appointment time allows the facility to refer these patients to other facilities.
2. Mammography for patients with breast implants will include imaging techniques that maximize the visualization of breast tissue, unless it is contraindicated or is modified by a physician. After April 28, 1999, technologists received specific instruction on imaging patients with breast implants during their 40 hours of required initial training. It is recommended by the FDA that technologists who qualified to do mammograms *before* the April 1999 date also receive this specific training.

Consumer Complaint Mechanism

The purpose of the consumer complaint mechanism is to provide a process for the patient to have their complaint heard if they believe they received seriously deficient mammography services and to ensure the complaint will be investigated and resolved. To understand the meaning behind the consumer complaint mechanism, it is important for technologists to know the definitions of words used relating to the law requirements.[9]

• Consumer: An individual who makes a complaint regarding the mammography services received at a facility (this may include the patient's representative, such as her family member or her referring physician).
• Adverse Event: An undesirable experience associated with the mammography services. Examples of an adverse event include poor image quality, mammography reports received more than 30 days after the date of the examination, or mammography technologists, interpreting

physicians, or medical physicists involved in mammography services without the proper credentials.

• Serious Adverse Event: An adverse event that may significantly compromise clinical outcomes, or for which sufficient corrective action is not taken in a timely manner.

• Serious Complaint: Is a report of a serious adverse event.

The consumer complaint mechanism provides a voice to the patient regarding serious concerns of mammography services she will receive or has received and to provide the facility with a mechanism to collect, resolve, and record patient complaints. Facilities are required to establish a process that addresses four areas of the consumer complaint mechanism[9]:

1. Provide written documentation of a system to collect and to resolve consumer complaints.
2. Maintain the records of each serious complaint for a period of 3 years (from the date the complaint was received).
3. If the consumer's complaint has not been satisfactorily addressed by the facility, provide consumers with sufficient instructions to file unresolved serious complaints with the facility's AB.
4. Report unresolved serious complaints to the AB according to the time specifications of the AB.

Facilities develop workplace policies to ensure the safety and quality of a mammography service. Policies are developed to ensure that all employees are aware of the defined practices of the mammography program and how each employee is required to approach these defined situations. Policies originate from many authoritative sources and often (although not always) are developed to ensure that personnel follow regulatory requirements. A list of regulatory agencies and professional organizations that may determine or influence policies that are developed for the particular needs of a mammography practice are listed below. Additionally, the facility may develop their own unique policies that affect the workplace.

• FDA-Mammography Quality Standards Act (MQSA)
  Signed into law October 27, 1992
• Nuclear Regulatory Commission (NRC)
  Signed into law October 11, 1974
• Occupational Safety and Health Administration (OSHA)
  Signed into law December 29, 1970
• Environmental Protection Agency (EPA)
  Established December 2, 1970 (By President Richard Nixon)
• Health Insurance Portability and Accountability Act (HIPAA)
  Signed into law August 21, 1996
• The Joint Commission (TJC)

Founded in 1951 as The Joint Commission on Accreditation of Hospitals (Name changed to The Joint Commission, 2007)

• American College of Radiology (ACR)
  (See Professional Organizations)
• State and Local Regulations

Policy examples that may be developed and included in the QA/QC manual for facilities that offer mammography services:

1. Radiation Safety Practices for the Employee and Patient
2. Required Mammography Reporting Practice
3. Communication of Mammography Results
   • To the patient
   • To the provider
   • Process for Patient Recalls
4. Image Storage and Retention
   • Image Loaning Process
5. Technologist Training Requirements and Orientation Program
6. Consumer Complaint Mechanism
7. Imaging the Patient with Breast Implants
8. Infection Control Processes
   • MQSA Standards
   • OSHA Standards
   • State and Local Standards
   • Manufacturer Standards
   • Facility Standards
9. Facility Medical Audit Process
10. Special Imaging Considerations for:
    • Pregnant Patient
    • Lactating Patient
    • Age of the Patient

The examples of policies provided in this chapter are included only to familiarize the reader with types of policies that may be contained in a QA/QC manual for mammography. It is understood that each individual facility determines the content of their QA/QC manual as well as the method of records organization to demonstrate compliance with the standards established by the MQSA.

Quality Assurance/Quality Control Manual

The Quality Assurance/Quality Control (QA/QC) manual is of paramount significance to the mammography program. Within its structure lies the description of the mammography program standards and the evidence of the facility's efforts to adhere to the defined standards established in the program. The QA/QC "manual" can actually be several "manuals" or possibly electronic information that serves to portray the performance and behavior of the facility, staff, and equipment through documentation. Whatever method is chosen to display the information, the QA/QC "manual" should provide an accurate account of all actions taken by the facility and staff to continually meet the established standards *of each segment of the program.* The QA/QC manual should be placed in a safe but accessible location for any member of the QA/QC team or facility authority to review at any time. QA/QC information developed electronically should be appropriately backed-up for security and must be available to the FDA inspector during the annual MQSA inspection. Examples of information contained in the QA/QC manual are listed below.

Quality Assurance Leadership

The development of the QA Program is a combined effort of the leadership team responsible for the mammography program: the lead interpreting radiologist, the medical physicist, and the quality control technologist. Together, these individuals establish a QA/QC program that addresses standards for each component of the mammography service and ensures that all involved personnel are informed of their accountability in meeting facility compliance. MQSA requires that each facility designate and provide identification of the lead interpreting physician, the medical physicist, and the quality control technologist. Additional authorities within the organization may wish to be apprised of the program and its contents. An example of leadership roles listed in the QA/QC manual might include the following:

- Organization CEO
- Radiology administrator
- Radiology/mammography manager
- Lead interpreting physician
- Medical physicist
- QC technologist
- Equipment service engineer
- Radiation safety officer

Equipment Information

Like the Facility Information document, the Equipment Information page is not required by MQSA, rather it acts as a courteous guide for the manager, other radiology personnel, or the FDA inspector. The Equipment Information page lists all equipment used for mammography services along with details such as manufacturer, model identification, serial number, date of purchase, date of installation, and service details. Additional helpful information includes equipment contact person, company address, and phone number of manufacturer or service individual, dates of most recent preventive maintenance or service performed on the equipment, and additional required medical physicist inspection if applicable. Examples of equipment that may be included on the Equipment Information page:

- All mammography units
- All Radiologist Workstations
- All Printers (if applicable)
- All densitometers (if applicable) used for the mammography service

Facility Information

The Facility Information document provides pertinent details about the mammography program. It should be kept in a convenient location so it is readily accessible to any personnel that may need the information quickly, especially in the absence of the QC Technologist or other member of the QC team. This information is particularly beneficial to radiology managers, service engineers, and FDA inspectors as it supplies both necessary details of the identification of the mammography service as well an account of significant changes occurring in the program. The Facility Information page is not required by MQSA, rather it acts as a courteous guide for the manager, other radiology personnel, or FDA inspector highlighting significant details about the program and alerting them of supporting documents addressing any major changes. Examples of what may be included on the Facility Information document:

- Facility name as it appears on AB material
- Facility identification number (accreditation ID-MAP ID)
- Facility identification number (FDA certificate)
- Certification/accreditation expiration date
- Most recent date of FDA inspection/name of inspector
- List of interpreting physicians—any changes to the roster (retirement, etc., include dates of last day of service)
- List of mammography technologists—any changes to the roster (retirement, etc., include dates of last day of service)
- Acquisition of new equipment—provide sequence of events and supporting documents for installation and applications and note first day of service
- Removal of equipment—provide sequence of events and supporting documents of activity and note last day of service
- Any major changes to existing equipment—provide sequence of events and supporting documents of activity
- Date of most recent medical physicist inspection
- Dates of equipment preventive maintenance

○ Mammography unit
○ Radiologist workstation
○ Laser printer (if applicable)

• Unusual occurrences such as providing continuing education for staff, positioning workshops, etc., that support quality improvement

Policies

A wide range of policies are required to meet Federal, State, and possibly local regulatory requirements, along with additional unique policies defined by the facility for the mammography service. These policies are described in detail earlier in this chapter.

Record

Documentation of QC Tests

The QC technologist is responsible for the specific testing of equipment used in the mammography service. To successfully perform this function, she must have comprehension of:

• Equipment testing requirements
• What component is being tested
• Testing frequencies
• Purpose of testing
• Acceptable parameters of testing results
• What actions to take if the testing results are outside of the acceptable parameters

In addition, there are several requirements relating to equipment that dictate its use if testing fails and allowable timeframes for corrective action. The QC technologist must be familiar with these requirements, aided by strong communication with the medical physicist responsible for the equipment aspect of the quality assurance program and the service engineers responsible for its repair and maintenance.

Organization, Neatness, and Transparency

Records for QC should be efficiently organized, neatly completed, and reflect factual occurrences of equipment function during testing procedures. There should be no "loose ends" in the testing process. If testing falls outside of acceptable limits, complete documentation of actions taken (and by whom) to correct the problem should be apparent to the person reviewing the records. Records related to the mammography service directly correlate to the facility's compliance of the MQSA. As such, complete transparency of QC records should be accessible to the responsible individuals of the facility such as the lead interpreting radiologist, radiology management, and administrators.

Corrective Action

Results that fall outside of acceptable limits during periodic QC testing by the QC Technologist require a process of correction. This process is known as "corrective action" and must be documented to illustrate the process used to correct the problem and ensure the equipment once again functions according to the standards of acceptance testing that was done by the medical physicist. This may include repeat testing, consultation with the medical physicist, calling for service, and potential repeat testing after the repair. All of these actions must be recorded along with supporting documents of actions taken. Ensuring all aspects of equipment repair and testing are corrected and documented can be time consuming for the QC technologist and stressful for the department. The QC technologist must be given the appropriate time to ensure the process for corrective action is followed and to ensure that documentation is complete for QC records. Minimizing the stress in the department can be accomplished by establishing clear processes and communication of what actions to take when equipment malfunctions. Corrective action measures are sometimes required for performance results such as repeat/reject analysis that may or may not involve equipment. Any performance indicators that fall below acceptance thresholds for the mammography service are the responsibility of the facility as they are indicators of performance reliability impacting image acquisition and patient safety. The lead interpreting physician has the general responsibility to ensure that the quality assurance program meets established MQSA requirements and should be consulted when corrective action measures are implemented.

Additional QC Records

In addition to the essential documentation of equipment QC, the QA/QC manual contains other testing results performed for the mammography service (which may also require corrective action documentation). Examples of additional documentation include the daily, weekly, and monthly QC forms that describe current repetitive QC tasks such as cleaning radiologist workstation monitors. Forms used routinely by technologists or other mammography personnel may be posted for easy access as they complete and initial the required tasks for QC. When completed, these forms should be retained in the QC manual until the next MQSA inspection for the facility.

Repeat/Reject Analysis

Records for the repeat/reject analysis should be available in the QA/QC manual. The repeat/reject analysis records should include documentation of analysis review and verification that the results were within acceptable parameters or whether corrective action was required. If corrective action was necessary, the corrective action process should be explained. Additionally, the records may include verification that each mammography technologist received her individual results of the Repeat/Reject Analysis for the quarter.

Equipment Service and Maintenance Records

Equipment service records should be organized and maintained to current status. The records, usually in the form of a service report, should be in dated order, easily located for each piece of equipment.

QA/QC Quarterly Review

Historically, the quarterly QA/QC review has not been addressed under the MQSA inspection process, rather it is a practice that has been described in previous ACR Quality Control Manuals, including the 2016 Digital QC Manual. One of the changes in the **ACR 2016 Digital Mammography Quality Control Manual** is the required quarterly "Facility QC Review" document included in the Radiologic Technologist's Section. The "Facility QC Review" form documents the required comprehensive review of the facility QC records by both the lead interpreting radiologist and the facility manager. Following this established ACR protocol helps the mammography service address the MQSA requirement for the lead interpreting physician to "ensure that the quality assurance program meets all MQSA QA requirements." The ACR Facility QC Review form is to be completed quarterly, ensuring that the following required actions of QC testing are followed[29]:

* QC tests are performed at the required frequencies.
* Data are collected as required.
* Documentation of results is complete.
* When necessary, appropriate corrective action is taken (and documented).
* Patient exams were suspended when MQSA compliance was not met and were resumed only upon appropriate corrective action taken.

Facilities who have elected to use of the ACR 2016 Digital Mammography Quality Control Manual are required to perform this quarterly review. Facilities who continue to follow the mammography machine manufacturer's Quality Control Manual are also required to implement a procedure to ensure the LIP is actively participating in the oversight of the QA/QC program due to changes made to the MQSA inspection process in September 2016.

The FDA announced EQUIP (Enhancing Quality Using the Inspection Program) in September 2016; EQUIP addresses the appropriate oversight of the facility quality assurance program. The following MQSA standard pertains to the responsibility of the lead interpreting physician:

900.12(d)(1)(i),(ii)(A)(B): (1) Responsible individuals. Responsibility for the quality assurance program and for each of its elements shall be assigned to individuals who are qualified for their assignments and who shall be allowed adequate time to perform these duties.

(i) Lead interpreting physician. The facility shall identify a lead interpreting physician who shall have the general responsibility of ensuring that the quality assurance program meets all requirements of paragraphs (d) through (f) of this section. No other individual shall be assigned or shall retain responsibility for quality assurance tasks unless the lead interpreting physician has determined that the individual's qualifications for, and performance of, the assignment are adequate.[9]

The EQUIP program requires facilities to address established oversight of the QA program by the lead interpreting physician by posing the following questions to the facility during the annual MQSA inspection[10]:

* Does the facility have a procedure for LIP oversight of QA/QC records and corrective actions? (Yes/No)
  ○ This requirement could be satisfied by a verbal answer by the LIP to the inspector, an answer in the form of an attestation signed by the LIP, or a Standard Operating Procedure (SOP) signed by the LIP, available at the time of the inspection.
* Does the procedure include LIP oversight of QA/QC records including review of the frequency of performance of all required tests? (Yes/No)
  ○ This question includes all QC tests performed by the QC technologist, medical physicist, or designated QC personnel performing these tasks.
* Does the procedure include LIP review to determine whether appropriate corrective actions were performed when needed? (Yes/No)

The EQUIP Program ensures the active participation of the LIP for oversight of the facility QA Program. Facilities may consult the ACR 2016 Digital Mammography Quality Control Manual to review the protocol in place for the quarterly review.

Physicist Annual Survey Report

Medical physicist reports must be kept until they have been reviewed by the MQSA inspector during the annual FDA inspection. A convenient location for the medical physicist report is in the QC manual. Additionally, documentation of corrective action (including service reports) undertaken due to recommendations made in the physicist report should be copied and attached to the report for members of the QA/QC leadership team, radiology managers, or FDA inspectors to review. Medical physicists may want to retain several years of facility reports for the purpose of comparing current equipment performance to previous findings. Check with the facility medical physicist prior to discarding reports.

Medical Audit

The annual medical audit must be available to the FDA inspector during the MQSA inspection. A convenient location for the medical audit is in the QA/QC manual; however, due to confidentiality considerations it may be placed in a separate location.

Most Recent FDA Inspection Report

The QA/QC manual is a convenient location for the FDA inspection report and is accessible to any member of the QA/QC team or radiology manager for review.

MQSA Annual Inspection

The FDA requires each facility offering mammography services undergo a **MQSA (FDA) annual inspection** for the purpose of verifying compliance with the standards defined in the MQSA. Certified MQSA inspectors from either the FDA or State agents acting on behalf of the FDA conduct the MQSA inspections. Facilities are given advance notice of the impending inspection when the inspector contacts the facility to schedule the inspection date. A confirmation notice is sent to the facility by the inspector; this notice informs the facility of the items that will be reviewed by the inspector. For a facility with one mammography machine, the average time to conduct an MQSA inspection is approximately 6 hours. Examples of records reviewed by the inspector include[9]:

- Equipment performance
  ○ Unit evaluation
  ○ Phantom image quality
- Technologist and physicist quality assurance and quality control (QA/QC) records
  ○ Repeat/reject analysis
  ○ Laser printer QC (if applicable)
  ○ Radiologist workstation monitor QC
  ○ Unit QC
- Medical records
  ○ Communication of patient results
  ○ Mammography report
- Quality assurance
  ○ Assigned personnel/responsibilities
  ○ Consumer complaint mechanism procedure
  ○ Infection control procedure

- Medical audit and outcome records
- Physicist annual survey
- Personnel records
  ○ Interpreting radiologists
  ○ Medical physicist
  ○ Radiologic technologist
- Records pertaining to additional off-site locations (if applicable)

When the inspection is completed, the inspector meets with the appropriate personnel at the facility to deliver the MQSA Facility Inspection Report. The FDA provides a gradient structure for noncompliant observations, recognizing that the quality impact to the service is dependent on the significance of the observation(s) identified. The report provided to the facility describes adverse inspection observations, dividing the observations into three categories or "levels":

- Level 1: The most severe of the adverse observations, this level indicates that the quality of mammography services could be seriously compromised. Requires written correspondence to the FDA within 15 working days of receiving the facility inspection report. The information to the FDA should include a complete description of the corrective action process and records, along with any supporting documents associated with the corrective action. Additionally, the facility should include a plan to ensure the deficient behavior will not be repeated.
- Level 2: This level indicates the facility performance is acceptable; however, deficient observations were identified that could compromise the quality of mammography services. A Level 2 observation requires written correspondence to the FDA within 30 working days of receiving the facility inspection report. The information to the FDA should include a complete description of the corrective action process and records, along with any supporting documents associated with the corrective action. Additionally, the facility should include a plan to ensure the deficient behavior will not be repeated.
- Level 3: Indicates a minor compliance deviation of the mammography service, with the facility meeting major factors affecting quality. This level does not require correspondence with the FDA, but does require corrective action for the deficient observations identified as soon as possible. The deviations noted for a Level 3 observation are reviewed during the facility's subsequent inspection to verify that corrective action was taken.
- When a facility demonstrates that all areas of the mammography service are in compliance, thereby meeting the quality standards of MQSA, they are given a report that indicates "All Items in Compliance."

A report indicating a Level 1, 2, or 3 adverse observations should be taken very seriously by a facility. The FDA implements thorough follow-up protocols to ensure that facilities who deviate from MQSA standards demonstrate they have taken measures of corrective action and that they are consistently followed. Additional action may be taken by the FDA, including conducting follow-up inspections, additional mammography review, and letters of warning to facilities that do not demonstrate satisfactory corrective action or behavior. Fortunately, noncompliant behaviors are not representative of US mammography practices. The ability of mammography facilities across the country to deliver quality mammography services is consistently demonstrated on the FDA/MQSA Web site on the MQSA National Statistics page. The most recent published information is from July 1, 2017:

Facilities inspected: 5,925

Total units at inspected facilities: 11,505

Percent of inspections where the highest noncompliance was a:

Level 1 violation: 0.8%

Level 2 violation[5]: 10.7%

Level 3 violation: 0.3%

Percent of inspections with no violation: 88.3%

Total annual mammography procedures reported, as of July 1, 2017[1]: 39, 279,737

---

[1]This number is an aggregate of the total number of procedures performed annually as reported by facilities to their accreditation bodies. Facilities are asked to disclose this information at their initial accreditation, and then at the time of their reaccreditation, which takes place once every 3 years. FDA began collecting these data in 1998. The aggregate does not reflect the current number of procedures performed at these facilities, but only the numbers reported by them during the 3-year period prior to the current date. We have aggregated only the numbers reported by certified, non-Veterans Administration facilities

[5]*Based on an analysis of the violation rates for all MQSA citations, the FDA has decided to elevate the five remaining Level 3 citations to Level 2 citations. This change took effect on October 27, 2016. Since all Level 3 citations, if repeated, could have been elevated to a Level 2 with a requirement of a 30-day response to FDA, they should not be viewed as minor in nature, and they should be initially cited as a Level 2. As a consequence, the Level 3 violation rates will approach zero, and the Level 2 violation rates may initially increase but should level off with time.*

(Source: FDA MQSA Web site: https://www.fda.gov/Radiation-EmittingProducts/MammographyQualityStandardsActand-Program/FacilityScorecard/ucm113858.htm)

MQSA GUIDANCE

The FDA provides organized, thorough, and easy to understand guidance documents in order to comply with the MQSA regulations. Guidance documents are developed using the requirements of Good Guidance Practices established by the FDA and are prepared for the FDA staff and the public to provide interpretation of regulatory issues. Guidance documents prepared by the FDA help to navigate the technologist new to mammography or the experienced radiology manager needing specific assistance on a regulatory issue. When using the FDA guidance resources, keep in mind that guidance documents are intended for guidance, and not to *mandate*; therefore, they are not legally binding. Their purpose is to assist facilities to comply with the regulations of the MQSA, which *does* have the force of the law. Guidance documents are helpful in that they represent the FDA's current thinking in regards to a regulation; therefore, if a facility follows FDA guidance for a specific MQSA requirement, it is considered to have met the requirement. Due to the broad scope of qualifications involved in mammography services, MQSA guidance contains a scope of documents that provide assistance, along with other documents that serve to inform the public of pertinent issues related to mammography. Becoming familiar with the MQSA Web site, "Mammography Quality Standards Act and Program," enables the user to easily navigate through a variety of guidance documents to answer questions associated with regulatory compliance. Only three of the many guidance documents available on the MQSA Web site are highlighted in this chapter. The reader is encouraged to visit "www.fda.gov" for comprehensive information regarding mammography information and compliance assistance.

Inspection Guidance

MQSA inspections for mammography facilities follow specific processes defined by the FDA and are carried out by FDA inspectors or qualified State inspectors to verify facility compliance of the MQSA. To properly address inspection preparation, however, a distinction should be made between *preparing for a facility inspection*, and the *continuous practice of quality assurance measures* by mammography personnel every day and for every patient for whom mammography services are offered. Good quality assurance practices that are established and continuously adhered to by all mammography personnel, along with appropriate documentation, essentially prepares the facility for a successful annual inspection. Beyond these practices, FDA inspection preparation guidance documents are provided to explain the inspection process in detail. This knowledge helps to minimize interruption to the mammography service and to provide notice of the documentation requirements that satisfy compliance that must be available on the date of the inspection. Documents on the FDA Web site that describe the inspection process include "Preparing for the Inspection" and "MQSA Inspection Procedures." Personnel familiar with the information contained in these documents assist in the inspection process to ensure a smooth and orderly MQSA inspection.

Policy Guidance Help System

Although all of the information published on the MQSA section of the FDA Web site is beneficial to the mammography community in some form, perhaps the most valuable portal to information concerning MQSA compliance is the PGHS. Just as its title implies, this informational system guides the visitor through an organized process to find specific material on any given subject relating to mammography compliance. The PGHS represents the FDA's current thinking on the regulations that enforce the MQSA and provides a clear interpretation of the regulations to ensure that facilities understand what is necessary to comply with each standard described in the law. The PGHS portal offers a table of contents that includes essential topics covering all aspects of the delivery of mammography services. Subtopics may be included for each subject and when appropriate will provide the citation for the regulation related to that topic. Terminology used in the PGHS is located under the section "Definitions," which defines the meaning of each term used, eliminating misinterpretation of requirements. And finally, a discussion is included for the regulation, which includes common questions related to the standard. The collection of questions is thorough for each subject or regulation, with answers from the FDA addressing the broad spectrum of concerns facilities may have in achieving compliance for a specific regulation. For any person involved in the leadership of a mammography practice, or for any mammography technologist interested in fully understanding the interconnection between the established standards of the MQSA, the required quality assurance and quality control, and the delivery of high quality mammography, the PGHS is highly recommended reading material.

Alternative Requirements (Standards)

The MQSA was passed into law by Congress in 1992. As such, each standard defined in the regulations must be met by every facility offering mammography services. To redefine or change a standard of the MQSA would require a lengthy process to amend the regulation. To ensure that the use of new technology or strategies developed in the mammography industry that improve or enhance patient care are not impeded due to the amendment process, an alternative requirement procedure was established within the MQSA. The alternative requirement standard provides the opportunity to evaluate advanced methods of technology within a reasonable time period through an application and approval process established by the FDA to determine if the proposed alternative standards would "provide at least as great an assurance of quality mammography as the original standards." Upon approval of a proposed alternative standard, the information is disclosed to the public and added to the list on the FDA Web site under "Approved Alternative Standards." As of this writing, there are currently twenty-four Approved Alternative Standards. The twenty-fourth Approved Alternative Standard became effective February 17, 2016 and describes the approval of the American College of Radiology 2016 Digital Quality Control Manual to be used in place of the mammography unit manufacturer's QC Manual when conditions described in the standard are met:

> #24: Approval of an Alternative Standard for Using the Quality Assurance Program Recommended by the ACR Digital Mammography Quality Control Manual for Full-Field Digital Mammography Systems, for Systems without Advanced Imaging Capabilities.[9]

Other examples of Approved Alternative Standards that are included on the FDA Web site page include the following:

- #3: Conducting the weekly phantom image test at facilities with intermittent mammography operation
- #8: Separate Assessment of Findings for Each Breast.

Each number and Approved Alternative Standard includes a description of the original standard and the Approved Alternative Standard for the subject indicated along with the date in which it becomes effective. This portal on the FDA Web site (www.fda.gov) is recommended reading material for all mammography technologists as well as those responsible for FDA mammography compliance to ensure that they are informed of the most recent MQSA standards.

ACR 2016 Digital Mammography Quality Control Manual

The quality assurance chapter for mammography has predominantly focused on the MQSA standards: what is contained in them and the practices and procedures that satisfy compliance. This chapter would not be complete without including additional materials developed by the American College of Radiology in their efforts to assist facilities, radiologists, medical physicists, and technologists in the effort to deliver high-quality mammography services to their patients.

• *The American College of Radiology 2016 Digital Mammography Quality Control Manual* (Figure 15-7)

Published on their Web site in August 2016, the ACR 2016 Digital Mammography QC Manual was included as an approved alternative standard. Facilities have the choice of using The ACR Digital QC Manual in place of following the manufacturer's digital QC manual. According to the MQSA, the following standard is required for imaging systems other than screen/film:

900.12(e)(6): Quality control tests—other modalities. For systems with image receptor modalities other than screen film, the quality assurance program shall be substantially the same as the quality assurance program recommended by the image receptor manufacturer, except that the

maximum allowable dose shall not exceed the maximum allowable dose for screen-film systems in paragraph (e)(5) (vi) of this section.[9]

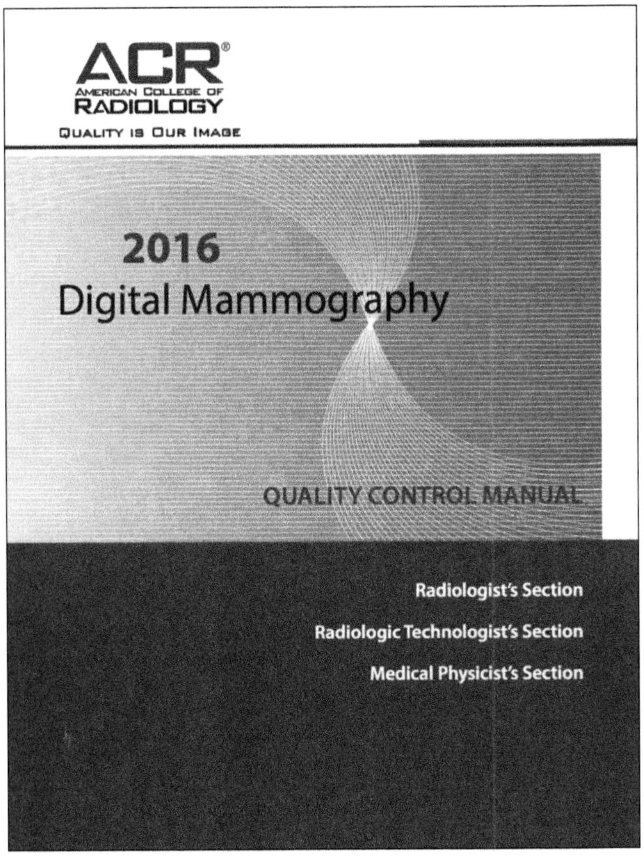

The first digital mammography unit was approved by the FDA in the year 2000, bringing with it the first FDA-approved manufacturer's QC manual. Sixteen years later, there were approximately twelve manufacturers representing several models of digital mammography equipment, all with QC manuals specific to the software applications currently being used with their digital mammography units. Adding to the confusion, some digital QC manuals included QC for the radiologist workstation and the printer, while other QC manuals would refer you to the manufacturer of the radiologist workstation and printer in order to comply with their recommended testing. Many of the digital QC manuals would refer the reader to the 1999 ACR Quality Control Manual (the screen/film manual) for quality control of some service components such as the viewbox and viewing conditions. The 2016 publication of the ACR Digital Quality Control Manual standardized quality control testing across all digital manufacturers, eliminating the variations of testing and results among mammography units, radiologist workstations, and printers. However, there were caveats: the new ACR 2016 Digital Quality Control Manual was only approved for use with the newly designed digital mammography phantom (Figure 15-8) and was reserved for 2D digital mammography only. Even so, for facilities that purchased 2D digital mammography equipment from different manufacturers, this was a welcome and overdue solution for the confusion. The new manual also

Figure 15-7
The 2016 ACR Digital Quality Control Manual standardizes quality control testing across all digital manufacturers. Approved for use for digital mammography systems without DBT or enhanced contrast options.

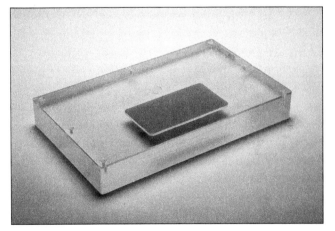

Figure 15-8
The FFDM FDA accreditation phantom developed for digital mammography for facilities following the standardized QC program structure using the 2016 ACR Digital Mammography QC Manual. (Photo: Mammo FFD™ Phantom, courtesy of Gammex, Inc., Sun Nuclear Corporation.)

introduces some changes in established mammography quality assurance practices[29]:

- The 2016 ACR Digital QC Manual refers to the radiologist designated to oversee the mammography program and to ensure all quality assurance requirements are met as the "lead interpreting radiologist," while the FDA terminology refers to him/her as the "lead interpreting physician."
- The new manual includes a "Facility QC Review" requiring the lead interpreting radiologist and the facility manager to review the facility's QC test results and the medical physicist reports at least quarterly (or more frequently if problems have been identified), while the original practice required the lead interpreting radiologist to review the QC tests and the medical physicist reports quarterly. Following this practice helps mammography services to address the FDA requirement stating that the lead interpreting physician has "the general responsibility of ensuring that the quality assurance program meets all MQSA QA requirements" while also ensuring that responsible individuals such as the facility manager are aware of the aspects of the QC practices which ultimately impact patient care and MQSA inspections.
- Radiologist Image Quality Feedback (optional) (Figure 15-9). This practice ensures the technologist performing mammography receives feedback regarding examinations that need improvement or that require patients to be called back for additional imaging to complete the exam or to receive positive feedback when deserved. Following this practice helps facilities to address the FDA requirement stating that "All interpreting physicians interpreting mammograms for the facility shall follow the facility procedures for corrective action when the images they are asked to interpret are of poor quality."

The ACR 2016 Digital Mammography Quality Control Manual can be electronically accessed on the ACR Web site by facilities offering mammography services or can be purchased directly from the ACR Web site if desired. A condition of the 2016 ACR Digital QC Manual was to exclude the section of "Clinical Image Quality Evaluation," keeping this publication consistent with other ACR QC Manuals in which image quality evaluation sections are not included. To address this critical component of mammography, the ACR announced its future intentions to update the clinical image quality material and make it available on their Web site.[29] Until that update is available, the ACR Mammography Quality Control Manual 1999 (film/screen) that includes **Patient Positioning and Compression**, and the **Clinical Image Evaluation** sections

have been placed on the ACR Web site and is accessible to any facility or individual. These sections cover important information on patient positioning/compression for the ACR routine and additional imaging projections, and the evaluation of clinical images to ensure maximum tissue coverage, adequate compression, adequate exposure, and labeling for the craniocaudal and mediolateral oblique projections.

■ NATIONAL MAMMOGRAPHY QUALITY ASSURANCE ADVISORY COMMITTEE

To assist in determining what measures should be contained within regulations, the FDA turns to outside experts in the particular field they are addressing. There are 50 FDA committees and panels that advise the FDA when making decisions; however, the final decisions are made by the FDA. The National Mammography Quality Assurance Advisory Committee advises the FDA on developing quality measures and regulations for facilities that offer mammography services.

On September 15, 2016, the National Mammography Quality Assurance Advisory Committee met to discuss a range of issues related to the delivery of mammography services. The recently published ACR 2016 Digital Quality Control Manual was presented and explained. Examples of additional topics that were discussed during the meeting that potentially could impact mammography quality assurance compliance are included below.[30] Decisions that are made by the FDA regarding these discussions could modify some topics included in this chapter and for this reason are mentioned here.

- Breast density reporting requirements
- Discussion of possible removal of Level 3 violations during the annual MQSA inspection
- Discussion of questions pertaining to infection control during the inspection process
- Discussion of facility readiness to supply personnel documentation
- Discussion of 2D images synthesized from DBT images
- Discussion of enhancing quality using the inspection program (EQUIP) initiative

At the time of this writing it is unknown how these discussions could subsequently change or modify the practices currently understood for facility compliance in these areas.

Optional - Radiologist Image Quality Feedback   *As Needed*
(For Quality Improvement)

Radiologist's Name: _____

Date: _____

Procedure	This report is to be completed by the Interpreting Radiologist when asked to interpret suboptimal cases requiring the patient to be called back. The form may also be used to provide feedback on excellent quality. The radiologists should complete this form as needed for each case. A system should be in place for analyzing feedback and taking measures for improvement as necessary.

Objective For the Radiologist to provide routine feedback to the technologists and manager on the quality of images.

Patient Identifier: _____
_____

Technologist's Name: _____
Date of Exam: _____

Overall Assessment

☐ Excellent   ☐ Good   ☐ Needs improvement, but do not repeat   ☐ Suboptimal, and should be repeated

Image Evaluation

	RCC	LCC	RMLO	LMLO	Other View	Other View
Positioning						
Missing tissue						
Laterally						
Posteriorly						
Medially						
Inferiorly						
Nipple not in profile						
Skin fold						
Pectoralis not down to PNL						
Tissue droopy (camel nose)						
Narrow/concave pectoralis						
Inframammary fold						
Not open						
Not shown						
Centering not correct						
Technical Issues						
Not enough compression						
Exposure Too Low (Excessive Noise)						
Exposure Too High (Image Saturation)						
Patient Motion						
Artifacts						
Incorrect Patient ID						
Other						
blank space (DELETE text)						

Additional Images Needed for Complete Breast Evaluation

Requested views ☐ RCC ☐ LCC ☐ RMLO ☐ LMLO ☐ Other View _____

Action Limits	**Recommended:** Patients should be called back for additional images if the quality is suboptimal according to the interpreting radiologist's request.
	Timeframe: Not applicable.

Figure 15-9
Optional Radiologic Technologist Image Quality Feedback form for quality improvement. (Source: Berns EA, Baker JA, Barke LD, et al. Digital Mammography Quality Control Manual. Reston, VA: American College of Radiology; 2016.)

WHERE TO FIND HELP WITH COMPLIANCE

All mammography personnel need to be informed of the regulations that govern the practice of mammography in the United States. This includes radiologists, medical physicists, radiology managers, lead mammography technologists, QC technologists, and staff technologists delivering mammography services to patients. For more than two decades, the MQSA has been in effect ensuring that mammography service standards are met. The information available regarding this subject is complete, easily accessible, and provided in an orderly manner on the FDA Web site, quickly guiding the reader to the subject of interest. In addition, State regulatory agencies, mammography equipment manufacturers, and countless professional individuals are available and willing to support facilities in their efforts to deliver high quality mammography and ensure all areas of compliance. The following list of people and places will help when there is a question regarding mammography compliance:

1. Mammography Quality Standards Act and Program (https://www.fda.gov/radiation-emittingproducts/mammographyqualitystandardsactandprogram/)
   • Guidance
     Policy Guidance Help System (PGHS)
   • Facility Certification and Inspection (MQSA)
     Preparing for an inspection
     Inspection Procedures
   • About the Mammography Program
     Get Notification of Mammography Updates (auto e-mail notification of MQSA updates)
   • Regulations
     – Alternative Standards
   • Consumer Information
   • MQSA Frequently Asked Questions (FAQ's)
   • Contact the MQSA Program
     FDA Hotline...1-800-838-7715
     Fax to MQSA Program...1-443-285-0689
     Email MQSA Program....MQSAhotline@versatechinc.com
2. American College of Radiology
   www.acraccreditation.org
   • 2016 ACR Digital Mammography QC Manual
   • Mammography Accreditation Program Requirements
   • Instructions for Uploading Images (for electronic image submission)
   • Clinical Image Quality Guide (ACR Mammography Quality Control Manual, 1999)
   • ACR Mammography Accreditation Program FAQ

• MQSA Requirements for Mammography Equipment Checklist
• Radiologic Technologist Quality Control Forms (FDA Approved Manufacturer's Mammography Units)
• Medical Physicist Evaluation Forms (FDA Approved Manufacturer's Mammography Units)
• DBT Initial Training FAQ
3. Your Facility Medical Physicist
4. Your Equipment Manufacturer

The purpose of the mammography QA program is to address each component of the mammography practice that impacts the end result of the service. Mammography services include the production, processing, and interpretation of mammographic images while ensuring safety, accuracy, and satisfaction to customers who use the service. The consequences of "falling short" of accuracy or customer satisfaction can have serious repercussions for the patient and for the facility. Establishing an effective quality assurance program can minimize the occurrence and therefore the undesirable consequences of inadequate performance through periodic testing and analysis. The quality assurance program reflects the goals of the facility to meet regulatory compliance standards that address the purpose of MQSA—to provide quality mammography services to all.

Review Questions

1. What significant action took place on October 27, 1992 that ensured all women nationwide would receive adequate quality mammography services?

2. What three categories does the MQSA address for interpreting physicians, medical physicists, and radiologic technologists to ensure that they are qualified and remain qualified to deliver mammography services?

3. Explain the role of the lead interpreting physician, the medical physicist, and the quality control technologist in the quality assurance program.

4. What valuable assistance portal is available on the FDA/MQSA Web site that represents the FDA's current thinking on the regulations that enforce the MQSA and provides a clear interpretation of the regulations to ensure that facilities understand what is necessary to comply with each standard described in the law?

References

1. Papp J. *Quality Management in the Imaging Sciences*. 4th ed. Missouri, MO: Mosby Elsevier; 2011.

2. Destouet JM, et al. The ACR's mammography accreditation program: ten years of experiences since MQSA. *J Am Coll Radiol*. 2005;2(7):585–594.

3. McLelland R, et al. The American College of Radiology Mammography Accreditation Program. *Am J Roentgenol*. 1991; 157:473–479.

4. www.acr.org Mammography Accreditation Program/Frequently Asked Questions K:\MammoMaster\1 MAP Policy-Proc Manual\1-General\Frequently Asked Questions.docx. Accessed October 10, 2016.

5. Department of Health and Human Services, Food and Drug Administration, 21 CFR Parts 16 and 900, Quality Mammography Standards; Final Rule, Title 21, Volume 8. Revised April 1, 2016.

6. ACR Mammography Accreditation Program Requirements (www.acr.org) Mammography. Accessed October 10, 2016.

7. Sickles EA, et al. ACR BI-RADS® mammography. In: *ACR BI-RADS® Atlas, Breast Imaging Reporting and Data System*. Reston, VA: American College of Radiology; 2013. 2013ACR BI-RADS Atlas, Breast Imaging Reporting and Data System.

8. Acraccreditation.org, Mammography, Clinical Image Quality Guide (from 1999 Mammography QC Manual).

9. www.fda.gov Home/Radiation-Emitting Products/Mammography Quality Standards Act and Program/Guidance (MQSA)/Policy Guidance Help System.

10. www.fda.gov/Home/Radiation-Emitting Products/Mammography Quality Standard Act and Program/Mammography Quality Standards Act (MQSA) Enhancing Quality Using the Inspection Program (EQUIP) Frequently Asked Questions—Facilities.

11. www.acraccreditation.org Mammography/Medical Physicist Evaluation Forms. Accessed October 10, 2016.

12. Burnside ES, et al. The ACR BI-RADS experience: learning from history. *J Am Coll Radiol*. 2009;6(12):851–860.

13. Sickles EA. Successful methods to reduce false positive mammography interpretations. *Radiol Clin North Am*. 2000;38(4):693–700; *Radiol Clin North Am*. 2010;48:859–878.

14. Yankaskas BC, et al. Effect of observing change from comparison mammograms on performance of screening mammography in a large community-based population. *Radiology*. 2011;261(3):762–770.

15. Roelofs AA, et al. Importance of comparison of current and prior mammograms in breast cancer screening. *Radiology*. 2007;242(1):70–77.

16. Thurfjell MG, et al. Effects on sensitivity and specificity of mammography screening with or without comparison of old mammograms. *Acta Radiol*. 2000;41:52–56.

17. Kleit AN, Ruiz JF. False positive mammograms and detection controlled estimation. *Health Serv Res*. 2003;38(4):1207–1228.

18. National Cancer Institute: Breast Cancer Surveillance Consortium. Performance Measures for 1,960,150 Screening Mammography Examinations from 2002 to 2006 by Time (Months) Since Previous Mammography—based on BCSC data as of 2009. Available at: www.breastscreening.cancer.gov. Accessed December 14, 2009.

19. Ryerson AB, Venard VB, Major AC. *National Breast and Cervical Cancer Early Detection Program: 1991–2002 National Report*. Centers for Disease Control and Prevention. Available at: http://www.cdc.gov/cancer/nbccedp/Reports/NationalReport/index.htm

20. *NHS Breast Screening Programme: Annual Review 2012*. U.K. National Health Service Breast Screening Web site www.cancerscreening.nhs.uk/breastscreen

21. Hubbard RA, et al. Cumulative probability of false-positive recall or biopsy recommendation after 10 years of screening mammography: a cohort study. *Ann Intern Med*. 2011; 155(8):481–492.

22. Burnside E, et al. The differential value of comparison with previous examinations in diagnostic versus screening mammography. *Am J Roentgenol*. 2002;179:1173–1177.

23. Sickles EA, D'Orsi CJ. ACR BI-RADS® follow-up and outcome monitoring. In: *ACR BI-RADS® Atlas, Breast Imaging Reporting and Data System*. Reston, VA: American College of Radiology; 2013.

24. Bassett LW, et al. *Quality Determinants of Mammography, Clinical Practice Guideline No. 13. AHCPR Publication No. 95-0632*. Rockville, MD: Agency for Health Care Policy and Research, Public Health Service, U.S. Department of Health and Human Services; 1994.

25. Linver MN, et al. The mammography audit: a primer for the Mammography Quality Standards Act (MQSA). *Am J Roentgenol*. 1995;165:19–25. doi:0361-803X/95/1651-19.

26. Linver MN. Audits measure practice quality of mammography. *Diagn Imaging (San Franc)*. 2000; 22(7):57–61, 79.

27. Jacobson DR. *Rad Tech's Guide to Mammography: Physics, Instrumentation, and Quality Control*. DABMP Blackwell Science; 2001.

28. Kopans DB. *Breast Imaging*. 3rd ed. Philadelphia, PA: Lippincott Williams & Wilkins; 2007.

29. Berns EA, et al. *Digital Mammography Quality Control Manual*. Reston, VA: American College of Radiology; 2016.

30. www.fda.gov Home/Advisory Committees/Recently Updated Advisory Committee Materials. Accessed October 10, 2016.

Mammography Quality Control

16

Objectives

- To understand the MQSA standards applicable to facility mammography quality control structures
- To understand the mammography unit equipment standards required in the MQSA and their relationship to image quality
- To understand the radiologist's mammography workstation equipment standards required by MQSA and their relationship to image quality
- To understand the purpose of quality control tests
- To understand testing variations between different FFDM QC program structures
- To understand the corrective action requirement and its process

Key Terms

- AAPM TG18 test patterns
- acquisition workstation (AWS)
- artifact evaluation test
- contrast-to-noise ratio (CNR)
- image quality phantom test
- mammography equipment evaluation (MEE)
- modulation transfer function (MTF)
- physicist annual survey
- radiologist workstation (RWS)
- signal-to-noise ratio (SNR)

INTRODUCTION

Screening mammography is the primary imaging procedure that has led to a reduction in the mortality rate associated with the diagnosis of breast cancer.[1-7] The ability to detect subtle indications of breast cancer, or to correctly interpret when breast cancer is not present, is dependent on the quality of the image provided for interpretation. Contributions that have led to an improvement in image quality can be isolated to two components: the technical performance of the equipment and the combined technical and artistic performance of the technologist. The technologist contributes the artistic component of high-quality positioning/compression; this topic is discussed in detail in Chapter 7, Parts 1 and 2. Chapter 11 provides an in-depth discussion of the equipment design approved for the process of mammography image production and display under the MQSA. Box 16-1 cites the mammography equipment requirement standard[8] according to the MQSA, while Figure 16-1 depicts the correlating MQSA Mammography Equipment Checklist requirement for the medical physicist (MP).[9] Chapter 15 addresses the importance of safeguarding image quality by establishing a quality assurance program that monitors the MQSA compliance of the mammography service (Box 15-1). An important aspect of the quality assurance program includes oversight of the equipment used to acquire, process, and display the mammography image. When mammography equipment functions as its unique design intended, it is possible to identify subtle characteristics associated with breast cancer on the resulting image. To ensure that all mammography equipment consistently performs at its established standards, a strict quality control program must be established and maintained. This chapter discusses the requirements established for mammography equipment prior to its use, and the rigorous quality control standards established to ensure that equipment performance remains accurate, reliable, and safe as prescribed by the MQSA. Assuring that facilities understand and comply with established equipment standards provides the patient and interpreting radiologist with confidence that the technical components contributing to image quality have been achieved.

MAMMOGRAPHY QUALITY CONTROL: OVERVIEW

Understanding the structure of quality control in today's mammography environment is complex. Radiology administration, lead interpreting physicians (LIPs), and quality control (QC) technologists must be familiar with federal laws governing quality control and understand how their QC program aligns with established MQSA standards. The MP bears the greatest burden to ensure the requirements of the MQSA are understood and followed. Table 15-4 lists the various FDA-approved digital mammography units. MPs must be prepared to provide quality control oversight to all of their customers—who may use any machine from this long list. When the technological differences for all mammography units in the United States are factored in, MPs may be required to perform QC testing of units offering film/screen mammography, CR–digital mammography, 2D FFDM mammography, and digital breast tomosynthesis (DBT or 3D) mammography, in addition to coordinating the QC program with the QC technologist and LIP. The technological differences of the mammography service setting are only one part of the complex landscape!

To navigate this complex landscape of mammography QC, Chapter 16 covers an overview of quality control procedures commonly performed across the manufacturers of 2D and 3D FFDM mammography units. Manufacturer-specific tests associated with DBT QC are not included in this chapter, and CR mammography has purposely been excluded.

QUALITY CONTROL PROGRAM STRUCTURE

Mammography QC Program Structure: Historical

The value of the quality control program in protecting image quality and human safety has consistently been recognized by the MQSA from its inception.

When the MQSA was passed into law in 1992, film/screen mammography was performed by all of the 11,000

BOX 16-1

MQSA General Equipment Standard Requirement

Citation:

900.12(b)(2): General. All radiographic equipment used for mammography shall be specifically designed for mammography and shall be certified pursuant to 1010.2 of this chapter as meeting the applicable requirements of §1020.30 and 1020.31 of this chapter in effect at the date of manufacture.

Discussion:

Facilities are required to accredit all of their x-ray units used for mammography by submitting both clinical and phantom images for each such unit to the accreditation body as specified in 900.4(c)(4)(i) and 900.4(d)(4).

Source: FDA PGHS/Equipment/General Equipment Requirement. Accessed December 9, 2016.

MEDICAL PHYSICIST'S CHECKLIST
MQSA REQUIREMENTS FOR MAMMOGRAPHY EQUIPMENT

Facility Name: _____

Unit Manufacturer: _____ Model: _____

Serial number: _____ Year Mfr: _____

Medical Physicist: _____ Room ID: _____

Signature: _____ Survey Date: _____

Feature	FDA Rule Section	Requirement	Applies to	Meets FDA Requirements? *(in NA, please explain)*
Motion of tube-image receptor assembly	3(i)	The assembly shall be capable of being fixed in any position where it is designed to operate. Once fixed in any such position, it shall not undergo unintended motion.	S-F & FFDM	☐ Yes ☐ No ☐ NA
	3(ii)	This mechanism shall not fail in the event of power interruption.	S-F & FFDM	☐ Yes ☐ No ☐ NA
Image receptor sizes	4(i)	Systems using screen-film image receptors shall provide, at a minimum, for operation with image receptors of 18 x 24 cm and 24 x 30 cm.	S-F	☐ Yes ☐ No ☐ NA
	4(ii)	Systems using screen-film image receptors shall be equipped with moving grids matched to all image receptor sizes provided.	S-F	☐ Yes ☐ No ☐ NA
	4(iii)	Systems used for magnification procedures shall be capable of operation with the grid removed from between the source and image receptor.	S-F & FFDM	☐ Yes ☐ No ☐ NA
Beam limitation and light fields	5(i)	All systems shall have beam limiting devices that allow the useful beam to extend to or beyond the chest wall edge of the image receptor.	S-F & FFDM	☐ Yes ☐ No ☐ NA
	5(ii)	For any mammography system with a light beam that passes through the X-ray beam-limiting device, the light shall provide an average illumination of not less than 160 lux (15 ft-candles) at 100 cm or the maximum source-image receptor distance (SID), whichever is less.	S-F & FFDM (except Fischer)	☐ Yes ☐ No ☐ NA
Magnification	6(i)	Systems used to perform noninterventional problem-solving procedures shall have radiographic magnification capability available for use by the operator.	S-F & FFDM	☐ Yes ☐ No ☐ NA
	6(ii)	Systems used for magnification procedures shall provide, at a minimum, at least one magnification value within the range of 1.4 to 2.0.	S-F & FFDM	☐ Yes ☐ No ☐ NA
Focal spot selection	7(i)	When more than one focal spot is provided, the system shall indicate, prior to exposure, which focal spot is selected.	S-F & FFDM	☐ Yes ☐ No ☐ NA
	7(ii)	When more than one target material is provided, the system shall indicate, prior to exposure, the preselected target material.	S-F & FFDM	☐ Yes ☐ No ☐ NA
	7(iii)	When the target material and/or focal spot is selected by a system algorithm that is based on the exposure or on a test exposure, the system shall display, after the exposure, the target material and/or focal spot actually used during the exposure.	S-F & FFDM	☐ Yes ☐ No ☐ NA
Application of compression	8(i)(A)	Each system shall provide an initial power-driven compression activated by hands-free controls operable from both sides of the patient.	S-F & FFDM	☐ Yes ☐ No ☐ NA
	8(i)(B)	Each system shall provide fine adjustment compression controls operable from both sides of the patient.	S-F & FFDM	☐ Yes ☐ No ☐ NA
Compression paddle	8(ii)(A)	Systems shall be equipped with different sized compression paddles that match the sizes of all full-field image receptors provided for the system.	S-F & FFDM	☐ Yes ☐ No ☐ NA
	8(ii)(B)	The compression paddle shall be flat and parallel to the breast support table and shall not deflect from parallel by more than 1.0 cm at any point on the surface of the compression paddle when compression is applied.	S-F & FFDM (except Fischer)	☐ Yes ☐ No ☐ NA
	8(ii)(C)	Equipment intended by the manufacturer's design to not be flat and parallel to the breast support table during compression shall meet the manufacturer's design specifications and maintenance requirements.	S-F & FFDM	☐ Yes ☐ No ☐ NA
	8(ii)(D)	The chest wall edge of the compression paddle shall be straight and parallel to the edge of the image receptor.	S-F & FFDM	☐ Yes ☐ No ☐ NA
	8(ii)(E)	The chest wall edge may be bent upward to allow for patient comfort but shall not appear on the image.	S-F & FFDM	☐ Yes ☐ No ☐ NA

Figure 16-1

MQSA Mammography equipment requirements checklist for the medical physicist. (Source: American College of Radiology Web site: Quality and Safety/Accreditation/Mammography/Medical Physicist Evaluation Forms/MQSA Requirements for Mammography Checklist. Accessed December 9, 2016.)

Feature	FDA Rule Section	Requirement	Applies to	Meets FDA Requirements? *(in NA, please explain)*
Technique factor selection and display	9(i)	Manual selection of mAs or at least one of its component parts (mA and/or time) shall be available.	S-F & FFDM	☐ Yes ☐ No ☐ NA
	9(ii)	The technique factors (kVp and either mA and seconds or mAs) to be used during an exposure shall be indicated before the exposure begins, except when AEC is used, in which case the technique factors that are set prior to the exposure shall be indicated.	S-F & FFDM	☐ Yes ☐ No ☐ NA
	9(iii)	Following AEC mode use, the system shall indicate the actual kVp and mAs (or mA and time) used during the exposure.	S-F & FFDM	☐ Yes ☐ No ☐ NA
Automatic exposure control	10(i)	Each screen-film system shall provide an AEC mode that is operable in all combinations of equipment configuration provided, e.g., grid, non-grid; magnification, nonmagnification; and various target-filter combinations.	S-F	☐ Yes ☐ No ☐ NA
	10(ii)	The positioning or selection of the detector shall permit flexibility in the placement of the detector under the target tissue. The size and the available positions of the detector shall be clearly indicated at the X-ray input surface of the breast compression paddle. The selected position of the detector shall be clearly indicated.	S-F	☐ Yes ☐ No ☐ NA
	10(iii)	The system shall provide means for the operator to vary the selected optical density from the normal (zero) setting.	S-F	☐ Yes ☐ No ☐ NA
X-ray film*	11	The facility shall use X-ray film for mammography that has been designated by the film manufacturer as appropriate for mammography.	S-F	☐ Yes ☐ No ☐ NA
Intensifying screens*	12	The facility shall use intensifying screens for mammography that have been designated by the screen manufacturer as appropriate for mammography and shall use film that is matched to the screen's spectral output as specified by the manufacturer.	S-F	☐ Yes ☐ No ☐ NA
Film processing solutions*	13	For processing mammography films, the facility shall use chemical solutions that are capable of developing the films used by the facility in a manner equivalent to the minimum requirements specified by the film manufacturer.	S-F	☐ Yes ☐ No ☐ NA
Lighting*	14	The facility shall make special lights for film illumination, i.e., hot-lights, capable of producing light levels greater than that provided by the view box, available to the interpreting physicians.	S-F & FFDM (for hardcopy comparison)	☐ Yes ☐ No ☐ NA
Film masking devices*	15	Facilities shall ensure that film masking devices that can limit the illuminated area to a region equal to or smaller than the exposed portion of the film are available to all interpreting physicians interpreting for the facility.	S-F & FFDM (for hardcopy comparison)	☐ Yes ☐ No ☐ NA

NA is acceptable for new units at existing facilities if these were previously evaluated and have not changed.

| **Figure 16-1** (*Continued*)

mammography facilities operating in the United States.[10] Mammography departments conformed to quality control requirements by following the MQSA standard, "Quality Control Tests Other Than Annual,"[11] which describes the QC testing requirements for the film/screen modality. The ACR published several editions of this quality control manual between 1992 and 1999. These manuals were thorough guides for mammography facilities and personnel that described in detail the equipment QC testing requirements for the mammography unit, film processor, and image display environment—the viewbox and viewing conditions. The FDA QC testing regulations in the film/screen environment were standardized for all mammography equipment manufacturers and for all facilities. All MPs and all QC technologists consulted the ACR Quality Control Manuals for analog imaging, the most recent being the ACR 1999 Quality Control Manual. The regulations applied to all and were clearly understood by all. The harmonious structure of mammography quality control would change with the introduction and FDA approval of digital imaging.

Mammography QC Program Structure: Current

In the year 2000, the first digital mammography system was approved for use in the United States, requiring facilities that adopted this new technology to follow an alternative MQSA standard for equipment quality control, different from that used in the film/screen environment. Quality control programs using digital equipment would adhere to the MQSA standard, "Other Modalities Quality Control Tests," that requires that "the quality assurance program shall be substantially the same as the quality assurance program recommended by the image receptor manufacturer."[12] Sixteen years after the FDA first approved digital mammography, the ACR 2016 Digital Mammography Quality Control Manual was approved by the FDA through the Alternative Standard process (refer to Chapter 15 for further explanation of the Alternative Standard), introducing a second quality control program structure for the digital environment. As a result, as of this writing, a facility may select one of the FDA-approved pathways to perform digital QC. Table 16-1 provides the two

Table 16-1 • Quality Control Program Structure Requirements under MQSA

QC REQUIREMENT	MQSA FFDM STANDARD	MQSA ALTERNATIVE STANDARD
	Other Modalities Quality Control Tests Citation: 900.12 (e)(6): Quality Control Tests—other modalities For systems with image receptor modalities other than film/screen, the quality assurance program shall be substantially the same as the quality assurance program recommended by the image receptor manufacturer, except that the maximum allowable dose shall not exceed the maximum allowable dose for film/screen systems in paragraph (e)(5)(vi) of this section.	Alternative Standard (MQSA) FDA may approve an alternative to a quality standard under section 900.12 when the agency determines that the proposed alternative standard will be at least as effective in assuring quality mammography as the standard it proposes to replace and is too limited in its applicability to justify an amendment to the standard or offers an expected benefit to human health that is so great that the time required for amending the standard would present an unjustifiable risk to human health. #24: Approval of an Alternative Standard for Using the Quality Assurance Program Recommended by the ACR Digital Mammography Quality Control Manual for Full-Field Digital Mammography Systems, for Systems without Advanced Imaging Capabilities: This alternative standard was approved and became effective on February 17, 2016. It has no time limit. The alternative standard allows mammography facilities to use the *ACR Digital Mammography Quality Control Manual* as an alternative to the quality assurance program recommended by the image receptor manufacturer. The FDA has determined that the ACR's quality control manual is, as required in 900.18 (a)(1): *Alternative Requirements,* "at least as effective in assuring quality mammography" as following the manufacturer's QC manuals.
Follows:	Image Receptor Manufacturer QC Manual (for FFDM DR units) Fuji (FDR) GE Lorad Siemens Giotto Philips Fischer Planmed	ACR 2016 Mammography Digital QC Manual (standardized for all image receptor manufacturers without advanced imaging capabilities [DBT])
Image Quality Phantom:	FDA—original approved accreditation phantom developed for film/screen	FDA-approved ACR FFDM mammography phantom
Medical Physicist Tests:	Image Receptor Manufacturer QC Manual ACR Web site: acr.org/accreditation/mammography/medical physicist forms	ACR 2016 Digital Mammography QC Manual
QC Technologist Tests:	Image Receptor Manufacturer QC Manual ACR Web site: acr.org/accreditation/mammography/radiologic technologist forms	ACR 2016 Digital Mammography QC Manual
Radiologist Workstation QC:	Follows Image Receptor Manufacturer QC Manual	ACR 2016 Digital Mammography QC Manual
Printer QC:	Follows Image Receptor Manufacturer QC Manual	ACR 2016 Digital Mammography QC Manual
Corrective Action Allowances:	Image Receptor Manufacturer QC Manual FDA Web site: fda.gov/PGHS/Alternative Standards/Requirements/Approved Alternative Standards/Individual Receptor Manufacturers	ACR 2016 Digital Mammography QC Manual

Facilities may choose to follow one of the two QC Programs defined under the MQSA. The two QC programs are prescribed for separate use, with no allowable interchange between the two.
Data Source: FDA MQSA PGHS (fda.gov); ACR Web site (http://www.acr.org); ACR 2016 Digital Mammography QC Manual.

different structures for FFDM DR QC along with the MQSA standards that each program must adhere to. The table defines the *MQSA FFDM STANDARD* QC pathway and its requirements in the center of the table and the *MQSA ALTERNATIVE STANDARD* and its requirements on the right side of the table. The two FDA-approved QC programs may not be used in conjunction with one another; rather they are intended to operate in isolation from one another.

Mammography QC Program Structure: FFDM Standard

Image Receptor Manufacturer

Facilities that choose to use the QC manual supplied by their FFDM image receptor manufacturer adhere to the "Other Modalities Quality Control Tests" described in Table 16-1, *MQSA FFDM STANDARD* to comply with quality control mandates. This choice requires the facility to follow all of the requirements contained in the image receptor manufacturer's QC manual. QC manuals supplied by image receptor manufacturers also address the QC testing requirements for the radiologist workstation (monitors) and the printer (if applicable). At the time of this writing, all of the image receptor manufacturers' QC manuals require the use of an FDA-approved accreditation phantom (Figure 16-2) for evaluating image quality. These are available from:

- Mammo 156™ Phantom—Gammex, a Sun Nuclear Company
- Nuclear Associates Model 18-220—Fluke Biomedical Corporation
- CIRS Model 015—Computerized Imaging Reference Systems, Inc.

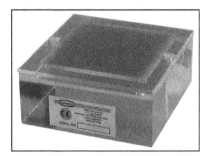

Figure 16-2
The original FDA accreditation phantom developed for film/screen mammography continues to be used for FFDM quality control and accreditation for facilities who follow the image receptor manufacturer's QC program structure. (Photo: Mammo 156™ Phantom, courtesy of Gammex, Inc., Sun Nuclear Corporation.)

Mammography QC Program Structure: Alternative Standard

2016 Standardized ACR Digital Mammography Quality Control Program

Facilities that choose to use the ACR 2016 Digital Mammography QC Manual adhere to the MQSA Alternative Standard described in Table 16-1. The Approved Alternative Standard that may replace the MQSA FFDM standard is the 24th approved alternative standard listed in the FDA PGHS, which is described under *MQSA ALTERNATIVE STANDARD* in Table 16-1. The publication of the ACR 2016 Digital Mammography QC Manual once again establishes standardized QA/QC procedures for all facilities offering 2D FFDM mammography. This option is offered to facilities regardless of the manufacturer of the image receptor they use as long as the facility meets the following conditions[13]:

- Only 2D FFDM equipment may adopt the use of the ACR 2016 Digital Mammography QC Manual. The ACR 2016 QC Manual is not approved for systems that utilize advanced imaging capabilities such as tomosynthesis (DBT).
- The facility follows all of the requirements contained in the ACR 2016 Mammography Digital QC Manual.
- The ACR Digital QC Manual also addresses the QC testing requirements for the radiologist workstation (RWS), the technologist acquisition workstation (AWS), and the printer (if applicable).

As of this writing, choosing to follow the ACR 2016 Mammography Digital QC Manual requires the use of the FDA-approved FFDM phantom[14] available from (Figure 16-3):

- CIRS Model 086—Computerized Imaging Reference Systems, Inc.
- Mammo FFDM™ Phantom, Gammex, a Sun Nuclear Company

It should be noted, however, that in a few circumstances, QC testing follows the established equipment manufacturer procedures and performance criteria due to a unique manufacturer-specific design of the component.

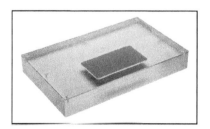

Figure 16-3
The FFDM FDA accreditation phantom developed for digital mammography. Facilities who follow the 2016 ACR Digital Mammography QC Manual use this new phantom. (Photo: Mammo FFDM™ Phantom, courtesy of Gammex, Inc., Sun Nuclear Corporation.)

Mammography QC Program Structure: Digital Breast Tomosynthesis

Facilities with advanced imaging capabilities such as DBT, or 3D digital imaging, are required to adhere to the *MQSA FFDM STANDARD* in Table 16-1. Facilities performing DBT must follow the image receptor manufacturer's QC manual for their quality assurance program in order to comply with MQSA.

▍ QUALITY CONTROL PERSONNEL STRUCTURE

MQSA mandates that qualified individuals be assigned the responsibility of the quality assurance program and each of its elements, which includes the quality control program. Within the framework of the QA program, the equipment used to produce the image, a major component of image quality, is addressed through its quality control program. Quality control is the part of the quality assurance program that focuses on instrumentation and equipment technical performance and reliability to ensure the quality and accuracy of the mammographic image and the safety of the patient. To ensure that regulatory equipment standards are met upon installation, and consistently achieved for daily operation, quality control testing and evaluation are required to be performed by qualified personnel. Quality control establishes standards (parameters) for equipment operation, periodically tests equipment components, and analyzes resultant data in an effort to detect problems that may negatively impact image quality prior to being observed on the mammographic image. Additionally, quality control practices include required "corrective action" when acceptable testing standards are not met. The FDA further requires that personnel identified for these responsibilities be given the time necessary to carry out associated QC tasks[15] (Box 16-2). An effective program includes invested personnel who plan, implement, and maintain all areas of quality control. There are three key personnel who are given specific mandated responsibilities for the QC program.[15] A successful QC program requires strong communication between the three entities.

1. The LIP

    The LIP is designated as the person responsible for the facility's QA program. Paramount among his/her responsibilities is to ensure there is an effective quality control program that meets the MQSA QA requirements. Individuals assigned responsibility for the QA/QC program are determined by the lead interpreting physician to be adequately qualified to perform tasks associated with the QA/QC program.

BOX 16-2

Quality Control Technologist Responsibilities

Citation:

900.12(d)(1)(iv): (1) Responsible individuals. Responsibility for the quality assurance program and for each of its elements shall be assigned to individuals who are qualified for their assignments and who shall be allowed adequate time to perform these duties.

(iv) Quality control technologist. Responsibility for all individual tasks within the quality assurance program not assigned to the lead interpreting physician or the medical physicist shall be assigned to a quality control technologist(s). The tasks are to be performed by the quality control technologist or by other personnel qualified to perform the tasks. When other personnel are utilized for these tasks, the quality control technologist shall ensure that the tasks are completed in such a way as to meet the requirements of paragraph (e) of this section.

Source: FDA MQSA PGHS/QualityControlTechnologistResponsibilities (fda.gov). Accessed December 9, 2016.

---

2. The MP

    MQSA guidance describes the minimum responsibilities of the MP: to manage the equipment-related activities of the QA/QC program, to conduct required annual equipment evaluations, and to provide reports to the facility regarding these evaluations.[16] MPs perform mammography equipment evaluations (MEEs) when new equipment has been installed; when major changes take place to the equipment, such as major repairs or major component replacements; or when annual equipment evaluations are due. Required annual MP evaluation of equipment requires many of the same tests as the MEE (Figure 15-5A–C). In addition to this significant role, the MP provides guidance to the facility for the QC program, as it is he/she who directly assists the quality control technologist as she carries out the routine responsibilities of ensuring continuous MQSA compliance. An MP who educates the QC technologist, elevating her understanding and performance of the quality control program, is invaluable to the QC technologist and to the facility.

3. The radiologic technologist (RT)

    According to MQSA guidance documents, the mammography QC technologist is responsible for all tasks that fall within the QA/QC program that are not assigned to the LIP or the MP. Among these responsibilities is the required performance of the periodic quality control testing to ensure the mammography equipment continues to meet standards of safety and quality that have been established during the MP's acceptance testing procedures. As such, the QC technologist has the responsibility of the routine obligations of the QC program and of all the communication that continuous oversight of the program requires. These responsibilities describe a commitment to the QC program that is deserving of further definition.

QC Technologist or Superwoman?

The above description of the technologist's role in the oversight of the QC program is an accurate account of just one facet of the program requirements. The commitment that is included in this responsibility reaches far beyond performing the required periodic testing—into abilities that demand meeting federal compliance, advanced technical knowledge, organization, detailed record keeping, problem-solving, and communication to name only a few. The role of the QC technologist in navigating the demands of an FDA-certified mammography facility is substantial, but successfully attaining the continuous goals of the program accomplishes a worthy task that is immensely rewarding. The technologist interested in this position should be open to the following broad applications of quality control in mammography:

1. Learning about federal regulations; what they mean, and how compliance is accomplished.
2. Understanding what contributes to mammography image quality and how those components are controlled and managed.
3. Understanding the role of the QC technologist in executing and coordinating the QC program under the direction and guidance of the MP and ultimately the LIP.
4. Strong communication skills ensuring all members of the QA/QC team, mammography staff, and biomedical engineering are provided critical information in a timely manner.
5. Accurate documentation of activities surrounding mammography equipment: installation, function, operation, corrective action, and inspections.

These five foundations of quality control management for mammography require exceptional skills in time management, organization, and communication. A successful quality control program includes a QC technologist motivated to accept unpredictable challenges, an accessible MP, and supportive LIP and radiology management.

ACCOUNTABILITY AND RECORD KEEPING

The following advice from basketball coach John Wooden, "Be prepared and be honest," is applicable to the process of documenting events involving the equipment in the mammography facility. In addition to performing the required QC testing, it is the QC technologist's responsibility to ensure that factual and accurate accounts of equipment incidents are recorded:

- Documentation of major equipment changes that take place during the year
- Performance and documentation of the periodic testing of mammography equipment
- Documentation of the corrective action process when applicable

Each of these incidents requires detailed records: date of occurrence, appropriate testing, who performed the test, test results, and supporting documents. Documentation should not have any loose ends; rather, every incident should have a full explanation with a finite ending. Supporting documents, such as an invoice from the biomedical engineer, recorded communication with the MP, or testing results from the MP, supply the ending of the incident. The documentation is used for a variety of circumstances and may be consulted by the biomedical engineer for troubleshooting or repair, reviewed by the MP for isolating a problem, or to validate MQSA compliance by an FDA inspector. Records that are complete provide all details surrounding the equipment incident. Timeliness of recording and factual accounting are necessary to ensure that the documented information is truthful and accurate. The information documented throughout the year is reviewed during the facility's annual MQSA inspection. The QC technologist should understand that the purpose of the inspection is to validate that the mammography service complies with the standards established in the MQSA, a federal law. As such, the technologist should recognize the confines of her role in the quality control program and receive support from appropriate authoritative sources such as the MP, the lead interpreting physician (Box 16-3), or radiology management when required. Because documentation of QC activities applies to a federal law, consequences exist to the facility or to individuals that falsify QA/QC documentation: the consequences may include possible fines and/or other severe penalties.

MAMMOGRAPHY STAFF OWNERSHIP AND TRANSPARENCY

Although the QC technologist has the primary responsibility of periodic equipment testing and documentation, all mammography technologists must abide by the requirements of the MQSA. An effective quality control program employs the efforts of all mammography technologists in order to ensure that the equipment quality control procedures take place as required. Examples of this may include daily QC of the radiologist workstation monitors, or documentation of equipment component malfunction, initiating the repair

---

BOX 16-3

Quality Assurance Records

Citation:

900.12(d)(2): Quality assurance records. The lead interpreting physician, quality control technologist, and medical physicist shall ensure that records concerning mammography technique and procedures, quality control (including monitoring data, problems detected by analysis of that data, corrective actions, and the effectiveness of the corrective actions), safety, protection, and employee qualifications to meet assigned quality assurance tasks, are properly maintained and updated. These quality control records shall be kept for each test specified in paragraphs (e) and (f) of this section until the next annual inspection has been completed and FDA has determined that the facility is in compliance with the quality assurance requirements or until the test has been performed two additional times at the required frequency, whichever is longer.

Source: FDA MQSA PGHS/General/QualityAssuranceRecords (fda.gov). Accessed December 9, 2016.

BOX 16-4

Mammography Equipment Evaluations

Citation:

900.12(e)(10): Mammography equipment evaluations. Additional evaluations of mammography units or image processors shall be conducted whenever a new unit or processor is installed, a unit or processor is disassembled and reassembled at the same or a new location, or major components of a mammography unit or processor equipment are changed or repaired. These evaluations shall be used to determine whether the new or changed equipment meets the requirements of applicable standards in paragraphs (b) and (e) of this section. All problems shall be corrected before the new or changed equipment is put into service for examinations or film processing. The mammography equipment evaluation shall be performed by a medical physicist or by an individual under the direct supervision of a medical physicist.

Source: FDA MQSA PGHS/General/QualityAssuranceEquipment/MammographyEquipmentEvaluation (fda.gov). Accessed December 9, 2016.

---

process. Appropriate forms that are accessible to all mammography technologists, perhaps placed on a designated QC bulletin board or online, readily apprise interested members of the QA committee, interpreting physician, or radiology managers of the status of completed QC tasks, upcoming QC tasks, or corrective action documentation. Placing this documentation in a communal location for interested staff members increases the likelihood that required QC responsibilities take place when they are due or are noticed should they be missed. Although MQSA requires a designated QC technologist for the supervision of the quality control program, ensuring that the mammography service continuously complies with all MQSA requirements is the responsibility of every technologist performing mammography.

REQUIRED QUALITY CONTROL TESTING

Topics discussed in this chapter include the mammography equipment used to produce, process, and display the mammography image for interpretation. Radiologic technologists who wish to obtain the ARRT Advanced Certification for mammography are expected to have a basic understanding of the tests performed by the MP and a detailed understanding of the tests performed by the QC technologist.[17] Required quality control procedures and processes are described for the following equipment used in the mammography service[12]:

- Mammography machine
- Radiologist workstation
- Printer (if applicable)

Acceptance Testing

New equipment that has been installed or existing equipment that has had major repairs or has been disassembled and reassembled are required to have acceptance testing performed prior to use for mammography. This testing must be done by a qualified MP, performing the tests described in the FDA **mammography equipment evaluation (MEE)** document (Box 16-4). During acceptance testing, the MP verifies that the equipment functions within the specifications set by the manufacturer and also looks for possible indications of defects in the equipment. All tests performed during the MEE must pass prior to using the mammography equipment to image patients. The baseline performance for specific equipment evaluations is established during acceptance testing and is included in the physicist's report to the facility. The baseline values are used as a reference point in subsequent periodic quality control testing performed by the QC technologist.[18]

Routine (Periodic) Performance Testing

Routine performance testing of the mammography equipment is performed by the QC technologist, with the exception of the **physicist annual survey** (Box 16-5), which is performed by the MP. Periodic equipment testing by the QC technologist is performed and documented at specific time intervals of daily, weekly, monthly, quarterly, and semiannually. Repetitively testing the equipment performance at required frequencies, and by exactly following the steps specific to each test, verifies that the equipment continuously performs within the predicted parameters established

BOX 16-5

Annual Physics Survey

900.12(e)(9)(i),(ii),(iii),(iv),(v) Surveys:

(i) *At least once a year, each facility shall undergo a survey by a medical physicist or by an individual under the direct supervision of a medical physicist. At a minimum, this survey shall include the performance of tests to ensure that the facility meets the quality assurance requirements of the annual tests described in paragraphs (e)(5) and (e)(6) of this section and the weekly phantom image quality test described in paragraph (e)(2) of this section.*

(ii) *The results of all rests conducted by the facility in accordance with paragraphs (e)(1) through (e)(7) of this section, as well as written documentation of any corrective actions taken and their results, shall be evaluated for adequacy by the medical physicist performing the survey.*

(iii) *The medical physicist shall prepare a survey report that includes a summary of this review and recommendations for necessary improvements.*

(iv) *The survey report shall be sent to the facility within 30 days of the date of the survey.*

(v) *The survey report shall be dated and signed by the medical physicist performing or supervising the survey. If the survey was performed entirely or in part by another individual under the direct supervision of the medical physicist, that individual and the part of the survey that individual performed shall also be identified in the survey report.*

Source: FDA MQSA PGHS/General/QualityAssuranceEquipment/AnnualPhysicsSurvey (fda.gov). Accessed December 9, 2016.

during the acceptance testing and reveals problems that may otherwise go unnoticed. Reducing the variables introduced into the testing environment by repeating the test in the same way at the same time allows the detection of possible problems that may degrade image quality prior to being observed on the mammographic image.[18]

Error Correction Testing

When routine testing results fall outside of the parameters established during acceptance testing, the equipment is examined to determine the cause. This evaluation to determine equipment malfunction may be performed by the biomedical engineer or the MP. When the cause has been determined, and the condition corrected, the equipment is tested by the biomedical engineer to ensure it meets the parameters established during acceptance testing prior to its use. When significant corrections or changes are made to the equipment, an additional inspection by a qualified MP is required prior to its use of performing mammography examinations.[18]

QUALITY CONTROL TOOLBOX

Mammography quality control requires an array of testing tools and devices that assist in determining equipment performance. The equipment evaluation performed by the MP involves complex testing using a variety of sophisticated measuring tools and devices. The QC technologist periodically performs a smaller-scale evaluation of the equipment using some of the same testing tools and devices used by the MP. An introduction to the *common* testing tools and devices used by the MP and the QC technologist provides insight to the mammography technologist considering a role as a QC technologist.

Quality Control Manual

The manufacturer QC manual and the ACR 2016 Digital Mammography QC Manual are comprehensive directives that describe the QC program, the QC testing procedures for the MP, and the QC testing procedures for the QC technologist. These QC manuals contain specific sections that provide a list of prescribed tests, the required test frequencies, and instructions on how to perform each test; these instructions must be followed precisely in order to comply with the MQSA. In addition to describing the testing procedures, the QC manual provides the appropriate QC forms for documentation of each test performed by the MP and by the QC technologist.

Quality Control Phantom Examples

Quality control testing involves the use of various QC phantoms that assist in the evaluation of specific features of the mammography unit and to evaluate image quality.

• To evaluate the presence or absence of artifacts and to perform detector calibration, a uniform 4-cm-thick acrylic phantom that covers the detector area is typically used (Figure 16-4).

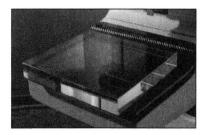

Figure 16-4
Uniform acrylic phantom; approximately 24 cm × 30 cm. Used to periodically calibrate the mammography machine's digital detector and to evaluate whether there are mammography machine artifacts. Due to the material the uniform phantom is made of, polymethylmethacrylate (PMMA), it is sometimes referred to as a PMMA phantom.

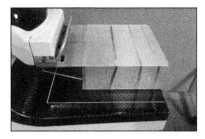

Figure 16-5
Proprietary tomosynthesis phantom developed by Hologic, Inc., for evaluation of specific tomosynthesis QC.

- Evaluation of 2D FFDM image quality is performed using only FDA-approved phantoms. MQSA regulations require facilities that use the image receptor manufacturer QC manual use the original FDA-approved phantom (Figure 16-2), while facilities using the ACR 2016 Mammography Digital QC Manual use the FDA-approved FFDM phantom (Figure 16-3).
- For facilities using DBT technology, tomosynthesis-specific QC tests are required using manufacturer-specific phantoms designed for DBT technology (Figure 16-5).
- Some manufacturers have developed proprietary phantoms that test specific features of their unit design, such as the GE Image Quality Signature Test (IQST) phantom and the Siemens PMMA phantom for artifact detection (Figure 16-6A,B).

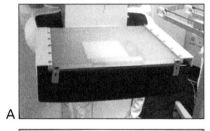

A

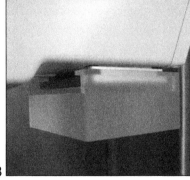

B

Figure 16-6
(A) Proprietary phantom developed by General Electric (GE). Used to perform MTF and CNR QC for GE digital mammography systems. **(B)** Proprietary uniform phantom, mounted on the tube head. Developed by Siemens to perform detector uniformity and artifact QC for Siemens digital mammography systems.

Generally, image receptor manufacturers of FFDM and DBT equipment supply the phantoms that are required for specific QC testing of their equipment, with the exception of the 2D FFDM image quality accreditation phantom, which must be purchased by the facility.

Cleaning Materials

Quality control requirements may include cleaning protocols for the radiologist workstation monitors and for technologist AWS monitors. Always follow the monitor manufacturer's recommendations for appropriate cleaning protocols due to the potential damage that can result from improper methods.

Medical Display Workstation Test Patterns

Workstation monitors used by the radiologist for mammography interpretation are a critical component in the imaging chain. The images displayed on these monitors are used for diagnostic and clinical purposes and therefore require that image quality not be compromised.[19] These electronic display devices typically utilize flat-panel liquid crystal display (LCD) monitors; this technology contributes to several specific factors that affect image quality. FDA recommends that only monitors specifically approved or cleared for FFDM use by FDA's Office of Device Evaluation be used.[20] To ensure that the radiologist workstation monitors are performing to the standards established by the manufacturer, extensive acceptance testing by a qualified MP is performed prior to use of the equipment for interpretation of mammography. There are several professional organizations that have developed guidelines for quality control procedures for medical display devices. The American Association of Physicists in Medicine (AAPM) Task Group 18 (TG18) has published guidelines for acceptance testing criteria and quality control for medical display devices. The specially designed **AAPM TG18 test patterns** are used in conjunction with testing procedures to evaluate a wide range of performance requirements. For complete information on all the TG18 patterns and testing purposes they are used for visit AAPM.org.[19] Although the range of testing performed by the MP requires the use of several of the TG18 test patterns to evaluate the radiologist workstation, only the TG18 QC test pattern is used for quality control by both the MP and the QC technologist. The Society of Motion Picture and Television Engineers (SMPTE) also developed a test pattern used to evaluate the performance of medical electronic display devices.[21] The SMPTE (pronounced sim-tee) is commonly used in the practice of quality control by the MP and the QC technologist.

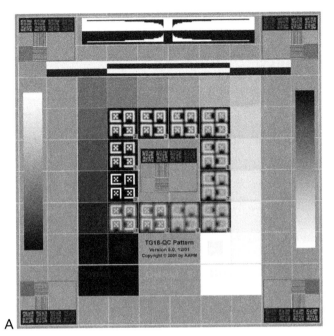
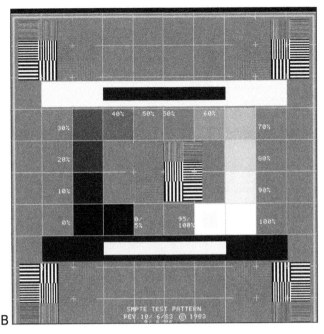

Figure 16-7
(A) AAPM TG18 QC test pattern developed by the American Association of Physicists in Medicine Task Group 18 for electronic display assessment. (Source: AAPM On-Line Report 03. Assessment of Display Performance For Medical Imaging Systems, 2005. (http://www. aapm.org/pubs/reports/OR_03.pdf).) **(B)** SMPTE test pattern developed by the Society of Motion Picture and Television Engineers for electronic display assessment. (Source: Society of Motion Picture and Television Engineers, http://www.SMPTE.org.)

To determine the appropriate test pattern to use for quality control, consult the QC manual that is used for the facility QC program. The mammography technologist's acquisition monitor is also used for the purpose of image quality evaluation and may require minimal QC testing using one of these two patterns. Figure 16-7A,B illustrates the differences between the AAPM TG18 QC pattern and the SMPTE pattern. Further explanation regarding the testing characteristics evaluated using these patterns can be found in this chapter under Radiologist Workstation Quality Control and Laser Printer Quality Control.

Quality Control Forms

Another responsibility of the QC technologist is the correct use of QC forms, as designated by the requirements of MQSA. The Mammography Accreditation Program section on the ACR Web site contains the QC forms for each manufacturer that has an FDA-approved mammography unit; these forms may be downloaded from acr.org/ accreditation/mammography Quality Control and Equipment Evaluation Forms.

The manufacturer-specific ACR Summary QC forms for the radiologic technologist list the periodic testing requirements for daily, weekly, monthly, quarterly, and semiannual intervals. These forms are used for the routine QC testing performed by the QC technologist; specific forms must be submitted with the facility's annual update requested by their AB; and some forms must be submitted during the triannual accreditation process.

Due to the numerous FDA-approved mammography machines, each with their own uniquely designed QC forms, only two examples are provided. Figures 16-8 and 16-9 display examples of the MP's MEE/Annual Survey form and the technologist's periodic QC forms used by mammography machine manufacturers.

The ACR 2016 Digital Mammography QC Manual has its own version of the MEE/Annual Survey forms for the MP and the periodic QC test forms for the radiologic technologist (Figure 16-10A–D).

Quality control forms used to verify individual equipment testing components range in their requirements for documentation:

- Forms may require minimal documentation, requiring only the technologist's initials and the testing date for QC verification (Figure 16-11).
- Forms may require several testing factors to be recorded—such as the kVp, mAs, target and filter combination, in addition to the QC testing results, and the technologist's initials (Figure 16-12).
- Forms may require the technologist to plot the resulting data on a control chart to track the performance of the equipment (Figure 16-13).

MEDICAL PHYSICIST'S MAMMOGRAPHY QC TEST SUMMARY
Full-Field Digital—Philips (Sectra)

Site Name _____   Report Date _____
Address _____   Survey Date _____
Medical Physicist's Name _____   Signature _____
X-Ray Unit Manufacturer [Philips (Sectra)]   Model _____
Date of Installation _____   Room ID _____

QC Manual Version # _____   *(use version applicable to unit tested; contact mfr if questions)*

Accessory Equipment

	Manufacturer	Model	Location	QC Manual Version #
Review Workstation*			☐ On-site ☐ Off-site	
Film Printer*			☐ On-site ☐ Off-site	

FDA recommends that only monitors and printers specifically cleared for FFDM use by FDA's Office of Device Evaluation (ODE) be used. See FDA's Policy Guidance Help System www.fda.gov/CDRH/MAMMOGRAPHY/robohelp/START.HTM.

Survey Type ☐ Mammo Eqpt Evaluation of new unit (include MQSA Rqmts for Mammo Eqpt checklist)   ☐ Annual Survey

Medical Physicist's QC Tests
("Pass" means all components of the test passes; indicate "Fail" if any component fails. Tests must be done for both on and off-site equipment.)

PASS/FAIL

1. **X-ray Tube Output (air kerma)**
2. **Air Kerma Reproducibility**
3. **Half Value Layer**
4. **AEC System: Breast Thickness and Exposure**
5. **AEC System: Density Compensation**
6. **Image Quality Evaluation**
   Phantom image scores: Fibers [____]   Specks [____]   Masses [____]
   Average glandular dose for average breast is 1 mGy (100 mrad)
7. **Contrast-to-Noise Ratio Reference Level**
   CNR *(value)* [____]
8. **Tube Voltage**
9. **Image Field and X-Ray Field Agreement**
10. **Missed Tissue and Chest Wall**
11. **Viewing Conditions**

*** YOUR MEDICAL PHYSICIST MUST SUMMARIZE HIS/HER RESULTS ON THIS FORM ***

A

Figure 16-8

Quality control forms for the FFDM Philips (Sectra) mammography unit. **(A)** Medical physicist's mammography QC test summary form—FFDM Philips (Sectra) mammography unit. (Source: ACR Web site (http://www.acr.org)/Quality and Safety/Accreditation/ Mammography/Medical Physicists Evaluation Forms.)

MAMMOGRAPHY QUALITY CONTROL CHECKLIST—FULL-FIELD DIGITAL PHILIPS (SECTRA)

Daily and Weekly Tests

Year																													
Month																													
Date																													
Initials																													
Daily Quality Control *(daily)*																													
Full Calibration *(weekly)*																													
Mammographic Accreditation Phantom *(weekly)*																													
Contrast-to-Noise Ratio *(weekly)*																													
Printer QC *(see FDA guidance)*																													
Display QC-AWS *(weekly)*																													
Review Workstation QC *(weekly)*																													

Year																													
Month																													
Date																													
Initials																													
Daily Quality Control *(daily)*																													
Full Calibration *(weekly)*																													
Mammographic Accreditation Phantom *(weekly)*																													
Contrast-to-Noise Ratio *(weekly)*																													
Printer QC *(see FDA guidance)*																													
Display QC-AWS *(weekly)*																													
Review Workstation QC *(weekly)*																													

B

Figure 16-8 (*Continued*)
(B) Mammography quality control checklist for the FFDM Philips (Sectra) mammography unit—daily and weekly tests for the radiologic technologist. (Source: ACR Web site (http://www.acr.org)/Quality and Safety/Accreditation/Mammography/Radiologic Technologist Quality Control Forms.)

MAMMOGRAPHY QUALITY CONTROL CHECKLIST—FULL-FIELD DIGITAL PHILIPS (SECTRA)

Monthly, Quarterly, and Semi-Annual
(date, initial and enter number where appropriate)

Year / Month	JAN	FEB	MAR	APR	MAY	JUN	JUL	AUG	SEP	OCT	NOV	DEC
Spatial Resolution *(monthly)*												
Visual Checklist *(monthly)*												
Repeat Analysis (≤2% change) *(quarterly)*												
Thickness Indication *(semi-annually)*												
Compression (25-45 lb) *(semi-annually)*												
Printer QC *(see FDA guidance)*												
Review Workstation QC *(See FDA guidance)*												

Date: _____ **Test:** _____ **Comments:** _____

C

Figure 16-8 *(Continued)*
(C) Mammography quality control checklist for the FFDM Philips (Sectra) mammography unit: monthly, quarterly, and semiannual tests for the radiologic technologist. (Source: ACR Web site (http://www.acr.org)/Quality and Safety/Accreditation/Mammography/Radiologic Technologist Quality Control Forms.)

MEDICAL PHYSICIST'S MAMMOGRAPHY QC TEST SUMMARY
Full-Field Digital—Planmed

Site Name		Report Date	
Address		Survey Date	
Medical Physicist's Name		Signature	
X-Ray Unit Manufacturer	Planmed	Model	
Date of Installation		Room ID	

QC Manual Version # [   ]   *(use version applicable to unit tested; contact mfr if questions)*

Accessory Equipment	Manufacturer	Model	Location	QC Manual Version #
Review Workstation*			☐ On-site ☐ Off-site	
Film Printer*			☐ On-site ☐ Off-site	

FDA recommends that only monitors and printers specifically cleared for FFDM use by FDA's Office of Device Evaluation (ODE) be used. See FDA's Policy Guidance Help System www.fda.gov/CDRH/MAMMOGRAPHY/robohelp/START.HTM.

Survey Type   ☐ Mammo Eqpt Evaluation of new unit (include MQSA Rqmts for Mammo Eqpt checklist)   ☐ Annual Survey

Medical Physicist's QC Tests
("Pass" means all components of the test passes; indicate "Fail" if any component fails. Tests must be done for both on and off-site equipment.)

PASS/FAIL

1. **Monitor Cleaning (AWS and RWS)** *(Mammography Equipment Evaluation only)*
2. **Monitor Quality (AWS)—TG-18 QC test phantom** *(Mammography Equipment Evaluation only)*
3. **Phantom Image Quality (AWS and RWS)** *(Mammography Equipment Evaluation only)*
   Phantom IQ Test on AWS   Fibers [   ]   Specks [   ]   Masses [   ]
   Phantom IQ Test on RWS
4. **Viewbox and Viewing Conditions** *(Mammography Equipment Evaluation only)*
5. **Signal Homogeneity** *(Mammography Equipment Evaluation only)*
6. **Uncorrected Defective Elements (DEL)** *(Mammography Equipment Evaluation only)*
7. **Large Focus Calibration** *(Mammography Equipment Evaluation only)*
8. **Small Focus Calibration (for mags only)** *(Mammography Equipment Evaluation only)*
9. **Signal-to-Noise (SNR)** *(Mammography Equipment Evaluation only)*
10. **Contrast-to-Noise (CNR)** *(Mammography Equipment Evaluation only)*
11. **Visual Checklist** *(Mammography Equipment Evaluation only)*
12. **Repeat Analysis** *(Mammography Equipment Evaluation only)*
13. **Defect Acceptance Test** *(Mammography Equipment Evaluation only)*
14. **System Fault Report** *(Mammography Equipment Evaluation only)*
15. **Review Workstation QC-Overall** *(Mammography Equipment Evaluation only)*
16. **Film Printer QC** *(Mammography Equipment Evaluation only)*
17. **Ghosting**
18. **Modulation Transfer Function (MTF)**
19. **Linearity/Noise Linearity**
20. **AEC**
21. **Compression Force**
22. **Mammographic Unit Assembly**
23. **Beam Quality Assessment—HVL Measurement**
24. **Breast Entrance Exposure and Average Glandular Dose**
    Average glandular dose for average breast is 3 mGy (300 mrad)   [   ] mrad

*** YOUR MEDICAL PHYSICIST MUST SUMMARIZE HIS/HER RESULTS ON THIS FORM ***

A

Figure 16-9
Quality control forms for the FFDM Planmed mammography unit. **(A)** Medical physicist's mammography QC test summary form—FFDM Planmed mammography unit. (Source: ACR Web site (http://www.acr.org)/Quality and Safety/Accreditation/Mammography/Medical Physicists Evaluation Forms.)

MAMMOGRAPHY QUALITY CONTROL CHECKLIST—FULL-FIELD DIGITAL
PLANMED   MODEL *(circle all that apply):*   NUANCE   NUANCE EXCEL
Daily and Weekly

Year	
Month	
Date	
Initials	
Monitor Cleaning (AWS & RWS) *(daily)*	
Monitor Cleaning (AWS) *(daily)*	
Phantom Image Quality (AWS & RWS) *(daily)*	
Viewbox and Viewing Conditions *(weekly)*	
Signal Homogeneity *(weekly)*	
Uncorrected DEL *(weekly)*	
Large Focus Calibration *(weekly)*	
Small Focus (Mag) Calibration *(weekly)*	
Review Workstation QC *(See QC Manual)*	
Laser Film Printer QC *(weekly)*	

Year	
Month	
Date	
Initials	
Monitor Cleaning (AWS & RWS) *(daily)*	
Monitor Cleaning (AWS) *(daily)*	
Phantom Image Quality (AWS & RWS) *(daily)*	
Viewbox and Viewing Conditions *(weekly)*	
Signal Homogeneity *(weekly)*	
Uncorrected DEL *(weekly)*	
Large Focus Calibration *(weekly)*	
Small Focus (Mag) Calibration *(weekly)*	
Review Workstation QC *(See QC Manual)*	
Laser Film Printer QC *(weekly)*	

B

Figure 16-9 *(Continued)*

(B) Mammography quality control checklist for the FFDM Planmed mammography unit—daily and weekly tests for the radiologic technologist. (Source: ACR Web site (http://www.acr.org)/Quality and Safety/Accreditation/Mammography/Radiologic Technologist Quality Control Forms.)

MAMMOGRAPHY QUALITY CONTROL CHECKLIST—FULL-FIELD DIGITAL
PLANMED   MODEL *(circle all that apply)*:   NUANCE   NUANCE EXCEL
Monthly, Quarterly, and Semi-Annual
(date, initial and enter number where appropriate)

Year / Month	JAN	FEB	MAR	APR	MAY	JUN	JUL	AUG	SEP	OCT	NOV	DEC
SNR *(monthly)*												
CNR *(monthly)*												
Visual Checklist *(monthly)*												
Repeat Analysis (≤2% change) *(quarterly)*												
Defect Acceptance Test *(semi-annually)*												
Compression Force (111–200 Newton) *(semi-annually)*												
System Fault Report *(when needed)*												
Review Workstation QC *(See QC Manual)*												

Date: **Test:**   **Comments:**

C

Figure 16-9 *(Continued)*
(C) Mammography quality control checklist for the FFDM Planmed mammography unit: monthly, quarterly, and semiannual tests for the radiologic technologist. (Source: ACR Web site (http://www.acr.org)/Quality and Safety/Accreditation/Mammography/Radiologic Technologist Quality Control Forms.)

Medical Physicist's DM QC Test Summary

Facility Name _____	Room ID _____
Address _____	Survey Date _____
_____	Report Date _____
_____	Date of Previous Survey _____
Map ID Unit # (00000-00) _____	Months Between Surveys _____ (must be ≤ 14)
X-Ray Unit Manufacturer _____	X-Ray Unit Model _____
X-Ray Unit Control Serial # _____	it Date of Manufacture _____
Date of Installation _____	
Cr Unit Mfr _____	CR Unit Model _____
CR Unit Serial # _____	
Medical Physicist _____	Telephone _____
Signature _____	

Quality Control Manual Used for Survey and Facility QC: *2015 ACR Digital Mammography Quality Control Manual*

Survey Type:	☐ Mammography Equipment Evaluation (MEE)—Acceptance Testing		☐ Routine Annual Survey
Equipment Tested:	☐ DM Unit ☐ AW Monitor	☐ RW Monitor ☐ Viewbox	☐ Printer Other _____
MP Oversight Level:	☐ Medical Physicist On-Site	☐ Medical Physicist Oversight	
Unit Description:	☐ Digital radiography (DR)	☐ Computed Radiography (CR)	☐ Tomosynthesis (DBT)
Unit Use:	☐ Diagnostic & Screening	☐ Diagnostic Only	☐ Screening Only

Medical Physicist's QC Tests

("Pass" means all components of test passes; "Fail" means any or all components fail; if "CA" checked, see Corrective Action Summary)

Medical Physicists Tests	Overall Pass/Fail/NA	CA	Tech QC Evaluation	Overall Pass/Fail/NA	CA
1. Mammography Equip Eval (MEE)			1. ACR DM Phantom Image Quality		
2. ACR DM Phantom Image Quality			2. CR Cassette Erasure *(if app)*		
3. Spatial Resolution			3. Comp Thickness Indicator		
4. AEC System Performance			4. Visual Checklist		
5. Average Glandular Dose			5. AW Monitor QC		
6. Unit Checklist			6. RW Monitor QC		
7. Computed Radiography *(if app)*			7. Film Printer QC *(if app)*		
8. AW Workstation Monitor QC			8. Viewbox Cleanliness *(if app)*		
9. RW Monitor QC			9. Facility QC Review		
10. Film Printer QC *(if app)*			10. Compression Force		
11. Site's Tech QC Program			11. Mfr Detector Calibration *(if app)*		
12. Display Device Tech QC Program			Optional—Repeat Analysis		

MEE or Troubleshooting	Overall Pass/Fail/NA	CA
Beam Quality (HVL) Assessment		
kVp Accuracy and Reproducibility		
Collimation Assessment		
Ghost Image Evaluation		
Viewbox Luminance		

ACR DM Phantom Summary

	Value	Limit
Fiber score		≥2.0
Speck group score		≥3.0
Mass score		≥2.0
SNR		≥40.0
CNR		≥2.0
AGD (mGy)		≤3.0

A

Figure 16-10

Quality control forms for the standardized FFDM quality control program using the ACR 2016 Digital Mammography Quality Control Manual. **(A)** Medical physicist's DM QC test summary form: FFDM mammography unit. (Source: ACR Web site (http://www.acr.org), Quality and Safety/Accreditation/Mammography/Medical Physicist Evaluation Forms.)

Medical Physicist's DM QC Test Summary
Medical Physicist's QC Tests *(continued)*

Facility Name _____   Map ID Unit # *(00000-00)* _____

Mfr & Model _____   Room ID _____

Survey Date _____

Corrective Action Summary*

Note: This is only a summary page, the Corrective Action Log Form may contain further details.

Required/ Recommended	Time Frame	Description	Utilize Corrective Action Log Form	Date Completed	Initials

B

Figure 16-10 *(Continued)*
(B) Quality control forms for the standardized FFDM quality control program: ACR 2016 Digital Mammography Quality Control Manual. Medical physicist's DM QC test summary form—FFDM mammography unit. (Source: ACR Web site (http://www.acr.org), Quality and Safety/Accreditation/Mammography/Medical Physicist Evaluation Forms.)

Digital Mammography Unit QC Summary Checklist

Facility _____   Room ID _____

MAP ID# *(00000-00)* _____   Unit Mfr & Model _____

Year						
Month	Jan	Feb	Mar	Apr	May	Jun
ACR DM Phantom Image Quality *(weekly)*						
CR Cassette Erasure, if app *(weekly)*						
Compression Thickness Indicator *(monthly)*						
Visual Checklist *(monthly)*						
AW Monitor QC *(monthly)*						
Compression *(semiannual)*						
Mfr Detector Calibration, if app Freq _____						
Overall *(only need to complete once for the facility)*						
Facility QC Review *(quarterly)*						
Repeat Analysis *(optional - as needed)*						

Key: Date and initial each test - | date |
                                        | initial |

Cross out boxes where mfr calibration test is not required - | X |
                                                                | X |

C

Figure 16-10 *(Continued)*
(C) Quality control forms for the standardized FFDM quality control program: ACR 2016 Digital Mammography Quality Control Manual. Digital mammography unit QC summary checklist—radiologic technologist. (Source: ACR Web site (http://www.acr.org), Quality and Safety/Accreditation/Mammography/Radiologic Technologist Quality Control Forms.)

Facility Display Device QC Summary Checklist

Facility _____   **MAP ID#** *(00000)* _____

Address _____

Address _____

QC Summary information for display devices at this MAP ID							
Physical Location at Facility/ ID Designation							
Device *(RW, film printer, viewbox)*							
Manufacturer							
Model							
Jan — Date							
Jan — Tech Initials							
Feb — Date							
Feb — Tech Initials							
Mar — Date							
Mar — Tech Initials							
Apr — Date							
Apr — Tech Initials							
May — Date							
May — Tech Initials							
Jun — Date							
Jun — Tech Initials							
Jul — Date							
Jul — Tech Initials							
Aug — Date							
Aug — Tech Initials							
Sep — Date							
Sep — Tech Initials							
Oct — Date							
Oct — Tech Initials							
Nov — Date							
Nov — Tech Initials							
Dec — Date							
Dec — Tech Initials							
Medical Physicist Survey Date							
Medical Physicist Name(s)							

D

Figure 16-10 (*Continued*)
(D) Quality control forms for the standardized FFDM quality control program: ACR 2016 Digital Mammography Quality Control Manual. Facility display device QC summary checklist—radiologic technologist. (Source: ACR Web site (http://www.acr.org), Quality and Safety/Accreditation/Mammography/Radiologic Technologist Quality Control Forms.)

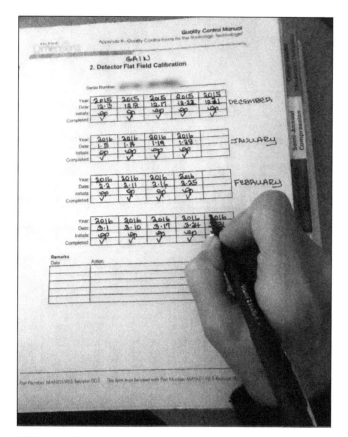

Figure 16-11
QC test form: specific component of mammography equipment QC, completion indicated with technologist initials, and performance date.

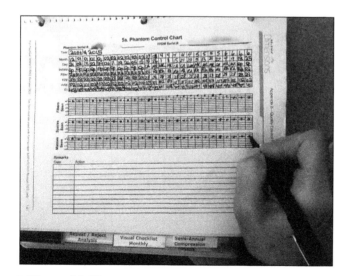

Figure 16-12
QC test form: specific component of mammography equipment QC, completion indicated with technologist initials, performance date, and additional exposure factor documentation.

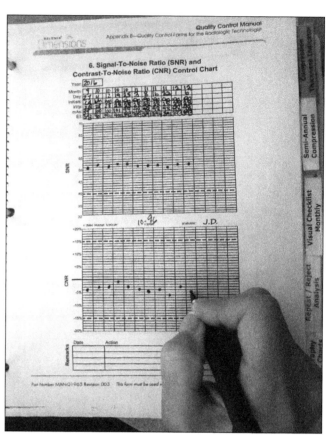

Figure 16-13
QC test form: specific component of mammography equipment QC requiring plotting of data in addition to technologist initials, performance date, and exposure factors. Note the *dotted lines* indicating established control limits.

Use of a control chart requires the technologist be familiar with quality control indicators such as baseline, control limit, and trending.

- The *baseline*, determined by acceptance testing performed by the MP, is represented by the central bold line, indicating the accepted norm.
- Determined *control limits* are indicated by the dotted lines placed above and below the baseline. Data points falling between the upper and lower control limits indicate stability. Data points falling outside the upper or lower control limits indicate instability, requiring corrective action.
- Control charts are used to quantitatively track equipment performance; they indicate stability, as well as they indicate a problem and when the problem occurred. When the collective data points are analyzed over a period of time, noticeable patterns or changes in equipment performance may be observed, such as *trending*, when plotted indicators show a trend in upward or downward patterns.

Identifying and correcting equipment problems before they are apparent on the image are the purposes of periodic QC testing.[18]

Densitometer (If Applicable)

Facilities that use a laser printer to print mammographic images for primary interpretation must perform established protocols for QC determined by the manufacturers' QC manual or the ACR 2016 Digital Mammography QC Manual. Laser printer QC requires the use of a densitometer, a device that measures the optical density (OD) of a printed test film. The densitometer evaluates areas on the test film to determine the amount of light transmitted through that portion of the film and assigns a numeric value ranging from 0 to 4 OD.[18] The laser printer characteristics evaluated using the densitometer can be found in this chapter under Laser Printer QC. Some facilities elect to print the weekly QC phantom image and may use the densitometer to measure the background density and the contrast of the image.

Corrective Action

Corrective action is initiated when:

- QC testing data falls outside of control limit parameters (for equipment or human factors)
- Trending data provides evidence of a potential equipment problem
- The realization that appropriate QC documentation is missing

When events reveal the need for corrective action, an accurate description of the process, from its initiation to its resolution, is recorded. The information should include:

- What incident triggered the corrective action
- Consultations, if any, with the LIP, MP, biomedical engineer, manufacturer, etc.
- Description of corrective action
- Actions taken, if necessary, that support MQSA compliance (such as stopping the use of equipment that has failed testing until corrective action is completed)
- Supporting documents of resolution

Detailed records describing the events of the corrective action process should be maintained. During the annual FDA inspection, this documentation provides organized records for the inspector that demonstrate that the facility consistently delivers quality mammography to its patients.

Communication

Throughout the year, the QC technologist is responsible for all communication that surrounds the activities associated with the mammography equipment: the MP annual inspection, preventive maintenance, and indications of potential problems. Through routine equipment QC testing, he/she is positioned to identify the first signs of problems that may require investigation or correction to comply with MQSA standards. Coordinating corrective action may involve contacting several individuals: consultation with the mammography manager, LIP, or MP; initiation of services from biomedical engineering; communication to the staff or information technology (IT) services. Protocols and policies that address QC equipment events that fall outside of the routine practice of service delivery assist in satisfactory recovery and documentation of occurrences and provide the QC technologist and staff with clear directives to follow.

MAMMOGRAPHY QUALITY CONTROL: MAKING SENSE OF THE CONFUSION

MQSA allows facilities to follow one of two standards to comply with equipment quality control mandates. The facility may follow the QC manual from their image receptor manufacturer (Table 16-1, center column), or they follow a standardized digital QC program developed by the ACR (Table 16-1, right column)—which uses the ACR 2016 Digital Mammography QC Manual (as long as they are **not** utilizing DBT technology). Both of these FDA-approved QC pathways describe periodic QC procedures for their mammography unit, radiologist workstation, and printer (if applicable). When all of the QC manuals are compared for QC procedures, the following differences are observed:

- Different QC tests are required for each established QC program.
- Manufacturers may use a different name for the same QC test.
- Required test frequencies may be different.
- Acceptance parameters/control limits may be different for some tests.

Table 16-2 provides a comparison of the FFDM DR mammography QC program procedures *performed by the technologist*. The table includes the technologist's QC test procedure name for each specific manufacturer's QC program. The frequency requirement is indicated in parenthesis next to the procedure name. Some of the QC requirements are common to some of the manufacturers, and some are requirements of

Table 16-2 • Technologists QC Tests Specific to FFDM (DR) Manufacturers and for Technologists Tests Included in the ACR 2016 Digital Mammography Quality Control Manual

DAILY/WEEKLY TECHNOLOGIST QC TESTS

QC TEST	FISCHER	FUJI (FDR)	GE	GIOTTO	LORAD	PHILIPS	PLANMED	SIEMENS	ACR 2016 DIGITAL QC MANUAL
Daily QC check		Good practice cleaning (weekly)	Monitor cleaning (daily)	Daily check (daily)		Daily quality control (daily)	Monitor cleaning (AWS and RWS) (daily)		
Detector/flat field	Detector calibration and flat-field test (weekly)		Flat field (weekly)	Flat-field homogeneity (weekly)	Detector flat-field calibration (weekly)	Full calibration (weekly)	Large focus calibration (weekly) Small focus calibration (weekly)	Detector calibration (Novation, weekly) (inspiration/fusion) (quarterly)	Manufacturer detector calibration (if applicable) Mfr. Recommendation
Phantom image quality	Phantom image quality test (weekly)	ACR phantom (weekly) 1st shot phantom (weekly)	Phantom image quality (weekly)	ACR phantom image quality (weekly)	Phantom image (weekly)	Mammographic accreditation phantom (weekly)	Phantom image quality (AWS and RWS) (daily)	Phantom image quality (daily)	ACR DM phantom image quality (weekly)
CNR/SNR			CNR (weekly)	Signal-to-noise (SNR) and contrast-to-noise (CNR) ratio (weekly)	SNR and CNR measurements (weekly)	CNR (weekly)	SNR/CNR (monthly) Signal homogeneity (weekly)	SNR/CNR measurement (weekly)	
Artifact				Artifact evaluation (weekly)	Artifact evaluation (weekly)		Uncorrected DEL (weekly)	Artifact detection (weekly)	
MTF			MTF (DS/essential/care—weekly)						
Compression thickness					Compression thickness indicator (biweekly)	Thickness indication (semiannually)			Compression thickness indicator (monthly)
AWS QC (technologist)	Phantom image acquisition test (weekly)	Monitor QC AWS (weekly)				Display QC AWS (weekly)	Monitor quality (AWS) (daily)		Acquisition workstation (AW) monitor QC (monthly)

								Radiologist
Review workstation (radiologist)	Review workstation QC (see QC Manual)	Review workstation QC (see QC Manual)	Review workstation QC (see QC Manual)	Review workstation QC (see QC Manual)	Diagnostic review *workstation QC* (see Lorad QC Manual)	Review workstation QC (see FDA guidance)	Review workstation QC (see QC Manual)	Review workstation QC (see QC Manual)	Workstation (RW) monitor QC (monthly) System QC for radiologist (optional) (as needed)
Laser printer QC	Laser image quality test (daily, if app)	Laser printer QC (see QC Manual)	Laser film printer QC (printer mfr rec)	Film printer QC (see QC Manual)	DICOM printer QC (weekly)	Printer QC (see FDA guidance)	Laser film printer QC (weekly)	Printer check (daily, when images printed)	Film printer (if applicable)
Viewbox/viewing conditions			Viewbox and viewing conditions (weekly)		Viewboxes and viewing conditions (weekly)		Viewbox and viewing conditions (weekly)		
Compression force	Compression force test (25–45 lbs) (semi-annually)	Compression device confirmation (111–200 Newtons) (semiannually)	Compression force (25–45 lbs) (semi-annually)	Compression force (25–45 lbs) (semi-annually)	Compression (25–45 lbs) (semiannually)	Compression (25–45 lbs) (semiannually)	Compression force (111–200 Newtons)	Compression force (25–45 lbs) (semi-annually)	Compression force (semiannual)
Repeat/reject analysis	Reject/repeat analysis (≤2% change) (quarterly)	Repeat analysis (≤2% change) (quarterly)	Repeat analysis (≤2% change) (quarterly)	Repeat/reject analysis (≤2% change) (quarterly)	Repeat/reject analysis (≤2% change) (quarterly)	Repeat analysis (≤2% change) (quarterly)	Repeat analysis (≤2% change) (quarterly)	Repeat analysis (quarterly)	Repeat analysis (optional) (as needed)
Visual checklist			Visual checklist (monthly)	Visual checklist (monthly)	Visual checklist (monthly)	Visual checklist (monthly)	Visual checklist (monthly)		Visual checklist (monthly)
System test	System operation (monthly)						System fault report (when needed)		

(Continued)

Table 16-2 • Technologists QC Tests Specific to FFDM (DR) Manufacturers and for Technologists Tests Included in the ACR 2016 Digital Mammography Quality Control Manual (Continued)

QC TEST	DAILY/WEEKLY TECHNOLOGIST QC TESTS								ACR 2016 DIGITAL QC MANUAL
	FISCHER	FUJI (FDR)	GE	GIOTTO	LORAD	PHILIPS	PLANMED	SIEMENS	
AEC			AOP mode and SNR (monthly)	Automatic exposure control system (AEC) (semi-annually)					
Spatial resolution	System resolution detector alignment/scan speed uniformity (monthly)		MTF (2000D) (monthly)			Spatial resolution (monthly)			
Defect acceptance test							Defect acceptance test (semiannually)		
Facility QC review									Facility QC review (quarterly)
Radiologist image quality feedback									Radiologist image quality feedback (optional) (as needed)

Data Source: Quality Control forms for the Radiologic Technologist listed on the ACR Web site (http://www.acr.org), Quality and Safety/Accreditation/Mammography/Radiologic Technologist Quality Control Forms.

all the manufacturers. The individual manufacturer QC tests performed by the technologist can be found:

- In the image receptor manufacturer QC manual
- On the ACR Web site (acr.org/accreditation/mammography/Radiologic Technologist Quality Control Forms)

Differences in equipment evaluations among image receptor manufacturers and the ACR FFDM QC program are also found in tests performed by the MP. The QC tests performed for individual image receptor manufacturers *by the medical physicist* can be found:

- In the image receptor manufacturer QC manual
- On the ACR Web site (acr.org/accreditation/mammography/MedicalPhysicistEvaluationForms)

The ACR FFDM QC program also specifies required QC tests performed by the MP and the radiologic technologist. Figure 16-10A–D describes the MP and the radiologic technologist QC test procedures included in the ACR 2016 Digital Mammography QC Manual.

- Common QC Tests
  Some periodic QC tests performed by the technologist are common to the image receptor manufacturer QC programs and to the standardized ACR Digital QC program. The following tests described in the MQSA Final Rule are currently included in all QC manuals for the technologist to perform:
  - Image Quality Phantom — weekly QC test
  - Repeat/Reject Analysis — quarterly QC test
  - Compression Force — semiannual QC test

  The corrective action for each of these tests is defined in the MQSA Final Rule and is included in the technologist's QC test section of this chapter.

- QC Test Corrective Action
  When QC test results fall outside of acceptable parameters, the facility must follow their specific QC program requirements for corrective action. The specific QC program the facility follows dictates the time frames for corrective action when equipment components fail quality control tests. Some mammography image receptor manufacturers have FDA approval for alternative standards for equipment correction periods when components of the system fail quality control tests. The PGHS includes the list of image receptor manufacturers with approved alternative standards. Each image receptor manufacturer describes the equipment component test and the correction period for their tests in the approved alternative standard on the FDA Web site in the PGHS. Corrective action requirements for failed test evaluations that are included in this chapter can be accessed using the following resources:

  - The image receptor manufacturer QC manual
  - The PGHS Alternative Standards (fda.gov/Policy Guidance Help System/Alternative Standards)
  - The ACR 2016 Digital Mammography QC Manual
- MEE and the Annual Survey
  - The MEE is performed for the purpose of acceptance testing when (Box 16-4):
    - New equipment has been installed.
    - Existing equipment has had major repairs or changes (disassembled and reassembled).

    According to the MQSA, all equipment components tested during the MEE must pass prior to using the equipment in the mammography service.[22]
  - The Annual Survey (Box 16-5) conducted by the MP includes the performance of the required quality control tests listed in the manufacturers' QC manual or the ACR 2016 Digital Mammography QC Manual. In addition to performing these tests during the annual survey, the MP is required to assess the **facility quality control program** to verify its compliance with MQSA. The periodic QC tests performed by the QC technologist and accompanying documentation are reviewed by the MP to verify the integrity of the program and to make appropriate recommendations for improvement. The MP must provide a report to the facility within 30 days of the inspection. It is strongly recommended that the physicist immediately communicate any equipment evaluation failures to the facility on the day of the inspection to assure that corrective action takes place within the allowable correction period for that component.

An observation for the reader: The radiologic technology student perceives the landscape of mammography QC as complex because they learn about several QC program requirements at the same time. However, the facility QC technologist greatly reduces this complexity by (normally) following the requirements of just one QC program!

MAMMOGRAPHY EQUIPMENT TESTS: MEDICAL PHYSICIST

The MP evaluates all the components of the FFDM imaging chain independently[23]: the mammography machine, the image receptor, the radiologist workstation, and the laser printer (if applicable). Depending on the QC manual that is followed, the MP equipment evaluation may include between 11 and 24 test procedures. The MP's evaluation of the mammography equipment is directed by the QC program manual selected by the facility (manufacturer-specific or the ACR 2016 Digital Mammography QC Manual) and includes specific procedures to test the following equipment functions:

- Mammographic Unit Assembly Evaluation
- Generator:
  - kVp Accuracy and Reproducibility
  - Beam Quality Assessment: Half-Value Layer Measurement
  - Breast Entrance Exposure, AEC Reproducibility, Average Glandular Dose, and Radiation Output Rate
  - Exposure Reproducibility
- System Performance:
  - AEC (automatic exposure control/phototimer)
  - System Resolution
  - System Artifact Evaluation
  - Image Quality Phantom
    - SNR
    - CNR
- System Hardware
  - Collimation Evaluation
  - Compression Paddle Alignment
  - Compression Force
- Radiologist Workstation
- Printer (if applicable)

Mammography Unit Tests: Medical Physicist

Mammography Unit Assembly Evaluation

The MP inspects the mammography unit assembly to ensure that the mechanical integrity of the unit, x-ray tube, and digital image receptor are in good and safe working condition. This inspection encompasses evaluating the stability of the equipment; smoothness of motion without obstruction to moving parts; that mechanical locks and detents work properly; and that the receptor is free from vibration. The inspection also verifies that the following requirements are in place to ensure safety and reliability to the patient and operator[24]:

- Compressed breast thickness scale is accurate.
  The importance of evaluating indicated breast thickness accuracy is significant, as this function can affect the tube voltage selection and resulting breast dose. MQSA requires the compressed breast thickness scale be accurate to ±0.5 cm and reproducible to ±0.2 cm. (Figure 16-14).
- Patient and operator are not exposed to sharp or rough edges.
- Operator technique control chart is posted.
- Adequate radiation shielding is provided to the operator.

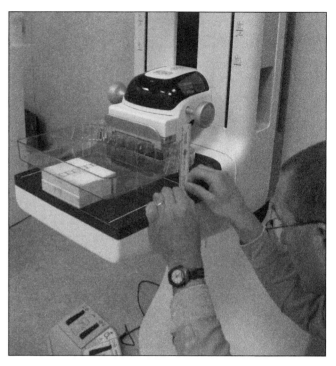

Figure 16-14
MP measures paddle deflection and evaluates compressed breast thickness accuracy.

- All indicator lights working properly.
- Autodecompression can be overridden to maintain compression (and status displayed).
- Manual emergency compression release can be activated in event of power failure.
- In case of power failure, tube stand and breast support are immobilized.
- Light field luminance is adequate.
- Breast compression paddles are flat and parallel to breast support (unless manufacturer-specific design).

Beam Quality Assessment: Half-Value Layer Measurement

Measuring the half-value layer (HVL) determines the amount of filtration that must be added to reduce the exposure rate to half of its original value[18] and is the determinant of beam quality. The HVL of the x-ray beam must be adequate to minimize the radiation dose delivered to the patient, but not so high that it reduces the contrast available for quality mammographic images. The HVL is determined by making x-ray exposures with and without an attenuator (aluminum sheets 0.1 mm thick) in the path of the x-ray beam (Figure 16-15). The x-ray exposure readings are measured with an ionization chamber. These recorded readings are then used to calculate the HVL. The HVL measurement is represented as millimeters of aluminum, so a typical HVL

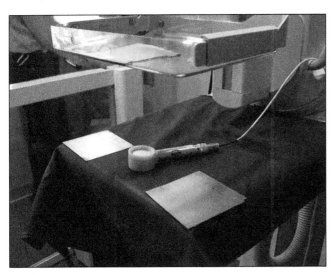

Figure 16-15
Half-value layer testing. Note the lead shield covering the detector, the ionization chamber, and aluminum sheets used to determine the HVL.

might read as "0.38 mm Al." The measured HVL is then used in the calculation to determine the average glandular dose.

Performance criteria: For tube voltages below 50 kVp, the calculated HVL must be at least (measured kVp/100) mm Al. For example, the HVL at 28 kVp must measure at least 0.28 mm Al.

Note: tests for the generator are performed with a lead shield covering the image receptor for protection from repeated exposures to the detector.

Breast Entrance Exposure, AEC Reproducibility, Average Glandular Dose, and Radiation Output Rate

AEC Reproducibility (Exposure Reproducibility) and Breast Entrance Exposure

The physicist performs this test to measure breast entrance exposure, or entrance skin exposure (ESE), using phototimed exposures of a phantom simulating an average patient (4.2 cm compressed breast thickness of 50% adipose and 50% glandular tissue composition). Air Kerma (AK) is used to describe the x-ray tube output and represents the amount of energy deposited per unit mass of air. The test also determines if the unit consistently and reproducibly delivers the same AK over several exposures.

To perform this test, the physicist makes several x-ray exposures with the mammographic phantom and an ionization chamber placed side by side within the x-ray field (Figure 16-16A,B). Compression is applied as in a clinical situation. The ionization chamber exposure reading (mR) and the mAs are recorded for

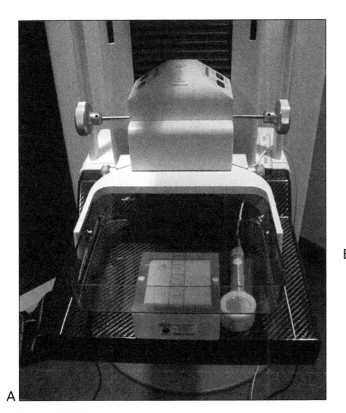

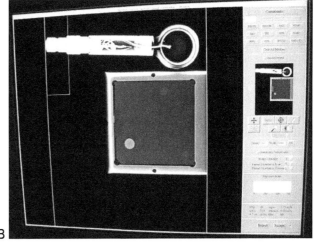

Figure 16-16
(A) Exposure measurements are collected using a phantom and ionization chamber to calculate mean glandular dose (MGD).
(B) Radiograph of the exposed phantom and ionization chamber.

each exposure. This measured ESE is used, along with the HVL measurement, to calculate the average glandular dose.

Performance criteria: Breast Entrance Air Kerma and AEC Reproducibility. The coefficient of variations for both air Kerma (exposure) and mAs shall not exceed 0.05.[25]

Average Glandular Dose

The average glandular dose is a calculated value derived from the measured HVL and the breast entrance exposure obtained from the two preceding tests. It represents the amount of energy absorbed by the glandular tissue in a breast of average size and tissue composition from one single x-ray exposure. It is expressed in units of milligrays (mGy) or millirads (mrad).

Performance criteria: The average glandular dose to an average breast (4.2 cm compressed, 50% glandular, 50% adipose) must not exceed 3.0 mGy (milliGrays), or 0.3 rad (300 mrad) per view.

Radiation Output Rate

The x-ray output is a measurement of the x-ray tube efficiency. It is expressed in mR/sec. The measurement of the output ensures that the unit produces a consistent beam with each exposure and that the x-ray tube can produce enough x-rays to produce a quality image in a reasonable amount of time.

The radiation output is measured with an ionization chamber positioned approximately 4.5 cm above the breast support surface—the height where the top of a compressed breast would be located. The compression device is placed within the beam, just above the probe. The measured output is the x-ray energy that reaches the breast during clinical imaging. A phantom is *not* placed in the beam with the probe, so that scatter will not affect the reading of the unit's output. The physicist makes an exposure long enough, but less than 3 seconds, to achieve an exposure reading of at least 2,400 mR.

Performance criteria: Mammography machines are required to produce a minimum output of 7.0 mGy/sec (800 mR/sec) when using Mo/Mo. For W/Rh units, the minimum x-ray output is 230 mR/sec. In addition, the unit must be able to maintain the minimum output averaged during a 3-second long exposure.

kVp Accuracy and Reproducibility

This test is performed to determine kilovoltpeak (kVp) *accuracy*: the kVp indicated on the control panel is the actual kVp that is produced by the x-ray tube and that it is consistently *reproducible*. A device known as a kVp

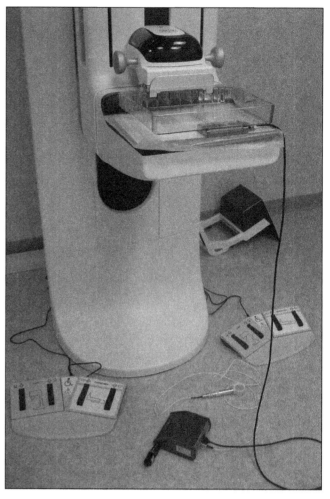

Figure 16-17
kVp accuracy and reproducibility testing. kVp measurement tool rests on the lead shield under the compression device. The device on the floor powers the kVp meter, transmitting the readings to the MP's display device.

meter is used to measure the kVp output of the unit (Figure 16-17). Exposures are made using clinically relevant kVp settings:

- Lowest kVp that the test equipment is able to record
- The most common clinically used kVp setting
- The highest kVp that is used clinically

The recorded measurements are evaluated to determine the accuracy and reproducibility of the kVp settings. Actual kVp typically varies from the indicated kVp, but cannot vary more than the standards set by MQSA.

Performance criteria[25]:

Accuracy: The kVp shall be accurate within ±5% of the indicated or selected kVp settings tested.

Reproducibility: At the most commonly used clinical settings of kVp, the coefficient of variation of reproducibility of the kVp shall be equal to or less than 0.02.

System (Spatial) Resolution

Image detail combines the quantitative measures of spatial and contrast resolution to describe image quality.[26] Spatial resolution refers to the ability of the imaging system to separate small objects that are close together and visually distinguish one from the other.[26,27] According to the MQSA, the focal spot performance should only be evaluated by determining the system resolution.[25] Spatial resolution can be evaluated for individual mammography systems by using a high-contrast resolution bar test pattern that determines a minimum resolution for the system (Figure 16-18A–C). The limiting spatial resolution for digital mammography is approximately 10 lp/mm[18] in the contact mode. When imaged, the bar test pattern must be oriented either parallel/perpendicular or at a 45° angle relative to the anode–cathode axis, as directed by the QC manual. Depending on the pattern placement relative to the anode–cathode axis, the system resolution will differ. The system resolution should be evaluated in both contact and magnification modes. The physicist evaluates the bar test pattern by examining the image and determining the smallest group of line pairs per millimeter (lp/mm) that can be resolved. The smallest group resolved represents the highest number of line pairs resolved. There is general agreement that evaluation of the system modulation transfer function (MTF) better evaluates resolution,[13,26,28] but it is acknowledged that the limiting spatial resolution evaluation (bar test pattern) is an easier testing technique and provides an acceptable method to evaluate detector performance.[13]

Performance criteria: Manufacturer specific

Modulation Transfer Function

The sharpness of an optical imaging system is characterized by a measurement called **modulation transfer function (MTF)**, also known as spatial frequency response. MTF is a measure of the transfer of contrast from the subject to the image. In technical terms, MTF is the *spatial* frequency response of an imaging system or a component; it is the contrast at a given spatial frequency relative to low frequencies. High spatial frequencies correspond to finite image detail. The more extended the response, the finer the detail, the sharper the image.[29] In other words, it measures how faithfully the detector reproduces detail from the object to the image. Currently, the only mammography units that include this as part of the MP QC program are those manufactured by GE and Planmed.

Automatic Exposure Control: AEC Performance (Phototimer)

The AEC design for FFDM DR imaging allows the detector to serve as a multielement sensor, fully absorbing the x-ray beam.[26,28] Operators of mammography equipment are dependent on AEC technology to provide consistent optimal exposure despite variations of breast thickness and tissue composition. The device works by automatically controlling kVp, mAs, and filtration to reach a desired amount of radiation exposure to the image receptor. When the device senses that the required amount of radiation has been delivered, it terminates the exposure. Because the detector is capable of sensing tissue composition in more than one area of the breast, it can assist in eliminating the potential of underexposure to dense regions.[26] While historical AEC evaluation described

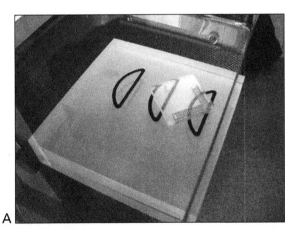
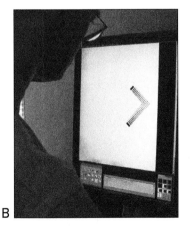
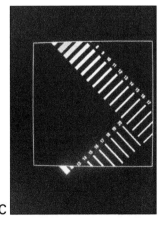

Figure 16-18
(A) Bar pattern positioned on top of the compression device, which compresses two uniform acrylic blocks on the detector. **(B)** The bar pattern image is acquired by the MP and displayed on the acquisition monitor. **(C)** The bar pattern image is evaluated by the MP using magnification to determine the resulting line-pair value for system resolution.

testing results in terms of *optical density*, AEC evaluation for modern FFDM DR detectors provides testing results in terms of signal. The advanced technology of FFDM DR detectors allows AEC evaluation methods to vary and may include density control function, exposure reproducibility, signal, exposure, and SNR or CNR. The AEC testing for FFDM DR detectors is manufacturer specific or follows the ACR 2016 Digital Mammography QC Manual. An example of AEC performance testing borrowed from several resources is included as an example for the reader:

The evaluation assesses the performance of the automatic exposure control function and also

- Verifies consistency in the detector signal-to-noise level for a range of breast thicknesses
- Evaluates exposure compensation of the AEC
- Evaluates AEC performance in all available operational modes (contact, magnification, tomography)

AEC Function Performance Using Different Phantom Thicknesses

To evaluate the ability of the AEC to provide consistent SNR for patients of all sizes, the MP tracks exposures using three or four acrylic phantom blocks, each 2.0 cm thick, that are large enough to cover the AEC area (Figure 16-19A,B). Exposures are acquired using the AEC mode and typical clinical factors. Separate exposures are acquired using the acrylic blocks of 2.0, 4.0, and 6.0 cm (sometimes 8 cm) thicknesses. The applicable exposure information is recorded on the QC test form: AEC mode (i.e., autofilter), kVp, target, filter, focal spot, density control step, mAs, and AEC sensor location. A variation of the

test is repeated for the magnification mode of operation. The MP calculates the results and analyzes the variances from the exposure index or SNR value for all tested breast thicknesses and operating modes to determine acceptable performance.

Performance criteria: Manufacturer specific

AEC Function Performance Using Different Density Compensation Steps

To evaluate the exposure compensation of the AEC, the MP makes several exposures using a 4-cm acrylic phantom, with the AEC sensor in a fixed position, in a selected AEC mode, using typical clinical factors. For each exposure, the AEC compensation step is changed until all of the density steps have been used for the exposures. The number of exposures is dependent on the image receptor manufacturer and as an example may include exposures using density steps from −3 to +3. The relevant factors for each exposure are recorded on the QC test form. The MP calculates the results and compares the outcome values for each exposure to the predetermined manufacturer value ranges for each density step to determine acceptable performance.

Performance criteria: Manufacturer specific

System Artifact Evaluation

FFDM system performance should produce a test image that is uniform in intensity and free of artifacts. During the **artifact evaluation test** performed by the MP, the integrity of the image receptor is established with continued periodic quality control performed by the QC technologist to monitor the established artifact-free system.

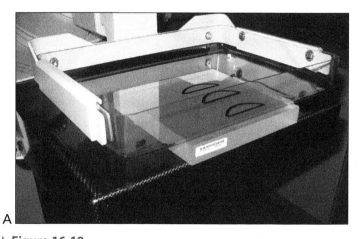
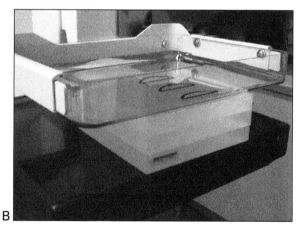

Figure 16-19
The AEC consistency is evaluated by the MP using uniform blocks 2.0 cm in thickness covering the AEC detector over a range of at least 2.0 to 6.0 cm. AEC tested at **(A)** 2.0 cm and **(B)** 6.0 cm.

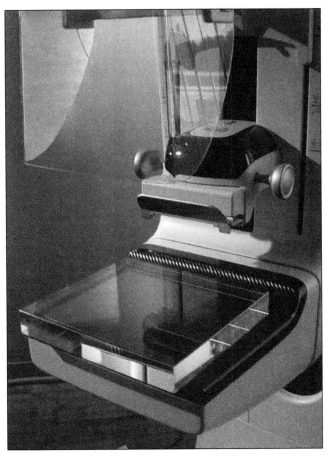

Figure 16-20
Acrylic uniform phantom measuring approximately 24 cm ×
30 cm covers the active detector on the mammography unit.

To test for artifacts, the MP uses a uniform attenuation phantom made of acrylic that is large enough to cover the imaging surface (Figure 16-20). The recommended type of phantom may vary between image receptor manufacturers. After ensuring that the surface of the detector and the phantom are clean, the phantom is placed on the detector and images are acquired using large and small focal spot sizes and all target/filter combinations.

Artifact sources may be the result of any abnormality in the path of the x-ray beam. Defects in the image receptor, dust within the tube head or on the filter (Figure 16-21A–D), or defects on the acrylic test device are just a few possibilities of artifact sources. If artifacts are observed during the testing procedure, it is possible for the MP to isolate the source of artifacts by analyzing the test results. The sources of artifacts are plentiful: the x-ray equipment, the image detector, the radiologist workstation, the DICOM printer (if applicable), or the phantom used for testing.

Ghosting Artifact

Direct conversion DR units that utilize selenium plates may experience difficulty in completely clearing the imaging detector of the previous image or images, which results in ghosting artifacts (Figure 16-22A,B). Outlines of previous mammogram images are visible as a ghosting artifact and are often seen on the flat-field test. The ghosting may get worse with detector age. It has not been determined to what extent ghosting noise interferes with the diagnostic quality of an image, if at all. However, testing by the physicist is recommended if ghosting is suspected.[30]

The performance criteria for phantom artifact evaluation are further discussed in this chapter under tests performed by the QC technologist.

Phantom Image Quality Test

- SNR
- CNR

The image quality test assesses the acquisition imaging chain to ensure that images produced by the system are of acceptable quality, to detect changes in quality over time, and to assess for artifacts. There are several elements that contribute to image quality that are evaluated during the image quality test, including SNR and CNR. Although the elements that are evaluated for image quality across all image receptor manufacturers and the ACR 2016 Digital Mammography QC Manual are similar, variations exist between the QC manuals for the MP tests of these elements:

- Testing in both operational modes: contact and magnification
- Scoring of the fibers, specks, and masses
- Acceptance parameters for the fibers, specks, and masses
- Type of FDA-approved accreditation phantom used for testing
- Methods of determining SNR and CNR

To perform this test, the MP acquires an image of an FDA-approved accreditation phantom. The phantom image is acquired using the imaging mode (i.e., autofilter) normally used for a screening exam for a 4.2-cm compressed breast with 50% adipose and 50% glandular tissue composition.

Scoring the structures visible on the phantom image, combined with acceptable evaluation of the SNR and CNR, confirms the unit's resolution and adequate SNR and CNR levels.

Signal-to-Noise Ratio

Signal-to-noise ratio (SNR) is defined as the ratio of a signal *power* to the noise power corrupting the signal. In less technical terms, SNR compares the level of a desired signal with the level of background noise. The higher the ratio, the less obtrusive the background noise is.

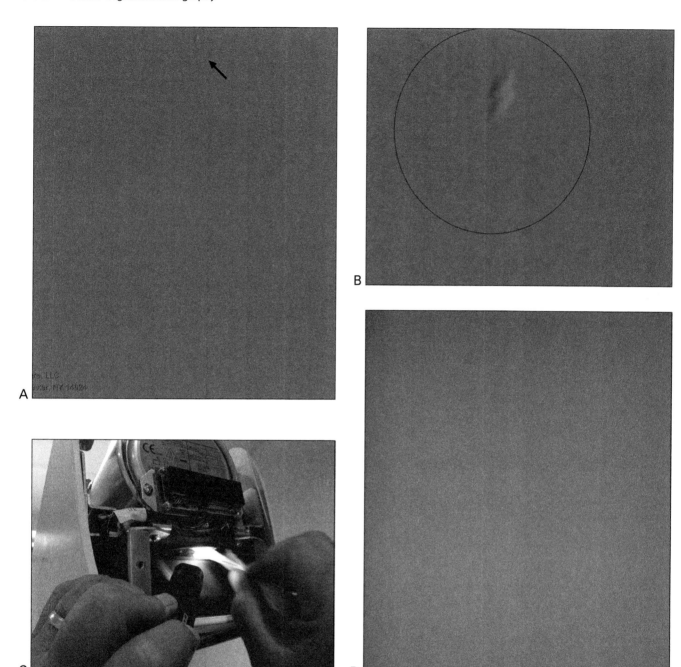

Figure 16-21
The uniform display of the flat-field test reveals dust and other artifacts in the path of the x-ray beam. **(A)** This flat-field image performed by the MP during acceptance testing reveals debris on the filter in the x-ray tube. **(B)** Close-up of the artifact. **(C)** Biomedical engineer removing debris from x-ray tube filter. **(D)** Corrected flat-field image without artifact.

Image quality is affected by the SNR. SNR is a quantitative description of the quality of the information carried by the radiographic image.[28] The quality of the image is increased when the signal is higher compared to the background noise. Background noise is made up primarily of quantum noise (which is determined by radiation exposure levels) and, with lesser, fixed amounts of electronic noise (which is inherent in the equipment design).

Contrast-to-Noise Ratio

Image contrast refers to the ability of an imaging system to distinguish between various structures on an x-ray image due to the perception of differences in their apparent signal intensities. The **contrast-to-noise ratio (CNR)** is similar to SNR in that both are a measurement of image quality. As with the SNR measurement, when the CNR ratio is higher, the background noise is less obtrusive,

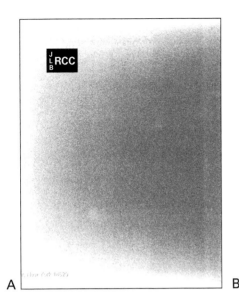
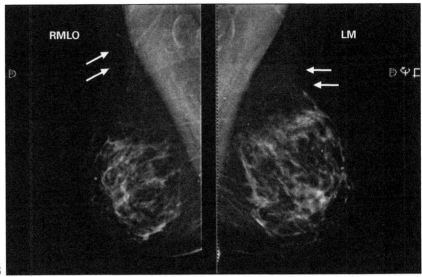

Figure 16-22
Ghosting artifacts are the result of incomplete clearing of the image receptor. **(A)** On the flat-field image, the homogenous appearance of the image is compromised. **(B)** On a patient image, there is shadowing, as if the image has been double exposed.

increasing the image quality. CNR measures the ratio of the difference between an object's signal intensity and its background to the noise corrupting the signal. It is a measurement that can help determine how well an object is seen in relation to its surroundings. An object within the breast tissue can be more difficult to see based on its size and density, when compared with the amount of noise interfering with the imaging of the tissue. For example, CNR indicates an imaging system's ability to detect subtle calcifications in dense breast tissue in relation to the background noise. The MP provides the baseline value of CNR for each individual mammography machine, defining acceptance parameters for subsequent periodic testing performed by the QC technologist. Subsequent periodic CNR evaluation by the QC technologist is recorded in terms of *a percentage of change* from the CNR baseline determined by the MP.[30]

To measure the SNR and CNR, regions of interest (ROI) are placed over designated locations within the image quality phantom by the physicist (or the software program supplied by the unit manufacturer) (Figure 16-23A–C). Values required to calculate the SNR are (a) the mean signal of the background and (b) the standard deviation (noise) of the background signal.

- To calculate SNR, the mean signal of the background is divided by the standard deviation of the background signal.
- Calculating the CNR requires the mean signal of the object in addition to the values needed for the SNR calculation. To calculate CNR, the difference between the object signal and the background signal is divided by the standard deviation of the background signal.

The software from some mammography machine manufacturers automatically calculates the SNR and CNR values within the ROI and provides the information to the MP. These same evaluations are repeated when the QC technologist conducts the periodic equipment performance test for image quality. Other machine manufacturers require the MP and the QC technologist to manually calculate SNR, CNR, and deviations from the baseline. The subject of SNR and CNR is covered more completely in Chapter 12.

Image Quality Phantom Type

Since its inception, the MQSA has required an FDA-approved accreditation phantom be used to evaluate image quality. The mammographic phantom approximates an average compressed breast thickness of 4.2 cm, with a 50% adipose and 50% glandular tissue composition. Embedded in the wax insert of the phantom are test objects consisting of fibers, speck groups, and masses that simulate calcifications and masses detected in breast tissue. Until 2017, the phantom developed for film/screen imaging was the only accreditation phantom available to evaluate image quality. This phantom (refer to Figure 16-2) measures 10.2 cm (L) × 10.8 cm (W) and 4.5 cm (H) and contains 6 fibers, 5 microcalcification speck groups, and 5 masses embedded in the wax insert of the phantom.

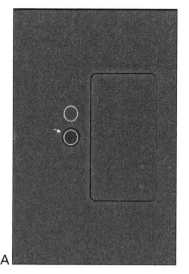
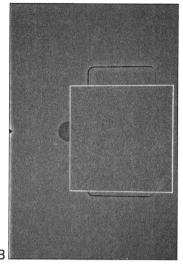
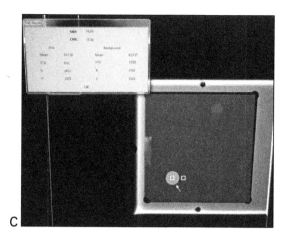

A   B   C

Figure 16-23
(A) Radiograph of FFDM phantom illustrating ROIs placed in the CNR cavity (*arrow*) and outside the CNR cavity (**circle**) to evaluate CNR and SNR. **(B)** FFDM phantom using magnification to evaluate test objects. **(C)** Radiograph of original accreditation phantom illustrating ROIs placed inside the acrylic disc (*arrow*) and outside the acrylic disc to evaluate CNR and SNR.

The test objects gradually decrease in size from largest to smallest, ranging in objects that should be visible on poorer performing imaging systems to objects that are difficult to see on even the best imaging systems. Figure 16-24A–C illustrates the original accreditation phantom, the schematic view of the test objects embedded in the wax insert, and a radiographic image of the phantom. Some manufacturers require the use of an acrylic disc when using this phantom; other manufacturers do not use the disk. The disk is 4 mm thick and 1 cm in diameter and is placed on top of the phantom (if applicable), positioned between the two largest fibers. To comply with the MQSA, facilities that follow a quality control program using the image receptor manufacturer QC manual are required to use the type of accreditation phantom pictured in Figure 16-24A to evaluate image quality as directed, with or without the acrylic disc.

Research conducted during the ACRIN DMIST study suggested that the mammography accreditation phantom developed for film/screen imaging was not appropriate for quality control with the new FFDM technology. The researchers recommended that a phantom be developed for FFDM that is more representative of image quality in FFDM.[31] In July 2016, the FDA approved a digital mammography accreditation phantom (refer to Figure 16-3). This accreditation phantom is required for use with the ACR 2016 Digital Mammography QC Manual published on the ACR Web site on July 29, 2016 (for facilities using 2D mammography imaging technology). Like the original analog accreditation phantom, the ACR digital mammography phantom approximates an average

compressed breast thickness of 4.2 cm compressed breast thickness, with a 50% adipose and 50% glandular tissue composition. In comparison to the original analog accreditation phantom, the ACR digital phantom measures 19.0 cm (L) × 31.0 cm (W) × 4.1 cm (H) and is designed to cover a majority of the active detector area of the IRSD. Due to its larger size, the uniform phantom can now also be used to evaluate the imaging system for artifacts. Embedded in the wax insert of the phantom are 6 fibers, 6 microcalcification speck groups, and 6 masses that simulate calcifications and masses detected in breast tissue. The test objects gradually decrease in size from largest to smallest, ranging in objects that should be visible on poorer performing imaging systems to objects that are difficult to see on even the best imaging systems. Located just above the wax insert is the CNR cavity. The CNR cavity is used to measure and calculate the SNR and CNR. Figure 16-25A–D illustrates the ACR Digital Mammography Phantom, the schematic view of the test objects embedded in the wax insert, a chart of the test object size specifications, and a radiographic image of the phantom.

According to the FDA, the phantom image shall achieve at least the minimum score established by the accreditation body and accepted by the FDA in accordance with 900.3(d) or 900.4(a)(8).[25]

- The ACR criteria for the original ACR accreditation phantom to pass accreditation scoring require the 4 largest fibers, 3 largest speck groups, and 3 largest masses be visible.[14]

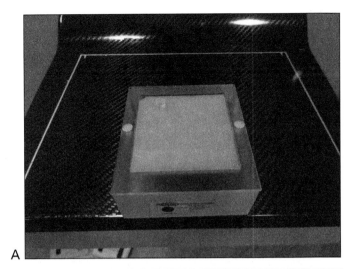

1.56 mm nylon fiber	1.12 mm nylon fiber	0.89 mm nylon fiber	0.75 mm nylon fiber
0.54 mm nylon fiber	0.40 mm nylon fiber	0.54 mm Al_2O_3 speck	0.40 mm Al_2O_3 speck
0.32 mm Al_2O_3 speck	0.24 mm Al_2O_3 speck	0.16 mm Al_2O_3 speck	2.00 mm thick mass
1.00 mm thick mass	0.75 mm thick mass	0.50 mm thick mass	0.25 mm thick mass

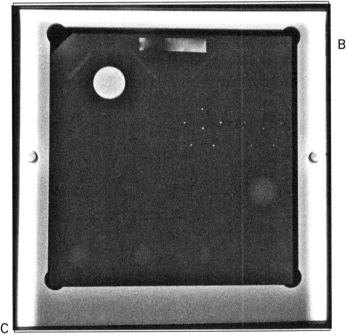

Figure 16-24

(A) Original ACR accreditation phantom positioned on the mammography image detector. Note size of phantom in relationship to the image detector. **(B)** Schematic illustrating the position and size of the different test objects embedded within the original ACR accreditation phantom. **(C)** Radiograph of the original ACR accreditation phantom illustrating visible test objects of fibers, speck groups, and masses. One centimeter disc location indicated between the two largest fibers; the mammography machine manufacturer specifies whether or not the disc is used when testing image quality.

• The ACR criteria for the digital mammography (DM) ACR accreditation phantom to pass accreditation scoring require the 2 largest fibers, 3 largest speck groups, and 2 largest masses be visible.[14]

The variation in the passing scores between the two phantoms is attributed to the accommodations made for the differences in test object size. The original accreditation phantom score of 4, 3, 3 is equivalent to the digital mammography phantom score of 2, 3, 2.[14]

Collimation Assessment: X-Ray Field to Light Field to Image Receptor Congruency and Compression Device Alignment

The x-ray field collimation apparatus/mechanism should be evaluated to ensure that all areas of the image receptor are exposed and that the patient is not exposed needlessly to scatter radiation.[26] Acceptable performance of this mechanism permits the operator to determine accurate tissue capture and to verify proper radiation safety

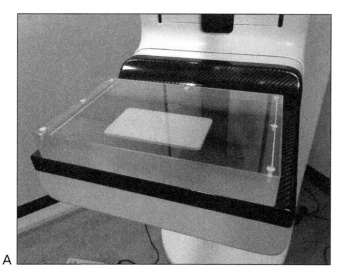

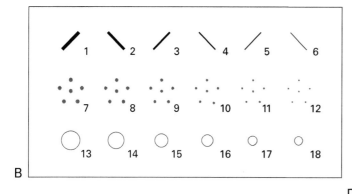

	Test Object Size Specifications					
Test Object	1	2	3	4	5	6
	mm	mm	mm	mm	mm	mm
Fiber Diameter	0.89 ± 0.05	0.75 ± 0.03	0.61 ± 0.03	0.54 ± 0.03	0.40 ± 0.03	0.30 ± 0.03
Speck Group Diameter	0.33 ± 0.0100	0.28 ± 0.0083	0.23 ± 0.0069	0.20 ± 0.0059	0.17 ± 0.0084	0.14 ± 0.0070
Mass Thickness	1.00 ± 0.05	0.75 ± 0.05	0.50 ± 0.05	0.38 ± 0.04	0.25 ± 0.03	0.20 ± 0.02

Figure 16-25
(A) ACR FFDM accreditation phantom positioned on the image receptor. Note size of phantom compared to the image receptor. Mammo FFDM™ Phantom manufactured by Gammex, a Sun Nuclear Company. **(B)** Schematic illustrating the position of the different test objects embedded within the FFDM FDA-approved accreditation phantom. (Image courtesy of Gammex, Inc., Sun Nuclear Corporation.) **(C)** Chart of size specifications of test objects embedded within the wax insert of the FFDM FDA-approved accreditation phantom. (Source: MQSA, FDA Web site (fda.gov), Recently Updated Advisory Committee Materials, National Mammography Quality Assurance Advisory Committee, 2016 Meeting Materials of the NMQAAC, Presentation Eric Burns, Ph.D., September 15, 2016.) **(D)** Radiograph of the ACR FFDM accreditation phantom illustrating visible test objects of fibers, speck groups, and masses. *Dark circle* indicates location of the CNR cavity.

for the patient. The MP performs this test by acquiring an "image" of the size and position of the x-ray field above the image receptor. This image can be acquired on a CR screen, GAF chromatic (self-developing) film strips, or an electronic x-ray detector (Figure 16-26). Comparison measurements are made between the border margin results to calculate the congruency of x-ray to light field, x-ray to image receptor alignment, and the chest wall compression device alignment. Evaluation is performed with both the small and large radiation field sizes. If the

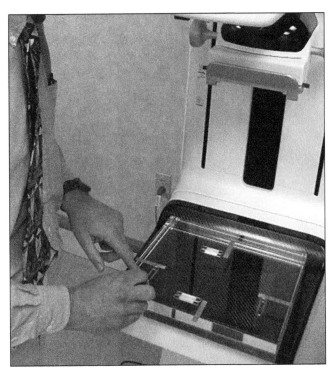

Figure 16-26
MP testing congruency of x-ray field, light field, and collimator alignment using small attenuators and self-developing film strips sensitive to exposure for digital QC testing environments.

18-cm × 24-cm compression device permits shifting to the right and to the left, evaluation must be performed in all positions.

Performance criteria: Acceptable levels of tolerance for the deviation of the light field, x-ray field, compression device, and image receptor have been established by the following MQSA standards[20]:

- Deviation between x-ray field and light field: The total of any misalignment of the edges of the light field and the x-ray field along either the length or width of the visually defined field at the plane of the breast support surface shall not exceed 2% of the SID.
- Deviation between x-ray field and edges of the image receptor: The collimation component shall allow the x-ray field to extend to the chest wall edge of the image receptor. The x-ray field cannot extend beyond any edge of the image receptor by more than 2% of the SID.
- Alignment of the chest wall edge of the compression device and the image receptor: The chest wall edge of the compression device shall not extend beyond the chest wall of the image receptor by more than 1% of the SID when tested with the compression device placed above the breast support surface at a distance equivalent to compressed average breast thickness. The shadow of

the vertical edge of the compression device shall not be visible on the image.

MQSA requires that should the test results fall outside of acceptable limits, the source of the problem shall be identified and corrective action shall be taken within 30 days of the test date.

Compression Force

The compression force test is included in the mammographic unit assembly evaluation performed by the MP. Using either an analog bathroom scale (the image receptor and compression device are protected with padding) or a calibrated foam compression block, maximum automatic compression force is applied and measured, and if applicable, manual compression force is tested, at least to 45 lbs.

Performance criteria: Maximum automatic compression force must be between 25 and 45 lbs (12 and 20 daN) (111 to 200 N).

Mammography Soft-Copy Display Tests: Monitors and Workstations (Medical Physicist)
Radiologist Review Workstation

The most important link in the digital imaging chain is the one between the image acquisition device and the Radiologist Review Workstation (RWS) for image display.[31] To ensure that the displayed image is a true representation of the subject and is free from artifacts, a thorough evaluation of monitor performance must be established by the MP[26] prior to clinical use (MEE) and evaluated annually thereafter. As with the mammography unit, major repairs or changes made to the RWS require an inspection by the MP prior to its return to clinical use. Quality control for the RWS used for mammography (most commonly LCD technology) adheres to the QC pathway that correlates to the appropriate MQSA standard described in Table 16-1. These standards require the MP and QC technologist to follow either the image receptor manufacturers' quality control manual or the ACR 2016 Mammography Digital QC Manual for performance evaluation. There are several factors that contribute to the quality of the image displayed on the RWS.[19,21,32–34] Display devices used in medical imaging are configured using the Digital Imaging and Communications in Medicine (DICOM) Grayscale Standard Display Function (GSDF), developed by the National Electrical Manufacturers Association (NEMA). These standards provide visual consistency across different display devices used for radiology interpretation.[35] The MP inspects the performance of the following monitor characteristics:

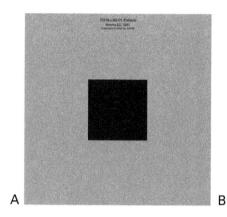
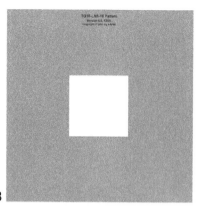
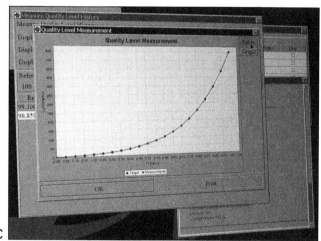

Figure 16-27
AAPM TG18 test patterns used to evaluate electronic soft-copy display for luminance by the MP with a photometer device. **(A)** AAPM TG18-LN8-01 test pattern evaluates Lmin, and **(B)** AAPM TG18-LN8-18 test pattern evaluates Lmax. (Source: AAPM On-Line Report 03. Assessment of Display Performance For Medical Imaging Systems, 2005. (http://www.aapm.org/pubs/reports/OR_03.pdf.) **(C)** Software supplied by manufacturers of soft-copy displays provides testing of luminance performance values with graph indicators of pass/fail.

Luminance, contrast, uniformity, resolution, and artifacts:

Luminance defines the amount of light emitted from a surface, or *from* the monitor screen. Luminance of the display is evaluated to determine how closely the gray-scale calibration of the monitor conforms with the DICOM GSDF.[31,35] Monitor luminance, L, is characterized by a range of luminance values from minimum (L_{min}) to maximum (L_{max}), with established white level standards of at least 420 cd/m^2 (candela/meter^2) for mammography displays.[36–40] Over the entire luminance range, the display must ensure a sufficient level of contrast to adequately appreciate image detail. This requires the contrast within the luminance range to deliver and maintain consistent values over time. Contrast values should comply with the AAPM Task Group 18 recommendations when evaluated by the MP[31,41] (Figure 16-27A–C). Each of the measured luminance levels of the GSDF test must be within 10% of the expected target luminance values. Professional medical grade mammography monitors typically have embedded technology that compensates for pixel luminance variation. Image uniformity performance across the display surface is also evaluated by the MP. Using a photometer and the AAPM TG18 UNL80 test pattern, variances in image luminance

across the entire display surface must be less than 15%[36] (Figure 16-28A,B). Additionally, the MP evaluates the resolution and artifacts of the display system using the AAPM Task Group 18 test patterns (Figure 16-29). Figure 16-7A illustrates the AAPM TG18 QC test pattern used to evaluate the RWS, while Figure 16-30 lists some of the parameters evaluated when using the TG18 QC test pattern.[19] Since the ACRIN DMIST study, the use of the more comprehensive AAPM TG18 QC test pattern, developed after the study began, is now recommended for display evaluation and is commonly used by MPs.[31] The SMPTE pattern is still commonly used by the QC technologist for display and printer evaluation and for this reason is included in the tests performed by the QC technologist in this chapter.

Radiologist Reading Room Environment

Illuminance is defined as light striking the surface, or the light that falls *on* the monitor. It is often described as ambient lighting and is an important factor in assessing reflection and glare and appropriate lighting for interpretation performance. For best performance, environments for mammography interpretation require a balance between luminance and illuminance. Ambient lighting that is too dark leads to radiologist eye strain, while ambient lighting

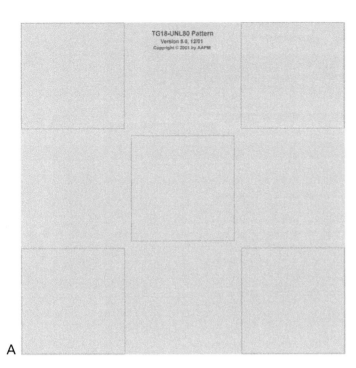

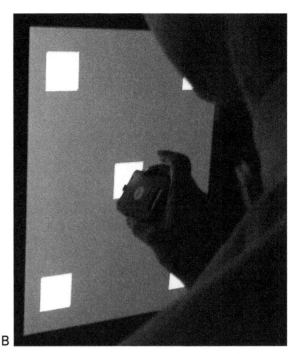

A   B

Figure 16-28
(A) AAPM TG18-UNL80 test pattern used to evaluate soft-copy display for uniformity by the MP with a photometer device. (Source: AAPM On-Line Report 03. Assessment of Display Performance For Medical Imaging Systems, 2005. (http://www.aapm.org/pubs/reports/OR_03.pdf.) **(B)** MP using photometer to measure luminance at the four corners and center of the monitor to evaluate display uniformity.

that is too bright reduces visible contrast. Ambient lighting should be consistently low. When tested by the MP using a photometer, readings should be in the 20- to 45-lux range[26,32] and reflection glare from other monitor surfaces kept to a minimum. The QC manual directives regarding RWS reading room conditions should be followed, typically requiring the MP to establish reading room configuration for glare and evaluating the ambient lighting.

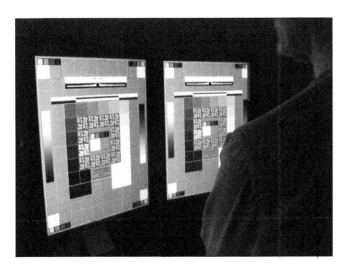

Figure 16-29
MP evaluates the RWS using the AAPM TG18 QC test pattern.

Acquisition Workstation (AWS)

The **acquisition workstation (AWS)** used by the technologist to acquire and assess the image may also be inspected by the MP. The information the technologist assesses, positioning/compression, contrast, and patient motion, is all displayed on the AWS. Although the AWS monitor is not used for interpretation, it should satisfy similar monitor requirements to the radiologist's monitor, and therefore, both displays should be similar to each other.[41] Technologist monitors (AWS) may be evaluated using the same testing procedures performed by the MP for the RWS. Depending on the requirements in the QC manual, the following tests may be included during the evaluation of the AWS monitor by the MP:

- Evaluation for cleanliness; ensuring the monitor surface is free from any dust, finger prints, or marks that may interfere with accuracy in viewing the image
- Evaluation of the AAPM TG18 QC or SMPTE pattern
  - 0% to 5% contrast patches apparent?
  - 95% to 100% contrast patches apparent?
  - Quality assessment of the alphanumeric indicators— How much is visible and how sharply apparent?
  - Sharpness of the line pairs in the four corners and center of the image
  - Assessment of the gray-scale ramp indicators—visible distinction between steps

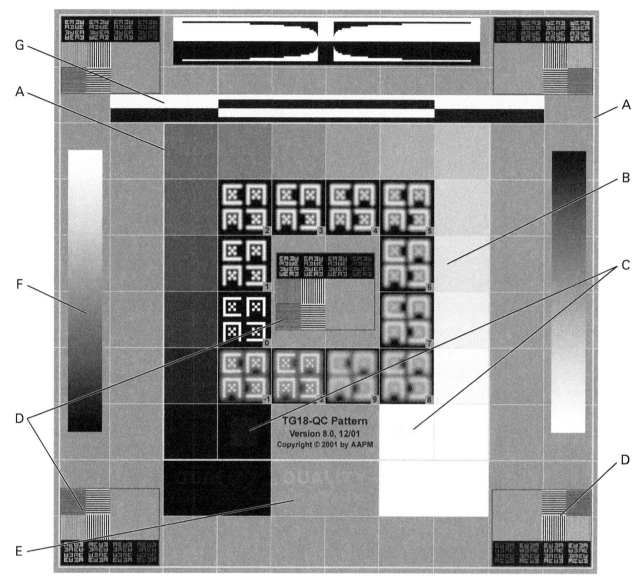

Verify:

- Straight lines evaluating geometric distortion (A)

- 16 luminance patches-varying pixel values for assessment of luminance response (B)

- Patches displaying 5% contrast at minimum and maximum pixel values (C)

- Line-pair patterns at center and corners for resolution assessment (D)

- "Quality Control" letters for evaluation of contrast detail (E)

- Vertical bars for evaluation of bit depth and artifacts (F)

- White and black bars to assess video signal artifacts (G)

Figure 16-30

Description of electronic display elements evaluated using the AAPM TG18 QC test pattern. (Source: American Association of Physicists in Medicine (AAPM) On-Line Report 03. Assessment of Display Performance For Medical Imaging Systems, 2005. (http://www.aapm.org/pubs/reports/OR_03.pdf).

- Luminance Testing

Using a photometer, the MP may include these tests in evaluating the AWS monitor:

- ○ Minimum and maximum luminance values
- ○ Luminance uniformity

Evaluation may also include verification of the DICOM GSDF conformance and artifact evaluation.

Laser Printer—Medical Physicist

On November 18, 2015, the FDA announced that the decision to maintain a laser printer for the purpose of printing hard-copy mammography images would be left to each individual facility.[42] Changes in the industry that included almost obsolete film/screen practices, and the increased use of DBT technology, interpreted solely using soft-copy interpretation, influenced the decision of the FDA to remove printer questions from the FDA inspection process.[43] If a facility chooses to maintain a laser printer, the QC for the printer must follow the appropriate QC pathway for the MQSA standards described in Table 16-1. The MP and QC technologist are required to follow either the image receptor manufacturers' QC, the laser printer manufacturers' QC, or the ACR 2016 Digital Mammography QC Manual for performance evaluation. Common tests for the laser printer performed by the MP include spatial resolution, geometric accuracy, and the OD measurements of the gray-scale pattern.

Mammography Equipment Tests: QC Technologist

Like the MP, quality control of the mammography equipment performed by the QC technologist is directed by the QC program manual selected by the facility (manufacturer-specific or standardized ACR 2016 Digital Mammography QC program) and includes methods to test operations of the mammography system. The names of the required QC tests and their frequencies performed by the QC technologist for various FFDM DR image receptor manufacturers and the ACR are listed in Table 16-2.

Compression Force

The use of adequate compression during the performance of the mammogram is essential to achieve image quality. Adequate compression ensures even penetration of the x-ray beam throughout the uniform breast tissue and reduces scatter radiation. The benefits of achieving adequate compression include the following:

- Minimizing motion
- Minimizing radiation exposure
- Increasing sharpness
- Increasing contrast
- Improved image quality for interpretation

For an in-depth discussion on the benefits of compression in mammography, see Chapter 11.

Purpose: The compression test is performed to ensure safety of the patient and accuracy of the examination. The test procedure separately evaluates the performance of the powered mode (foot pedal operation) and the manual mode (fine adjustment). Test results verify three important requirements of compression[13]:

- That adequate compression can be applied in the powered mode and manual mode of operation for accuracy
- That the system does not allow too much compression in the powered mode causing harm to the patient

- That compression can be maintained throughout the acquisition process

Frequency: Semiannually

Procedure: Using towels to protect the IRSD and the compression device, an analog bathroom scale is placed on the IRSD. Follow the QC manual directions for applying maximum powered compression and for applying manual compression (Figure 16-31). An example of this may be to first apply compression in the powered mode until it stops, recording the resulting compression force on the appropriate QC form. Next, apply compression in the manual mode until the amount of maximum compression force is achieved, again recording the resulting information. Depending on the image receptor manufacturer, results may reflect various examples of compression force units: pounds (lb), kilograms (kg), Newtons (N), or deca-Newtons (daN).

Performance criteria: According to the MQSA, for the powered compression mode a minimum compression force of at least 25 pounds (111 Newtons) shall be provided. The maximum compression force for the powered compression mode must be between 25 and 45 pounds (111 and 200 Newtons).[20]

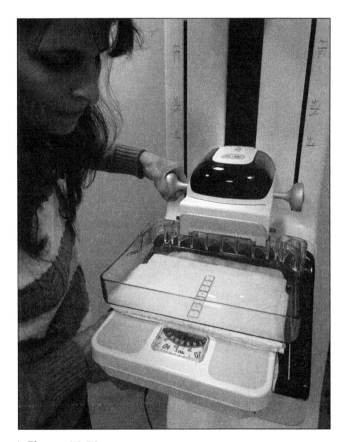

Figure 16-31
QC technologist tests manual compression force during required semiannual mammography unit testing.

Please note: technologists should not confuse this quality control test of compressing a bathroom scale with the art of applying compression to a patient's breast. The 25- to 45-lb range describes the acceptance range for testing automatic compression force. For the mammography procedure, the correct method of determining adequate compression is for the technologist to ensure the breast is taut, by tapping the breast when compression is complete. Some technologists incorrectly associate the 25- to 45-lb testing compression force range as the required amount of compression force that must be achieved when compressing a patient. As of this writing the correct method of evaluating adequate compression is described above. The application of compression is further explained in Chapter 7, Part 1.

Corrective action: According to the MQSA, if compression test results fall outside of the established action limits, the source of the problem shall be identified and corrective action shall be taken before any further examinations are performed or any films are processed using the component of the mammography system that failed the test.[20]

Compression Thickness

Compression thickness is a simple test to verify that the indicated breast thickness is correct (Figure 16-32) (also refer to MP test Figure 16-14). Some manufacturers use compression thickness as a function of the automatic exposure control. Verification that the indicated breast thickness correlates correctly to the compression parameters established during the MP acceptance testing:

• Confirms that the technical factors used during patient exposures are correct
• Ensures appropriate x-ray beam filtration selection for image quality and dose
• Protects the patient from unnecessary radiation

Follow the QC manual instructions to evaluate compression thickness. The values for compression thickness and for compression force are recorded. The frequency and corrective action specifications are determined by the QC Manual that is used.[30]

Detector Calibration (Flat Field or Gain Calibration)

Detector calibration prepares the detector for clinical use by addressing the sensitivity variances within the detector. Some FFDM DR detectors may have a nonuniform response due to variations in pixel sensitivity or faulty pixels. Variations in detector uniformity may also be a result of inherent conditions of the imaging system such as the anode heel effect or x-ray beam divergence.[28,44] The flat-field correction

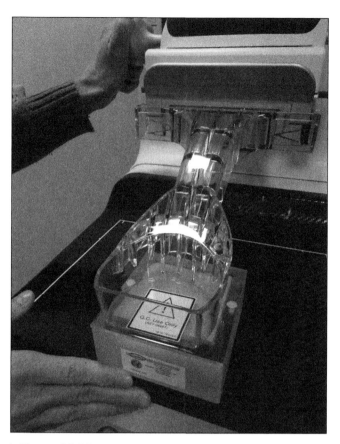

Figure 16-32
QC technologist tests the accuracy of the compression thickness indicator during manufacturer-specific periodic testing of the mammography machine.

process applied in FFDM DR systems should produce images that are uniform in intensity and free of artifacts.[28] This capability is determined by the detector design and established parameters of the manufacturer. At installation, the service engineer verifies the detector calibration, which is tested for acceptance by the MP prior to clinical use. Flat-field correction or detector calibration re-establishes the expected performance of consistent detector uniformity if drifting of the established parameters has occurred. This calibration is periodically performed by the technologist, making it not so much a quality control test as a housekeeping requirement. Variations of sensitivity can be corrected by using a uniform acrylic block large enough to cover the detector and then making prescribed x-ray exposures. The technologist makes several exposures using various target/filter combinations and focal spot sizes (Figure 16-33A,B). After making the required number of exposures, software provided by the manufacturer completes the calibration process. The temperature of the detector is an important consideration when performing calibration; this QC requirement must be performed within a specific temperature range as specified by the manufacturer.[30]

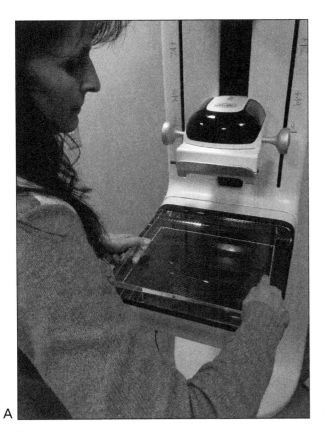 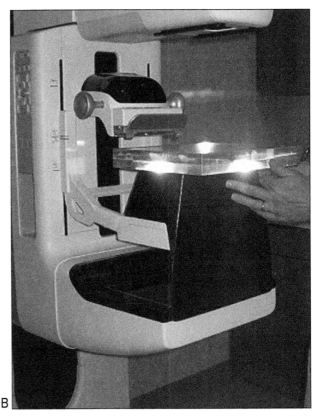

A B

Figure 16-33
QC technologist performs detector calibration using acrylic uniform phantom in the **(A)** contact mode and in the **(B)** magnification mode.

Follow the QC manual for the frequency, procedure, and corrective action requirements for detector calibration.

Artifact Evaluation

The QC technologist periodically assesses the system for artifacts to ensure that the image remains blemish free. The test can assist in isolating the origin of the artifact so that it can be eliminated. A uniform block of acrylic large enough to cover the image receptor is used to perform the test. The QC manual directions are followed for artifact testing. This may involve exposing the uniform acrylic phantom using various combinations of exposure factors and available filters. The first exposure is acquired and viewed on the monitor at a predetermined brightness index, which permits easier visibility of artifacts. The image is evaluated in full resolution, which displays the image in actual pixel size. Panning through each section of the image detector, the technologist looks for artifacts on what should be a uniform flat-field image with no blemishes (Figure 16-34A,B). When evaluation of the first exposure is complete, the acrylic block is rotated 180° for the subsequent exposure and evaluation acquired using the remaining filter(s). Rotation of the acrylic block allows the technologist to easily trace observed artifacts

to the phantom or to the system. If artifacts are traced to the image detector, the technologist should consider performing a flat-field calibration (detector calibration) before repeating the artifact test.

- Types of artifacts
  ○ Dead Pixels
  A common artifact observed in DR systems is a consistent black or white spot seen on all images in exactly the same location (Figure 16-35A–D). This represents what is known as a dead pixel—one that does not respond properly when exposed to radiation. A single or even a few widely spaced dead pixels may not be a cause for concern; however, when many become apparent, they can interfere with the radiologist's interpretation or can become distracting. Calibration procedures for locating and removing dead pixels are usually accomplished through a remote service performed by the service engineer.
  ○ Detector Artifact
  Careful evaluation of the flat-field image is necessary to recognize artifacts that are uncommonly observed in the detector. Figure 16-36A,B illustrates a minus density artifact observed during the artifact evaluation test performed by the technologist. Subsequent testing performed by the MP verified a minus density

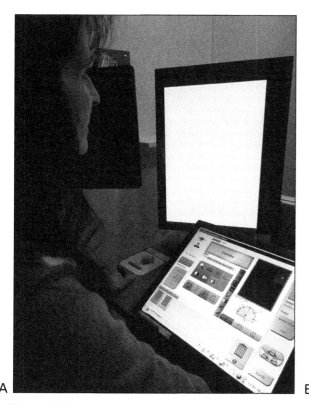

Figure 16-34
(A) QC technologist performs artifact test using the image from the uniform phantom QC test. **(B)** Each section of the flat-field image is evaluated using actual pixel size or one-to-one pixel evaluation.

Figure 16-35
(A) Dead pixels are seen as consistent black or white spots on the image. **(B)** On the magnified flat-field image, they are relatively easy to discern. **(C)** On a patient image, it can mimic a calcification. **(D)** Close up image of the artifact.

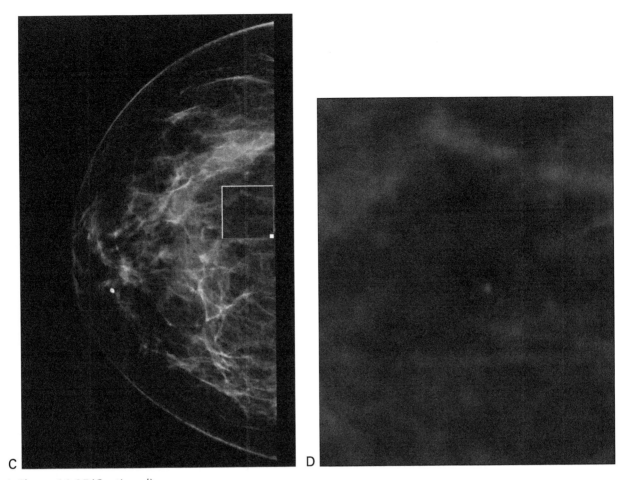

| **Figure 16-35** (*Continued*)

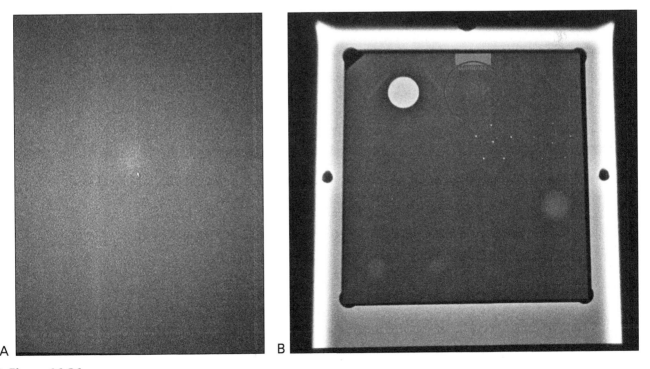

Figure 16-36
(A) Minus density artifact revealed during artifact evaluation for acceptance testing by MP. **(B)** Further investigation confirmed detector artifact demonstrated on the accreditation phantom image. This resulted in replacement of the detector.

artifact that could not be eliminated by service. Due to the location of the artifact, it was necessary to replace the detector.

Follow the QC manual for the frequency, procedure, and corrective action requirements for the artifact evaluation test. Refer also to the MP tests for ghosting artifact. Note that the first action taken by the technologist in the discovery of an artifact is to isolate the source and repeat the test for verification when appropriate. Artifacts isolated to the acrylic block should not be ignored.

Phantom Image Quality

The **image quality phantom test** is performed weekly by the technologist for all FFDM DR manufacturers with the exception of one manufacturer, which requires the technologist to perform daily QC for the phantom image. The purpose of performing the phantom image evaluation is to verify that the components of the imaging chain consistently produce images of adequate quality. The QC test is divided into three parts: SNR/CNR evaluation, image quality scoring objects, and artifact evaluation. The phantom image quality test performed by the MP highlights the basic differences inherent in MQSA QC programs. The QC technologist's periodic tests of phantom image quality verifies the consistent performance of the SNR and CNR values within the ranges established during the MP acceptance testing. The SNR and CNR values are recorded on a control chart to determine if the values fall within the acceptance parameters.

Phantom Image Quality Scoring—Original ACR Accreditation Phantom

The phantom image must achieve the minimum score established by the facility's accrediting body and the FDA (Figure 16-24A–C). The accrediting body's rules for scoring the objects within the wax insert of the phantom image should be reviewed to determine the score of an object that is only partially visible. For QC programs using the original ACR accreditation phantom, at minimum, the four largest fibers, the three largest speck groups, and the three largest masses must be visible to pass accreditation. This is a subjective judgment; different people will see different numbers of test objects in the same image. For this reason, the same technologist performs and evaluates the phantom image under the same viewing conditions each week. Consult the QC manual for instructions on how the phantom should be reviewed for soft copy evaluation. When the scoring is completed for each object: fibers, speck groups, and masses, the phantom is reviewed for artifacts. If artifacts are found in the phantom that mimic the test object (i.e., fibers, specks, or masses), the last counted test object for that artifact description is deducted (i.e., if the artifact looks like a fiber, the last fiber is deducted from the total fiber score). Each test object score is compared to the previous analysis to determine if the image quality has changed. The fibers, speck groups, and masses are recorded on the QC phantom form. It should be noted that there are differences between FFDM image receptor manufacturers regarding passing scores for fibers, speck groups, and masses for *quality control purposes* (example: some manufacturers may require 5 fibers, 4 speck groups and 4 masses to pass periodic QC testing), but for accreditation purposes, *all* manufacturers must visualize at minimum 4 fibers, 3 speck groups, and 3 masses. The exposure factors are recorded on the QC phantom form: mAs, kVp, target/filter, manufacturer exposure indicator, SNR, and CNR change. These values can be compared with previous phantom exposures for additional detection of potential generator problems. In addition to exposure and test objects, the phantom image can be used to note any grid artifacts or nonuniformity in the image.

Phantom Image Quality Scoring—ACR Digital (DM) Accreditation Phantom

The differences in the configuration of the ACR DM phantom used in the ACR Standardized Digital QC Program compared to the original ACR accreditation phantom are discussed in the QC image quality tests performed by the MP (Figure 16-25A–D). Notable differences include the size and additional purpose of the DM phantom to evaluate a larger detector area for artifacts as well as evaluate image quality. Other differences include the number of test objects embedded in the wax insert and the CNR cavity used to calculate the CNR value. The accrediting body's rules for scoring the objects within the wax insert of the phantom image should be reviewed to determine the score of an object that is only partially visible. For QC programs using the DM accreditation phantom, the two largest fibers, the three largest speck groups, and the two largest masses must be visible to pass accreditation. Unlike the original ACR phantom, deductions are not made for object-like artifacts found within the pink wax insert. Similarities also exist between the original ACR accreditation phantom and the ACR DM accreditation phantom:

- The test objects visible in the wax insert are counted from the largest to the smallest.
- Phantom test object scores must achieve the minimum score established by the facility's accrediting body and the FDA.
- The same technologist performs and evaluates the phantom image under the same viewing conditions each week.

Consult the ACR 2016 Digital Mammography QC Manual for instructions on how the phantom should be reviewed for soft copy evaluation. Each test object score is compared to the previous analysis to determine if the image quality has changed. The fibers, speck groups, and masses are recorded on the QC phantom form. The exposure factors are recorded on the QC phantom form: mAs, kVp, target/filter, manufacturer exposure indicator, SNR, and CNR change. These values can be compared with previous phantom exposures for additional detection of potential generator problems. In addition to exposure and test objects, the phantom image can be used to note any grid artifacts or nonuniformity in the image.

It should be noted that the ACR DM phantom covers a majority of the detector (Figure 16-3) in comparison to the original ACR accreditation phantom (Figure 16-2). Due to this advantage, the weekly QC performed by the technologist that adheres to the ACR 2016 Digital Mammography QC Manual, produces an image of the ACR DM phantom that allows simultaneous evaluation of image quality and evaluation of artifacts.[13]

CNR and MTF Measurement

The sharpness of an optical imaging system is characterized by a measurement called **modulation transfer function (MTF)**, also known as spatial frequency response. MTF is a measure of the transfer of contrast from the subject to the image. In technical terms, MTF is the *spatial* frequency response of an imaging system or a component; it is the contrast at a given spatial frequency relative to low frequencies. High spatial frequencies correspond to fine image detail. The more extended the response, the finer the detail, the sharper the image.[45] In other words, it measures how faithfully the detector reproduces detail from the object to the image. Currently, the only available mammography units that utilize this QC test are those manufactured by GE. The QC technologist's procedure to test the MTF and the CNR are combined. An exposure is made using the manufacturer-specific IQST phantom (Image Quality Signature Test Phantom) (Figure 16-6A). When the exposure is completed the Quality Assurance Program software yields MTF values in lp/mm and the change in CNR value that are compared to acceptance parameters. Planmed includes the MTF test for the MP to perform, but does not require the technologist to perform periodic tests for MTF.

Radiologist Workstation QC

The crucial elements of the RWS for mammography interpretation and the stringent requirements of quality control for this equipment are discussed in the MP QC tests in this chapter for soft-copy displays. These standards require the MP and QC technologist to follow either the image receptor manufacturers' QC manual, the RWS monitor manufacturers' QC manual, or the standardized ACR 2016 Digital Mammography QC Manual for the RWS. The QC procedures performed by the technologist, the frequency, and the pass/fail criteria for the RWS are specific to the requirements described in the QC manual. During the MP inspection of the RWS, extensive evaluation ensures that the equipment components perform to established standards (see RWS QC: Medical Physicist in this chapter). The technologist's responsibility is to periodically evaluate these same components verifying that the equipment consistently performs within the established parameters. This is accomplished by performing tests on the RWS that are a scaled-down version of the MP's tests to verify that monitors maintain consistent performance. Common RWS QC responsibilities of the technologist include:

- Verify monitor cleanliness, free from dust, fingerprints, and smudges that interfere with image accuracy (follow protocols described in the QC manual—often describing the use of dry, lint-free cloths)
- Evaluation of luminance, contrast, uniformity, resolution, and artifacts as displayed on either the SMPTE or TG18 QC test patterns
- Verify manufacturer software requirements for calibration and other automated evaluations (DICOM GSDF) are performed with satisfactory results
- Verify RWS room configuration and lighting is consistent with established requirements described in the QC manual and by the MP

To evaluate the RWS luminance, contrast, uniformity, and resolution, the technologist may either be directed to analyze the AAPM TG18 QC test pattern or the SMPTE pattern (Figure 16-37). The MP most often prefers the

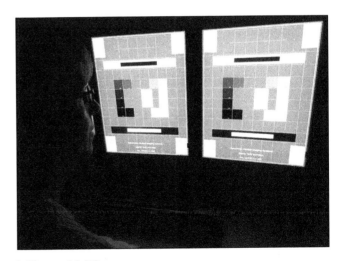

Figure 16-37
During periodic RWS QC, the QC technologist uses the SMPTE pattern to evaluate the electronic display.

AAPM TG18 QC test pattern if available during testing, and for this reason, the analysis of the AAPM TG18 QC pattern was included in the Medical Physicist RWS QC section. To ensure the reader understands the application of each pattern to RWS QC, the SMPTE pattern (see medical physicist soft-copy display, Figure 16-7B) analysis is included in the technologist's RWS QC section. Figure 16-38 illustrates the parameters of the SMPTE pattern used to evaluate the RWS performance. In addition to evaluating the RWS using the AAPM TG18 QC or SMPTE pattern, the technologist's responsibility includes verifying the results from the automated software QC provided by the manufacturer that further ensures consistent performance of the RWS. Finally, periodic QC responsibilities for the technologist

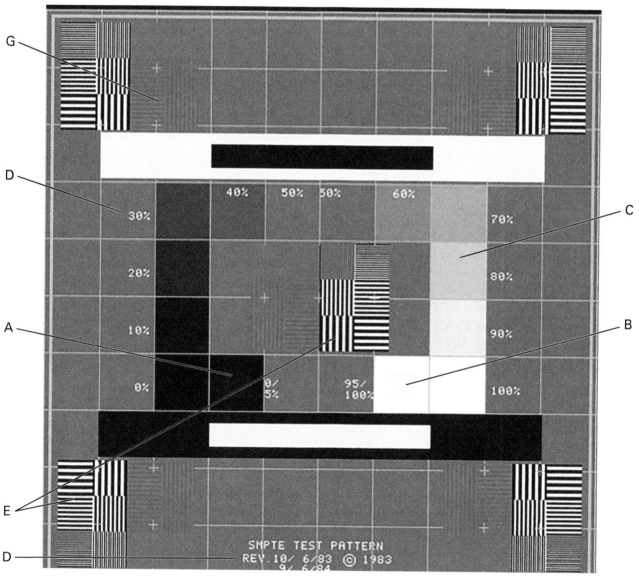

Verify:

- 0%–5% contrast patches (A)

- 95%–100% contrast patches (B)

- Each gray-level step can be distinguished between 0%–100% (C)

- Alphanumeric characters can be distinguished (D)

- Visibility of high contrast line-pairs in the center and corners (E)

Figure 16-38

Description of electronic display elements evaluated using the SMPTE test pattern. (Source: Society of Motion Picture and Television Engineers (http://www.SMPTE.org).)

may include verification of room configuration and lighting requirements as well as specific intervals of maintaining monitor cleanliness (using only products recommended for use by the manufacturer) and inspection for obvious monitor artifacts.

Corrective action requirements are defined by the determinants described in the QC program manual.

Acquisition Workstation QC

QC protocols for the AWS may follow similar QC practices for those of the RWS. Specific AWS QC is determined by the QC program manual for the image receptor manufacturer or by the ACR 2016 Digital Mammography QC program. Because the technologist uses the AWS to evaluate image quality and accuracy of tissue representation, QC practices for the AWS are a common quality control procedure. Like the RWS, the technologist's monitor may be evaluated for monitor cleanliness, brightness and contrast, resolution, and artifacts. Electronic display test patterns such as the AAPM TG18 QC or the SMPTE pattern may be selected to evaluate the monitor (see Soft-Copy Display QC: Medical Physicist). Additionally, the technologist may be asked to verify automated software QC performance was performed and completed satisfactorily.

Corrective action requirements are defined by the determinants described in the QC program manual.

Laser Printer—QC Technologist

Refer to Medical Physicist Laser Printer QC section.

Digital Breast Tomosynthesis Quality Control

At the time of this writing, there are three manufacturers with approved DBT units for use in mammography facilities in the United States:

- Hologic (2011)
- GE (2014)
- Siemens (2015)

Currently, no standardized QC program exists for DBT; rather, quality control for DBT follows the "image receptor manufacturer" QC program standard described in Table 16-1, *MQSA FFDM STANDARD*. Typically, the MP and the technologist perform the 2D FFDM QC requirements for the specific equipment components defined in the QC manual and then perform the DBT QC for each specific equipment component if it is required. Manufacturers may have proprietary DBT phantoms that have been developed for specific quality control tests. The Hologic Dimensions unit, for example, has a specific phantom to use for semi-annual DBT geometry calibrations (Figure 16-39A–C).

Repeat/Reject Analysis

The repeat/reject analysis is a quarterly QC evaluation that is included in all FFDM DR image receptor manufacturer QC programs. The ACR standardized program includes this test as an optional QC evaluation. Table 16-2 provides the test title used for the repeat/reject analysis depending on the manufacturer. Consult the QC manual for specific instructions on how to conduct the analysis and the forms required to calculate the repeat/reject rates.

The purpose of the repeat/reject analysis evaluation is to determine the number and the cause of repeated/rejected mammograms. Analyzing the data gathered at the end of the analysis period identifies department performance that may impact efficiency and cost. Additionally, the analysis provides indications of technologist performance that may impact patient exposures.

In order to conduct the analysis, there must be a method to collect:

- Total number of patient exposures during the analysis period
- Total number of repeated exposures during the analysis period (this includes repeated mammograms filed with the examination)
- Means to sort the images that have been repeated (reasons why)

Meaningful data collected for the analysis must consist of at least 250 patients. At the end of the analysis period, the images are sorted into categories as to why they were repeated. Reasons for repeated images generally are due to patient related repeats, equipment-related repeats, or miscellaneous reasons for repeats. A partial list of reasons for repeated images may include:

- Positioning
- Patient motion
- Exposure too high (exposure saturation)
- Exposure too low (excessive noise on the image)
- Incorrect patient ID
- Software failure
- Blank image

Determine the overall percentage of the repeat rate by dividing the total number of repeated images by the total number of patient exposures during the analysis period. Multiply this number by 100 for the overall department repeat rate. Figure 16-40 illustrates the calculations used to determine the overall department repeat rate of 2.0%:

Total number of repeats = 83
Total number of patient exposures during analysis = 4,092
$83 \div 4,092 = 0.020 \times 100 = 2.0\%$

The reject rate is determined using the same calculation.

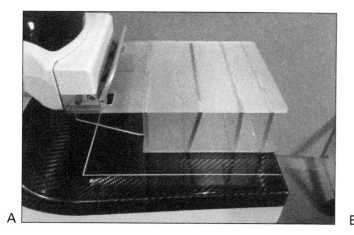

A

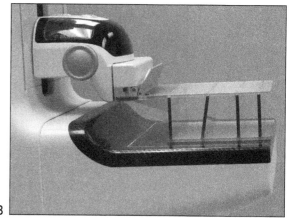

B

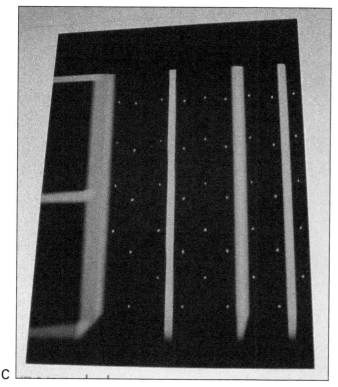

C

Figure 16-39
(A) Manufacturer-specific phantom used for DBT image quality and **(B)** side view of phantom. **(C)** Radiograph of DBT phantom displays metallic BBs.

To determine the percentage of repeats in each individual reason category, divide the number of images in the reason category by the total number of repeats. The "positioning" category in Figure 16-40 has a total of 42 repeated images. The total number of repeated images during the analysis period is 83. The following calculation, 42 ÷ 83=0.506 × 100 = 51%, indicates that approximately half of the department reasons for repeats were due to positioning.

Most FFDM units are equipped with software that collects and analyzes the repeat/reject data at the end of the analysis period for the QC technologist. Facilities may choose to conduct ongoing repeat/reject analysis by gathering this data quarterly.

There is a distinction between a repeated image and a rejected image. A "repeated" image indicates that a second projection was acquired, but the original image is kept with the exam because it contains some diagnostic value. A "rejected" image indicates that the original image contained no diagnostic value and it was rejected from the examination file. Although it is time consuming to calculate the individual repeat/reject rates for each technologist in addition to the overall department analysis, information

From: <u>January 1</u> to <u>January 31</u>

Reason	Number of Exposures						Subtotals	% of repeats
	Left CC	Right CC	Left MLO	Right MLO	Left Other	Right Other		
1. Positioning	10	7	7	10	3	5	42	51.0%
2. Patient motion							0	—
3. Good images (no reason)	2		3				5	6.0%
4. Improper Detector Exposure (Saturation)				1			1	1.0%
5. Detector Underexposure (Excessive Noise)						1	1	1.0%
6. Incorrect Patient I.D.		1			1		2	2.0%
7. Artifacts	1	2	2	1		2	8	10.0%
8. Equipment Failure							0	—
9. Patient Failure	5	4	6	6	2	2	24	29.0%
10. Software Failure							0	—
						Totals	83	100%

Total repeats with reasons:	83
Total exposures:	4,092
Ratio %	2.02%

Remarks:_____

_____

_____

_____

Corrective Action:_____

_____

_____

_____

Figure 16-40
Example of quarterly repeat analysis conducted for mammography quality assurance. Note the overall department repeat rate and the percentage of repeats for each category.

revealed by this practice can be beneficial in targeting specific areas for improvement.

A desirable overall repeat rate is approximately 2% or less. A rate of 5% may be considered adequate if the LIP and the MP agree that this is reasonable.

Performance criteria: If the total repeat or reject rate is different than the previous quarter's determined rate by more than 2.0% (either positively or negatively), the cause of the change should be determined and corrective action initiated. Documentation and assessment of corrective action is a requirement of MQSA.[46]

Visual Checklist

The visual check of the mammography machine and the mammography room is designed to ensure that the unit is mechanically stable and working properly, that patient safety during the procedure is maintained, and that accessories necessary for examinations are available and in good condition. Consult the QC manual for requirements listed for the visual checklist and the QC forms supplied by the QC program.

Examples of equipment and room assessment requirements for safety and patient care may include:

- Unit indicator lights, locks, and detents
- Compression devices (all) and magnification stand
- Equipment cables

The visual check is a practice to periodically take inventory of the equipment and mammography room to ensure that patient and operator safety, comfort, and convenience are not compromised. Observances of malfunctioning equipment should be reported immediately following the protocols established by the facility. The visual check is also useful as a communication tool between several technologists working in the same mammography room.

Using the visual check form to document minor conditions of wear in accessories (such as compression devices) assists in ensuring that replacements are available should the component fail, thus avoiding downtime. The visual checklist is also a convenient location to include the date of evaluation and to note the condition of lead aprons used in the mammography department. Including the lead aprons on the list of items to be reviewed ensures they will be available and in good condition when their use is necessary.

QUALITY ASSESSMENT OF IMAGE QUALITY (QA)

In October 2016, the FDA announced the Enhancing Quality Using the Inspection Program (EQUIP) initiative. The EQUIP requirements emphasize inspection questions that address the responsibility of the facility to ensure ongoing reviews of image quality and to ensure the LIP oversight of the QA/QC program. The FDA plan is to provide EQUIP education to facilities beginning January 2017, with expectation of facility EQUIP compliance by January 2018. Since EQUIP specifically affects the QA/QC facility program in regard to implementing policies or procedures for image quality review, it is appropriate to discuss this subject amidst other MQSA regulations that require periodic reviews such as the repeat/reject analysis. The LIP provides oversight of the QA/QC component of EQUIP for image quality. Facilities are required to provide the following minimum documentation during the FDA inspection.

Clinical Image Quality

The facility must have a procedure to ensure that clinical images continue to comply with the clinical image quality standards established by the facility's accrediting body. The facility must establish a mechanism for periodic reviews of image quality attributes from a sample of mammograms performed by each radiologic technologist and for a sample of mammograms accepted for interpretation by each interpreting physician. The facility must supply the inspector written documentation that the reviews took place at least once since the last inspection, although a more frequent periodic review is encouraged.[43]

Quality Assurance—Clinical Image Corrective Action

The facility must establish a procedure for corrective action when clinical images are of poor quality.[43] Facilities must show that a process is in place that provides ongoing IP feedback, and a process to document corrective action when implemented, and documentation of the effectiveness of the corrective action. The ACR 2016 Digital Mammography QC Manual supplies a form for ongoing feedback to the technologist from the IP (Figure 16-41). Feedback from the IP to the technologist communicates valuable information about exam specifics, providing quality improvement when necessary and complements for exceptional performance.

QA Quarterly Review

Radiologist Quarterly Review is discussed in Chapter 15.

Chapter Summary

For radiologists to consistently receive mammography images that meet quality standards for interpretation, variables that impact image quality must be controlled. The mammography equipment used to produce the image, and the electronic display used for interpretation purposes, must be carefully and periodically monitored to verify that performance continues to meet initial acceptance standards of operation. Once the MP has accepted the equipment for use in mammography service, it is the QC technologist who actively safeguards image quality. The familiarity she develops through routine QC testing allows her the opportunity to observe shifts in equipment performance that may indicate problems. Adequate training for the technologist preparing to perform the equipment evaluations for QC is essential and should include not only *how* to perform the tests, but also *why* the tests are performed. Ensuring that potential problems are addressed prior to being detected on a clinical image is the goal of the quality control program, which can best be achieved when the QC technologist is fully engaged in the QC program.

Optional—Radiologist Image Quality Feedback   *As Needed*
(For Quality Improvement)

Radiologist's Name _____

Date _____

Procedure	This report is to be completed by the Interpreting Radiologist when asked to interpret sub-optimal cases requiring the patient to be called back. The form may also be used to provide feedback on excellent quality. The radiologist should complete this form as needed for each case. A system should be in place for analyzing feedback and taking measures for improvement as necessary.

Objective   For the Radiologist to provide routine feedback to the technologists and manager on the quality of images.

Patient Identifier: _____

_____

Technologist's Name: _____

Date of Exam: _____

Overall Assessment

☐ Excellent   ☐ Good   ☐ Needs improvement, but do not repeat   ☐ Sub-Optimal, and should be repeated

Image Evaluation

	RCC	LCC	RMLO	LMLO	Other View	Other View
Positioning						
Missing tissue						
Laterally						
Posteriorly						
Medially						
Inferiorly						
Nipple not in profile						
Skin fold						
Pectoralis not down to PNL						
Tissue droopy (camel nose)						
Narrow/concave pectoralis						
Inframammary fold						
Not open						
Not shown						
Centering not correct						
Technical Issues						
Not enough compression						
Exposure Too Low (Excessive Noise)						
Exposure Too High (Image Saturation)						
Patient Motion						
Artifacts						
Incorrect Patient ID						
Other						

Additional Images Needed for Complete Breast Evaluation

Requested views   ☐ RCC   ☐ LCC   ☐ RMLO   ☐ LMLO   ☐ Other View _____

Action Limits	**Recommended:**	Patients should be called back for additional images if the quality is suboptimal according to the interpreting radiologist's request.
	Time frame:	Not applicable.

Figure 16-41

Example of image quality feedback form used to inform technologist of ongoing exam performance. Radiologist quality feedback form developed for ACR 2016 Digital Mammography QC Manual. (Source: Berns EA, Baker JA, Barke LD, et al. Digital Mammography Quality Control Manual. Reston, VA: American College of Radiology; 2016.)

Review Questions

1. According to MQSA, there are two quality control program structures that facilities may follow. Explain the MQSA standards that direct each program and the QC manuals that correlate to the MQSA standard.

2. Explain the primary goal of performing periodic QC equipment evaluation.

3. Describe the purpose of the EQUIP program and how facilities may comply with EQUIP requirements.

4. In digital mammography, what values provide information regarding adequate exposure and appropriate dose to the patient?

5. To pass the FDA accreditation process, the phantom submitted to the accrediting body must demonstrate how many fibers, speck groups, and masses?

6. Explain what triggers a "corrective action" process and what supportive documents may prove resolution of the event.

7. Describe the purpose of the repeat/reject analysis and how the overall percentage of the repeat rate is determined.

8. Explain the important distinction between:

   a. Conducting the compression force test for quality control purposes
   b. Appropriate application of compression force during the mammography procedure

Case Study 16-1

1A. Refer to Figures 16-2 and 16-3. Describe the differences inherent in the original accreditation phantom designed for film/screen mammography (Figure 16-2) and the ACR digital (DM) accreditation phantom (Figure 16-3) designed for digital mammography.

1B. Refer to Figures 16-24 and 16-25. Who uses the phantom in Figure 16-24? Figure 16-25? What are the passing scores for the objects for both phantoms for accreditation? Why are the scores different? Why are the number of objects different in the two phantoms?

Case Study 16-2

1. Refer to Figure 16-7. Describe the two test patterns commonly used for electronic display evaluation by the MP and the QC technologist and some of the technical elements they evaluate.

Case Study 16-3

1. Refer to Figure 16-13. Several tests the QC technologist performs require plotting data on a form. Why do the plotted data points vary in position on the chart? What criteria signify a trend in results? What do the dashed lines on the CNR section of the chart signify?

Case Study 16-4

1. Refer to Figure 16-22. What is ghosting? What causes ghosting? How do image receptor manufacturers counteract this effect?

References

1. ACR Practice Parameter for the Performance of Screening and Diagnostic Mammography (American College of Radiology) Revised 2013 (Resolution 11)*.
2. Duffy SW, et al. The impact of organized mammography service screening on breast carcinoma mortality in seven Swedish counties. *Cancer.* 2002;95:458–469.
3. Hellquist BN, et al. Effectiveness of population-based service screening with mammography for women ages 40 to 49 years: evaluation of the Swedish Mammography Screening in Young Women (SCRY) cohort. *Cancer.* 2011; 117:714–722.
4. Smart CR, et al. Benefit of mammography screening in women ages 40 to 49 years. Current evidence from randomized controlled trials. *Cancer.* 1995;75:1619–1626.
5. Tabar L, et al. Recent results from the Swedish Two-County Trial: the effects of age, histologic type, and mode of detection on the efficacy of breast cancer screening. *J Natl Cancer Inst Monogr.* 1997:43–47.
6. Tabar L, et al. Update of the Swedish two-county program of mammographic screening for breast cancer. *Radiol Clin North Am.* 1992;30:187–210.
7. Tabar L, et al. Swedish two-county trial: impact of mammographic screening on breast cancer mortality during 3 decades. *Radiology.* 2011;260:658–663.
8. Policy Guidance Help System (PGHS): fda.gov/Equipment/General Equipment Requirement. Accessed December 9, 2016.

9. American College of Radiology Website: Quality and Safety/ Accreditation/Mammography/Medical Physicist Evaluation Forms/MQSA Requirements for Mammography Equipment Checklist. Accessed December 9, 2016.

10. Department of Health and Human Services, Office of Inspector General. Lessons from Inspections of Mammography Facilities, June Gibbs Brown, Inspector General, MAY MM OEI-05-92-00300.

11. Policy Guidance Help System (PGHS), fda.gov/Mammography Quality Standards Act and Program/PGHS/Quality Assurance/Equipment/Quality Control Tests Other Than Annual. Accessed December 9, 2016.

12. Policy Guidance Help System (PGHS), fda.gov/Mammography Quality Standards Act and Program/PGHS/Quality Assurance/Equipment/Other Modalities Quality Control Tests. Accessed December 9, 2016.

13. ACR 2016 Digital Quality Control Manual Mammography manual/acr.org

14. ACR website: acr.org/Quality and Safety/Accreditation/ Mammography/Mammography Accreditation Program Requirements.

15. Policy Guidance Help System (PGHS), fda.gov/Mammography Quality Standards Act and Program/PGHS/Quality Assurance/General/Responsible Individuals for Quality Assurance Program.

16. Policy Guidance Help System (PGHS), fda.gov/Mammography Quality Standards Act and Program/PGHS/Quality Assurance/General/Medical Physicist Responsibilities.

17. The American Registry of Radiologic Technologists 2017 Post-Primary Discipline Handbook/Mammography. Accessed December 9, 2016.

18. Papp J. *Quality Management in the Imaging Sciences*. 4th ed. St. Louis, Missouri: Mosby/Elsevier; 2010.

19. Assessment of Display Performance for Medical Imaging Systems © 2005 by American Association of Physicists in Medicine One Physics Ellipse College Park, MD 20740-3846 /AAPM On-Line Report No. 03/American Association of Physicists in Medicine Task Group 18 Imaging Informatics Subcommittee.

20. Policy Guidance Help System (PGHS) fda.org.

21. Gray JE. Use of the SMPTE test pattern in picture archiving and communications systems. *J Digit Imaging*. 1992; 5(1):54–58.

22. Policy Guidance Help System (PGHS): fda.gov/Mammography Quality Standards Act and Program/PGHS/Mammography Equipment Evaluation.

23. Parikh J, Fanus D. Implementing digital quality control in a breast center. *J Am Coll Radiol*. 2004;1(11), 854–860. doi:10.1016/j.jacr.2004.05.006

24. American College of Radiology (ACR). *Mammography Quality Control Manual*. Reston, VA: American College of Radiology Committee on Quality Assurance in Mammography; 1999.

25. Department of Health and Human Services, Food and Drug Administration. 21 CFR Parts 16 and 900 Quality Mammography Standards, Final Rule (Tuesday, October 28, 1997).

26. Minigh J. Quality assurance in digital mammography. *Radiol Technol*. 2008;79(5).

27. Jacobson DR. *Mammography, Physics, Instrumentation, and Quality Control*. Blackwell Science; 2001.

28. Pisano ED, Yaffee MJ, Kuzmiak CM. *Digital Mammography*; 2004.

29. Koran N. Digital imaging: understanding image sharpness part 1: Introduction to resolution and MTF curves. Available at: http://www.normankoren.com/Tutorials/MTF.html. Accessed June 26, 2010.

30. Andolina VF, Lillè SL. *Mammographic Image. A Practical Guide*. 3rd ed. Philadelphia, PA: Wolters Kluwer; 2010.

31. Yaffe MJ, et al. Quality Control for Digital Mammography: Part II. Recommendations from the ACRIN DMIST Trial. *Med Phys*. 2006;33(3).

32. ACR-AAPM-SIIM Practice Parameter for Determinants of Image Quality in Digital Mammography (American College of Radiology) Amended 2014 (Resolution 39)*.

33. Burgess AE, Kang H. Incomplete skin representation in digital mammograms. *Med Phys*. 2004;31:2834–2838.

34. Goo JM, et al. Effect of monitor luminance and ambient light on observer performance in soft-copy reading of digital chest radiographs. *Radiology*. 2004;232:762–766.

35. National Electrical Manufacturers Association. *Digital Imaging and Communications in Medicine (DICOM) Part 14: Grayscale Standard Display Function*.

36. Krupinski EA, Flynn M, Hirschorn DS. *IT Reference Guide for the Practicing Radiologist*. Reston, VA: American College of Radiology; 2013.

37. Norweck JT, et al. ACR-AAPM-SIIM technical standard for electronic practice of medical imaging. *J Digit Imaging*. 2013;26:38–52.

38. Silverstein LD, et al. Paradigm for achieving color-reproduction accuracy in LCDs for medical imaging. *J Soc Imag Display*. 2012;20:53–62.

39. Andriole KP, et al. ACR-AAPM-SIIM practice guidelines for digital radiography. *J Digit Imaging*. 2013;26:26–37

40. Kanal KM, et al. ACR-SIIM practice guidelines for digital radiography. *J Digit Imaging*. 2013;26:26–37.

41. Practice Guideline for Determinants of Image Quality in Digital Mammography (American College of Radiology) 2007 (Resolution 35)*.

42. Mammography Quality Standards Act and Program: fda.org, MQSA Insights/Printers and the Evolution of Mammography. Accessed November 18, 2015.

43. Mammography Quality Standards Act and Program: fda. org, MQSA Insights/EQUIP: Enhancing Quality Using the Inspection Program, October 21, 2016/ A Message from the Director, Division of Mammography Quality Standards (DMQS): EQUIP, December 2, 2016.

44. Routine Quality Control Tests for Full-Field Digital Mammography Systems Equipment Report 1303: Fourth Edition, October 2013/NHS Cancer Screening Programmes (The National Office of the NHS Cancer Screening Programmes is operated by Public Health England).

45. FDA American College of Radiology. *ACR Practice Guideline for the Performance of Screening and Diagnostic Mammography*; 2008 (Resolution 24)*. Available at: http//www.org/SecondaryMainMenuCategories/quality_safety/guidelines/breast/ Screening/Diagnostic.aspx. Accessed September 6, 2010.

46. Policy Guidance Help System (PGHS): fda.gov/Mammography Quality Standards Act and Program/PGHS/Quality Assurance/Equipment/Repeat Reject Analysis and Fixer Retention-Quarterly Quality Control Tests.

Diagnostic Procedures and Breast Cancer Treatment

Diagnostic Procedures

17

Objectives

- Describe the procedure for preoperative wire localization and specimen radiography

- Describe the procedure and identify specialized equipment used in cyst aspiration and pneumocystography

- Explain the ductography procedure and its mammographic presentation

- Gain an appreciation for FNAC because it is not expensive and is quick and easy to perform. Unfortunately, it is not widely used; why?

Key Terms

- ductography
- fine-needle aspiration cytology (FNAC)
- preoperative wire localization
- sonographic imaging

INTRODUCTION

Many diagnostic procedures are helpful in the diagnosis of breast disease. When these ancillary procedures are combined with mammography, diagnosis becomes timely and more accurate. The 20-year survivability for tumors less than 1.5 cm is 88% and 71% if 1.5 to 2 cm in size.[1] Earlier detection is always better.

All of the procedures in this chapter can be performed online, meaning they can be performed during the same appointment as a diagnostic mammogram, except for preoperative wire localization. Online procedures reduce the patient's stress level because she does not wait for her next appointment and battery of tests, rather everything is done immediately; there is no time for her to worry. Working online is done at the discretion of the radiologist.

The procedures and protocols described in this chapter are used at the Elizabeth Wende Breast Clinic in Rochester, New York. Each facility and radiologist has a unique protocol to fit the needs of their patients, but the basic procedures will be similar to those described in this chapter.

This chapter covers the most common additional diagnostic procedures. Other procedures, such as stereotactic core biopsy, MRI, and problem-solving mammography, are covered in other chapters in this book.

 PREOPERATIVE WIRE LOCALIZATION

With the advent of screening mammography, **preoperative wire localization** of nonpalpable lesions became a necessity. Every surgeon today recognizes the need for preoperative localization under mammographic guidance. In addition to directing the surgeon to the area requiring biopsy, wire localization helps the surgeon excise a smaller specimen. With four out of five biopsies proving benign, the patient achieves better cosmetic results if her lesion is localized preoperatively and a smaller amount of breast tissue is removed.

Localization also assists the pathologist. Not only does a radiograph of the specimen verify removal of the lesion, but it also localizes the suspected lesion within the specimen. The pathologist does not have to search through an abundance of extra breast tissue to find it.

Preoperative wire localization is usually performed on a nonpalpable lesion or a suspicious area that was found mammographically. Because the surgeon cannot feel the suspicious area, the radiologist assists the surgeon by implanting a wire in the suspected tissue using radiographic guidance. This wire guides the surgeon to the tissue that needs to be biopsied.

Patient Preparation for Mammographic Wire Localization

Some surgeons may prescribe premedication for their patient to help reduce her anxiety over the wire localization and surgical procedures. Because the patient's active participation is usually required during the localization process and because many medications cause hypotension, which makes the patient susceptible to fainting,[2] it is preferable that she not be premedicated until *after* the wire localization procedure has been completed.[3,4]

Preoperative wire localizations can be performed at radiology facilities that are not physically connected or adjacent to the hospital or clinic where the surgery will be performed. When the localization is performed at this type of facility, the patient should be informed so she can make appropriate arrangements:

• She will leave the mammography facility and travel to another building where the surgery is to be performed; thus, she should have a companion with her who can drive her to the next location.

• She should wear a large, loose blouse that buttons down the front because she should not lift her arms over her head following the procedure to avoid loosening or moving the localization wire. Also, she will have a wire and dressing on her breast and will not be able to wear a bra immediately after the procedure.

• The patient should also be advised to wear dark blue slacks or skirt as a precaution because a blue dye (methylene blue) may be used during the procedure. In the rare event of an accidental drip, it will be less evident on her blue clothes.

Each step of the wire localization procedure should be explained to the patient. If a woman does not speak English or is hearing impaired, use of an interpreter or signer is recommended so that she can understand the procedure. Most facilities require a consent form be signed before performing any invasive procedure; after the procedure has been explained adequately, the patient can sign the form. More importantly, once the patient understands the procedure, she is usually more cooperative.

Because the procedure is stressful, it is possible that the patient will feel faint.[5] The technologist assisting with the wire localization should be compassionate and attentive to the patient's needs and keep a watchful eye on her condition. To prevent the patient from feeling faint, some radiologists position the patient so she cannot see the needle,[2,6,7] or the patient is given an eye shade to wear so she cannot see. If the patient does feel faint, she should be allowed to lie down and rest. Once she feels well enough, the procedure can continue at the discretion of the radiologist.

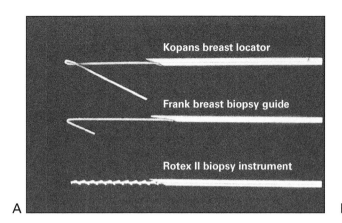

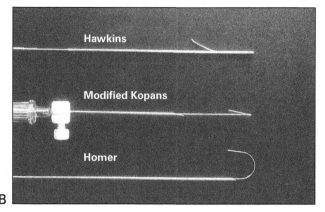

Figure 17-1

Examples of some of the needle/wire and needle/trocar sets used for preoperative wire localization of a mammographically detected lesion. **(A)** The Kopans, Frank, and Rotex II. **(B)** The Hawkins, Modified Kopans, and Homer breast localizers.

Equipment and Technique

Several needle/wire localization sets are on the market today (Figure 17-1). The Kopans,[6] Sadowsky, Urrutia,[8] Hawkins,[9] Frank,[10] and Homer[11] sets are some of the more popular commercially available combinations. These sets consist of a hollow needle through which a thin wire is inserted into the breast tissue. Some radiologists may prefer to customize their equipment, such as Wende Logan-Young, M.D. of the Elizabeth Wende Breast Clinic who sometimes uses the stiff inner trocar from a Rotex II Screw Needle Biopsy Instrument passed through a Cook Modified Kopans 21 gauge needle.[2] A hook wire set may be more useful in fatty tissue as trocars, which are straighter, do not grip adipose tissue as well. The straight screw trocars are more useful for denser, more fibrous breasts where the screw-type tip can better grip the tissue.

A stiffer wire or trocar is usually more helpful to the surgeon; its interior tip is easy to locate. If the surgeon moves the outer tip back and forth, she/he can feel the inner tip of the wire moving and can locate the lesion. This helps the surgeon make an incision that is closer to the inner tip, leaving a smaller scar. When the radiologist uses a wire that is not as stiff, the surgeon may need to cut where the wire enters the skin and follow it down to the lesion, leaving a larger scar (Figure 17-2).

When directed inward toward the patient's body (perpendicular to the chestwall), wires and trocars can migrate into the pectoral muscle. When the muscle contracts, its pumping motion can draw wires and trocars toward the muscle, perforating the thorax or pericardial sac.[12] Thus, the needle and wire are always placed *parallel* to the pectoral muscle, so that it cannot enter the muscle.

During the localization procedure, a narrow compression device (approximately 9 cm) is usually used. Patients find the smaller device less intimidating and more

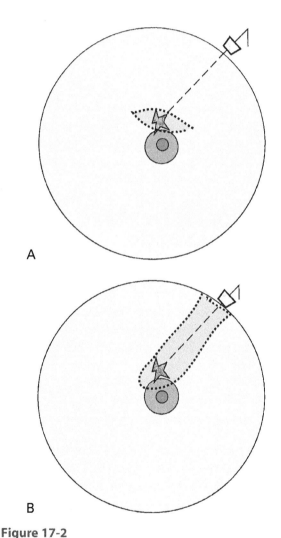

Figure 17-2

(A) The surgeon can feel the inner tip of the stiffer trocar/needle combination localization set. She/he removes a much smaller specimen by making an incision in the area of the lesion. **(B)** When using the thinner, more malleable wire localization set, the surgeon must incise where the needle enters the skin and dissect the tissue by following the wire to the lesion. This results in a larger specimen and also a larger postoperative scar.

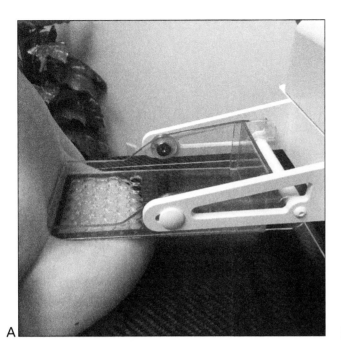 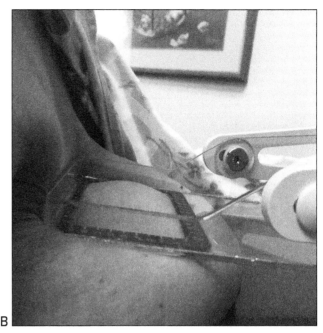

A

B

Figure 17-3
The two designs of localization compression devices. **(A)** The fenestrated compression device is usually found to be more beneficial during preoperative wire localization because the technologist can further compress the tissue in the questionable area, which permits the lesion to be visualized more clearly. **(B)** A localization compression device with a large cutout window produces pillowing of the tissue that results in three problems: (1) greater distance for the needle to travel to the lesion, (2) the protruding tissue not as firmly fixed, and (3) the questionable area less resolute because the breast tissue is thicker and uncompressed.

comfortable. Most equipment manufacturers provide some type of grid system on the compression device as a reference for identifying the location of the lesion on the image in relation to its location in the breast. This usually consists of lead numbers and letters embedded in the plastic to designate the anterior to posterior location (nipple to chestwall) and the lateral to medial location on the craniocaudal projection or superior to inferior location on the Lateral projection.

Most equipment manufacturers offer two designs of localization compression devices (Figure 17-3): one, which is perforated with a number of concentric holes large enough for a needle hub to pass through but small enough to prevent the tissue from bulging out through the holes, and the second, which has only one large opening. The perforated compression device provides compression of the abnormal area and, because it is narrower, provides compression only at the specified area. Thus, the characteristics of the lesion are often better visualized than on routine images using the full-size compression device. The compression device with the single large opening is not thought to work as well.[2] During compression, the breast tissue "pillows up" through the hole; therefore, the area to be localized is less resolute. Additionally because the part of the breast where the region of interest (ROI) is located is not compressed, when the radiologist inserts the needle

set, it is more difficult for the radiologist to direct the needle accurately. Also, the needle must pass through more tissue to reach the lesion.

Localization Procedure

The Routine Localization

Preoperative localization of a nonpalpable breast lesion is performed by a radiologist, with the assistance of a mammography technologist. The radiologist uses mammographic x-ray guidance to position the needle and then inserts the hook wire in the area of the detected lesion. The technologist's responsibilities include setting the x-ray technique, positioning the patient, and assisting the radiologist throughout the procedure.

Prior to beginning the procedure the radiologist reviews the images to determine the approach to each patient's lesion (how the technologist should position the patient for the procedure). Each radiologist will have his/her own protocol for performing localizations, and most radiologists use a technique similar to the one described in the following paragraphs, with the patient's breast minimally compressed and needle insertion parallel to the pectoral muscle; however, some use a more "freehand" approach.[13]

Before beginning the localization procedure, the technologist should assemble a basic prep tray for the radiologist

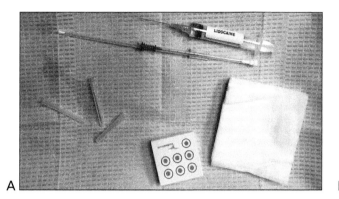
A

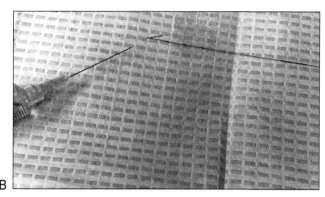
B

Figure 17-4
Prep tray. **(A)** A basic wire localization prep tray for the radiologist. **(B)** A close up of the hook wire next to a 25-gauge straight needle.

(Figure 17-4) and should make certain that accessory devices are installed on the mammography machine and that the settings on the machine are adjusted for this procedure. When performing localizations, she must confirm that the automatic compression release on the machine has been deactivated so that it does not inadvertently pull the localization needle/wire out of the breast. During the localization procedure, the technologist should always manually raise up the compression device after each exposure.

After the patient is seated (Figure 17-5), position her breast on the image receptor support device (IRSD). The patient must sit with her breast compressed throughout the procedure, so compression should be firm but not uncomfortable. Place a small lead BB on the compression device at the approximate site of the lesion, mark the skin with ink at the center of an aperture adjacent to the lead marker, and take a scout image (Figure 17-6). The ink is important because if the patient inadvertently moves between the scout image and needle placement, you will know because the inked area will also shift. From the scout image, the radiologist can see the proximity of the lead marker to the location of the lesion. The needle is inserted through the hole in the compression device closest to the position of the lesion, or at the intersection of the letters and numbers.

The skin over the lesion is cleansed with an alcohol or Betadine wipe, and the radiologist introduces the needle through the skin perpendicular to the IRSD. The needle should pass beyond the lesion, as it may retract slightly once the compression is released. A check image should be taken before removing compression. When taking this image, the radiologist and technologist should try to have the shadow of the hub superimposed directly over the insertion point of the needle; this avoids confusion as to the exact path of the needle (Figure 17-7A). If this image indicates that the needle is in the correct location over the lesion, the compression is carefully lifted, making certain that the hub of the needle doesn't catch on the edge of

the compression device. Next, the breast is compressed at a right angle to the original image and another exposure is made. Again use moderate compression as the patient must sit with her breast compressed until this image is reviewed by the radiologist. This second check image verifies the depth of the needle, so the radiologist knows to either withdraw or insert it further toward the lesion. If the needle is repositioned, another check image is taken to verify its position before the hook wire is introduced.

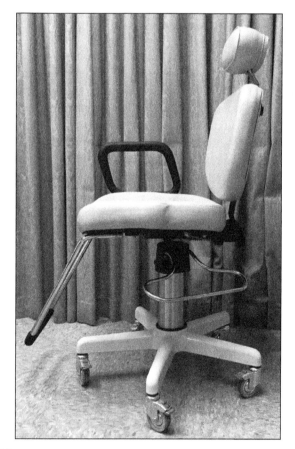

Figure 17-5
A mammography positioning chair offers stability to the patient and options for positioning to the technologist.

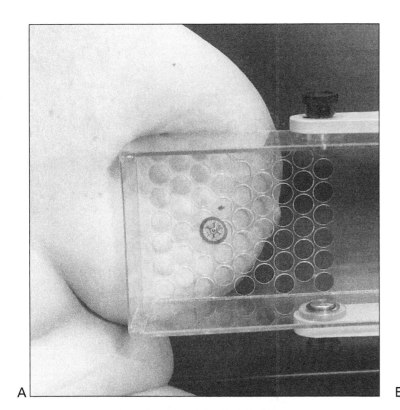

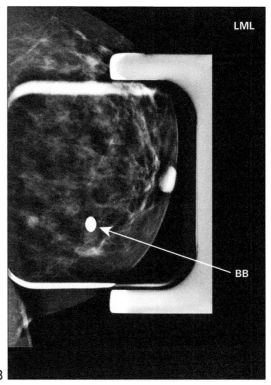

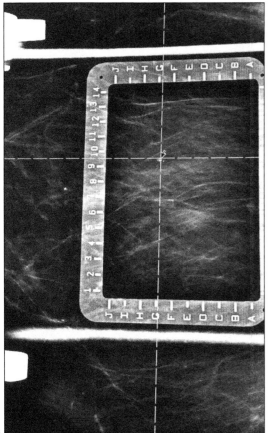

Figure 17-6

Two designs of wire localization compression devices. **(A)** The technologist marks the center of one opening with an *ink dot* and places a lead BB in front of one of the fenestrated compression device's openings. **(B)** The lead BB is visible on the LML scout image indicating the distance between the opening closest to the BB and the location of the lesion. Any migration of the *ink dot* indicates the patient moved. **(C)** The compression device with the cutout uses a grid pattern of lead letters and numbers to ascertain the exact location of the ROI. The crosshair device indicates the location of the ROI is at the intersection of the *lines*.

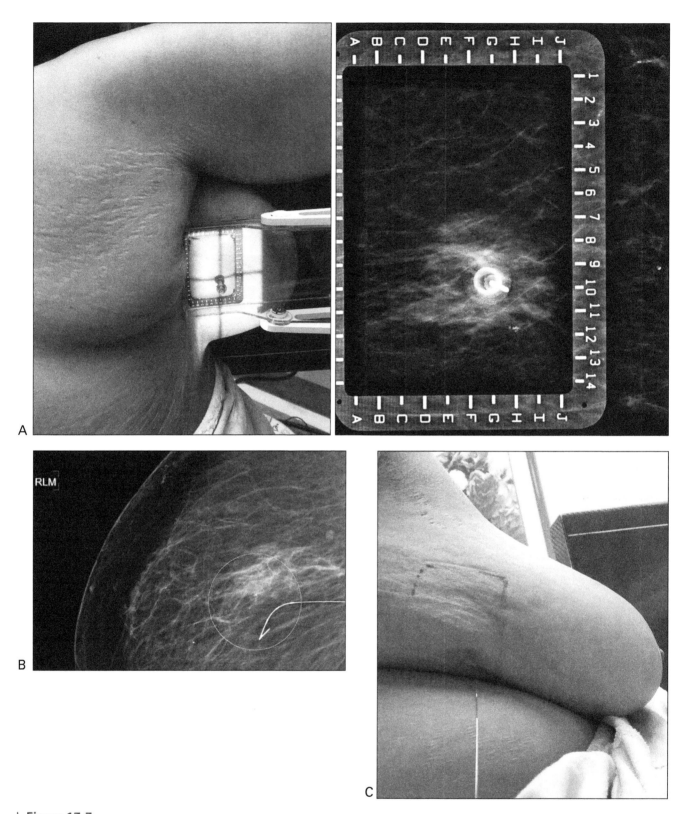

Figure 17-7
The scout image identified the exact location of the area to be biopsied. **(A)** The wire localization set is inserted perpendicular to the IRSD, or parallel to the chestwall. **(B)** After the hook wire has been deployed, images are taken to show the relationship of the **tip of** the wire to the ROI. **(C)** The hook wire anchors into the breast tissue. The wire that protrudes from the breast is taped to the skin. The patient is taken to the operating room.

At this point, some radiologists and surgeons inject methylene blue dye as a marker for locating the lesion in case the needle or trocar becomes dislodged. Before injecting the dye, add 0.1 cc of air to 0.1 cc of methylene blue in the syringe and shake it; the air identifies the dye's position on follow-up images. Also, a small amount of lidocaine solution can be injected to anesthetize the area, if the patient is not allergic.

The wire or trocar is now introduced into the breast tissue. Depending on which localization needle set is used, and the radiologist's preference, the needle may or may not be removed. Now, two more images at 90° angles should be taken to verify the final position of the wire or trocar in relation to the lesion (Figure 17-7B). These final images should be sent with the patient to the surgical unit. The protruding wire or trocar is then covered and the covering is taped to the patient's skin (Figure 17-7C).

Positioning for a Routine Localization

During localization, the site of the lesion determines the position and angle of the breast and compression. For needle placement, the breast should always be compressed in the position in which the lesion is closest to the compression device. This ensures that the needle travels the shortest distance from skin to lesion, leaving less room for error. This is helpful to the radiologist as there is less chance of needle misalignment, and helpful to the surgeon because less dissection will be necessary to find the end of the needle within the breast.

In approximately 90% of patients undergoing preoperative wire localization for a nonpalpable lesion, the abnormality is visible on both routine (CC and MLO) mammographic views. An additional Lateral view should be taken to avoid confusion over the exact location of the lesion. When the lesion is visible on two right-angled views, it is usually localized in the following manner (Figure 17-8):

- If the lesion is in the upper half of the breast, position the breast and C-arm for a CC view, compress, and introduce the needle from cephalad to caudad.
- If the lesion is in the lower inner quadrant, introduce the needle from the medial side of the breast, which is compressed in the ML position, with the compression device centered over the lower half of the breast.
- If the lesion is located in the lower outer quadrant, compress the breast in an LM position, with the compression device compressing the lower half of the breast, and introduce the needle from the lateral side of the breast.
- Rarely, a caudocranial view (FB or reverse CC) may be indicated to localize a centrally located mass in the lower half of the breast.

By adjusting the position of the breast and angle of compression, you can make certain that the needle travels the shortest distance from the skin to the lesion, which leaves less margin for error.

Case Study **17-1**

Refer to Figure 17-8 and the text and respond to the following questions:

1. Why are CC and MLO views not sufficient to locate a lesion?

2. What views are necessary to pinpoint the location of a lesion?

3. Almost three-fourths of all lesions are located in the upper half of the breast. For the preoperative wire localization procedure, how would the patient be positioned?

4. If a lesion is located at 7:00 o'clock in the right breast, what position places the lesion in the shortest skin-to-lesion distance?

Localizing a Lesion Visible on Only One Standard View

If a lesion is visible on only one of the two standard views, it can still be localized. Although some mammographers use complex stereotactic computerized systems for localization of these lesions, Evans and Cade reported that the "standard localizing technique may be as accurate as the stereotactic technique."[14]

To localize the lesion, select the view on which the lesion was originally detected. Then, with the nipple in profile, take two additional radiographs: one with the C-arm angled 15° from the original view and the second with the C-arm angled 15° in the opposite direction of that view. Be careful not to twist or roll the breast tissue when obtaining these views. From these three images, select the two in which the lesion is most identifiable. The lesion must be visible on at least two of these images or it cannot be localized.

To determine the lesion's exact position, perform the following for each of the two angled views that were chosen: on a sketch of the breast, draw the position of the IRSD for the first view. On the image, measure the distance of the lesion to the nipple; mark that point on the sketch. Draw a line through that point perpendicular to the IRSD. The lesion must be located somewhere on this line. Repeat these computations for the second image; the lesion lies at the intersection of the two lines (Figure 17-9).

The localization procedure for a lesion seen on only one standard view is the same as it would be for a standard localization with one exception—the two views that will be taken during the procedure will not be at right angles, but more likely will be at a 15° to 30° angle from each other.

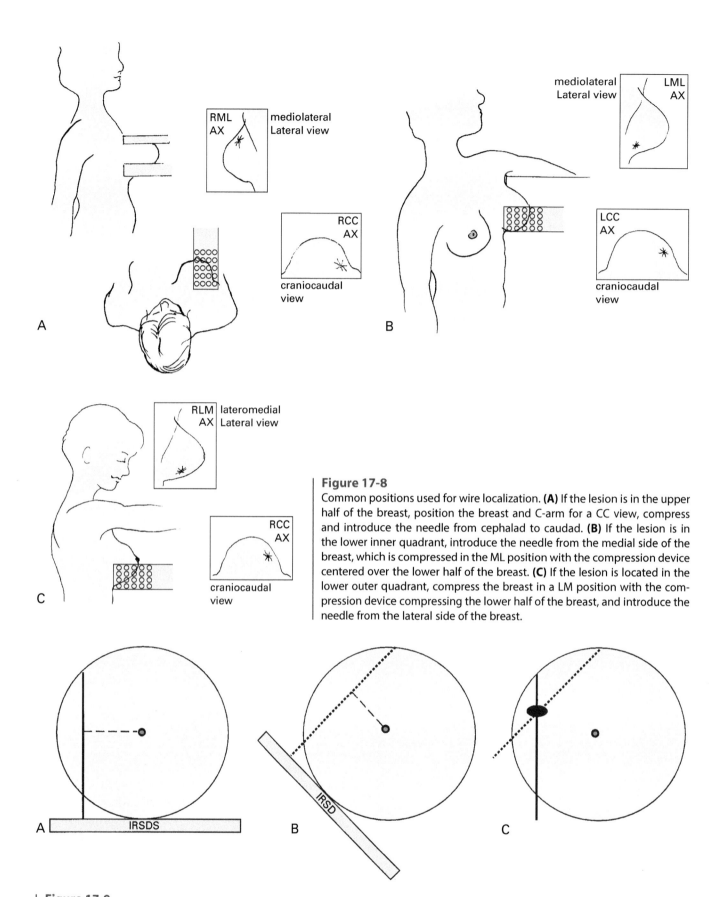

Figure 17-8
Common positions used for wire localization. **(A)** If the lesion is in the upper half of the breast, position the breast and C-arm for a CC view, compress and introduce the needle from cephalad to caudad. **(B)** If the lesion is in the lower inner quadrant, introduce the needle from the medial side of the breast, which is compressed in the ML position with the compression device centered over the lower half of the breast. **(C)** If the lesion is located in the lower outer quadrant, compress the breast in a LM position with the compression device compressing the lower half of the breast, and introduce the needle from the lateral side of the breast.

Figure 17-9
(A) The distance from the nipple to the lesion is measured on one of the views (*dashed line*). The lesion must lie on the line drawn through the point perpendicular to the IRSD (*solid line*). **(B)** The distance from the nipple to the lesion is measured on the other view (*dashed line*). The lesion must lie along the line drawn through the point perpendicular to the IRSD (*dotted line*). **(C)** The location of the lesion is determined to be at the intersection of the dotted and solid lines. (Modified from Logan-Young W, Hoffman NY. *Breast Cancer: A Practical Guide to Diagnosis, Vol. 1: Procedures.* Rochester, NY: Mt. Hope; 1994.)

Localizing a Lesion Located in a Duct

If a lesion is identified and is visible only through ductography, it can be localized in the usual manner, with one addition. Before the localization procedure begins, ductography is again performed using a mixture of equal parts of methylene blue and contrast agent. The contrast agent identifies the lesion localized on the mammogram for the radiologist, and the methylene blue indicates the correct duct to the surgeon.

Ultrasound or Palpation Localization

Whenever possible, localizing a lesion under sonographic guidance or through clinical palpation is preferable to localizing it mammographically. These methods are faster, so it is easier for the patient to tolerate the discomfort. If the lesion can be localized through palpation, localize it in the usual way with the localization needle, the dye, lidocaine, and the wire, with one exception to the procedure: x-ray images at each step are not necessary—only the needle's final position is verified mammographically. Infrequently, the surgeon can palpate a lesion but may prefer to localize it because she/he is uncertain whether the lesion will be palpable through surgical gloves.

Occasionally, a lesion is clinically ill defined, yet ultrasound reveals a definite area of attenuation. In such instances, locate the lesion sonographically by holding the transducer over the lesion. After cleansing the area adjacent to the transducer with alcohol or Betadine, place the needle in the lesion using ultrasound as a guide. Again, the steps of the procedure remain the same, except that only the needle's final position is verified mammographically.

Localizing a lesion clinically or under sonographic guidance works well with lesions in the lower half of a large breast because mammographic guidance is more awkward and unwieldy in this location.

SPECIMEN RADIOGRAPHY

The specimen should always be radiographed after the biopsy to ensure the lesion was removed.[2,15] The radiologist should have the original diagnostic images to compare them with the specimen radiograph and should show them to the pathologist to make sure she/he knows what to look for.

Some hospital pathology departments or diagnostic radiology departments use a small x-ray unit that has a soft x-ray beam and is specifically designed for radiography of biopsy specimens (Figure 17-10A). If a specimen imager is not available, a specimen can be radiographed using the mammography machine (Figure 17-10B). To x-ray the

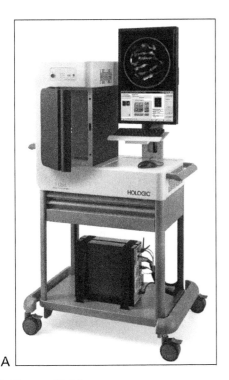
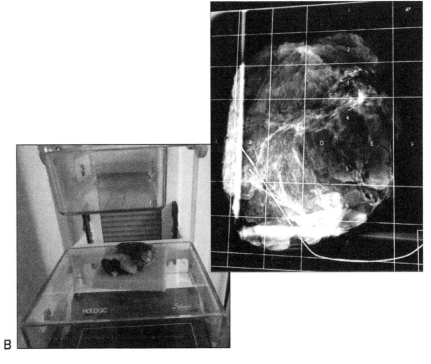

Figure 17-10
Imaging the specimen. **(A)** A dedicated specimen imager. This can be used in the operating room. (Courtesy Hologic, Inc., and affiliates.) **(B)** Imaging the specimen in the mammography room. Use the magnification mode. Note the grid pattern on the x-ray for easy identification of the location of the ROI for the pathologist.

specimen with the mammography machine, use 1.5 to 2 times magnification, coned down to the specimen's size. The specimen is compressed to prevent the appearance of a "pseudomass" caused by compiled tissue. The lesion should be circled on the image, and the radiograph should be sent to the pathologist with the specimen.

FOLLOW-UP ON PATHOLOGY REPORTS

According to the Mammography Quality Standards Act (MQSA), mammography facilities must attempt to procure a pathology report when a biopsy is recommended. Occasionally, you may have a patient whose mammogram shows a nonpalpable lesion suggestive of cancer, yet the pathology report is normal. When this happens, Wende Logan-Young suggests a protocol to maintain optimum care of the patient (Figure 17-11). She first reviews the radiograph of the specimen to be certain the lesion was removed. If the lesion is not identified with certainty on the specimen radiograph, the patient returns for a repeat mammogram 2 months after the surgery. If the lesion is still visible mammographically, the patient is advised to undergo a second biopsy. However, if postsurgical changes obscure the biopsy area, the mammogram is repeated in 4 months, and again at 6 month intervals for the next 2 years until the lesion can be identified, and rebiopsy recommended.

If the lesion is discernible on the radiograph of the biopsy specimen, Logan-Young reviews the excised tissue with the pathologist. With a large biopsy specimen, only a portion of the tissue is submitted in paraffin blocks, while the rest remains in formalin. The tissue in formalin is x-rayed first to determine if the lesion can be identified within it. If so, it is given to the pathologist to submit in paraffin for further examination. If the lesion is not in the tissue that remains in formalin, the paraffin blocks are x-rayed. If the lesion is in one of the blocks, the block is then submitted to the pathologist for more slides.

Because most pathology departments keep the tissue in formalin for only a short period, the mammography facility should obtain pathology reports quickly.

ULTRASOUND

Indications and Contraindications for Ultrasonography of the Breast

Sonographic imaging of the breast can help determine the nature of many problematic findings. Ultrasound's primary contribution is in its ability to distinguish a cyst from a solid lesion. Ultrasound also helps the radiologist evaluate palpable areas of thickening or lumps in dense breast tissue, and it is valuable in assessing a woman with an exceedingly posterior palpable mass with a normal mammogram. Ultrasound is helpful in determining the nature of the following problematic findings:

• Fluid—cyst, intracystic lesion, abscess, hematoma, oil cyst, and silicone gel leaks in patients with implants
• Solid mass—smoothly outlined masses such as benign tumors, hamartomas, lymph nodes, smoothly outlined cancer, and irregularly outlined masses

Although ultrasonography is a helpful adjunctive tool when used with mammography, it is not as sensitive as mammography and should not be used as a replacement for a mammogram. Ultrasound does not image the fine calcifications that accompany 35% to 45% of breast cancers, a particularly important marker for identifying cancer in younger women. Only when examining dense breast tissue does ultrasonography come close to mammography's accuracy in detecting hidden cancer.[16-19] Ultrasound is often recommended as an addition to routine mammographic screening for patients with dense breast tissue (BIRADS C and D categories).

The Basics of Breast Ultrasonography Interpretation

Ultrasonography of the breast should be performed by the radiologist, an ultrasound technologist, or a specially trained mammography technologist. Because this text is designed for mammography technologists, the basic physics of ultrasound may not be familiar to the reader. However, the use of ultrasound for breast disease diagnosis is not uncommon. The following paragraph offers a basic understanding of the images produced during breast ultrasonography.

On an ultrasound image, fluid appears as a dark circumscribed area; a solid mass shows internal echoes, which appear as white specks within the area. When using ultrasound to determine if a lesion is a solid mass or a fluid-filled cyst, the ultrasonographer should watch the monitor carefully as she increases the gain setting of the unit. If the lesion is a cyst, echoes appear first in the part of the cyst closest to the transducer. With a soft tissue mass, a sprinkling of white echoes distributed throughout the mass will suddenly appear (Figure 17-12). This is a crucial, but sometimes subtle, sign of possible cancer.

Ultrasound cannot determine if a solid mass is cancerous or benign. Some cancers, particularly papillary adenocarcinoma and medullary carcinoma, can resemble a smoothly outlined benign mass on ultrasound.

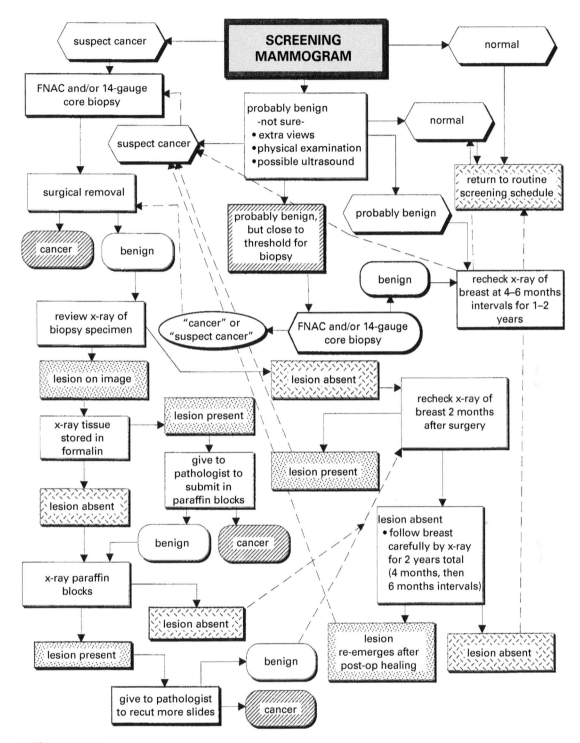

Figure 17-11
Flowchart showing recommended follow-up of a screening patient with a nonpalpable lesion. (Reprinted from Logan-Young W, Hoffman NY. *Breast Cancer: A Practical Guide to Diagnosis, Vol. I Procedures.* Rochester, NY: Mt. Hope; 1994, with permission.)

▌▌ CYST ASPIRATION

A radiologist or surgeon may decide to aspirate a patient's cyst if it is large and painful or if it conceals an area of breast tissue on the mammogram that is significant for an accurate diagnosis. Cyst aspiration can be performed under ultrasound guidance if the cyst is not palpable or under clinical guidance for larger, palpable cysts.

Each physician has his/her personal protocol for performing an aspiration, which is a simple procedure.

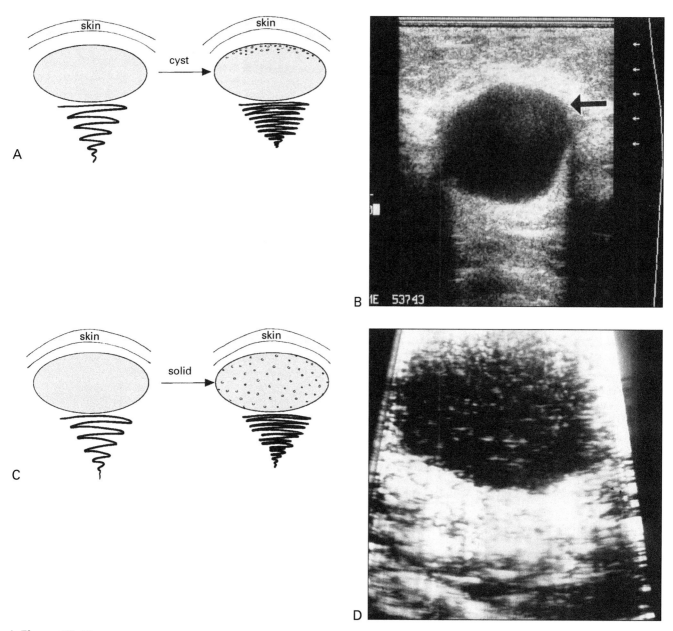

Figure 17-12
During ultrasonography, if the lesion is a cyst, echoes will appear first in the part of the cyst closest to the transducer **(A, B)**. With a soft tissue mass, a sprinkling of echoes distributed throughout the entire mass will suddenly appear **(C, D)**.

A butterfly or standard needle attached to a syringe is inserted through the alcohol-cleansed skin into the cyst. The physician or an assistant applies negative pressure by pulling back on the syringe plunger to withdraw the fluid from the cyst (Figure 17-13). The needle is then removed, and pressure is applied to the area for 3 to 5 minutes to reduce the chance of hematoma.

To reduce the patient's discomfort, a smaller gauge needle such as a 21 gauge butterfly can be used. Occasionally, a larger gauge (19 gauge or 20 gauge) needle is necessary if the cyst is filled with thicker, more viscous fluid.

Cystic fluid that is aspirated usually does not need to be sent for cytologic analysis, but the radiologist may wish to have it assessed under the following circumstances:

1. If the cyst refills within 1 month after aspiration, the fluid from a second aspiration should be sent for analysis. An intracystic cancer or a papilloma can cause fluid to reaccumulate quickly.
2. If the fluid appears to contain blood.
3. If an intracystic lesion is discernible on ultrasound or on a pneumocystogram.
4. If a solitary, palpable cyst is identifiable on a postmenopausal patient.

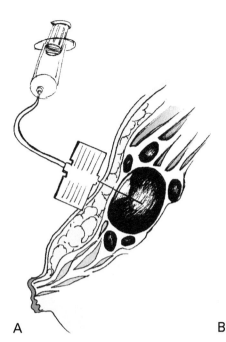

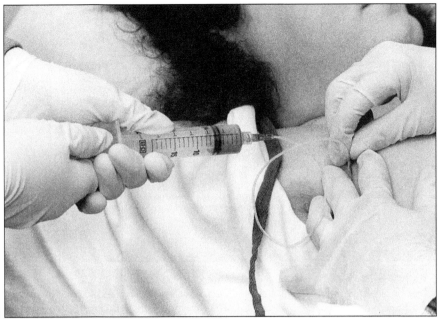

A   B

Figure 17-13
Cyst aspiration. **(A)** A butterfly or standard needle attached to a syringe is inserted through the alcohol-cleansed skin to the cyst. **(B)** The physician or an assistant applies negative pressure by pulling back on the syringe plunger to withdraw the fluid from the cyst.

Pneumocystography

The decision to perform pneumocystography is made on the same basis as the decision to send cyst aspirate for cytological evaluation. Pneumocystography provides an image with better vizualization of the cyst wall than may be obtainable with ultrasound.

The procedure is performed in conjunction with cyst aspiration. Before the needle is withdrawn from the cyst after an aspiration, the syringe with the cystic fluid is detached from the needle. A syringe filled with air, equal to the amount of fluid that was withdrawn from the cyst, is reattached to the needle, and the air is injected into the cyst. The needle is withdrawn, and a CC and Lateral view mammogram are taken (Figure 17-14). The air does not cause discomfort to the patient and is reabsorbed into the breast tissue within a week. If the patient does feel discomfort following the procedure, some of the air can be reaspirated from the cyst.

▌ DUCTOGRAPHY

Ductography is also known as galactography or contrast-assisted mammography. It outlines the ductal system, provides information on the reason for production of nipple discharge, and locates the site within the duct where the discharge is produced.

Ductography is indicated in patients who have a unilateral spontaneous discharge from the nipple that is either bloody

or clear and watery. Bloody or clear, watery discharge can be associated with a ductal carcinoma that is mammographically invisible; however, a papilloma is more frequently the cause (Figure 17-15). The ductogram can help the radiologist determine the cause and location of the discharge.

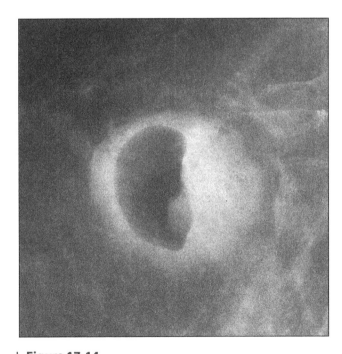

Figure 17-14
This pneumocystogram was performed to verify an intracystic lesion seen on ultrasonography. On biopsy, this was proven to be an intracystic cancer.

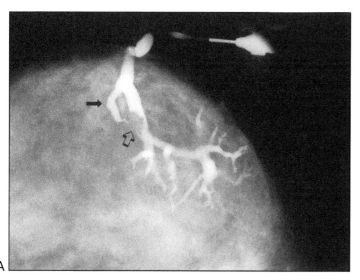
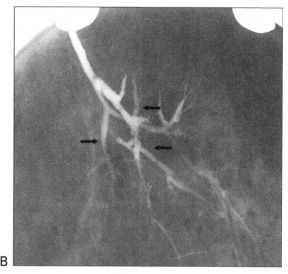

A B

Figure 17-15
Ductogram images. **(A)** A typical dilated duct associated with a sessile papilloma (*open arrow*). Without the ductogram, the surgeon might probe and dissect the wrong branch of the duct (*closed arrow*). **(B)** A magnification view ductogram visualized filling defects (*arrows*), which proved to be an intraductal carcinoma on open surgical biopsy.

Case Study **17-2**

Refer to Figures 17-15 to 17-17 and the text and respond to the following questions.

1. What is another common term used to denote ductography?

2. Why do we perform a ductogram?

3. Who performs the ductogram?

4. What type of x-ray imaging is done during a ductogram?

Ductography is not indicated in patients who have a bilateral discharge from the nipple, or discharge that is present only if expressed from the breast. Constant expression of discharge stimulates the breast to secrete fluids within the tissue and ducts, which compounds the condition. Bilateral discharge is generally caused by hormonal changes or is drug related. Many medications, such as cardiovascular and antihypertensive drugs, can produce or exacerbate cystic disease, which may produce a bilateral discharge.

Ductography Equipment

During ductography, the duct that produces the discharge is located and cannulated with a small gauge cannula. Several cannulae and kits are available that are suitable for

ductography, but the smaller gauged cannulae work best because they facilitate placement in the duct—a larger gauge makes cannulation more difficult.

Two of the more popular types of cannulae are the straight cannula and the right-angle–bent cannula. Examples of these include the Ranfac end-port 30 gauge sialographic straight cannula and the Jabczenski end-port 30 gauge right-angle ductographic cannula (Figure 17-16). Each of these has distinct advantages. The Ranfac cannula is longer and can drop further into the duct; therefore, the pressure of injecting the contrast makes it less likely to be expelled from the duct. Another advantage of its length is that it can be used to cannulate ducts in a deeply inverted nipple. In most instances, the Jabczenski is more convenient to use because its right angle can be taped into place after cannulation.

Other equipment necessary for a ductogram includes a nonionic contrast agent, a small syringe (generally less than 5 cc), a 19 gauge needle for extracting the contrast agent, cytology slides and fixative, tape, magnifying glasses, and a bright light to illuminate the nipple area. A nursing pad is used as a dressing following the procedure.

Ductography Procedure

In most facilities that perform ductography, the radiologist performs the procedure. However, the technologist can perform the procedure under a radiologist's supervision.[2]

Before the duct can be cannulated, a small amount of fluid must be elicited from the nipple to locate the correct duct (Figure 17-17A). The fluid can usually be

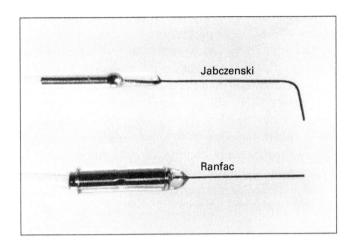

Figure 17-16
The Ranfac end-port, 30-gauge, disposable, sialographic straight cannula **(bottom)** and the Jabczenski end-port, 30-gauge, right-angle ductographic cannula **(top)** are typical of those commonly used for ductography.

expressed by stroking the breast with firm pressure from the outer perimeter of the breast toward the nipple, covering all quadrants until a drop of discharge is visible. If eliciting discharge is difficult, ask the patient to try this herself; she knows how much pressure to apply without discomfort.

Once the fluid has been expressed and the duct has been identified, a slide of the fluid can be made to send to a cytology lab. Gently touching a slide to the expressed discharge will cause some of the fluid to adhere to the slide. This is smeared with a second slide, and fixed in the manner recommended by the cytology lab.

Next, the cannula is inserted into the duct from which the discharge was expressed (Figure 17-17B and C). The patient should be lying on her back during cannulation. Because the ductal opening is small and difficult to perceive, a bright light and high-powered magnifying glasses are used to better visualize the area. Once found, it usually

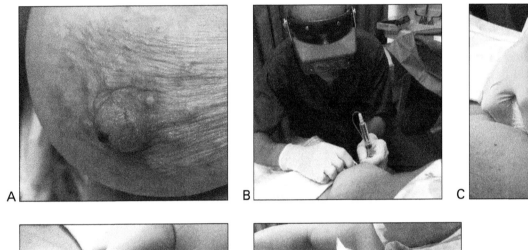

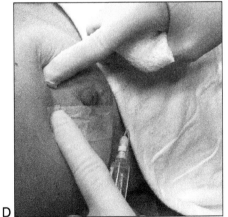

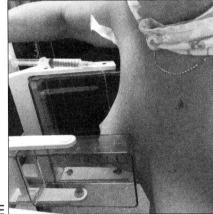

Figure 17-17
A ductogram procedure. **(A)** Elicit a drop of discharge fluid to see which duct to cannulate. **(B, C)** The radiologist needs a magnifying device to see the miniscule opening on the nipple. The patient lies supine as the radiologist inserts the cannula into the duct. **(D)** Inject 1 cc or less of an iodine contrast agent. Then tape the cannula in place in case more contrast needs to be injected. **(E)** Magnified CC and Lateral images are taken. Apply **minimal** compression to the breast so the contrast material is not expelled. Note the syringe resting on the magnification stand platform.

takes less than a minute to cannulate the duct; however, small ducts or ones located in difficult to cannulate areas (such as a fissure within the nipple) may take much longer. Once the cannula passes beyond the sphincter of the orifice, it will suddenly drop into the duct's lactiferous sinus. The cannula must be placed here, as the contrast will not flow retrogradely until it passes the sphincter.

The contrast agent is now injected into the duct. Because the patient is lying on her back, gravity helps the contrast agent flow easily into the duct. If the duct is filled with fluid, the contrast agent will replace it, and fluid the same color as the discharge may flow out of the ductal opening. Because the cannula gauge is so small, it is difficult to inject the contrast agent. Only 1 cc of contrast should be injected before an image is taken.

Once the contrast is injected, the cannula is taped to the patient's nipple (Figure 17-17D), the syringe is taped to her chest, and she is escorted to the mammography machine where a CC view is taken. Use only mild compression to prevent the contrast from being expelled from the duct. Once the CC image verifies that the duct has been adequately filled with contrast, a Lateral image is also taken (Figure 17-17E).

When the ductogram is complete, the cannula is removed and a dressing is placed over the nipple. The dressing consists of a nursing pad saturated with water and a Saran wrap covering. The wet dressing helps drain the contrast agent from the breast and dilutes it so that it is less irritating to the patient's skin and nipple; the Saran wrap covering prevents the patient's clothes from becoming wet from the dressing. Without the wet dressing, the contrast may dry on the nipple, plugging the duct and preventing drainage of the remaining contrast agent. If this happens, the patient may develop a bacterial infection. The patient should continue to wear a dressing for 12 to 36 hours after the ductogram, depending on the amount of contrast agent injected.

▍▍ FINE-NEEDLE ASPIRATION CYTOLOGY

Fine-needle aspiration cytology (FNAC) of the breast is often used to verify a suspected malignancy on a mammogram or to confirm a benign impression of a lesion visible on a mammogram or an ultrasound scan.

The use of FNAC on benign-appearing lesions can eliminate the need for a patient to undergo an open surgical biopsy or can indicate the need for one on a patient whose lesion appears benign on mammography, but whose cytology returns as positive for cancer or atypical cells. FNAC is particularly helpful in evaluating women younger than age 28 who have a palpable mass; these women usually have a

benign condition, but they are frequently sent for surgical biopsy if FNAC is not performed.

Although FNAC can be helpful in evaluating patients, there are pitfalls in performing the procedure. For FNAC to be accurate, skill in needle placement and slide preparation is essential. In addition, the cytopathologist who reads the slides must be adept at interpreting FNACs. Because of these pitfalls, the decision to biopsy or monitor a patient should never be made solely on the outcome of the FNAC. This decision should be made by the radiologist before performing the FNAC procedure, based on the patient's imaging and clinical evaluations.[2]

FNAC Procedure

FNAC can be performed under clinical, ultrasound, or mammographic guidance. The method selected depends on whether the lesion is palpable or nonpalpable and under which imaging modality a nonpalpable lesion is best seen. Several techniques for FNAC have been published.[2,20–23] The following is a basic protocol that is frequently used.

Clinical and Sonographic Guidance

During clinically or ultrasound-guided FNAC of a lesion, the patient may sit or may be supine—whichever position is best for the radiologist to palpate or image the mass and fix it in place. Local anesthesia is not used; the procedure takes approximately 5 seconds. Placement of the transducer over the lesion is the only difference between a clinically and ultrasound-guided FNAC procedure.

The radiologist stretches the skin tightly over the lesion with one hand. After wiping the skin with alcohol, a disposable 2-cm-long 23 gauge butterfly needle is inserted through the skin to the palpable mass. The tubing of the butterfly needle is attached to a 20-cc syringe, held by an assistant. As soon as the needle passes through the skin, the assistant pulls back on the plunger of the syringe to apply negative pressure. This draws the cellular material into the lumen of the needle (Figure 17-18A). While the assistant applies negative pressure, the radiologist slides the needle in and out of the lesion ten to twenty times, angling it in several directions, to obtain cellular material samplings from all areas of the mass (Figure 17-18B and C).

When the radiologist finishes "peppering" the needle in the lesion, the assistant slowly and smoothly releases the syringe's negative pressure. This slow release is important because if pressure is released too quickly, the sudden force of pressure could push the cellular material in the needle back into the breast. Once the barrel of the syringe is in the neutral position, the radiologist removes the needle from the breast. The assistant firmly presses gauze on the insertion site

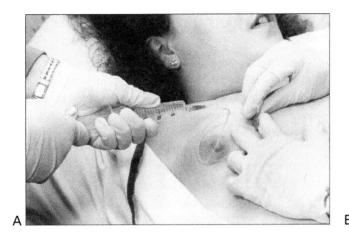

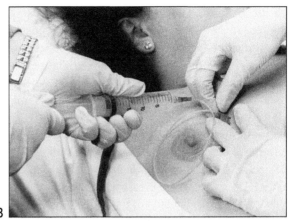

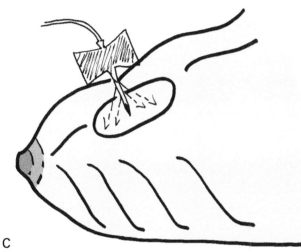

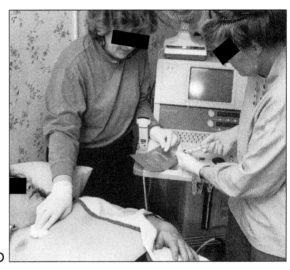

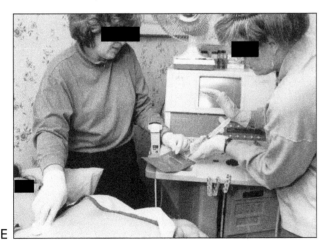

Figure 17-18
(A) The radiologist introduces a 23-gauge needle into the lesion to perform FNAC. The assistant then withdraws the plunger of the syringe to provide negative pressure, aspirating cellular material into the lumen of the needle. **(B)** The radiologist moves the needle back and forth within the mass **(C)** to obtain cellular material from all areas of the lesion. **(D)** With one hand, the assistant applies firm pressure to the area that has been aspirated while with the other hand she assists the physician by pointing the needle toward the slide. **(E)** Meanwhile, the radiologist removes the syringe from the tubing. After filling the barrel with air, she reattaches it to the tubing. She pushes the barrel, which forcibly expels the cellular material onto one of the slides.

to prevent a hematoma as the radiologist prepares the slides for cytologic evaluation. The radiologist detaches the syringe from the needle, fills it with air, and reattaches it, pushing forcefully on the plunger. The force of the air expelled from the syringe will push the cellular material out of the needle and onto the cytology slide (Figure 17-18D and E).

Preparing and fixing the slides quickly prevents the cells from air-drying, which could prevent an accurate diagnosis.

The method of fixation depends on the specifications of the laboratory where the sample will be sent.

Mammographic-Guided FNAC

FNAC can be performed under mammographic guidance with the aid of a stereotactic device or by using a similar technique to that used during preoperative wire localization. The breast is compressed using the same fenestrated compression device and is positioned using the same logic as described for preoperative localization of a nonpalpable lesion (see Figure 17-3A). A scout image is taken to locate the lesion. The breast remains under minimal compression while this image is reviewed.

If the lesion is close to the skin, a 23 gauge butterfly needle is used; for deeper lesions, the radiologist uses a 21 gauge skinny needle, which is available in several lengths. After wiping the breast with alcohol, the needle is inserted perpendicular to the IRSD (Figure 17-19). A second radiograph is taken to make sure the needle has been inserted into the lesion. Once this is confirmed, a 20-cc syringe is attached to the needle and an assistant pulls back on the plunger to apply negative pressure as the radiologist moves the needle in the lesion to obtain the cellular sample. Again, the negative pressure is slowly released before the needle is removed from the breast, and the slides are prepared the same way as described in the clinical FNAC procedure.

 ## FLOW CYTOMETRY

Some cancers release circulating tumor cells, or cancer stem cells, into the bloodstream or the lymphatic system of the patient. These cells are likely involved in metastatic development of secondary tumors as well as they enable the tumor to reconstitute itself after therapy is completed. These cells are more resistant to the effects of chemotherapy and to radiation therapy. Their presence is a predictor of poor outcome for the patient, with a direct relationship with their prevalence: a higher presence equates to a lower chance of survival. These cells are rare, perhaps one in a million cells; thus, flow cytometry is a valuable diagnostic tool to determine their presence.

Flow cytometry rapidly analyzes large numbers of cells, one at a time, for light scatter features and fluorescence characteristics. Cells are analyzed by passing a single-cell suspension through a laser light and measuring the light scatter and/or fluorescence from each individual cell, one after the other. The flow cytometer processes thousands of cells in a few seconds or minutes. Flow cytometry analysis is used

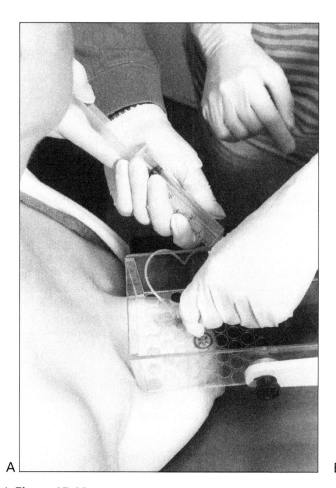

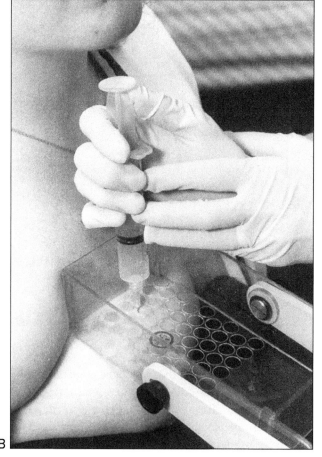

A

B

Figure 17-19
(A) A 23-gauge butterfly needle is introduced into the breast to perform FNAC under mammographic guidance. **(B)** A longer 21-gauge needle used for FNAC on deeper lesions.

to detect the surface features of cells, which may include molecules expressed by cells, by using antibody stains that specifically recognize these structures and molecules.

Viable cells are collected in a single-cell suspension (saline or tissue culture medium) and stained with monoclonal antibodies that are tagged with fluorescent compounds. A continuous flow of a fine stream (approximately the diameter of one cell) is passed through a laser beam, and both scattered light and fluorescence are detected using photodetector technology. Because the antibodies used in the analysis are directly linked to the fluorescent molecule, as each cell passes through the beam, it fluoresces at a specific color (or wavelength) that is unique to the fluorescent compound. The flow cytometer can measure each of several different parameters simultaneously for individual cells and store these on a computer disk. Computer software is then used to specifically analyze selected populations of cells for their expression of the proteins or antigens of interest.

Although flow cytometry is being studied as a means to detect micrometastases in axillary lymph nodes,[24] its primary use is to analyze lymphomas and leukemias. Two applications may be relevant to breast cancer: the analysis of lymph node suspensions for carcinoma cells (micrometastases) that might not be detected through standard techniques[2] and DNA analysis of the primary cancer for cell cycle or ploidy, which may be relevant to determining a patient's risk of relapse.[3,25] The first of these is experimental; some data indicate that it is probably not of practical clinical use.[26] The second technique is primarily used by the pathologist analyzing the original tumor resection and may be useful in predicting which tumors are likely to relapse or metastasize.

Cellular DNA ploidy evaluates the number of chromosomes in a cell. A tumor is less aggressive if it is diploid, having the standard number of chromosomes. When tumors are tetraploidy, polyploidy, or aneuploidy, the cells have an abnormal number of chromosomes; these tumors are more aggressive. In addition to ploidy, determining the S phase of the cancer cells alerts the diagnostician to the percent of active DNA synthesization. A lower S phase yields a better prognosis for the patient.

The use of flow cytometry combined with mammography is usually restricted to those patients whose mammograms demonstrate enlarged axillary lymph nodes, indicating possible lymphoma or leukemia. Cells are acquired from the lymph nodes using FNAC and are immediately placed in saline or tissue culture media (as recommended by the reference flow cytometry lab). Cells must be received in the laboratory in a viable (living) state because cell death can cause cells to lyse and may alter their staining qualities, thus rendering them nonanalyzable by flow cytometry.

Flow cytometry results are used to determine the prognosis of the patient, to monitor therapy response, and to document recurrence.

Review Questions

1. Why do we perform preoperative wire localization?

2. If the pathology report is discordant with the radiologist's interpretation, what follow-up steps are suggested?

References

1. Porter GJR, et al. Influence of mammographic parenchymal pattern in screening detected and interval invasive be cancers on pathologic features, mammographic features and patient survival. *AJR Am J Roentgenol.* 2007;188:676–683.
2. Logan-Young W, Hoffman NY. *Breast Cancer: A Practical Guide to Diagnosis. Vol. 1: Procedures.* Rochester, NY: Mt. Hope; 1994.
3. Homer MJ, Pile-Spellman ER. Needle localization of nonpalpable breast lesions: the importance of communication. *Appl Radiol.* 1987;November:88–98.
4. Homer MJ. Breast imaging: pitfalls, controversies and some practical thoughts. *Radiol Clin North Am.* 1985;23:466–467.
5. Helvie MA, et al. Localization and needle aspiration of breast lesions: complications in 370 cases. *Am J Roentgenol.* 1991;157:711–714.
6. Kopans DB, DeLuca S. A modified needle-hookwire technique to simplify preoperative localization of occult breast lesions. *Radiology.* 1980;134:781.
7. Kopans DB, Meyer JE. Computed tomography guided localization of clinically occult breast carcinoma–the 'N' skin guide. *Radiology.* 1982;145:211–212.
8. Urrutia EJ, et al. Retractable-barb needle for breast lesion localization: use in 60 cases. *Radiology.* 1988;169:845–847.
9. Hawkins IF Jr, et al. *Wide Range of Applications of a New 22-Gauge Needle which Permits Placement of Larger Catheters of Needles (Including Spring Barb Needle for Breast Lesion Localization).* Las Vegas, NV: American Roentgen Ray Society; 1980.
10. Frank HA, et al. Preoperative localization of nonpalpable breast lesions demonstrated by mammography. *N Engl J Med.* 1975;295:259–260.
11. Homer MJ. Nonpalpable breast lesion localization using a curved-end retractable wire. *Radiology.* 1985;157:259–260.
12. Davis PS, et al. Migration of breast biopsy localization wire. *Am J Roentgenol.* 1988;150:787–788.
13. Roux S, Logan-Young W. Private practice interdisciplinary breast centers-their rationale and impact on patients, physicians, and the health care industry: a bicoastal perspective. *Surg Oncol Clin N Am.* 2000;9(2):177–198.
14. Evans WP, Cade SH. Needle localization and fine-needle aspirations of nonpalpable breast lesions with use of standard stereotactic equipment. *Radiology.* 1989;173:53–56.
15. Rebner M, et al. Two-view specimen radiography in surgical biopsy of non-palpable breast masses. *Am J Roentgenol.* 1987;149:283–285.

16. Maturo VG, et al. Ultrasonic appearance of mammary carcinoma with a dedicated whole-breast scanner. *Radiology.* 1982;142:713–718.

17. Logan WW. The radiologist's increasing role in breast cancer diagnosis. In: Margulis AR, Gooding CA, eds. *Diagnostic Radiology.* San Francisco, CA: University of California Printing Department; 1982.

18. Logan WW. Ultrasonography: its role in the diagnosis of breast carcinoma. In: Margulis AR, Gooding CA, eds. *Diagnostic Radiology.* San Francisco, CA: University of California Printing Department; 1982.

19. Sickles EA, et al. Breast cancer detection with sonography and mammography: comparison using state-of-the-art equipment. *Am J Roentgenol.* 1983;140:843–845.

20. Wilkinson EJ, et al. Cytological needle sampling for the breast: techniques and end results. In: Bland KI, Copeland EM III, eds. *The Breast: Comprehensive Management of Benign and Malignant Diseases.* Philadelphia, PA: WB Saunders; 1991.

21. Fornage BD, et al. Breast masses: US-guided fine-needle aspiration biopsy. *Radiology.* 1987;162:409–414.

22. Hall FM. US-guided aspiration biopsy of the breast. *Radiology.* 1987;164:285–286.

23. Novak R. Method for control of the target at aspiration biopsy of nonpalpable breast lesions. *Acta Radiol Diagn (Stockh).* 1986;27:65–70.

24. Donegan WL. Tumor-related prognostic factors for breast cancer. *CA Cancer J Clin.* 1997;47:28–51.

25. Greve B, et al. Flow cytometry in cancer stem cell analysis and separation. *Cytometry A.* 2012;81:284–293. doi:10.1002/cryo.a.22022. Accessed December 30, 2016.

26. Van Diest PJ, et al. Pathological investigation of sentinel lymph nodes. *Eur J Nucl Med.* 1999;26:S43–S49.

Minimally Invasive Needle Breast Biopsy

18

Objectives

- Explain the principles of a stereotactic biopsy
- Define needle gauge, stroke margin, stereo pair, and biopsy
- Relate 3D thinking to *X*, *Y*, and *Z* coordinates
- Compare and contrast needle core biopsy and vacuum-assisted biopsy
- Name the parts and describe the process for using a biopsy instrument

---

Key Terms

- biopsy device
- Cartesian coordinate system
- core biopsy
- planar images
- polar coordinate system
- reference point

- stereo pair
- stereotactic breast biopsy
- stroke
- stroke margin
- targeting

INTRODUCTION

This chapter familiarizes the reader with current methods of breast needle biopsy (BNB), emphasizing stereotactic large gauge needle (core) biopsy.

Approximately 39 million mammograms are performed in the United States each year; as a consequence, approximately 1.6 million breast biopsies are done.[1] Statistically:

1,000 mammograms are done.
100 will be recalled for additional imaging.
10 to 15 will be referred for biopsy.
3 to 4 cancers will be diagnosed.

Needle biopsy has replaced surgical excisional biopsy for diagnosing most breast abnormalities. Currently, 70% of breast biopsies are via percutaneous methods.[2–4]

The two methods used for BNB are fine-needle aspiration cytology (FNAC) and large-core automated needle biopsy (**core biopsy**). The ease with which clinicians obtain, preserve, and interpret the sample distinguishes the methods.[5–12]

Fine-needle Aspiration Cytology

FNAC provides a sampling of cells (cytological material). Compared with core biopsy, it is more difficult to become proficient in the FNAC technique because of the sparse amount of material collected. The false-negative rate with FNAC is reported to be between 5% and 20%, with those proficient in the technique at the lower rate.[13] The preparation and interpretation of the cytological sample also demands meticulous technique and, most importantly, a pathologist trained in cytopathology of the breast.

A small gauge needle is used to increase the aspirate sample amount. FNAC is performed with a 20 to 23 gauge needle attached to a syringe directly or with connective tubing. A variety of needle types are used; however, Chiba or spinal needles are the most common. Needle length varies depending on the depth of the abnormality in the breast and the biopsy modality.

Once the needle is inserted into the abnormality, negative pressure is applied by pulling back on the syringe, allowing the aspiration of material for sampling. The cytological or cellular material is preserved on slides for interpretation by a cytopathologist. Depending on the modality used for biopsy, FNAC can be accomplished in a relatively short period of time: 3 to 30 minutes. (See Chapter 17 for a further discussion on FNAC.)

Core Biopsy

Core biopsy yields a large core of tissue (histological material). A specially designed 8- to 14-gauge needle or probe is placed in a rapid-fire automated biopsy instrument (commonly called a gun) or vacuum-assisted driver. Once the **biopsy device** is placed at the appropriate depth, the spring-loaded, double-action gun rapidly advances a two-stage needle and acquires a core of tissue during its excursion. The vacuum-assisted devices use a rotating cutter and suction to acquire the sample. Histological or tissue samples procured with core biopsy are preserved in formalin for a histopathologist to interpret. Depending on the modality used, the core biopsy procedure takes 20 minutes to 1 hour or more to perform. In most cases, core biopsy offers a more definitive diagnosis when compared with FNAC.[5–10] The false-negative rate is between 2% and 6.7%. A false negative is usually associated with a suspicious area of microcalcifications.[13]

 BIOPSY MODALITIES

To perform BNB, physicians use *clinical* or *image* guidance. Imaging methods for biopsy include ultrasound, MRI, and **stereotactic breast biopsy** (SBB). These methods require varying degrees of training, experience, procedure time, and equipment; each provides a different degree of accuracy.

Clinical Guidance

Clinically guided BNB is useful for palpable abnormalities that may or may not be mammographically and sonographically evident. The biopsy instrument is handheld and hand-guided, which may negatively affect accuracy. Other negative aspects of clinical guidance are the lack of confirmation and evidence of accurate needle placement. If the needle biopsy is positive, the patient can avoid excisional biopsy and make appropriate choices regarding definitive treatment. However, negative results may pose a dilemma; depending on the initial level of clinical concern, the choice with negative results is between open excisional biopsy and follow-up interval mammography.

Ultrasound-Guided Biopsy (Sonographic)

Sonographic biopsy can be used with palpable or nonpalpable abnormalities and is a quick and efficient means to acquire tissue samples. Although the biopsy device is handheld, as in clinically guided biopsy, real-time ultrasound images monitor needle movement. This is especially true when performing FNAC, yielding exceptional accuracy in trained hands. Ultrasound-guided interventional procedures account for the primary biopsy technique employed by most imaging centers today.[14] Calcifications,

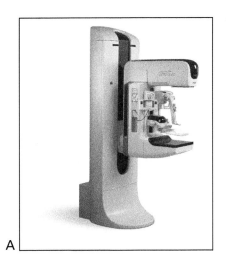 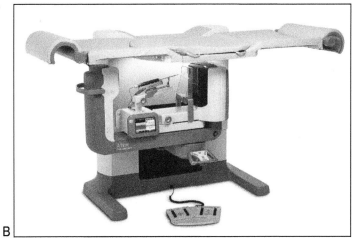

Figure 18-1
Biopsy equipment. **(A)** Add-on unit to existing mammography machine; for upright stereotactic core biopsy. (Hologic Dimensions with Affirm.) **(B)** Dedicated prone table for stereotactic core biopsy. (Hologic Affirm Prone Biopsy System; 2D/3D imaging capability.) Images courtesy of Hologic, Inc. and affiliates.

architectural distortions, and small masses measuring 6 mm or less pose the greatest difficulty for this modality.

Stereotactic Guidance

SBB requires specially designed equipment to calculate the location of an abnormality by using two angled radiographs approximately 30° apart (usually ±15° from center) and a coordinate system. Studies have shown that obtaining the exact location of an abnormality is possible in three dimensions and is accurate to within 1 mm tolerances.[15,16] In fact, the Greek and Latin root words comprising stereotactic mean "touching in space." There are few exceptions to the types of abnormalities amenable to stereotactic guidance. Calcifications, masses, and architectural distortions are identifiable in most cases.

The stereotactic procedure is less dependent on clinician skills than ultrasound or clinically guided methods because the breast is immobile. Consequently, the abnormality is less likely to move. In addition, a guidance system holds the biopsy instrument and the needle or probe as it enters the breast for sampling. The two types of stereotactic equipment used today are upright add-on units and dedicated prone tables (Figure 18-1). Add-on units allow the patient to be upright, or semi-reclined in a sitting position, or lying on her side during the procedure; prone tables allow the patient to be recumbent.

▌ PRINCIPLES OF STEREOTACTIC LOCALIZATION

The primary tasks of SBB are positioning and imaging by the technologist and targeting and sampling by the clinician.

This section describes the principles of stereotactic localization, stereotactic imaging, and the fundamentals of stereotactic core biopsy to accomplish safe, efficient, and successful sampling. Most stereotactic procedures are straightforward, requiring an understanding of the biopsy process. Others are complex and require an awareness of stereotactic principles to appropriately position and target the abnormality. Although a computer performs the mathematics necessary to calculate target location, computations depend on information from those performing the procedure. If the input information is inaccurate, errors will occur. Unsuccessful localization of the abnormality is rarely a malfunction of the stereotactic system or computer but more often results from human error. A review of basic principles can prevent or help recognize an error, preferably before the needle is inserted.

The most valuable skill for the technologist to acquire is the ability to "see" the approximate 3D location of an abnormality in the breast from the two-view mammogram (see Chapter 9). This proficiency and other illustrated visual clues below can help avoid faulty positioning, procedural difficulties, and incorrect sampling.

Stereology

Stereology is the science of determining 3D information about an object based on planar (2D) views. A simple and familiar comparison is the stereoscopy the brain accomplishes through the human visual system. Each eye gives a different perspective of an object; our brain then reconstructs the object three dimensionally. This is simple to demonstrate: hold an object in front of your eyes and alternately close one eye and then the other, realizing the different perspective each eye is relaying to the brain. Take this one step further—alternately look at this object with one eye and then the other in reference to a more distant (or near) object. The distance of the apparent "shift" of the object in relation to the reference object is *parallax.* The brain solves the parallax problem (i.e., the difference in relation to the reference) and accurately perceives the distance of the object. The resulting depth perception allows us to know how far to reach out to accurately touch the object. Depth perception is severely inhibited (in the absence of other visual or familiar clues) with vision loss in one eye or only one perspective of the object. This problem is evident with the mammogram, where vertical and horizontal measurements are fairly easy to determine but the accurate depth measurement is elusive.

Stereotactic breast localization involves the same visual principles that the brain and eyes use to accurately see a 3D object. The object under consideration is the nonpalpable breast abnormality. For our purposes, the 3D result is not reconstruction but accurate, quantitative computation of the location of the abnormality in the breast in three dimensions: horizontal, vertical, and depth. Swift and accurate location of the abnormality is possible using the following:

Stereo pair—consisting of two **planar x-ray images** of the abnormality from different perspectives

Reference point or *points*—providing the relative comparison of shift of the abnormality to determine depth and other coordinates

Computer—for solving the mathematics of the parallax effect and determining location to within 1 mm

In 2016, the FDA approved the first 3D imaging system for BNB. This biopsy system works in the 2D mode as well as 3D, and with an upright mammography machine or with a prone dedicated biopsy table. Abnormalities found on a tomosynthesis exam but not well visualized on 2D images can now be successfully biopsied. It has been reported that a 2D prone stereotactic core biopsy takes, on average, 29 minutes to complete, while a 3D biopsy requires only 13 minutes due to the ease of identifying and targeting the abnormality.[17]

Overview of the Stereotactic Procedure

A scout image properly demonstrating the abnormality within the biopsy window is a prerequisite. Two images, acquired with the x-ray tube at two different positions (typically +15° and −15°), are projected side by side on a computer monitor to form the stereo pair (Figure 18-2). The clinician places target marks on the abnormality on both

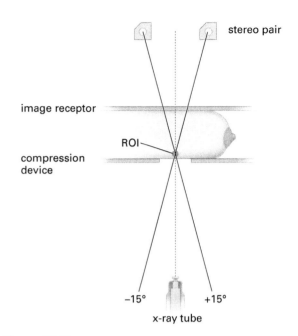

Figure 18-2
Three-dimensional localization. When two images with a separation of 30° are acquired, a computer can calculate the location of a structure inside the breast with pinpoint accuracy.

Case Study **18-1**

Refer to Figure 18-2 and the text and respond to the following questions.

1. What is a prerequisite in order to do a stereotactic biopsy procedure?

2. What is a stereo pair?

3. What is the purpose of the stereo pair?

stereo images. The computer bases coordinate calculation on the abnormality's shift from the reference point(s) on these images.

The computer also provides a coordinate system for the results to be translated for practical use. After coordinate determination, a needle or probe is placed in the breast for sampling, and a confirmation (or prefire) stereo pair is acquired. If the prefire stereo pair demonstrates accurate needle placement, the next step is sampling of the abnormality. Subsequent samples are possible with or without additional stereo images. The following detailed discussion of 3D localization provides technical information and visual clues that are helpful during the procedure. Because variations among units are inevitable, each biopsy team should endeavor to discover a unit's unique characteristics.

Coordinate Systems

The primary purpose of a coordinate system is to identify a unique visual point in the breast that will be used as the target for the biopsy needle. The coordinate system, regardless of type, gives the location of the abnormality in three dimensions (Figure 18-3). The horizontal plane is expressed by X or H, the vertical plane by Y or V, and depth by Z or D.

The two types of coordinate systems are Cartesian and polar. A **Cartesian coordinate system** defines a point by its distance from three axes that intersect at right angles. The familiar X, Y, Z coordinates are the distances from the reference point in the X (left–right axis), Y (up–down axis), and Z (depth) directions (Figure 18-4). An example of abnormality location would be as follows: $X = +4$ mm, $Y = 10$ mm, $Z = 22$ mm. Perhaps, the most obvious advantage of the Cartesian method is that it is familiar and easy to adapt to its use. The simplicity of this coordinate system permits users to easily adjust needle position. For example, if analysis of the prefire stereo pair suggests that the needle is 5 mm too far to the left, visualize repositioning the biopsy needle 5 mm to the right for correction. A Cartesian system also allows easier correlation with other aspects, such as scale and reference, described in the next section.

A **polar coordinate system** defines a target by the distance from a fixed point and the angular distance from a reference line (Figure 18-5). Coordinates are most often given as H, V, D. Horizontal and vertical coordinates are set in angles rather than millimeters. While this system is accurate, recognizing errors is more difficult for the user, unless they are gross in nature. Correcting an error requires trigonometric calculations too complex to be practical

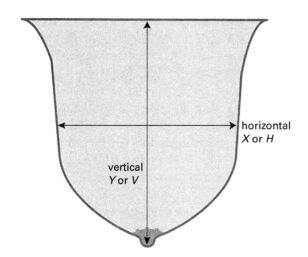

Frontal or Superior View
(prone unit) (upright unit)

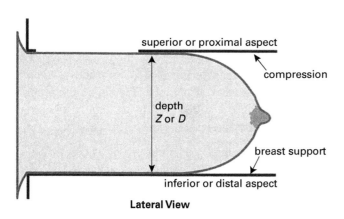

Lateral View

Figure 18-3
Three-dimensional coordinates. A coordinate system gives the location of the abnormality in three dimensions: X or H represents the horizontal plane, Y or V the vertical, and Z or D the depth. (From Willison KM. Fundamentals of stereotactic breast biopsy. In: Fajardo LL, Willison KM, Pizzeutiello RJ, eds. A Comprehensive Approach to Stereotactic Breast Biopsy. Cambridge: Blackwell Science; 1996:15. Copyright © 1996 Wiley-Blackwell. Reproduced with permission from John Wiley & Sons.)

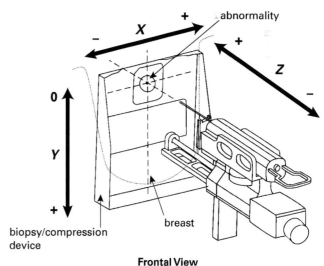

Frontal View

Figure 18-4
Cartesian coordinates. A Cartesian system identifies the location of a unique point by three axes intersecting at right angles. (From Willison KM. Fundamentals of stereotactic breast biopsy. In: Fajardo LL, Willison KM, Pizzeutiello RJ, eds. A Comprehensive Approach to Stereotactic Breast Biopsy. Cambridge: Blackwell Science; 1996:16. Copyright © 1996 Wiley-Blackwell. Reproduced with permission from John Wiley & Sons.)

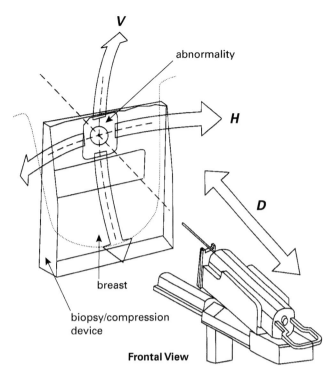

Figure 18-5
Polar coordinates. A polar system identifies the location of a unique point by the distances from a fixed point and the angular distances from a reference line. (From Willison KM. Fundamentals of stereotactic breast biopsy. In: Fajardo LL, Willison KM, Pizzeutiello RJ, eds. A Comprehensive Approach to Stereotactic Breast Biopsy. Cambridge: Blackwell Science; 1996:16. Copyright © 1996 Wiley-Blackwell. Reproduced with permission from John Wiley & Sons.)

during a procedure. Because the needle travels on an arc, a correction of *H*, *V*, or *D* may change the accuracy of the other coordinates. Thus, acquiring a new stereo pair and retargeting the abnormality is the most effective method to correct an error.

Scale

Although the coordinate system is not visible on the biopsy window, an applicable scale exists for the horizontal, vertical, and depth axes. The coordinate scale, usually expressed in millimeters, defines the location of point "0" for the vertical and horizontal axes and divides the biopsy window into positive and negative halves or quadrants. Figure 18-6A demonstrates the biopsy window from two different stereotactic units.

Although both use Cartesian systems, point 0 is in a different location for each unit. This information is useful in checking calculated coordinates against the scout image. The scout image demonstrates an abnormality at a specific point on the scale of the biopsy window; coordinate calculation should match this position. If abnormality location is

in a negative quadrant, coordinates should be negative and so on (Figure 18-7).

Correlation of coordinates and scout position may be difficult with the scale of a polar system because the angles that define target location are not easily related to its position on the scout image. However, the biopsy window is divided into negative and positive halves. The clinician can detect an error before needle insertion when the set position of the biopsy needle is contrary to the position of the target on the scout image.

Scale and Depth

The scale also defines point 0 for the depth axis. Figure 18-6B illustrates 0 (or the zero plane) for the depth axis at either the distal or proximal surface of the breast. The depth coordinate of an abnormality is expressed in millimeters from 0 to the abnormality. A depth coordinate that differs greatly from the expected depth should raise curiosity and at least a recheck of parameters. With at least one stereotactic unit, an arbitrary scale defines the depth coordinate. This scale does not directly relate to the distance of the abnormality from either the proximal or distal skin surface. With an arbitrary scale, the clinician has no correlative data to ensure that the depth coordinate is accurate. In fact, no direct visible information exists to correlate coordinate depth with expected abnormality depth before needle insertion. However, during needle insertion, the clinician can correlate centimeter markings on the needle with the expected depth of the abnormality.

The Reference

All coordinates are determined from measurements based on a reference point or points. The shift of a targeted abnormality on the stereo pair, in relation to this established recognized reference, provides for an exact 3D position to within 1 mm.

Location of the Reference

The equipment manufacturer determines the location of the reference point(s). For some units, the established reference is located on the biopsy compression device between the compressed breast and the x-ray tube. Because the biopsy/compression device is removable, accurate placement is critical. If the centering of the biopsy/compression device is in error, reference placement and coordinate determination will be in error. Other manufacturers locate the reference point(s) on the breast support platform, between the compressed

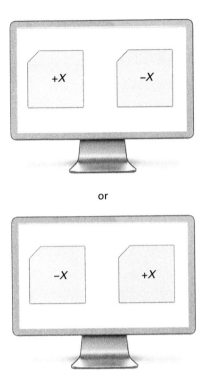

Figure 18-9
Display of the positive/negative 15° images is specific for each breast biopsy system manufacturer. The positive image should be displayed to the right (or left) on the monitor and the negative image on the opposite side.

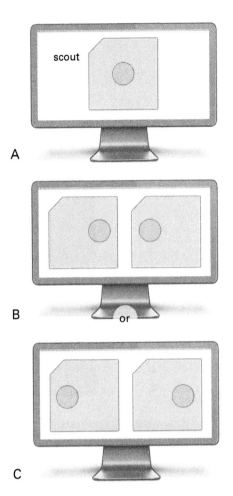

Figure 18-10
Display of the positive/negative 15° images is specific for each breast biopsy system manufacturer; the display of the planar images determines the direction of the shift of the abnormality. **(A)** Ideally, the ROI should be in the center of the biopsy window on the scout image. Depending on the manufacturer, the abnormality will appear to move **(B)** toward or **(C)** away from one another on the stereo pair.

display. Viewing the stereo pair appropriately (as recommended by manufacturer), the projected image of the abnormality will move either *toward* or *away* from each other in the horizontal plane only (Figure 18-10). This directional shift remains constant for a specific unit. The display of the planar images also determines the appearance of the biopsy needle after it is positioned in the breast; the needle tips are directed either toward or away from one another.

The technologist and clinician should be familiar with the circumstances of placement and directional shift as this offers correlative visual confirmation. For example, visual clues such as errant directional shift or misdirected needle tips indicate mistakes early in the procedure. X-ray tube or acquisition order errors are possible causes. Coordinate calculations will be in error with incorrect acquisition (Figure 18-11).

Distance of Shift and Centering

The distance of abnormality shift on the positive/negative planar images from the scouted projection will vary from one patient to another due to variable breast compression thicknesses and various abnormality depths relative to the breast support or compression device. However, in *all* cases, the abnormality should shift equally from the scouted position on both planar images (Figure 18-12A).

For example, from the scouted projection, if the abnormality shifts 10 mm on the (+) X image, then it will also shift 10 mm on the (–) X image. However, abnormality shape may change with different projections. This equal shift may not be as evident if the abnormality is not centered in the biopsy window (Figure 18-12B). The projected abnormality might shift outside the confines of the image receptor or x-ray field. Proper centering of the abnormality (Figure 18-13) in the horizontal plane (left-to-right axis) on

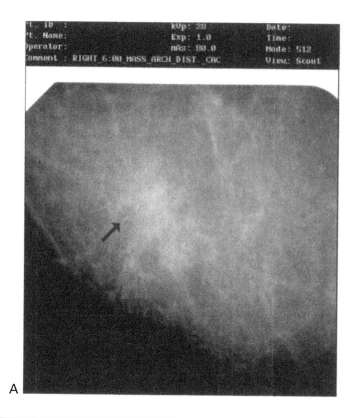

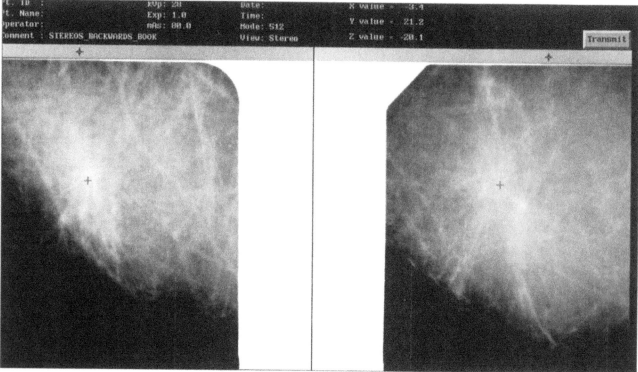

Figure 18-11

Direction of shift. **(A)** Note the position of the abnormality on the scout image (*arrow*). **(B)** The inward shift of the abnormality (for this system, the abnormality should have shifted outward) on the stereo images is a visual clue that alerts the technologist to inappropriate order of stereo acquisition. The error is also evident in the negative depth coordinate (upper right-hand corner). (From Willison KM. Fundamentals of stereotactic breast biopsy. In: Fajardo LL, Willison KM, Pizzeutiello RJ, eds. A Comprehensive Approach to Stereotactic Breast Biopsy. Cambridge: Blackwell Science; 1996:21. Copyright © 1996 Wiley-Blackwell. Reproduced with permission from John Wiley & Sons.)

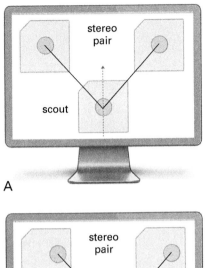

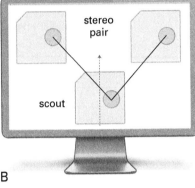

Figure 18-12
Equal shift of the abnormality. In the stereo pair, the abnormality shifts equally from the scouted position. **(A)** This equal shift is easily seen when the abnormality is well centered in the biopsy window. **(B)** When the abnormality is off-centered on the scout image, the equal shift is less apparent on the stereo pair.

the scout image will in most cases prevent nonvisualization (see section "Shift and Nonvisualization"). Centering in the vertical plane is not necessary; however, it may facilitate access by the biopsy team.

Distance of Shift and Depth

The distance of abnormality shift depends on the depth of the abnormality relative to either the breast support or the biopsy/compression device and the stereotactic geometry of each manufacturer's system. The two scenarios for abnormality shift are as follows:

1. In one system, an abnormality in closer proximity to the biopsy/compression device will move less distance in the imaging field than an abnormality closer to the breast support (Figure 18-14A). The closer the abnormality is to the compression device, the less it will move. As compression thickness increases, so will the abnormality shift (Figure 18-14B)

2. In another system, an abnormality in closer proximity to the compression device will move a greater distance in the imaging field than an abnormality closer to the breast support (Figure 18-14C). The closer the abnormality is to the biopsy/compression device, the more it will move. As compression thickness increases, abnormality shift increases (Figure 18-14D).

An awareness of shift distance relative to depth is a useful guide for the biopsy team. For example, depending

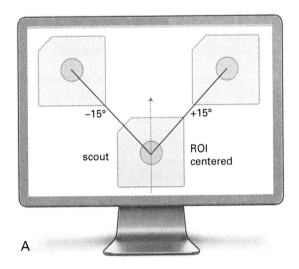

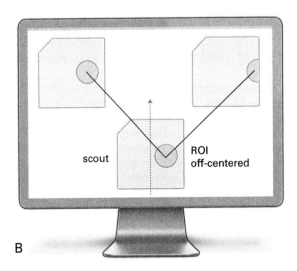

Figure 18-13
Ideally, the ROI should be centered in the biopsy window. **(A)** Centering the ROI on the scout image maintains visualization on the stereo pair. **(B)** Poor centering has the potential for the ROI to shift outside the biopsy window on the stereo images.

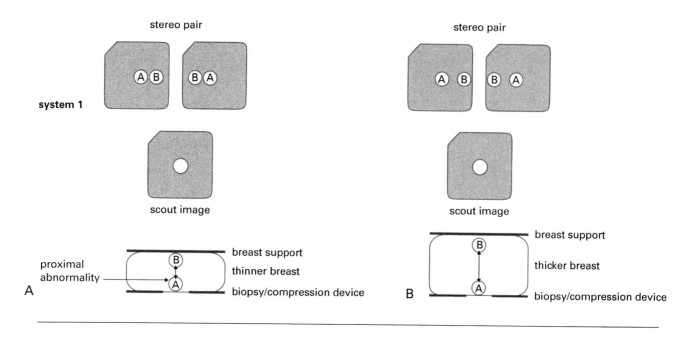

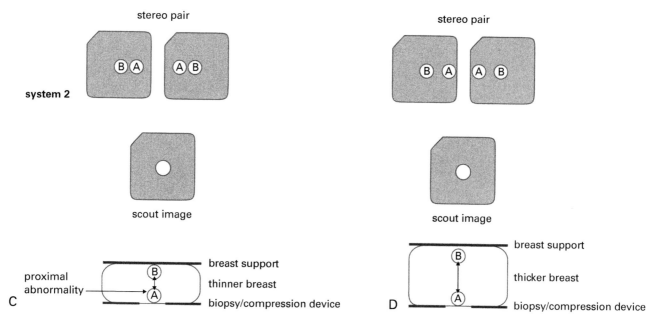

Figure 18-14

Distance of shift of two systems. **(A)** In System 1, an abnormality located closer to the biopsy/compression device will shift a *lesser* distance than an abnormality located closer to the breast support. **(B)** In System 2, an abnormality located closer to the biopsy/ compression device will move a *greater* distance than an abnormality located closer to the breast support. **(C and D)** Increasing breast thickness increases the distance of the shift. This is the result of the stereotactic geometry of each system. (From Willison KM. Fundamentals of stereotactic breast biopsy. In: Fajardo LL, Willison KM, Pizzeutiello RJ, eds. A Comprehensive Approach to Stereotactic Breast Biopsy. Cambridge: Blackwell Science; 1996:26. Copyright © 1996 Wiley-Blackwell. Reproduced with permission from John Wiley & Sons.)

on the unit, extensive abnormality shift on the stereo images may indicate improper positioning (Figure 18-15), contributing to negative **stroke margin** (discussed later in this chapter). For the clinician, understanding the distance and direction of shift is useful when identifying ill-defined abnormalities to target. When examining the stereo images for the abnormality, search only that portion of the image where the abnormality will shift (Figure 18-16).

Shift and Nonvisualization

The breast support design and field limitations of some units may reduce the ability to sample an abnormality

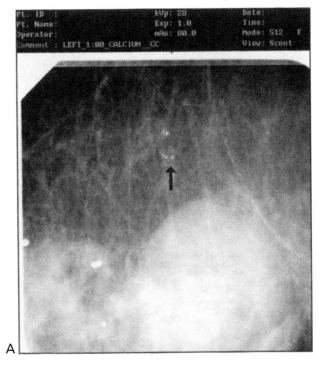

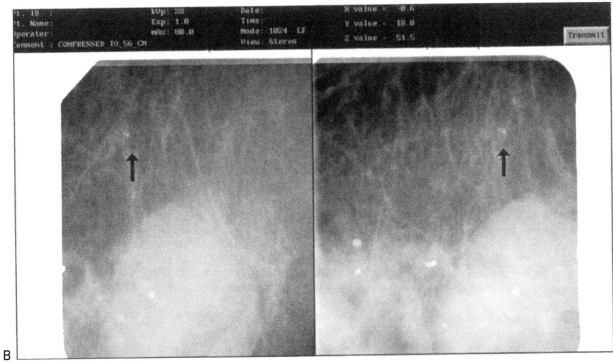

Figure 18-15
Shift and depth. **(A)** The scouted abnormality (*arrow*) in the CC projection **(B)** shifts a great distance on the stereo images (*arrow*), indicating that the abnormality is positioned *distal* to the biopsy/compression device for this SBB system.

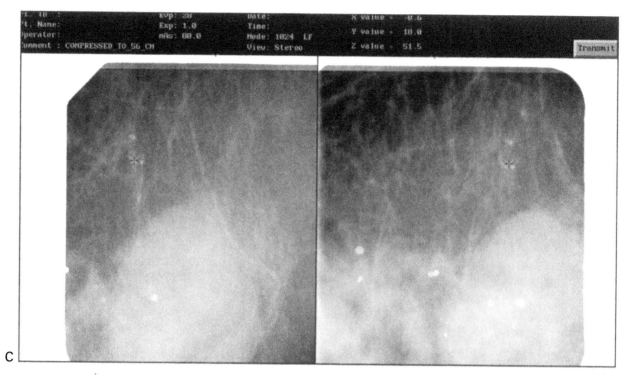

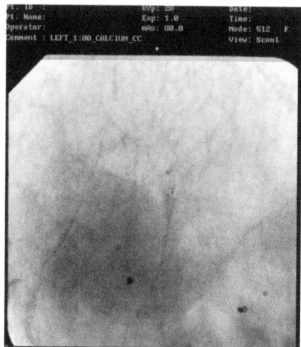

Figure 18-15 (*Continued*)
(C) Coordinate calculation (upper right-hand corner) indicates a depth of 51 mm with a total breast compression of 56 mm, inadequate for the stroke of the biopsy instrument. **(D)** The breast is repositioned in a FB projection.

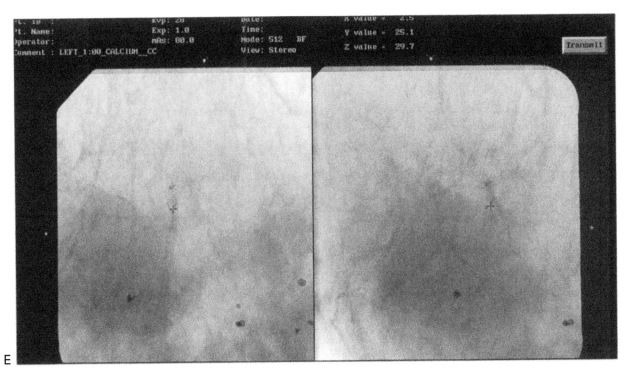

E

Figure 18-15 (*Continued*)
(E) The new stereo pair demonstrates minimal shift, which (in this SBB system) means that the abnormality is more *proximal* to the biopsy/compression device. Coordinate calculation indicates depth to be 29.7 for the compression of 56 mm, allowing ample room for stroke, with a 5 mm prefire position. (From Willison KM. Fundamentals of stereotactic breast biopsy. In: Fajardo LL, Willison KM, Pizzeutiello RJ, eds. A Comprehensive Approach to Stereotactic Breast Biopsy. Cambridge: Blackwell Science; 1996:27–29. Copyright © 1996 Wiley-Blackwell. Reproduced with permission from John Wiley & Sons.)

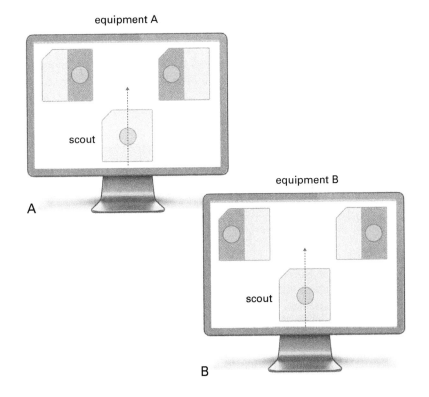

A

B

Figure 18-16
When trying to locate an ill-defined ROI, the physician should search only in the area to which the abnormality characteristically shifts. **(A)** With equipment A, abnormalities shift *toward* one another on the stereo pair; therefore, the search should be confined to the shaded areas. **(B)** With equipment B, abnormalities shift *away* from one another; thus, the search should be confined to the shaded areas.

because it is only partially visualized, or it is outside the field of view on one or both stereo images, despite accurate centering. Appropriate centering of the abnormality in the imaging field is critical with this equipment; however, the geometry of the unit is the limiting factor. If both stereo images do not show the abnormality, or the same portion of the abnormality, then appropriate targeting is not possible. The clinician has two choices: cancel the biopsy or use a "target on scout" method.

Case Study 18-2

Refer to Figure 18-13 and the text and respond to the following questions.

1. What effect on the abnormality occurs when the x-ray tube is shifted ±15°?

2. Is the degree of abnormality shift the same for all patients?

3. Is it possible for an abnormality to shift out of view on the stereo pair?

Nonvisualization is more likely to occur if the SBB equipment allows a proximal abnormality (positioned closer to the biopsy/compression device) to shift a greater distance compared with a distal abnormality (Figure 18-17). Core biopsy requires positioning of the abnormality as close to the biopsy/compression device as possible (for easier access, accuracy, and stroke margin), thereby increasing the possibility of nonvisualization. Furthermore, the occurrence of nonvisualization increases in those units with a fixed breast support, while systems with a movable breast support maintain the abnormality in the field of view.

Nonvisualization also occurs when breast thickness is greater, usually 6 cm or more, depending on the geometry of the unit. Determining the compression thickness at which nonvisualization occurs allows the clinician and technologist to choose a viable projection that provides compression thickness within the imaging confines of the SBB unit.

The mathematical algorithms for 3D localization are designed for a particular set of stereo angles; therefore, never change the angle of stereo acquisition for coordinate calculation unless recommended by the manufacturer.

■■ THE CORE BIOPSY PROCEDURE

Before discussing instrumentation and expanding on principles, a rudimentary understanding of the biopsy procedure is necessary. Step-by-step illustrations of a typical biopsy procedure are outlined in Figure 18-18. The core biopsy procedure is a "clean" procedure rather than a sterile procedure.

Initial Preparation

1. Verify calibration: A daily quality control test to check calibration of the targeting system is necessary before beginning the scheduled biopsies (Figure 18-19).
2. Review the mammogram: The clinician and technologist should decide the most effective approach for accessing

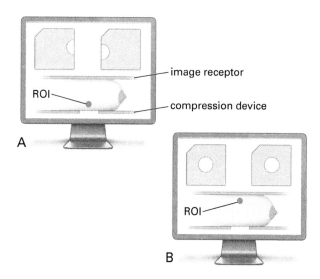

Figure 18-17
(A) A ROI that is closer to the compression device shifts a greater distance on the stereo pair. As the compressed breast thickness increases, the ROI is likely to shift out of view on the stereo pair, preventing a biopsy from being performed. A moveable breast support/image receptor helps maintain visualization. **(B)** When the ROI is closer to the image receptor, there is less shifting; however, it is more difficult to biopsy a ROI deep in the breast.

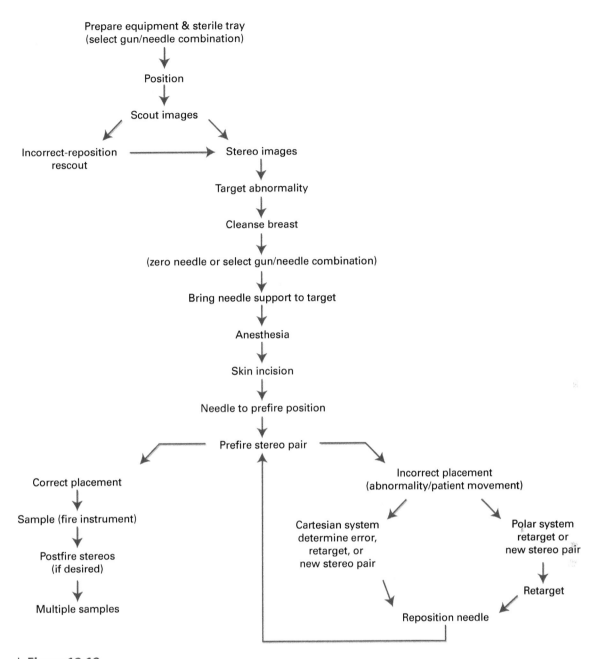

Figure 18-18
Work flow chart. Flow chart for a typical stereotactic core biopsy procedure. (From Willison KM. Fundamentals of stereotactic breast biopsy. In: Fajardo LL, Willison KM, Pizzeutiello RJ, eds. A Comprehensive Approach to Stereotactic Breast Biopsy. Cambridge: Blackwell Science; 1996:31. Copyright © 1996 Wiley-Blackwell. Reproduced with permission from John Wiley & Sons.)

the abnormality. This initial projection may be modified during actual patient positioning.

3. Prepare the equipment for the patient and the procedure.
4. Program the unit for needle length and the stroke of the biopsy instrument. This step may be done at this point, or later in the procedure, depending on the manufacturer's recommendations.

When the Patient Arrives

1. Prepare biopsy tray (Figure 18-20).
2. Complete necessary paperwork and requisitions.
3. Obtain consent.
4. Have patient change clothes and use the bathroom.
5. Remove eyeglasses, earrings, hearing aids, necklaces, empty pockets, and such.

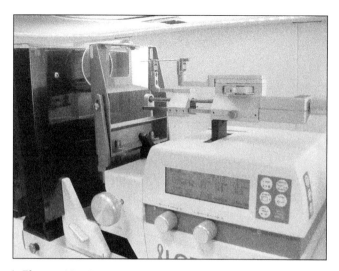

Figure 18-19
Check calibration. QC is required before the first case of the day is done.

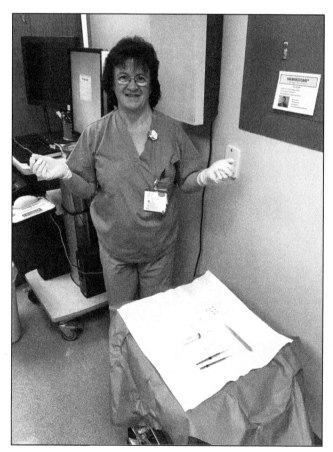

Figure 18-20
The technologist sets up the sterile biopsy tray before the procedure begins. There are basic items common to this tray; however, each clinician wants something unique on her/his tray.

Position and Scout

1. Position the patient (Figure 18-21A): Selecting the appropriate approach to the abnormality can be simple or complicated, depending on several factors (the position of the patient's body, C-arm rotation, and visualization of the abnormality in both scout and stereo images). These are all issues that require attention. Providing positive stroke margin is critical.
2. Obtain the scout image (Figure 18-21B): The first step in the imaging process is to ensure adequate centering and visualization of the abnormality in the biopsy window. Acquire the scout image with the x-ray tube perpendicular to the image receptor. Repositioning the breast, adjusting technical factors, and repeating the scout image a few times may be necessary to obtain the final working image.

Acquire the Stereo Pair

Acquire the two images that form the stereo pair according to the manufacturer's recommendations (Figures 18-21C and D). If the abnormality is not identifiable on either one of these images, the technologist can vary the technique accordingly or reposition the patient, rescout, and repeat the stereo images.

Determine Coordinates

Each manufacturer specifies the steps to target the abnormality for coordinate calculation (Figure 18-21E).

Transfer Coordinates

The task of transferring the target coordinates is electronic (Figure 18-21F). Electronic transfer provides for the display of all three coordinates, with subsequent positioning of the biopsy platform or stage at a later point. Verification by the biopsy team of the transfer of coordinates from the targeting computer to the needle guidance system is critical.

Sampling

1. Take precautions: Follow universal precautions as defined by OSHA standards. If necessary, drape the equipment and the patient in case of blood spatter (especially important with upright systems).
2. Clean with antiseptic: Lightly cleanse the skin within the biopsy window using alcohol or a povidone–iodine solution (Figure 18-21G). Remove excess solution with a sterile sponge.

3. Place the needle guide: Place sterile needle guide on the needle guidance system, according to the manufacturer's instructions (Figure 18-21H).
4. Secure the biopsy instrument: Secure the loaded biopsy instrument in the holder on the needle guidance platform or stage (Figure 18-21I).
5. Program needle length: Program the unit for needle length and the stroke of the biopsy instrument (Figure 18-21J). Depending on the manufacturer's recommendations, this task can be completed now or it could have been done earlier while setting up the equipment for the procedure.

6. Guide the needle: The biopsy team uses an automated or manual control to match the needle guidance device with the target coordinates for the X and Y axes, targeting the abnormality (Figure 18-21K).
7. Administer anesthesia: The needle is brought forward, accurately indicating the site for anesthesia (Figure 18-21L). Local anesthesia is administered to the skin and subcutaneous tissues. An excessive amount of anesthesia can interfere with the visualization of the abnormality on subsequent images. Anesthetic volume may also displace the abnormality. To minimize the volume injected per

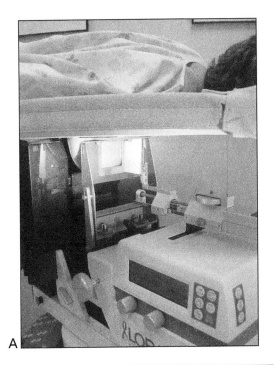

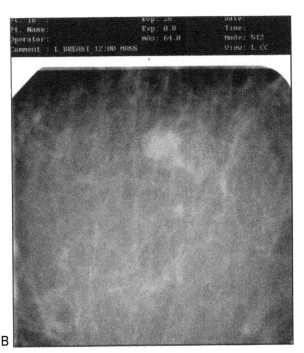

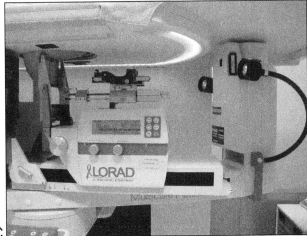

Figure 18-21
Steps of the biopsy procedure. **(A)** Position the patient. **(B)** Obtain the scout image. This scout image demonstrates a smoothly outlined abnormality, well centered in the biopsy field. **(C)** Acquire the stereo images. Acquire two stereo images with the tube at different source positions. Note the shift of the C-arm.

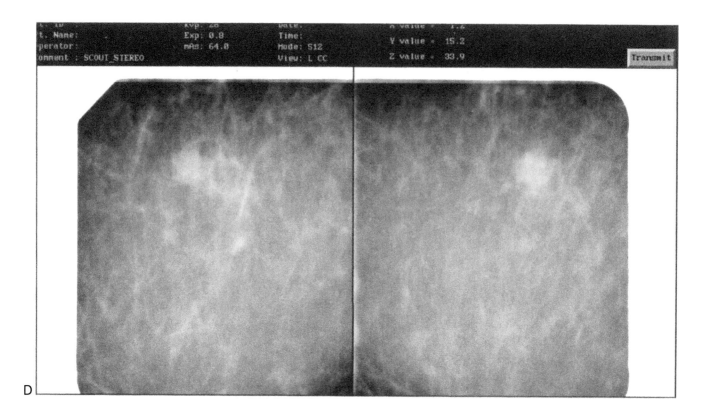

D

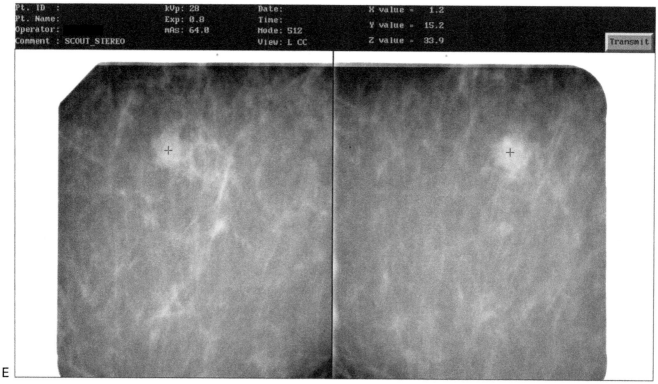

E

Figure 18-21 *(Continued)*
(D) Stereo images. The abnormality is easily seen on the stereo images, demonstrating proper directional shift. **(E)** Coordinate determination. Based on targeting *(cursors)*, the computer determines coordinates (upper right hand corner) for the abnormality.

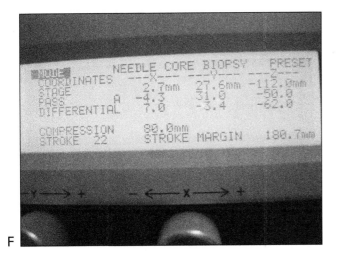

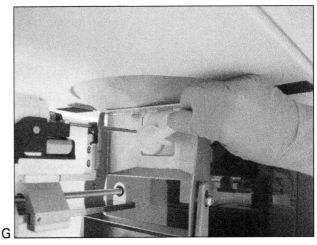

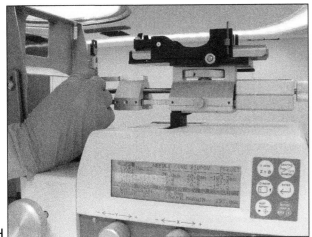

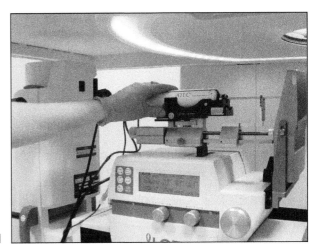

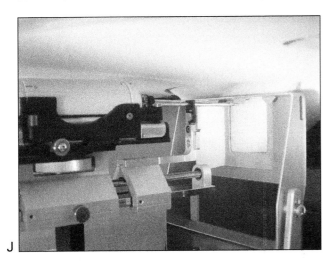

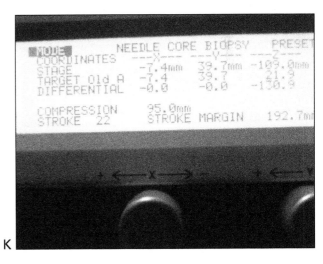

Figure 18-21 (*Continued*)
(F) Transfer coordinates to the needle guidance system. **(G)** Apply antiseptic conservatively. **(H)** Affix the needle guide. The forward needle guide maintains accuracy of needle placement. **(I)** Mount the biopsy instrument. Secure the biopsy instrument into the holder. **(J)** Calibrate needle length. Calibration for needle length ensures accuracy in reaching the depth coordinate. **(K)** The clinician matches the platform needle-guidance stage with the abnormality coordinates.

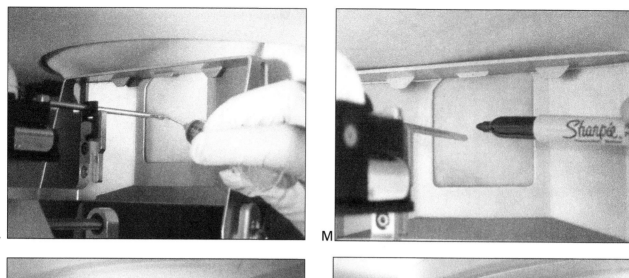

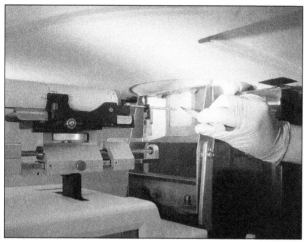

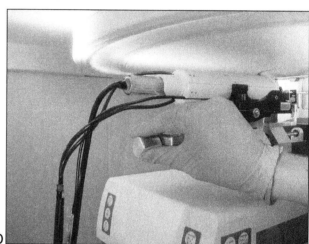

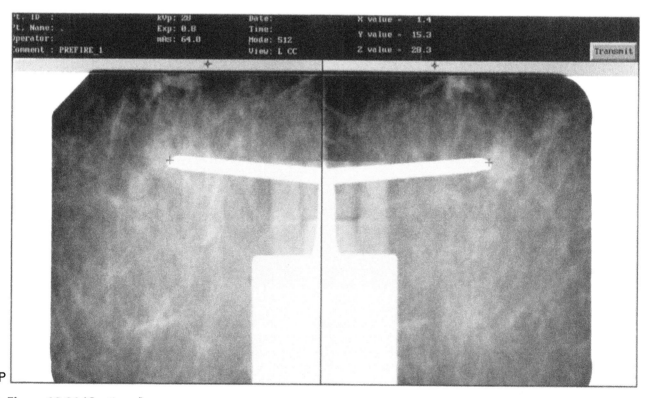

Figure 18-21 (*Continued*)
(L) Anesthesia. Move the needle forward to indicate the site for anesthesia of superficial and subcutaneous tissue. **(M)** Mark the skin. Once a skin welt has been raised, bring the needle forward just far enough to make a mark on the skin. **(N)** Make a skin incision. A small skin incision allows smooth passage of the biopsy needle through the skin. **(O)** Placement of the biopsy needle. The clinician advances the biopsy needle into the breast to the appropriate depth. **(P)** Prefire.

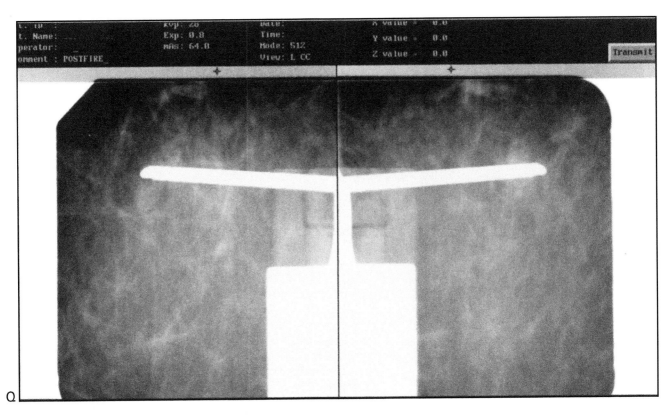

Figure 18-21 (*Continued*)
(Q) Postfire. (From Willison KM. Fundamentals of stereotactic breast biopsy. In: Fajardo LL, Willison KM, Pizzeutiello RJ, eds. A Comprehensive Approach to Stereotactic Breast Biopsy. Cambridge: Blackwell Science; 1996:33–39. Copyright © 1996 Wiley-Blackwell. Reproduced with permission from John Wiley & Sons.)

anesthetic dose, 2% lidocaine hydrochloride can replace a 1% formulation.

8. Mark the skin: Mark the skin for an incision (Figure 18-21M).
9. Make the skin incision: Bring the needle forward again, accurately indicating the site for incision. For core biopsy, a 3 to 4 mm skin incision facilitates entry of the biopsy needle, reducing skin drag on the outer cannula during advancement of the biopsy instrument (Figure 18-21N). Access to multiple targets is possible through the same skin incision; however, the limit in any direction is about 4 mm. Most clinicians make a skin incision parallel to the widest axis of the needle.

Placement of the Biopsy Needle

The clinician guides the needle into the breast, advancing to the desired depth (Figure 18-21O). See later discussion on determining prefire depth.

Confirmation (Prefire Stereo) Images

Acquire a prefire stereo pair before the final firing or advancing of the biopsy instrument to the targeted lesion location to ensure correct needle placement and to check for abnormality movement (Figure 18-21P). Retract the anterior needle guide while acquiring the prefire images to prevent superimposition over the area of interest.

First Sample

1. Check for proper seating of the biopsy instrument.
2. Ensure that the anterior needle guide is forward to provide accurate needle placement.
3. Ensure positive stroke margin, discussed later in this chapter.
4. Fire the biopsy instrument or begin sampling.

Postfire Stereo Images

Acquire postfire images, if desired, immediately after firing the biopsy instrument to verify that the needle has pierced the abnormality (Figure 18-21Q). Lesion movement and needle deflection are two possible problems commonly encountered on postfire images. This information may alter subsequent needle position.

Tissue Marker Clips

Multiple specimen sampling often removes all radiographic evidence of the abnormality (this frequently occurs

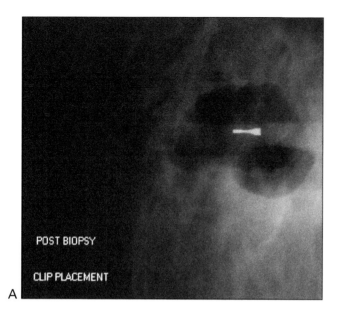

POST BIOPSY

CLIP PLACEMENT

A

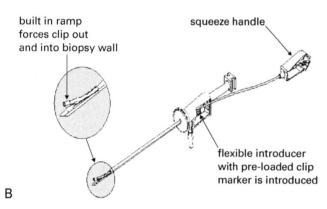

built in ramp
forces clip out
and into biopsy wall

squeeze handle

flexible introducer
with pre-loaded clip
marker is introduced

B

Figure 18-22
Clip placement. **(A)** Removal of all radiographic evidence of an abnormality during biopsy requires placing a tissue marker clip to mark the area for follow-up localization. **(B)** A line drawing to explain deployment of the clip inside the biopsy cavity.

with small groupings of calcifications); this necessitates the physician place a tissue marker clip to identify the location of the abnormality (Figure 18-22). The literature illustrates this to be a safe and effective method for later localization and follow-up.[18,19]

Tissue marker clips are also useful to mark the location of a large cancerous mass for which the patient will undergo induction chemotherapy to shrink the tumor before surgery. In some cases, induction chemo removes all radiographic and sonographic evidence of disease. The tissue marker clip is useful to mark the location for later breast conservation therapy or to monitor tumor shrinkage.

Clip deployment is possible with a "straight needle" method or a through probe method[19] depending on the initial mode of biopsy. An upright two-view mammogram is recommended after deployment.[20]

Specimen Radiography

Specimen radiography ensures removal of calcifications. Reviewing this image before releasing the patient from compression allows further sampling, if necessary. Typically, a standard mammography unit using the magnification mode provides the necessary image. Always use caution in handling and transferring core specimens (Figure 18-23A and B).

Poststudy Image

Acquiring a poststudy image with the x-ray tube perpendicular to the breast support documents access to the abnormality. A recognizable reduction in the number of calcifications or a mass with a section removed confirms successful sampling (Figure 18-23C).

Complications After a Biopsy

Complications following a needle biopsy occasionally happen, although the likelihood is much greater when the patient has an open surgical biopsy. With a needle biopsy, the patient could have:

- An allergic reaction to the local anesthetic. This is more likely to occur with patients who have congestive heart failure or liver disease. The symptoms to watch for include flushing or redness of the skin, itching skin, unusually warm skin, and small red or purple spots on the skin.
- Bleeding or hematoma. When positioning the patient for the biopsy procedure, the technologist is responsible for inspecting the scout image for the presence of blood vessels overlying the area to be biopsied. If blood vessels are seen near this area, either the breast or the C-arm should be rotated to position the area of interest away from blood vessels. Hematomas cause irritation and possibly infection. To reduce complications resulting from a hematoma, pressure should be directed over the biopsy site immediately at the conclusion of the biopsy procedure. This pressure should be constant for several minutes. A cold compress should be applied to the breast for the next 12 hours. Hematomas resolve over time.
- Infection. Anytime the skin is pierced, the opportunity for infection exists. A bacterial cleaning solution is applied to the surface of the skin before the clinician makes a small incision to introduce the biopsy needle. The biopsy needle is sterile, and the biopsy team practices a sterile technique. Yet infections happen. The patient should be advised to contact the clinician if symptoms of

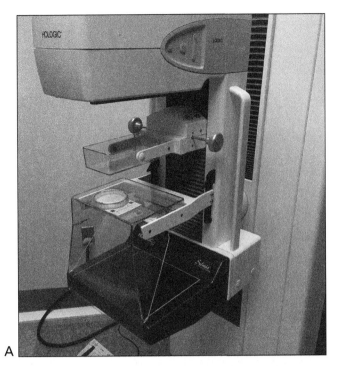

A

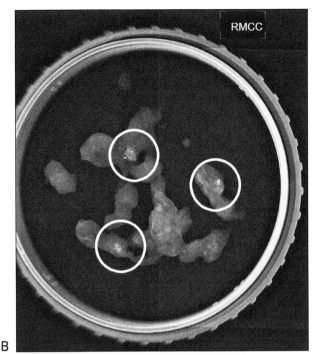

B

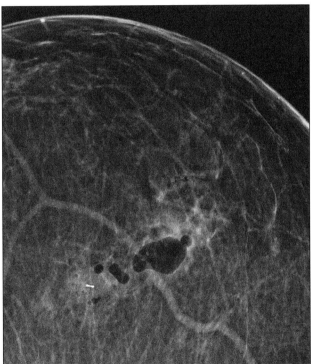

C

Figure 18-23

Specimen radiography. **(A)** Specimen radiography, using the magnification mode, provides proof of calcium in the biopsy specimen. **(B)** Use of the magnification mode makes it easier to look for microcalcifications. **(C)** Post exam mammogram shows evidence of tissue removal as well as clip placement.

infection appear at the biopsy site: redness, discomfort, and fever. A prescription for antibiotics usually resolves the infection.

When the biopsy is scheduled, patients should be quarried about blood thinners. If the patient does use blood thinner medication, they may be advised to discontinue this medication for several days before the procedure.

PRINCIPLES AND INSTRUMENTATION OF CORE BIOPSY

The Biopsy Instrument

Each biopsy device ("gun" or "driver") is a spring-loaded system with a cocking device and firing button (Figure 18-24);

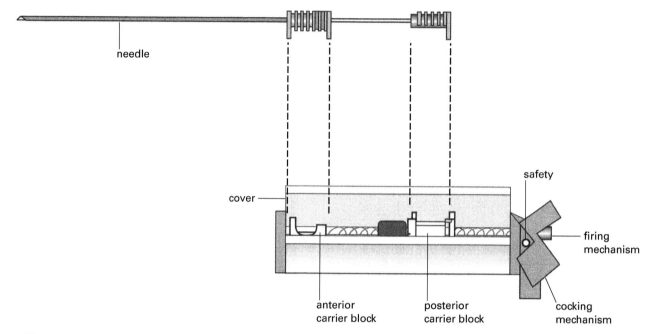

Figure 18-24
Spring–loaded biopsy instrument/needle combination. (From Willison KM. Fundamentals of stereotactic breast biopsy. In: Fajardo LL, Willison KM, Pizzeutiello RJ, eds. A Comprehensive Approach to Stereotactic Breast Biopsy. Cambridge: Blackwell Science; 1996:44. Copyright © 1996 Wiley-Blackwell. Reproduced with permission from John Wiley & Sons.)

some systems may be multidirectional, vacuum assisted, with a powered rotating cutter (Figure 18-25). An automatic or manual safety feature is standard on all instruments to prevent premature or accidental firing.

Anterior and posterior carrier blocks hold the hubs of each part of a biopsy needle or probe (Figure 18-24). The design of the mechanism allows high-velocity firing of the carrier blocks carrying the needle and probe to sample

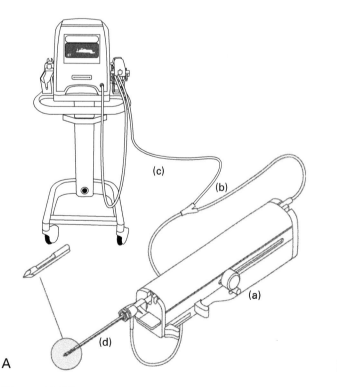

A

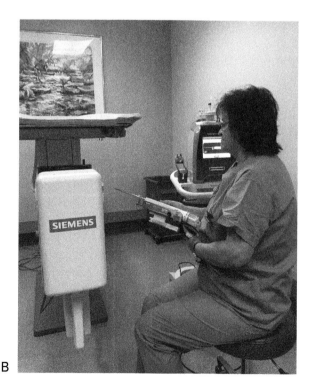

B

Figure 18-25
A multidirectional vacuum-assisted biopsy system. **(A)** A line drawing showing the biopsy probe, tubing, and the vacuum control module. **(B)** The technologist prepares to attach the biopsy system to the stage of the stereotactic table.

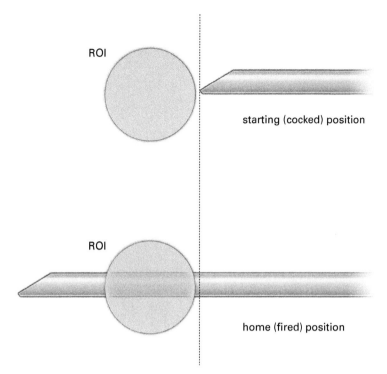

Figure 18-26
The stroke of the biopsy device is the distance the needle travels from the starting (cocked) position to the home (fired) position.

the abnormality. The distance the gun moves the needle or probe, from the starting (or cocked) position to the home (or fired) position, is the **stroke** (or throw) of the instrument (Figure 18-26). Stroke varies between 11 and 23 mm, depending on the manufacturer and the model. With shorter throw instruments, less of the sample notch is available for sampling. Strokes of 19 to 23 mm are most popular.

The efficiency of the biopsy instrument depends on spring force, its velocity of movement, maintenance, weight, cocking mechanism, safety features, and most critically the firing mechanism. Spring-loaded devices differ from multidirectional vacuum-assisted devices in many ways. The greatest difference is the size and continuity of the biopsy specimens (Figure 18-27); the vacuum-assisted device is more proficient in acquiring larger, unfragmented specimens. The multidirectional devices also do not require removal of the biopsy probe to retrieve the specimen as the vacuum transfers the sample out of the breast for collection (Figure 18-28). Another advantage of this device is that samples may be taken without firing the biopsy gun. A disadvantage of the vacuum device is that the entire biopsy collection chamber must be within the breast for effective operation, reducing the type of breast amenable to this device. The vacuum-assisted biopsy device is more expensive as are the required probes (needles) and tubing.

Needles and Probes

The gauge of the needle affects the size of the biopsy specimen and has a direct correlation with the effectiveness of sampling and the histologic interpretation.[6,21,22] Biopsy needles and probes used for core biopsy are typically 8 to 14 gauge.

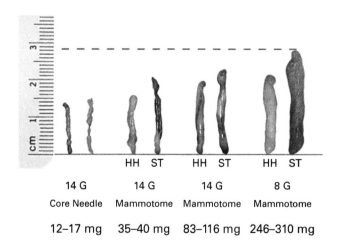

Figure 18-27
Specimen comparison. Comparison of specimen continuity and size between the spring-loaded and vacuum-assisted devices. (Courtesy Mammotome, Leica Systems.)

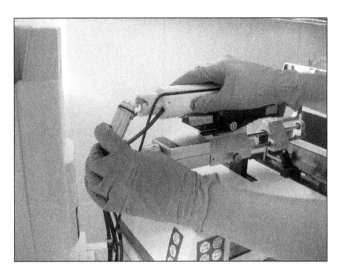

Figure 18-28
Removal of specimen. Vacuum-assisted devices transfer the specimen for retrieval without removing the biopsy instrument from the breast.

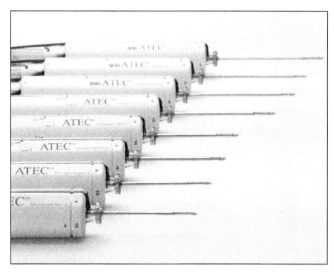

Figure 18-29
Various length ultrasound devices displayed.

• *Spring loaded*
  14 gauge = 17 mg; typical size of the specimen
• *Vacuum assisted*
  14 gauge = 35 to 40 mg
  11 gauge = 83 to 110 mg
  8 gauge = 250 to 310 mg

The length of the needle is a consideration also, as the needle length directly correlates with accessible depth, superimposition of the biopsy instrument in the biopsy window, and the amount of available working space (Figure 18-29). The biopsy needles for spring-loaded devices have two parts: an inner stylet, cut with a sample notch for specimen acquisition, and an outer cutting cannula (Figure 18-30). The needles have a beveled tip.

Needles (probes) for vacuum-assisted devices consist of three parts: an outer cannula, inner rotating cutter, and a central vacuum stylet (Figure 18-31). Generally, these probes also have a specimen collection chamber and gear that allows rotation of the cutting stylet.

Sampling Sequence

Spring-Loaded Instruments

The firing of the biopsy instrument occurs in two stages. The posterior carrier block holding the notched stylet portion of the needle fires first. This triggers the anterior carrier block to drive the cutting cannula forward over the stylet. The sample or "core" of tissue is taken during this excursion (Figure 18-32). If for some reason the posterior block does not make its full movement, the anterior block that holds the cutting cannula will not fire. The open sample notch is left in the breast, causing complications to the procedure. This may occur from mechanical failure

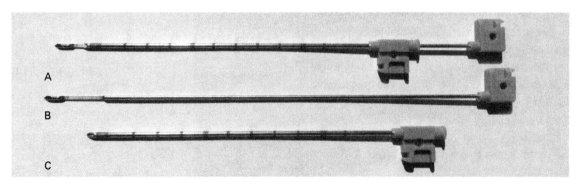

Figure 18-30
(A) The core biopsy needle has two parts, **(B)** the inner stylet with sample notch and **(C)** the outer-cutting cannula.

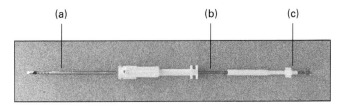

Figure 18-31
A probe for vacuum-assisted biopsy. The probe device showing three-part construction: (*a*) outer cannula (*b*) inner-rotating cutter and (*c*) a central vacuum stylet.

or negative stroke margin. Hard or fibrous tissue may also "heap up" in front of the bevel, which may stop the movement of the needle in cases of very minimal stroke margin.

Removal and reinsertion for multiple samples is necessary, emptying the sample notch after each pass. The sample notch is unidirectional.

Vacuum-Assisted, Multidirectional Devices

These devices also have a spring-loaded firing mechanism but differ in ways that improve the facility of sampling. The driver (gun apparatus) is powered electrically, allowing a cutter to rotate to collect the sample. The driver also connects via tubing to a suction device. The probe (needle) is either "fired" or manually driven into the breast, depending on physician preference, and narrow or negative stroke margin. After switching the driver on, the physician opens the sample notch allowing the vacuum to pull the tissue into the chamber. Slowly advancing the inner rotating cutting stylet through the outer cannula cuts the specimen (Figure 18-33). The vacuum stylet then draws the specimen through the outer cannula to the specimen collection chamber (Figure 18-28). Before removing the sample, the physician rotates the sample notch to another position to access multiple areas for sampling (Figure 18-34). After sampling, the clip is deployed through the probe (Figure 18-35).

Case Study **18-3**

Refer to Figure 18-33 and the text and respond to the following question.

1. List several advantages of the vacuum-assisted biopsy device.

Stroke Margin

The compressed breast must be of sufficient thickness to accept the forward motion of the needle from the prefire to postfire position, without exiting the far side of the breast and striking the breast support platform. *The distance from the postfire position of the tip of the needle to the breast support, usually allowing 4 mm for safety, is known as stroke margin* (Figure 18-36).

Positive stroke margin indicates ample thickness for needle excursion. *Negative* stroke margin indicates that the needle will exit the backside of the breast, causing injury, complication, or termination of the procedure.

The radiologist may manually calculate stroke margin, or the computer of the SBB unit will calculate it. Regardless, the team, including the technologist, must be aware of the calculation of stroke margin. Visual indicators are equally important. For example, if the computer or manual calculations determine positive stroke margin but visual clues indicate otherwise, recheck the calculations; incorrect information keyed into the computer or a misread number could be the reason. The following general formulas help determine stroke margin; however, always follow the manufacturer's recommendations:

- When depth is determined from the proximal aspect of the compressed breast:
  Stroke margin = (compression thickness – 4 mm) – (prefire depth + stroke).
- When depth is determined from the distal aspect of the compressed breast:
  Stroke margin = (prefire depth – stroke) – 4 mm.

  To counter a negative stroke margin:

- Alter the prefire position of the needle tip.
- Use a shorter stroke biopsy instrument.
- Reposition the breast (see Chapter 9).
- Vacuum-assisted biopsy instruments allow the needle to be manually advanced into the breast in the uncocked position. Biopsy is possible because sampling with these instruments does not depend on the spring-loaded movement but rather on the cutting cannula and the suction of the vacuum. Where stroke margin is an issue, and because the vacuum-assisted device can pull from up to 0.5 to 1 cm from the collection chamber, it is possible to place the needle at a shorter depth than indicated and still biopsy the abnormality.

Programming Needle Length and Stroke

Programming needle length (sometimes expressed by the length of the needle/gun combination) and biopsy instrument

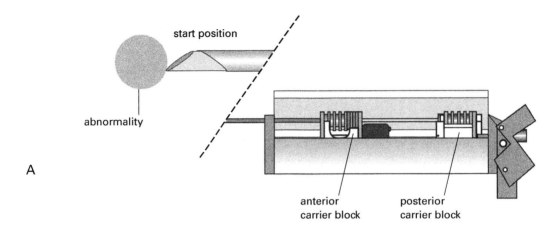

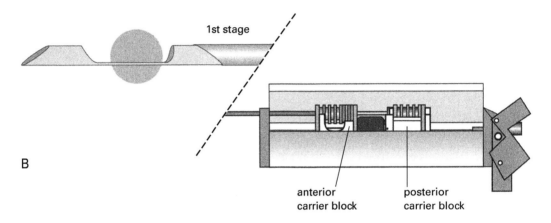

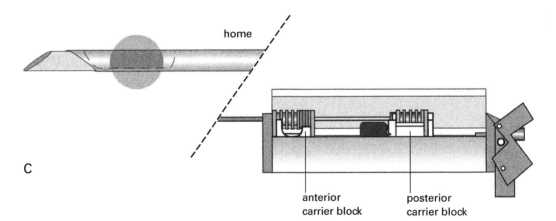

Figure 18-32
Two-stage firing mechanism. Firing the biopsy instrument occurs in two stages. **(A)** The posterior carrier block holding the stylet fires first, **(B)** advancing the sample notch into the abnormality. **(C)** This triggers the firing of the anterior carrier block that holds the cutting cannula, allowing the removal of tissue. (From Willison KM. Fundamentals of stereotactic breast biopsy. In: Fajardo LL, Willison KM, Pizzeutiello RJ, eds. A Comprehensive Approach to Stereotactic Breast Biopsy. Cambridge: Blackwell Science; 1996:47. Copyright © 1996 Wiley-Blackwell. Reproduced with permission from John Wiley & Sons.)

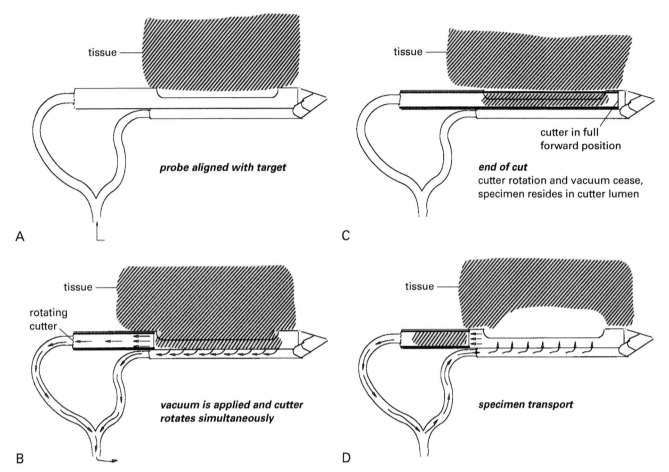

Figure 18-33
Sampling sequence for a vacuum-assisted device. **(A)** The biopsy device may be fired or placed in the breast at the correct depth. **(B)** The suction pulls the tissue into the sample notch. **(C)** The rotating cutter shears the specimen. **(D)** The vacuum transports the sample for retrieval.

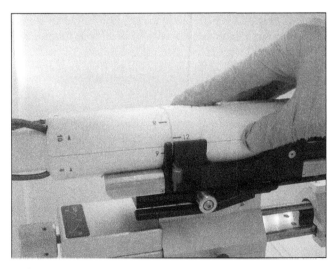

Figure 18-34
Multisampling with a vacuum-assisted device. Rotating the hand piece to mark clock time allows multidirectional sampling.

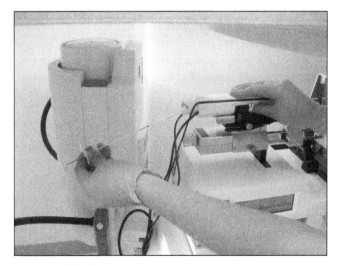

Figure 18-35
Clip deployment. After multisampling, a tissue marker clip is deployed through the biopsy probe.

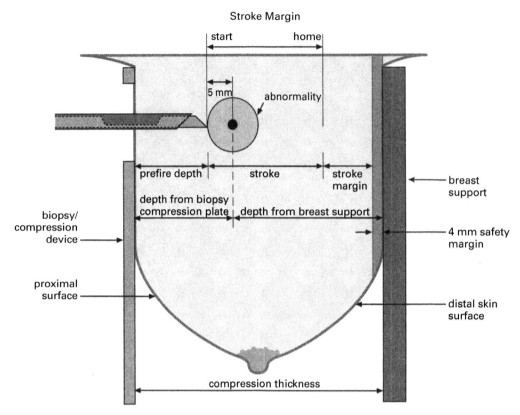

Figure 18-36
Stroke margin. (From Willison KM. Fundamentals of stereotactic breast biopsy. In: Fajardo LL, Willison KM, Pizzeutiello RJ, eds. A Comprehensive Approach to Stereotactic Breast Biopsy. Cambridge: Blackwell Science; 1996:49. Copyright © 1996 Wiley-Blackwell. Reproduced with permission from John Wiley & Sons.)

stroke are necessary to arrive at an accurate depth coordinate and ensure accurate calculation of stroke margin. Programming the stroke simply requires entering a number into the computer or into the stroke margin calculation. Programming needle length is slightly more complicated.

Factoring the needle length into the system is either done as a one-time default setting or requires a zeroing process during each procedure. Needle calibration is specific to each unit; follow the manufacturer's instructions.

Determining Prefire Position

Ideally, firing of the biopsy instrument will place the center of the abnormality in the center of the sample notch, allowing maximum capture of the abnormality. To achieve this result requires placing the needle proximal to the depth coordinate before firing. This is the prefire or back-off position.

Calculating the prefire position, or "back-off," depends on the following criteria:

1. Stroke of the biopsy instrument.
2. Distance from the tip of the needle to the sample notch (Figure 18-37).

3. Length of the sample notch when measured at the inferior aspect (Figure 18-37). Measurement should be made by the clinician rather than relying on printed package measurements, as manufacturers differ in how they measure the sample notch.

The formula to determine prefire back off is as follows:

$$\text{Pre-fire back-off} = S - (L/2 + NT)$$

Where: S = Stroke
L = Length of available sample notch
NT = Length of needle tip

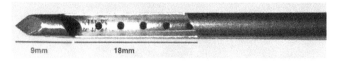

Figure 18-37
The collecting chamber of the biopsy device measures 18 mm, while the needle tip measures 9 mm. When targeting a ROI, we must always take into account the 9-mm measurement.

Parker[23] and Hendrick[24] recommend placing the needle 5 mm proximal to the depth coordinate. For example, if the depth coordinate were 24 mm, the prefire position would be 19 mm. Although this standard is adequate for most of the longer stroke (22 to 23 mm) biopsy instruments, it is inaccurate for shorter throw instruments. Figure 18-38 illustrates a comparison. Parker and Hendrick also report that the abnormality will move forward with needle impact.

Calibration of the Stereotactic System

The manufacturer calibrates the stereotactic system at installation of the unit. However, daily *verification* is necessary. The QC testing procedure analyzes the accuracy of the biopsy system, including the targeting device, digitizing system, and coordinate calculation. Daily QC (or more frequent if necessary) testing by the technologist, before the first procedure of the day, ensures the unit's accuracy. Deviation from normal limits requires at least one repeated test. If retesting confirms the error, service is necessary. Neglecting this important test can complicate and jeopardize procedures.

Targeting

Accurate **targeting** of the abnormality is critical for precise stereotactic localization. The essence of stereotactic

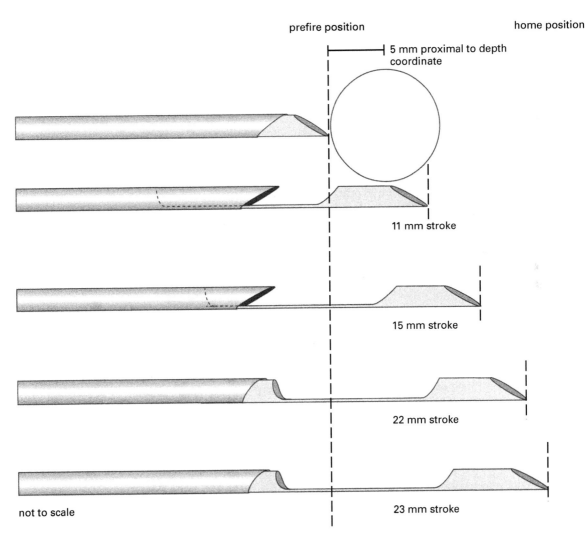

Figure 18-38
A comparison of biopsy instrument prefire positions. Prefire position, or "back-off", will vary with the stroke of the biopsy instrument and needle measurements. The accepted 5 mm prefire position proximal to the depth coordinate will be satisfactory for 22 or 23 mm throw instruments, but not for shorter throw instruments. This figure illustrates how the abnormality could be missed with shorter throw instruments. (From Willison KM. Fundamentals of stereotactic breast biopsy. In: Fajardo LL, Willison KM, Pizzeutiello RJ, eds. A Comprehensive Approach to Stereotactic Breast Biopsy. Cambridge: Blackwell Science; 1996:52. Copyright © 1996 Wiley-Blackwell. Reproduced with permission from John Wiley & Sons.)

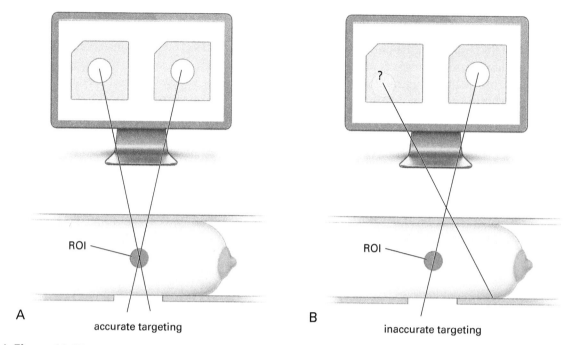

Figure 18-39
Targeting the ROI. **(A)** The ROI is well visualized on both stereo images, providing for accurate targeting and yielding accurate results. **(B)** The ROI is not seen with certainty on the left-hand image of the stereo pair. Guessing the position of this ROI for targeting yields incorrect horizontal and depth coordinates.

localization involves targeting the same point in space (or as near to it as can be estimated) on both planar images (Figure 18-39). This necessitates proper *display, shift,* and *identification* of the abnormality on both planar images. The physician must also identify a unique point within the abnormality on both planar images. The identification process is not always easy (Figure 18-40). For example, identifying a unique point within a well-rounded mass presents little challenge. However, choosing a unique point for odd-shaped masses, diffuse areas of distortion, or calcifications may be difficult. Principles of shift and display aid in appropriate targeting (Figure 18-41). *Under no circumstances should the biopsy continue if the clinician cannot identify the abnormality, or a unique point, on both stereo images.* Selecting alternative projections may solve this dilemma.

Target on Scout

An alternative method to use with nonvisualization of the region of interest on one of the stereo pair images is the "target on scout" feature. This allows the scout to replace one of the stereo images in targeting and coordinate calculation. The abnormality must be visible on the scout and at least one stereo image in order to utilize this feature.

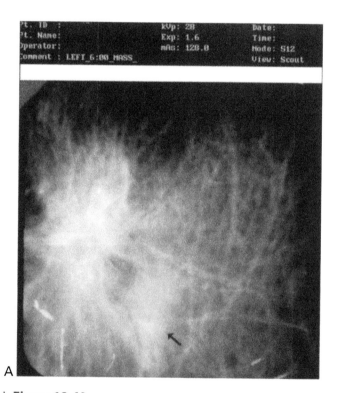

Figure 18-40
Targeting and abnormality identification. Following lumpectomy and irradiation, this patient has a new mass. **(A)** The scout image demonstrates this abnormality (*arrow*) well.

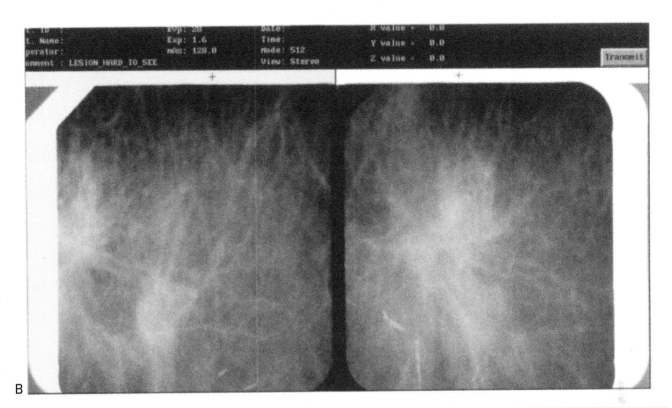

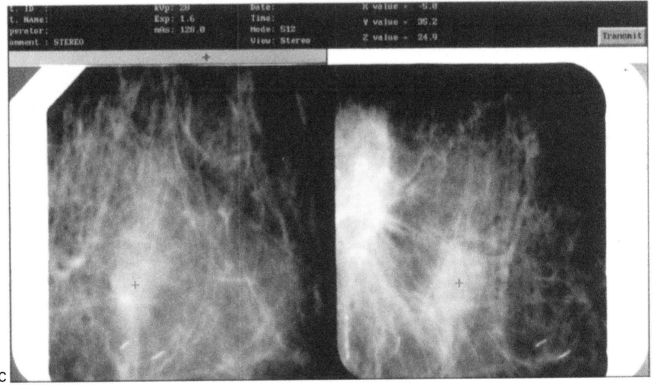

Figure 18-40 (*Continued*)
(B) On the stereo images, the abnormality is well-visualized on the left-hand image but not on the right. **(C)** Repositioning in a new projection provides a stereo pair that demonstrates the abnormality on both the left and right images, allowing for accurate targeting. Histology is positive for recurrence. (From Willison KM. Fundamentals of stereotactic breast biopsy. In: Fajardo LL, Willison KM, Pizzeutiello RJ, eds. A Comprehensive Approach to Stereotactic Breast Biopsy. Cambridge: Blackwell Science; 1996:54–55. Copyright © 1996 Wiley-Blackwell. Reproduced with permission from John Wiley & Sons.)

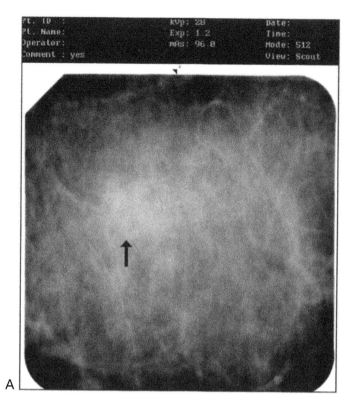

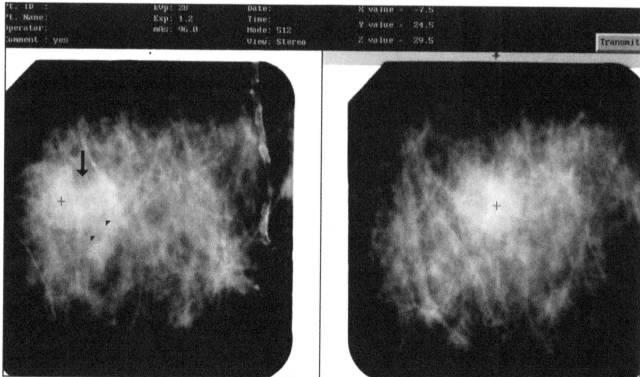

Figure 18-41

Applying principles of shift for accurate targeting. Failed aspiration of a cyst in the right breast under ultrasound guidance in a patient post left breast mastectomy resulted in a hematoma. The aspiration was then attempted under stereotactic guidance. **(A)** The scout image demonstrates the cyst (*arrow*) to the left of the reference cursor (*arrowhead*). **(B)** On the stereos, the right-hand image demonstrates the cyst well; *note the wide shift of the abnormality.* The wide area of density on the left stereo image makes it difficult to correctly identify the abnormality. The edge effect (*arrowheads*) seems to indicate this area to be the cyst (*arrow*). However, the distance of shift should be the same in each stereo image, alerting the clinician that this density is not the cyst. The cyst is actually to the left of this density (*cursor*). (From Willison KM. Fundamentals of stereotactic breast biopsy. In: Fajardo LL, Willison KM, Pizzeutiello RJ, eds. A Comprehensive Approach to Stereotactic Breast Biopsy. Cambridge: Blackwell Science; 1996:56. Copyright © 1996 Wiley-Blackwell. Reproduced with permission from John Wiley & Sons.)

Targeting Procedure

The mammography equipment manufacturer recommends the targeting *sequence* for accuracy; the computer program maintains sequencing. In most cases, there is a prompt for sequencing within the computer software program. When targeting the abnormality, adhere to the following specific rules:

1. With some units, it is necessary to identify the reference point(s) and mark them with a cursor. Never attempt to complete targeting if the reference points are not visible or are incorrectly marked because the calculations will be wrong (Figure 18-42).
2. Maintain the same vertical axis. Between stereo image acquisitions, the abnormality will not shift in the vertical direction unless the patient moves between images. Therefore, when identifying or targeting, always remain on the same vertical axis (Y-axis) from one planar image to the other (Figure 18-43). A horizontal locus line appears on the monitor to maintain the same vertical plane.
3. Use the cursor to locate the targets on both planar images.

Targeting Accuracy

Several methods ensure safe, effective biopsy and improve and verify targeting accuracy. Before targeting, review the scout and stereo images:

1. Check the scout image for superimposed blood vessels that may be punctured during sampling (Figure 18-44).
2. Check the scout image for proper centering.
3. Check both stereo images for the abnormality (Figure 18-45). *If the abnormality is not visualized*, recheck the centering on the scout image and also check the technical factors.
4. Check stereo images for direction of abnormality shift.

   After targeting:

1. Verify accurate transmission or transference of target coordinates.
2. Check the scout image for abnormality position in the biopsy window and correlate with the calculated X and Y coordinates; they should match.
3. Compare the depth coordinate with mammographic information. If the depth coordinate of the abnormality is outside the expected depth, it is possible that identification of the abnormality and/or targeting might be incorrect.
4. With most SBB systems, the depth coordinate should be a positive number, in which case a negative depth coordinate would indicate an error.

Confirmation (Prefire) Stereos

Acquire the confirmation stereo pair with the needle at the exact depth coordinate or at the prefire position. These images verify accurate placement of the needle. Figure 18-46 demonstrates possible errors; these visual errors may have several causes: faulty targeting, patient or abnormality movement, and/or calculation errors.

X (H) or Y (V) errors are readily discernible but are not measurable due to the magnification factor on the prefire images; additionally foreshortening of the needle gives a false impression of the actual position of needle depth (Z or D). Rather than rely on the appearance of the stereo image to estimate an error, use the computer to check for inaccuracies by targeting the needle tips. If the coordinates of the needle position do not match the original calculated coordinates (allowing for prefire back-off), then a needle placement error is most likely due to a mechanical or computer error (Figure 18-47).

In some cases, the error will be in millimeters. This errant needle position is actually useful as an offset target; most vacuum-assisted biopsies done today target *below* the lesion as this allows visualization of the lesion in the prefire stereo pair. Other errors are not intentional and require repositioning of the needle. A correction factor can be calculated by determining the difference between the coordinates of the needle and the abnormality coordinates. If the needle position is accurate but an error is visible, then abnormality movement is most likely the reason (Figure 18-48).

Multidirectional vacuum-assisted devices allow the biopsy chamber to rotate 360°. This permits some leeway in the accuracy of needle placement. Simply rotating the biopsy chamber in the direction of the abnormality often resolves many targeting issues.

Less common is errant targeting of the abnormality. Again, this needle position may be useful as an offset target. If the abnormality is visible on both of the prefire stereo images, then retargeting is possible to determine the abnormality's new location. If the abnormality is not visible on one or both images (sometimes the needle obscures the abnormality), then it is necessary to repeat the stereo pair after removing the needle from the breast. Retargeting will give the new location of the abnormality. A new set of confirmation stereos will confirm needle placement.

Multiple Area Sampling

With a multidirectional vacuum-assisted device, rotation of the collection chamber allows multiple area sampling. Probe removal in between samples is not necessary as the

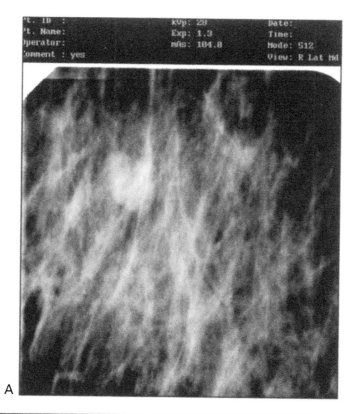

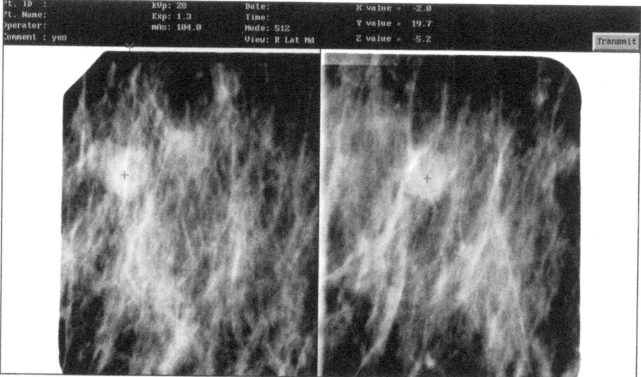

Figure 18-42

Identification of reference points. Reference points incorrectly marked on stereo images yield inaccurate coordinates. Comparing the position of the abnormality on the scout image to the resulting coordinate will ensure accurate targeting. **(A)** In this case, the abnormality is positioned in the scout image in the negative half of the biopsy window, at approximately −9 mm. **(B)** The horizontal coordinate (upper right-hand corner) determined from the stereo images yields an inaccurate −2.8 mm position. The depth coordinate also yields a negative number, which is another indication that the targeting was inaccurate. The depth coordinate will not always be a negative value in false reference marking, so it is best to check all coordinates. (From Willison KM. Fundamentals of stereotactic breast biopsy. In: Fajardo LL, Willison KM, Pizzeutiello RJ, eds. A Comprehensive Approach to Stereotactic Breast Biopsy. Cambridge: Blackwell Science; 1996:59. Copyright © 1996 Wiley-Blackwell. Reproduced with permission from John Wiley & Sons.)

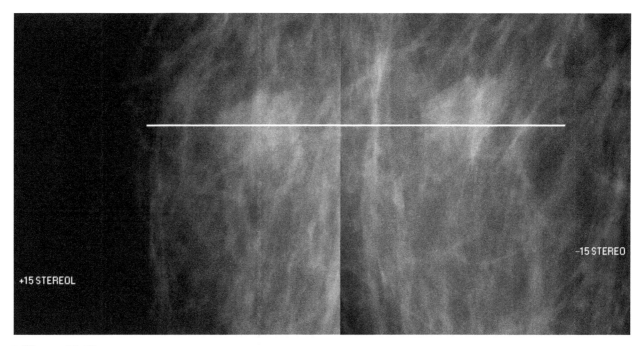

Figure 18-43
Maintaining a vertical axis. Unless the patient or abnormality has moved a great distance between stereo images, the abnormality will remain on the same vertical axis. A *horizontal line* appears on the monitor to maintain the same vertical axis.

collection chamber closes for rotation and the suction stylet transports the sample for retrieval.

Various methods exist for multiple area sampling with a spring-loaded device, which requires removal and reinsertion of the biopsy device to retrieve each sample.

- The clinician can choose *multiple passes* simply by varying the horizontal and vertical position of the needle while maintaining the same depth. Some digital systems require identification of the "offsets" as part of the targeting process yielding new X (H) and Y (V) coordinates.
- The clinician may choose *multiple targets* resulting in new horizontal, vertical, and depth coordinates by targeting many unique points on both planar images. Multitargeting is especially useful for calcifications that may be at different depth planes.

POSITIONING FOR STEREOTACTIC BIOPSY

The goal of SBB positioning is to appropriately center and visualize an abnormality while at the same time allowing adequate needle sampling. Positioning is multifaceted, ranging from the relatively simple task of positioning the abnormality in the projection of discovery to more challenging issues. The complex conditions that exist in positioning for mammography also apply to stereotactic biopsy. Even though the focus is imaging a specific area of the breast rather than the entire breast, the same factors that complicate routine mammography apply: body habitus, location of the breast on the body, and breast tissue composition. Additionally, and perhaps even more critical and demanding, are the factors that influence the ultimate approach to positioning for SBB:

- Ensuring positive stroke margin.
- Accessibility to an abnormality's location may be difficult.
- The technologist must identify the abnormality on the scout image and maintain clarity on the stereo projections
- Overlying blood vessels.
- Patient comfort.

This arduous set of tasks can be overcome with a positive attitude, an open mind, and motivation to master new techniques. The technologist achieves proficiency in a variety of circumstances; she can facilitate the positioning process and shorten the learning curve by adhering to the following guidelines:

- Be knowledgeable about the stereotactic unit by learning both its advantages and limitations.

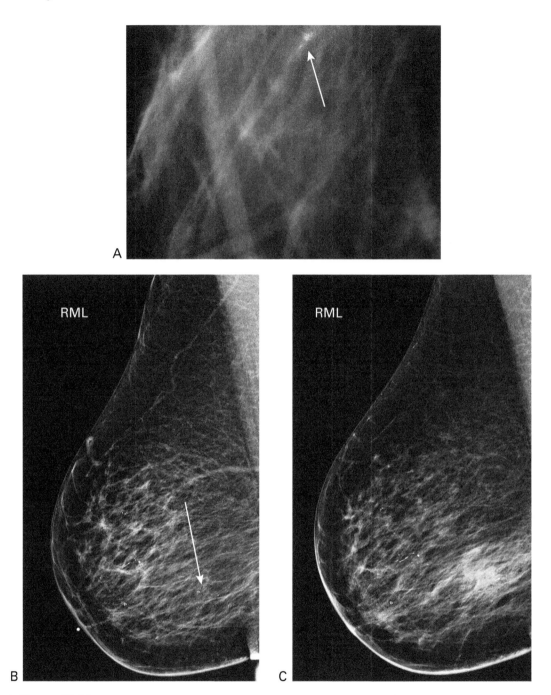

Figure 18-44
Avoid blood vessels. The stereo scout image should always be inspected for blood vessels overlapping the tissue to be excised. **(A)** Numerous blood vessels are in the area of calcifications (arrow) to be biopsied. **(B)** The pre-biopsy mammogram with calcifications (arrow) indicated. **(C)** Blood vessel punctured at needle insertion causing a hematoma. This not only increases patient bleeding but also can obscure the area of interest during the procedure.

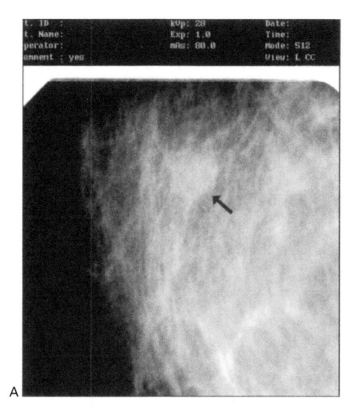

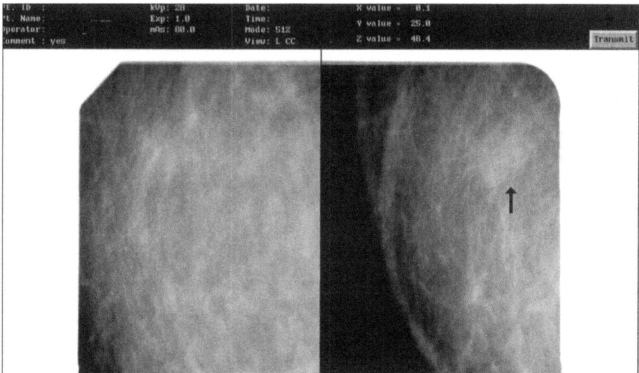

Figure 18-45
Check both stereo images for abnormality visualization. **(A)** A low-density abnormality well visualized on the scout image (*arrow*) **(B)** can only be seen on one side of the stereo pair (*arrow*).

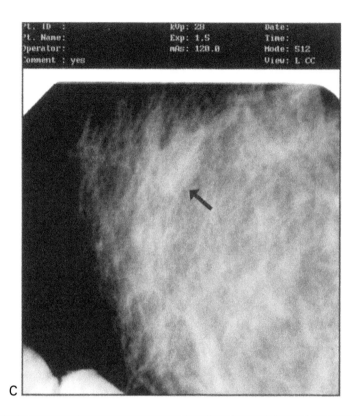

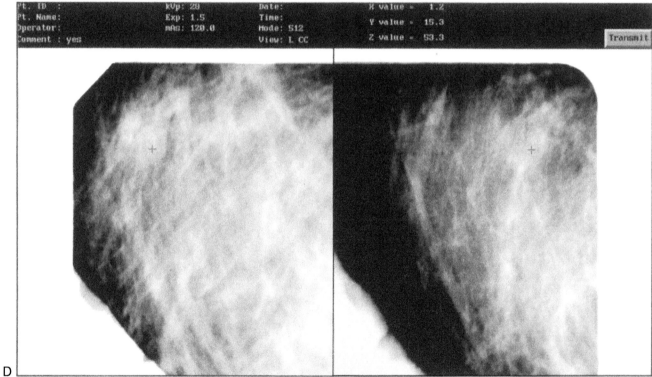

Figure 18-45 (*Continued*)
(C) Repositioning and rescouting (*arrow*) **(D)** allows visualization on both stereo images (*cursors*). (From Willison KM. Fundamentals of stereotactic breast biopsy. In: Fajardo LL, Willison KM, Pizzeutiello RJ, eds. A Comprehensive Approach to Stereotactic Breast Biopsy. Cambridge: Blackwell Science; 1996:62–63. Copyright © 1996 Wiley-Blackwell. Reproduced with permission from John Wiley & Sons.)

- Understand the rudiments of stereotactic biopsy, grasping the concepts of stroke and the calculation of stroke margin.
- Become adept at approximating abnormality location in the breast based on the two-view mammogram.

Understanding these elements and the positioning basics discussed below will provide a strong foundation to develop and build positioning skills.

Positioning Basics

Patient Motion

Movement of the breast can increase dose, add extensive time to the procedure, and can complicate the biopsy process. To minimize motion, inform the patient of the steps of the biopsy, the noises she will hear, and the sensations she will feel.

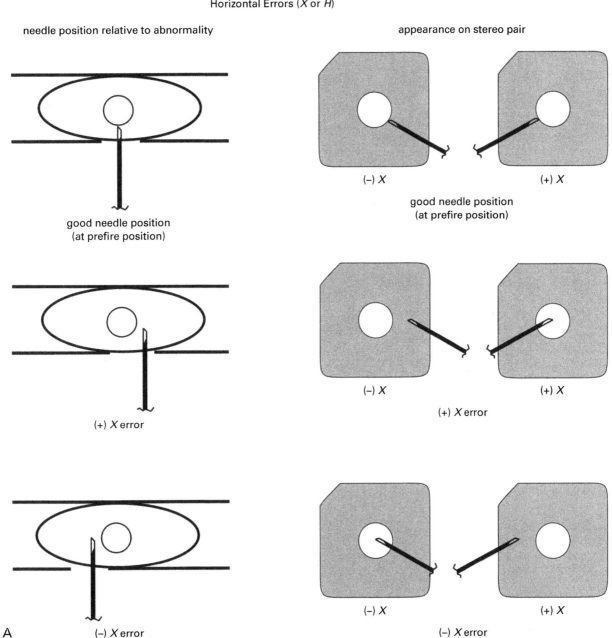

Horizontal Errors (*X* or *H*)

needle position relative to abnormality

appearance on stereo pair

good needle position
(at prefire position)

(–) *X*   (+) *X*

good needle position
(at prefire position)

(+) *X* error

(–) *X*   (+) *X*

(+) *X* error

A   (–) *X* error

(–) *X*   (+) *X*

(–) *X* error

Figure 18-46
(A) Examples of horizontal errors.

Depth Errors (*Z* or *D*)

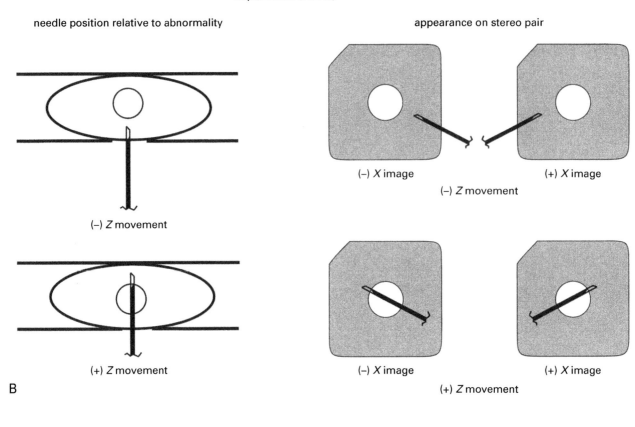

Vertical Errors (*Y* or *V*)

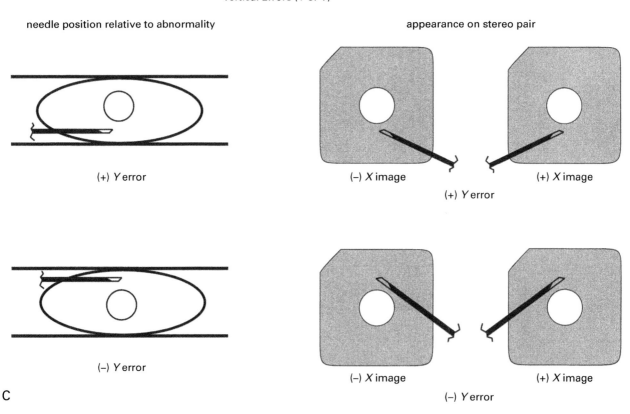

Figure 18-46 (*Continued*)
(B) Examples of depth errors. **(C)** Examples of vertical errors. (From Willison KM. Fundamentals of stereotactic breast biopsy. In: Fajardo LL, Willison KM, Pizzeutiello RJ, eds. A Comprehensive Approach to Stereotactic Breast Biopsy. Cambridge: Blackwell Science; 1996:64–65. Copyright © 1996 Wiley-Blackwell. Reproduced with permission from John Wiley & Sons.)

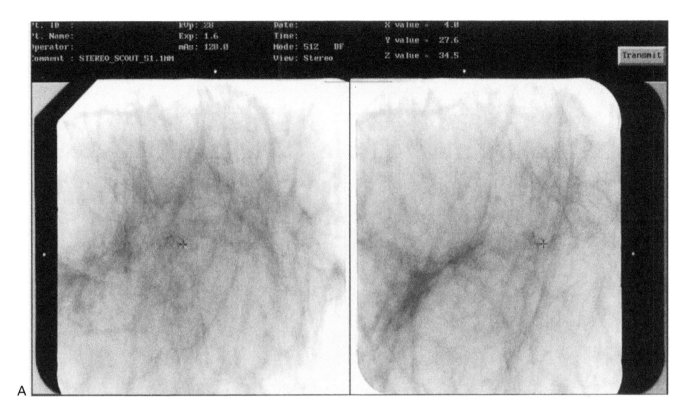

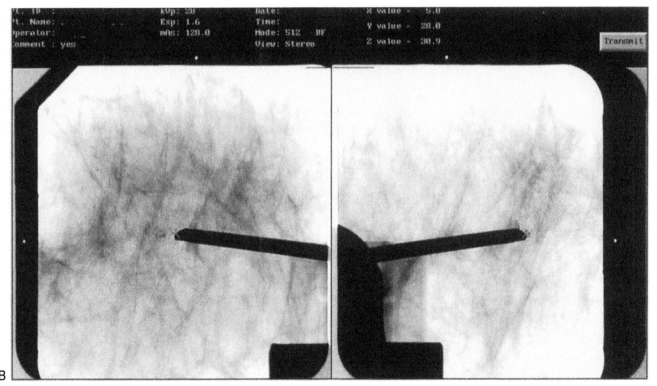

Figure 18-47

Inaccurate needle placement. **(A)** The stereo images yield coordinates as shown (upper right-hand corner). **(B)** Confirmation stereos demonstrate a horizontal error. Targeting over the needle tips (*cursor*) indicates the needle guidance system is inaccurate (upper right-hand corner). The biopsy/compression device was not placed correctly. A correction factor was determined and sampling completed. (From Willison KM. Fundamentals of stereotactic breast biopsy. In: Fajardo LL, Willison KM, Pizzeutiello RJ, eds. A Comprehensive Approach to Stereotactic Breast Biopsy. Cambridge: Blackwell Science; 1996:66. Copyright © 1996 Wiley-Blackwell. Reproduced with permission from John Wiley & Sons.)

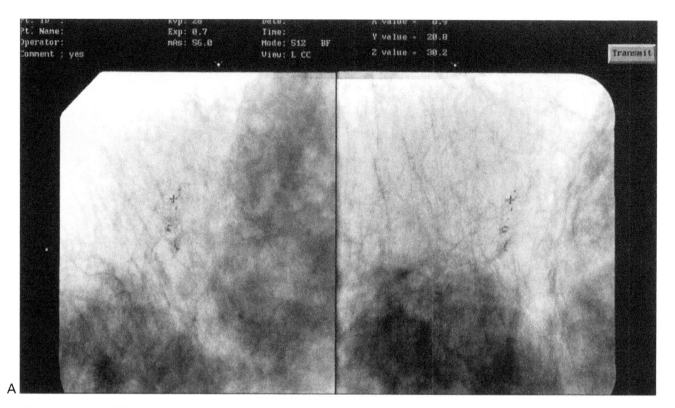

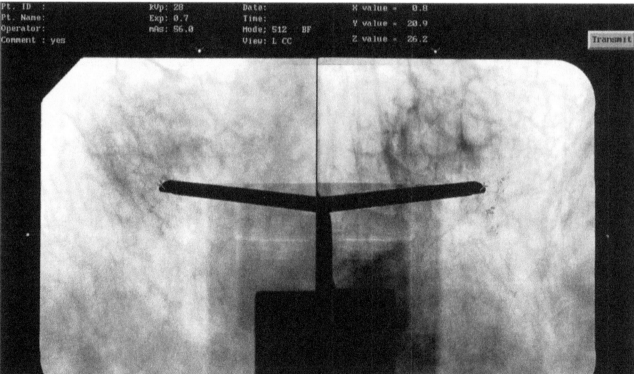

Figure 18-48

Abnormality movement. **(A)** Stereo images demonstrate abnormality coordinates (upper right-hand corner). **(B)** Confirmation stereos indicate a horizontal error. Targeting the needle indicates accurate placement (upper right-hand corner). The abnormality has moved. The stereos were repeated after removal of the needle and new coordinates obtained. (From Willison KM. Fundamentals of stereotactic breast biopsy. In: Fajardo LL, Willison KM, Pizzeutiello RJ, eds. A Comprehensive Approach to Stereotactic Breast Biopsy. Cambridge: Blackwell Science; 1996:68. Copyright © 1996 Wiley-Blackwell. Reproduced with permission from John Wiley & Sons.)

If the patient moves her breast at any time after acquisition of the stereo images, the abnormality will move, and the targeting coordinates may no longer be accurate. If movement is suspected, reposition the breast in the biopsy window, retake the scout and stereo images, and retarget the abnormality. Additional prefire stereo images are necessary to again check for correct needle placement. With the use of a Cartesian coordinate system, reacquiring stereos may not be necessary; a simple measurement and adjustment may be possible. However, prefire stereo images are always necessary to verify accurate needle placement.

Patient Comfort

For most patients, the most uncomfortable part of the biopsy procedure is remaining in one position for an extended period of time. Explain this to the patient in advance and make every effort to make her comfortable. The extended procedure time means that the patient should use the lavatory before beginning the procedure. Also, have her remove earrings, necklaces, glasses, and any apparel that might interfere with her comfort or the x-ray beam. Before final positioning of the breast, allow the patient to remain in position for a few minutes so she can identify an awkward position or points of pressure. Offer a blanket to keep her warm. Approximately 8% of cancelled procedures are due to the patient's inability to tolerate the procedure.[25]

Prone Table

With a prone table, the patient is usually in a slight right anterior oblique (RAO) or left anterior oblique (LAO) position, depending on the breast and the location of the abnormality. Pressure points often include the ipsilateral shoulder and inferior ribs. When addressing comfort issues, be judicious with padding for the shoulder or ribs when dealing with a posterior lesion in a small breast. Excessive padding will raise the breast up, limiting posterior access. Place a soft but thin sponge or other material between the shoulder, ribs, and table to help alleviate discomfort. A thin gel pad creates a nice cushion between pressure points and the table without excessively raising the breast out of the table aperture.

The neck is another area that may be uncomfortable during prone biopsy. A thin, warm water bottle, supportive sponges or a rolled towel placed beneath the hollow formed by the neck and table can offer support and comfort. Do not place anything beneath the head (Figure 18-49). This causes additional stress and strain on the neck and shoulder. However, if access to the posterior breast is not necessary, offer a small, thin pillow to give both head and neck support in the same plane. Be sure that the

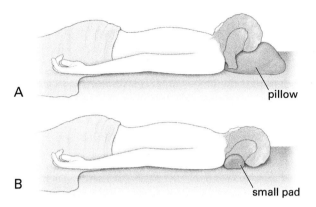

Figure 18-49
Neck support. **(A)** Placing a pillow under the head when the patient is prone may cause discomfort to the neck and shoulder. **(B)** Placing a small cushion to support the neck is more appropriate.

contralateral breast is also comfortably positioned and out of the way. If the contralateral breast needs to be over the table opening, a sling can be made from the patient's gown to hold the breast up and out of the way. During the procedure, if the patient complains of stiffness or loss of sensation in the neck or arm, the technologist can massage the area to alleviate discomfort.

The lower back may also need support to prevent an uncomfortable lordotic curve. Place a small pillow beneath the abdomen to prevent discomfort, or provide a pillow for support beneath the bent leg.

Add-On Units

Adapting a dedicated mammography unit with add-on stereotactic equipment presents many challenges for the technologist. The biopsy team should first make a complete analysis of the positioning situation before the patient arrives. This may shorten procedural time and reduce complications. Speed is important with upright procedures. Awareness of the following issues will help provide the best possible environment for the patient while maintaining the requirements of stereotactic biopsy.

Support: For the patient to remain motionless in an upright position during the entire biopsy procedure, the technologist must ensure her comfort. Little effort should be expected of the patient to maintain the biopsy position. Back support is particularly important. Pillows or other similar props can provide the necessary support. Sufficient back support holds the patient in position, diminishes fatigue, and reduces the opportunity for motion. Support for the feet and legs also provide stability. Without foot support, the legs suspend freely, which counters the patient's ability to lean forward for breast positioning. This also places unnecessary stress on the lower back, making it increasingly uncomfortable and difficult for the patient to remain motionless during the biopsy procedure. The floor can provide foot support if the chair is low enough, or use a footstool if the biopsy chair does not provide a footrest. Although it might be advantageous for the biopsy chair to be on wheels, this may be a hindrance if the wheels do not lock for final positioning.

Bleeding: Extensive bleeding at the biopsy site is not common; however, always drape the lower half of the patient's body to prevent staining clothes or skin.

Vasovagal response: A vasovagal response should always be a concern in any procedure where the patient is upright. Diminishing the likelihood of a vasovagal response with upright procedures depends on several factors. Make every effort to position the patient in a way that shields her view of the biopsy procedure and sterile tray. Assure the patient is comfortable and well supported. The clinician and technologist should communicate with her at all times during the examination. A likelihood of a vasovagal response may also increase with limitations on food intake. There is no need to limit food intake for core biopsy or FNAC, unless the patient will proceed directly to a surgical suite postbiopsy.

TECHNICAL CONSIDERATIONS FOR SBB POSITIONING

X-Ray Field Size

Biopsy Field

Each stereo unit has a specified x-ray field size. The technologist should be aware of the actual dimensions of the field, as this may differ from the size of the biopsy window available on the compression device. The imaging field is typically 50 mm × 50 mm, although one table manufacturer now offers an additional 60 mm × 70 mm imaging field. This wider field of view is helpful when scouting the breast for the abnormality, especially when having difficulty locating the area of concern.

Centering and Abnormality Shift

Projectional shift of the abnormality occurs in the horizontal plane with stereo acquisition. Centering the abnormality in the horizontal plane (X or H axis) of the biopsy window is critical to maintain visualization during stereo acquisition. However, nonvisualization of the abnormality can still occur on one or both stereo images despite proper centering. The abnormality may not remain within the confines of the image receptor or x-ray field. The probability of

nonvisualization also increases as compression thickness increases. Nonvisualization becomes more critical when the image receptor field size is limited. The abnormality may also elude visualization as a result of system design. This can occur on systems that do not allow for increased compression thickness, usually above 6 cm.

Centering in the vertical plane (Y axis) is not necessary as the stereo projections do not affect vertical placement. However, a certain vertical placement within the biopsy window may facilitate the examination by creating easier access for the biopsy team.

Compression Thickness and the Breast Support

As described above, nonvisualization of the abnormality can occur when the abnormality is outside the field of view when the tube head is in place for stereo acquisition. This effect increases with compression thickness. A movable breast support prevents this phenomenon from occurring, so that there is never a failure to image an abnormality as a result of compression thickness. The technologist adjusts the breast support on the basis of compression thickness.

Some units do not have an adjustable breast support. In this instance, the technologist must reposition the breast to decrease compression thickness. Another method is to "target on scout." The technologist can off-center the abnormality in the biopsy box and use the scout and the stereo image that maintains visualization of the abnormality. Never reduce the angle of stereo acquisition to maintain visualization, unless recommended by the manufacturer.

Tissue Coverage within the Biopsy Window

When positioning, always strive to cover the biopsy compression device window completely with breast tissue (Figure 18-50). Compression of the breast on all sides of the biopsy window reduces the possibility of motion. Coverage of the biopsy window increases stability of the breast for needle insertion and better tissue sampling. Window coverage also ensures coverage of the entire x-ray field, thereby diminishing scatter. With digital reconstruction, the computer interprets the uncovered portion of the biopsy window as a structural part of the breast resulting in extremely poor latitude for subsequent image processing (window and level functions), which inhibits visualization of the abnormality. Images of retroareolar abnormalities are especially susceptible to incomplete filling of the biopsy window. If possible, it is best to rotate the breast upward or downward to fill the biopsy window rather than profiling

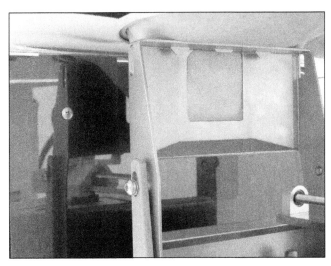

Figure 18-50
Coverage of the biopsy window. Coverage of the biopsy window with breast tissue prohibits breast movement and provides stability for needle insertion.

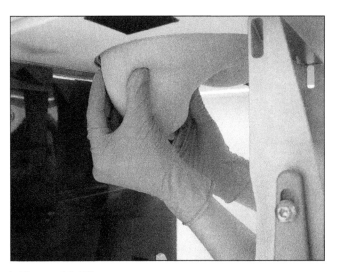

Figure 18-52
Tightening the skin. The technologist spreads the skin with both thumbs while compressing to tighten the skin surface. This minimizes "tenting" and facilitates needle insertion.

the nipple. When this is not possible, place a small amount of single-use putty, modeling clay, or aluminum foil in the uncovered portion of the imaging field to act as a wedge filter, which will decrease pixel overexposure (Figure 18-51).

Compression

Compression has a twofold purpose in stereotactic biopsy. It immobilizes the breast to prevent motion and tightens the skin surface to facilitate passage of the needle through the skin. The vigorous compression force associated with routine mammography is not necessary for stereotactic biopsy, rather compression should be applied until there

is a "spring" to the skin when touched. Because compression over the biopsy area is not possible due to the open biopsy window, the technologist should spread the skin over the area, using her thumbs to make the skin tight (Figure 18-52). This creates tension on the skin surface and minimizes inward "tenting" with needle insertion. Breast or abnormality movement may be caused by inward tenting and may prohibit the cutting edge of the biopsy needle from passing through the skin. Affixing Tegaderm over the compression device opening is another positioning aid that helps provide stability when compressing the breast and inserting the needle.

Visualizing the Abnormality

The circumstances of stereotactic biopsy are sometimes in direct conflict with the technical factors that apply to efficient routine mammographic imaging. Fine microcalcifications and low-density masses may be susceptible to nonvisualization as a result of the following factors:

1. Loss of subject contrast from decreased compression and increased breast thickness
2. Use of higher kVp settings to shorten the exposure time results in a less contrasty image
3. A grid is not used when imaging with the magnification mode. Grids clean up scatter
4. Increased geometric unsharpness from increased object-to-image receptor distance

The technologist must be aware of these compromises to apply the necessary technical skills to image the abnormality. The best the technologist can do in positioning is to

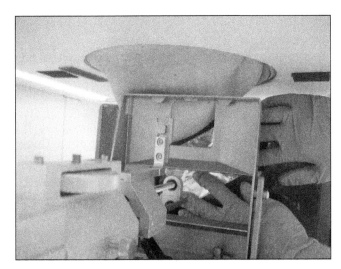

Figure 18-51
Noncoverage of the biopsy window. The technologist can place aluminum foil in the uncovered portion of the biopsy window to provide better image quality.

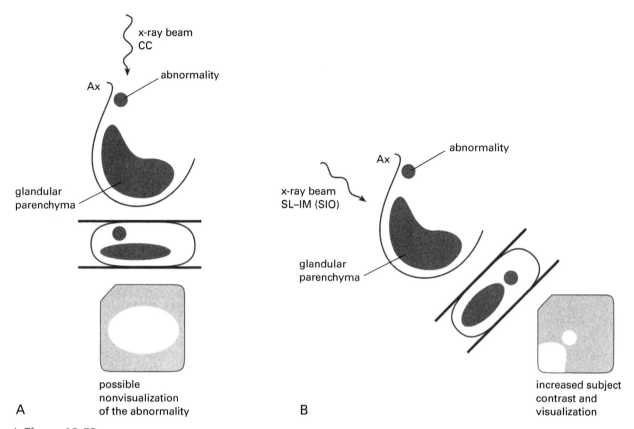

Figure 18-53

Increasing subject contrast. Demonstrating an abnormality against a fatty background increases subject contrast. **(A)** In this example, the CC projection superimposes the abnormality over glandular structures, resulting in possible nonvisualization. **(B)** A superolateral to inferomedial (SIO) projection projects the abnormality over the fatty portion of the medial breast, increasing subject contrast and visualization. (From Willison KM, Saunders DA. Positioning in stereotactic procedures. In: Fajardo LL, Willison KM, Pizzeutiello RJ, eds. A Comprehensive Approach to Stereotactic Breast Biopsy. Cambridge: Blackwell Science; 1996:147. Copyright © 1996 Wiley-Blackwell. Reproduced with permission from John Wiley & Sons.)

select the projection that allows the thinnest compression while maintaining a positive stroke margin. Thinner breast compression decreases geometric unsharpness and scatter.

Increased subject contrast improves abnormality visualization.

Positioning the abnormality against a background of adipose tissue improves subject contrast (Figure 18-53). The majority of breast tissue lies in the subareolar region and in the upper outer quadrant. This characteristic pattern allows the technologist to take advantage of the adipose-replaced areas of the breast. If the technologist and clinician consider the distribution of a patient's glandular parenchyma, they can select a projection that allows imaging of an abnormality against a background of fat (Figure 18-54).

Logistics for Add-On Units

C-Arm Rotation

When selecting a position for biopsy, the technologist must be aware of the logistics of the C-arm swing for stereo images. The patient should be unencumbered by the x-ray tube housing and the image receptor mount of the mammography machine during stereo rotations. The technologist learns to avoid projections that inhibit C-arm movement. For example, when the technologist positions the patient for a CC projection, she may have to move the patient's head to accommodate tube rotation for stereo acquisition. This increases the likelihood of breast and abnormality movement. Even if the source-image distance (SID) of the unit allows stereo rotation without interference with the patient's head, her head may still interfere with the path of the x-ray beam. The inferior aspect of the C-arm has to clear the patient's lower body with stereo rotation. The technologist should consider a different projection if the patient has to move to accommodate tube shift. For example, in the above case, a 20° oblique in the ML or LM projection would replace the CC projection. This new projection should be sufficient to allow clearance for tube shift.

The technologist must also consider efficiency and ease of access from the clinician's perspective. For example, any oblique projection, where the clinician is working from the inferior aspect of the breast, may introduce difficulty into the biopsy procedure.

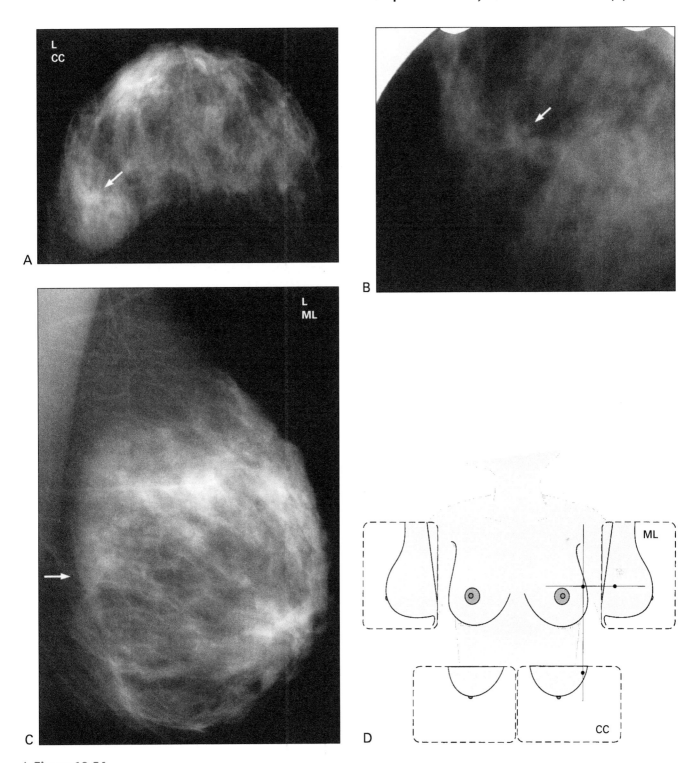

Figure 18-54
Subject contrast. **(A)** The CC mammogram demonstrates an area of architectural distortion (*arrow*) in the lateral aspect of the left breast. **(B)** A coned-down magnified view acquired in an SIO projection demonstrates this abnormality (*arrow*) in fat, increasing the subject contrast and substantiating a real abnormality rather than a pseudo mass. **(C)** A ML projection localizes the abnormality (*arrow*) at approximately 2 o'clock in the left breast. **(D)** For biopsy, the team did not attempt a CC or FB due to abnormality depth from the skin surface.

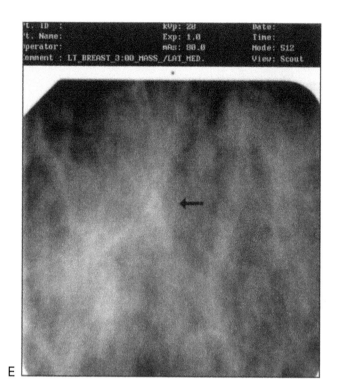

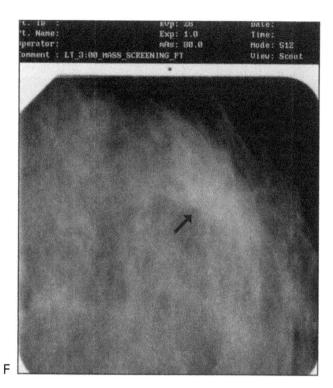

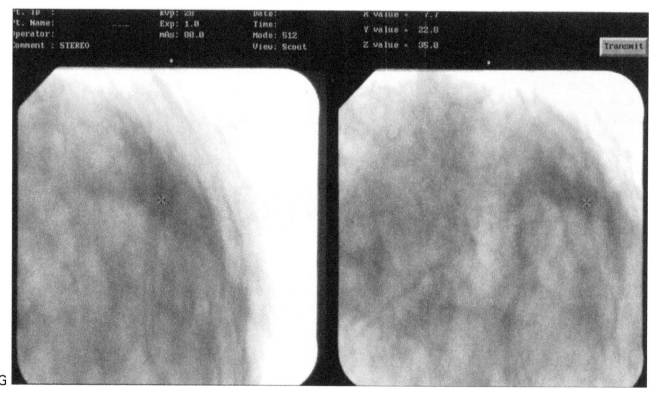

Figure 18-54 (*Continued*)

(E) An LM scout projection demonstrates the abnormality (*arrow*). However, visualization is not maintained on the stereo images, preventing localization. **(F)** Reproduction of the SIO projection, where the abnormality is imaged against a background of fat, demonstrates the abnormality (*arrow*) on the scout projection. **(G)** Visualization of the abnormality is maintained on both stereo images (*cursors*) (Carcinoma). (From Willison KM, Saunders DA. Positioning in stereotactic procedures. In: Fajardo LL, Willison KM, Pizzeutiello RJ, eds. A Comprehensive Approach to Stereotactic Breast Biopsy. Cambridge: Blackwell Science; 1996:148–149. Copyright © 1996 Wiley-Blackwell. Reproduced with permission from John Wiley & Sons.)

Positioning the Breast

Once the patient is comfortable, the technologist can focus on positioning the breast. This section discusses the various positioning factors for stereotactic biopsy, focusing primarily on prone positioning. However, many of these methods also apply to upright positioning. Positioning can be straightforward, requiring minimal planning. For example, if an abnormality is well demonstrated in one of the routine mammographic projections and this projection allows for positive stroke margin for needle core biopsy, then use that projection. Conversely, some situations require flexibility and application of all the technologist's skills. The technologist's creativity is critical in difficult cases where convention does not work. Generally, a solution for a difficult set of circumstances is possible with some work and patient cooperation, but there will also be cases where needle core biopsy is not possible for any number of reasons. The following section provides a basis on which to build positioning skills.

Purpose

The task of positioning for BNB is to visualize the abnormality on the scout image and to maintain visualization on both stereo images or at least one stereo image in order to use the "target on scout" feature of the equipment. If the abnormality is not visualized on either one or both of the stereo images, and subsequent repositioning fails to remedy the situation, biopsy is not possible. Positioning that achieves a positive stroke margin is just as important.

Team Approach

The clinician and technologist, together as a team, should decide on a starting projection for biopsy. However the technologist should have the freedom to alter the projection when necessary. When in doubt, the technologist needs the clinician to confirm identification of the abnormality on the scout image. The scout image might demonstrate the abnormality but escape identification on one or both stereo images. The technologist may want to consult with the clinician before abandoning the projection.

Altered Perspective with Prone Units

When using a prone unit, the technologist may at first find positioning disorienting because of the altered perspective of the breast and the disassociation of the breast from the body (Figure 18-55). For example, the 12:00 area of the breast may shift more medial or lateral when the breast is dependent, or the breast will seem to pull or turn in one

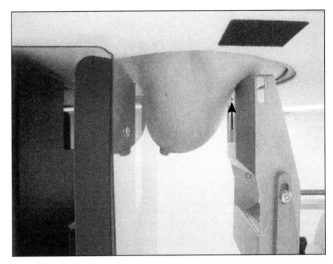

Figure 18-55
Altered perspective with prone units. The technologist may experience disorientation with prone positioning. In this *oblique* projection, the *arrow* indicates 2:00 and not 12:00, as it seems to appear.

direction or the other. Positioning can be especially perplexing when using a projection other than CC or Lateral. In addition, the abnormality location in reference to breast landmarks may change when the breast is dependent. For example, when the breast is dependent in a Lateral or near Lateral projection, the abnormality will consistently appear more inferior than expected.

Reorientation takes some adjustment. Placing a marker on the breast at the approximate location of the abnormality can help maintain one's perspective (Figure 18-56). The technologist can also reorient the breast, as it would be for the CC projection, noting the 12:00 position and the approximate location of the abnormality from this point.

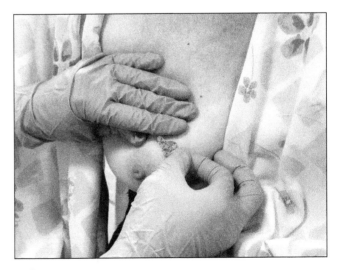

Figure 18-56
Placing a lead marker at the approximate location of the abnormality can aid the technologist in the positioning process.

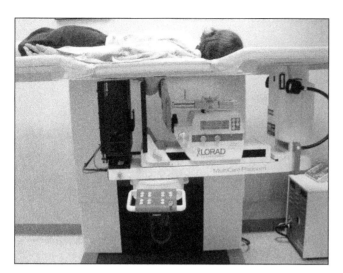

Figure 18-57
The CC projection.

Choosing the Biopsy Approach

Projections for SBB

Once the clinician and technologist determine the approximate location of the abnormality, they can identify the appropriate C-arm approach. To maximize the use and effectiveness of the stereotactic unit, the team must be aware of the positioning choices available with the system and the application of each projection.

Eight projections and endless possible oblique angles that the team can use in stereotactic biopsy are available with a system providing 360° access. Figures 18-57 to 18-64 demonstrate each of these projections on a prone system.

If the system offers 180° access, only the following five projections are available for positioning: CC, ML, LM, SIO, and MLO. While upright units mechanically provide 360°

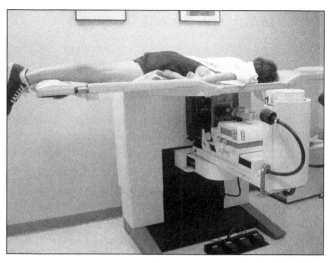

Figure 18-59
The LM projection as demonstrated on the right breast.

access, other limitations may prohibit use of the full rotation. For example, the unit may have the capability to provide a FB approach, but the patient would have to straddle the tube head; additionally, the biopsy team would have to work upside down (Figure 18-65).

Blood Vessels

The technologist must look for blood vessels near the abnormality on the scout image. An examination of the mammogram can help determine the proximity of blood vessels. Blood vessels that project over the abnormality may be at risk for puncture, creating unnecessary complications during needle biopsy (Figure 18-44). Targeting first the abnormality and then the blood vessel can also reveal where the blood vessel is located in relation to the abnormality. If necessary, roll or reposition the breast. The

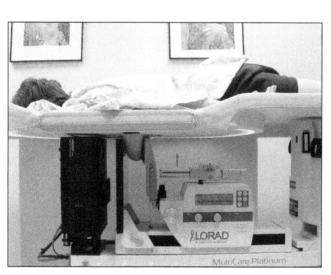

Figure 18-58
The FB projection.

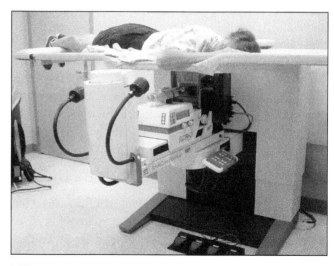

Figure 18-60
The ML projection as demonstrated on the left breast.

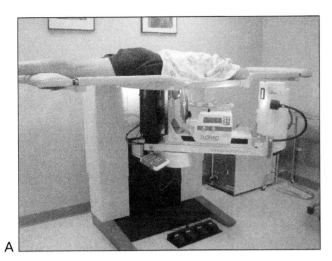 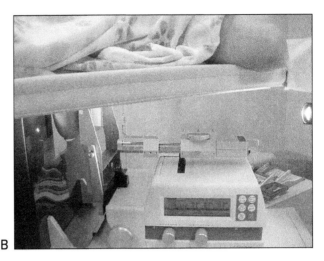

Figure 18-61
The MLO projection. **(A)** The MLO projection demonstrated on the left breast and **(B)** close-up.

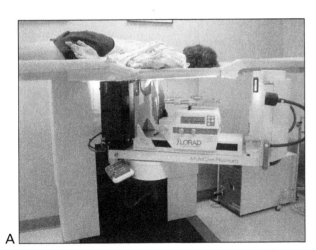 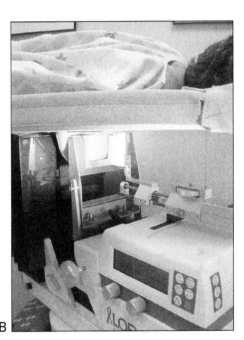

Figure 18-62
The SIO projection. **(A)** The SIO projection demonstrated on the right breast and **(B)** close-up.

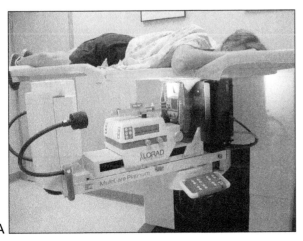 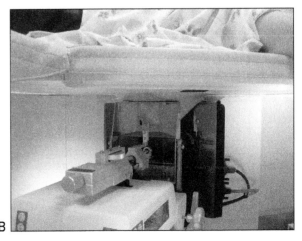

Figure 18-63
The inferomedial to superolateral oblique (IM-SL) projection. **(A)** The IM-SL demonstrated on the left breast and **(B)** close-up.

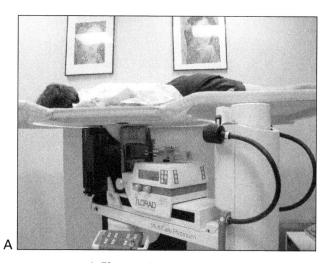
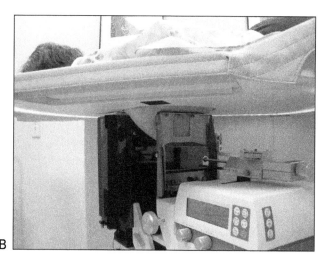

Figure 18-64
The LMO projection. **(A)** The LMO projection demonstrated on the left breast and **(B)** close-up.

technologist can simply rotate the breast or C-arm slightly, 5° to 10°, to modify the projection and eliminate the risk of vessel puncture.

Full Breast Scout

When visualization is elusive, a larger field of view scout image to locate an abnormality can be done in the mammography room. This single large scout view replaces doing a number of small-field scout images, diminishing the technologist's frustration in finding the abnormality and minimizing the patient's discomfort. The ample-sized scout is especially helpful with extremely posterior abnormalities, fine microcalcifications, low-density abnormalities that are difficult to define from the surrounding glandular structures, and when dealing with a very large breast.

An alternative scouting capability is available from one prone table manufacturer who now provides a 60 mm × 70 mm exposure field. Larger than the standard 50 mm × 50 mm exposure field, this longer and wider exposure

Stereotactic Projections								
	Cranio-caudal	Caudal-cranio	Medio-lateral	Latero-medial	SM–IL (ACR–MLO)* Superomedial to Infero-lateral Oblique	IL–SM (ACR–LMO or reverse)* Infero-lateral to Supero-medial Oblique	SL–IM (ACR–SIO)* Supero-lateral to Infero-medial Oblique	IM–SL* Infero-medial to Supero-lateral Oblique
location of abnormality	*(diagram)*	*(diagram)*	*(diagram)*	*(diagram)*	*(diagram)*	*(diagram)*	*(diagram)*	*(diagram)*
upper-outer quadrant	X			X	X slight oblique only	X	X	
upper-inner quadrant	X		X		X		X	X
lower-inner quadrant		X	X		X	X		X
lower-outer quadrant		X		X		X	X	X

*The degree of obliquity depends on the location of the abnormality.

Figure 18-65
This table correlates access to the four quadrants with the possible projections available. (From Willison KM, Saunders DA. Positioning in stereotactic procedures. In: Fajardo LL, Willison KM, Pizzeutiello RJ, eds. A Comprehensive Approach to Stereotactic Breast Biopsy. Cambridge: Blackwell Science; 1996:157. Copyright © 1996 Wiley-Blackwell. Reproduced with permission from John Wiley & Sons.)

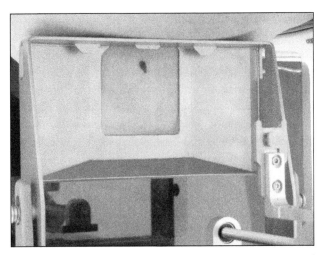

Figure 18-66
Once the larger scout image is acquired, the approximate abnormality location is marked. The technologist reacquires the scout with the smaller biopsy/compression device to ensure proper centering.

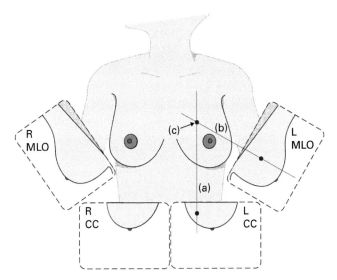

Figure 18-67
Triangulation. The technologist can use this simple method to approximate the location of an abnormality. Since the x-ray beam always remains perpendicular to the image receptor in routine mammography, follow a perpendicular line back through the breast from the abnormality on both the (*a*) CC and (*b*) MLO projections (or any two projections). (*c*) The two lines will intersect at the approximate location of the abnormality. (From Willison KM, Saunders DA. Positioning in stereotactic procedures. In: Fajardo LL, Willison KM, Pizzeutiello RJ, eds. A Comprehensive Approach to Stereotactic Breast Biopsy. Cambridge: Blackwell Science; 1996:161. Copyright © 1996 Wiley-Blackwell. Reproduced with permission from John Wiley & Sons.)

area displays more breast tissue. When searching for an abnormality in a dependent breast, this wider exposure field results in fewer exposures for the patient.

Technologists who are new to stereotactic biopsy may want to use the larger scout method routinely until they become adept at dependent positioning. The scout image may also be useful in providing a comparison for the clinician who is new to the SBB procedure, especially in cases where the breast structures provoke perceptual difficulties.

After the technologist determines the proper approach and location through use of the larger scout image, mark the skin with ink or a lead marker to provide a landmark when positioning with the smaller biopsy window. The technologist should always repeat the scout image using the smaller biopsy window to ensure adequate centering of the abnormality before stereo acquisition (Figure 18-66).

Locating the Abnormality for Positioning

One of the most effective skills the technologist can develop is to fully understand the 3D information available from the two-view mammogram. In doing so, she can determine the quadrant and approximate clock-time location of the abnormality. This skill greatly assists the technologist in choosing the appropriate projection for biopsy, optimizing the SBB equipment, and countering other difficult positioning tasks.

Abnormality Demonstrated on Two Views

If any two mammographic projections demonstrate an abnormality, the technologist can determine an approximate location by using triangulation. Figure 18-67 demonstrates a

simple method of triangulation, showing direct correlation with the mammogram. This method renders the quadrant and approximate clock time of the abnormality. The technologist can also estimate the approximate depth of the abnormality by measuring from the nipple to the abnormality on either mammographic image. These localization techniques render an approximate location and serve only as a guideline. Once the technologist determines the location, it might be useful to place a BB or make an ink mark on the patient's skin to correlate to the approximate location of the abnormality. Note that when the breast is dependent in the prone position, location of the abnormality usually moves inferiorly due to gravity.

Abnormality Demonstrated on One View

If the abnormality is visible on only one mammographic image, triangulation is not possible. In these cases the stereotactic unit is especially useful because it accurately calculates the location of the abnormality—most importantly, the depth coordinate. Under these circumstances, the projection that demonstrates the abnormality is also the scout position. After stereo acquisition, the team targets the abnormality and determines stroke margin. A positive stroke margin allows biopsy. A negative stroke margin indicates repositioning in the reverse projection (Figure 18-68). For example, an MLO projection demonstrates an abnormality not readily identifiable on the CC projection. For stereotactic biopsy, replicate the MLO projection (superomedial to inferolateral). If the depth coordinate does not allow for a positive stroke margin, then reposition in the reverse projection (inferolateral to superomedial); this should provide the shortest skin-to-abnormality distance and positive stroke margin.

Stereotactic biopsy is not a replacement for a diagnostic workup of the patient. Proving that the abnormality is real before placing the patient on the biopsy table is best. Indistinct abnormalities visible on only one view require angled oblique views, magnification, spot compression, or the like to prove they are real. Do not depend on the stereo unit to decide pseudo mass; the imaging parameters of the SBB system may not reveal a real abnormality that is low density and ill defined.

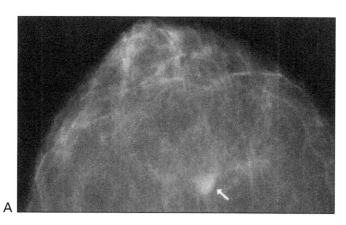

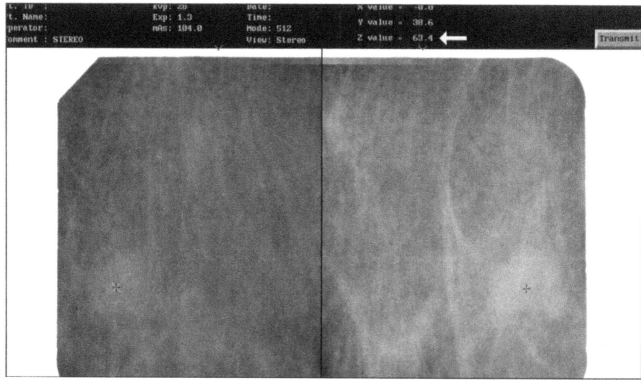

Figure 18-68

Abnormality on one view. **(A)** The CC mammogram demonstrates an ill-defined mass density (*arrow*). The abnormality was not demonstrated on either the MLO or Lateral projections. **(B)** The scout CC projection for stereotactic core biopsy demonstrates this abnormality, which maintains visualization on both stereo images (note the wide shift, typical of deep abnormalities on this unit) (*cursors*). Coordinate calculation (*arrow*) renders a depth coordinate of 63.4 mm with total breast compression measuring 72 mm, producing a negative stroke margin.

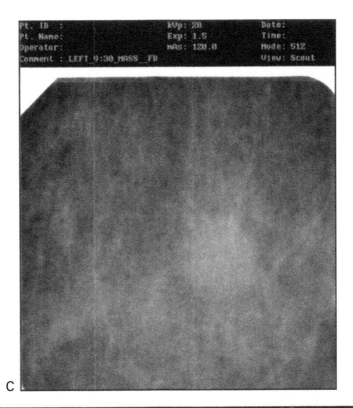

C

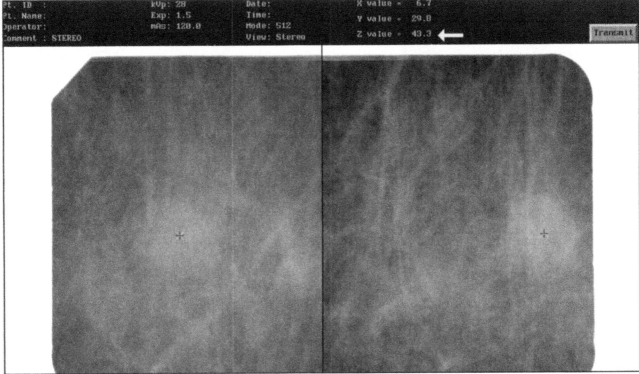

D

Figure 18-68 (*Continued*)
(C) Reversing the position of the C-arm for a FB approach demonstrates the abnormality on the scout image. **(D)** The abnormality maintains visualization on both stereo images (note reduced shift, indicating, for this unit, a more superficial location). Retargeting renders a depth coordinate (*arrow*) of 43.3 mm (with a total compression approximately the same as previously indicated), resulting in a positive stroke margin. (From Willison KM, Saunders DA. Positioning in stereotactic procedures. In: Fajardo LL, Willison KM, Pizzeutiello RJ, eds. A Comprehensive Approach to Stereotactic Breast Biopsy. Cambridge: Blackwell Science; 1996:163. Copyright © 1996 Wiley-Blackwell. Reproduced with permission from John Wiley & Sons.)

Shortest Skin-to-Abnormality Distance and Positive Stroke Margin

When possible, limit positioning choices to those projections that provide the shortest skin-to-abnormality distance and that also allow abnormality visualization on the scout and stereo images (Figure 18-69). The shorter skin-to-abnormality distance minimizes trauma to the breast, provides for positive stroke margin, and ensures minimal excursion of the biopsy needle into the breast. The deeper into the breast the needle travels, the greater the length available for deflection. This is especially important with the smaller needle gauges in use with FNAC.

Sometimes, the projection providing the shortest skin-to-abnormality distance does not demonstrate the abnormality. In this case, choose the projection that allows visualization and at least a positive stroke margin, regardless of the shortest skin-to-abnormality distance. It is not always possible to determine positive stroke margin before final positioning. The technologist should perform a cursory targeting of the abnormality to determine stroke margin; repositioning may be necessary.

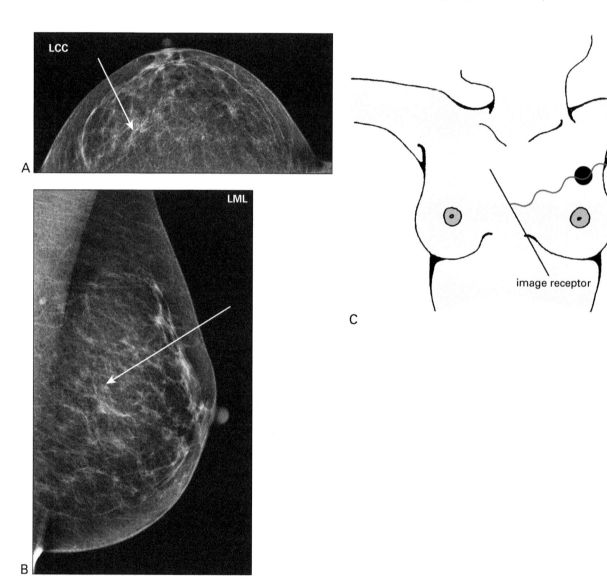

Figure 18-69
Shortest skin-to-ROI distance and positive stroke margin. The **(A)** CC and **(B)** ML projections triangulate the ROI to be at 1:00 in the left breast. Although the LM would be an appropriate approach for biopsy, in this projection, the breast compresses to only 3 cm, resulting in a negative stroke margin. **(C)** An SIO projection provides the shortest skin-to-ROI distance. In this projection, the breast compresses to 4 cm, providing a positive stroke margin.

Table with a Center Aperture

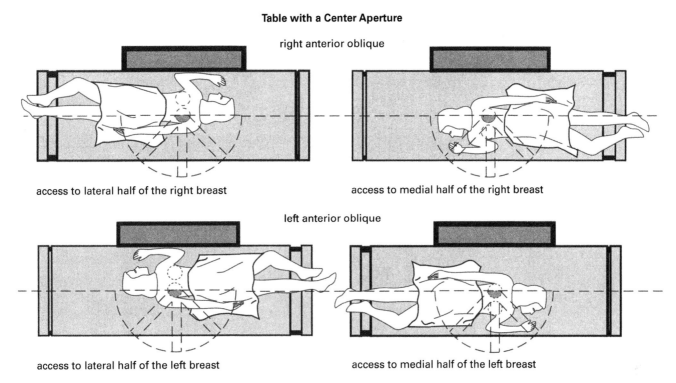

Figure 18-70
Prone positioning. In general, the patient is placed in the right anterior oblique (RAO) position for access to the right breast and a left anterior oblique (LAO) position for access to the left breast. (From Willison KM, Saunders DA. Positioning in stereotactic procedures. In: Fajardo LL, Willison KM, Pizzeutiello RJ, eds. A Comprehensive Approach to Stereotactic Breast Biopsy. Cambridge: Blackwell Science; 1996:166. Copyright © 1996 Wiley-Blackwell. Reproduced with permission from John Wiley & Sons.)

Prone Positioning

The technologist facilitates positioning by placing the patient appropriately on the table. In general, placing the patient in a RAO provides access to the right breast, whereas the LAO provides access to the left breast (Figure 18-70). With a center table aperture, the technologist should position the patient so that the half of the breast containing the abnormality is available for 180° rotation. This allows the maximum number of projections for accessing the breast. Place the ipsilateral arm at the patient's side and flex the contralateral arm at the elbow, resting the hand near the patient's head. This allows the breast to hang suspended through the table opening. Typically, the technologist gains greater access if she centers the breast in the table aperture, permitting the patient's chestwall to fully descend into the table aperture, allowing greater maneuverability of the breast. Accessing some posterior abnormalities requires the patient to be completely flat; others require further adjustments, depending on the location of the abnormality and the selected C-arm approach.

Recommendations for SBB Positioning

The methods described below aid the technologist in effectively positioning the breast for stereotactic biopsy. Not all methods will be successful with all patients, but having many methods to select from will help to achieve success. Some of these methods are specific to prone units; others have application for both prone and upright units.

Maximizing Breast Support Placement

In general, the technologist achieves greater access, especially for posterior abnormalities, by moving the breast support as close to the breast as possible and by overemphasizing this maneuver. This tactic is the same principle that Eklund[26] describes in elevating the inframammary fold for routine mammography. For stereotactic positioning, perform this maneuver in *any* projection by moving the breast support forward behind the breast, allowing the availability of greater amounts of breast tissue. Sacrificing breast tissue nearer the breast support (Figures 18-71 to 18-73) increases chestwall access proximally.

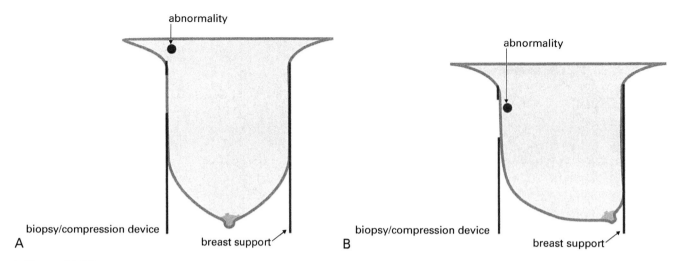

Figure 18-71

Maximizing breast support placement. Greater access to posterior abnormalities is possible by **(A)** moving the breast support forward behind the breast, **(B)** sacrificing distal breast tissue. (From Willison KM, Saunders DA. Positioning in stereotactic procedures. In: Fajardo LL, Willison KM, Pizzeutiello RJ, eds. A Comprehensive Approach to Stereotactic Breast Biopsy. Cambridge: Blackwell Science; 1996:167. Copyright © 1996 Wiley-Blackwell. Reproduced with permission from John Wiley & Sons.)

Position Parallel with the Clock Time

To gain optimal maneuverability of the breast, select the projection where the x-ray beam is parallel to the clock-face location of the abnormality (Figure 18-74). For example, if the abnormality is at 12:00, use a CC projection; if the abnormality is at 10:00 in the right breast, use a 45° SIO projection (Figure 18-75). This method allows greater mobility of the breast and better placement of the breast support platform.

Posterior Abnormalities

The technologist can successfully image what seem to be inaccessible posterior abnormalities that are near the chestwall. The team should never base the decision not to biopsy solely on the location of the abnormality on the mammogram. For example, a posterior location on the mammogram does not always indicate difficulty with stereotactic positioning.

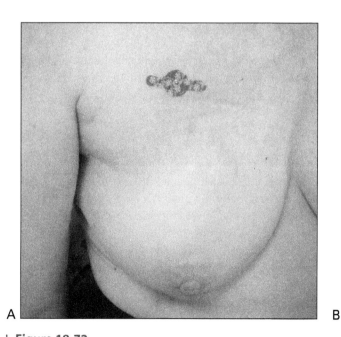
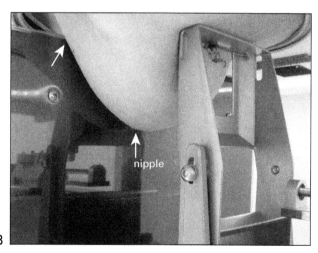

Figure 18-72

Breast support placement. **(A)** Moving the breast support forward behind the breast allows greater access to the chestwall abnormalities nearer the biopsy/compression device, usually causing the nipple to roll under. **(B)** Demonstrates completed positioning of this abnormality. Note how the tissue near the breast support trails off (*arrow*), allowing greater proximity to the chestwall abnormalities.

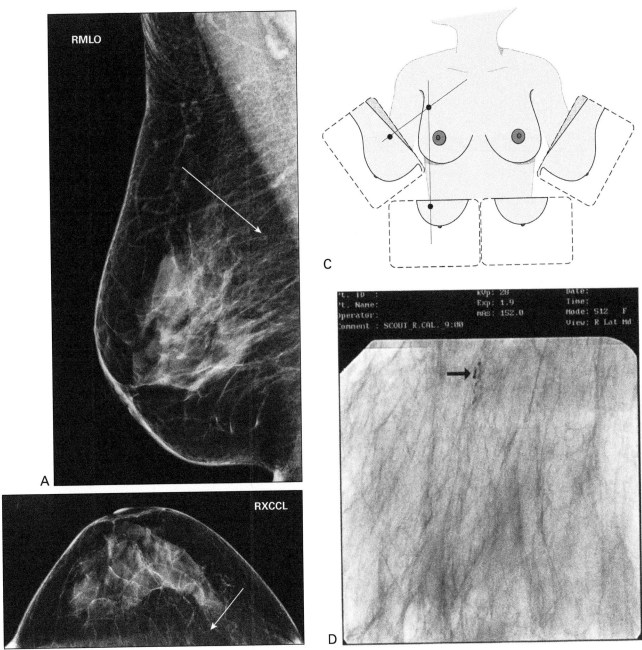

Figure 18-73
Abnormality access. **(A)** The routine screening mammogram demonstrates an area of calcifications in the superior aspect of the right MLO projection (*arrow*). **(B)** An XCCL localizes these calcifications (*arrow*) in the upper-outer quadrant at about 10:00. **(C)** With extreme forward movement of the breast support, sacrificing medial tissue, an LM projection allows access to this abnormality. **(D)** The scout image demonstrates these calcifications for biopsy. (C and D reprinted from Willison KM, Saunders DA. Positioning in stereotactic procedures. In: Fajardo LL, et al., eds. A Comprehensive Approach to Stereotactic Breast Biopsy. Cambridge: Blackwell Science; 1996:168–169. Copyright © 1996 Wiley-Blackwell. Reproduced with permission from John Wiley & Sons.)

Enlist the patient's cooperation. For example, request that she relax her ribcage into the table aperture. Gentle manipulation and downward pulling of the breast and adjacent tissue can extend more posterior tissue through the opening. With large, heavy breasts, the weight of the breast in the pendulous position aids in lowering the posterior portions of the breast through the table aperture for greater access. The technologist will have greater success at imaging posterior abnormalities by varying the biopsy approach. Try the appropriate following methods before abandoning the biopsy procedure.

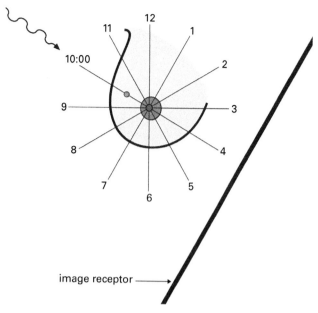

Figure 18-74
Positioning parallel to clock time. The technologist gains greater posterior access and breast mobility by choosing a projection that parallels the x-ray beam with the clock time of the abnormality. (From Willison KM, Saunders DA. Positioning in stereotactic procedures. In: Fajardo LL, Willison KM, Pizzeutiello RJ, eds. A Comprehensive Approach to Stereotactic Breast Biopsy. Cambridge: Blackwell Science; 1996:169. Copyright © 1996 Wiley-Blackwell. Reproduced with permission from John Wiley & Sons.)

Shoulder Placement

When positioning the patient on the table, the technologist can place the ipsilateral shoulder at the very rim of the table opening or allow the shoulder to drop through the opening (Figure 18-76). This allows the patient's torso and breast to drop lower into the table aperture, providing greater access to posterior tissue.

Steeper Oblique

Situations may arise in which placing the ipsilateral arm up near the head rather than at the side, and rolling the patient into a steeper oblique, nearly on her side, will be beneficial. Abnormalities that are extremely posterior and lateral in location may be easier to access with this maneuver. The amount of tissue accessible in this position depends on the total volume of lateral breast tissue.

Lowering the Arm Through the Table Aperture

For truly posterior abnormalities, especially in the tail of Spence, place the affected breast and the ipsilateral arm through the table opening (Figure 18-77). Use an arm sling as support for both comfort and the reduction

of motion. The technologist should demonstrate the abnormality free of the pectoral muscle. Puncture of the pectoral muscle may cause the patient unnecessary discomfort.

Tincture of Benzoin

Applying tincture of benzoin (before compression) to the skin in contact with the surface of the biopsy compression device may prevent the breast from slipping out of compression.

Subareolar Abnormalities

With abnormalities located in the subareolar region, complete tissue coverage of the biopsy window may be difficult. With just a portion of the biopsy compression device in contact with the skin, patient and abnormality movement may occur during the procedure. If the breast is large enough, choose a projection that allows nipple rotation upward or downward to cover the biopsy window (Figure 18-78). This upward or downward rotation can also increase stroke margin by bringing more breast tissue behind the abnormality.

If complete coverage of the biopsy window is not possible, use aluminum foil as a wedge filter to enhance imaging.

Breast Size

Breast size can impede accessibility and visualization. The suggestions listed below are useful for breasts that provide a challenge.

The Small Breast

In general, the technologist can apply the same methods that achieve good results for posterior abnormalities to the small breast. Gently manipulate the breast to pull a maximum amount of tissue through the table opening. Request the patient relax her upper torso into the table aperture. Overemphasizing the movement of the breast support platform behind the breast also increases the volume of available breast tissue.

The Large Breast

Large breasts can present challenges:

- In locating and visualizing an abnormality; the full breast scout image is especially helpful in these circumstances.
- Extra vigilance is necessary to prevent pain or injury when a large breast is of sufficient length to touch or rest on the C-arm.

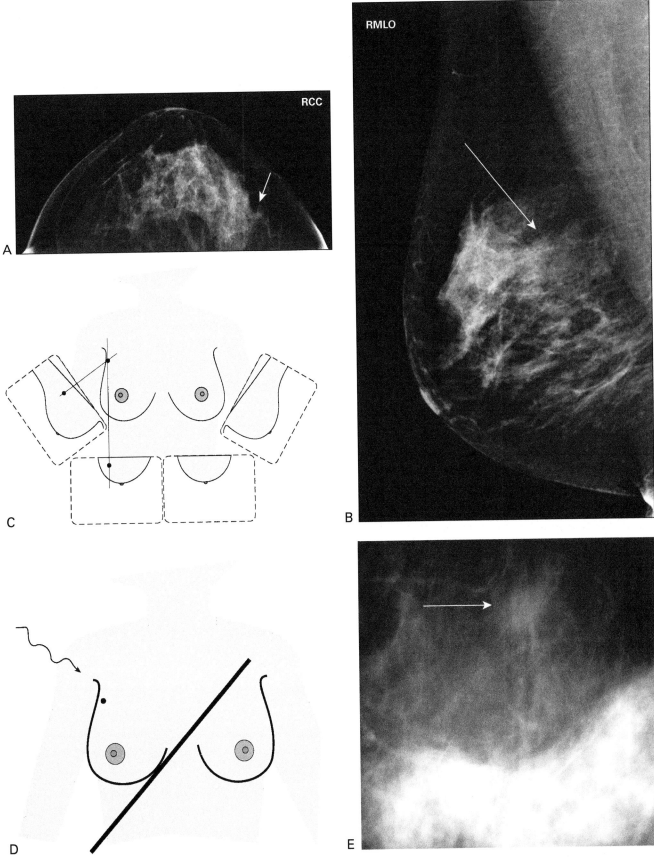

Figure 18-75
Parallel to clock time. **(A, B)** This routine screening mammogram demonstrates a mass density (*arrows*) in the **(C)** extreme posterior aspect of the upper outer quadrant at about 10:00 in the right breast. A LM fails to access the abnormality. **(D)** Positioning the x-ray beam parallel to the clock time of the abnormality results in a SIO projection, allowing greater mobility of the breast and access to this extremely posterior abnormality. **(E)** The scout image demonstrates the abnormality for biopsy (this was cancer on biopsy). (C and D reprinted from Willison KM, Saunders DA. Positioning in stereotactic procedures. In: Fajardo LL, et al., eds. A Comprehensive Approach to Stereotactic Breast Biopsy. Cambridge: Blackwell Science; 1996:170–171. Copyright © 1996 Wiley-Blackwell. Reproduced with permission from John Wiley & Sons.)

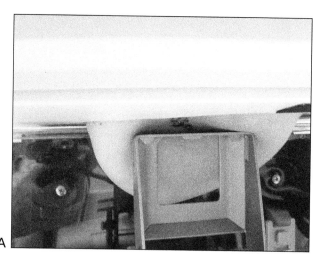
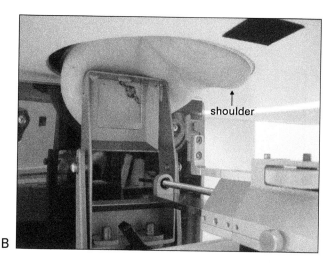

Figure 18-76
Shoulder placement. Placing the patient's shoulder in, or near, the table aperture can aid the technologist in accessing posterior abnormalities. **(A)** Shown in an LM projection with the shoulder normally placed, prohibiting access to this posterior abnormality. **(B)** Dropping the shoulder (*arrow*) into the table aperture allows access to this abnormality.

- Stroke margin is rarely an issue with breasts that compress to a thickness greater than 6 cm. However, two problems arise as a result of increased compression thickness:
  - ○ The area of interest is farther away from the image receptor, increasing blur.
  - ○ The thickness of the breast creates more scatter, thereby reducing image contrast.

The most effective ways to mitigate these problems are to (a) choose a C-arm projection that makes the breast as thin as possible (maintaining stroke margin) and (b) position the abnormality over adipose tissue for easier visualization. If the breast is not only thick but also is dense, overlapping breast structures may prohibit visualization of the abnormality, either on the scout or stereo images. The technologist may use alternative projections. For example, simply rotating the breast or the C-arm 10° to 15° may make the previously occult abnormality visible.

The Thin Breast

The thin breast can pose stroke margin difficulties.

- If breast compression is marginally close to allowing positive stroke margin, slightly releasing the force of compression may provide the few millimeters of additional breast tissue necessary to produce a positive stroke margin.

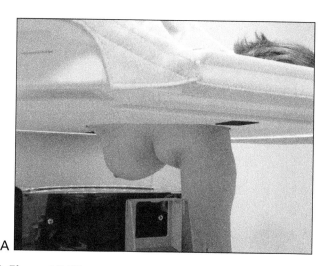
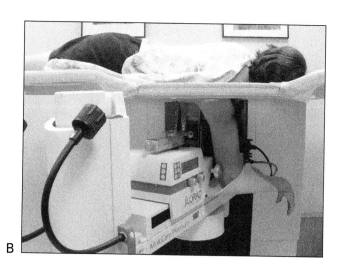

Figure 18-77
Positioning arm through the opening. **(A)** Greater access to posterior abnormalities can be achieved by lowering the ipsilateral arm and breast through the table aperture. **(B)** The arm is supported in a sling. This is a difficult position for the patient to maintain so the biopsy team must be experienced and work quickly.

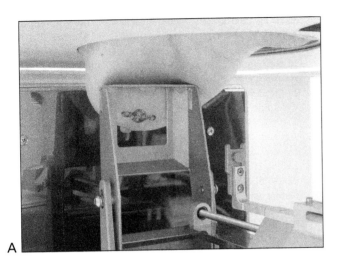

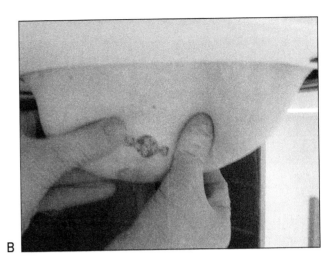

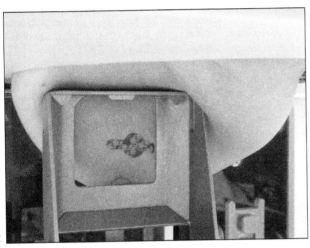

Figure 18-78
Nipple rotation for subareolar abnormalities. **(A)** Leaving the nipple in profile results in incomplete coverage of the biopsy window. **(B)** Rotating the nipple out of profile increases the surface area of the breast, **(C)** providing almost complete coverage of the biopsy window.

- Rolling the breast up and toward the breast support may offer increased breast thickness.
- Alternative projections may also increase the thickness of the compressed breast. For example, positioning the breast in an oblique angle may produce greater thickness than the CC or Lateral projections.
- Multidirectional vacuum-assisted devices allow alternative placement of the biopsy device that may be useful in cases of negative stroke margin.
- The instrument is not fired inside the breast; instead, it is fired outside the breast and is then dialed into the breast.
- The vacuum biopsy device has the ability to pull upward of 0.5 to 1.0 cm from the probe's collection chamber.
- Another option is to use a biopsy instrument with a smaller stroke, decreasing the necessary stroke margin; however, these samples tend to be small and fragmented.
- Many biopsy instruments permit partial closure of the collecting chamber. Placing the abnormality in the distal

half rather than in the center of the collecting chamber results in fewer cancelled procedures.

Side Arm (Orthogonal Arm)

Another alternative solution to negative stroke margin requires use of an orthogonal arm (Figure 18-79), which allows imaging of the abnormality from one perspective and biopsy from another projection. The biopsy team should ensure that the excursion of the needle does not pierce the opposite side of the breast; this is more likely to happen with a subareolar abnormality.

When employing a sidearm device, the technologist should choose the projection that allows adequate centering in the biopsy window and provides the shortest skin-to-abnormality distance from the side approach. For example, if the abnormality is at 12:00, position the breast for a MLO view, rather than the CC, to minimize the amount of breast tissue the needle will traverse. If visualization is not possible on both stereo images, then use the "target on scout" method.

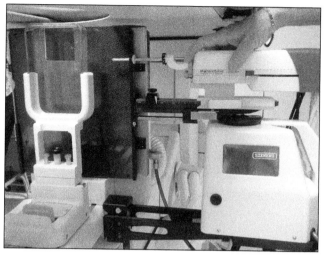

Figure 18-79
Orthogonal arm. Positioning of the patient for a side-arm approach to counter negative stroke margin. (Photo courtesy of Sarasota Memorial Hospital, Sarasota, FL.)

Review Questions

1. In stereotactic breast biopsy, the purpose of the coordinate system is to identify a unique visual point in the breast that will be used as a target for the biopsy needle. The coordinate system gives the location using either the Cartesian or the polar system. Describe the differences between the two systems.

2. When performing a stereotactic breast biopsy, do we want a positive or negative stroke margin?

3. When is it appropriate to use the "target on scout" feature?

4. List several factors that make stereotactic breast biopsy positioning challenging.

References

1. Angarita FA, et al. Perioperative measures to optimize margin clearance in breast conserving surgery. *Surg Oncol.* 2014;23(2):81–91.
2. Crowe JP, et al. A prospective review of the decline of excisional breast biopsy. *Am J Surg.* 2002;184(4):353–355.
3. Stolier AJ, Rupley DG. The impact of image-directed core biopsy on the practice of breast surgery: a new algorithm for a changing technology. *Am J Surg.* 1997;63(9):827–830.
4. Eberth JM, et al. Surgeon influence on use of needle biopsy in patients with breast cancer: a national medicare study. *J Clin Oncol.* 2014;32(21):2206–2216.
5. Gent HJ. Stereotaxic needle localization and cytological diagnosis of occult breast lesions. *Ann Surg.* 1986;204:580–585.
6. Elvecrog EL, et al. Nonpalpable breast lesions: correlation of stereotaxic large-core needle biopsy and surgical results. *Radiology.* 1993;188:453–455.
7. Lofgren M, et al. X-ray guided fine needle aspiration for the cytologic diagnosis of non-palpable breast lesions. *Cancer.* 1988;61:1032–1037.
8. Azavedo E, et al. Stereotactic fine needle biopsy in 2594 mammographically detected non-palpable lesions. *Lancet.* 1989;1:1033–1036.
9. Ciatto S, et al. Non-palpable breast lesions: stereotaxic fine needle aspiration cytology. *Radiology.* 1989;173:57–59.
10. Parker SH, et al. Nonpalpable breast lesions: stereotactic automated large core biopsies. *Radiology.* 1991;180(2):403–407.
11. Parker SH, et al. Stereotactic breast biopsy with a biopsy gun. *Radiology.* 1990;176(3):741–747.
12. Logan-Young W, et al. The cost effectiveness of fine needle aspiration cytology and 14-gauge core needle biopsy compared with open surgical biopsy in the diagnosis of breast carcinoma. *Cancer.* 1998;82:1867–1873.
13. Singhal H, Davis L. *Breast stereotactic core biopsy/fine needle aspiration.* Available at: http://eMedicine.Medscape.com/article/1845123-overview. Updated October 21, 2013. Accessed January 29, 2017.
14. Hooley RJ, et al. Breast ultrasonography: state of the art. *Radiology.* 2013;268(3):642–659.
15. Nordenstrom B. Stereotaxic screw needle biopsy of nonpalpable breast lesions. In: Young WW, ed. *Breast Carcinoma: The Radiologists Expanded Role.* New York: Wiley; 1977.
16. Bolmgren J, et al. Stereotaxic instrument for the needle biopsy of the mamina. *Am J Roentgenol.* 1977;129(1):121–125.
17. Schrading S, Distelmaier M, Dirricks T, et al. Digital breast tomosynthesis guided vacuum-assisted breast biopsy: initial experiences and comparison with prone stereotactic vacuum-assisted biopsy. *Radiology.* 2015;274(3):654–662.
18. Liberman L, et al. Clip placement after stereotactic vacuum-assisted breast biopsy. *Radiology.* 1997;205:417–422.
19. Burbank F, Forcier N. Tissue marking clip for stereotactic breast biopsy—initial placement accuracy, long-term stability, and usefulness as a guide for wire localization. *Radiology.* 1997;205:407–415.
20. Fajardo LL, et al. Placement of endovascular embolization microcoils to localize the site of breast lesions removed at stereotactic core biopsy. *Radiology.* 1998;206:275–278.
21. Liberman L, et al. Calcification retrieval at stereotactic, 11-gauge, directional, vacuum-assisted breast biopsy. *Radiology.* 1998;208:251–260.
22. Dowlatashahi D, et al. Non-palpable breast lesions: findings of stereotaxic needle core biopsy and fine needle aspiration cytology. *Radiology.* 1991;81:745–750.
23. Parker SH, Jobe WE. *Percutaneous Breast Biopsy.* New York: Raven Press; 1993.
24. Hendrick RE, Parker SH. *Stereotaxic imaging.* In: *Syllabus: A Categorical Course in Physics, Technical Aspects of Breast Imaging.* Oak Brook, IL: Radiologic Society of North America; 1994.
25. Venta LA. Image-guided biopsy of non-palpable breast lesions. In: Harris JR, ed. *Diseases of the Breast.* 2nd ed. Philadelphia, PA: Lippincott Williams & Wilkins; 2000:149–164.
26. Eklund GW, Cardenosa G. The art of mammographic imaging. *Radiol Clin North Am.* 1992;30:1.

Breast Cancer Treatments

19

Objectives

- List surgical options for a patient diagnosed with breast cancer
- Enumerate why mastectomy or lumpectomy would be an appropriate surgical choice
- Explain the significance of lymph node sampling
- Describe why axillary node dissection versus sentinel lymph node (SLN) would be an appropriate choice
- Describe the differences between chemotherapy and hormone therapy
- Describe and prioritize the various breast reconstruction options available
- Identify conditions when external radiation therapy versus brachytherapy would be an appropriate choice

---

Key Terms

- chemotherapy
- hormone therapy
- lumpectomy
- lymphatic system

- mastectomy
- radiation therapy
- reconstructive surgery

▌▌ INTRODUCTION

Survival: The Goal

With the introduction of dedicated mammography machines and recording systems in the early 1970s, modern mammography began. A decade later, beginning in 1984–2013, breast cancer incidence increased likely as a result of better detection (Figure 19-1).[1] Advancements in specialized equipment and clinical techniques brought great strides not only in the early detection of breast cancer but also in treatment methods: radiation therapy, chemotherapy, hormone therapy, and targeted drugs.[2]

These imaging and treatment improvements resulted in increased survival rates of all people with breast cancer and with all stages of the disease.

- In 2016, there were approximately 3.75 million breast cancer survivors in the United States.
- The peak incidence for developing breast cancer occurs between ages 55 and 64; the median age at diagnosis is 62.[1]
- Before the widespread adoption of screening mammography began in the United States in the mid-1980s, DCIS accounted for 3% of disease; today, it constitutes 25%.
- From 1989 to 2014, there was a 38% decrease in mortality due to breast cancer.[3]
- Today, 61% of all breast cancers are considered local disease because it is confined to the breast; 31% is regional disease—it has spread outside the confines of the breast.
- Overall survival statistics show 89% of patients are alive 5 years after diagnosis; at 10 years, it is 83%; 15 years is 78%.[4]
  - If the disease is localized, the 5-year survival rate is an incredible 99%, with 93.5% at the 10-year mark. If the disease is regional, the 5-year figure is 85%, with the 10-year mark reduced to 67%.[1,4]

The goal for treatment of all life-threatening disease is survival—survival without recurrence. There are different types of treatments for patients with breast cancer: surgery, **chemotherapy**, **hormone therapy**, and **radiation therapy**. Surgery and radiation therapy are considered local treatments, while chemotherapy and hormone therapy are systemic therapies used to treat the entire body because breast cancer cells have spread outside the breast.

Location, Location, Location

Most breast cancers arise in the epithelial cell layer that lines the milk ducts or that lines the lobules (Figure 19-2). Epithelial carcinogenesis is a process that requires time for a cascade of events to occur that ultimately results in cancer.

Field carcinogenesis results as an accumulation of genetic changes to a single cell line that leads to a progressively dysplastic appearance of cells, deregulated cell growth, and finally cancer. Multistep carcinogenesis is a series of neoplastic changes evolving over time with the cells starting out as normal, devolving into hyperplasia, atypical hyperplasia, in situ, and finally invasive breast cancer. In this process, tumor suppressor genes and proto-oncogenes become altered so they no longer function to control replication and division of the cell.

The first stage of disease development begins with *initiation*, a rapid and irreversible alteration of DNA by a carcinogen. Spanning decades, *promotion* leads to a premalignant stage. And finally, there is *progression* to cancer. With the pathologist's declaration, "the biopsy shows breast cancer," a woman's world quickly changes. The emotional impact is immediate and frightening. The patient needs answers to deal with her fears and all the negative images this diagnosis conjures up. She needs to quickly understand her treatment options, as well as all the nuances related to her specific cancer type and stage of disease. She will spend many sleepless nights at her computer searching

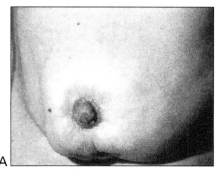 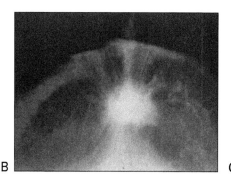 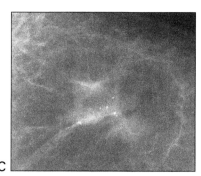

Figure 19-1
(A) This photo captures the clinical signs of advanced breast cancer. **(B)** The x-ray of this breast clearly demonstrates the advanced cancer as well as the clinical signs of skin thickening and retraction of the skin line. **(C)** This is an example of the "typical" breast cancer found today. This minimal tumor is completely occult clinically.

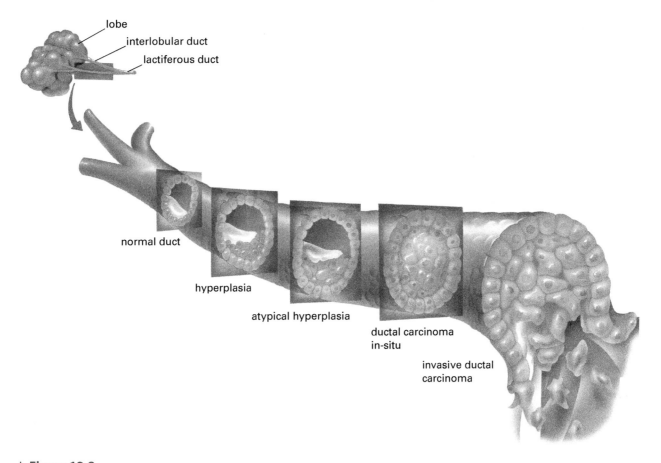

lobe
interlobular duct
lactiferous duct

normal duct

hyperplasia

atypical hyperplasia

ductal carcinoma
in-situ

invasive ductal
carcinoma

Figure 19-2
Understanding breast cancer. Cellular progression to breast cancer. (From: ACC Atlas of Pathophysiology, 1st Edition; Lippincott Williams & Wilkins (2001))

for information about breast cancer. Much of what she will read should give her hope.

TREATMENT OPTIONS: SURGERY

What a difference a decade (or two) makes. When the authors began working in this field over 40 years ago, we only performed mammograms on women who had secondary clinical signs of advanced breast cancer. Because the disease was advanced, treatments were harsh; all decisions about treatment were left entirely to the doctor. The woman with clinical symptoms went into the operating room not only *not* knowing if she had breast cancer but also not knowing if she would wake up with her breast intact or removed by mastectomy. Chemotherapy was brutal and radiation therapy was equally harsh. Thankfully, "time heals everything." Today, because the tumors we deal with are smaller, treatments are less extensive, and treatment regimes are not as severe. Also, today, there are many pharmaceutical agents that ameliorate the side effects brought about by the various treatments.

Surgery

When a person is diagnosed with breast cancer, the usual first step is surgery to eradicate the tumor bulk. **Mastectomy** is the total removal of the breast; **lumpectomy** is considered breast conservation surgery (BCS) because only the portion of the breast containing the tumor is removed (Figure 19-3). Some patients may have a choice of lumpectomy with radiation therapy versus mastectomy; the size, location, and type of breast cancer determine if there is a choice. When women do have a choice, they most often choose lumpectomy because it is less invasive.[5]

Generally, a woman has a choice when there is only one site of cancer; this means no multifocal or multicentric disease is identified; the tumor is smaller than 4 cm, and the pathologist identifies clear or negative margins, which means no cancer cells are identified in the tissue surrounding the tumor (Figure 19-4).

Among women diagnosed with stage I or II breast cancer, 61% undergo BCS (with the majority also receiving additional therapy) and 36% undergo mastectomy. Stage III patients tend to have a mastectomy (72%), with a much

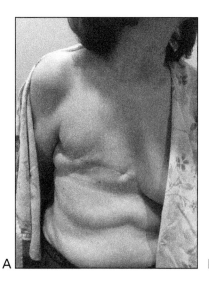
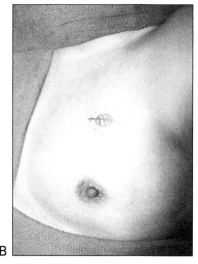

Figure 19-3
(A) Mastectomy. **(B)** Lumpectomy. Extent of tumor (*diagonal lines*) and extent of resection (*dotted line*) are marked on the skin to determine appropriate incision size.

smaller percentage undergoing BCS (21%). Women diagnosed with stage IV disease most often receive radiation and/or chemotherapy alone (48%).[6]

Lumpectomy versus Mastectomy

For the patient who has a choice between lumpectomy versus mastectomy, the decision-making process includes answers to the following considerations:

- Do you want to keep the breast?
- Do you want your breasts to match in size? If mastectomy is selected, reconstruction is an option. When lumpectomy is the choice, if the surgery on the involved breast results in an obvious distortion, reconstruction will make the breasts once again symmetrical in size and shape.
- How anxious are you about recurrence? Recurrence is always possible; however, this is less likely with a mastectomy.
- Some women do not want to undergo radiation therapy treatments that accompany lumpectomy. These women should have a mastectomy.[7]

- Where do you live? Mastectomy is more common in the United States than in other countries. Within the borders of the United States, more mastectomies are done in the South and midwestern states.
- In what type of facility will you undergo treatment? Mastectomies are more commonly performed in community hospitals; lumpectomies are more common in university-based hospitals.
- How old is your surgeon? Older surgeons are more likely to perform a mastectomy, especially if the patient is older. An "older surgeon" is a doctor who had their surgical training prior to 1981.

Lumpectomy

Lumpectomy is breast preservation surgery, where only the tumor plus some surrounding healthy tissue is removed (Figure 19-5). Technically, it is a partial mastectomy with a variable amount of tissue removed; thus, the categories of lumpectomy are the following: partial mastectomy, reexcision, quadrantectomy, and wedge resection.

Lumpectomy is combined with a course of radiation therapy, usually 5 to 7 weeks in length for external beam or

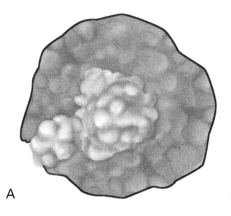
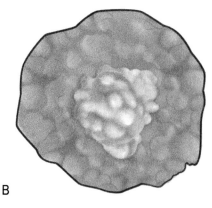

Figure 19-4
(A) Tumor extends to the margin of the specimen; this is a "positive" margin. The surgeon will continue to remove tissue until negative margins are identified. **(B)** Negative margins. The tumor is surrounded by 1 to 2 cm of normal tissue.

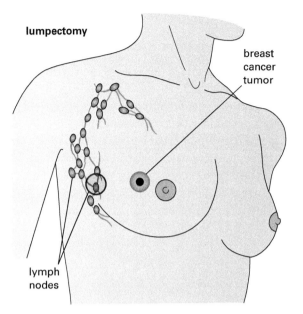

lumpectomy

breast
cancer
tumor

lymph
nodes

Figure 19-5
Lumpectomy removes the tumor plus a small amount of healthy tissue surrounding the cancer. The lymph nodes are evaluated as well.

a shorter course with internal radiation. Radiation is used to kill any cancer cells left behind after surgery. If chemotherapy is also necessary, it is usually administered after surgery but before the radiation therapy sessions begin.

The advantages of lumpectomy include preservation of the appearance of the breast, preservation of sensations within the breast, and a shorter and easier recovery period because the surgery is not extensive. The disadvantage is the higher risk of recurrence; if the tumor recurs, the woman would then have to have a mastectomy. Local recurrence with lumpectomy is approximately 9% to 14%.[8] The 20-year survival rate is the same for lumpectomy and for mastectomy.[5,6,9]

Since lumpectomy is combined with radiation therapy, sometimes there may be difficulty in complying with the radiation treatment schedule for the entire 5- to 7-week process, or perhaps, the woman is not a candidate for the shorter-course brachytherapy. If compliance with radiation therapy treatments will be a problem, mastectomy may be the better choice. Additionally, if a woman has lumpectomy with radiation therapy and then has a recurrence, or if she subsequently develops a separate primary breast cancer in that same breast, the breast cannot tolerate additional radiation therapy. Mastectomy is her only choice.

Lumpectomy with radiation is *not* recommended:

- If the woman has recurrence and had previously been treated with lumpectomy and radiation. Radiation cannot be administered to the same area twice.
- If the tumor is multicentric or multifocal. Extensive tumor bulk cannot be effectively targeted with radiation therapy; radiation works best within a targeted area.

- For cosmetic reasons. If removal of a large tumor plus some surrounding healthy tissue in a small breast results in gross disfigurement, with the two breasts now very asymmetric in size, mastectomy with reconstruction may be the better option.
- If multiple attempts by the surgeon to achieve negative margins are unsuccessful.
- If the woman has certain connective tissue disease such as lupus, scleroderma, or vasculitis. These women are too sensitive to the side effects associated with radiation, thus are not candidates for lumpectomy with radiation therapy.
- If pregnant.
- If the patient is unwilling or unlikely to go to daily radiation treatments for 5 to 7 weeks. Sometimes, this may be due to the distance that must be traveled daily to the radiation facility
- If the patient would have greater peace of mind with having a mastectomy. Local recurrence is more likely with lumpectomy.

Mastectomy

Mastectomy is removal of the breast. This surgical procedure may be a requirement for some patients based on the size, location, and type of breast cancer, while others may have a choice between mastectomy and lumpectomy. Women who have a choice and select mastectomy usually do so "for peace of mind"; with virtually all the breast tissue removed, there is very little tissue left for a recurrence of breast cancer. Additionally, a person may also select mastectomy to avoid radiation therapy that accompanies lumpectomy surgery. Many breast cancer patients who have a mastectomy do not need radiation therapy, but lumpectomy candidates *always* have radiation in addition to surgery.

The disadvantages of having a mastectomy are permanent loss of the breast and more extensive surgery so recovery takes longer, and often, the patient has additional **reconstructive surgery** to replace the missing breast.

Mastectomy versus Lumpectomy

Mastectomy would be the surgery of choice:

- If the tumor is larger than 4 cm.
- For some tumors under 4 cm, depending on the type and stage.
- Younger women (less than 40 years) and patients with larger and/or more aggressive tumors are more likely to be treated with mastectomy.[7,10]
- If the breast is small. A lumpectomy on a small-breasted woman often results in a virtual mastectomy.
- If the surgeon makes multiple attempts to remove the tumor with lumpectomy but continues to have positive margins of tumor extension.

- If the patient had prior radiation treatments for breast cancer and has recurrence, or if another primary breast cancer appears. The breast can only be treated once with radiation therapy.
- If there is the presence of connective tissue disease such as lupus, scleroderma, or vasculitis. Lumpectomy with radiation is not an option for these patients.
- If pregnant.
- If the patient is not likely to commit to the daily treatments required with radiation therapy.
- If the patient seeks "more peace of mind" to be rid of this breast cancer by denying it a place to return.

Types of Mastectomy

There are five types of mastectomies:

1. Simple mastectomy (Figure 19-6A). This surgery concentrates on the breast tissue itself. The surgeon removes the entire breast but does not perform axillary lymph node dissection (removal of lymph nodes in the underarm area) nor are the muscles beneath the breast disturbed. Occasionally, however, intramammary lymph nodes are removed because they happen to be located within the breast tissue taken during surgery. This type of surgery is appropriate for women with multiple or large

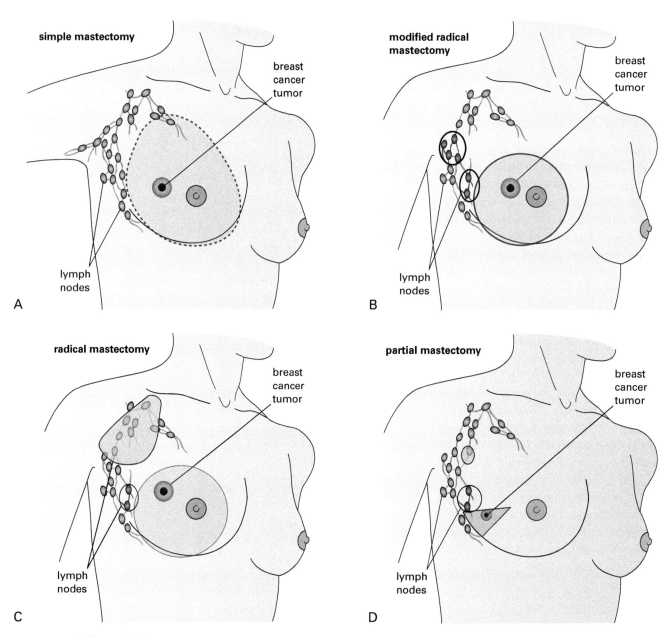

Figure 19-6
(A) Simple mastectomy **(B)** Modified radical mastectomy **(C)** Radical mastectomy **(D)** Partial mastectomy.

areas of DCIS and for high-risk women who have opted for prophylactic mastectomy—that is, breast removal in order to reduce the possibility of breast cancer from occurring. With prophylactic mastectomy, there is up to a 97% reduction in risk. This elective surgery is done only for women who meet specific profiles, test positive for BrCA 1 or 2; have a very strong family history of breast cancer; or have been diagnosed with LCIS. Some women with unilateral nonmetastatic breast cancer choose to undergo contralateral prophylactic mastectomy. This elective surgery has increased rapidly, from 5% of total mastectomies in 1998 to 30% in 2011.[11]

2. Modified radical mastectomy (Figure 19-6B). Most people with invasive breast cancer, who decide to have a mastectomy, have a modified radical mastectomy. A modified radical mastectomy involves removal of the breast tissue and a sampling of the level I and II lymph nodes; examining the lymph nodes helps to identify whether cancer cells may have spread beyond the breast. No muscles are removed from beneath the breast.

3. Radical mastectomy (Figure 19-6C). The most extensive of all the types. The surgeon removes the entire breast along with the pectoral muscles and three levels of lymph nodes. Formerly known as the Halsted radical mastectomy, named after the American surgeon of the 1800s, this surgery was common in the past when the only cancers "discovered" were clinically well advanced. Today, this type of surgery is only done when a breast cancer has spread to the chest muscles. Radical mastectomy is now rarely performed because in most cases, modified radical mastectomy has proven to be just as effective and is less disfiguring.

4. Partial mastectomy (Figure 19-6D). Partial mastectomy is the removal of the cancerous part of the breast tissue and some normal tissue surrounding the tumor bed. While lumpectomy is technically a form of partial mastectomy, more tissue is removed in partial mastectomy than in lumpectomy.

5. Subcutaneous or nipple-sparing mastectomy (NSM). The most controversial of all the types. The surgeon removes the breast tissue but preserves the nipple. This surgery typically is not performed on patients diagnosed with breast cancer because it retains some breast tissue; recurrence is possible. The technique of NSM continues to gain popularity as a prophylactic procedure in high-risk patients. NSM offers an opportunity to preserve the native breast envelope without mutilation of the nipple–areola complex and avoids multiple surgical procedures required for reconstruction. The current indications for NSM, if any, in the treatment of early invasive breast cancer remains uncertain and requires rigorous scientific scrutiny.[12]

Case Study 19-1

Describe the differences between the various types of mastectomies shown in Figure 19-6.

Side Effects and Risks Associated with Mastectomy

All surgery has risks as well as side effects; the benefits must outweigh the risks. As mammography improved in its ability to detect early breast cancer, the surgery required by these smaller and earlier stages of cancer changed. The radical and extensive surgery required by the larger and more advanced tumors was refined.

However refined, surgery is invasive and has its risks. The side effects and risks associated with mastectomy include:

- Numbness along the incision site and tenderness in the tissue adjacent to the scar. The reason for this is the nerves are cut.
- Touch sensitive along the scar. The cut nerve endings are constantly irritated. As healing progresses, these sensations lessen.
- Fluid often collects along the scar. This is known as a hematoma or seroma. This condition will resolve itself over time, or the surgeon can insert a needle in this area and drain the fluid.
- Formation of scar tissue. People heal differently. Some form adhesions, abnormal membranous surfaces along the scar site, while others heal wonderfully well.
- Delayed wound healing. People heal differently; some quickly rebound while others having the same surgery struggle to recover. During surgery, blood vessels are cut; the healing process involves blood flow into the area to bathe the injured tissue
- Increased risk of infection. Surgeons counsel their patients to be alert for the earliest signs and symptoms of infection and to contact them immediately if present.

TREATMENT OPTIONS: LYMPHATIC SYSTEM AND LYMPH NODES

Lymph is a clear fluid in the blood stream; it passes out of the arteries and into the capillaries. From the capillaries, it bathes and cleanses the tissues in the body, ultimately draining away through the lymphatic system. The **lymphatic system** filters disease, bacteria, viruses, and other impurities. Lymph nodes are filters found along the lymphatic system (Figure 19-7A); they trap and eliminate these unwanted substances by a process known as phagocytosis.

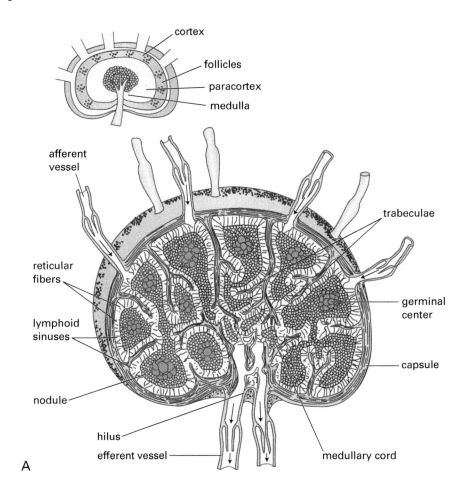

A

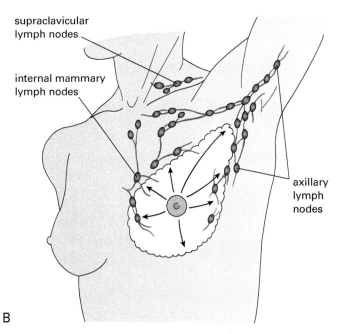

B

Figure 19-7
(A) Structural features of a lymph node. (Reprinted from Porth CM. *Pathophysiology Concepts of Altered Health States*. 7th ed. Philadelphia, PA: Lippincott Williams & Wilkins; 2005.) **(B)** Lymphatic drainage of the breast.

Although breast cancer is not easily controlled, the spread of breast cancer is fairly predictable. The cancer cells spread through a customary path, out from the tumor and into the surrounding lymphatic system and/or vascular system, and then it progresses throughout the body. The breast is primarily drained via the axillary lymph node basin, with the internal mammary and supraclavicular regions being secondary routes (Figure 19-7B). Cancer cells can bypass the lymphatic system and circulate via the blood stream, but the usual route is through the lymphatic system.

Once breast cancer has been diagnosed, checking the status of the lymph nodes is the next very important step.

Axillary Lymph Node Dissection

In the past, because tumors were so advanced, surgeons surveyed the lymph nodes by a procedure known as axillary node dissection. The surgeon removes the axillary fat pad, which contains the lymph nodes. The pathologist locates the lymph nodes in the excised fat pad and examines 2 to 3 sections per node. This procedure was done not only to check the status of the nodes but also to remove cancer cells from the lymphatic system in order to prevent further dissemination of the disease.

There are three levels of lymph nodes under the arm (Figure 19-8). Level I is at the lower edge of the pectoralis minor muscle; level II is found underneath the pectoralis minor muscle; and level III is found above the pectoralis minor muscle. A typical dissection removes level I and II nodes. If the woman is having a mastectomy, this is done at the time of surgery; with a lumpectomy, this procedure can be done concurrently or later. With a lumpectomy, the axillary node dissection is a separate incision. The number of lymph nodes in the axilla varies between individuals. Typically 5 to 30 lymph nodes are removed during an axillary dissection. The importance of the removal of lymph nodes is not the number removed, rather those that contain cancer cells are removed.

As a consequence of surgery to the lymphatic system, the normal flow of lymphatic fluid is disrupted. A common deleterious side effect is lymph edema; this condition occurs in 20% of women who undergo axillary lymph node dissection and in about 6% of women who undergo SLN biopsy.[13] Lymph edema is a chronic condition (Figure 19-9). There is no cure for lymphedema, but with early diagnosis, proper health care, good nutrition, and exercise, it may be possible to reduce the effects.

With the advanced cancers found in the past, the surgeon had to be certain that all nodes were removed; the belief being, the more lymph nodes removed, the better the prognosis. Today, we recognize that if breast cancer cells

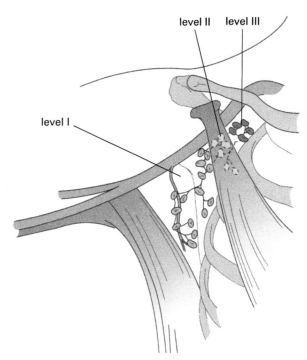

Figure 19-8
The axillary lymph nodes are divided into three levels by the pectoralis minor muscle. The level I nodes are inferior and lateral to the pectoralis minor, the level II nodes are below the axillary vein and behind the pectoralis minor, and the level III nodes are medial to the muscle against the chestwall. (Reprinted with permission from Mulholland WM, Lillemoe KD, Doherty GM, et al. *Greenfield's Surgery: Scientific Principles and Practice.* 4th ed. Philadelphia, PA: Lippincott Williams & Wilkins; 2006.)

are identified in even one lymph node (the sentinel node), then we are dealing with a systemic disease, not a localized process; in these cases, treatment for the entire body is pursued.

The Case for Sentinel Lymph Node Dissection

Screening mammography routinely discovers nonpalpable and impalpable breast cancers, in which no lymph node involvement is identified. Performing axillary node dissections on all of these node-negative people will result in disruptions to the flow of lymphatic fluid and perhaps lymph edema.

Sentinel Lymph Node (SLN)

Sentinel lymph node (SLN) dissection is an alternative to axillary node dissection. The SLN (Figure 19-10) is the first node "downstream" from the cancer in the lymph circulatory system. If the cancer were to travel away from the breast tumor and into the lymphatic system, this node would be the first one to show evidence of disease. If this node contains cancer cells, then the disease is systemic;

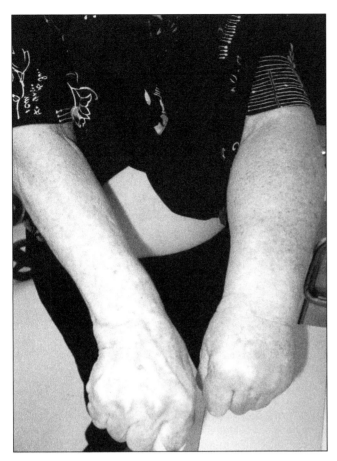

Figure 19-9
Lymphadenopathy: arm, after breast cancer surgery and lymph node removal. (Courtesy of Dr. Benjamin Barankin.)

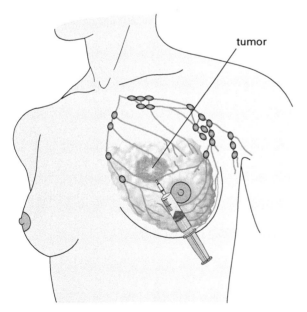

Figure 19-10
The SLN is the first node that receives lymphatic drainage from the tumor bed.

if "clean," then it is localized disease. If the SLN contains cancer cells, then axillary dissection is done.

The SLN dissection technique is not appropriate for everyone; several conditions rule out its use:

- If the tumor is larger than 2 cm.
- If the surgeon can feel hard/firm lymph nodes upon physical examination, this procedure is not recommended.
- If the cancer is multifocal or multicentric.
- If the patient had previous breast surgery, including reduction surgery.
- If the patient had radiation therapy to the breast.
- If inflammatory breast cancer.
- If the patient is pregnant, the procedure is not advised.

Factors that influence the prognosis for patients diagnosed with breast cancer include tumor size, hormone receptor status, lymph node involvement, and the age of the patient, with lymph node status the most powerful predictor. The 5-year survival rates are 99% if the disease is localized, 85% if the lymph nodes are positive, and 26% with distant metastases.

Effective in the mid-2012, the standard of care was changed to no longer require women with early-stage breast cancers to have a full dissection and removal of the axillary lymph nodes. Instead, radiation to the axilla can be planned.

Sentinel Lymph Node Mapping

In a developing embryo, the breast and its lymphatic system arise from a central breast bud. The breast is drained primarily by the axillary drainage basin, with 97% of lymph passing through the axillary region; the internal mammary lymph drainage basin, located beneath the sternum, accounts for the remaining 3%. The SLN technique examines only the axillary nodes, even if the tumor is located in the medial aspect of the breast, since the drainage pattern is predominately up and out.

The road to SLN mapping of the breast was actually the connection of many smaller trails through the body. Cabanas, who advanced the SLN technique with his work in penile carcinoma during the 1970s, is generally credited with developing the technique.[14] However, it was Gould and his colleagues who coined the term SLN. Gould and colleagues investigated cancer of the parotid gland in the 1950s.[15] They observed that certain lymph nodes were always first in line to drain the tumor bed. In 1992, Morton reported success using the SLN technique with melanoma; he used blue dye to make the lymphatic channels and nodes visible.[16] In 1994, the literature recorded the use of a radiotracer to identify the SLN.[17] In 1994, we have the first documented use of SLN with breast cancer.[18]

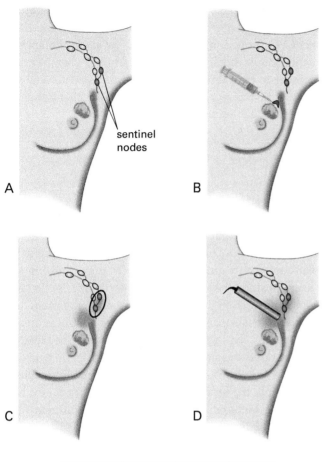

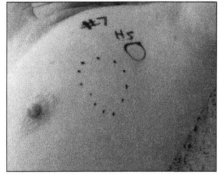

Figure 19-11
(A) The sentinel nodes are the first lymph nodes that drain the tumor. **(B)** A radioactive material is injected into the tumor bed. **(C)** The breast is gently massaged to promote uptake of the radioactive material by the lymphatic system. **(D)** A Geiger counter passes across the breast searching for the SLN. **(E)** The skin covering the tumor is marked. The "hot spot," denoting the location of the SLN, is clearly identified.

SLN Procedure

A radiotracer such as Technetium-99m is injected into the area surrounding the tumor. A blue dye, which makes visual identification of the lymphatic system easier, is frequently used in conjunction with the radiotracer. This combination results in 99% accuracy in locating the sentinel node. The breast is gently massaged to help disperse the injected materials into the lymphatic system. A gamma detector is passed across the breast to find the "hot spot," an area with a high radioactive count (Figure 19-11).

Macrophages line the inside of the lymph node. By a method known as phagocytosis, the macrophages attempt to digest the radiotracer because it is a foreign substance in the body; digestion leads to the removal of the material by the body's efficient cleaning crew. However, if the macrophages have been destroyed and replaced by disease, then the radiotracer cannot be cleared out of the lymphatic system. The absence or presence of a radiotracer provides additional information about the prognosis of the patient.

Lymphatic drainage is orderly; if the first 1 to 2 nodes are disease-free, then it is assumed the cancer is localized. With only a couple lymph nodes to examine with the SLN technique, the pathologist is able to evaluate each lymph node in greater detail; typically, the pathologist examines 60 sections per node to look for micrometastases. Whereas with the classic axillary dissection, 5 to 30 lymph nodes are harvested for the pathologist; typically 2 to 3 sections per lymph node are examined. In this case, it would be easy to miss micrometastases.

TREATMENT OPTIONS: RADIATION THERAPY

Radiation therapy uses high-energy wavelengths, in the mega-volt range, to kill cancer cells (Figure 19-12). It affects cells only in the part of the body that is treated with radiation. Radiation is used to destroy undetectable cancer cells and to reduce the risk of cancer recurring in the affected breast. Radiation therapy will be part of the treatment plan for a patient who has had a

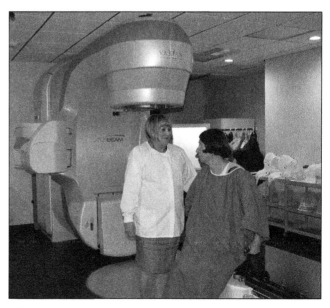

Figure 19-12
A radiation therapy machine.

lumpectomy; it may or may not be done for a patient who has a mastectomy. Radiation therapy is recommended after mastectomy[19]:

- If the tumor was larger than 5 cm
- If the tissue removed during the mastectomy does not have clear margins
- If cancer was found in four or more lymph nodes
- If the disease is multicentric or multifocal

Radiation therapy destroys cancer cells left behind after surgery, reducing recurrence by up to 70%. Radiation's high-energy wavelength damages DNA in a cell; DNA is the material the cell uses to maintain its functions and to repair itself when damaged. Radiation harms healthy tissue adjacent to the tumor as well as the targeted diseased cells in the tumor; however, the more rapidly dividing cancer cells are affected to a greater extent than the slower growing healthy cells. Also, since cancer cells are disorganized, it is more difficult for them to repair the damage caused by radiation; healthy cells are able to repair themselves.

Radiation treatments are delivered over time, as the cells are continuously replicating and dividing. Delivery over time maximizes the likelihood that the radiation treatments will be successful. Small-dose delivery also permits time for healthy cells that suffer less damage to recover and repair themselves.

Radiation therapy is appropriate for some patients with stage 0 (DCIS), most patients with stage I invasive cancer and higher who have had lumpectomy, and some patients who have had a mastectomy. It is also used to help control stage IV disease, where cancer has spread to other parts of the body. Sometimes, hyperthermia is combined with radiation therapy. Hyperthermia uses an energy source like ultrasonic waves or microwaves to heat the cancer cells to 113°F. This may make the cancer cells more sensitive to radiation. The hyperthermia treatment is done within 1 hour prior to the radiation therapy session.

Radiation can be a form of *primary* treatment for breast cancer; after surgery, the patient has only radiation treatments. Or radiation can be used as *adjuvant* therapy; radiation can be combined with surgery and chemotherapy in order to treat any residual cancer cells. With adjuvant therapy, first surgery is done, followed by chemotherapy, and then radiation therapy.

Simulation (Planning Session)

Before radiation therapy treatment begins, the patient undergoes a planning session to maximize the effect radiation will have on the tumor and to minimize its effects on healthy tissue (Figure 19-13). A radiation oncologist calculates the total dose to be given, while a medical dosimetrist plans out the treatment area and uses the simulation session to position the angles of radiation delivery to limit the effects of radiation to the healthy tissue. Small tattoos, or a special indelible marking pen, define the treatment area by putting dots, the size of a freckle, on the skin. The radiation therapist uses the markings to align the radiation field during each visit. Beam-shaping blocks and multileaf collimators protect the healthy tissue adjacent to the tumor bed. Use of an immobilization device on the treatment table ensures stability during treatment sessions.

Dosimetry

The amount of radiation used to treat the disease depends upon the type of cancer, the size of the tumor, the type of surgery the patient had, whether clear margins were attained during surgery, and whether or not the lymph nodes are involved.

The total radiation dose is divided into daily doses, called fractions. A fraction typically is 180 to 200 rads or centiGrays per session; the cumulative dose is usually 4,500 to 5,000 centiGrays delivered over 5 weeks, followed by an

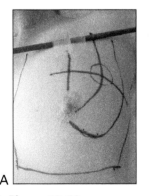
A

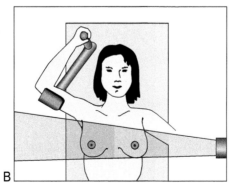
B

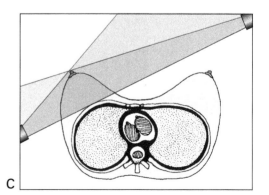
C

Figure 19-13
(A) Simulation planning session determines the area for treatment. **(B)** Shows the path of the external radiation field. **(C)** Illustrates a cross section of targeting to maximize the dose to the desired area and minimize radiation to other body parts.

additional 1,000 to 2,000 centiGrays over a 1-week period, targeted specifically at the tumor site.

There are two main kinds of radiation therapy that may be considered, and some people have both. External radiation treatments are delivered once a day, 5 days a week, for approximately 1 month. Internal radiation treatments are usually given twice per day for 1 week. A linear accelerator produces external radiation, while radioactive pellets or seeds are used for internal radiation.

External Beam Breast Cancer Radiation

External beam radiation (also known as traditional or whole breast radiation therapy) uses x-rays, like that used in a regular x-ray exam, but the beam is high energy and highly focused and targets the cancerous area for 2 to 3 minutes per treatment session. This form of treatment usually involves multiple appointments at an outpatient radiation center—as many as 5 days a week for 5 to 6 weeks. Accelerated radiation therapy requires a slightly higher dose of radiation over a shorter course of treatment, usually 3 to 4 weeks. Since 2011 the American Society of Radiation Oncology has recommended the shorter-course intensity-modulated radiation therapy plan. This higher treatment dose plan limits the adverse effects to the healthy tissue.

External radiation treatments begin approximately 4 to 6 weeks after surgery. This time gap allows the patient to heal following surgery.

Internal Breast Cancer Radiation (Brachytherapy)

In 1901, Pierre Currie loaned a rubber-coated radium sulfate capsule to a Paris physician to treat Lupus, using it as a skin applicator.[20] In the United States, Robert Abbe was the first physician who urged treating tumors using radium brachytherapy.[21] Today's brachytherapy for breast cancer uses Iridium-192 pellets.

The Greek word *brachios* means short. Brachytherapy/accelerated partial irradiation/intracavity therapy is the newer type of radiation therapy, with a duration of up to 1 week. Rather than external radiation, where radiation passes through healthy skin and healthy breast tissue before it reaches the tumor site, brachytherapy places the radiation *at* the tumor site.

Internal radiation is delivered one of two ways, via an implantable device. This type of radiation therapy may be only one treatment—delivered in the operating room. The surgeon places a highly radioactive device inside the tumor bed/lumpectomy site to kill any possible remaining cancer cells. More likely, though, this therapy is done as an outpatient procedure.

With the outpatient procedure, radiation is delivered to the tumor bed via an implanted balloon catheter that was positioned in the tumor bed during the patient's lumpectomy surgery (Figure 19-14). This device stays in this cavity until her treatments are finished. Twice a day, for 3 to 5 days, the patient visits the radiation oncology center; there must be a 4- to 6-hour interval between treatment sessions. A radioactive seed is attached to a guide wire that is inserted into the catheter. Over several minutes, the pellet is moved to various points within the balloon, following a pattern to ensure all areas of the tumor bed are exposed to radiation.

Brachytherapy allows a higher dose of radiation to treat a smaller area in a shorter time than is possible with external radiation.[22] Not every patient is a candidate for this treatment; patients must meet specific criteria.

Radiation Therapy Side Effects

All cancer treatments produce side effects. Side effects can be immediate or delayed. With external radiation therapy, side effects usually present 3 to 4 weeks into the treatment cycle; they typically resolve 4 to 6 weeks after the treatment regime is finished. Other side effects can take months or years to develop; these are usually permanent. If a patient

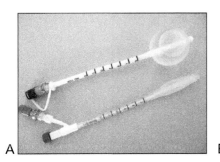 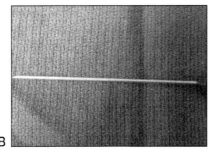 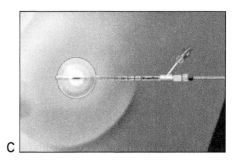

Figure 19-14
(A) This brachytherapy device is positioned in the lumpectomy cavity and is left in place for the duration of treatment. **(B)** The radium seeded probe is inserted twice daily throughout the week of outpatient treatments. **(C)** The balloon catheter is easily removed when treatment is concluded. (Image courtesy of Hologic, Inc. and affiliates)

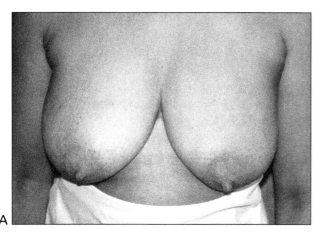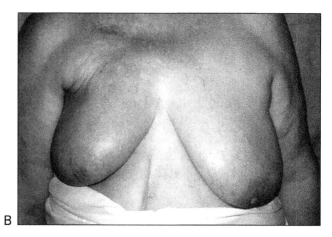

A   B

Figure 19-15
Cosmetic outcome after breast-conserving surgery with radiation therapy. **(A)** Excellent cosmetic outcome. The treated breast (**left**) is identical to the untreated breast. **(B)** Fair cosmetic outcome. Significant shrinkage and ptosis is evident in the treated (**right**) breast. (Reprinted with permission from Mulholland WM, Lillemoe KD, Doherty GM, et al. *Greenfield's Surgery: Scientific Principles and Practice*. 4th ed. Philadelphia, PA: Lippincott Williams & Wilkins; 2006.)

will have reconstruction surgery, she is advised to wait until the radiation treatments are finished in order to minimize unfavorable cosmetic results.

Temporary side effects from radiation therapy to the breast can include fatigue, which can last from a few weeks to a few months after treatment ends. Often the skin turns pink, red, or tan and becomes sensitive and irritated; this can range from mild to intense. Applying creams and other medicines can often soothe this. There may be a puckering of the skin around the scar site, and the breast may shrink in size and become firm. Lymph edema may be present if an axillary dissection was done, and especially if radiation treatments included the axillary region (Figure 19-15).

Rare conditions may develop months to years later: rib fracture, heart injury, and radiation pneumonitis due to inflammation of the lung if it received radiation. Brachial plexopathy is radiation damage to the nerves in the chest; the higher the dose to the lymph nodes in the axilla, the more likely this side effect will be permanent.

Recurrence

Sometimes, despite the surgeon's best efforts, the radiation treatments the patient completes, and the chemotherapy side effects she endures—sometimes the cancer recurs:

- Lumpectomy with radiation therapy: the chance for local recurrence within the first 10 years is 3% to 15%.[23]
- Mastectomy with negative lymph nodes is 6%.[24]
- Mastectomy with positive lymph nodes, no radiation therapy: 23%.[24]
- Mastectomy with positive lymph nodes, with radiation therapy: 6%.[24]

If there is a recurrence and the patient was previously treated with radiation, the breast cannot again be treated with radiation. The healthy breast cells have had as much radiation as they can safely handle.

Recurrence after mastectomy is more likely:

- If the tumor was 5 cm or larger
- If there was tumor invasion of the blood vessels or lymphatic system
- If upon resection of the tumor positive margins were identified
- If four or more positive lymph nodes are identified in a pre or post menopausal woman or at least one positive lymph node in a premenopausal woman was involved
- If the cancer has invaded the skin, as happens with inflammatory breast cancer or with locally advanced disease
- local: confined to the breast
- regional: in the axillary or clavicular lymph nodes
- distant (metastatic): in another part of the body

With metastatic disease, breast cancer tends to spread to the lung, liver, bone, and brain. If the breast cancer metastasizes, for example, to the spine, it is still a breast cancer; it is not classified as a bone cancer. It is a breast cancer that has escaped the confines of the breast. It will respond to breast cancer treatment protocols.

There are many different treatments available to the woman with recurrence. These treatments can be used alone, in combination, or used in a sequence.

- If the patient had a lumpectomy with radiation therapy and has a local recurrence, she will be treated with a mastectomy. Hormone therapy and/or chemotherapy may also be given.

- If the patient had a mastectomy and has a local recurrence, she will have the new tumor removed plus radiation therapy. Hormone therapy and/or chemotherapy may also be given.
- If the patient has distant metastatic disease, she will be treated with chemotherapy, hormone therapy, or both.

TREATMENT OPTIONS: RECONSTRUCTION SURGERY

Reconstruction Following Mastectomy

When a breast cancer patient has a mastectomy, several options for reconstructive surgery are available: a silicone or saline implant; tissue from a donor site such as the back, belly, or buttocks; a reconstructed mound with a tattooed nipple or a nipple constructed from her own transplanted tissue; or a reconstructed mound with a smooth surface, sans nipple.

Approximately 75% of women who have a mastectomy opt for reconstructive surgery, with half choosing implants.[25] Most of the other half select TRAM Flap surgery. Reconstructive surgery can be immediate, meaning the procedure is done at the time of mastectomy. Other patients will elect a delay of months or years between their mastectomy and reconstructive surgery. Some never have reconstructive surgery. Reconstruction is usually performed by a plastic surgeon.

Women who opt for a lumpectomy may or may not need reconstructive surgery. If the lumpectomy surgery leaves them cosmetically imbalanced, they may opt for reconstruction. Reconstruction surgery may be done at the same time as a lumpectomy. This is called oncoplastic surgery, and many breast surgeons can do this without the help of a plastic surgeon. Surgery on the healthy breast is also often done so both breasts have a similar appearance.

Implant Reconstruction

A breast implant uses saline-filled or silicone gel–filled forms to reshape the breast. The outside of a saline-filled implant is made up of silicone, and it is filled with sterile saline. Silicone gel–filled implants are filled with silicone instead of saline.

Insertion of an implant for a patient who had a skin-sparing mastectomy is rather straightforward, with an implant replacing the excised breast tissue inside the remaining breast skin pouch. Women who have non–skin-sparing mastectomies are still able to have implant reconstruction after having a skin-stretching procedure known as tissue expansion. The surgeon inserts a device, a tissue expander, under the skin and gradually adds fluid to the empty implant over a course of approximately 6 months. The gradual increase in the size of the tissue expander causes the skin and soft tissue to stretch to the desired size that will accommodate an exchange of expander with a permanent implant (Figure 19-16).

Autologous Reconstruction

Autologous reconstruction involves taking "spare" tissue from a donor site in the patient's body: from the back, belly, or buttocks. The donor tissue can be detached as a free piece of tissue and moved to the location of the breast, or it can be grafted as a "flap." With most flap reconstruction, the donor tissue remains attached and is slid under

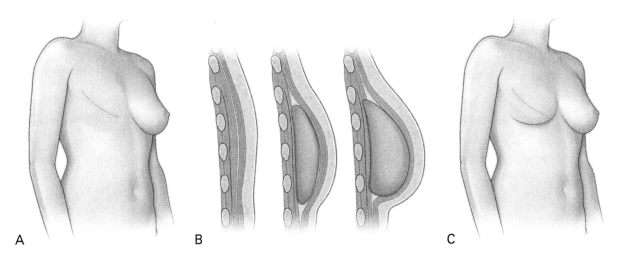

A   B   C

Figure 19-16
Breast reconstruction with tissue expander. **(A)** After mastectomy, a tissue expander is inserted to prepare for reconstruction. **(B)** The expander is gradually filled with saline solution through a tube to stretch the skin enough to accept an implant beneath the chest muscle. **(C)** The breast mound is restored. Although permanent, scars will fade with time. The nipple and areola are reconstructed later.

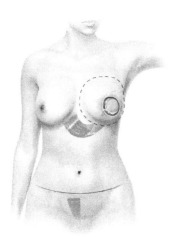

Figure 19-17
Breast reconstruction: TRAM flap. A flap of the transrectus abdominis muscle is tunneled through the abdomen to the breast area. (Image from Sabel M, Mulholland MW, eds. *Operative Techniques in Breast, Endocrine, and Oncologic Surgery.* 1st ed. Philadelphia, PA: Wolters Kluwer; 2015.)

the skin to become a breast replacement. There are many advantages for this procedure:

- It maintains the blood supply to the tissue.
- There is no rejection of the donated tissue so the encapsulation side effect often associated with silicone or saline implants is not encountered.
- Natural tissue from the body lasts, whereas silicone or saline implants must be replaced every 10 to 15 years.
- Looks natural because it is body tissue, as opposed to fluid encased in an implant envelope.

Because blood vessels are involved with flap procedures, they are usually not recommended for a woman with a history of diabetes or connective tissue or vascular disease, or for a woman who smokes, as the risk of problems during and after surgery is much higher.

Flap Reconstructive Surgery

There are four types of flap reconstructive surgery, each determined by the donor site.

1. TRAM Flap—transverse rectus abdominis muscle
    The most popular of the reconstruction options, especially if the woman has excess belly fat or an abdomen stretched by pregnancy. She receives a "tummy tuck" as a fringe benefit. Skin, fat, and muscle from the lower abdomen are slid up through a tunnel under the skin to the breast area; the blood supply for the tissue is maintained (Figure 19-17).
    A TRAM Flap is *not* possible if:
    - The woman is thin and does not have enough abdominal tissue.
    - The patient is a smoker, because blood vessels will be narrowed and less flexible.
    - The woman already has a surgical scar(s) on the abdomen. An exception is made for a C-section scar.
2. DIEP Flap—deep inferior epigastric perforator
    This surgery derives its name from the main blood vessel running through the tissue used to reconstruct the breast. The skin, fat, and the blood vessel from the lower abdomen are used. Since no abdominal muscle is used, recovery time is faster than with the TRAM Flap. The DIEP tissue is completely removed and then reinserted; there is no tunneling under the skin. The surgeon must reconnect the blood vessels, so this procedure takes longer than the TRAM Flap. The woman also receives a bonus "tummy tuck" (Figure 19-18).

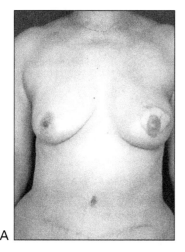 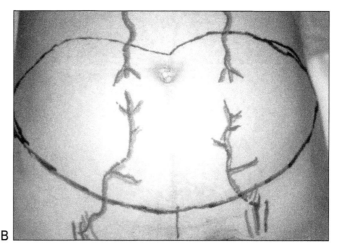

A   B

Figure 19-18
Breast reconstruction: DIEP flap. **(A)** After deep inferior epigastric perforator flap reconstruction. **(B)** Deep inferior epigastric perforator flap; illustrating blood supply from the superior and inferior epigastric vessels.

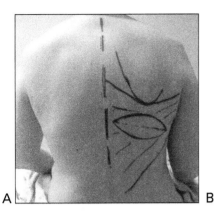 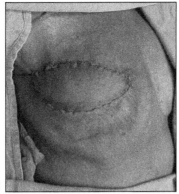 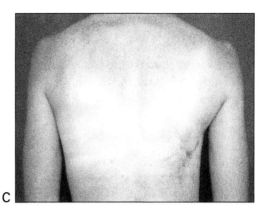

Figure 19-19
Breast reconstruction: Latissimus dorsi flap. **(A)** Tissue taken from the back is tunneled to the front of the chestwall to support the reconstructed breast. **(B)** The transported tissue forms a flap that can hold a breast implant if there is not enough tissue to form a breast mound. **(C)** Scar on the back after latissimus harvest. (Images **A** and **B** from Sabel M, Mulholland MW, eds. *Operative Techniques in Breast, Endocrine, and Oncologic Surgery*. 1st ed. Philadelphia, PA: Wolters Kluwer; 2015.)

3. Latissimus dorsi flap
This option is named after the latissimus dorsi muscle, which is located in the back, below the shoulder, and behind the armpit. The skin, fat, and a portion of the muscle are tunneled under the skin to the chest area. The blood supply is maintained (Figure 19-19).

There are several considerations as well as a few disadvantages for this option:
- This technique works well with small-breasted women.
- There is not much donor fat in this part of the body to make it a viable option for women with larger breasts. The new breast will not match the size of the remaining breast unless an implant is also included.
- The skin from the back tends to be a different color than the chest skin.

- The surface of the back is no longer smooth; it is obvious where the muscle was removed.

4. SGAP/IGAP Flap
The skin, fat, and gluteus maximus muscle are removed from the buttocks and inserted on the chest. Blood vessels must be reconnected to keep the transplanted tissue viable. This type of surgery is rare because it is complex and has a high failure rate (Figure 19-20).

Case Study **19-2**

Describe the basic differences between the four types of flap reconstructive surgery shown in Figures 19-17 to 19-20.

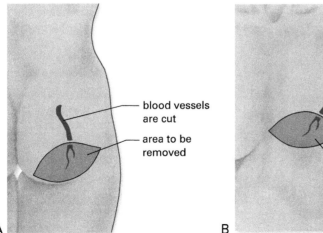 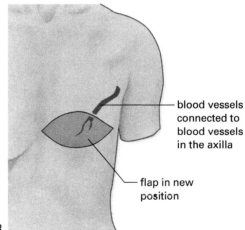

blood vessels are cut

area to be removed

blood vessels connected to blood vessels in the axilla

flap in new position

Figure 19-20
Breast reconstruction: SGAP/IGAP flap. **(A)** Donor site is the buttocks. **(B)** Donated tissue in position on chestwall.

Prophylactic Surgery

Some people at high risk for developing breast and/or ovarian cancer choose to be proactive and reduce their risk by having prophylactic mastectomy as well as prophylactic ovary removal.

Prophylactic Mastectomy

For people at high risk of developing breast cancer, removal of both breasts can reduce their risk by approximately 90%. Although this surgery removes both breasts, a small amount of breast tissue remains; however, their risk is greatly diminished (Figure 19-21). Generally, reconstructive surgery follows. The valid reasons for selecting this elective surgery include the following:

- A strong family history of breast cancer, especially if the family members were premenopausal when diagnosed.
- Testing positive for the BrCA1 or BrCA2 gene mutation.
- A personal history of breast cancer.
- A diagnosis of LCIS; this person has an increased risk for developing invasive breast cancer.
- If the patient had radiation treatments to the chest before the age of 30.

Prophylactic Ovary Removal

This elective surgery removes the ovaries and fallopian tubes and may be done for people at an increased risk of developing ovarian and/or breast cancer. If a woman is at high risk for developing breast cancer, she is also at a higher-than-average risk for developing ovarian cancer. However, to be effective, removal must be done before age 30. The side effects from this surgery are hot flashes, depression, difficulty sleeping, lessened sex drive, and decreased bone strength.

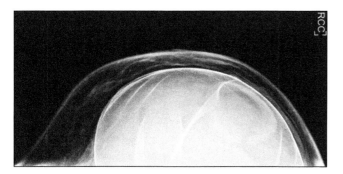

Figure 19-21
This patient had bilateral prophylactic mastectomies due to a strong family pedigree for breast and ovarian cancer. Saline implants replaced the 90% of her breast tissue that was removed.

BrCA1 and BrCA2 Gene Mutation

Women who test positive for the BrCA1 gene tend to develop ER negative tumors, which are not influenced by estrogen. BrCA1 carriers reap great benefits from removal of their ovaries, which reduces their risk for developing ovarian cancer by 85%; but this surgery does not influence their risk of developing breast cancer.

BrCA2 carriers tend to develop ER-positive tumors. BrCA2 carriers who have their ovaries removed decrease their risk of developing breast cancer by 72%, but this surgery does not affect their risk of developing ovarian cancer. Removal of the ovaries before menopause provides the maximum benefit.

▌▌▌ TREATMENT OPTIONS: ADJUVANT THERAPY

Systemic Therapy

After a diagnosis of breast cancer is established, many factors are considered before surgery begins. Surgery is just the beginning of a treatment process, not the end. The surgeon and oncologist evaluate the patient and the cancer to determine a treatment plan. Some of the considered factors include characteristics of the tumor:

- Tumor size
- Grade of the tumor
- Hormone receptor status
- Rate of tumor cell growth
- Oncogene expression
- Human epidermal growth factor receptor 2 (HER2/ERBB2) status
- Lymph node involvement

Together the physicians evaluate the patient's age, general health, location of the tumor, and menopausal status to construct a risk/benefit assessment. The considerations include:

- If the tumor is in situ, no chemotherapy is required because the disease is localized.
- If the tumor is invasive and is larger than 1 cm, chemotherapy is usually recommended.
- If the tumor is invasive, hormone receptor negative, and HER2/ERBB2 positive, chemotherapy is necessary.
- If the woman is premenopausal with invasive disease, chemotherapy is required because tumors in this age group tend to be more aggressive.
- If the lymph nodes are positive, chemotherapy is required regardless of the size of the tumor or the menopausal status of the woman.

New molecular classifications of early-stage breast cancer loom on the horizon. Gene expression microarrays appear to predict the risk of disease recurrence as well as the potential benefit of chemotherapy. Gene expression profiling techniques demonstrate that breast cancer is a molecularly heterogeneous disease, meaning the presence of multiple subtypes of breast cancer comprise a tumor. These subtypes are associated with differences in clinical outcome:

- Longest survival times—luminal A tumors
- Intermediate survival times—luminal B tumors
- Shortest survival times—basal-like and HER2/ERBB2-positive tumors

Clinical trials underway in Europe and in North America will improve the ability to tailor therapy on an individual basis.[26]

Systemic therapy is treatment that gets into the bloodstream via oral ingestion or by way of injection; the bloodstream delivers medication to the cancer cells wherever they are throughout the body. There are three general categories of systemic therapy used for breast cancer: chemotherapy, hormonal therapy, and targeted therapy. Treatment options are based on information about the cancer and the patient's overall health and treatment preferences.

Chemotherapy

Chemotherapy is the use of cytotoxic (toxic to cells) drugs to destroy cancer cells that may have spread from the breast to other parts of the body via the lymphatic system and/or the blood stream. This is a form of systemic therapy that affects every part of the body, whether healthy or diseased. It works by interfering with the cancer cell's ability to grow and divide. Chemotherapy is prescribed by a medical oncologist, a doctor who specializes in treating cancer with medication.

Not every person diagnosed with breast cancer needs chemotherapy. The oncologist considers several factors when deciding if chemotherapy is an appropriate option, including:

- The type of breast cancer
- The grade of the disease
- The size of the tumor
- The stage of the disease
- The types of receptors and status
- The number of lymph nodes involved
- The risk for cancer to spread elsewhere in the body
- How likely is it that chemotherapy will be effective
- The overall goals of treatment

Chemotherapy may be given *before* surgery to shrink a large tumor and make surgery easier, called neoadjuvant chemotherapy. It may also be given *after* surgery to reduce the risk of recurrence, called adjuvant chemotherapy. Most often, it is treatment that follows surgery. Chemotherapy may also be given if a patient has a metastatic breast cancer recurrence.

Surgery to remove the tumor is the first step on the path to recovery. If chemotherapy is necessary, there is usually a 2- to 4-week recovery sojourn between chemotherapy and radiation therapy regimes. If chemotherapy is not required, then radiation therapy sessions begin 3 to 6 weeks after surgery.

Chemotherapy treatment plans are very individualistic, depending upon lymph node involvement, tumor size, hormone receptor status, grade of the tumor, and oncogene expression. There are approximately 90 chemotherapy agents approved for use with breast cancer patients:

- Alkylating agents work on all phases of a cell's cycle; this slows or prevents the cancer cell from reproducing.
- Nitrosources are similar to alkylating agents; this interferes with the enzymes that repair DNA.
- Antimetabolites interfere with DNA and ribonucleic acid growth during the S-phase of the cell cycle.
- Antitumor antibiotics interfere with the DNA by altering the membranes that surround the cell, which stops enzyme production and mitosis.
- Mitotic inhibitors stop mitosis by preventing enzymes from making proteins needed for cell reproduction during the M-phase of the cell cycle.
- Corticosteroid hormones kill cancer cells or slow their growth.
- Sex hormones alter the production of male/female hormones to slow the growth of hormone receptors and cells.

Usually, chemotherapy consists of a combination of lower doses of multiple drugs rather than a high dose of one powerful drug; the combination approach results in less severe side effects for the patient.

What Is Chemotherapy?

Healthy cells grow and divide in an orderly fashion, while cancer cells exhibit uncontrolled growth. Chemotherapy works by interfering with the growth and replication of fast-growing cells. Cells that divide rapidly are cancer cells and cells in the blood, mouth, GI tract, nose, nails, vagina, and hair. The underlying premise of chemotherapy is that it will kill more cancer cells than healthy cells. Chemotherapy is a tool we use to destroy the killer before it destroys us (Figure 19-22).

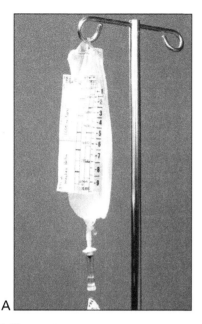
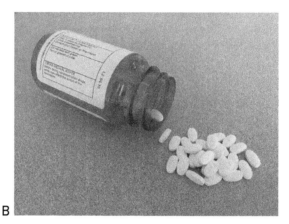

Figure 19-22
Chemotherapy. **(A)** IV drip is one way to introduce chemotherapy medication. (Image courtesy of *Nursing Procedures*. 4th ed. Ambler, PA: Lippincott Williams & Wilkins; 2004.) **(B)** Chemotherapy can also be in pill form.

Vascular access for delivery of chemotherapy is via a PICC line (peripherally inserted central catheter) which is implanted in a large vein such as the subclavian vein, or in the arm. A chemotherapy regimen consists of a specific treatment schedule of drugs given at repeating intervals for a set period of time. Chemotherapy is given on many different schedules; it may be once a week, once every 2 weeks (also called dose-dense), once every 3 weeks, or even once every 4 weeks. A patient may receive one drug at a time or combinations of different drugs at the same time. Research has shown that combinations of certain drugs are sometimes more effective than single drugs for adjuvant treatment. The medications used to treat cancer are continually being evaluated.

Myth: More Is Better

A *cycle* of chemotherapy is a one-time, one round of drugs administered to a patient. A *course* of chemotherapy is the total number of cycles administered during the entire treatment plan. A course typically consists of 4 to 8 cycles. The course of treatment usually lasts 3 to 6 months because the body is allowed time to recover between cycles. Treatment usually involves a combination of two to three different drugs. The oncologist determines the types of agents used, the amount used in each cycle, and the number of cycles that comprise the course. Taking more chemotherapy, the "more is better" theory, is a myth because "more" does not offer an advantage. The patient needs the right amount, not more.

Side Effects

Chemotherapy is well known for its side effects, with some patients suffering severe physical discomfort while others experience mild reactions. The side effects of chemotherapy depend on the individual, the drug(s) used, the schedule, and dose. Some side effects are temporary and fade quickly once treatment is finished; others may take months to disappear.

Supportive medications help ameliorate some side effects, while cosmetic devices help other conditions:

- Hair loss (alopecia): this side effect has an emotional impact because the loss of head hair is so visible. Wigs, hats, and scarves provide disguises for the 2 to 3 months for hair to grow back after treatments are finished. Hair loss happens to all parts of the body. The use of some drugs, specifically doxorubicin and epirubicin, cause the loss of hair.
- Nausea and vomiting: the severity depends upon which chemotherapy drugs are taken. Anthracycline drugs have more severe side effects. Fortunately, antinausea medications help reduce this discomfort. The younger the patient, the more nauseated they become. Fortunately, the nausea trigger zone in the brain decreases as we age.
- Fatigue: a reduction in the production of red blood cells occurs during treatment. Patients develop anemia. To combat this side effect, a patient can be given a transfusion of growth factors which will stimulate the production of red blood cells.

- Suppressed immune system: leukopenia/neutropenia is a reduction in the production of white blood cells. Opportunistic infections are easily acquired.
- Nails: taxane drugs cause nails on the hands and feet to become sore and brittle. They break easily and sometimes fall out.
- Neuropathy: pain from damage to the nerves. Chemotherapy with taxanes often leads to neuropathy, which usually involves the hands and feet. Usually, this is a temporary side effect; however, it can persist long after treatment ends.[27]
- Bone loss: osteoporosis. Treatment with aromatase inhibitors, which is generally reserved for postmenopausal women, can cause osteoporosis as well as myalgia and arthralgia.[28]
- Mouth sores.
- Changes to taste and smell.
- Memory loss: "chemo brain." Cognitive function difficulties present as memory and concentration problems. This condition is more difficult to quantify because the stress, anxiety, and depression from dealing with having cancer cause the same symptoms as the chemotherapy drugs.

Long-term and/or permanent side effects include:

- Early menopause: some drugs damage the ovaries. This can lead to impaired fertility and premature menopause, which increase the risk of osteoporosis.[29] If a woman is over 40 years of age, this usually is permanent; if she is younger than 40, the effect often is temporary.
- Weight gain: this is common, especially if the woman enters menopause as a result of chemotherapy. The more weight gained, the less likely the patient is to lose the weight. Weight gain can be caused by changes in metabolism as well as not being physically active during the months of chemotherapy treatments.
- Heart disorders and leukemia: these are rare but possible side effects of chemotherapy; approximately 1% to 2% of patients are affected. Anthracyclines and HER2-targeted drugs can lead to cardiomyopathy and congestive heart failure.[30] This side effect is dose dependent. Sometimes it can be reversed if chemotherapy is stopped at the first sign of symptoms.

Just as with radiation therapy, chemotherapy affects healthy cells as well as diseased cells. However, healthy cells will repair the damage over time: hair grows back, mouth sores heal, nausea ends, and appetites return.

Hormonal (Antiestrogen) Therapy

After breast cancer surgery, many people will be treated with a combination of chemotherapy and hormone therapy.

Others will have only chemotherapy or only hormone therapy. Among women with hormone receptor positive breast cancer of any stage, 79% receive hormonal therapy.[6]

Hormonal therapy is an effective treatment for most tumors that test positive for either estrogen or progesterone receptors (called ER positive or PR positive), in both early-stage and metastatic breast cancer. 75% of breast cancers are ER positive and/or PR positive. This type of tumor uses hormones (estrogen) to fuel its growth.

Estrogen and progesterone are natural hormones produced by the body and are found in the bloodstream. Cancers secrete an angiogenesis factor, a substance that causes development of a bizarre vascular system. As estrogen and progesterone move throughout the vascular system, the cancer cell's receptors latch onto the free-floating hormones. Estrogen and progesterone stimulate the cancer cell, causing it to grow. Blocking the hormones from entering the cell can help prevent a cancer occurrence or recurrence.

Hormone therapy works in one of two ways:

1. Tamoxifen/raloxifene: receptors on the surface of the cancer cells prefer tamoxifen or raloxifene over estrogen or progesterone. Tamoxifen and raloxifene bind with the receptors, leaving no openings for estrogen and progesterone. The tumor then "starves" (Figure 19-23).
2. Aromatase inhibitor (AI): these agents cause the body to produce less estrogen and progesterone. With less of these free-floating natural hormones in the blood stream, the tumor is forced to go "on a diet."

Tamoxifen and Raloxifene

Tamoxifen and raloxifene are selective estrogen receptor modulators (SERM). Tamoxifen is a first-generation SERM, while raloxifene is second generation. Tamoxifen has been in use for almost 45 years. It has been shown to:

- Reduce the risk of recurrence (tertiary prevention) by 42%
- Reduce the likelihood of developing a contralateral breast cancer by 47%[31] (100% would make tamoxifen a true primary prevention agent)
- Reduce the risk of distant recurrence
- Reduce the risk of breast cancer in women at high risk for developing breast cancer
- Lower the risk of a local recurrence for women with DCIS who have had a lumpectomy

Tamoxifen is effective with ER-positive, PR-positive tumors; it does not work with either ER-negative or PR-negative tumors.

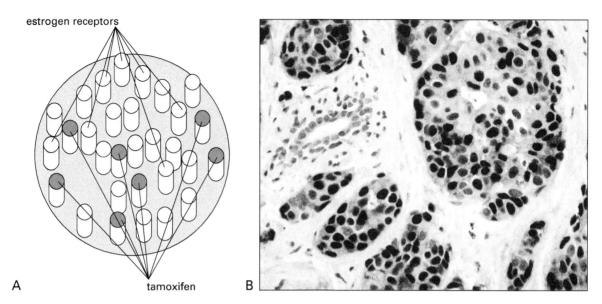

Figure 19-23
(A) Estrogen receptors are found on the surface of many breast cancer cells. **(B)** Immunohistochemistry demonstrates that estrogen receptor (ER) expression in breast cancer is very heterogeneous (dark-staining nuclei are ER positive). In some invasive breast cancers (IBCs), nearly every tumor cell contains high levels of ER.

In 1992, the National Surgical Adjuvant Breast and Bowel Project launched their landmark Breast Cancer Prevention Trial (BCPT). As many as 13,388 women age 35+ who were considered at high risk for developing this disease were enrolled in this study. They were randomly assigned to take tamoxifen or a placebo daily for 5 years. The results showed an almost 50% reduction in developing breast cancer in the tamoxifen group. The unwanted side effects from taking tamoxifen: blood clots, hot flashes, vaginal dryness, discharge or bleeding, and an elevation in the risk of developing endometrial cancer.[32–34] However, tamoxifen may improve bone health and cholesterol levels.

Raloxifene, the second-generation SERM, was developed to treat osteoporosis in postmenopausal women. Doctors noted their patients using raloxifene developed fewer breast cancers. STAR (Study of Tamoxifen and Raloxifene) found raloxifene to be equivalent in effectiveness to tamoxifen in high-risk postmenopausal women, but that raloxifene has fewer side effects.

Tamoxifen and raloxifene report a 50% reduction in developing invasive breast cancer. Tamoxifen also reduces the likelihood of developing LCIS and DCIS, while raloxifene has no effect on these types of breast cancer. Tamoxifen is the only agent approved by the FDA for use with premenopausal women at high risk. Postmenopausal women have the option of using either tamoxifen or raloxifene. Tamoxifen is used for only 10 years, although side effects are also increased with this longer duration of therapy; no clinical benefit has been found with its continued use. Raloxifene can be used indefinitely.

Options for hormonal therapy for premenopausal women include the following:

* Five or more years of tamoxifen, with switching to an AI after menopause begins.
* Either tamoxifen or an AI combined with suppression of ovarian function. One of the oldest hormone treatments for hormone receptor–positive breast cancer is to stop the ovaries from making estrogen, called ovarian suppression; this causes temporary menopause.

Aromatase Inhibitors (AI)

In postmenopausal women, AI decreases the amount of estrogen made by tissue other than the ovaries; AI accomplishes this by blocking the aromatase enzyme, which changes weak male hormones (androgen) into estrogen when, during menopause, the ovaries have stopped making estrogen. Women who have not gone through menopause should not use AI because this medication cannot block the effects of the large amount of estrogen made by the ovaries.

There are three AI medications; all three are thought to work equally well and all have similar side effects. If a woman has serious side effects from one AI, she should try one of the other types. The side effects of AI include muscle and joint pain, hot flashes, vaginal dryness, an increased risk of osteoporosis and broken bones, and increased cholesterol levels.

A woman may be treated with AI only, or she may be prescribed with an AI at the conclusion of tamoxifen treatment. Treatment with an AI plus tamoxifen is more effective than tamoxifen alone at reducing the risk of recurrence in postmenopausal women. Breast cancer recurrence rates with tamoxifen at 5 years is 12.6%; at 8 years, it is 19.2%; with AI at 5 years, it is 9.6%; and at 8 years, it is 15.3%.[35] Postmenopausal women who are prescribed hormonal therapy have several options: start therapy with an AI for up to 5 years, begin treatment with tamoxifen for 2 to 3 years, and then switch back to an AI for 2 to 3 years; or take tamoxifen for 5 years then switch to an AI for up to 5 years, in what is called extended hormonal therapy.

Studies are underway in Canada and the United Kingdom to evaluate AI as a breast cancer prevention agent. Currently in the United States, the FDA has approved AI for treatment purposes only; it is not approved for prevention. Chemoprevention of cancer is defined as the "use of natural, synthetic, or biologic chemical agents to reverse, suppress, or prevent carcinogenic progression to invasive cancer."[36]

Chemotherapy and Hormone Therapy Together

Premenopausal women with ER-positive, PR-positive tumors can be treated with chemotherapy only, with hormone therapy only, or with a combination of both. The combination may help decrease the chance of recurrence the most. Postmenopausal women with ER-positive, PR-positive tumors may or may not be advised to do the combination therapy, but they are always advised to use hormone therapy.

If a woman has an ER-negative tumor, she will do equally well taking chemotherapy only or chemotherapy and hormone therapy combined. Since the result is the same, most elect chemotherapy only.

Targeted Therapy

Targeted therapy works differently than chemotherapy to limit the growth and spread of cancer cells while reducing damage to healthy cells. These therapy treatments target the cancer's specific genes, proteins, or the tissue environment that contributes to cancer's growth and survival. These treatments are very focused because not all tumors have the same targets.

The first approved targeted therapies for breast cancer were antiestrogen hormonal therapies. Then HER2-/ERBB2-targeted therapies were approved to treat HER2-positive breast cancer. Targeted therapy is also used for metastatic hormone receptor–positive breast cancer, for osteoclast-targeted therapy (bisphosphonate drugs) that blocks the cells that destroy bone, and the list goes on. These therapies are unique for each patient and are very specific, depending on her own tumor.

Many research studies are ongoing to find out more about specific molecular targets and new treatments directed at them.

THE FUTURE: PREVENTION

Humans are fortunate: we can prevent some types of disease and have learned how to cure others. The polio and measles vaccines are classic examples of prevention. We attempt to cure and/or prevent all disease—from the common cold to every chronic and life-threatening illness. People have rallied around the pink ribbon to find a cure for breast cancer and to spread the word on the need for early detection (Figure 19-24).

Primary Prevention

This is prevention of de novo malignancies in a healthy population. Primary prevention is what the polio and measles vaccines do. It is what we eventually hope to do for breast cancer. We have not yet discovered a vaccine for breast cancer, but we do have some medications that can be taken by people at high risk in order to reduce their risk of developing this disease. This is where we need the breakthrough, to have the greatest impact on prevention. Stay tuned, some exciting developments are happening here. See Chapter 21.

Secondary Prevention

This level of prevention is directed to those patients who have a known premalignant lesion. Prevention here involves taking medicines that keep the disease from

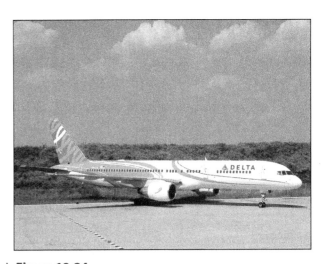

Figure 19-24
Delta Airlines' pink ribbon plane is painted pink! (Image courtesy of Delta Airlines.)

progressing. An example would be someone who tests positive for HIV and who takes drugs to prevent HIV from developing into AIDS. With breast cancer, chemoprevention is the administration of pharmacological agents to prevent, delay, or slow the development of cancer in women with a precancerous condition or with significant risk factors for malignancy.

Tertiary Prevention

This level of prevention is focused on the recurrence of breast cancer. Today, we are successful in treating breast cancer. We cannot yet cure someone of breast cancer, but for many women diagnosed with breast cancer, this is now a chronic disease, not a terminal one.

Review Questions

1. Describe the sentinel lymph node procedure.

2. What are the differences between (1) radiation therapy (Figures 19-13 and 19-14), (2) chemotherapy (Figure 19-22), and (3) hormone therapy?

References

1. Howlader N, et al., eds. *SEER Cancer Statistics Review, 1975–2013*. Bethesda, MD: National Cancer Institute. Available at: http://seer.cancer.gov/csr/1975_2013/, based on November 2015 SEER data submission, posted to the SEER web site, April 2016.

2. Berry DA, et al. Effect of screening and adjuvant therapy on mortality from breast cancer. *N Engl J Med.* 2005;353:1784–1792.

3. Siegel RL, et al. Cancer statistics 2017. *CA Cancer J Clin.* 2017;67(1):7–30.

4. Miller KD, et al. Cancer treatment and survivorship statistics 2016. *CA Cancer J Clin.* 2016;66(4):271–289.

5. *Mastectomy vs. Lumpectomy*. Available at: www.breast-cancer.org/treatment/surgery/mast_vs_lump.jsp. Accessed July 29, 2008.

6. American College of Surgeons, Commission on Cancer. *National Cancer Database, 2013 Data Submission*. Chicago, IL: American College of Surgeons; 2015.

7. McGuire KP, et al. Are mastectomies on the rise? A 13-year trend analysis of the selection of mastectomy versus breast conservation therapy in 5865 patients. *Ann Surg Oncol.* 2009;16:2682–2690.

8. Brett S. More long-term follow-up from breast cancer trials. *J Watch General.* 2002. [N Engl J Med. 2002;347:1227–1232].

9. Litiere S, et al. Breast conserving therapy versus mastectomy for stage I-II breast cancer: 20 year follow-up of the EORTC 10801 phase 3 randomised trial. *Lancet Oncol.* 2012;13:412–419.

10. Freedman RA, et al. Receipt of locoregional therapy among young women with breast cancer. *Breast Cancer Res Treat.* 2012;135:893–906.

11. Kummerow KL, et al. Nationwide trends in mastectomy for early-stage breast cancer. *JAMA Surg.* 2015;150:9–16.

12. Murthy V, Chamberlain RS. Nipple sparing mastectomy in modern breast care. *Clin Anat.* 2013;26 (1):56–65.

13. DiSipio T, et al. Incidence of unilateral arm lymphoedema after breast cancer: a systematic review and meta-analysis. *Lancet Oncol.* 2013;14:500–515.

14. ACS. *Breast Cancer Facts & Figures 2005–2006*. Atlanta, GA: American Cancer Society; 2006.

15. Cabanas RM. An approach for the treatment of penile carcinoma. *Cancer.* 1977;39(2):456–466.

16. Gould EA, et al. Observations on a "sentinel node" in cancer of the parotid. *Cancer.* 1960;13:77–78.

17. Morton DL, et al. Technical details of intraoperative lymphatic mapping for early stage melanoma. *Arch Surg.* 1992;127(4):392–399.

18. Veronesi U, et al. Sentinel node biopsy to avoid axillary dissection in breast cancer with clinically negative lymph nodes. *Lancet.* 1997;349(9069):1864–1867.

19. Giuliano AE, et al. Lymphatic mapping and sentinel lymphadenectomy for breast cancer. *Ann Surg.* 1994;220(3):391–398.

20. RadiologyInfo.org. *Brachytherapy*. Available at: http://www.radiologyinfo.org/en/info.cfm?pg=brachy.Accessed March 23, 2009.

21. Silverstone R. Robert abbe: founder of radium therapy in America. *Bull N Y Acad Med.* 1956;32(2):157–167.

22. RT Answers. *Answers to Your Radiation Therapy Questions*. Fairfax, VA: Society for Radiation Oncology. Available at: www.rtanswers.org/treatmentinformation/index.aspx. Accessed March 23, 2009.

23. Arnold ND, et al. Age, breast cancer subtype approximation, and local recurrence after breast conserving therapy. *J Clin Oncol.* 2011;29(29):3885–3891.

24. Carlson RW. Chapter 67: Surveillance of patients following primary therapy. In: Harris JR, et al., eds. *Diseases of the Breast.* 5th ed. Philadelphia, PA: Lippincott Williams & Wilkins; 2014.

25. American Cancer Society 2008. Study quantifies risk of breast cancer recurrence. *CA Cancer J Clin.* 2008;58(6):322.

26. BreastCancer.org. *Why Reconstruction*. Available at: http://www.breastcancer.org/treatment/surgery/reconstruction/why/. Accessed June 24, 2008.

27. Rivera E, Cianfrocca M. Overview of neuropathy associated with taxanes for the treatment of metastatic breast cancer. *Cancer Chemother Pharmacol.* 2015;75:659–670.

28. Conte P, Frassoldati A. Aromatase inhibitors in the adjuvant treatment of postmenopausal women with early breast cancer: putting safety issues into perspective. *Breast J.* 2007;13:28–35.

29. Howard-Anderson J, et al. Quality of life, fertility concerns, and behavioral health outcomes in younger breast cancer survivors: a systematic review. *J Natl Cancer Inst.* 2012;104:386–405.

30. Curigliano G, et al. Cardiovascular toxicity induced by chemotherapy, targeted agents and radiotherapy: ESMO clinical practice guidelines. *Ann Oncol.* 2012;23(suppl 7): vii155–vii166.

31. NCI, US NIH SEER Program. *SEER 17 Incidence and Mortality 2000–2003, NCI, DCCPS, Surveillance Research Program, Cancer Statistics Branch*. Bethesda, MD: National Cancer Institute.

32. Cianfrocca M, Grandishar W. New molecular classifications of breast cancer. *CA Cancer J Clin*. 2009;59:303–313.

33. Davies C, et al. Early Breast Cancer Trialists' Collaborative Group (EBCTCG), Relevance of breast cancer hormone receptors and other factors to the efficacy of adjuvant tamoxifen: patient-level meta-analysis of randomised trials. *Lancet*. 2011;378:771–784.

34. Schover LR, et al. Sexual dysfunction and infertility as late effects of cancer treatment. *EJC Suppl*. 2014;12:41–53.

35. Fisher B, et al. Tamoxifen for prevention of breast cancer: report of the national surgical adjuvant breast and bowel project P-1 study. *J Natl Cancer Inst*. 1998;90:1371–1388.

36. Susan G. Komen for the cure. *Types of Treatment*. Available at: http://Ww5.komen.org. Accessed March 23, 2009.

Breast MR

Objectives

- List at least three strengths for breast MR, and two limitations.
- Label the parts in a drawing of an MRI unit.
- Define precessing, steady-state, and magnetic moment.
- Describe at least three medical conditions for referring a patient for breast MR services.
- List the major safety precautions for the magnet; list some of the safety precautions for the patient.

Key Terms

- coil
- gradients
- hydrogen
- magnetic moment
- precession
- radiofrequency (RF)

█ INTRODUCTION

A Century (Almost)

Scientists are a restless lot. From 1915 through the 1940s, they were not merely content with simply studying the elements from the periodic table; they examined their composition down to the level of atoms. These scientists were interested in subatomic particles and the properties of radiation, magnetism, light, sound, and more. Scientists created a new language for this new field known as quantum mechanics; they quantified everything: they measured, weighed, and timed these unseen particles and their phenomena.

Chemical elements with an odd number of protons in the nucleus were singled out for investigation because of their unique potential. Intriguing to the scientists was the most simple and most abundant element in our universe: **hydrogen**, with its single positive charge in its nucleus. Hydrogen and heavy elements with magnetic properties were studied and amazingly applied both to healthcare for *saving* lives and to the military for making bombs that *destroy* life. Such is the background for the beginning of MRI development.[1]

What is it about hydrogen that fascinated the scientists and motivated years of study and experimentation? Two particles (electrons and protons) in lightweight hydrogen gas, and their ability to create a weak magnetic state that hums as a radiofrequency (RF) signal. The heavier nucleus, at the center of the atom, has one proton. The hydrogen atom also has one rapidly orbiting lightweight electron. While both particles exhibit weak magnetism, it is the heavier proton in the nucleus that is measured; the electron is too small, light, and too difficult to individually measure in a volume of material with thousands of other electrons. The mass of an electron is 9.1×10^{-28} g while a proton is $1,836 \times$ electron mass.

A proton spins like a top, and like a top, it has a spin-intrinsic angle that changes as its spin speed changes. It moves in wide orbits of fast spins, and then, it wobbles and falls with slower reduced energy, an event called **precession**. These oscillations create noise from the wobble. As the proton gains strength, it suddenly and briefly returns to its high-energy state with a humming resonance. With a release of energy, the higher-energy state returns the positively charged proton to its former natural state and creates 6 excess protons for every 10,000 protons in the area of matter where the hydrogen atoms reside. It is these 6 excess protons that create the weak magnetic signal that is picked up as an RF signal.

Radiofrequency (RF) is an electromagnetic wave propagated by an antenna. This transmits data invisibly through the air. Such is the basis for MRI.

Felix Bloch of Stanford University picked up on the spin in 1946. He theorized that any spinning charged particle (like a hydrogen atom) creates an electromagnetic field, and he quantified this. His work in quantum theory earned him the Nobel Prize in physics and put the emphasis on the words nuclear and magnetic, the basis for nuclear magnetic resonance (NMR), 30 years before it was applied to imaging humans.

By 1977, Raymond Damadian, a physician and experimenter, and his colleagues produced the first NMR scan of a human. Sixty percent of the human body is composed of water; water (H_2O) is composed primarily of hydrogen. They studied the hydrogen atoms inside a human lying in a narrow tunnel surrounded by this massive magnet. They assembled an image of his tissue, fat, bone, muscles, and organs. The reward for being first—their NMR machine resides in the Smithsonian. Two years later, 1979, the first in vivo breast NMR scan was produced.

Rapid advancements during the 1980s and 1990s improved MRI scanning: the introduction of faster and more powerful computers, a host of improvements in the use of magnets, innovative **coils**, and modified RF pulse sequences to excite the hydrogen protons to make them obey complicated sequences of radio pulse commands delivered by a computer.[1,2] By 1982, there were only a few NMR machines in the world used for diagnostic imaging; today, they are found in virtually every medical diagnostic center. Magnetic resonance (MR) has been used in the radiology department for more than 40 years; breast applications have gained a place in the diagnostic/screening mix.[3–6]

The name has changed from NMR to magnetic resonance imaging (MRI) because of the negative connotations from the word nuclear. In current medical papers referencing the use of MRI technology for a body part, it is simply called MR, as in breast MR. But it is still the progeny from scientists (Pauli, Rabi, Lauterbur, Mansfield, Heywang, and others), and of observations and experiments with spinning atoms and magnetism, along with a century of innovations.

Mammographic Imaging Advances

Articles, studies, reports, and editorials from recent medical journals routinely extol the virtues of screening mammography, especially in regard to the newer 3D digital technologies; most recognize the unique advantages of computer-acquired and processed images. The consensus is that mammography remains the gold standard for breast imaging.[3–12] That may change, and soon.

We have witnessed changes in medical imaging systems: from film to digital imaging using x-rays to digital imaging using MR. Why the interest in MRI technology for breast imaging? Why now?

Eight major reasons[3,4,12–24]:

1. After more than four decades of clinical use, MRI has demonstrated that it is effective; that it can accomplish more of the difficult imaging tasks, particularly with soft tissue body parts; and that it has a wider range of applications than digital mammography that includes detection, localization, biopsy, and treatment planning for cancers.

2. MRI does its best work in the most challenging imaging conditions: for women with *BrCA1* and *BrCA2* genes who are at high risk of developing cancer and for women who have proven breast cancer and are therefore at an increased risk for recurrence.

3. For patients who undergo neoadjuvant chemotherapy, MRI has the best correlation with pathology, better than mammography or ultrasound.

4. Availability. Virtually all hospitals and outpatient imaging centers provide MRI services.

5. The ability of radiologists to display all the images acquired in various digital formats relevant to the patient, for comparison before making a diagnosis or planning treatment.

6. MRI has postprocessing capabilities not possible with digital mammography.

7. MRI does not use ionizing radiation.

8. Fibroglandular tissue does not affect the sensitivity/specificity of the examination.

In its earliest clinical use, breast MR was considered primarily as an adjunctive problem-solving tool to mammography and ultrasound in diagnosing anomalies in soft tissue. Currently, it plays a more central, yet still adjunctive, role for the diagnosis, staging, and treatment planning for breast cancer in selected groups of patients.[3,25,26] One caution: some controversy exists as breast MR defines its role in the larger context of the available radiology services.[27–31]

BREAST MR OVERVIEW: CHEMISTRY MEETS PHYSICS AND BIOLOGY

Magnetic Materials

Magnetism is a property of matter, which results from orbiting electrons (a negative charge) interacting with protons (a positive charge) in the nucleus of an atom. The orbiting electrons cause the atoms to have a **magnetic moment** associated with an intrinsic angular momentum called *spin*. A magnetic moment occurs when an object is placed into a magnetic field; all the atoms align in the direction of the magnetic force. Materials that have magnetic properties may interfere with MRI scanning. Let's see what they are.

Ferromagnetic materials generally contain iron, nickel, or cobalt. Examples of ferromagnetic materials include magnets and various objects that one might find in a patient, such as aneurysm clips, pacemakers, shrapnel, and such. These materials have a large positive magnetic susceptibility; that is, when they are placed in a magnetic field, the field strength is much stronger inside the material than outside.

Ferromagnetic materials are also characterized by their clusters of 10^{17} to 10^{21} atoms called magnetic domains; they all have their magnetic moments pointing in the same direction. The moment of the domains is random in unmagnetized materials and points in the same direction in magnetized materials. The ability of a material to remain magnetized when an external magnetic field is removed is a distinguishing factor compared with paramagnetic, superparamagnetic, and diamagnetic materials. These materials cause susceptibility artifacts characterized by loss of signal and spatial distortion on MRI images. This can occur even with fragments that are too small to be seen on a plain radiograph.

Paramagnetic materials include oxygen and ions of various metals like iron (Fe), magnesium (Mg), and gadolinium (Gd). These ions have unpaired electrons, resulting in a positive magnetic susceptibility. The magnitude of this susceptibility is less than 1/1,000 of that of ferromagnetic materials. The effect on MRI is increased in the T1 and T2 relaxation rates (decreased in the T1 and T2 times).

Superparamagnetic materials consist of individual domains of elements that have ferromagnetic properties in bulk. Their magnetic susceptibility is between that of ferromagnetic and paramagnetic materials. Examples of superparamagnetic materials include iron-containing contrast agents for bowel, liver, and lymph node imaging.

Diamagnetic materials do not have intrinsic atomic magnetic moments, but when placed in a magnetic field, they weakly repel the field, resulting in a small negative magnetic susceptibility. Materials such as water, copper, nitrogen, barium sulfate, and most tissues in the human body are diamagnetic.

MRI takes advantage of the magnetic properties of hydrogen nuclei (protons) in breast tissue. A small fraction of the total number of protons in the body are brought into alignment inside the strong magnetic field within the MRI scanner. Then, the protons are exposed to a brief pulse of RF energy, which displaces their magnetic vectors. As the protons "relax" and realign along the applied magnetic field, excess energy is released. This energy, the electromagnetic MR signal, is detected and electronically processed to construct an image, exploiting the various "relaxation times" of the different tissue composition of the breast to generate image contrast.

Hydrogen, a lightweight gas with atomic #1, is the (chemical) element most widely used in MR imaging. It has

Overview MRI Process

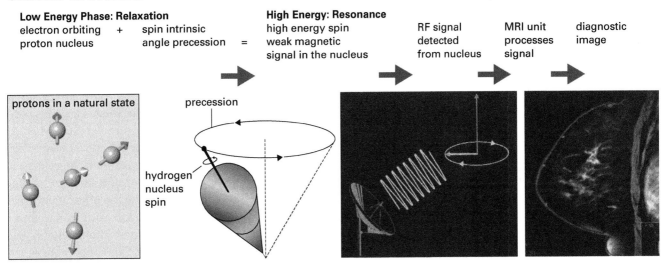

Low Energy Phase: Relaxation
electron orbiting + spin intrinsic
proton nucleus angle precession =

High Energy: Resonance
high energy spin
weak magnetic
signal in the nucleus

RF signal
detected
from nucleus

MRI unit
processes
signal

diagnostic
image

protons in a natural state

precession

hydrogen
nucleus
spin

Figure 20-1
Overview of MRI process.

electromagnetic properties (physics) and is present in the water found in 60% of the human body's tissues (biology). It is the best candidate to exploit to find changes within body tissues—if you have the right tools and smart practices to coax hydrogen atoms to signal the presence of breast cancers. Figure 20-1 provides a set of illustrations to follow the exploitation of hydrogen atom's natural properties to produce a weak magnetic signal that MRI processes into clinical images.

The properties of hydrogen atoms are as follows:

1. *Spin.* The electron orbiting its proton particle. In a two-phase cycle of resonance and relaxation, spin creates magnetism in the proton particle's nucleus.
2. *Magnetic nucleus.* The positively charged proton always is involved in the spin.
3. *A 1-second pause.* Length of time of relaxation, off-phase, or out-of-phase slower spinning with precession.
4. *Attraction to a stronger magnetic field.* Just as orbiting bodies in space (the sun, moon, and planets) influence each other, the Earth's magnetic field influences the naturally spinning hydrogen atom. The strongest oscillation and magnetic signal occurs when it has a loss of coherence during its resonance phase and falls 90°.
5. *Precession movements that oscillate.* Hydrogen atoms wobble, or precess. They transition their spin orientation to the opposite orientation; that is, they flip 90° or 180°. These larger movements create RF signals. The MRI unit detects these signals emitted from the proton's magnetic nucleus during its noisiest millisecond peak of resonance phase, just before the hydrogen atom recovers its natural magnetism and repeats the two-phased cycle.

MRI Equipment: Cancer-Hunting Tools

Let's take a look at an MRI unit (Figure 20-2):

1. The parts we can see and touch
2. Then relate how these tangible "real" parts we can see and touch work together with the "invisible" parts: RF pulses and magnetic signals
3. Smart practices—computer algorithms that create an image of the inside of the body

An MRI machine is more than a big noisy magnet with a long tube through its center and a sliding table for the patient. To the millions of patients worldwide who benefit from its performance, it is the most beautiful machine on the planet.

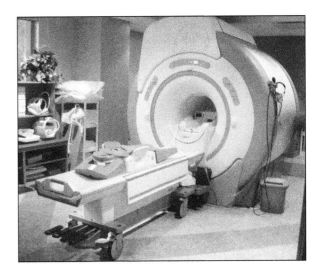

Figure 20-2
MRI unit with the breast coil in position on the patient bed. (Image courtesy of Richard Goldberg, MD. Partners Imaging Center. Sarasota, FL.)

An MRI system includes a magnet and an RF system of specialized antennas. The antennas are actually loops of wires bundled together and shaped into coils (gradient coils, RF coils, and shim coils) that send and receive radio signals between a patient, signal detectors, and the computer. This two-way exchange carries and shares information about the condition of the hydrogen nuclei in a human body. Other components include smaller specialized body coils, an active RF shield, power supply, RF amplifier and synthesizer, NMR probes (receiver coil interface), computer, display unit (monitor), and a refrigeration unit (cryogens).[32–36] Computers in MRI units link with other computers, PACS, and networks for administrative and medical record functions[37] (Figure 20-3).

Magnets

The magnet is the largest and most important component in an MRI system because its magnetic strength defines what it can and cannot do. To be useful in diagnostic medicine, a magnet must be able to produce a stable magnetic field in a defined area. In MRI, that area of magnetism must be strong enough to penetrate throughout the selected volume of the body part being imaged and strong enough to detect weak magnetic signals from the hydrogen protons in the selected body part. An MRI magnet with the brute strength of 1.5 T (15,000 G) meets these requirements for breast MR.

The MRI unit concentrates its strongest force inside the magnet's bore, yet it still influences all the space inside the MRI room and adjacent areas. Large magnets in the shape of a cylindrical tube are used for MRI. Its magnetism creates magnetic poles at either end of the open tube. Figure 20-4 shows the magnetic alignment in a linear flow through the tube: out one end and looping back to reenter the magnetic bore at the other. These lines represent the paths for magnetic forces in and around a magnet and are known as flux lines. The magnetic field from the unit reaches well beyond the open bore of the MRI unit.

Superconducting electromagnets are the most frequently used magnets in medical MRI systems because they are powerful enough and flexible enough to perform many different types of examinations on virtually any part of the human body. Electromagnets consist of a long wire with a current running through it to create a magnetic field; this is a commonly used design form for

Typical Magnetic Resonance System

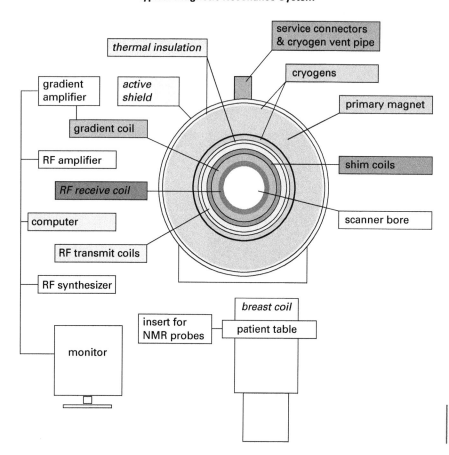

Figure 20-3
Annotated MRI machine: its parts and functions.

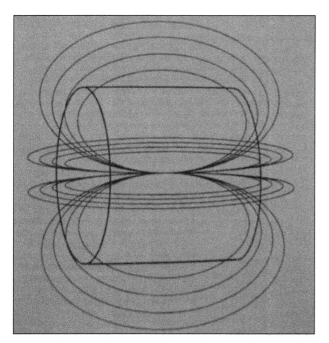

Figure 20-4
Magnetic field flux lines. Flux lines display the direction of movement of magnetism: in at its south pole and out at the north pole. The magnetic field encompasses the area in and around the magnet that is influenced by the magnetic force.

MRI magnet bathed in cryogens

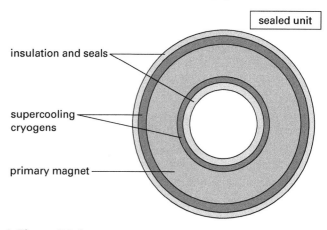

Figure 20-5
MRI magnet bathed in cryogens. A 1.5-T MR unit is more efficient when the wire coils that constitute the magnet are bathed in supercooled cryogens at 452.4° below zero. At these low temperatures, there is almost no resistance to the flow of electricity through the wires.

many electromagnetic devices that carry electricity. The laws of electromagnetism state that moving electrical charges induce magnetic fields around themselves. For imaging objects as large as a human, this type of magnet would be prohibitively expensive to operate without using cryogens to supercool the wires of the magnet to greatly reduce electrical resistance. Cryogens bathe the wires and provide many system benefits for efficient operations beyond the more efficient use of electricity; they also help maintain magnetic field shapes and assist in maintaining homogeneity of the magnet.

Cryogens: The Supercoolant

There are three basic types of magnets used in clinical MRI systems: resistive, permanent, and superconducting, each with its own electrical power requirements. Only the latter with a minimum magnetic field strength of 1.5 T is suitable for breast MR scanning. Generally, high-resolution medical imaging requires a strong magnet to consistently find and image the magnetic nuclei of the hydrogen atom.[32,35,38]

Superconducting 1.5-T MRI units use cryogens: liquid nitrogen and/or liquid helium inside an insulated vacuum, an industrial strength version of a thermos bottle. Cryogens supercool the coil wires (Figure 20-5). Note that insulation holds the cryogens and the primary magnet coils inside

a sealed and shielded area of the MRI unit.[5] A 1.5-T MRI unit becomes more efficient when it is supercooled.[32,33,35] The wires are bathed in liquid helium at 452.4° below zero. Cryogens are expensive, refilled every 1 to 3 years depending on the MRI machine use. Yet the operating cost for this type of magnet is less expensive than for lower-strength magnets powered by electric but without this supercooling feature.

Magnetic Flux Lines and Magnet Safety

Superconductive flux lines are parallel with and encase the bore of the magnet; this is the magnetic field outside the bore of the magnet (Figure 20-4). A strong magnetic field outside the MRI machine can be potentially dangerous to patients, staff, and visitors in a medical facility. How can a facility control the invisible magnetic flux lines? Not with ordinary walls, windows, or doors; the fringe fields of magnetism are contained by several types of magnetic field shielding.[32,33,35]

The fringe field from a high-strength magnet can extend well outside the MRI room unless proper magnetic shielding is in place. Many years ago, high-field systems were installed into huge suites, about four times the size of today's MRI room. The farther away you are from the magnet, the less pronounced the effects from its magnetic field. These big rooms incorporated *passive shielding*, where the walls, floor, and ceiling are lined with steel. This is usually a one-time build-out cost and offers effective shielding in medical imaging centers or hospitals where space is at a premium. *Active shielding* uses small magnets outside the cryogen bath to restrict and direct the magnetic field lines to an acceptable location. Active shielding is provided by the manufacturer. This method allows MRI magnets to be installed in trailers for mobile imaging and in temporary sites with no passive shielding.

Magnetic Fields

The large magnetic field inside the MRI bore affects a volume of space, not a specific point; it must be focused into a smaller defined area to image a specific body part. Magnetic fields useful for imaging are shaped by smaller custom-designed areas placed close to the specific body part to be scanned. These focused magnetic fields, while small, are powerful enough to detect the signals from the few excess protons that resonate. Small, specialized magnetic fields are created and shaped using RF pulses that carry encoded protocols to gradient coils inside the magnet. The magnetic field "fits" the patient; it complements the pulse sequences that carry examination protocols for various images (2D, 3D, volume examinations) and works hard to serve the purpose of the scan. Shim coils assure homogeneity in the magnetic field during the examinations and throughout changing pulse sequences (Figure 20-6).

Coils

All coils are bundled loops of wires that carry RF signals; all coils are part of an RF system.[34] Each set of coils has a specific role in the detection, manipulation, transmission, and processing of the hydrogen atom's signal, and all sets of coils receive and send data through the RF system computer. The computer coordinates the data sent to and received from the coils. RF signals are either on or off, with each condition sending an RF signal.

MRI machines have four major types of coils: (a) shim, (b) gradient, (c) surface, and (d) RF. The overall purpose of this system of wires is to detect the exchange of energy between spin states in hydrogen nuclei and produce an image from the protons' nuclear resonance.

The RF system sends and receives radio signals that:

1. Control the magnet's stability and homogeneity (shim coils)
2. Alter its magnetism to form custom-made magnetic fields near the patient to maximize signal acquisition for examinations and pulse sequences (gradient coils, X–Y–Z coils for slice thickness, and volume studies)
3. Receive/detect magnetic signals from the hydrogen protons (transmitter/receiver, surface/body, breast coils)[39]
4. Relay these proton signals to the computer for processing (RF coils)

It's all in a day's work. All RF coils, whatever their function, send their specialized information to the computer for processing into an image.

Gradients

Gradients are coils of wire within the magnet that make gradual or graded changes to the shape of the strong linear magnetic field inside the MRI bore. There are three independent gradients. They are oriented in three dimensions, X–Y–Z, to influence changes to the magnetic field during an examination. Gradients also determine the orientation plane for imaging. Gradients can be activated independently, in pairs for oblique examinations, or all excited simultaneously to acquire a volume sample. A volume sample can be shaped for thin or thick slices. A side-by-side review of thin-slice images in various planes through a volume of selected tissue illustrates the usefulness of using specialized MRI coils for evaluation, surgical planning, and other applications (Figure 20-7).

How do gradient coils function within the powerful 1.5-T magnet? In addition to shaping the image slices,

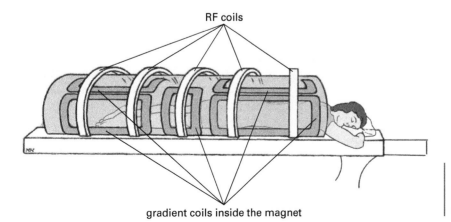

RF coils

gradient coils inside the magnet

Figure 20-6
MRI coils: RF and gradient. Gradient and RF coils shape and focus the main magnetic field.

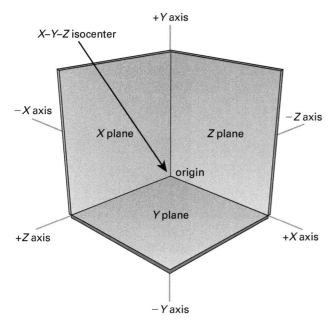

Figure 20-7

Gradient *X–Y–Z* coils. Gradient coils are found inside the magnet. They apply variable magnetic fields at the discretion of the MRI technologist. Various combinations of gradients produce differing images.

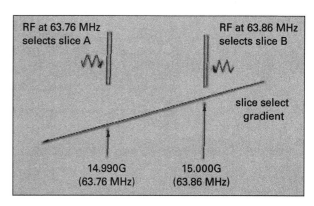

Figure 20-8

Gradients: moving the isocenter. The Larmor equation states a reciprocal relationship between RF signals and the strength of the magnetic gradient. From the magnet isocenter to the edge of the magnet in one direction, the gradient field increases, while from the isocenter to the opposite end, the strength of the gradient field decreases.

gradients can also influence a shift in the magnetic field of the main magnet from its reference point in the center of the bore. The magnetic isocenter is the center point of a magnetic field; it is the origin and reference point of the coordinate system in the center of the bore. An *X–Y–Z*-oriented magnetic center shifts toward one end or the other of the magnet's bore when gradient coils are activated.

The laws of electromagnetic induction state that when you pass a current through a gradient coil, you induce a magnetic or gradient field. This gradient field interacts with the main magnetic field, whereas the magnetic field strength along the axis of the gradient coil is altered linearly. This means that from the magnet's isocenter to one end of the magnet in one direction, the gradient field increases, while from the isocenter to the opposite end, the strength of the gradient field decreases[32,35] (Figure 20-8).

Gradients use changes detected in the magnetic strength of the proton signal as the proton changes its state from low energy to high energy and precesses. The Larmor equation states: "The processional frequency of the magnetic moments increases or decreases, depending on the magnetic field strength they experience at different points along the gradient. Therefore, the precessional frequency increases when the magnetic field increases and decreases when the magnetic field decreases." In other words, the precessional frequency is equal to the magnetic field strength of the magnet multiplied by the gyromagnetic ration. At 1.5 T, the precessional frequency of hydrogen is

63.86 MHz. At 1.0 T, the precessional frequency of hydrogen is 42.57 MHz; and at 0.5 T, the precessional frequency of hydrogen is 21.28 MHz.

RF System and Other Coils

RF coils transmit and receive the pulses to begin and end intricate commands to the magnet for collecting information about the targeted tissue; they provide a connection to a wired network for communication of other machine functions and activities. An RF system comprises a synthesizer, amplifier, and transmitter, usually built into the MRI unit. See Figure 20-3.

The MRI frequency range is from 3 to 100 MHz.[34] The RF transmitter power is variable. Newer scanners may have a peak power of up to 35 kW and are capable of sustaining average power of 1 kW. A recent development in MRI technology has been the sophisticated multielement phased array: 18 coils capable of acquiring multiple channels of data in parallel. These transmit-and-receive RF coils are built into an MRI unit.[32,34]

Shim coils detect inhomogeneity in the magnetic field and make adjustments to restore homogeneity to the magnetic field. Specialty coils within this group are designed for a particular function, such as the birdcage coil, which produces a homogeneous *B1* field for volume studies.

Surface coils. Breast MR has its specialty surface coil placed close to the breasts to restrain movement while at the same time picking up the magnetic signal from the hydrogen protons. NMR probes, specialized electronic signal pickup devices, are a vital component of instrumentation linked to the acquisition of hydrogen protons' signal. The RF frequency and pulse sequence selected for a specific diagnostic protocol is matched to the RF from

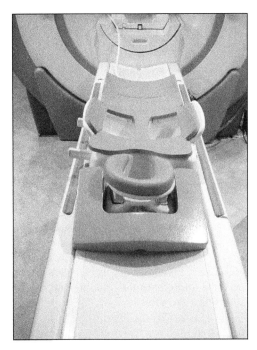
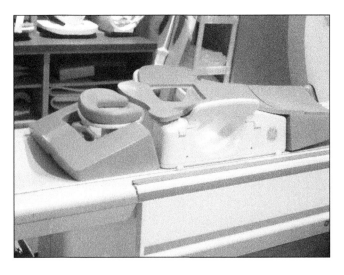

Figure 20-9
Breast MR coil. A look at a breast coil. (Images courtesy of Richard Goldberg, MD. Partners Imaging Center. Sarasota, FL.)

the protons and the length of the relaxation period that can be expected for the targeted material. Probes are specific to a type of study such as volume, 2D, or 3D.[36] They receive, in real time, the signals that the nuclei return to the instrument for digitization, thus allowing an exact image of the tissue sampled. The size of the coil's sensitive volume extends to the circumference of the coil and to a depth equal to the radius of the coil. This is how breast MR coils are able to retrieve signals from the chestwall and the patient's axilla. Beyond this area, signal drop-off is present, relative to the distance from the coil. If the system uses the surface coil to transmit and receive, less outside tissue is excited and the image quality and SNR are much higher. Using a body coil to transmit the signal can cause artifacts because of signal resonating from other tissue in the magnet bore, whose protons also have been excited by the RF signal. Generally, current models have RF capabilities to transmit only, receive only, or transmit and receive RF signals[32,35] (Figure 20-9).

MRI TECHNOLOGY: SMART PRACTICE

The Basics

MRI uses a property of atoms called "spin" to distinguish small differences in energy between a lower-energy relaxation phase and the high-energy resonance phase. This is what the MRI system works hard to exploit.[1,2,26,32,35]

Our hydrogen atom has one proton, a positive-charged particle in the nucleus, and one electron, a negative-charged particle spinning around its center. Together, they spin like a bar magnet with a positive-charged north pole and a negative-charged south pole. Their bonded spin produces a weak magnetism during its two-phase cycle called resonance and relaxation. How can MRI exploit this natural property of spin? Consider the parts of Figure 20-10.

A. Illustrates hydrogen protons in their free-spinning natural state. The orientation of each proton is pointing toward its north pole. Notice that they are free to spin independently of each other in Earth's magnetic field of 0.5 G, which is equal to 0.5 T in MRI magnetic strength.

B. The larger movement of the spinning proton is called precession. This diagram illustrates the slowing spinning spiral of an atom. Like a spinning top that slows and wobbles, sometimes, it falls sideways 90° or 180°, changing its orientation.

As the atom loses spin energy and begins to wobble, it is now that the atom is most influenced by the Earth's stronger magnetic force. The Earth's magnetic force creates torque, or a twisting pull on the slower-spinning

Case Study 20-1

Describe what is happening in Figure 20-10, Parts A to D.

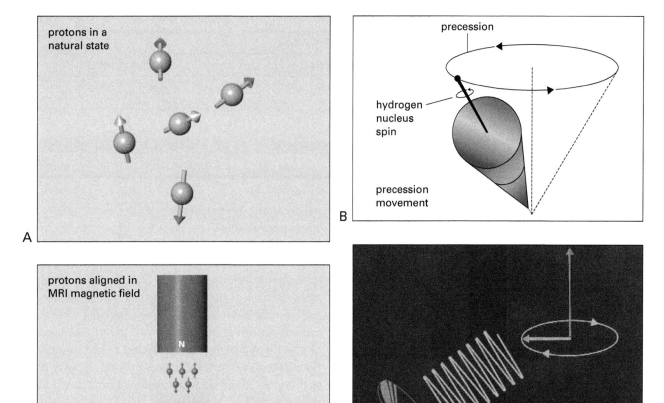

Figure 20-10

Basics of MRI. **(A)** In the low-energy (relaxation) phase, electrons orbit around the proton in the nucleus. **(B)** The hydrogen atom precesses about the magnetic axis. **(C)** When placed into an MRI unit, the protons align with the direction of the magnetic field (magnetic moment). The same number of protons align "north" as align "south," so these forces cancel each other. It is the excess protons that ultimately provide the signal to create the image. **(D)** The MRI unit emits a pulse specific to hydrogen; this causes the protons to absorb the energy required to precess in a different direction (this creates the resonance). The RF pulse forces the excess protons to spin at a particular frequency (Larmor frequency) and in a particular direction. When the RF pulse is turned off, the protons return to their natural alignment within the magnetic field and release their excess energy. The surface coil picks up the signal and sends it to the computer to create an image.

atom. An off-phase or out-of-phase precessing proton creates a faint humming noise that is detected as an RF signal.

C. When a patient is placed inside a strong MRI magnetic field of 1.5 T, three times the strength of the Earth's magnetic field, the hydrogen proton's weak magnetism is overcome. The protons succumb to the force of the stronger MRI magnet and line up in a parallel or antiparallel direction to the axis of the MRI magnet. The protons are held in a steady state.[32,35]

D. When the hydrogen nuclei are aligned, an RF transmitter bombards the protons with an RF pulse, which flips the protons transversely or on their sides. When the RF pulse is turned off, the protons relax back to their original aligned state thereby giving back the energy that was used to knock them down. It is through this process

of turning RF pulses on and off (pulse cycle) that we are able to create an image. Some RF pulse sequences can last up to 10 minutes or more. The hydrogen proton's weak magnetic signal in selected tissues is accessed with a matching RF, and the proton's signal is interrogated to produce a variety of images such as 2D, 3D, volume, and (T1,T2, PD) MIPS. The result is a detailed view of the anatomy of breast tissue.

***The hydrogen atom's property of spin with its two-phase cycle is** the basis for MRI.* Table 20-1 illustrates a more detailed explanation of what happens during relaxation and resonance.

The importance of using the hydrogen atom includes the density of hydrogen atoms inside body tissue; the predictability of its cycle from slow and fast spins; differences

Table 20-1 • Effects from RF signal off

	CHANGES TO CURRENT	
RELAXATION PHASE	**IN MRI RECEIVER COIL**	**RESONANCE PHASE**
Low-energy state	Weak to strong signal	High-energy state
Slower spins		Faster spins
Loss of phase	More "wobble"	
One second	Duration/time	Milliseconds
Orientation change 90° or 180°	Oscillation increases FID signal	Return to magnetic field
T1		T2

in the times between the cycles, particularly the 1-second pause for relaxation; and finally, the signals it emits from changes between its loss of coherence and return to a stronger magnetic state in order to begin another cycle. The signal is detected as RF. When the RF pulse is turned off, an oscillating magnetic field induces a small current in the receiver coil. This signal is called the free induction decay (FID).[32,35] Consider this as the proton's signal for the pickup microphone. T1 is a measure of the time for the loss of its magnetism to a buildup of its magnetic peak from precession. T2 is the very brief time it spins fastest during its strongest oscillation and while sending its signal.

A key strategy in MRI is to exploit resonance from a loss of phase, which has a tendency to oscillate at a larger amplitude at some frequencies than at others. Increasing the strength of the MRI magnet amplifies a signal. At 1.5 T, the precessional frequency of hydrogen is 63.86 MHz. At 1.0 T, the precessional frequency of hydrogen is 42.57 MHz; and at 0.5 T, the precessional frequency of hydrogen is 21.28 MHz. These frequencies are known as resonant frequencies (resonance frequencies). At these frequencies, even small forces can produce large vibrations, like small electric bursts can cause loud and annoying static on a radio speaker.[32,34,35]

Combining RF pulse sequences, and strong magnetism, the MRI unit provides a very smart, flexible, and virtually inexhaustible approach to exploit the characteristics of the hydrogen proton for scanning patients. Pulses of radiofrequencies for breast MR range from 15 to 80 MHz for hydrogen atoms, with many common breast sequences close to the 63.87 MHz. Pulse sequences can be sent in a variety of timed and/or repeated patterns—like a series of musical notes. The following section contains a brief list of pulse sequences common to breast MR. They illustrate the richness and possibilities for innovation with MRI to tease out information from the hydrogen atoms in various types of body tissues. Keep in mind that RF pulses carry the various instructions through the gradient coils to shape the magnetic field near the patient, thus assuring the strongest magnetic pull from the weak magnetism in the proton. RF coils send the pulse sequences to tailor the desired image as slices, 2D, or 3D. The interplay between the magnet and RF pulses and the ability to produce new

pulse combinations truly boggles the mind. That is truly a smart performance.

In a way, it is ironic to compare the banging noise from an MRI unit to music, but the MRI system really does play life-saving music. A pulse sequence, like a good musical arrangement, satisfies its particular purpose. A pulse sequence that lasts several minutes, then, can be compared with an entire musical performance of a song with selected RF signals sent in a well-structured order, activated at precise times, and lasting for a prescribed duration with sly or clever nuances to produce a desired image. Protocols for breast MR differ dramatically.[35,38,40] Many commercial products, books, posters, charts, and computer programs are directed at simplifying and standardizing protocols.[41] Interventional real-time MRI techniques related to pulse sequencing are yet another attempt to simplify and enhance complex choices for an examination. Yet radiologists are known to experiment and to modify protocols for examinations, so the possible number and variations of protocols used in facilities can vary.

Pulse Sequences and Techniques

Let's begin with the basic pulse sequences for T1 and T2 and note that T1 and T2 times are different for breast tissue, brain tissue, blood, and other tissues. Each type of tissue has its own starting and ending point for changes in phase in the hydrogen proton spins; each type of tissue requires a different RF setting and possibly its own specialized NMR probe.[32,34,35]

The following is a list of the most common sequences for breast MR.

- *Pulse cycle* is a repeating unit composed of a series of one or more RF *pulses* with a measurement of one or more MR signals.
- *Pulse sequence* is a series of *pulse cycles.*
- *TR* (time-to-repetition) is the time interval between two successive *pulse cycles* and is usually measured in milliseconds.
- *TE* (time-to-echo) is the time interval from one-pulse cycle (or series of pulses in a more complicated pulse cycle) to the measurement of the MR signal (echo) and is usually measured in milliseconds.

- *Relaxation* is the process that occurs after terminating the RF pulse, in which the physical changes that were caused by the RF pulse return to the state they were in before the application of the RF pulse.
- *T1 recovery* is caused by the nuclei giving up their energy to the surrounding environment (lattice). Energy released to the surrounding lattice causes nuclei to recover their longitudinal magnetization (magnetization in the longitudinal plane). The rate of recovery is an exponential process, with a recovery time constant called T1. This is the time it takes 63% of the longitudinal magnetization to recover in the tissue.
- *T1-weighted* image is an image in which the intensity contrast between any two tissues in an image is due mainly to the T1 relaxation properties of the tissues. To produce a T1-weighted image, a short TE is used to eliminate the effect of T2 and a short TR is used in order not to eliminate the effect of T1.
- *T2 decay* is caused by nuclei exchanging energy with neighboring nuclei. The energy exchange is caused by the magnetic field of each nucleus interacting with its neighbor. T2 decay results in a decay or loss of transverse magnetization (magnetize the transverse plane).
- *T2-weighted* image is an image in which the intensity contrast between any two tissues in an image is due mainly to the T2 relaxation properties of the tissues.
- *2D imaging*—A method of acquiring images slice by slice. Usually, there is a minimal gap between slices. By exciting tissue at a certain frequency, the linear slope of the gradient spatially encodes the tissue signal, thus creating the slices at a predetermined location.
- *3D imaging*—A method of acquiring images in a volume. This volume can be divided into slices at any slice thickness and in any plane. Good for high-resolution images of small-slice thickness. Also allows manual manipulation of images as a three-dimensional object, depending on the system's software capabilities. This can be a benefit in surgical planning.
- *Spin-echo sequence*—To produce a T2-weighted image, a long TR is used to eliminate the effect of T1, and a long TE is used in order *not* to eliminate the effect of T2. The spin-echo is the most commonly used pulse sequence. The pulse sequence timing can be adjusted to give T1-weighted images. Dual-echo and multiecho sequences can be used to obtain both proton density and T2-weighted images simultaneously. Figure 20-11 shows the pulse relationships in a spin-echo sequence.

The two interesting variables in spin-echo sequences are the repetition time (TR) and the echo time (TE). All spin-echo sequences include a slice-selective 90° pulse followed by one or more 180° refocusing pulses (Figure 20-11).

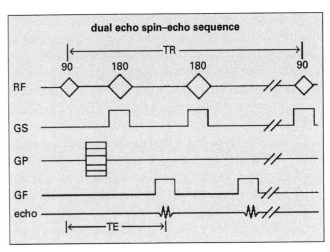

Figure 20-11
Suppression techniques. Fast spin-echo pulse cycle.

The following abbreviations are used:

- *RF* = Radiofrequency
- *GS* = Gradient slice
- *GP* = Gradient phase
- *GF* = Gradient frequency

Gradient-Echo Pulse Cycle

Gradient-echo sequences show a range of variations compared with spin-echo sequences. Not only is the basic sequence varied, by adding dephasing or rephasing gradients at the end of the sequence, but also there is a significant extra variable to specify to things like the TR and TE. This variable is the flip (or tip) angle of the spins. For the basic gradient-echo sequence, illustrated in Figure 20-12, the larger flip angles give more T2 weighting to the image, and smaller flip angles give more T1 weighting.

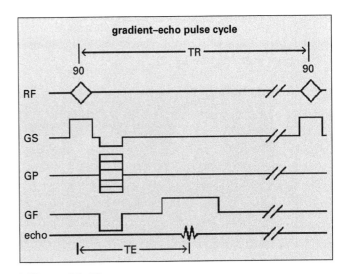

Figure 20-12
Gradient-echo pulse cycle.

There are two important conditions that make MR imaging very useful and at the same time very challenging. First, that various types of tissue will exhibit different T1 and T2 values differently. For example, gray matter in the brain has a different T1 and T2 value than blood or bone. Using three variables (proton density, T1, and T2 values), a highly resolved image can be constructed. Next, the state of hydrogen protons in diseased tissue differs from healthy tissue of the same type, making MRI particularly good at identifying tumors and other lesions. Great care, skill, and expertise are required to obtain MRI's great benefits. Pulse sequences have undergone an evolution with constant emergence of new and novel acquisition schemes.

Suppression Techniques

MRI protocols can tailor pulse sequences to suppress acquisition of a tissue to allow greater influence from another, such as fat/water separation to image a cyst or evaluate an implant.

Fat Saturation Techniques

Fat saturation (or fat suppression) has many uses in MR imaging; however, distinguishing between fatty and nonfatty tumor components is the most important use. Fat suppression or fat saturation can be performed in many different ways.

Even echo (also known as gradient-moment rephasing) rephasing is used primarily in T2-weighted or T2 imaging. This method reduces artifacts from intravoxel dephasing by acquiring the second and succeeding even echoes at a multiple of the first echo.

Presaturation is used primarily in T1-weighted imaging. This method uses additional RF pulses to nullify the signal from fat. The system will place a large saturation pulse at the resonant frequency of fat, relative to the system's field strength and based on the resonant frequency of water: at 1.5 T, fat resonates at 220 Hz from the water peak. At 1.0 T, the fat peak is at 147 Hz from water; and at 0.5 T, fat is 73 Hz from water (Figure 20-13).

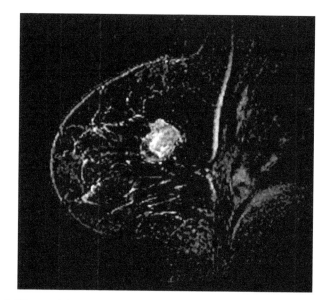

Figure 20-14
Subtraction technique demonstrating tumor enhancement. Pre- and postcontrast images were superimposed and the computer subtracted the similar areas to leave the differentiated tumor highlighted for improved viewing. The subtraction technique demonstrates tumor enhancement.

Other methods include but are not limited to the following:

- Binomial pulse
- Dixon method
- Chemical shift/chem sat
- Off resonance
- Subtraction

Subtraction Techniques

The subtraction method is a postprocessing technique that involves overlaying an image without contrast with an image of the target area taken with contrast. The computer aligns the images and "subtracts" the precontrast image from the postcontrast image, leaving only the enhanced areas visible. An example of this subtraction reconstruction technique is shown in Figure 20-14. The images are

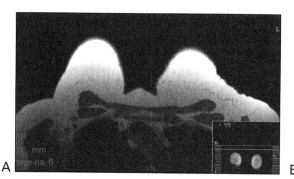
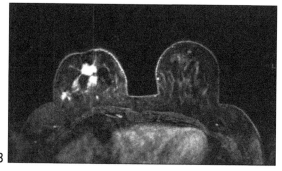

Figure 20-13
Fat suppression. **(A)** Unsuppressed. This makes it easy to see why fat suppression makes it easier to find lesions. **(B)** Spectrally selective fat suppression. Now it is easy to see the tumor. (Images courtesy of EWBC. Rochester, NY.)

filmed by the technologist and presented to the radiologist for interpretation. MRI studies are usually interpreted with comparison made to the patient's mammogram, ultrasound, and any other previous imaging performed on the breasts.

CURRENT BREAST MR

What Breast MR Contributes

Physicians cite professional publications and case examples from their clinical experience to illustrate the use and benefits of breast MR. Medical journals are replete with studies that compare mammography and MRI.[4,8,11,12,19,22–24,42] Currently, physicians find many reasons to refer a patient for a breast MR examination. They include the following[31]:

- Induction of chemotherapy
- Determine the extent of disease
- Patients who present with lobular CA
- Patients who present with infiltrating ductal CA
- Postlumpectomy patients
- Axillary lymphadenopathy
- Patients with implants: silicone gel–filled, saline-filled, soybean oil–filled, and free silicone injections
- Patients with involvement of tumor extending to the chestwall

Studies have shown that breast MR evaluation in women with a newly diagnosed breast cancer identifies *additional areas of tumor* in 27% to 37% of patients.[43] Clinical experience at a high-volume breast center from 2003 to 2007 indicated that 89% of all examinations were done for two reasons: to determine the extent of disease (60%) and screening patients at high risk (29%).

Case Examples

1. *MRI detects cancers missed by mammography and ultrasound for persons at high risk of developing breast cancer.*

   Current applications of breast MR include scanning women with a strong family history of breast and ovarian cancers, who may be susceptible to breast cancer due to inherited BrCA genes. Also at high risk for breast cancer are patients with dense breast tissue and those with ambiguous mammogram results. All may benefit from having a breast MR. MRI has high sensitivity that is improved with the use of contrast agents.[12,15,19,44,45] Sensitivity in MRI ranges from 71% to 100% versus mammography at 16% to 40%.[46]

Mammography does not image dense breasts well; MRI is effective in imaging dense breast tissue. At least 25% to 45% of women have dense breasts.[47] Several studies report women with increased breast density have a four- to sixfold increased risk for developing breast cancer[5–7,23,48] (Figure 20-15).

2. *MRI detected biopsy-proven satellite lesions in women recently diagnosed with breast cancer.*

   Breast MR scanning of both breasts often discovers occult ipsilateral and/or contralateral cancers.[11,15,19,46,48–50] Testing is useful in the early detection of occult breast cancers (Figure 20-16).

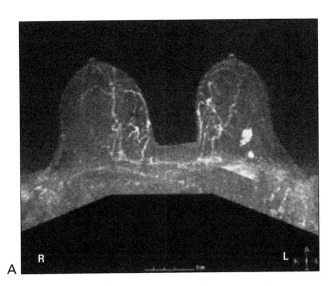

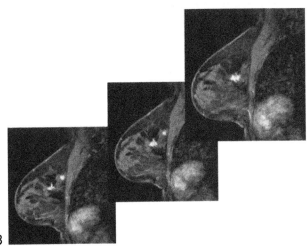

Figure 20-15
High risk: unsuspected cancer. **(A)** The patient presents for an MRI due to her high-risk status; her mother, at age 47, was diagnosed with breast cancer. Two areas within the left breast enhanced, so she was brought back for further evaluation. **(B)** Diagnosis: the area 6 cm from the nipple is invasive ductal carcinoma, nuclear grade 2. The area 8 cm behind the nipple is also IDC, but nuclear grade 1. (Images courtesy of EWBC. Rochester, NY.)

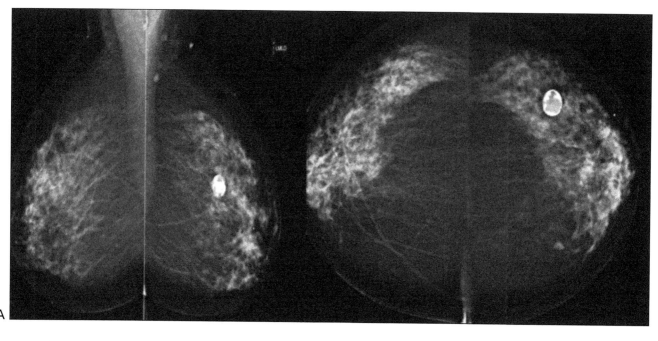

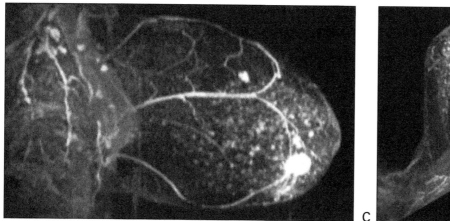

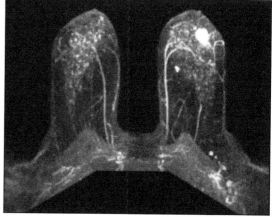

Figure 20-16
Satellite lesions: extent of disease. **(A)** A 66-year-old presents with a left breast lump × 2 weeks. **(B)** and **(C)** demonstrate the satellite lesions within the left breast. Diagnosis: Invasive ductal carcinoma, nuclear grade 1 in the 3:00 site and grades 1 to 2 in the 11:00 location. (Images courtesy of EWBC. Rochester, NY.)

3. *A growing body of evidence suggests that breast MR may be better at detecting DCIS than mammography.*[5–7,13,51]

DCIS is an early stage of breast cancer that lines the ducts and is likely to become invasive cancer. It accounts for approximately 30% of all breast cancers.[13] In August 2007, German researchers reported in the medical journal *Lancet* that they detected almost twice as many cases of DCIS using MRI. They studied the cases of more than 7,000 women who had mammography and MRI examinations. They found that MRI detected 92% of DCIS cases (153 of 157) while mammography detected 56% (93 of 167).[5–7] This report along with others from the University of Washington in Seattle found that MRI is better in detecting DCIS.[15]

This is a turnabout from the earlier belief that mammography is better at detecting DCIS (Figure 20-17).

4. *Evaluation of chemotherapy.*
Breast MR can be used to detect biological and chemical changes by monitoring the response to chemotherapy; tracking tumor volume is important in the follow-up of treatment[42,52] (Figure 20-18).

5. *Evaluation of breast implants.*
This noncontrast examination is solely to evaluate the implant for rupture. MRI is effective in imaging intracapsular ruptures. Referring physicians and patients need to be aware it does not evaluate the breast tissue. The examination may incidentally see gross pathology. MRI is the most accurate modality in the evaluation of

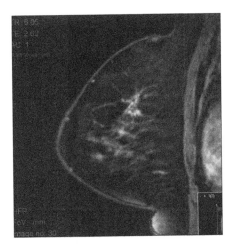

Figure 20-17
DCIS/LCIS. The architectural distortion was biopsied under MRI guidance. Pathology yielded DCIS and LCIS. (Image courtesy of EWBC. Rochester, NY.)

breast implant integrity.[53–56] A European study reported MRI accuracy of 92%, sensitivity of 89%, and specificity of 97% for implant evaluation.[57] Evaluation of breast implants is an important service that has a large patient pool of younger women with dense breast tissue. Many sites use contrast, even when simply checking implant integrity, to evaluate the breast tissue in front of or behind the implant. Differentiation between silicone and water requires postimaging processing using suppression techniques[53,57] (Figure 20-19).

6. ***Evaluation of the extent of disease: tumor size and surgical planning.***
Monitoring tumor size with breast MR is playing a more important role in surgical planning.[8,12,58–61] Mammography cannot match the capability of MRI to estimate the extent of a tumor. For lesions identified by mammography, the size of the tumor is routinely underestimated;

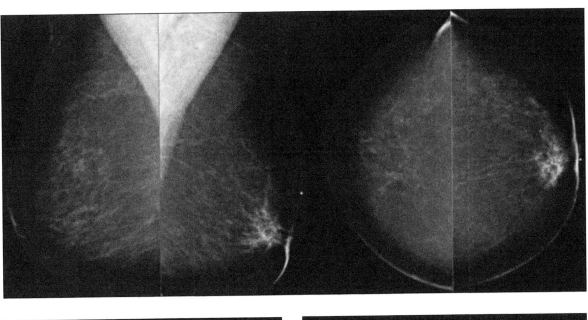

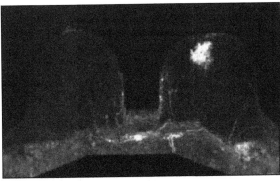

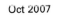
Oct 2007

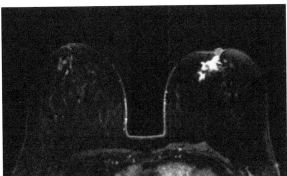
May 2008

Figure 20-18
Evaluation of chemotherapy. In October 2007 (mammogram and MRI images), this patient presented with left breast pain plus a lump. After chemotherapy, note the reduction in the tumor bulk on her May 2008 MRI scan. Diagnosis: Invasive ductal carcinoma, nuclear grade 3. (Images courtesy of EWBC. Rochester, NY.)

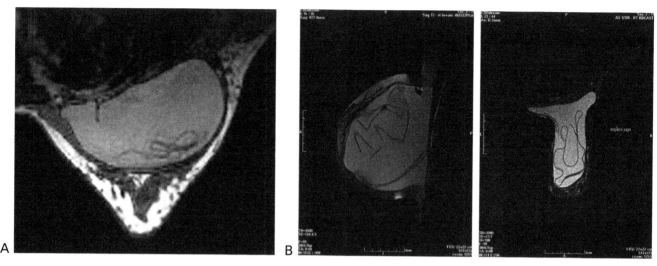

Figure 20-19
Breast implant evaluation. Both sets of images display intracapsular rupture or the linguine signature. (Images for set B courtesy of EWBC. Rochester, NY.)

Case Study **20-2**

What do the breast MR images in Figure 20-19 illustrate?

for lesions found with MRI, the majority is overestimated. On the basis of the biopsy results, many surgeons routinely order a breast MR prior to surgery to identify the extent of the disease. At times, this may make the difference in selecting between a lumpectomy and a mastectomy. Size matters in surgical planning.[8,12]

Patients who present with lobular cancer or infiltrating ductal cancer are prime candidates for investigation of the extent of their disease. Both breasts are routinely scanned during surgical planning as the ipsilateral breast may present with additional pathology (multifocal or multicentric) not demonstrated on the mammogram, as well as the contralateral breast may have occult disease.[11,13,15,19,26,43,44,58] Patients with suspected recurrence alert physicians to review the extent of prior surgery and to evaluate adjunctive therapy for subsequent planning.

Controversy over the outcome, specifically whether it improves patient care, is the issue. Moving away from a tradition of breast conservation surgery established in recent decades, back toward the more radical surgery employed in the past, is viewed as problematic and even counterproductive by some[27-31] (Figure 20-20).

7. ***MRI can visualize deep into the chestwall and into the axilla.***
MRI is not limited to imaging only the breast tissue that fits into the surface coil. It also visualizes deep into the

chestwall and the axilla.[62-65] Mammography can image only the tissue that rests atop the imaging platform. Detecting deep axial tumors is considered one of breast MR's strengths[26,59,60,65] (Figure 20-21).

8. ***Postoperative follow-up.***[43,66,67]
Breast MR may also play a significant role in the treatment of postlumpectomy patients.[12,26,68] What happens if unclear tumor margins were identified on the biopsy specimen? Often, residual tumor in the biopsy cavity can be visualized with contrast-enhanced MRI. Preliminary reports show that quantification of tumor features may improve the specificity of MRI breast images. This can be achieved with dynamic scanning (repeated scanning over a determined area of tissue) with a contrast agent and then plotting a time versus intensity curve.

9. ***Lesion segmentation.***
Lesion segmentation provides important clinical characteristics of a tumor (such as shape, size, texture, borders, and signal heterogeneity). This is where breast MR has become an important adjunct to mammography. MRI can image the subtle differences between soft tissues, and it clarifies borders adjacent to each other in exquisite detail. Because the breast is a soft tissue organ, interest in applying this nonionizing imaging modality to the detection of breast disease was almost immediate.[1]

Since its introduction into clinical use, MRI has been a proven medical technology that demonstrates biological, chemical, and anatomical changes in soft tissue. This is where breast MR, with its greater sensitivity, has advantages over mammography.[17,25,26,45,51,69]

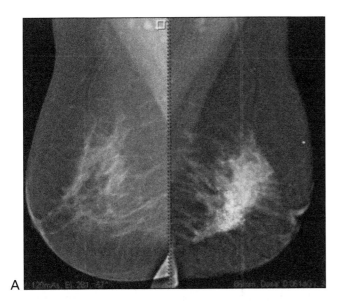
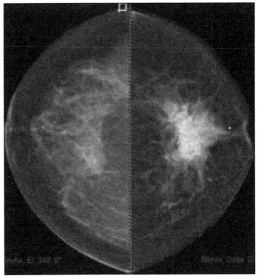

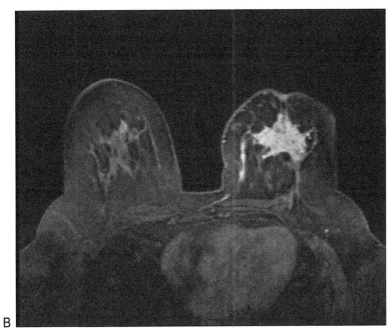

Figure 20-20
Lobular carcinoma—treatment planning. **(A)** Patient presents for evaluation of a lump plus nipple inversion of the left breast. Diagnosis: Invasive lobular carcinoma, nuclear grades 2 and 3. **(B)** The mass extends over an 89 × 71 × 67 mm area. Skin thickening and nipple inversion area also present. (Images courtesy of EWBC. Rochester, NY.)

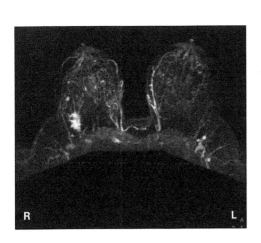
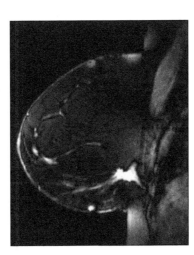

Figure 20-21
Axillary–chestwall extension. 3-cm breast cancer with evidence of extension to involve the chestwall. Diagnosis: Invasive ductal carcinoma. (Images courtesy of EWBC. Rochester, NY.)

Case Study 20-3

What do the breast MR images in Figure 20-21 illustrate?

MRI Limitations

The COMICE Trial, with a cohort study of 1,623 women, was the first prospective review of breast MR. Findings revealed no differences in survival or quality of life between its two groups. MRI accurately detected additional lesions but did not reach statistical significance.[70] Some concluded breast MR does more harm than good.[27–31] Others suggested technology and techniques have improved since this early study.

While there is much evidence to favor breast MR, there also are limitations to this procedure that require further consideration. These limitations suggest a few reasons behind the cautious move by the American Cancer Society toward recommendations for screening breast MR in clinical practice.[3] One MRI weakness is *specificity* for anomalies. MRI *sensitivity* excels, visualizing virtually all anomalies; however, unambiguous images are required for a diagnosis. Is the annotated area on the image a cancer or something else? The doctor needs to know and orders a biopsy to be certain. Breast MR often requires biopsy and is so directed in the ACS guidelines. MRI has a higher correlation with biopsies than mammography or ultrasound, so the current controversy and cautious approach continue in tandem.

With breast MR, both breasts should be imaged simultaneously using special protocols allowing for a thin-slice thickness to be obtained. Just as there are no documented or substantiated claims cleared by the FDA for diagnosing the disease multiple sclerosis on a brain MR scan, there will be no definitive claims made regarding the actual benefits of breast MR until more clinical studies have been performed.

MRI Technology Issues

1. Sensitivity may be "too good." The *sensitivity* of breast MR has approached 100% in some studies; MRI identifies most anomalies, including some that may not be cancer.[71] These false-positives result in a biopsy recommendation.
2. The *specificity* of MR is lower than mammography, resulting in more recalls and biopsies.[16,17]
3. Interpretation of MRI scans is highly variable. As expected, specialization improves yields and improves detection. Diagnosis by practitioners with experience and specialization in breast care imaging is better than that of practitioners with general MRI and breast imaging experience.[3,19,72]

MRI-Related Issues

1. False-positive results from breast MR can leave women feeling anxious about undergoing future breast examinations. In a UK study, 4% of women left distressed and 47% reported intrusive thoughts about the examination 6 weeks afterward.[73]
2. Cost and reimbursement are important issues related to screening breast MR. A much higher cost is associated with breast MR scanning when compared with routine x-ray mammography; MRI fees range between $500 and $1,300. A Mayo Clinic Web page featured Blue Cross Blue Shield information on breast MR insurance coverage. The advice included as follows: expect to pay about $1,000 for the service and check with your insurance company for utilization and payment policies.[74] Insurance carriers often impose conditions and restrictions. Recent policy guidelines from Blue Cross Blue Shield cite only a few medically necessary indications for breast MR and recommend prior authorization for the service.

Breast MRI Guidelines: Careful Progress

The 2003 American Cancer Society efforts to approve a recommendation for breast MR screening included favorable discussions for specific guidelines but ended with not enough compelling evidence to issue guidelines at that time. Meanwhile, breast MR with an approach to staging cancers was widely adopted in other countries with developed health care systems, while there were very different views on the merits and ramifications of preoperative MRI examinations.[3,12,26,27,43,50,75] ACS 2007 meetings resulted in the first US guidelines specific to breast MR screening. In April 2009, the ACS released a supplement to their existing guidelines. Current guidelines include the following key recommendations:

The Guidelines[3]

- MRI is in addition to, not a substitute for, routine screening or diagnostic mammography and, when indicated, diagnostic breast ultrasound. MRI supplements the use of these standard imaging tools in appropriately selected clinical situations.
- Women who have a first-degree relative with a BrCA1 or BrCA2 mutation and are untested themselves are candidates for MRI.
- Women who have a lifetime risk of developing breast cancer of 20% to 25% or more using standard risk assessment models. Estimates for the level of risk consider family history, clinical factors, and expert consensus where evidence for certain groups is lacking.

- Females who, between ages 10 and 30, received radiation treatment to the chest for conditions such as Hodgkin disease.
- Women who carry or have a first-degree relative who carries a genetic mutation in the TP53 or PTEN genes (Li–Fraumeni syndrome and Cowden and Bannayan–Riley–Ruvalcaba syndromes).
- For women with diagnosed breast cancer. MRI provides enhanced detection in both the breast known to have cancer and the opposite, or contralateral, breast.
- Surgical decisions should not be based solely on MRI findings because not all suspicious lesions on MRI are cancer. Suspicious lesions should be biopsied before a surgery plan is devised in order to avoid surgical overtreatment.
- In the rare instance where cancer is found in the lymph nodes but not the breast, an MRI finds the cancer in nearly 60% of the cases.
- Recommendations are conditional. An acceptable level of quality MRI screening should be performed by experienced providers in facilities that provide MRI-guided biopsy.

▮▮ BREAST MR EXAM: CLINICAL PRACTICE

Preparation Checklist

Examination preparation for each facility will be guided by its own policies and practices for the MRI examination. A brief checklist is provided as a guide for your consideration when establishing or evaluating a breast MR service.[76,77]

Yes	No	
☐	☐	Staff trained in MRI and mammography
☐	☐	Support staff and materials for contrast infusion in place: IV access right antecubital unless contraindicated 24-gauge angiocath, butterfly 22-gauge angiocath
☐	☐	Facility safety policies, practices, and emergency code procedures in place
☐	☐	Monitoring equipment in place
☐	☐	Safety program in place
☐	☐	Scheduled time for patients and staff. Contrast enhancement varies with cycle; whenever feasible, schedule in the second week of the menstrual cycle.
☐	☐	Pregnant women policies for various diagnostic examinations

Patient Interview

The most important acronym in breast MR is TLC. A knowledgeable, supportive staff with good communication skills is essential to ensure high-quality imaging from a cooperative patient. Breast MR is a stressful examination. Many candidates for breast MR have a history of breast disease, are at high risk for breast cancer, or have a specific medical problem that qualifies them for the service. Their doctors have referred them.[73] Unlike conventional radiographic imaging that may take several quick exposures in a short time span, MRI imaging can be 30 to 60 minutes of several series of acquired images, with each series lasting anywhere from 1 to 15 minutes, depending on the MRI system. This can seem like an eternity for the patient who may be apprehensive. Take time to explain the examination. Answer all patient questions. The following item checklist covers the basics of an interview, but by no means is it all inclusive or designed to reflect your facility's policies or practices.

- Noise. There will be noise, thumping, or banging when the MRI machine is scanning. Don't move when the machine is scanning. The patient can listen to music or can be provided earplugs that help reduce the noise.
- Remain still and follow commands such as hold your breath. The slightest movement of the patient can cause an entire series of images to not be of diagnostic quality.
- Claustrophobia. 1 in 20 patients (1% to 5%) may be claustrophobic. Patients in a prone position are able to see the light, and for many, this transforms their feelings of confinement. Their physician may provide a mild sedative to take before the examination.[78]
- Metallic eye shadow/mascara and tattoo eyeliner can irritate the patient's eyes due to metallic properties of the tattoo ink; this causes localized heating on the eyelid. Some sites use cool gel eye masks during the scan if warranted.
- Patients who have recently undergone surgery and may have titanium surgical staples in their body must wait a minimum of 6 weeks before entering a magnetic field.
- Patients who are breast-feeding should refrain from having a breast MR. This is due to high activity of the breast tissue. Small tumors or lesions may be obscured during this time.
- Verify patients do not bring any metallic items into the MRI room.
- Set the room up prior to the arrival of the patient. The MRI technologist places the appropriate NMR probe on the patient table, attaches monitoring equipment, positions the patient for comfort over the long scanning sequences, and inserts a needle in the forearm for contrast infusion. An IV stand with contrast should be in place and ready for the second series of scans with contrast (Figure 20-22).

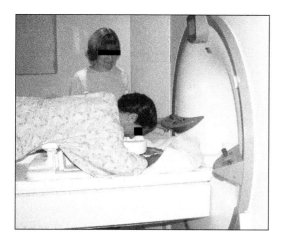 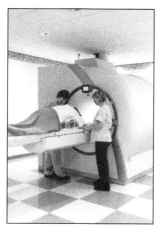

Figure 20-22
Prescan setup. Precise instructions prior to positioning: mainly to remain still when the magnet is actively scanning. Provide earplugs and a call button for the patient. Document scars, moles, skin lesions, and prior biopsy sites. (Images courtesy of EWBC. Rochester, NY.)

- Some facilities invite the patient for a dry run of the examination to acquaint them with the unit and the sounds they will hear.

Positioning

A dedicated breast MR examination consists of the patient lying prone with the breasts hanging pendulous in the breast coil. She faces the open end of the magnet bore.[38–42,65] The technologist inserts a butterfly needle or IV into the patient's arm for contrast administration at a later time during the scanning process.

The patient table slides into place inside the magnet bore until the breast tissue is at the center of the magnet. This centering point is usually obtained under a marking or centering light while the patient is outside of the bore (Figure 20-23).

The scanner performs its prescanning calculations to ensure the best possible image. During prescan, adjustments are made for flip angle, center frequency, and transmit gain. Unlike mammography QC, this prescan is performed on every patient at the beginning of their examination. This prescan optimizes the system according to the size and density of the breast tissue. Following the prescan adjustments, several scans, in axial and sagittal planes, are performed. These scans are performed both before and after contrast administration. The scan time for each series varies from 1 to 15 minutes, depending on the pulse sequence selected. Overall, a routine breast MR with and without contrast should take less than 1 hour. This time is field strength dependent as well.

Screening mammography consists of a single-volume image of each breast in at least two different projections: mediolateral oblique (MLO) and craniocaudal (CC) (Figures 20-24 and 20-25). The MLO projection in mammography is similar to the sagittal view in MRI while the CC projection is similar to the axial view.[26,32,35] As you may already know, there are many additional views that may be necessary during a mammogram, including spot compression and magnification views, just to name a few. Have all relevant images available for the physician's review.

Breast MR Exam with Contrast

MRI should not be performed without contrast. Contrast is the key factor in determining several disease processes and is required in most breast MR sequences. Many sites will use contrast, even when simply checking implant integrity, to evaluate the breast tissue in front of or behind the implant. Adverse reaction to the contrast media is usually insignificant, such as headache or injection site coldness and sensitivity; however, thorough patient screening before the contrast is administered is advised.[75]

Gadolinium (Gd-DTPA), a paramagnetic substance, is a common MR contrast agent. At the proper concentration, Gd contrast agents cause preferential T1 relaxation enhancement, causing an increase in the signal on T1-weighted images. Caution: At high concentrations,

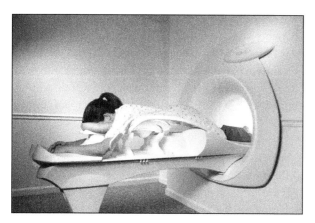

Figure 20-23
Patient positioning in breast MR. The patient lies prone, facing forward in the magnetic bore of the MRI unit. She is positioned to remain comfortable for long periods without movement. Note the surface coil mounted on the table.

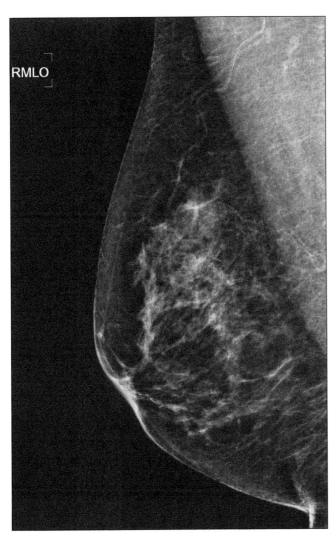

Figure 20-24
Mediolateral oblique mammogram.

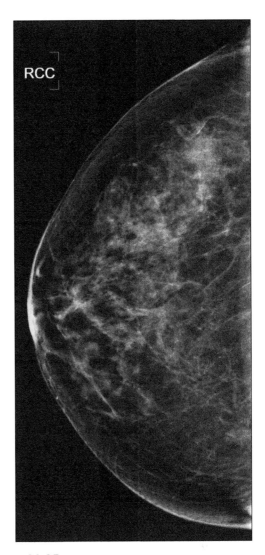

Figure 20-25
Craniocaudal mammogram.

loss of signal is seen instead—a result of the T2 relaxation effects dominating. Without the administration of a contrast such as gadolinium, much of the breast tissue can appear isointense.

While the morphologic information (border, shape, size, and texture) about a tumor or lesion is critical to the interpretation, dynamic contrast scanning with time intensity curves can demonstrate the quick uptake and washout associated with malignant tumors. Contrast enhancement provides information such as tumor angiogenesis and vascularity.

Current applications of breast MR include scanning women with dense breast tissue, those at high risk for breast cancer, or those with ambiguous mammogram results. All may benefit from having a breast MR. Surgical planning and implant integrity are also indications for breast MR. Pre- and postcontrast images of both breasts are included in the breast MR scan.

Display: Many Images

A computer interprets the data and creates images *that display the different resonance characteristics of different tissue types.* A typical breast MR examination will have about 100 images for the physician to review (Figure 20-26). We see images in shades of gray detailing differences between water, fat, and other tissue types. The RF signals that are used in creating breast MR images are derived from the energy released by hydrogen protons precessing from their high-energy to their low-energy state and from the protocol (magnetic field and pulse sequence) applied. Both CT and breast MR use digital computing to process images. But unlike CT where a high-energy source (x-rays) pass through the breast tissue leaving photons to be counted and reassembled as an image, MRI collects the weak magnetic signals from hydrogen protons from a specific area within a crafted magnetic field. The signal is a collection of all the

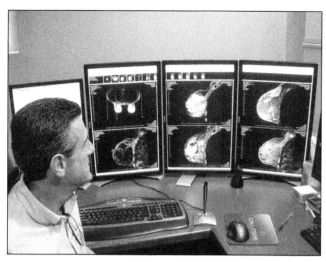

Figure 20-26
Display of images. The radiologist reviews breast MR images. (Image courtesy of Richard Goldberg, MD. Partners Imaging Center. Sarasota, FL.)

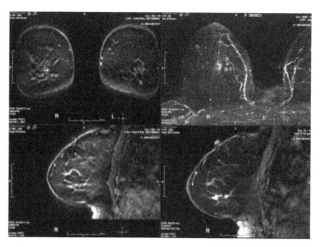

Figure 20-27
Reformatting. You are able to take a 3D scan (axial T1 3Ds in this case) and reformat into a coronal, sagittal, and MIP that yields information to localize a lesion without having to actually scan in those planes. (Images courtesy of EWBC. Rochester, NY.)

hydrogen atoms since it is not possible to demonstrate what an individual atom is doing in that large volume. MRI works with subatomic particles to report changes in energy and precessing. The changing resonance signals present in a volume are the basis for the image. When it comes to the information a computer assembles as an image, MRI is finesse; CT is brute force. Yet both need dense targets for better images. In CT and in digital mammography, more pixels make a better image; in MRI, more voxels (volume elements) dense with hydrogen protons improves the MRI image. Breast images can be displayed in all three planes (x, y, and z) as a series of thin slices, or the data can be used to reconstruct and image anomalies inside a volume of tissue. Cross-sectional slices can range from 1.0 to 10.0 mm in slice thickness. With cross-sectional imaging, the issue of having overlying parenchyma obscuring an area is not a concern.

Postimage Processing

Breast MR offers many options for postimage processing beyond suppression and subtraction techniques: maximum intensity projection (MIP); 3D volume of the brightest voxels in each slice that rotates/spins for accurate assessment; reformats; axial, sagittal, and coronal without imaging for localizing; CAD for angio/color maps; and the list goes on. Angio map is a spatial representation of time/intensity data and acts as an overlay to unite kinetics and morphology in one data set. Kinetic curves demonstrate enhancement signal intensity over time. Figure 20-27 illustrates the reformat capability.

MRI Safety: For Patients and the Machine

Initial concerns for safety near a powerful magnet include *keeping the area free of metallic objects and screening patient and staff for medical implants before attempting entry into the MRI room.* Table 20-2 is a general guide. For official requirements, refer to the *ACR Guidance Document for Safe MRI Practices: 2013* to evaluate the safety of your MRI room or to establish a new MRI room. This document citation was current as of August 2016.[79]

Remember, the Magnet Is Always On!

Become familiar with the items identified on this chart (Figure 20-28) or similar charts available in your facility with similar warnings. Medical facilities all have emergency codes and procedures, policies, departmental practices, specialized training, and rules regarding safety for MRI services. Licensure and accreditation demand periodic review and adherence to such rules.

Although MRI is generally considered safe, pregnant patients will not be scanned without the approval of the radiologist. The benefits must outweigh the risks before

Case Study **20-4**

The MRI room can be a dangerous place for the patient as well as the magnet. Why?

Table 20-2 • MRI Safety

NOT ELIGIBLE	DEPROGRAM	DANGEROUS
Cardiac pacemakers	Neurostimulators	Metal bone implants
Aneurysm clips	Bone growth stimulators	Rods
Implanted clips	Implanted defibrillators	Screws
Intracranial clips	Cochlear implants	Plates
	Watches	
MAY BE CONTRAINDICATED	Cell phones	**POSSIBLE ARTIFACTS**
	Credit cards	
Some cardiac valves	IV pumps	Patient monitoring equipment
Stapedectomy implants	Magnetic dental implants	Pulse oximeters
Vena cava filters	Tattoo eyeliner	EKG devices
Halo collars	Beepers/pagers	Radios
Breast tissue expanders	Keyless car starters	Cellular phones
Implant expanders	Door openers	IMED/VAC pumps
Hairpins	iPods, CD players	Excessive dental work
Barrettes	Computer discs	Metal zippers
Bobby pins		Metal buttons
Clips		Tattoos
Metallic eye shadow		

scanning a pregnant female. Usually, if the patient's MRI findings would indicate immediate medical attention to the mother during her pregnancy, the patient's physician and the radiologist will make the decision whether to scan her. If the results would indicate the mother could wait until after delivery for the medical treatment, she should not be scanned.

Emmanuel Kanal, MD, and Frank Shellock, PhD, reported that even when a manufacturer states their aneurysm clip is MRI compatible, several nonferromagnetic aneurysm clips have become magnetized and torqued in a magnetic field. The reason for concern is that the brain does not form scar tissue, so the twisting or torquing action of the magnetic field on ferromagnetic items can possibly dislodge an aneurysm clip, which can cause bleeding, stroke, or death if the torqued clip ruptures the artery.[80,81] Patients and any accompanying family members need to be thoroughly screened before entering the magnetic field.

MRI-GUIDED BIOPSY

MRI-guided breast biopsy is a fast and safe alternative to surgical biopsy. Lesions detected only by breast MR must be biopsied by this same modality. MRI-guided biopsy can use many techniques, including needle core and vacuum-assisted devices. Histologic correlation is necessary to ensure lesion sampling.[3,14,26,82,83]

We have witnessed a remarkable evolution in surgical treatment from Halstead's first radical mastectomy in 1882 to current medical practice favoring breast conservation procedures. Changes in biopsy techniques and staging of breast cancer have contributed to this evolution.[14,26,61,71,84,85] Now, needle core biopsy takes another step forward to allow both MRI acquisition of a tissue sample coexistent with a diagnostic evaluation during the same visit and without a surgical procedure.[66,82] Current ACS guidelines recommend MRI-guided biopsy.

A breast surface coil utilizes an immobilization (not compression) device to secure the breast tissue for needle biopsy or FNAC (Figure 20-29). Fiducial markings aligned on the grid plates assist the physician in guiding the biopsy needle to the area of interest. Chestwall lesions that can be inaccessible with mammographic compression plate techniques can be localized. A variety of free-hand approaches,

Figure 20-28
MRI safety sign. Caution must be exercised in the MRI room—for the sake of the patient as well as the expensive machine. (Image courtesy of Richard Goldberg, MD. Partners Imaging Center. Sarasota, FL.)

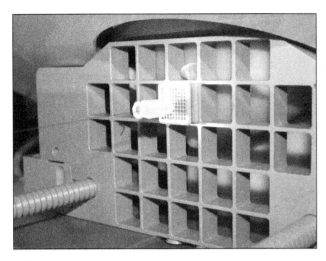 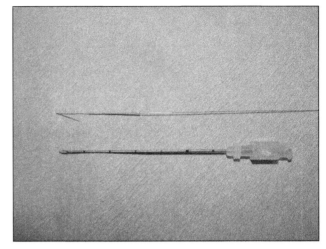

Figure 20-29
Localization for breast MR examination. Preoperative wire localization using the MRI unit. (Images courtesy of EWBC, Rochester, NY.)

including tangential needle paths designed to avoid punctures to breast implants, are available.

The breast surface coil is placed on top of the patient table; the patient is positioned on the unit in the same manner as the breast imaging scan, lying prone with breasts hanging pendulous.[25,26,32,35] An immobilization device with screens that allow an opening for core needle access is applied to firmly hold the breast in place for the biopsy while maintaining the accuracy of the biopsy device stroke. A physician trained in its use sets up the biopsy device and aligns the biopsy device to the center of the target tissue, guided by the image on the display monitor. The $X–Y–Z$ coils reconstruct the ROI within a volume of tissue; pulse sequences display a visual path to the target and guide the biopsy needle placement. A 3D guidance procedure is used to verify the settings before a biopsy sample is taken from the breast (Figure 20-30). Tissue samples are taken and sent to the pathologist for examination and report; the patient is briefed on the process for a diagnosis and released.

A SUMMARY WITH A FUTURE FOCUS

Breast MR has potential to play a more important role in diagnosing breast cancer. Close tracking of breast MR techniques and clinical results from trials in the United States and from other countries are necessary to generate a greater public awareness. Perhaps screening breast MR will become valuable to more women in the future. Time will tell if a more aggressive approach for women at higher risk of developing this disease or for detecting recurrence is in order given the number of women and men affected by breast cancer each year.

Biopsy is critical as many lesions have been detected through MRI that were occult on mammography and ultrasound. Stereotactic biopsy or ultrasound-guided biopsy may not be able to visualize some tumors that are demonstrated on MRI.

A review of articles from medical journals, newspapers, and popular magazines and topics from medical seminars and conferences suggest that the following issues, among others, are the most likely candidates to become the focus of the future study from the medical community, health care advocates, government agencies, and medical insurance companies.

Technology Issues

- New and improved equipment/imaging techniques[61,69,80,81]
- Alternatives to MR breast—nuclear medicine options[86–88]
- Equipment safety issues[79,89]

Facility/Radiologist Issues

- Staffing and MRI accreditation changes[90–92]
- Interpretation and experience with MRI and mammography[27,41,88]
- Treatment planning/oncology surgery[52,91,93–97]
- MRI-guided biopsy and false positives[75,82]
- New techniques: contrast materials, pulse sequences, software, and real-time interactive MRI[34,37,98]

Patient Issues

- Patient selection/older women/broaden the base[7,62,92,97]
- Patient safety[79,81,89]
- Access to breast MR services/coordination[64]
- Cost and reimbursement[74,99]

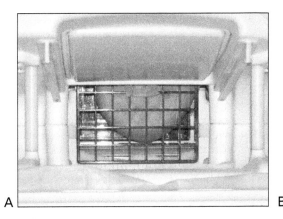
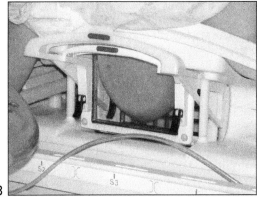
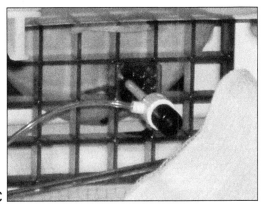
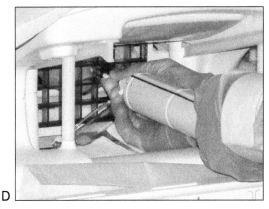

Figure 20-30
Breast MR biopsy and localization. Vacuum-assisted breast biopsy using the MRI unit. **(A)** Medial access for biopsy approach. **(B)** Lateral view of back plate. **(C)** Suspicious area localized. **(D)** Biopsy device introduced into the breast. (Images courtesy of EWBC. Rochester, NY.)

Review Questions

1. Name four of the eight reasons for the interest in using breast MR imaging.

2. What are gradients and what is their function in an MRI system?

References

1. Matson J, Simon M. *The Pioneers of NMR and Magnetic Resonance in Medicine: The Story of MRI.* Bar-Ilan University Press; 1996.
2. Lauterbur PC. Image formation by induced local interactions: examples employing nuclear magnetic resonance. *Nature.* 1973;242:190–191.
3. Saslow D, et al. American cancer society guidelines for breast screening with MRI as an adjunct to mammography. *CA Cancer J Clin.* 2007;57:75–89.
4. Krieg M, et al. Efficacy of MRI and mammography for breast cancer screening in women with familial or genetic predisposition. *N Engl J Med.* 2004;351:427–437.
5. Boyd NE, et al. Quantitative classification of mammographic densities and breast cancer risk: results from the Canadian National Breast Screening Study. *J Natl Cancer Inst.* 1995;87:670–675.
6. Brisson J, et al. Mammographic features of the breast and breast cancer risk. *Am J Epidemiol.* 1982;115:428–437.
7. Byrne C, et al. Mammographic features of the breast and breast cancer risk: effects with time, age, and menopause status. *J Natl Cancer Inst.* 1995;87(21):1622–1629.
8. Dummin LJ, Cox M, Plant L. Prediction of breast tumor size by mammography and sonography. A breast screen experience. *Breast.* 2007;16(1):46.
9. Chapter news: MR & nuclear medicine. ASRT Scanner; 1996:14.
10. Coons T. MRI's role in assessing and managing breast disease. *Radiol Technol.* 1997;67(4):311–325.
11. Deurloo EE, et al. Additional breast lesions. *Eur J Cancer.* 2005;41:1393–1401.
12. Berg WA, et al. Diagnostic accuracy of mammography, clinical breast examination, US, and MR imaging in pre-operation assessment of breast cancer. *Radiology.* 2004;233:830–849.
13. Houssami N, et al. Accuracy and surgical impact of magnetic resonance imaging in breast cancer staging: systematic review and meta-analysis in detection of multifocal and multicentric cancer. *J Clin Oncol.* 2008;26:3248–3258.
14. Sumkin J. Transitions in breast imaging: digital mammography, MRI-guided-biopsy in aid in battle against breast cancer. *RT Image.* 2006;19:41.
15. Lehman CD, et al. MRI evaluation of the contralateral breast in women with recently diagnosed breast cancer. *N Engl J Med.* 2007;356(13):1295–1303.

16. Hussman K, et al. MR mammographic localization: work in progress. *Radiology.* 1993;189:915–917.
17. Bluemke DA, et al. Magnetic resonance imaging of the breast prior to biopsy. *JAMA.* 2004;292:2735–2742.
18. Stout NK, et al. Rapid increase in breast magnetic resonance imaging use: trends from 2000 to 2011. *JAMA Intern Med.* 2014;174:114–121.
19. Sardanelli F, et al. Sensitivity of MRI versus mammography for detecting foci of multifocal, multicentric breast cancer in fatty and dense breasts using the whole–breast pathologic examination as a gold standard. *Am J Roentgenol.* 2004;183:1149–1157.
20. Wernli KJ, et al. Patterns of breast magnetic resonance imaging use in community practice. *JAMA Intern Med.* 2014;174:125–132.
21. Kuhl CK, et al. Mammography, breast ultrasound, and magnetic resonance imaging for surveillance of women at high familial risk for breast cancer. *J Clin Oncol.* 2005;23:8469–8476.
22. Leach MO, et al. Screening with magnetic resonance imaging and mammography of a UK population at high familial risk of breast cancer; a prospective multicentre cohort study (MARBIS). *Lancet.* 2005;365:1769–1778.
23. Lehmman C, et al. Screening women at high risk for breast cancer with mammography and magnetic resonance imaging. *Cancer.* 2005;103:898–905.
24. Gabriel H, et al. Breast MRI for cancer detection in a patient with diabetic mastopathy. *Am J Roentgenol.* 2004;182:1081–1083.
25. Pfleiderer S, et al. Dedicated double breast coil for magnetic resonance mammography imaging, biopsy, and preoperative localization. *Invest Radiol.* 2003;38(1):1–8.
26. Kopans DB. Magnetic resonance imaging of the breast. In: Kopans DB, ed. *Breast Imaging.* 3rd ed. Philadelphia, PA: Lippincott Williams & Wilkins; 2006:691–728.
27. Winer E. Role of MRI in breast cancer detection unclear for majority of women. *HemOnc Today.* Available at: http://www.hemoncltoday.com. Accessed September 21, 2009.
28. Warner E, et al. Surveillance of BrCA1 and BrCA2 mutation carriers with magnetic resonance imaging, ultrasound mammography and clinical breast examination. *JAMA.* 2004;292:1317–1325.
29. CancerConsultants.com. MRI does not improve staging compared with conventional methods in early breast cancer. Available at: www.p4healthcare,com/go/pbis/news/aspx. Accessed August 6, 2009.
30. Newly diagnosed early breast cancer MRI may cause more harm than good. *Medical News Today.* Available at: http://www.medicalnewstoday.com. Accessed August 13, 2009.
31. Morrow M. Magnetic resonance imaging in the breast cancer patient: curb your enthusiasm. *J Clin Oncol.* 2008;26(3):352.
32. Hashemi R, Braddley WG Jr, Lisanti C. *The Basics of MRI.* Philadelphia, PA: Lippincott Williams & Wilkins; 1997.
33. Mallard JR. Magnetic resonance imaging (MRI)—The odyssey of one contributor to its birth. Engineering in Medicine and Biology Society. Proceedings of the Annual International Conference of the IEEE. Aberdeen; June 1992;7:2860–2862.
34. Hardy CJ, et al. Large field-of-view real-time MRI with 32 channel system. *Magn Reson Med.* 2004;52(4):878–884.
35. Bradley W. Fundamentals of MRI: part II. Available at: http://www.radiography.net/mri/fund%20mr2. Accessed September 7, 2009.
36. Burum D. Guide to selecting an NMR probe. MR Resources. Available at: www.mrr.com/parts/measurement. Accessed September 21, 2009.
37. IT policies—networks. Materials Research Institute. Available at: http://www.mri,psu/internetpolicy/networks.asp. Accessed September 7, 2009.
38. Hyton NM, Kinkle K. Technical aspects of breast magnetic resonance imaging. *Magn Reson Imaging.* 1998;9:13–16.
39. Sun L, Olsen JO, Robitaille PM. Design and optimization of a breast coil for magnetic resonance imaging. *Magn Reson Imaging.* 1993;11:73–80.
40. Hyton NM, Frankel SD. Imaging techniques for breast MR imaging. *Magn Reson Imaging Clin N Am.* 1994;2:511–525.
41. New Software for MR breast imaging simplifies diagnosing biopsies. Siemens; September 10, 2009. Available at: http://www.ehealthnews.eu. Accessed September 21, 2009.
42. Yeh E, et al. Perspective comparison of mammography, sonography, and MRI in patients undergoing neoadjuvant chemotherapy for palpable breast cancer. *Am J Roentgenol.* 2005;184:868–877.
43. Bilimoria KY, et al. Evaluating the impact of preoperative breast magnetic resonance imaging on the surgical management of newly diagnosed breast cancers. *Arch Surg.* 2007;142:441–445.
44. Berg W, et al. Detection of breast cancer with addition of annual screening ultrasound or a single screening MRI to mammography in women with elevated breast cancer risk. *JAMA.* 2012;307(13):1394–1404.
45. Turnbull LW. Dynamic contrast-enhanced MRI in the diagnosis and treatment of breast cancer. *NMR Biomed.* 2009;22:28–29.
46. Schnall M. MR imaging evaluation of cancer extent. *Magn Reson Imaging Clin N Am.* 2006;14:379–381.
47. Barlow WE, et al. Prospective breast cancer risk prediction model for women undergoing screening mammography. *J Natl Cancer Inst.* 2006;98:1204–1214.
48. Friedman P, et al. Breast MRI: the importance of bilateral imaging. *Am J Roentgenol.* 2006;187:345–349.
49. Heron DE, et al. Bilateral breast carcinoma: risk factors and outcomes for patients with synchronous and metachronous disease. *Cancer.* 2000;88:2739–2750.
50. Jobsen JJ, et al. Synchronous, bi-lateral breast cancer: prognostic value and incidence. *Breast.* 2003;12:3–8.
51. Kuhl CK. MRI is better for early breast cancer detection. *Lancet Study.* 2007. Available at: http://cancergenetics.com/2007. Accessed May 18, 2010.
52. Thibault F, et al. MRI for surgical planning in patients with breast cancer who undergo preoperative chemotherapy. *Am J Roentgenol.* 2004;183:1159–1168.
53. Middleton MS, McNamara MP. *Breast Implant Imaging (Chapters 9 and 10).* Philadelphia, PA: Lippincott Williams & Wilkins; 2003.
54. Scaranelo AM, et al. Evaluation of rupture of silicone breast implants by mammography, ultrasonography and magnetic resonance imaging in asymptomatic patients: correlation with surgical findings. *Sao Paula Med J.* 2004;122:41–47.
55. Huch RA, et al. *MR Imaging of the Augmented Breast.* Vol. 3. Berlin, Germany: Springer; 1998:371–376.
56. Gorczyca D, Brenner RJ. *The Augmented Breast: Radiologic and Clinical Perspectives.* 1st ed. New York, NY: Thieme Medical Publishers; 1996.

57. Holmich L, et al. The diagnosis of breast implant rupture: MRI findings compared with findings at explantation. *Eur J Radiol.* 2005;53(2):213–225.

58. Al-Hallaq HA, et al. Magnetic resonance imaging identifies multifocal and multicentric disease in breast cancer patients who are eligible for partial breast irradiation. *Cancer.* 2008;113:2498–2514.

59. Ojeda-Fournier H, Comstock C. MRI breast cancer: current indications. *Indian J Radiol Imaging.* 2009;19(2):161–169.

60. Wurdinger S, et al. Differentiation of phyllodes breast tumors from fibroadenomas on MRI. *Am J Roentgenol.* 2005;185: 1317–1321.

61. Penn A, et al. Morphologic blooming in breast MRI as a characterization of margin for discriminating benign from malignant lesions. *Acad Radiol.* 2006;13(11):1344–1354.

62. Kozlowski K. Breast MRI: a case for wider use. *Radiol Today.* 2008;9(20):20.

63. Yu J, Morris E, Park A. Efficacy of breast MRI in elderly women. *Am J Clin Oncol.* 2007;25(185):608.

64. Mann RM, et al. Breast MRI: guidelines from European Society of Breast Imaging. *Eur Radiol.* 2008;18(7):1307–1318.

65. Ko EY, et al. Breast MRI for evaluating patients with metastatic axillary lymph node and initially negative mammography and sonography. *Korean J Radiol.* 2007;8(5):382–389.

66. Houssami N, Hayes DF. Review of preoperative magnetic resonance imaging (MRI) in breast cancer: should MRI be performed on all women with newly diagnosed, early stage breast cancer? *CA Cancer J Clin.* 2009;59:290–302.

67. Fisher B, et al. Effect of preoperative chemotherapy on the outcome of women with operable breast cancer. *J Clin Oncol.* 1998;16:2672–2685.

68. Poggi MM, et al. Eighteen-year results in the treatment of early breast carcinomas with mastectomy versus breast conservation therapy: the National Cancer Institute Randomized Trial. *Cancer.* 2003;98:697–702.

69. Orenstein B. Think small—Mayo Clinic researchers retool scintimammography to target small lesion. *Radiol Today.* 2005;6:8.

70. Turmbull L. Magnetic resonance imaging in breast cancer: results of the COMICE Trial. *Breast Cancer Res.* 2008; 10(3):10.

71. Orel SG, Schnall MD. MR imaging of the breast for the detection, diagnosis and staging of breast cancer. *Radiology.* 2001;10(220):13–30.

72. Tozaki M, Fukuda K. High-spatial-resolution MRI of non-masslike breast lesions: interpretation model based on Bi-Rads descriptors. *Am J Roentgenol.* 2006;187:330–337.

73. Anderson J, Walker LG, Leach MO. Magnetic resonance imaging: an acceptable way of screening women with a family history of breast cancer. *Breast Cancer Res Treat.* 2004;88(Suppl):S188.

74. Mayo Clinic Health Solutions Staff. Mayo website. Blues cost advice for breast MR. Available at: http://www.blue.regence.com/trgmedpol/radiology/rad5

75. Sandep G, et al. Non-enhancing breast malignancies on MRI: sonographic and pathologic correlations. *Am J Roentgenol.* 2005;185:481–487.

76. Radiological Society of North America. MRI-guided breast biopsy. Radiology Info.org. *RSNA 2010*; July 10, 2009.

77. Magnetic resonance breast imaging (MRI, MR). Available at: http://www.imaginis.com/breasthealth/mri. Accessed September 28, 2009.

78. Hricak H, Amparo E. Body MRI: alleviation of claustrophobia by prone positioning. *Radiology.* 1984;152:819.

79. Kanal E, Barkovich AJ, Bell C. ACR guidance document on MR safe practices: 2013. *J Magn Reson Imaging.* 2013;37:501–530.

80. Dorfman GS, et al. Translational research working group. *Clin Cancer Res.* 2008;14(18):5678–5684.

81. Berrie C. New pacemaker system safe for use with MRI: presented at ESC, September 1, 2008.

82. Liberman L, et al. MRI guided 9 gauge vacuum breast biopsy: initial clinical experience. *Am J Roentgenol.* 2005;185:183–193.

83. Lehman C, et al. Clinical experience with MRI-guided vacuum-assisted breast biopsy. *Am J Roentgenol.* 2005;184: 1782–1787.

84. Schelfout K, et al. Contrast-enhanced MR imaging and the staging of breast lesions. *Eur J Surg Oncol.* 2004;30:501–507.

85. El Khouli Riham H, et al. MRI-guided vacuum-assisted breast biopsy: a phantom and patient evaluation of targeting accuracy. *J Magn Reson Imaging.* 2009;30(2):424–429.

86. Tozaki M. Diagnosis of breast cancer: MDCT versus MRI. *Breast Cancer.* 2008;15(3):205–213.

87. MRI technology breaks new ground in molecular imaging. Available at: http://www.azonaro.com/news. Accessed September 18, 2009.

88. Hardy K. Functional breast imaging modalities—breast surgeons explore their routes in improving cancer diagnosis. *Radiol Today.* 2009;10(14):22.

89. Evans JC, Smith ET, Nixon TE. A national survey of attitudes towards the use of MRI in patients known to have intracranial aneurysm clips. *Br J Radiol.* 2001;74:1118–1120.

90. American College of Radiology. ACR develops modular MRI accreditation program. Available at: http://www.acr.org.accreditation/featured categories. Accessed September 21, 2009.

91. Hardy K. Breast MRI's evolving role. *Radiol Today.* 2008;9(19):6.

92. Gradishar WJ, et al. Invasive breast cancer version 1.2016, NCCN clinical practice guidelines in oncology. *J Natl Compr Canc Netw.* 2016;14:324–354

93. Morrow M, Freedmann G. A clinical oncology perspective on the use of breast MR. *Magn Reson Imaging Clin N Am.* 2006;14:363–378.

94. Godinez J, et al. Breast MRI in the evaluation of eligibility for accelerated partial breast irradiation. *Am J Roentgenol.* 2008;191:272–277.

95. Pengel KE, et al. The impact of preoperative MRI on breast-conserving surgery of invasive cancer: a comparative cohort study. *Breast Cancer Res Treat.* 2009;116(1):161–169.

96. Veronesi U, et al. Twenty-year follow-up of a randomized study comparing breast-conserving surgery with radical mastectomy for early breast cancer. *N Engl J Med.* 2002;347:1227–1232.

97. Ma J, et al. SU-F-I-16: short breast MRI with high-resolution T2-weighted and dynamic contrast enhanced T1-weighted images. *Med Phys.* 2016;43:3390.

98. Yutzy S, Deurk J. Pulse sequences and system interfaces for interventional and real-time MRI. *J Magn Reson Imaging.* 2009;27(2):267–275.

99. Plevritis SK, et al. Cost effective for selected women with BrCA 1 and BrCA 2 mutations. *JAMA.* 2006;295:2374–2384.

Breast Cancer Diagnostic Technologies: Today and Tomorrow

21

Objectives

- To become familiar with adjunctive technologies already FDA approved and others in various stages of development
- To understand their potential benefits and limitations
- To understand the meaning of FDA approval and how it is obtained
- To understand the issue of breast density and its effect on imaging and interpretation

---

Key Terms

- 510(k)
- breast density
- causal risk
- cone-beam breast CT
- contrast-enhanced mammography
- Food and Drug Administration (FDA)

- Institutional Review Board (IRB)
- masking risk
- premarket approval (PMA)
- sensitivity
- specificity

INTRODUCTION

It seems that every time we read or watch the news, we hear about another test for breast cancer that is better than mammography. Patients are always asking if you have "that new machine that doesn't squeeze the breast." As technology marches on, there is no limit to the innovative approaches scientists and engineers dream up to detect breast cancer earlier, less invasively, and less painfully.

Thankfully, there are processes in place for required testing on new medical devices. These requirements are there to assure the public that any equipment used to examine or perform any procedure is safe and will not cause harm to either the patient or the operator.

 FIRST, DO NO HARM...

FDA Approval Process

Many people, both medical professionals and the public, think that U.S. **Food and Drug Administration** (FDA) approval means that a technology "works" and insurance providers will reimburse for medical examinations using that technology. Unfortunately, this is not the case. FDA approval simply means that it is safe to use for its intended purpose, not necessarily that it works better than anything that has come before. Once FDA approval is granted, insurance companies require a multitude of studies with statistical proof that the technology is worthwhile on its own and does not duplicate the results of another accepted technology before they will agree to pay for its use.

Before a new technology can be sold to the medical community, it must pass the FDA approval process. The FDA regulates the safety and effectiveness of all medical products sold in the United States. Technologies for the early detection of breast cancer most likely will involve imaging or clinical laboratory devices, and these are overseen by the Center for Devices and Radiological Health of the FDA. Some technologies, such as scintimammography, may also require review by FDA's Center for Drug Evaluation and Research because they use injections of radionuclide agents.

Before undergoing approval, a new device is classified into one of three categories:

- Class I: General Controls—Devices that require little more than proper labeling or production practices to ensure safety and effectiveness.
- Class II: Performance Standards and Special Controls— These devices must comply with performance standards that have been established for the device, and special controls may include things such as labeling requirements or performance standards that the FDA deems necessary for the product.

- Class III: **Premarket Approval** (PMA)—These are often life-sustaining or life-supporting devices or are important in preventing impairment of human health; thus, they are associated with a higher risk. All new devices are placed in class III until they are proven to be equivalent to a device already on the market. All class III devices require premarket authorization from FDA.

Once classified, a new medical device must undergo an FDA review before being introduced into the market. There are two main pathways to FDA approval: known as PMA (premarket approval) and "**510(k)**" (premarket notification). Most medical devices in the United States are cleared through the 510(k) process. This involves submission of a plan explaining how clinical trials will be conducted, the objectives for the trial, what results are expected, and what risks and precautions may be involved. If the request is considered sound, the FDA will grant an investigational device exemption (IDE), which allows the device to be used on patients, with informed consent, only for the purpose of gathering clinical data in a trial. An **Industrial Review Board** (IRB) may be required to approve and oversee the clinical trial to protect the health and the rights of the study participants.

Rating Performance: Sensitivity and Specificity of New Technologies

Sensitivity and **specificity** are the most widely used statistics to describe a diagnostic test and predict its usefulness. Sensitivity measures the proportion of actual positives that are correctly identified as such, or the probability of a positive test among patients with disease (i.e., the percentage of breast cancers that are correctly identified as breast cancer), and specificity measures the proportion of negatives that are correctly identified, or the probability of a negative test among patients without disease (i.e., the percentage of negative mammography examinations that are correctly identified as not having breast cancer). Therefore, sensitivity is the measurement of how often the technology successfully finds lesions within the tissue. Specificity is the measurement of how accurately it can determine what the lesion is.

Some technologies are very sensitive—they can find everything. However, once you can see a lesion, there needs to be a way to determine if what you see is suspicious enough to warrant biopsy, or not.

 DIAGNOSTIC TECHNOLOGIES

Mammography: 2D FFDM and DBT

Mammography has long been considered the "gold standard" of breast imaging. Whether it is performed on a 2D FFDM machine or is a DBT exam, mammography is the most accurate and cost-effective method of screening for breast cancer. Using NCI's PDQ summary of breast cancer statistics, mammography's sensitivity is 85% and specificity is 90%,[1] with a proven record of decreasing mortality rates. Another government agency, the Breast Cancer Surveillance Consortium (BCSC), is a collaborative network of mammography and pathology registries; it is a resource for studies designed to assess the delivery and quality of breast cancer screening and related patient outcomes. BCSC reports statistics about women who had mammograms between 1996 and 2009 (Figure 21-1). Many women follow the advice to have yearly mammograms. The combination of mammography screening examinations that find breast cancers in their early stages, along with advances in treatments, has made it possible for 98% of breast cancers that are found *early* to be cured.

However, mammography is not perfect; it does not find all cancers. There are some types of cancers that are not visualized on a mammogram. Additionally, there is the human element; due to the nature of breast tissue and how it is imaged on a mammogram, it is possible for a cancer to be overlooked by the radiologist or for a cancer to not be pulled onto the image by the technologist. Because of these weaknesses, new technologies and methods continue to be devised to aid radiologists and technologists to perform at an even higher degree of perfection.

Breast Tissue Density

From the earliest days of mammography, radiologists have recognized that the radiographic composition of the breast varies widely between individuals. Breast composition is a function of x-ray attenuation—the absorption of x-rays by tissue as they pass through the breast—and is important because an appreciation of breast composition can "help indicate the relative possibility that a lesion could be obscured by normal tissue."[2] Put even more simply, dense breast tissue reduces the sensitivity of screening mammography, *and* it can be an independent risk factor for breast cancer as well. This section of the chapter endeavors to take some of the mystery out of breast tissue density, defining breast density with more particularity, explaining known influencers over an individual's breast density, discussing the impact of **breast density** on interpretation of mammograms and the relationship between breast density and risk of breast cancer, and examining the evaluation of breast density. Finally, this section explores some of the utilization of breast density in the development of new tools for breast health surveillance and the management of breast disease.

Breast Density: Defined

Breast tissue density is a *radiological* term that refers to the appearance of fibroglandular tissue on the mammographic image. It is the supportive structure in the breast, as well as the ductal system. Fatty tissue is virtually transparent to x-rays and appears black on a mammogram, providing good contrast for cancers (which appear white on the mammogram); fibroglandular, or dense, tissue also appears white and therefore can disguise or mimic cancers. Dense tissue presents particular difficulty in that even a small region of high density can obscure a small cancer.

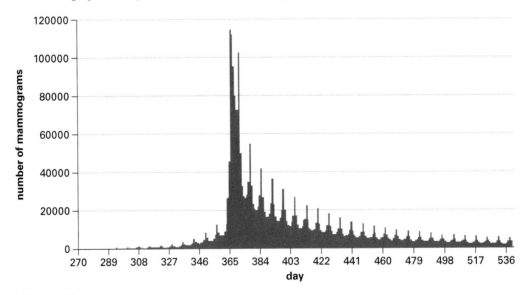

Figure 21-1

For women with two or more screening mammograms that are 9 to 17 months apart, we computed the lag time in days between these screening mammograms. The mode is actually 366 days. The peaks occur every 7 days because women often come back on the same day of the week as their earlier mammogram. The distribution of lag time is important for the definition of sensitivity. (Source: Data collection and sharing was supported by the National Cancer Institute-funded Breast Cancer Surveillance Consortium (HHSN261201100031C). A list of the BCSC investigators and procedures for requesting BCSC data for research purposes are provided at: http://breastscreening.cancer.gov/.)

An individual woman's breast tissue density is simply the percentage of her breast that is composed of fibroglandular tissue, a percentage that will vary over her lifetime, increasing and decreasing during periods of child bearing and lactation and generally decreasing with menopause.[3] Notwithstanding this generality, however, breast density varies widely between individuals, across populations, and between ethnic groups.[4]

Other than age, the major impact on breast density in an individual is from changes in body mass index (BMI),[5,6] hormone replacement therapy,[7–9] and from tamoxifen or other aromatase inhibitors utilized as breast cancer prevention drugs.[10,11] Breast density has also been found to be a heritable condition.[12]

The Importance of Breast Density

Scientists have long recognized that breast cancers develop primarily in the lobular and ductal systems and that it is also these systems that cause the mammographic image of a breast to appear dense. This realization led many to believe that density was related to the disease itself and to a woman's risk for developing the disease.[13,14] However, because density also serves to mask or hide cancers, the determination that density was an independent risk factor, as well as lowering sensitivity of the mammogram, took many years of research and had to wait for improvements in the technology of mammography and other imaging modalities.

Masking Risk

Full-field digital mammography (FFDM) was developed in large part to address the reduction in sensitivity of analog mammography observed when screen-film imaging was used with patients having high breast tissue density.[15,16] Separation of the acquisition and display of the mammographic image in FFDM allows the optimization of both.[17] Generally, image optimization is accomplished by increasing the contrast in dense areas of the mammogram through image processing.[18] Although FFDM materially improved the sensitivity of screening patients with dense breast tissue over analog mammography, research continues to show that sensitivity remains low for patients with dense breast tissue.[19]

Sensitivity is, of course, the ability to detect breast cancers from the mammographic image, and breast sensitivity is affected inversely with density, reducing with increasing density. Sometimes referred to as masking, or **masking risk**, the lowered sensitivity caused by high tissue density has been found to be the cause of the delayed diagnosis of many interval cancers.[20–22]

Causal Risk

In 1975, John Wolfe, MD, presented a paper[23] to the American Roentgen Ray Society (ARRS) in which he described a retrospective study of over 7,000 breast cancer patients. In this study, the parenchymal patterns of the subjects, as depicted by the images obtained by the new imaging modality of mammography, were classified into four groups, and the incidence of breast cancer at least 6 months following the mammogram was tracked. Wolfe's classifications involved both the ductal patterns that were observed and the density of the tissue that, it was noted, often obscured visibility of the ductal system, in which breast cancers were believed to originate.

It proved difficult to replicate Wolfe's research, but research concerning breast density has evolved to where breast tissue density is generally accepted as an *independent* risk factor for cancer itself, rather than just confusing the interpretation of the mammogram.[24–28] The understanding of high tissue density as a risk factor has reached the level of consensus, with the American Cancer Society (ACS) quantifying the relative risk of breast cancer due to extremely dense breast tissue (BIRADS D) density at 2.1 to 4.0 times the normal risk. Extremely dense breast tissue is ranked as equivalent with having one first-degree relative with breast cancer and just behind a personal history of breast cancer or two to three first-degree relatives with premenopausal breast cancers.[29]

It is important to note that the cited line of research clearly differentiated the *causal* risk of a breast cancer from the risk of a breast cancer being missed on interpretation because of the confounding effect of density on the mammographic image (masking). This difference is an important one, for while masking and causal risk are independent of one another, in the woman with dense breast tissue the two risks serve to create a "perfect storm," magnifying the impact of each on the detection of breast cancer.

The implications of breast density on causal risk continue to be discovered through ongoing lines of research.[30] Breast density has been linked to risk for postmenopausal women sufficient to warn against the use of hormone therapy[31]; tissue density has been associated with risk of cancer in the contralateral breast for women who have previously been treated for ductal carcinoma in situ (DCIS)[32]; and density has been differentiated as a risk factor in cases of lobular involution.[33] As breast density research continues, it is probable that relationship between tissue density and the fundamental biology of breast cancer will be clarified.[34]

Evaluating and Classifying Breast Density

With breast density linked to risk for breast cancer (masking and causal), and the prospect of being able to utilize breast density in the surveillance and management of breast disease, ease and uniformity of measurement becomes increasingly important and challenging. Categorization of density is an *integral* part of mammographic interpretation, and it has traditionally been considered as being only incidental to the process of image assessment. As this section describes, the evolution of understanding of the implications of breast density increases the importance of density evaluation. A woman's breast density has now become a serious matter requiring attention to both accuracy and uniformity of approach.[35]

BIRADS Breast Tissue Categorization

With breast density linked to risk for breast cancer, and the prospect of being able to use breast density to manage the surveillance and management of breast disease, ease and uniformity of measurement becomes increasingly important. In the late 1980s, the American College of Radiology (ACR) promulgated the Breast Imaging Reporting and Data System (BIRADS) to provide a uniform lexicon for reporting mammography. BIRADS is best known for its assessment categories, but it also included *tissue density categorization* in recognition of the fact that density was being associated with increased risk of breast cancer,[36,37] as well as reflecting reduction in mammographic sensitivity with increasing breast tissue density.[38–40] The importance of tissue density was reflected in BIRADS through expanded tissue composition descriptions, and the use of percentage ranges in BIRADS 4th Edition to help inform referring physicians of the relative predicted performance of mammography, as well as breast cancer risk.[41,42]

In its 4th Edition, BIRADS used quartile-based percentage density ranges to describe density, for example, a BIRADS density 3 breast was defined as "the breast is heterogeneously dense, which could obscure detection of small masses (approximately 51% to 75% glandular)." The quartile ranges proved to be confusing, however, as they failed to correspond to the percentage of women who were classified in each category, and the historic distributions of density as reflected in BCSC mammography reports remained virtually unchanged over almost 4 million mammograms covering the period from 1996 through 2008.[2] See Table 21-1

for several additional studies that help to define the relative numbers by breast density assessment category.

BIRADS density categories *can* serve the purpose of identifying patients whose mammograms may be lower in sensitivity or who may be at increased risk for breast cancer. However, determination of the BIRADS density category in clinical practice has been almost entirely subjective—a scoring of density provided by a rapid visual assessment by a single interpreting physician. Studies have shown that radiologists tend to overestimate tissue density on visual examination of mammographic images, with reported overestimation in one study ranging from 37% for MQSA certified, but inexperienced radiologists, to 6% for experienced breast radiologists who have just received specialized training in estimating density.[43]

In a 2006 study out of the University of Virginia,[44] an institution that has been historically active in density research, researchers compared interreader performance with the performance of a quantitative assessment system that has become a research standard.[45] Using three breast radiologists with one, five, and ten years of mammography interpretation experience, respectively, the readers evaluated 200 mammograms and independently assigned BIRADS density grades to each. The qualitative BIRADS grades were then compared with quantitative assessments produced by an interactive thresholding system.[45] The study found that the range of reader assigned qualitative BIRADS density grades at the two ends of the scale (BIRADS 1 and 4) were much narrower than the ranges established by BIRADS (0% to 25% and greater than 75%) when evaluated quantitatively, but that the ranges for scattered densities and heterogeneous density (BIRADS 2 and 3) assigned by the readers were much broader than are encompassed by the BIRADS density categories, with considerable overlap in physician density assessments.

The Nicholson et al.'s[44] study cited above clearly demonstrated the weakness of ascribing percentages to density

Table 21-1 • BIRADS Density Distributions Reported in Major Studies

	N	BIRADS 1	BIRADS 2	BIRADS 3	BIRADS 4
Kerlikowske et al., 2011[a] (FFDM)	231,034	8.8%	39.4%	45.4%	6.3%
Kerlikowske et al., 2011[a] (FSM)	638,252	7.4%	44.7%	40.3%	7.7%
Kerlikowske et al., 2007[b] (FSM)	301,955	8.9%	44.8%	35.8%	7.8%
Pisano et al., 2008 (DMIST)[c]	49,333	10.5%	43.0%	38.7%	7.5%
Carney et al., 2003[d] (FSM)	463,672	9.1%	47.0%	36.0%	7.8%
Elmore et al., 2004[e] (FSM)	100,153	8.6%	40.6%	39.4%	11.4%
Weighted Average	1,784,399	8.4%	44.4%	39.0%	7.8%

[a]Kerlikowske K, et al. Comparative effectiveness of digital versus film screen mammography in community practice in the United State. *Ann Int Med.* 2011;155:493–502.
[b]Kerlikowske K, et al. Longitudinal measurement of clinical mammographic breast density to improve the estimation of breast cancer risk. *J Natl Cancer Inst.* 2007;99:386–395.
[c]Pisano ED, et al.; Digital Mammographic Imaging Screening Trial (DMIST) Investigators Group. Diagnostic performance of digital versus film mammography for breast-cancer screening. *N Engl J Med.* 2005;353(17):1773–1783.
[d]Carney PA, et al. Individual and combined effects of age, breast density, and hormone replacement therapy use on the accuracy of screening mammography. *Ann Int Med.* 2003;138:168–175.
[e]Elmore JG, et al. The association between obesity and screening mammography accuracy. *Arch Int Med.* 2004;164(10):1140–1147.

quantification when density is utilized qualitatively. As indicated in the introductory paragraph for this breast density section of the chapter, breast density provides a relative measure of the risk that a cancer might be missed in the interpretive process. While the *quantitative* measure of density is important to the understanding or calculation of causal risk, the *qualitative* appreciation of density also reflects upon the value of the underlying mammogram in an individual's surveillance program.

A basic challenge of human breast density determination is that it is inherently two dimensional, while the breast is a three-dimensional object. The dense tissue being imaged on a mammogram is distributed throughout the breast, but the visual appraisal sees only the two-dimensional "distribution," which may not account for layering of tissues or changes in relative density as may be reflected by differing absorption of x-rays by the fibroglandular tissue. For example, is a particularly dense-appearing region of a mammographic view caused by a particularly dense lesion, or is it the summation of many "layers" of fibroglandular tissue?

In 2013, the ACR released its 5th Edition of BIRADS[2] and, for the first time, referred to the classification of breast density as the "overall assessment of the *volume* of attenuating tissues in the breast."[2] For classification of breast tissue density, BIRADS 5th Edition renumbered the tissue classifications (A–D) to avoid confusion with the numerical assessment categories (0–6), adopted minor wording changes, and eliminated the percentages that had been added to the previous edition of BIRADS in 2003.[42] With these changes came a renewed emphasis on use of specific BIRADS language in the report to avoid confusion. The BIRADS 5th Edition breast composition categories are:

A. The breasts are almost entirely fatty.
B. There are scattered areas of fibroglandular density.
C. The breasts are heterogeneously dense, which may obscure small masses.
D. The breasts are extremely dense, which lowers the sensitivity of mammography.

BIRADS 5th Edition specifically recognizes that category C often includes regions of high density in an otherwise low tissue density breast. In contrast with the general requirement that the specific breast tissue descriptive language be used in the report, BIRADS 5th Edition specifically recommends a second descriptive sentence, such as "The dense tissue is located anteriorly in both breasts, and the posterior portions are mostly fatty"; or, "Primarily dense tissue is located in the upper outer quadrants of both breasts; scattered areas of fibroglandular tissue are present in the remainder of the breasts." This recommendation represents a notable departure from earlier reporting practice.

Sprague et al.[35], cited in the introduction to this section, emphasized the chief difficulty with breast density categorization by physicians—the subjective nature of that determination. This study analyzed the performance of 83 radiologists in three programs, reading a total of 216,783 screening mammograms, and found wide variation (6.3% to 84.5%) in the performance of radiologists in categorizing women with dense breasts (BIRADS category C-D). Participating radiologists interpreted a minimum of 500 mammograms, but the study is silent as to the training of participants or the median number of mammograms interpreted by the participant group. Earlier studies of radiologist performance in density classification have found large differences in results that could be attributed to differences in training or volume.[43,44]

The conclusion of the Sprague et al.'s study was that, in the absence of consensus guidelines,[46] physicians relying on density assessments in making referral decisions for supplemental breast imaging due to high tissue density should exercise caution because the "findings suggest that a woman's likelihood of being told she has dense breasts varies substantially on the basis of which radiologist interprets her mammogram." There is more to be gleaned from Sprague et al., however. Notably, the data included many instances when consecutive screening mammograms were available for individual patients, and, when consecutive mammograms were interpreted by different radiologists, the study found 17.2% discordance in the dense versus nondense findings. Even when the consecutive mammograms for a single patient were reviewed by the same radiologist, the discordant rate was 10.0%.

This last statistic is perhaps the most important of the study for, while it might be possible to decrease the interpretive variability between radiologists with appropriate training, the 10% single reader, or *intra*-reader discordant rate implies variability that is too large to be explained by change in patient menopausal status, starting or discontinuing hormone replacement therapy, or other changes that would explain a difference other than variability in the interpretation. Intrareader variability may, in this instance, be considered as an inherent threshold for the reliability of physician analysis and reporting of breast density.

Objective Density Assessment

The correlation between breast density and both causal and masking risk has been discussed previously in this section. These relationships have led many commentators to suggest that density be used as a tool to individualize breast screening for the needs of specific women, as contrasted with reliance on the "one-size-fits all" approach of traditional screening.[47,48] Before breast density can be utilized to vector patients to or between screening modalities in a multimodality surveillance program, however, there must be some effective system for objectively determining breast density. The kind of human reader variability that has consistently been found in studies over two decades cannot support a large-scale supplemental screening program.[33,43,44]

As previously discussed briefly in this section, breast density is a three-dimensional phenomenon, while physician density assessment is performed in two dimensions using the standard four views of a conventional digital mammogram. Digital breast tomosynthesis (DBT) provides a little more perspective with respect to layering of breast tissues, but there are no studies to date that address improvement of *density* assessment using DBT versus conventional 2D digital mammography. The breast may be considered as being composed of fat and nonfat, and the determination of density may be considered as a comparison of the amount of nonfat tissue divided by the total volume of breast tissue.

$$\frac{\text{Nonfat}}{\text{Total Breast Tissue(Fat + Nonfat)}}$$

Fat is radiographically transparent, appearing on the mammogram as black, while the nonfat, or more particularly the fibroglandular tissue of the breast, appears white. Unfortunately, cancers also appear white, and this is the reason that tissue density can cause confusion or even completely frustrate the detection of a cancer. Figure 21-2 illustrates four levels of breast tissue density from fat replaced (A) to almost completely dense (D).

Viewing Figure 21-2, it is easy to understand that the difficulty interpreting from these images increases from (A) through (D) in a fairly predictable manner as the breast density increases. While the resolution of the images on paper is nowhere near as high as on a high-resolution monitor, it should be evident that the dense (white) areas

can obscure cancers. It is difficult, however, to determine where in the *continuum* of density it is that *material impairment* of the radiologist's ability to detect cancers in otherwise asymptomatic women begins. This difficulty partially explains the extreme variability in density assessment of Sprague et al.[35] The quartile basis of BIRADS breast density quantification is not precise enough to discriminate patients within categories, particularly in density category C. As technologies become more sensitive, there is also no capability within BIRADS (e.g., C-1, C-2, C-3, etc.) to reflect a more granular determination of density upon which appropriate patients could be vectored on to supplemental screening.

Breast density must reflect the volumetric nature of density. One might struggle with the concept of gleaning volumetric information from the two-dimensional images that comprise a "mammogram." Even tomosynthesis provides information from only a small angular shift in the image. It is important, however, to remember that the two-dimensional image is rendered in gray, and the third dimension of a grayscale image is provided by the relative "grayness" of each pixel in the image. In other words, the x- and y-axes are provided by the pixel array, with the z-axis being available in gray scale with over *16-thousand* individual gradations to provide the third dimension. As an interesting aside that may also contribute to subjectivity issues, it is important to note that the human eye is only able to discriminate 700 to 900 shades of gray using contemporary medical displays.[49]

Without delving too deeply into the science of assessing breast density objectively, the basic requirement for objective determination is *reproducibility*. Other than by operation of one of the conditions itemized earlier that can affect an individual's tissue density (e.g., age, changes in BMI, use

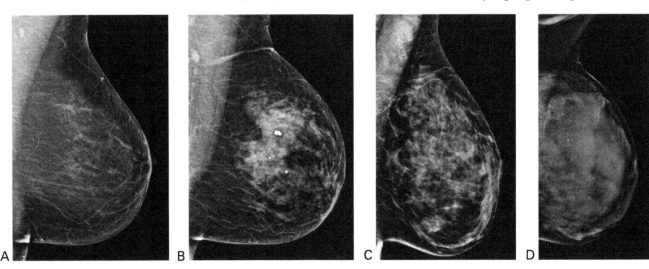

Figure 21-2
The four levels of breast density. **(A)** Almost entirely fatty **(B)** Scattered areas of fibroglandular density **(C)** Heterogeneously dense **(D)** Extremely dense

of hormones, etc.), a woman's breast density assessment should be the same without regard to the mammography equipment utilized, the date or location of the exam. Accomplishing this task requires that density be measured in a manner that quantifies density *relative* to the amount of fat in the individual woman's own breast.

Relative physics requires that the grayscale pixel value for pure fatty tissue be determined for each woman, and that value is then compared to the grayscale value for each pixel in the image of the breast within the skinline. The information gathered will cumulatively provide the overall density and can also be utilized to inform about regions of particularly high density. Because density is determined relatively, the assessment will not be affected by differences in mAs or other imaging parameters between units or between years (assuming no actual temporal change in the breast). Table 21-2 illustrates the concept of relative breast density.

Determining the pixel value for pure fat in an individual woman's breast was not easy, but was solved through the work of Prof. Martin Yaffe, PhD, of the University of Toronto, and his colleagues[50] and applied to the calculation of breast density in a landmark paper presented by Ralph Highnam, PhD, at the International Workshop on Digital Mammography in 2010.[51]

The term "relative" is important in other respects. First, because dense tissue has been quantified in reference to the actual composition of the patient's own breast, rather than some other standard; her density can be compared with her density as determined using the same objective measurement technology in prior years. Second, the patient's breast density can be compared with the density of other women. Third, the density of one subgroup, for example, ethnic, socioeconomic, etc., can be compared with other such groups.

From a practical perspective, objective measurement of breast density provides the ability to begin to individualize breast screening, using supplemental imaging modalities for women whose breast density is high enough to materially affect the sensitivity of the screening mammogram. The prospect of individualizing screening, as now occurs for women who are at highest risk under the American Cancer Society breast MRI recommendations,[52] has the potential of expansion through other adjuvant screening to increase the proportion of breast cancers that are detected, diagnosed, and treated at smaller tumor sizes, decreasing both morbidity and mortality.[53]

Individualizing Breast Screening

Table 21-1 displays the density findings in several large studies. Historically, patients have been classified as "not dense" if they were BIRADS 5th Edition A–B (BIRADS 4th Edition 1–2) and "dense" if they were BIRADS 5th Edition C–D (BIRADS 4th Edition 3–4), and, under this criteria, approximately 47% of women receiving mammograms are considered as mammographically dense. These terms take on additional meaning when one considers the prospect of individualizing breast screening to add supplemental imaging for women with dense breasts, although there continues to be debate about which women with dense tissue will benefit from such additional imaging.[54,55] Masking risk is, in effect, the risk of having an interval cancer—one that is discovered during the *interval* between a normal screening mammogram and a woman's next regularly scheduled screening exam—or a delayed detection of a cancer that can be identified retrospectively on a previous mammogram. Interval cancers typically have poorer prognosis than screen-detected cancers,[56] as do cancers that are diagnosed during subsequent screenings, but that were missed on an earlier screening exam due to masking.

The goal of individualized screening is to reduce the size of tumors at detection/diagnosis, and thereby increase the effectiveness of treatment.[53] It is especially important to diagnose and treat cancers *before* they grow larger than 2 cm in size, because at 2 cm, or if they are node positive, these cancers are designated as stage II, and the recommended treatment includes chemotherapy and/or targeted drug therapy.[57] As treatment extends beyond surgery and radiation therapy, morbidity increases dramatically, impacting patients' ability to cope with day-to-day activities. Postchemotherapy cognitive impairment (PCCI), commonly referred to as "chemo brain," has now been identified in the brain using functional MRI[58] and affects approximately 17% to 34% of women receiving chemotherapy.[59,60]

Table 21-2 • Relative Breast Density Measurement

MAMMO UNIT	YEAR	FAT GRAYSCALE	AVG PIXEL GRAYSCALE	TISSUE DENSITY	
				%[a]	BIRADS
Unit 1	1	3,500	3,902	11.5	3
Unit 1	2	4,200	4,683	11.5	3
Unit 2	1	2,800	3,122	11.5	3
Unit 2	2	2,400	2,676	11.5	3

The concept of relative density. A grayscale pixel value for pure fatty tissue is determined for each woman; this value is then compared to the grayscale value for each pixel in the image.
[a]Note that these percentages are actual.

While research indicates that the effects of PCCI can be mitigated somewhat by exercise, there is also evidence of PCCI persisting for up to 20-year posttherapy.

For women with dense breast tissue, individualization of screening to include supplemental imaging can mean the difference between finding a cancer when it is small and provides a wide range of treatment options and delaying its detection until after the cancer has grown to where more intense therapy is required. As this chapter is being written, objective breast density is in the process of being incorporated in several evaluation programs that are in common use for assessing the breast cancer risk of individual women. Objective breast density is also being used to determine which mammography patients should be offered supplemental breast ultrasound to augment their screening mammography.

Like so much in medicine, breast density remains an unfinished story. Its importance is unmistakable, however, in the continuing effort to minimize the effects of breast cancer through early detection and treatment of the disease. Understanding breast density remains important for women and all who are privileged to care for them.

Ultrasound

Ultrasound is the most frequently utilized of all the adjunctive imaging technologies for characterization of breast tissue (Figure 21-3). Initially, its value was in determining the characteristics of known lesions, whether the ROI was a fluid-filled cyst or a solid mass. Today, the quality of ultrasound images has improved to the extent that it can, in many cases, visualize even the spiculated borders of cancers (Figure 21-4). This is largely due to technological advances such as compound imaging and the Doppler effect.

Historically, there was only one ICD-9 (International Classification of Diseases, 9th revision) code for breast ultrasound. This code did not have the word "diagnostic" in its description, but it was understood that a breast ultrasound exam was done to discover if a palpable lump, or a mass found on a mammogram, was cystic or solid. Although not labeled as a diagnostic procedure, this examination was only performed on symptomatic patients.

With the 2008 publication of the ACRIN 6666 Study results, physicians began requesting whole-breast ultrasound screening exams on their patients with dense breast tissue. The American College of Radiology Imaging Network (ACRIN) conducted a multicenter trial of whole-breast ultrasonography for screening women with dense tissue; to enrich the study results, a requirement for inclusion as a study participant required the woman not only have dense breast tissue, but she also had to be at high risk for developing this disease. The 2008 results showed breast ultrasound

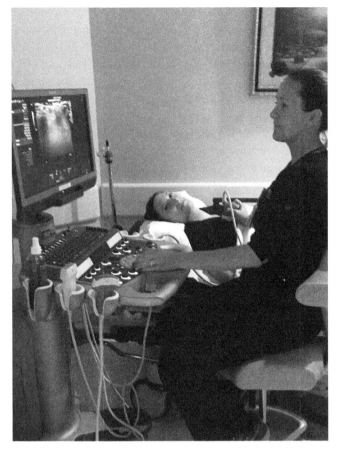

Figure 21-3
Ultrasound is the most frequently used adjunctive modality with mammography. It can be used in a diagnostic setting to focus on a specific ROI, or it can be used in the screening environment to scan the entire breast of a woman with dense breast tissue.

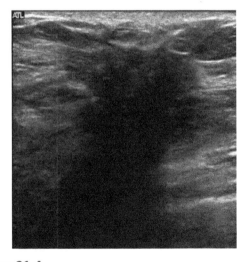

Figure 21-4
Ultrasound reveals a hypoechoic mass with irregular borders. On biopsy, this proved to be an infiltrating ductal carcinoma.

increased detection of cancers in these women by 36%, but in return, it takes a big toll on the rate of benign biopsies.[61] Subsequent to the ACRIN Study, additional papers reported the use of whole-breast ultrasound examinations resulted in the detection of an additional 3 to 4 cancers/1,000 women, cancers not detected by the mammogram.[62–65]

Due to increased use of the single-breast ultrasound ICD-9 code, in 2009, CMS amended the billing code so it could also be used for an asymptomatic woman whose mammogram was incomplete due to the amount of dense breast tissue. In short course, confusion arose from the single ICD-9 code being used for *both* diagnostic and screening purposes, so in 2015, two new codes were developed. One code is used when scanning the entire unilateral breast; the other code is used when scanning less than the entire unilateral breast. Both are unilateral but provide for a 50% decrease in payment when the 2nd breast is scanned.

Today, women with dense breast tissue are often requested to undergo bilateral screening ultrasound examinations in addition to their mammogram. However, because ultrasound is very operator dependent and still not able to detect microcalcifications, it is not recommended as a screening tool for the general population, and it does not replace the need for screening mammography.

Hand-held ultrasound scanning of all women with dense breast tissue is impractical. This exam is:

- Time-dependent—19 minutes/patient.[61]
- Operator dependent—the quality of the exam depends on the skill and experience of the technologist performing the scan.
- Not reproducible—scanning is conducted in real-time; patient positioning is impossible to replicate once she moves from the position she was scanned in.
- Radiologists often repeat the scan the technologist did, although in a limited fashion. This requires more time of the radiologist.

To accommodate the increase in volume of screening ultrasound exams, ultrasound companies now manufacture large field-of-view transducers mounted on automated breast ultrasound machines (ABUS) (Figure 21-5).

New Ultrasound Methods: 3D, ABUS

Automated breast ultrasound (ABUS) is technology originally developed by U-Systems (San Jose, CA); U-Systems is now a division of the GE Healthcare Company (Figure 21-6). The transducer of any high-resolution compound ultrasound equipment is attached

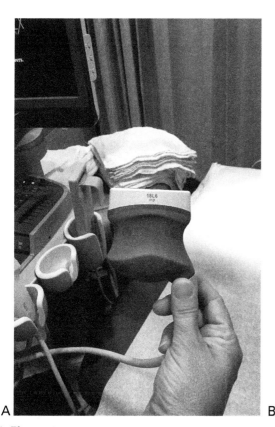
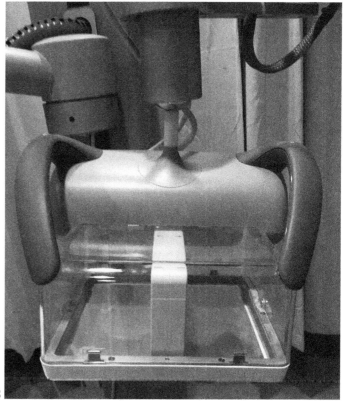

Figure 21-5
Breast ultrasound transducers. **(A)** Hand-held, small field-of-view transducer operated by the technologist. **(B)** Automated breast ultrasound transducer. Position the membrane on the breast, press the "scan" button, and sit back and relax because the unit performs the scan automatically.

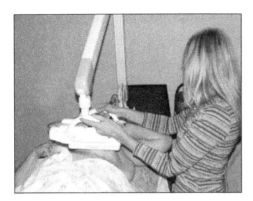

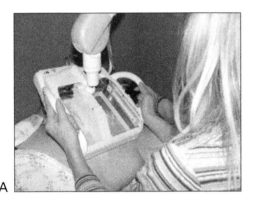

A

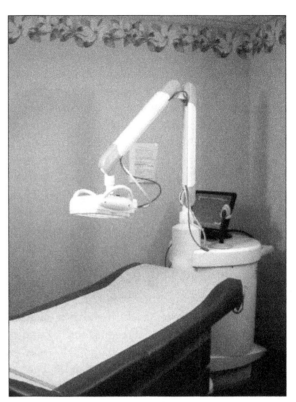

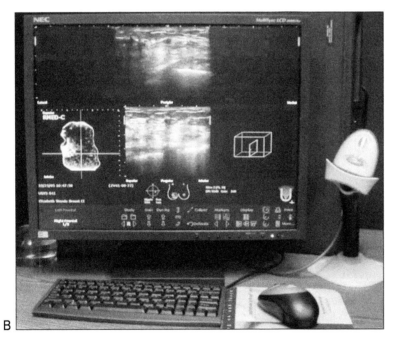

B

Figure 21-6

ABUS, developed by U-Systems (San Jose, CA). **(A)** The technologist images the breast using the large-field transducer that systematically scans the breast. **(B)** The ABUS workstation. The radiologist is able to reconstruct the images into 3D rendering or view slices in transverse, sagittal, and coronal planes.

to a mechanical arm guided by computer, and images are acquired in longitudinal rows, overlapping to assure complete coverage. The mechanical arm controls transducer speed and position, with a technologist maintaining appropriate contact pressure and orientation vertical to the skin. The ABUS unit methodically scans a woman's breast, capturing up to 350 ultrasound images that can be rendered and reviewed in 3D. The ABUS software creates a continuous ciné loop of the images, creating the appearance of real-time scanning. It combines several ultrasound frames together to determine and cancel out random variation (noise) and increase signal-to-noise ratio. The resulting image quality and improved contrast resolution allows for visualization throughout the breast. The positioning and images are very reproducible so that scans can be compared from one date to another for changes. This, combined with automated acquisition, wide field of view, and rapid point of reference (RPR), provides the clinician many real-time options for reviewing the acquired data.

ABUS records the complete exam for review by a radiologist. There is no need for the radiologist to repeat the scan, as often happens with a hand-held ultrasound exam. On average, a whole-breast scan takes 7 minutes for the technologist to complete, and 4 minutes for the radiologist to review and report the results.

Case Study **21-1**

Automated Breast Ultrasound

This 51-year-old patient was recalled for asymmetry seen in the left breast. The radiologist requested a Lateral magnified view using a quad paddle for compression.

A. MLO.

B. CC.

C. The area of asymmetry partially resolves on the magnified view.

D. ABUS shows cysts and a hypoechoic nodule in the left UIQ. This was found to be consistent with the patient's known fibroadenoma.

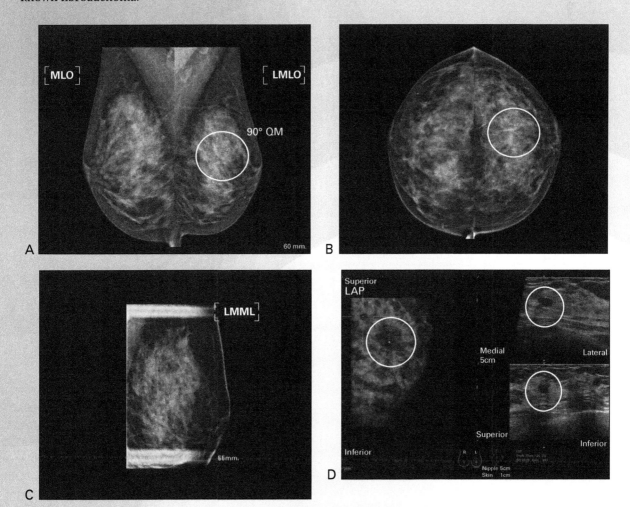

Case Study **21-2**

Automated Breast Ultrasound

This 51-year-old female was recalled for nodularity in the right breast. She had a past history of cysts.

A. MLO views.
B. CC views.
C. The density partially resolves on a magnified view.
D. ABUS shows a hypoechoic nodule laterally in the right breast, consistent with the patient's known fibroadenoma. Cysts are also noted.

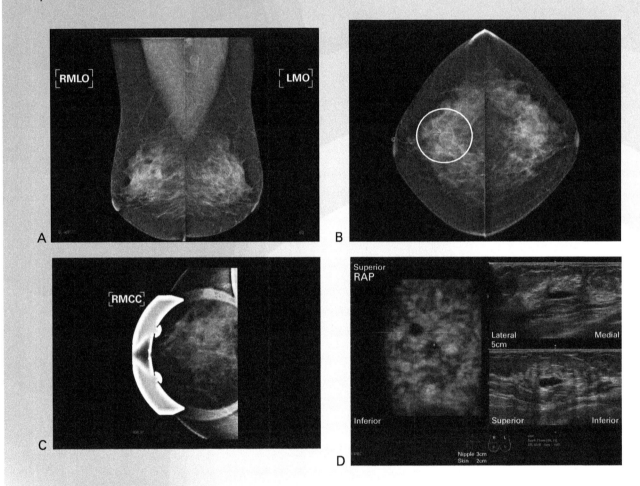

New Ultrasound Methods: Compound, Doppler, 3D, Elastography

Compound and Doppler technologies are available on many of today's sonography units. Compound ultrasound imaging uses several ultrasound beams that strike the tissue from different angles. This significantly reduces speckle and improves the contrast and definition of small masses and even some microcalcifications. Doppler technology allows the assessment of tumor vascularity. It is potentially useful for predicting the biological activity of a tumor and

predicting responses to treatment. One hope for 3D ultrasound imaging is to permit a display of the volume of tissue rather than for measurements of a single slice. This could then be used to measure tumor volume and changes in tumor size over time.

Elastography detects differences in tissue stiffness and other mechanical properties. Cancerous tissue is usually more rigid and less easily deformable than normal breast tissue. In elastography, the mechanical properties of breast tissue are measured from point to point within the breast by ultrasound. A mathematical equation is then inferred, giving a quantitative analysis of the tissue. The hope is that this technology may help to decrease the number of biopsies performed on benign lesions.

Indications for Use

Ultrasound is often used as a diagnostic tool in women with dense tissue, following a mammogram that is indeterminate, and for women with palpable areas of concern. Second-look ultrasound is common following breast MRI when unsuspected lesions appear in areas of the breast that are clear on the mammogram. These lesions must be biopsied, and if they are able to be seen on ultrasound, it is much easier for the patient and less expensive to perform the biopsy under ultrasound guidance rather than MRI guidance.[66]

Ultrasound is:

- Widely available
- Inexpensive
- No contrast agent injection
- No radiation
- Well-tolerated by the patient
- Used for staging, response to therapy, and to detect recurrence

CEM: Contrast-Enhanced Mammography

Contrast-enhanced mammography (CEM) is an adjunctive imaging technique to mammography. The foundation principles of CEM are the same as any of the functional-based imaging techniques that rely on the increased vascularity of tumors: MRI, use of Gadolinium; CT, use of a nonionic iodine contrast agent; PEM, use of FDG; and scintimammography, use of sestamibi.

Like any living tissue, breast cancers require blood flow to sustain the tumor. Rapidly developing tumors create a bizarre vascular system with "leaky" capillaries. When a contrast agent is injected into the vascular system, the agent collects in the metabolically active, hypervascular tumor as well as in the extracellular space around the tumor due to the nonpatent capillaries. The contrast agent used in CEM is the same standard non-ionic–iodinated contrast agent used in CT.

Dual Energy

There are two basic approaches to CEM: (1) background subtraction and (2) dual-energy imaging.

1. In background subtraction, a preinjection image is acquired; a contrast agent is injected; then postinjection images are acquired. A computer then subtracts the preinjection image information from all postinjection images. The concept is very similar to subtraction angiography in the Special Procedures Suite.

2. After injection of a contrast agent, dual-energy imaging acquires two images in rapid succession, using two different x-ray energies: one at a high photon energy level and one at low energy. A computer then subtracts breast parenchymal structures common on both images to enhance visibility of the contrast agent. Most research is done using this method because it is not affected by patient motion and because there is enough time to image both breasts with a single injection of contrast (Figure 21-7).

With dual-energy CEM, the high- and low-energy x-ray exposures record the differences in uptake of a contrast agent, displaying areas of increased vascularity that provide physiological information that may complement morphological information on a mammogram or DBT. At this time, there does not appear to be an advantage to adding a coregistered DBT image, except for localization purposes or for a better look at enhancing areas seen on the CEM image but not readily perceived, even in retrospect, on a 2D FFDM image.

The contrast agent accumulates in metabolically active lesions and is not affected by breast density. It accumulates with sufficient concentration for an x-ray image of its distribution; however, the amount of accumulated contrast agent is low, even in tumors. The amount of background agent disbursed throughout the vascular system of the entire breast is almost the same signal strength as the amount of contrast agent that accumulates in the tumor. To enhance the difference between the background and the tumor, dual-energy x-ray images are taken. The CEM images are *not* looking at the breast structures to identify a cancer; instead, these exposures display the differences in the concentration of iodine. The iodine in the contrast agent absorbs x-rays differently than normal tissue.

A low-energy exposure is acquired; this is the standard mammographic image we routinely produce. With a molybdenum target tube, this would be acquired in the 25 to 30 kVp range, and with a tungsten target tube with a rhodium or silver filter the typical kVp range would be 28 to 33. These low kVp, low-energy images are below the k-edge of iodine (33 keV). Iodine from the contrast agent does not attenuate the low-energy x-ray photons; therefore, the image displays only the breast parenchyma.

In rapid succession, the high-energy exposure is taken. A molybdenum or rhodium target tube would perhaps use a copper or aluminum filter, at 45 to 49 kVp; a tungsten target tube uses a copper filter, at 45 to 49 kVp. These x-ray energies are above the k-edge of iodine so they are

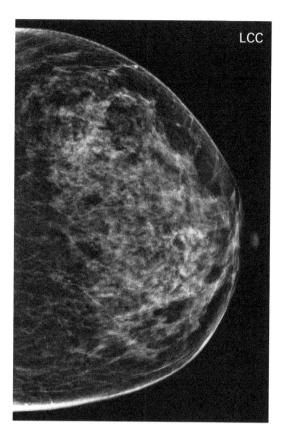
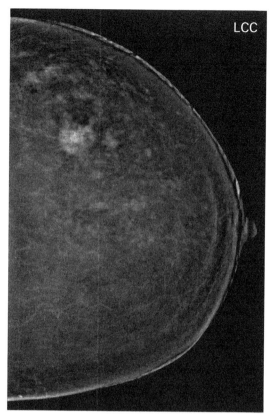

Figure 21-7
LCC mammogram and CE image. Marked enhancement of an invasive lobular carcinoma in the UOQ. (Images courtesy of Hologic, Inc. and affiliates.)

attenuated by the iodine, with the resultant image displaying both the breast parenchyma and the iodine disbursement throughout the breast. The computer subtracts the breast parenchyma, present in both the low- and high-energy images, and displays just the information about the distribution of the iodine (Figure 21-8).

The dose to the patient for the low-energy image is that of a standard mammogram. The high-energy image is half of the standard dose. So for a CEM exam, the patient receives a dose 1.5× that of a standard mammogram.

To perform this examination, a facility needs additional accessory equipment and personnel trained to respond to a reaction to the contrast agent. The following is a list of necessary items:

- Power injector
- Check for renal sufficiency
- Observe the patient for a reaction to the contrast agent/iodine
- Crash cart
- Medicine for allergic reaction
- Personnel trained for an emergency response

The patient is injected in the antecubital vein of the arm contralateral to the breast of concern. The amount of contrast administered depends on body weight, typically 1.5 mL/kg. The patient is seated for the 30-second power injection of the contrast agent; the breast is not in compression as normal blood flow is needed in order for the iodine to travel throughout the breast. Imaging begins 2 minutes after the start of the injection; the imaging window is approximately 6 minutes in which to acquire standard images of the affected breast as well as whatever additional projections the radiologist deems necessary; the left over time is consumed by imaging the nonaffected breast. As time progresses, the iodine concentration diffuses due to washout, and the concentration of iodine in the tumor diffuses so that the background enhancement is the same as the enhancing lesion. Standard compression force is used.

An example of a CEM protocol:

- One-hour appointment
- Nurse interviews and screens patient
- Nurse inserts IV
- Technologist loads contrast agent into the power injector
- Radiologist on standby
- Inject patient and wait 2 minutes
- Start imaging of affected side 1st, unaffected side 2nd

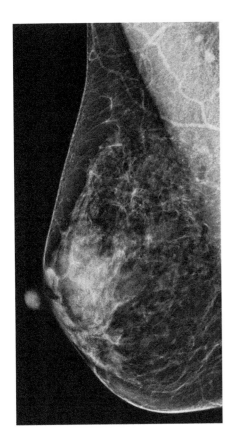
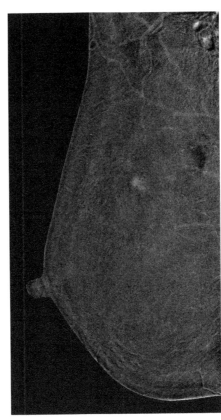

Figure 21-8
RMLO mammogram and CE image. Marked enhancement of an invasive ductal carcinoma located at 12:00. (Images courtesy of Hologic, Inc. and affiliates.)

Indications for use of CEM:

- Adjunct to mammography
- Patient with dense breast tissue and an inconclusive diagnostic mammogram
- Ultrasound with complex masses
- Localize a known or suspected lesion
- For patients who are unable to have an MRI
- More affordable than MRI
- Evaluate extent of disease
- Monitor effectiveness of drug therapy on the tumor

Scintimammography aka Molecular Breast Imaging or Breast-Specific Gamma Imaging

Scintimammography, also known as molecular breast imaging (MBI) and breast-specific gamma imaging (BSGI), is a nuclear medicine approach to breast imaging. It uses a radioactive tracer to produce images with a high-resolution, small field-of-view gamma camera. BSGI and MBI differ primarily in the number and type of detectors used (e.g., multicrystal arrays of cesium iodide or sodium iodide or nonscintillating semiconductor materials such as cadmium zinc telluride).

The radioactive tracer that is injected concentrates more in breast cancer cells than in normal breast tissue. This spatial concentration of the tracer is detected by the gamma camera to form an image; imaging must begin immediately upon injection and takes approximately 40 minutes. The radiotracer typically used is technetium Tc-99m sestamibi. MBI and BSGI image blood flow, much like MRI does; they do not evaluate the architecture of a lesion but rather its metabolic activity. Planar single photon emission radionuclide imaging produces a one-dimensional image (like mammogram).

The dose to the patient and also to the technologist who positions the patient immediately after they have been injected with the radioisotope has always been an issue. The dose is approximately 830 mR. The Mayo Clinic, where much research on this technology takes place, is trying a lower-dose version.

Scintimammography imaging is not affected by dense breast tissue, breast implants, or scarring. However, it does have a limited ability to detect cancers smaller than 1 cm, thus is less accurate in detecting nonpalpable abnormalities.[67,68] FDA approved in 1999, it has shown potential as an adjunct to mammography, but technical limitations such as low resolution of the images have kept it from becoming used more widely. Investigations continue with newer higher-resolution gamma cameras (Figure 21-9) and new radiopharmaceuticals, with promising results, showing a sensitivity exceeding 90% and specificity of about 50%.[69]

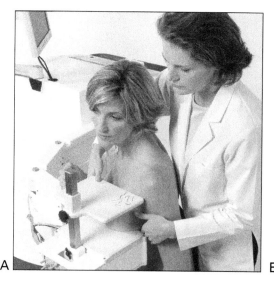
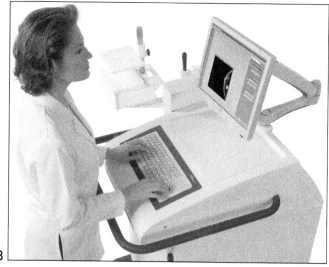

Figure 21-9

(A) A patient is intravenously injected with a small dose of 99mTc-sestamibi, the same pharmaceutical used in cardiac stress tests. Imaging can begin immediately and continue as needed for up to 2 hours. Patients are seated throughout the imaging process and each view takes between 6 and 10 minutes to acquire. **(B)** The Dilon Technologies 6800 BSGI gamma camera allows imaging in all mammographic positions, plus selective studies of hard to reach areas such as the axilla. (Photos courtesy of Dilon Technologies Inc.)

BSGI and MBI have been suggested for a variety of applications:

- Initial staging for patients recently diagnosed with breast cancer
- To monitor tumor response to determine the impact of therapy
- To evaluate suspected recurrence
- For patients with indeterminate breast abnormalities
- When mammography is limited due to dense breast tissue, implants, free silicone, or paraffin injections
- For patients at high risk for malignancy
- Among patients for whom breast MRI is contraindicated

Positron Emission Tomography, Positron Emission Mammography

Positron: a positron emitting radionuclide labeled to a sugar-like molecule is injected into the body. This tracer accumulates throughout the body according to each tissue-type's affinity for the tracer.

Emission: the source of the radioactive signal is emission of photons from within the body.

Tomography: 3D volume image reconstruction.

PET uses a radioactive tracer to identify regions in the body with increased metabolic activity. Researchers have used PET to discern malignant from benign lesions in many parts of the body, including the breast; FDA approved PEM in 2003. Studies indicate that PEM scans have a sensitivity of 90% and a specificity of 86%.[70]

Positron emission mammography (PEM) is a specialized form of PET technology that provides radiologists, breast surgeons, oncologists, and nuclear medicine, a new tool to image and characterize the scope of breast disease at a metabolic rate. CMR Naviscan Corporation, a CMR Company (Carlsbad, CA), has designed the PEM Flex Solo II (Figure 21-10). It is an organ-specific, high-resolution PET

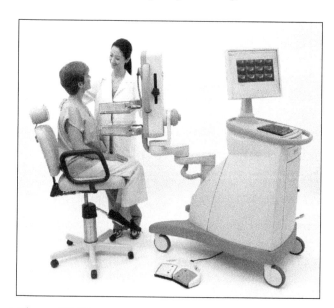

Figure 21-10

The Naviscan PEM Flex Solo II. Images are obtained about an hour after the injection of a glucose radiotracer. Cancer cells absorb and accumulate sugar faster than healthy tissue. Essentially, PEM captures a "snapshot" of the cellular activity occurring within a mass or cancerous tissue. (Photo courtesy of CMR Naviscan Corporation.)

scanner. Solo II is intended for use as an adjunct imaging modality. It yields higher count rate sensitivity while maintaining resolution capabilities that image cancers as small as 1.5 to 2.0 mm.

The dedicated PEM unit provides much higher spatial resolution images than a whole-body PET scanner because the dual detectors are mounted inside mammography compression devices, so they are in close proximity to the breast. Having the detectors so close to the breast tissue allows for an in-plane spatial resolution of 1.5 mm full width half maximum. The lesion size that can be detected with a PEM unit is as small as 1.6 mm.

Patients are requested to fast at least 4 hours prior to the PEM scan to reduce blood glucose. When the patient arrives for the scan, serum blood is drawn to determine the patient's blood glucose level. Then 5 to 10mCi FDG is injected. FDG (fluorodeoxyglucose) accumulates in glucose avid cells. Inflammatory and cancerous cells have a higher metabolic rate than normal cells, so their uptake of FDG should be higher. Wait 1 hour, then image. The patient is positioned similar to a mammogram, and slight compression (10 to 15 lb) is used. It takes approximately 8 minutes for 1 million coincident counts to be acquired. Typically 4 views are taken so the scan time is 32 minutes; the patient is seated for this lengthy procedure.

Tumor size and cell type are factors that affect PEM scan accuracy. PEM is more likely to identify invasive ductal carcinoma but is likely to miss invasive lobular carcinomas. Although the basic mechanism of uptake is via glucose metabolism, factors that result in this variation in glucose uptake in breast tumors have not been clearly identified. When positive, however, the intensity of PEM uptake in a primary breast tumor has been shown to correlate with the degree of tumor aggressiveness. As sites of inflammation or infection will also display increased uptake of FDG, care must be taken in interpreting PEM scans of patients after biopsy or surgery. With these limitations, PEM is not useful as a screening tool. It may, however, provide some benefit when used for problem solving.[69]

Indications for use:

- Presurgical planning
- Staging
- Evaluate lymph nodes
- Evaluate tumor response to therapy
- Watch for recurrent disease
- Differentiate post-op scarring from local recurrence
- Check for extent of disease: multifocal/centric

Case Study 21-3

Positron Emission Mammography

- History: 40-year-old, dense-breasted female presenting with palpable abnormality in the right breast
- Findings: Ultrasound-guided biopsy showed expected IDC from mammogram but with unexpected DCIS intertwined in lesion. MRI and PEM found expected IDC lesion and greater than expected extensive DCIS

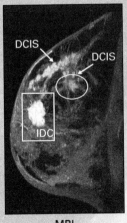
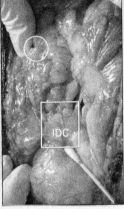
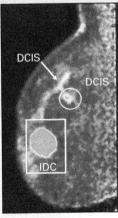

MRI   Pathology   PEM

(Images courtesy CMR Naviscan Corporation (James Rogers, MD, Swedish Cancer Center, Seattle, WA))

Case Study 21-4

Positron Emission Mammography

- History: 46-year-old with suspicious 1 cm mass overlying right pectoral muscle on screening mammogram
- Findings: Ultrasound-guided biopsy confirmed IDC at 12:00 position. PEM correlate was found as well as a second site suspicious for malignancy. MRI was performed and found known index IDC but no additional abnormality prospectively. Retrospective comparison to PEM showed the possible secondary site of centrally clumped enhancement. MRI guided biopsy found DCIS.

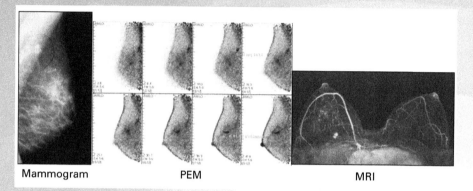

Mammogram   PEM   MRI

(Images courtesy CMR Naviscan Corporation (Marie Tartar, MD, Scripps Cancer Center, La Jolla, CA).)

Dedicated Cone-Beam Breast CT

Breast imaging has evolved over the last 100 years since the first imaging of mastectomy specimens was performed in 1913 by Albert Salomen, M.D. in Berlin, and in 1930, in vivo breast imaging using Kodak film was reported by Warren Stafford, M.D. at the University of Rochester. Screening mammography found acceptance in the 1980s.

Film-screen mammography evolved into FFDM after the results from ACRIN/DMIST in 2005 showed advantages for certain groups of women: those with dense breasts, and pre- and perimenopausal women. DBT became widely adopted after FDA approval in 2011. At about the same time, there were frequent lay media discussions about the importance of breast density, in large part due to public advocacy groups such as "are you dense.org." Because of this, breast density notification is now mandatory in the majority of states in the United States.

With approval of DBT, the concept of 3D breast imaging became popular. The advantages of 3D imaging for screening or supplemental screening became obvious, mainly because of false-positive and false-negative mammograms due to dense breast tissue on mammography. Initially, the available modalities employing 3D imaging included tomosynthesis, whole-breast ultrasound, and MRI. MRI is recommended for high-risk (greater than 20% lifetime risk) screening and for evaluation of the breasts for extent of malignant disease and for occult malignancy, but not for routine screening.

The newest technology developed for breast imaging is dedicated **cone-beam breast CT** (CBCT); Koning Corporation (Rochester, NY) Cone Beam CT for the breast was introduced at RSNA 2006. Utilizing a cone-shaped x-ray beam and a digital flat panel detector for volumetric data capture, cone-beam CT combines the advantages of tomosynthesis with the 3D display of MRI. It also allows easy addition of contrast enhancement, when indicated. Significantly, it can also be used to biopsy findings seen only on the CBCT.

It may seem logical that 3D imaging is the obvious way to image the breast, since the breast is inherently a 3D structure. However, currently in conventional mammography we begin by compressing and deforming the breast into a 2D shape and then we image it. In addition, a big drawback to current mammographic imaging is the fact that most normal tissue and almost all abnormalities we are looking for in the breast are displayed as white structures. This is obviously challenging when hoping to find small lesions that have the same "density" as the surrounding tissues. Tomosynthesis was developed to overcome some of these problems. Tomosynthesis is marketed as "3D"; however, it is really a 2D modality reconstructed to 3D. Essentially, it is a better mammogram.

CBCT, in contrast, is true 3D with 360° imaging and true isotropic imaging. This results in true isotropic resolution. This means identical resolution in all planes: sagittal, transverse, and coronal. The standard resolution is 0.273 mm, with high-resolution reconstruction being 0.122 mm. Since a large percentage of breast cancers, especially DCIS, are associated with microcalcifications, which measure 0.2 mm or less, the ability to detect these small calcifications is very important.

In addition and very significantly, dedicated breast CT is performed without compression, which is a huge advantage for comfort and therefore acceptability and compliance for the patient. In fact, compression, while it is extremely important for excellent images in mammography, also contributes to structural overlap and anatomic noise. This leads to both false-positive (such as asymmetry which turns out to be nothing) and false-negative mammograms (where a true lesion is masked by surrounding dense tissue). For the woman being imaged, the CBCT is much easier and more comfortable. I like to call it "the no pressure mammogram." Some women, however, cannot get comfortable on the examining table because of preexisting shoulder or neck problems. Women with large abdomens may also not be suitable candidates for this procedure.

Breast CT is performed by imaging each breast individually (Figure 21-11). The patient lays on the horizontal

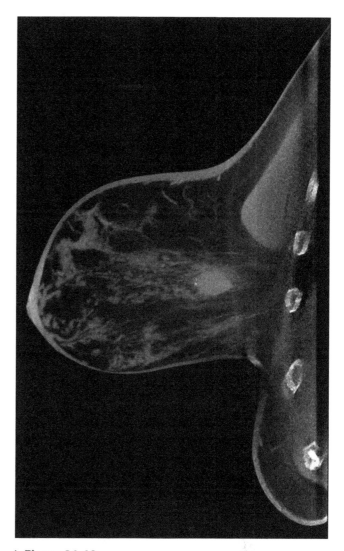

Figure 21-12
Sagittal image showing posterior tissue including ribs. (Image courtesy Avice O'Connell, MD, University of Rochester Medical Center. Rochester, NY.)

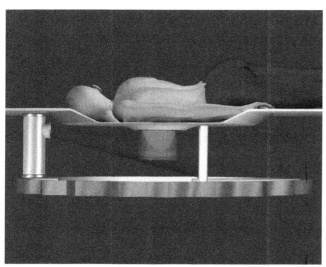

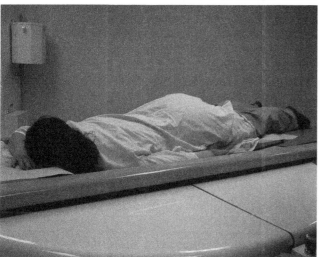

Figure 21-11
Image of table and patient. (Image courtesy Avice O'Connell, MD, University of Rochester Medical Center. Rochester, NY.)

gantry in a slightly obliqued prone position in order to include posterior tissue down to the chestwall and superior tissue into the axillary tail (Figure 21-12). The technical details include a high-power mammography source and a high-resolution flat panel detector. The kVp is 49, with 50 to 100 mA. Average glandular dose is 6 to 9 mGy.

The images are acquired in a 360° rotation around the breast, one breast at a time. In one 10 second sweep, 300 low-dose projection images are obtained. These are then reconstructed with a 3D algorithm for easy display. Image viewing is both 2D multislice, multiplanar viewing, and full 3D visualization (Figure 21-13).

The ability to perform contrast imaging is another advantage of CBCT over mammography and tomosynthesis. Many other parts of the body utilize contrast for cancer imaging; the breast also needs contrast imaging for tumor detection and also for optimal evaluation of known tumors. Currently, high-risk screening and evaluation of known cancer are

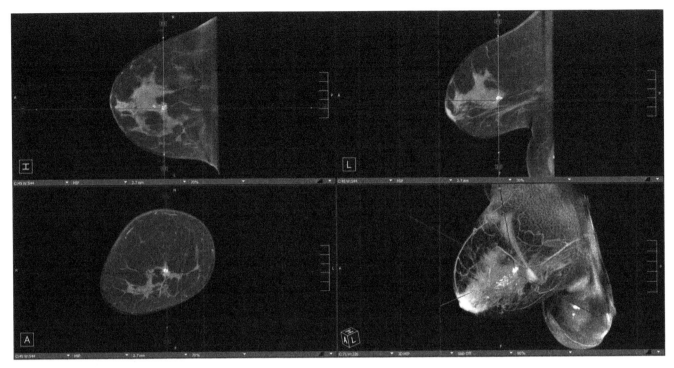

Figure 21-13
Easy to read 4 on 1 presentation. Note isotropic coronal view—not possible on any other modality. (Images courtesy Avice O'Connell, MD, University of Rochester Medical Center. Rochester, NY.)

performed with contrast-enhanced MRI. Contrast enhancement with conventional mammography is being tried in several centers; however, for many reasons, CBCT is better suited for this. Contrast is indicated for high-risk screening and for the same indications as contrast-enhanced breast MRI. Pre- and postcontrast images of each breast are performed, a total of 2 "views" per breast. We use nonionic contrast, 1 mg/kg at 2 cc per second. A power injector is ideal but not essential. Scanning is started at 90 seconds.

Compared to MRI, the CBCT exam usually takes 10 minutes of table time, compared to up to 40 minutes for contrast-enhanced breast MRI. Figure 21-14A and B shows pre- and postcontrast images of a malignant mass.

Finally, biopsy capability is essential for any modality. It is extremely important to be able to biopsy findings on the modality that shows it most accurately. The FDA has approved the biopsy bracket for the Koning CBCT. In many ways, the CBCT biopsy is performed like a stereotactic biopsy (Figure 21-15A–C).

BIOLOGICAL CHARACTERIZATION TECHNOLOGY

Genetic Testing (BrCA1, BrCA2)

A breast cancer (BrCA) gene test is a blood test to check for specific mutations in genes that help control normal cell growth. BrCA1 and BrCA2 produce tumor suppressor proteins. These proteins help repair damaged DNA; they play a role in ensuring the stability of the cell's genetic material. When either of these genes are mutated so that its protein product either is not made or does not function correctly, DNA damage may not be repaired properly. As a result, cells are more likely to develop additional genetic alterations that can lead to cancer.

A BrCA gene test does not test for cancer itself, it tests for the likelihood of developing this disease. Finding changes in the genes called BrCA1 and BrCA2 can help determine a woman's risk of developing breast cancer and ovarian cancer. The BrCA test is only done for people with a strong family history of breast cancer or ovarian cancer and sometimes for those who already have one of these diseases. Genetic counseling before and after a BrCA test is very important to help understand the benefits, risks, and possible outcomes of the test.

A woman's risk of breast or ovarian cancer is higher if she has BrCA1 or BrCA2 gene changes. Breast cancer is extremely rare in men, but BrCA2 gene changes have been linked to male breast cancer and possibly prostate cancer. The risk of some other cancers, including pancreatic and colon cancer, may also be higher. The gene changes can be inherited from either the maternal or paternal parent.

The cost for genetic testing can range from several hundred to several thousand dollars. Insurance policies vary with regard to whether the cost of genetic testing is covered. However, a positive genetic test result may affect a person's

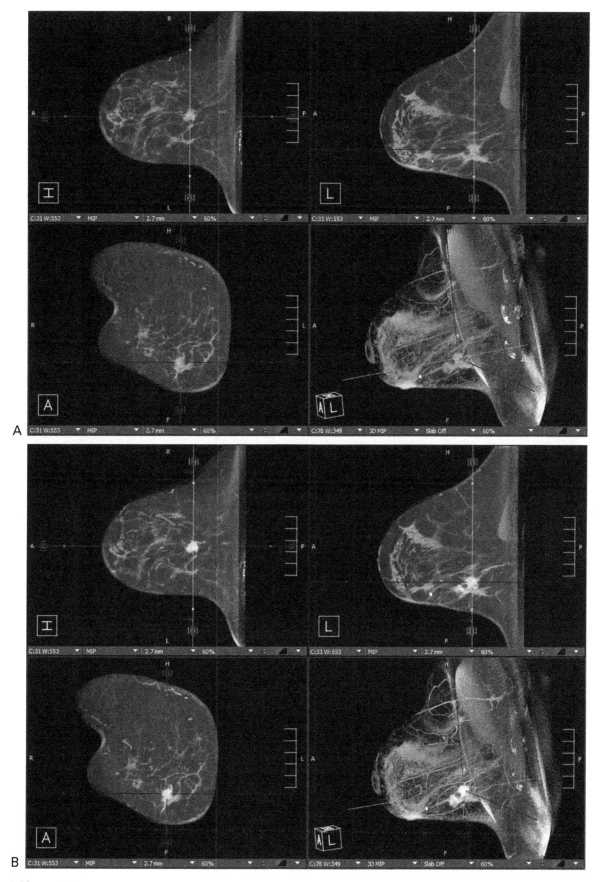

Figure 21-14
(A) Precontrast and **(B)** postcontrast images of a malignant mass. The exam is completed in approximately 10 minutes. (Images courtesy Avice O'Connell, MD, University of Rochester Medical Center. Rochester, NY.)

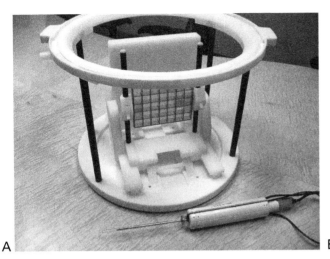
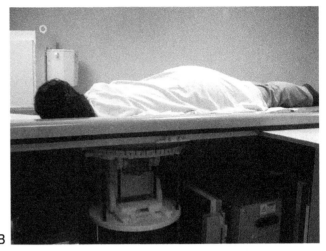
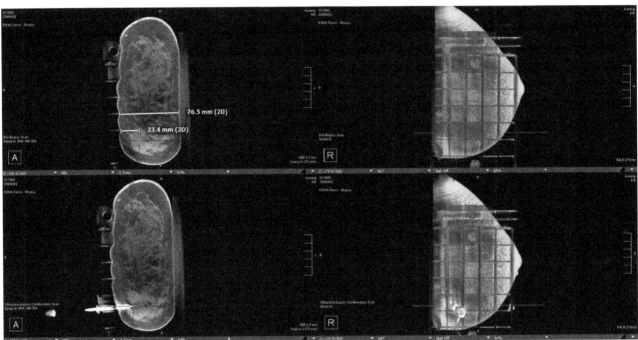

Figure 21-15
Biopsy capability. **(A)** Koning CBCT biopsy bracket can work with any vacuum-assisted biopsy device. **(B)** Patient lies prone on the table for the biopsy. **(C)** Koning CBCT provides measurement and lesion location in real 3D. Biopsy is done accurately. (Images courtesy Avice O'Connell, MD, University of Rochester Medical Center. Rochester, NY.)

insurance coverage, particularly their health insurance, or their potential success in finding employment. A person with a positive result may be denied coverage for medical expenses related to their genetic condition, dropped from their current health plan, or be unable to qualify for new insurance, and some employers may view the affected individual as a potential cancer patient whose expensive medical treatments could drive up the cost of the company's health insurance plan. Therefore, many patients choose to make out-of-pocket payment for the testing, regardless of their coverage. Since 1995, there have been laws that prohibit employers or health insurance companies from using genetic testing results to discriminate against a person. Proving discrimination is difficult.

Several approaches are available for managing cancer risk in individuals with alterations in their BrCA1 or BrCA2 genes. These include but are not restricted to the following:

- **Surveillance**—If cancer develops, it is important to detect it as soon as possible. Careful monitoring for symptoms of cancer may be able to catch the disease at an earlier stage. Surveillance methods for breast cancer may include clinical breast examination (CBE), breast self-examination (BSE), screening mammography, and screening MRI.
- **Prophylactic surgery**—This type of surgery involves removing as much of the at-risk tissue as possible in order

Case Study 21-5

Cone-Beam Breast CT

This 43-year-old female presents after a PET scan. She has a mass in her right breast. She had a personal history of breast carcinoma in the left breast at age 37. No history of lymph node involvement. The right breast mass was proven to be invasive ductal carcinoma with lobular features and intraductal carcinoma, solid-type NG 1.

A. CC and MLO views.
B. Lateral and magnified views show a posterior lesion.
C. Ultrasound shows a solid mass.
D and E. CBCT shows multiple areas of enhancement.
F. 3D rendering of CBCT shows vascular components feeding several lesions.

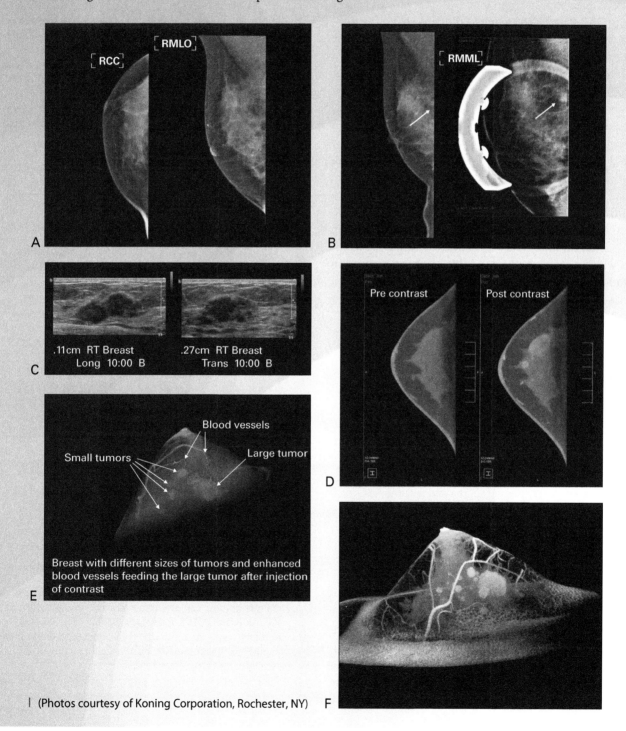

A [RCC] [RMLO]

B [RMML]

C .11cm RT Breast Long 10:00 B .27cm RT Breast Trans 10:00 B

D Pre contrast   Post contrast

E Small tumors   Blood vessels   Large tumor
Breast with different sizes of tumors and enhanced blood vessels feeding the large tumor after injection of contrast

F

(Photos courtesy of Koning Corporation, Rochester, NY)

to reduce the chance of developing cancer. Preventive mastectomy (removal of healthy breasts) does not, however, offer a guarantee against developing breast cancer. Because not all at-risk tissue can be removed, some women have developed breast cancer even after prophylactic surgery.[71,72]

- **Risk avoidance**—Behaviors that may decrease breast cancer risk include exercising regularly and limiting alcohol consumption. Research results on the benefits of these behaviors are based on studies in the general population; the effects of these actions in people with BrCA1 or BrCA2 alterations are not yet known.

- **Chemoprevention**—This approach involves the use of natural or synthetic substances to reduce the risk of developing cancer or to reduce the chance that cancer will come back. For example, the NCI-supported Breast Cancer Prevention Trial[73] found that the drug tamoxifen reduced the risk of invasive breast cancer by 49% in women at increased risk for developing the disease. Few studies have been performed to test the effectiveness of tamoxifen in women with a BrCA1 or BrCA2 alteration. One study found that tamoxifen reduced the incidence of breast cancer by 62% in women with alterations in BrCA2.[74] However, the results showed no reduction in breast cancer incidence with tamoxifen use among women with BrCA1 alterations. Additional chemoprevention studies with tamoxifen and other substances in women with an altered BrCA1 or BrCA2 gene are anticipated.

Review Questions

1. Discuss the effect of breast density on the ability to image the patient, the ability to detect breast cancer, and the effect on her risk to develop breast cancer.

2. Discuss technologies that have been FDA approved and how they may be used within a practice, along with their strengths and weaknesses.

3. Genetic testing has become more commonplace for women at high risk of developing breast cancer. Discuss how knowing BrCA status can affect an individual's imaging and treatment decisions.

References

1. *PDQ® Screening and Prevention Editorial Board. "PDQ Breast Cancer Screening"*. Bethesda, MD: National Cancer Institute. Updated March 4, 2016. Available at: http://www.cancer.gov/types/breast/hp/breast-screening-pdq. Accessed June 5, 2016. (PMID: 26389344).
2. Sickles EA, et al. ACR BI-RADS® mammography. In: *ACR BI-RADS® Atlas, Breast Imaging Reporting and Data System*. Reston, VA: American College of Radiology; 2013.
3. Checka CM, et al. The relationship of mammographic density and age: implications for breast cancer screening. *AJR Am J Roentgenol.* 2012;198(3):W292–W295.
4. McCarthy AM, et al. Racial differences in quantitative measures of area and volumetric breast density. *J Natl Cancer Inst.* 2016;108(10). doi:10.1093/jnci/djw104.
5. Hart V, Reeves KW, Sturgeon SR, et al. The effect of change in body mass index on volumetric measures of mammographic density. *Cancer Epidemiol Biomarkers Prev.* 2015;24(11):1724–1730.
6. Phipps AI, Buist DS, Malone KE, et al. Breast density, body mass index, and risk of tumor marker-defined subtypes of breast cancer. *Ann Epidemiol.* 2012;22(5):340–348.
7. Martin LJ, Minkin S, Boyd NF. Hormone therapy, mammographic density, and breast cancer risk. *Maturitas.* 2009;64(1):20–26.
8. Litherland JC, et al. The effect of hormone replacement therapy on the sensitivity of screening mammograms. *Clin Radiol.* 1999;54(5):285–288.
9. Laya MB, et al. Effect of postmenopausal hormonal replacement therapy on mammographic density and parenchymal pattern. *Radiology.* 1995;196(2):433–437.
10. Mullooly M, et al. Mammographic density as a biosensor of tamoxifen effectiveness in adjuvant endocrine treatment of breast cancer: opportunities and implications. *J Clin Oncol.* 2016;34(18):2093–2097.
11. Megglorini ML, et al. Tamoxifen in women with breast cancer and mammographic density. *Eur J Gynaecol Oncol.* 2008;29(6):598–601.
12. Boyd NF, et al. Heritability of mammographic density, a risk factor for breast cancer. *N Engl J Med.* 2002;347(12):886–894.
13. van Gils CH, et al. Changes in mammographic breast density and concomitant changes in breast cancer risk. *Eur J Cancer Prev.* 1999;8(6):509–515.
14. Yaffe MJ, et al. Breast cancer risk and measured mammographic density. *Eur J Cancer Prev.* 1998;7(Suppl 1):S47–S55.
15. Carney PA, et al. Individual and combined effects of age, breast density, and hormone replacement therapy use on the accuracy of screening mammography. *Ann Intern Med.* 2003;138:168–175.
16. Kerlikowske K, Grady D, Barclay J, et al. Effect of age, breast density, and family history on the sensitivity of first screening mammography. *JAMA.* 1996;276:33–38.
17. Pisano ED, et al.; Digital Mammographic Imaging Screening Trial (DMIST) Investigators Group. Diagnostic performance of digital versus film mammography for breast-cancer screening. *N Engl J Med.* 2005;353(17):1773–1783.
18. Pisano ED, Yaffe MJ. Digital mammography. *Radiology.* 2005;234:353–361.
19. Pisano ED, et al. Diagnostic accuracy of digital versus film mammography: exploratory analysis of selected population subgroups in DMIST. *Radiology.* 2008;246(2):376–383.
20. Kerlikowske K, et al. Identifying women with dense breasts at high risk for interval cancer: a cohort study. *Ann Intern Med.* 2015;162(10):673–681.
21. Choi WJ, et al. Analysis of prior mammography with negative result in women with interval breast cancer. *Breast Cancer.* 2016;23(4):583–589.

22. Boyd NF, et al. Mammographic features associated with interval breast cancers in screening programs. *Breast Cancer Res.* 2014;16(4):417.

23. Wolfe JN. Breast patterns as an index of risk for developing breast cancer. *Am J Roentgenol.* 1976;126:1130–1139.

24. Boyd NF, et al. Mammographic density and the risk and detection of breast cancer. *N Engl J Med.* 2007;356(3):227–236.

25. Barlow WE, et al. Prospective breast cancer risk prediction model for women undergoing screening mammography. *J Natl Cancer Inst.* 2006;98(17):1204–1214.

26. Harvey JA, Bovbjerg VE. Quantitative assessment of mammographic breast density: relationship with breast cancer risk. *Radiology.* 2004;230(1):29–41.

27. Vacek PM, Geller BM. A prospective study of breast cancer risk using routine mammographic breast density measurements. *Cancer Epidemiol Biomarkers Prev.* 2004;13(5):715–722.

28. Yaffe MJ, et al. Breast cancer risk and measured mammographic density. *Eur J Cancer Prev.* 1998;7(Suppl 1):S47–S55.

29. American Cancer Society. *Breast Cancer Facts & Figures 2015-2016.* Atlanta, GA: American Cancer Society, Inc.; 2015.

30. Boyd NF, et al. Breast tissue composition and susceptibility to breast cancer. *J Natl Cancer Inst.* 2010;102:1224–1237.

31. Kerlikowske K, Cook AJ, Buist DS, et al. Breast cancer risk by breast density, menopause, and postmenopausal hormone therapy use. *J Clin Oncol.* 2010;28(24):3830–3837.

32. Habel LA, Capra AM, Achacoso NS, et al. Mammographic density and risk of second breast cancer after ductal carcinoma in situ. *Cancer Epidemiol Biomarkers Prev.* 2010;19(10):2488–2495.

33. Ghosh K, et al. Independent association of lobular involution and mammographic breast density with breast cancer risk. *J Natl Cancer Inst.* 2010;102:1–8.

34. Douglas JA, et al. Mammographic breast density—evidence for genetic correlations with established breast cancer risk factors. *Cancer Epidemiol Biomarkers Prev.* 2008;17(2):3509–3516.

35. Sprague BL, et al. Variation in mammographic breast density assessments among radiologists in clinical practice: a multicenter observational study. *Ann Intern Med.* 2016;165(7):457–464. doi:10.7326/M15-2934.

36. Hainline S, Myers L, McLelland R, Newell J, Grufferman S, Shingleton W. Mammographic patterns and risk of breast cancer. *AJR Am J Roentgenol.* 1978;130:1157–1158.

37. Carlile T, et al. Breast cancer prediction and the Wolfe classification of mammograms. *JAMA.* 1985;254:1050–1053.

38. Fajardo LL, et al. Correlation between breast parenchymal patterns and mammographers' certainty of diagnosis. *Invest Radiol.* 1988;23:505–508.

39. Van Gils CH, et al. Effect of mammographic breast density on breast cancer screening performance: a study in Nijmegen, the Netherlands. *J Epidemiol Community Health.* 1998;52:267–271.

40. Mandelson MT, et al. Breast density as a predictor of mammographic detection: comparison of interval- and screen-detected cancers. *J Natl Cancer Inst.* 2000;92:1081–1087.

41. Burnside ES, et al. The ACR BI-RADS® experience: learning from history. *J Am Coll Radiol.* 2009;6:851–860.

42. D'Orsi CJ, Bassett LW, Berg WA, et al. *Breast Imaging Reporting and Data System (BI-RADS): Mammography.* 4th ed. Reston, VA: American College of Radiology; 2003.

43. Martin KE, et al. Mammographic density measured with quantitative computer-aided method: comparison with radiologists' estimates and BI-RADS categories. *Radiology.* 2006;240(3):656–665.

44. Nicholson BT, et al. Accuracy of assigned BI-RADS breast density category definitions. *Acad Radiol.* 2006;13:1143–1149.

45. Byng JW, et al. Analysis of mammographic density and breast cancer risk from digitized mammograms. *Radiographics.* 1998;18:1587–1598.

46. Haas JS, Kaplan CP. The divide between breast density notification laws and evidence-based guidelines for breast cancer screening laws: legislating practice. *JAMA Intern Med.* 2015;175:1439–1440.

47. Kerlikowske K. Evidence-based breast cancer prevention: the importance of individual risk. *Ann Intern Med.* 2009;151(10):750–752.

48. Cummings SR, et al. Prevention of breast cancer in postmenopausal women: approaches to estimating and reducing risk. *J Natl Cancer Inst.* 2009;101:384–398.

49. Kimpe T, Tuytschaever T. Increasing the number of gray shades in medical display systems—how much is enough? *J Digit Imaging.* 2007;20(4):422–432.

50. Highnam R, et al. Robust breast composition measurement—Volpara™. In: J Marti, et al., eds. *IWDM 2010. LNCS,* vol. 6136. Girona, Spain: International Workshop on Digital Mammography; 2010:342–349.

51. *Volpara Density.* Wellington, NZ: Volpara Solutions.

52. Salslow D, et al. American Cancer Society guidelines for breast screening with MRI as an adjunct to mammography. *CA Cancer J Clin.* 2007;57:75–89.

53. Duffy SW, et al. Tumor size and breast cancer detection: what might be the effect of a less sensitive screening tool than mammography. *Breast J.* 2006;12(Suppl 1):S91–S95.

54. Kerlikowski K, et al. Identifying women with dense breasts at high risk for interval cancer: a cohort study. *Ann Intern Med.* 2015;162:673–681.

55. Burkett BJ, Hanemann CW. A review of supplemental screening ultrasound for breast cancer: certain populations of women with dense breast tissue may benefit. *Acad Radiol.* 2016;23(12):1604–1609. Pii: S1076-6332(16)30096-4. doi:10.1016/j.acra.2016.05.017.

56. Lehtimaki T, Lundin M, Linder N, et al. Long-term prognosis of breast cancer detected by mammography or other methods. *Breast Cancer Res.* 2011;13(6):R134. doi:10.1186/bcr3080.

57. Breast Cancer Treatment (PDQ®), Stage I, II, IIIA, and Operable IIIC Breast Cancer, National Cancer Institute. Available at: http://www.cancer.gov/cancertopics/pdq/treatment/breast/healthprofessional, Accessed August 22, 2016.

58. Miao H, et al. Long-term cognitive impairment of breast cancer patients after chemotherapy: a functional MRI study. *Eur J Radiol.* 2016;85(6):1053–1057.

59. Myers JS, et al. Potential factors associated with perceived cognitive impairment in breast cancer survivors. *Support Care Cancer.* 2015;23(11):3219–3228.

60. Vearncombe KJ, et al. Predictors of cognitive decline after chemotherapy in breast cancer patients. *J Int Neuropsychol Soc.* 2009;15(6):951–962.

61. Berg WA, et al. Combined screening with ultrasound and mammography versus mammography alone in women at elevated risk of breast cancer. *JAMA* 2008;299(18):2151–2163.

62. Weigert J, Steenbergen S. The Connecticut experiment: the role of ultrasound in the screening of women with dense breasts. *Breast J.* 2012;18(6):517–522.

63. Kelly K, et al. Breast cancer detection using automated whole breast ultrasound and mammography in radiographically dense breasts. *Eur Radiol.* 2010;20:734–742.

64. Bae MS, et al. Breast cancer detected with screening ultrasound: reasons for nondetection at mammography. *Radiology.* 2014;270(2):369–377.

65. Brem RF, et al. Screening breast ultrasound: past, present, and future. *AJR Am J Roentgenol.* 2015;204(2):234–240.

66. Destounis SV, et al. The role of MRI and "second-look" ultrasound for evaluation of breast cancer. *Appl Radiol.* 2006;35(10).

67. Edell SL, Eisen MD. Current imaging modalities for the diagnosis of breast cancer. *Del Med J.* 1999;71:377–382.

68. Ziewacz JT, et al. The difficult breast. *Surg Oncol Clin N Am.* 1999;8:17–33.

69. Hruska C. Molecular breast imaging to screen for breast cancer in women with mammographically dense breasts and increased risk. *American Society of Clinical Oncology, Breast Cancer Symposium; September 4, 2008; Washington, DC.*

70. Shirazi P. Pros and cons of molecular breast imaging. *Imaging Technology News.* July 25, 2012. Available at: http://itnonline.com

71. Rebbeck TR, et al. Bilateral prophylactic mastectomy reduces breast cancer risk in BRCA1 and BRCA2 mutation carriers: The PROSE Study Group. *Am J Clin Oncol.* 2004;22(6):1055–1062.

72. Rebbeck TR, et al. Prophylactic oophorectomy in carriers of BRCA1 or BRCA2 mutations. *N Engl J Med.* 2002;346(21):1616–1622.

73. Fisher B, et al. Tamoxifen for prevention of breast cancer: report of the national surgical adjuvant breast and bowel project P−1 study. *J Natl Cancer Inst.* 1998;90(18):1371–1388.

74. Thull DL, Vogel VG. Recognition and management of hereditary breast cancer syndromes. *Oncologist.* 2004;9(1):13–24.

■■ INDEX

Note: Page numbers followed by "*f*" indicate figures; those followed by "*t*" indicate tables; those followed by "*b*" indicate boxes.

A

AAPM (American Association of Physicists in Medicine), 521
AAPM Task Group 18 (TG18) QC test pattern, 558–559, 559*f*, 588*f*
AAPM TG18-UNL80 test pattern, 588, 589*f*
Abdomen, protruding, 202, 309*t*–310*t*, 310*t*, 316–317, 317*f*
Abnormalities. *See* Mammographic abnormalities
Abscess, 123
  breast, 379
ABUS. *See* Automated breast ultrasound (ABUS)
Accessory nipple, 85
Accreditation programs in stereotactic breast biopsy (SBBAP), 514
Acquisition workstation (AWS), 432, 433*f*, 434, 439, 589–590, 599
  digital mammography room, 421
  of mammography machine, 387–388, 387*f*
ACR. *See* American College of Radiology (ACR)
ACR 2016 Digital Mammography Quality Control Program, 553
ACR 2016 Digital Mammography Quality Control Manual, 542–544, 543*f*, 545*f*
ACR Basic Clinically Relevant Audit, 531–532, 532*b*
ACR Practice Parameter, 73
ACR Standardized Projections, 149, 151*t*–152*t*
ACRIN. *See* American College of Radiology Imaging Network (ACRIN)
ACRIN/DMIST study. *See* American College of Radiology Imaging Network/Digital Mammographic Imaging Screening Trial (ACRIN/DMIST) study
Acrylic uniform phantom, 581, 581*f*
ACS. *See* American Cancer Society (ACS)
Actual quality, 70, 70*f*
ADC. *See* Analog-to-digital converters (ADC)
Adenosis, 120, 120*f*

Adequate compression devices, 136
Adequate exposure assessment, 135
Adjuvant therapy
  for breast cancer, 714–719
  chemotherapy, 715–717, 716*f*
  hormonal (antiestrogen) therapy, 717–719, 718*f*
  systemic therapy, 714–715
AEC. *See* Automatic exposure control (AEC)
2010 Affordable Health Care Act, 29
Age, breast cancer and, 19, 19*t*, 20*f*, 20*t*, 65*b*, 66
AI (aromatase inhibitors), 717–719
AIDET method, 45–46
Air Kerma (AK), 577
  and AEC reproducibility, 577
Airgap
  craniocaudal projection, 243–246, 245*f*
  MLO
    axillary, thin patient, small breast, 214, 215*f*
    elimination, 216–219
    inferior breast, 216, 218*f*
    management, 215
    superior breast, 215–216, 217*f*, 218*f*
Algorithms, defined, 428
Alignment, 388
Alopecia (hair loss), with chemotherapy, 716
Aluminum, in antiperspirants and powders, 11, 13
American Association of Physicists in Medicine (AAPM), 558–559
American Cancer Society (ACS), 18, 753
  annual *vs.* biennial screening, 32–33, 33*t*
  "C" recommendation rating, 31–32
  chemotherapy, 33
  decreased anxiety, 33
  for early breast cancer detection in women without breast symptoms, 29, 30*b*
  guidelines, 25, 25*t*
  "I" recommendation rating, 32
  increased anxiety, 33
  mortality reduction in age, 31, 31*t*
  mortality reduction statistics, 30–31, 31*t*
  screening *vs.* palpation detection, 33
  SEER data report, 32
  statistical errors and assumptions, 30
  task force membership, 30
American College of Radiology (ACR), 3, 46, 91, 301, 511–512, 514

  Mammography Accreditation Program of, 385
  phantom image quality control test
    digital accreditation phantom, 584, 586*f*, 596–597
    original accreditation phantom, 583–584, 585*f*, 596
  thyroid shielding, 51, 51*b*
American College of Radiology Imaging Network (ACRIN), 758–759
American College of Radiology Imaging Network/Digital Mammographic Imaging Screening Trial (ACRIN/DMIST) study, 422–423
American Registry of Radiologic Technologists (ARRT), 62, 304
American Society of Radiologic Technologists (ASRT), 62, 304, 521
Americans with Disabilities Act, 53
Amorphous selenium (a-Se), 450–451, 450*f*
Analog imaging, transition
  to 2D FFDM, 496–497, 496*f*
  to FFDM, 474, 474*t*
Analog mammograms
  digital *vs.*
    client's viewpoint, 427
    technologist's viewpoint, 427
Analog mammography, 7
  circumstances for breath holding in, 13
  image collection, 436–437
  image display, 436–437
  image processing, 436–437
  image storage, 436–437
  vs. xeroradiography, 7, 7*t*
Analog-to-digital converters (ADC), 432
Anatomy, breast, 84–89
  internal, 85–89
Anode angle, 399*f*
Anterior compression modifier, 180–181, 180*f*
Antiestrogen therapy, 717–719, 718*f*
Antiperspirants
  mammography examination and, 47–48, 49*f*
  xeroradiography and, 11–13, 12*f*
Anxiety, in patients, 39
Apex of, breast, 84, 84*f*
Apocrine metaplasia, 122
Appointment scheduling
  automated, 40–43
  direct patient contact, 43
  face-to-face or phone call, 43
  first impression model, 40